Parasitic Diseases of Wild Mammals

SECOND EDITION

Parasitic Diseases of Wild Mammals

SECOND EDITION

Edited by William M. Samuel
Margo J. Pybus
A. Alan Kocan

Iowa State University Press / Ames

William M. Samuel, Ph.D., is a professor in the Department of Biological Sciences at the University of Alberta. He is also the coordinator for the Challenge Grants in Biodiversity Program, which provides research funds to graduate students studying conservation biology and ecology.

Margo J. Pybus, Ph.D., is a wildlife disease specialist with the Alberta Natural Resources Service—Fisheries and Wildlife. She has over 20 years of experience in field and experimental investigation of disease and parasites in free-ranging wildlife.

A. Alan Kocan, Ph.D., is a professor of pathobiology in the College of Veterinary Medicine at Oklahoma State University. His major research interests are parasitic and infectious diseases of wild and domestic animals, with recent emphasis on tick-transmitted diseases.

© 2001, 1971 Iowa State University Press
All rights reserved

Iowa Sate University Press
2121 South State Avenue, Ames, Iowa 50014

Orders: 1-800-862-6657
Office: 1-515-292-0140
Fax: 1-515-292-3348
Web site: www.isupress.com

Authorization to photocopy items for internal or personal use, or the internal or personal use of specific clients, is granted by Iowa State University Press, provided that the base fee of $.10 per copy is paid directly to the Copyright Clearance Center, 222 Rosewood Drive, Danvers, MA 01923. For those organizations that have been granted a photocopy license by CCC, a separate system of payments has been arranged. The fee code for users of the Transactional Reporting Service is 0-8138-2978-X/2001 $.10.

♾ Printed on acid-free paper in the United States of America

First edition, 1971
Second edition, 2001

Library of Congress Cataloging-in-Publication Data

Parasitic diseases of wild mammals / edited by William M. Samuel, Margo J. Pybus, and A. Alan Kocan.—2nd ed.
       p. cm.
    Rev. ed. of: Parasitic diseases of wild mammals / John William Davis. 1st ed. 1971.
    Includes bibliographical references and index (p.).
    ISBN 0-8138-2978-X (alk. paper)
    1. Wildlife diseases. 2. Mammals—Parasites. 3. Veterinary parasitology.
    I. Samuel, William M. II. Pybus, Margo J. III. Kocan, A. Alan. IV. Davis, John William.
    Parasitic diseases of wild mammals.

    SF996.4 P37 2001
    639.9'64—dc21
                                                    00-047257

The last digit is the print number: 9 8 7 6 5 4 3 2 1

CONTENTS

PREFACE

When the first edition of *Parasitic Diseases of Wild Mammals* was published in 1971, the field of wildlife parasitology was, for the most part, in the stage of documenting the presence and identity of parasites in mammalian hosts. Few had challenged the idea that parasites were so well adapted to their hosts that they seldom caused disease (but see coverage of lungworms and elaeophorosis in the first edition). Nonetheless, *Parasitic Diseases of Wild Mammals* served many years as a reference book for parasitologists, veterinarians, professors, senior students, wildlife biologists, public health workers, and others. With chapters arranged in similar and uniform format, the first edition provided current information on 17 selected parasites, or related groups of parasites, of wild mammals.

The field of wildlife parasitology, particularly as it relates to mammals, has changed dramatically since publication of the first edition, moving well beyond the case report and parasite survey stage of development. Much information has accrued on the ecology and epidemiology/epizootiology of parasites of wild mammals, as well as the significance of parasites in conservation biology. This information explosion has clearly illuminated the complexity of the host-parasite relationship for those few parasites of wild mammals studied in detail and has revealed that some parasites are able to cause severe disease and death of hosts in certain situations. Reasons for this information explosion are many and include establishment of

1. strong research programs on specific parasites with disease-causing propensities,

2. teaching/research curricula at the university level,

3. data-gathering and disseminating facilities around the world (for example, Canadian Cooperative Wildlife Health Centre, U.S. National Wildlife Health Center, Southeastern Cooperative Wildlife Disease Study) and disease monitoring programs in Scandinavia and France that are specific to wildlife disease, and

4. growth and maturation of the Wildlife Disease Association and its major publication, the *Journal of Wildlife Diseases.*

In summary, today it is commonplace to use integrated approaches to better understand host-parasite interactions and the inherent role of parasitic organisms within natural ecosystems.

This book updates information on several important parasites or parasitic groups covered in the first edition and adds information on groups not covered previously. It will become immediately obvious that the second edition is long overdue. As one brief example, *Trichinella* is no longer considered a monospecific zoonotic organism, but rather comprises a suite of different isolates, ecotypes, subspecies, or species infecting mammals worldwide. Virtually all aspects of the epidemiology of trichinosis have changed in recent years.

The second edition of *Parasitic Diseases of Wild Mammals* will serve as a benchmark reference for parasites or parasitic groups

1. with members that are significant pathogens of mammals (for example, see Chapter 9 on lungworms and Chapter 5 on sarcoptic mange),

2. that normally do not have pathogenic tendencies, or are difficult to assess, but nonetheless have potential to cause problems (examples include Chapter 8 on gut nematodes of ungulates, Chapter 7 on taeniid tapeworms, and Chapter 14 on hepatic capillariasis),

3. with zoonotic importance (examples include Chapter 17 on giardiasis, Chapter 15 on trichinellosis, and Chapter 11 on *Baylisascaris*),

4. that we might temptingly refer to as emerging diseases (examples include crytosporidians in Chapter 18 and new forms in Chapter 22, on toxoplasmosis), and

5. that are conspicuous organisms that evoke management concerns or public interest (examples include Chapter 4 on ticks, and Chapter 6 on liver flukes).

This volume presents up-to-date summaries of five groups of ectoparasites (lice, biting flies, bot flies, ticks, and mange mites), ten groups of helminths or endoparasites (liver flukes, taeniid tapeworms, gastrointestinal nematodes of ruminants, lungworms of terrestrial and marine mammals, baylisascarids, filarioid nematodes, kidney worms, hepatic nematodes, and *Trichinella*), and nine groups of protozoans including enteric forms (*Amoeba, Giardia,* coccidia), tissue-invaders (amoebae, hepatozoons, *Besnoitia,* and *Toxoplasma* and relatives), and blood-inhabiting forms (trypanosomes and relatives, piroplasms). The format is, for the most part, uniform, although in some cases authors had freedom to arrange the presentation to best present the information.

It is hoped that the contents here will be worthwhile for both novices and experts in wildlife parasitology and also for those with other expertise in need of a reference on parasitic diseases of wild mammals.

The editors acknowledge the Wildlife Disease Association, the membership of which initiated the idea for this volume. We also acknowledge the many members who contributed to this volume. Royalties that will accrue from sales go to the Wildlife Disease Association.

Parasitic Diseases of Wild Mammals

SECOND EDITION

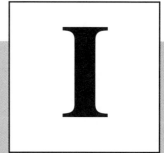

PART I

ECTOPARASITES

1

LICE (PHTHIRAPTERA)

LANCE A. DURDEN

INTRODUCTION. Lice are small (0.35–10 mm long as adults), wingless, dorsoventrally flattened insects with a simple (hemimetabolous) life cycle. They are ectoparasites of mammals and birds throughout the world. Typically, they parasitize individual mammals in small numbers and cause no apparent discomfort. However, large populations of lice are sometimes encountered, and these may affect the host detrimentally. Small louse populations can also debilitate their hosts by causing hypersensitivity, and for lice that vector pathogenic organisms, the bite from a single infected ectoparasite can be significant. Detailed study of the host-parasite relationships between lice and wild mammals is largely in its infancy, and much of our current knowledge stems from studies of louse-infested domesticated mammals. Infestation by lice is termed pediculosis.

CLASSIFICATION, TAXONOMY, AND MORPHOLOGY. Lice can be divided into sucking lice (Anoplura) and chewing (i.e., biting) lice (Mallophaga). Traditionally, the Anoplura and Mallophaga have been treated as separate insect orders but many authors now treat these two groups as suborders of a single order, the Phthiraptera. Further, some authors assign equivalent subordinal taxonomic rank to the Anoplura and each of the three major groups of chewing lice (Amblycera, Ischnocera and Rhyncophthirina), sometimes rejecting the name Mallophaga altogether (Lyal 1985). A neutral approach will be taken in this chapter by using the terms "sucking lice" and "chewing lice."

The generic assignments of some lice, as sometimes reported in the literature, are not always taxonomically correct. For example, usage of the generic names *Bovicola, Damalinia, Tricholipeurus,* and *Werneckiella* has not been consistent. Currently accepted generic combinations for sucking lice are provided by Durden and Musser (1994a) with an additional change by Chin (1998), and for chewing lice of mammals by Emerson and Price (1981).

About 550 valid species of sucking lice have been described, and Durden and Musser (1994a) provide a taxonomic list of the species described through 1993. The sucking lice are currently separated into 16 families and 49 genera (Kim and Ludwig 1978; Durden and Musser 1994a; Chin 1998). Ferris (1919–1935, 1951) provides descriptions and synopses of those species described through 1950, whereas Kim et al. (1986)

provide illustrations, keys, and synopses of the 76 North American species. Kim (1987) provides an identification guide to the immature stages of several species of sucking lice.

About 2700 valid species of chewing lice have been described, and several hundred more species probably await discovery. Partly because of the larger number of species involved and the greater host diversity, the chewing lice are taxonomically less well known than are the sucking lice. However, checklists of world and North American chewing louse species have been prepared by Hopkins and Clay (1952) and Emerson (1972), respectively. Hellenthal and Price (1994) provide an identification key to species of the diverse assemblage of chewing lice associated with pocket gophers. Price (1987) provides a guide to the immature stages of some chewing lice. Although taxonomic interpretations differ, the chewing lice are often divided into 3 suborders, 11 families, and 205 genera.

Scanlon (1960) prepared a guide to the sucking and chewing lice of mammals inhabiting New York state which can also be used to identify lice collected in adjacent states. Price and Graham (1997) have prepared a guide to the sucking and chewing lice of mammals and birds with emphasis on species parasitizing domestic animals.

All lice are dorsoventrally flattened, although engorged individuals of some species can temporarily appear more cylindrical. As indicated by their vernacular names, the sucking lice have piercing-sucking mouthparts while the chewing lice have mandibular, chewing mouthparts. The head is narrower than the thorax in the sucking lice (Fig. 1.1) but wider than the thorax in the chewing lice (Fig. 1.2). Chewing lice can be easily separated into three main groups (suborders of some authors): the Amblycera (Fig. 1.2A), Ischnocera (Fig. 1.2B-E) and Rhyncophthirina (Fig. 1.2F). Members of the Amblycera possess maxillary palps and 4-segmented antennae concealed in grooves along the side of the head. Members of the Ischnocera lack maxillary palps and have 3- to 5-segmented antennae, which are free from the head. Members of the Rhyncophthirina have a distinctly elongate rostrum with tiny mandibles at the tip. Eyes are reduced or absent in most lice, although distinct ocular points or eyes are present in some of the larger sucking lice such as the hog louse, *Haematopinus suis* (Fig. 1.1F), and the peccary sucking louse, *Pecaroecus javalii* (Fig. 1.1E).

Each of the three thoracic segments of lice bears a pair of legs that terminate in claws. These are highly modified as tibiotarsal claws in sucking lice, and the diameter enclosed by the largest (hind) claws typically conforms to the diameter of the host hair shaft. The elongate louse abdomen bears sclerotized plates in many species, which impart some rigidity to the expandable body. Finger-like gonopods, which aid in egg manipulation and deposition, are situated terminally on the female abdomen, and adults of both sexes bear distinctive genitalia in this region.

LIFE HISTORY. Sucking lice are obligate hematophagous (blood-feeding) ectoparasites of placental mammals. As a group, the chewing lice have more diverse feeding habits ranging from hematophagy to the ingestion of host fur, feathers, or sloughed skin of mammals or birds. The skin-piercing, stylet-like mouthparts of the sucking lice are better adapted for a hematophagous diet than are the mandibular mouthparts of chewing lice. Sucking lice have a powerful pharyngeal (cibarial) pump that creates suction for imbibing blood and the midgut typically has discrete structures called mycetomes that harbor microorganisms for aiding blood meal digestion.

Female lice glue their eggs onto the hair shafts of their mammalian hosts. Eggs are distinctively shaped in many louse species, and although they are small, they glisten as the host fur is parted and are therefore easier to find than the lice themselves. Louse eggs are glued so permanently to host hair that they typically remain attached after they have hatched until the hair is lost during a host molt. After several days of embryonic development the first instar nymph emerges from the egg. Another two nymphal instars follow, with each stage lasting 2–8 days, depending on species, and each stage being terminated by a molt that precedes the next stage. Nymphs can be distinguished from adults because they are smaller, lack genitalia, are less sclerotized, and have fewer body setae.

Adult stages of most lice can live ~30 days if they do not succumb to host grooming or other causes of mortality; generation time averages about 45 days. Mating occurs on the host with the smaller male louse crawling beneath the female and curving his abdomen upward to initiate copulation. A few species of chewing lice in the genus *Bovicola* (Fig. 1.2C) are parthenogenetic.

With few exceptions, lice transfer from one individual mammal to another when the hosts are in close physical contact such as during mother-offspring contacts (in burrows and nests or during suckling), mating, or aggressive behaviors (Durden 1983). A few lice can cling to winged hematophagous flies, which they use for transport (phoresy) when the fly disperses to a new host (Durden 1990). At least one species of sucking louse, the sheep foot louse (*Linognathus pedalis*), can crawl short distances on pasture to infest new hosts (Durden 1983). Because most lice are host specific and host mammals typically interact with other members of their own species, transfers to heterospecific hosts are rare. However, this phenomenon has been recorded in a few wild mammals, especially for lice infesting different species of deer (Brunetti and Cribbs 1971; Westrom et al. 1976; Foreyt et al. 1986).

Lice of rodents and other small mammals appear to undergo more or less continuous generations although host hibernation, molting, and pregnancy (estrogens imbibed with the blood meal adversely affect some ectoparasites) may curtail louse reproduction. In temperate climates, lice of larger mammals such as deer, cattle, and horses usually multiply to large numbers

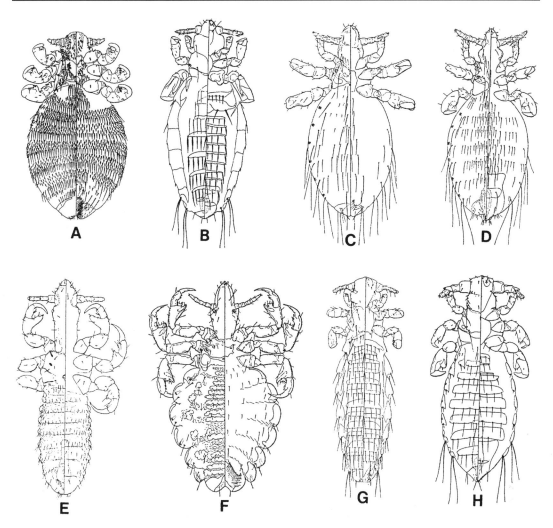

FIG. 1.1—Representative sucking lice showing dorsal morphology to left of midline and ventral features on right: (A) *Echinophthirius horridus,* ♀, ex harbor seals (Phocidae), Holarctic region; (B) *Hoplopleura hesperomydis,* ♂, ex deer mice (*Peromyscus* spp.), N. America; (C) *Solenopotes ferrisi,* ♀, ex deer (*Odocoileus* and *Cervus*), N. America; (D) *Linognathus africanus,* ♂, ex sheep and goats (*Ovis* and *Capra*) [but see Brunetti and Cribbs (1971) and Foreyt et al. (1986) for deer as hosts], Cosmopolitan; (E) *Pecaroecus javalii* (posterior claws omitted dorsally), ♂, ex peccary (*Pecari*), USA to S. America; (F) *Haematopinus suis,* ♀ ex swine (*Sus*), Cosmopolitan; (G) *Neohaematopinus sciuropterii,* ♀, ex flying squirrels (*Glaucomys* spp.), N. America; (H) *Polyplax spinulosa,* ♂, ex domestic rats (*Rattus* spp.), Cosmopolitan. Not to scale. [A–D, F–H redrawn from Ferris (1919–1935); E redrawn from Ferris (1951.)]

during the winter and early spring but are present as small populations during the summer. Samuel and Trainer (1971) and Westrom and Anderson (1983) demonstrated this phenomenon for *Tricholipeurus parallelus* (Fig. 1.2B) on white-tailed deer, and for *Solenopotes ferrisi* (Fig. 1.1C) infesting Columbian black-tailed deer, respectively, in North America.

HOST ASSOCIATIONS. Lice are typically host specific with most species parasitizing a single host species, or a few closely related species. Lice of some mammals such as hyraxes, cattle, sheep, and some squirrels are further specialized in that they are segregated onto distinct body regions of the host. Lice are so committed to an ectoparasitic existence, often on a single host species, that they cannot survive more than a few hours (or a few days in rare cases) away from their host.

Lice are intimate ectoparasites that, barring dislodgement, live permanently in the host pelage. They have generally evolved with their hosts, which

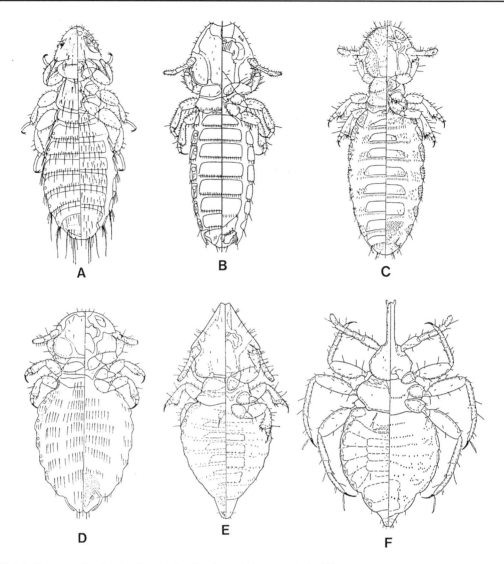

FIG. 1.2—Representative chewing lice showing dorsal morphology to left of midline and ventral features on right: (**A**) *Heterodoxus spiniger,* ♀, ex carnivores, Cosmopolitan (Amblycera); (**B**) *Tricholipeurus parallelus,* ♂, ex deer (*Odocoileus* spp.), Canada to S. America (Ischnocera); (**C**) *Bovicola ovis,* ♀, ex sheep (*Ovis*), Cosmopolitan (Ischnocera); (**D**) *Trichodectes canis,* ♀, ex canids, Cosmopolitan (Ischnocera); (**E**) *Felicola subrostrata,* ♂, ex felids, Cosmopolitan (Ischnocera); (**F**) *Haematomyzus elephantis,* ♂, ex African and Indian elephants (*Loxodonta* and *Elephas*), Africa and Indian subcontinent (Rhyncophthirina). Not to scale. [A–E redrawn from Emerson and Price (1975); F redrawn from Werneck (1950.)]

accounts for the close host-parasite interrelationships and congruent phylogenies that they often exhibit (Kim 1985; Emerson and Price 1985; Hafner and Nadler 1988). Certain groups of mammals such as rodents, hyraxes, artiodactyls, and old-world primates are parasitized by diverse assemblages of sucking lice, whereas monotremes, marsupials, bats, edentates, pangolins, elephants, whales, and sea cows are not parasitized by any sucking lice (Durden and Musser 1994a). As a group, the rodent family Sciuridae (squirrels, chip-munks, susliks, and marmots) are parasitized by many more genera (ten) of sucking lice than any other mammal group, which may reflect an ancient host-parasite association.

Table 1.1 provides information on each of the 50 sucking louse genera that have been reported from mammals; many species are known from mammals of North America (Table 1.2). Sucking and chewing lice have almost certainly accompanied wild ungulates introduced to North America (Table 1.3). In addition to

TABLE 1.1—Sucking lice (Anoplura) parasitic on mammals

Louse Family/Genus	No. of Species	Host(s)	Distribution
Echinophthiriidae			
Antarctophthirus	6	Seals, sea lions, walrus	Worldwide—marine
Echinophthirius	1	Seals	Holarctic—marine
Latagophthirus	1	River otter	N. America
Lepidophthirus	2	Seals	Old World—aquatic
Proechinophthirius	2	Sea lions	Old World—marine
Enderleinellidae			
Atopophthirus	2	Flying squirrels	S.E. Asia
Enderleinellus	46	Squirrels	Almost worldwide
Microphthirus	1	Flying squirrels	N. America
Phthirunculus	1	Flying squirrels	S.E. Asia
Werneckia	5	Squirrels	Africa
Haematopinidae			
Haematopinus	21	Ungulates	Worldwide
Hamophthiriidae			
Hamophthirius	1	Colugo	Borneo
Hoplopleuridae			
Ancistroplax	5	Shrews	Southern Asia
Haematopinoides	1	Moles	N. America
Hoplopleura	146	Rodents, pikas	Worldwide
Paradoxophthirus	1	Squirrel	People's Republic of China
Pterophthirus	5	Echimyid and caviid rodents	Neotropics
Schizophthirus	9	Dipodid and myoxid rodents	Old World
Hybophthiridae			
Hybophthirus	1	Aardvark	Africa
Linognathidae			
Linognathus	51	Artiodactyls, canids	Worldwide
Prolinognathus	9	Hyraxes	Africa
Solenopotes	9	Artiodactyls	Worldwide
Microthoraciidae			
Microthoracius	4	Camels, llamas	Asia, N. Africa, S. America
Mirophthiridae			
Mirophthiris	1	Platacanthomyine rodent	People's Republic of China
Neolinognathidae			
Neolinognathus	2	Elephant shrews	Africa
Pecaroecidae			
Pecaroecus	1	Collared peccary	New World
Pedicinidae			
Pedicinus	16	Cercopithecid primates	Old World
Pediculidae			
Pediculus	3	Primates, including humans	Worldwide
Polyplacidae			
Abrocomaphthirus	2	Abrocomid rodents	S. America
Ctenophthirus	1	Echimyid rodent	Paraguay
Cuyana	1	Chinchilla	Argentina
Docophthirus	1	Tree shrew	India
Eulinognathus	29	Rodents	Old World, S. America
Fahrenholzia	12	Heteromyid rodents	New World
Galeophthirus	1	Caviid rodent	Argentina
Haemodipsus	6	Rabbits and hares	Almost worldwide
Johnsonpthirus	5	Squirrels	Africa
Lagidiophthirus	1	Chinchilla	S. America
Lemurpediculus	2	Lemurs	Madagascar
Lemurphthirus	3	Bushbabies	Africa
Linognathoides	11	Sciurid rodents	Holarctic region
Neohaematopinus	31	Squirrels, woodrats	Almost worldwide
Phthirpediculus	3	Lemurs	Madagascar
Polyplax	82	Rodents	Worldwide
Proenderleinellus	1	Cricetomyine rodent	Africa
Sathrax	1	Tree shrews	S.E. Asia
Scipio	3	Rodents	Africa
Typhlomyophthirus	2	Platacanthomyine rodents	People's Republic of China
Pthiridae			
Pthirus	2	Gorilla, humans	Worldwide
Ratemiidae			
Ratemia	3	Equids	Old World

TABLE 1.2—Sucking lice (Anoplura) parasitic on North American mammals

Host(s)	Louse/Lice	Distribution
Moles	*Haematopinoides squamosus*	Eastern and Central USA
Canids (general)	*Linognathus setosus*	Cosmopolitan
River otter	*Latagophthirus rauschi*	Northwestern N. America
Otariid seals and sea lions	*Proechinophthirus fluctus*	N. Pacific and Bering Sea
	Antarctophthirus spp.	Various distributions
Walrus	*Antarctophthirus trichechi*	Arctic region
Phocid seals	*Echinophthirius horridus*	Holarctic region
Equids	*Haematopinus asini*	Cosmopolitan
Feral and domestic swine	*Haematopinus suis*	Cosmopolitan
Peccary	*Pecaroecus javalii*	Southwestern USA to S. America
Deer (*Odocoileus* spp.)	*Solenopotes binipilosus*	N., Central and S. America
American elk	*Solenopotes ferrisi*	Across N. America
Caribou	*Solenopotes tarandi*	Northern Holarctic region
Mountain goat	*Linognathus pedalis*	Cosmopolitan
Domestic sheep	*Linognathus africanus*	Cosmopolitan
	Linognathus ovillus	Worldwide in temperate regions
	Linognathus pedalis	Cosmopolitan
Feral and domestic goats	*Linognathus stenopsis*	Cosmopolitan
	Linognathus africanus	Cosmopolitan
Cattle	*Haematopinus eurysternus*	Worldwide in temperate regions
	Haematopinus quadripertusus	Worldwide in tropics and subtropics
	Linognathus vituli	Cosmopolitan
	Solenopotes capillatus	Holarctic; introduced elsewhere
Prairie dogs	*Enderleinellus suturalis*	Most of N. America
	Linognathoides cynomyis	South Dakota
Marmots (groundhogs)	*Enderleinellus marmotae*	Northeastern and North-central USA
	Linognathoides marmotae	Western N. America
Flying squirrels (*Glaucomys* spp.)	*Hoplopleura trispinosa*	Across N. America
	Neohaematopinus sciuropteri	Across N. America
	Microphthirus uncinatus	N. America
Eastern gray squirrel	*Enderleinellus longiceps*	N. America; introduced to Europe
	Hoplopleura sciuricola	N., Central and S. America; introduced to Europe
	Neohaematopinus sciuri	Holarctic region
Western gray squirrel	*Enderleinellus kelloggi*	California
	Hoplopleura sciuricola	N., Central and S. America; introduced to Europe
	Neohaematopinus griseicolus	Western USA and Mexico
Kaibab squirrel	*Enderleinellus kaibabensis*	Arizona
Fox squirrel	*Enderleinellus longiceps*	N. America; introduced to Europe
	Hoplopleura sciuricola	N., Central and S. America; introduced to Europe
	Neohaematopinus sciurinus	Across N. America
Red squirrels (*Tamiasciurus* spp.)	*Enderleinellus tamiasciuri*	Across N. America
	Hoplopleura sciuricola	N., Central and S. America; introduced to Europe
	Neohamatopinus semifasciatus	N. America to northern S. America
Ground squirrels (*Spermophilus* spp.)	*Enderleinellus osborni*	Western N. America and Mexico
	Enderleinellus suturalis	Most of N. America
	Linognathoides laeviusculus	Holarctic region
Eastern chipmunk	*Hoplopleura erratica*	Eastern N. America
Other chipmunks	*Enderleinellus osborni*	Western N. America and Mexico
	Hoplopleura arboricola	Central and western N. America
	Neohaematopinus pacificus	Western N. America
Kangaroo rats and pocket mice	*Fahrenholzia* spp.	Southwestern Canada to Central America
Voles and lemmings	*Hoplopleura acanthopus*	Holarctic region
	Polyplax alaskensis	Across N. America, especially northern regions
	Polyplax borealis	Northern Holarctic region
Woodrats	*Neohaematopinus* spp.	Western N. America
Grasshopper mice	*Hoplopleura onychomydis*	Western USA
Peromyscus spp.	*Hoplopleura hesperomydis*	Across N. America and Mexico
	Polyplax auricularis	Canada to Central America
Rice rats	*Hoplopleura oryzomydis*	Southern USA to northern S. America
Cotton rats	*Hoplopleura hirsuta*	N., Central and S. America
	Hoplopleura arizonensis	Southwestern USA to S. America
House mouse	*Hoplopleura captiosa*	Cosmopolitan
	Polyplax serrata	Cosmopolitan
Domestic rats	*Hoplopleura pacifica*	Worldwide in warmer climates
	Polyplax spinulosa	Cosmopolitan
Hares and jackrabbits	*Haemodipsus setoni*	Holarctic region
Domestic (laboratory) rabbit	*Haemodipsus ventricosus*	Cosmopolitan

TABLE 1.3—Lice parasitic on some wild mammals (Ungulates) introduced into North America[a]

Host(s)	Louse/Lice	Origin
Axis deer (chital)	*Damalinia forficula forficula*	Asia
Blackbuck antelope	*Trichlipeurus balanicus balanicus*	India
	Linognathus cervicaprae	India
	Linognathus pithodes	India
Fallow deer	*Bovicola tibialis*	Europe
Muntjac	*Damalinia forficula forficula*	Asia
	Tricholipeurus indicus	Asia
	Solenopotes muntiacus	S. Asia
Red deer	*Bovicola longicornis*	Europe
	Solenopotes burmeisteri	Eurasia
	Solenopotes ferrisi	N. America[b]
Sika deer	*Damalinia maai*	Eurasia
	Solenopotes burmeisteri	Eurasia
Roe deer	*Damalinia meyeri*	Eurasia
	Solenopotes capreoli	Eurasia

[a]Although not all of the lice listed have been recovered from these hosts in North America, it is suspected that all or most of them have accompanied their hosts as introductions into this continent.

[b]Presumably this louse transferred from American elk to European red deer, two cervids that some mammalogists now treat as a single species.

references already cited, useful synopses of various groups of sucking lice include works by Séguy (1944) and Beaucournu (1968) for western Europe, Johnson (1960, 1964) for species of Africa and southeast Asia, respectively, Kühn and Ludwig (1967) for the primate-infesting genus *Pedicinus,* Johnson (1972) for sucking lice of Venezuelan rodents, Ledger (1980) for lice of sub-Saharan Africa, Mishra (1981) and Adhikary and Ghosh (1994) for the Indian fauna, Durden (1991) for the rodent-infesting genus *Neohaematopinus,* and Méndez (1990) for the Panamanian fauna. Hopkins (1949), Kim (1985), and Durden and Musser (1994b) provide overviews of the host associations of sucking lice.

Although most species of chewing lice are ectoparasites of birds, about 500 described species, representing 43 genera in seven families (Table 1.4) parasitize mammals; many species are known from mammals of North America (Table 1.5). Representatives of the Amblycera (four families associated with mammals), Ischnocera (two families associated with mammals), and Rhyncophthirina (one family) all parasitize mammals. Emerson and Price (1981) provide a host-parasite list for chewing louse–mammal associations documented through 1980. Some additional guides to various groups of chewing lice associated with mammals include works by Séguy (1944) for western European species; Werneck (1948, 1950) for the world fauna; Kéler (1971) for the Australasian fauna; Ledger (1980) for the fauna of sub-Saharan Africa; Emerson and Price (1975) for the fauna of Venezuela; Scanlon (1960) and

Whitaker (1982) for the faunas of New York state and Indiana (USA), respectively; Emerson and Price (1988) for the three species of *Haematomyzus;* Barker (1991) for taxa associated with Australian rock wallabies; Hellenthal and Price (1991) for taxa associated with pocket gophers; Rékási (1994) for the fauna of central Europe; and Timm and Price (1994a,b, 2000) for the genera *Eutrichophilus* and *Felicola,* respectively. Hopkins (1949) and Emerson and Price (1981, 1985) provide overviews of the host associations of the chewing lice of mammals.

EPIZOOTIOLOGY, CLINICAL SIGNS, AND PATHOLOGY. Small inconsequential louse infestations are the norm on most parasitized wild mammals. In fact, large louse infestations on mammals often reflect host senility, illness, an immunocompromised state, nutritional deficiencies, or the inability to groom efficiently. Lice can detrimentally affect their mammalian hosts in several ways such as by causing anemia, dermatitis, pruritis (itching), skin sensitization and other allergic reactions, intense grooming, fur-matting and alopecia (fur loss), inflamed or scaly skin, unthriftiness, decreased growth rates, secondary infections at bite sites, and the transmission of parasites and pathogens (Nelson et al. 1975, 1977). However, even when louse infestations on wild mammals are large, they have rarely been implicated as the cause of serious pathological conditions (Nelson et al. 1975, 1977). For example, the primary cause of death of 19 radio-tracked wolves (*Canis lupus*) and coyotes (*Canis latrans*) in Minnesota and Wisconsin that were infested with chewing lice, *Trichodectes canis* (Fig. 1.2D), was never deemed to have been a result of louse infestation, and in only two cases were lice considered to be a possible secondary cause of mortality (Mech et al. 1985). However, gray wolves with severe infestations of *T. canis* in Alaska had varying degrees of alopecia accompanied by broken guard hairs, matted underfur, and skin lesions, which lowered the commercial value of their pelts and possibly also resulted in compromised overwinter survival (Schwartz et al. 1983).

Notwithstanding the above statements, louse infestations can cause serious health problems in wild mammals. Foreyt et al. (1986) reported severe alopecia, depression, and poor growth (compared to uninfested animals) in fawns of mule deer (*Odocoileus hemionus*) and white-tailed deer (*Odocoileus virginianus*) caused by heavy infestations of the sucking louse *Linognathus africanus* (Fig. 1.1D). Similarly, Brunetti and Cribbs (1971) reported deaths of mule deer and Columbian black-tailed deer (*Odocoileus hemionus columbianus*) caused by exsanguination anemia due to massive infestations of this louse. Both of these reports are intriguing, not only because of the associated pathology, but also because *L. africanus* normally parasitizes sheep and goats (Table 1.2). Another two reports of severe pediculosis involve alopecia and fur-matting in coyotes caused by the chewing louse *T. canis* (Foreyt et al.

TABLE 1.4—Chewing lice (Mallophaga) parasitic on mammals

Louse Suborder/Family/Genus	No. of Species	Hosts	Distribution
RYNCOPHTHIRINA			
Haematomyzidae			
Haematomyzus	3	Elephants, suids	Africa, Asia
ISCHNOCERA			
Trichophilopteridae			
Trichophilopterus	2	Lemurs, aye-aye	Madagascar
Trichodectidae			
Bovicola	31	Ungulates	Worldwide
Cebidicola	3	Primates	Neotropics
Damalinia	19	Ungulates	Almost worldwide
Dasyonyx	15	Hyraxes	Africa
Eurytrichodectes	2	Hyraxes	Africa
Eutrichophilus	19	Porcupines	New World
Felicola	55[a]	Carnivores, loris	Almost worldwide
Geomydoecus	84[b]	Pocket gophers	N. and Central America
Lutridia	3	Otters	Old World, S. America
Lymeon	2	Sloths	Neotropics
Neofelicola	4	Viverrids	S.E. Asia
Neotrichodectes	10	Raccoons, mustelids	N., Central and S. America
Parafelicola	6	Viverrids	Old World
Procavicola	32	Hyraxes	Africa
Procaviphilus	7	Hyraxes	Africa
Stachiella	9	Mustelids	Almost worldwide
Thomomydoecus	20[b]	Pocket gophers	N. and Central America
Trichodectes	16	Carnivores, ungulates	Worldwide
Tricholipeurus	23	Ungulates	Worldwide
AMBLYCERA			
Boopiidae			
Boopia	16	Marsupials	Australasia
Heterodoxus	17	Carnivores, marsupials	Australasia[c]
Latumcephalum	3	Macropodid marsupials	Australia
Macropophila	4	Macropodid marsupials	Australia
Paraboopia	1	Macropodid marsupials	Australia
Paraheterodoxus	3	Potoroid marsupials	Australia
Phacogalia	2	Dasyurid marsupials	Australia
Gyropidae			
Abrocomophaga	3	Abrocomid and octodontid rodent	S. America
Aotiella	2	Howler monkeys	Neotropics
Gliricola	39	Rodents	Neotropics
Gyropus	19	Rodents	Neotropics
Macrogyropus	4	Rodents, peccaries	Neotropics
Monothoracius	2	Rodents	Neotropics
Phtheiropois	8	Rodents	Neotropics
Pitrufquenia	1	Myocastorid rodent	Neotropics[d]
Protogyropus	1	Caviid rodents	Neotropics
Trimenoponidae			
Chinchillophaga	1	Chinchillas	S. America
Cummingsia	10	Rodents, marsupials	S. America
Harrisonia	1	Echimyid rodent	Neotropics
Hoplomyophilus	1	Echimyid rodent	Neotropics
Philandesia	3	Chinchillas	S. America
Trimenopon	1	Caviid rodent	Neotropics

[a]*Lorisicola*, *Suricatoecus* and *Paradoxuroecus* are here treated as subgenera of *Felicola* following Timm and Price (1994b).
[b]These species have been segregated into several subspecies (Hellenthal and Price 1994).
[c]*Heterodoxus spiniger* now parasitizes carnivores throughout the world.
[d]Introduced to North America, Europe, and elsewhere.

1978). One of the coyotes was estimated to have an infestation of 50,000 lice. Severe infestations of canids by *T. canis* and *Linognathus setosus,* and of felids by *Felicola subrostrata* (Fig. 1.2E), can cause restlessness, scratching, skin inflammation and alopecia (Kim et al. 1973). Severe pediculosis due to *Echinophthirius hor-*

ridus (Fig. 1.1A) infestations can cause alopecia in harbor seals (Conlogue et al. 1980; Skirnisson and Olafsson 1990).

In India, severe infestations of *Microthoracius cameli* can cause unthriftiness and weakness in camels (Lodha 1964). In South America, a closely related

TABLE 1.5—Chewing lice (Mallophaga) parasitic on North American mammals.

Host(s)	Louse/Lice	Distribution[a]
Canids (general)	*Heterodoxus spiniger*	Cosmopolitan
	Trichodectes canis	Cosmopolitan
Red fox	*Felicola vulpis*	Holarctic region
Gray fox	*Felicola quadraticeps*	Across N. America
Lynx	*Felicola spenceri*	Western N. America
Domestic cat	*Felicola subrostrata*	Cosmopolitan
Bobcat	*Felicola americanus*	Western and Central USA
Mountain lion, ocelot, Florida panther	*Felicola felis*	Across N. America
Ermine (i.e., short-tailed weasel or stoat)	*Stachiella ermineae*	Holarctic region
	Stachiella kingi	Holarctic region
Long-tailed weasel, black-footed ferret	*Neotrichodectes minutus*	Across N. America
Least weasel	*Stachiella mustelae*	Holarctic region
Mink	*Stachiella larseni*	Across N. America; introduced elsewhere
Marten	*Stachiella retusa martis*	Northern N. America
American badger	*Neotrichodectes interuptofasciatus*	Western and Central N. America
Striped skunk, hooded skunk	*Neotrichodectes mephitidis*	Across N. America
Spotted skunk	*Neotrichodectes osborni*	USA to Central America
Hog-nosed skunk	*Neotrichodectes arizonae*	Southwestern USA to Central America
Ringtail	*Neotrichodectes thoracicus*	Southwestern USA to Central America
Raccoon	*Trichodectes octomaculatus*	Across N. America
Black bear	*Trichodectes pinguis euarctidos*	Across N. America
Grizzly bear	*Trichodectes pinguis pinguis*	Western N. America
Donkey	*Bovicola ocellata*	Cosmopolitan
Horse	*Bovicola equi*	Cosmopolitan
	Bovicola ocellata	Cosmopolitan
Elk	*Bovicola longicornis*	Holarctic region
	Bovicola concavifrons	N. America
Caribou	*Bovicola tarandi*	Holarctic region
Deer (*Odocoileus* spp.)	*Tricholipeurus lipeuroides*	Canada to S. America; introduced elsewhere
	Tricholipeurus parallelus	Canada to S. America; introduced elsewhere
Cattle	*Bovicola bovis*	Cosmopolitan
Bison	*Bovicola sedecimdecembrii*	Holarctic region
Goat	*Bovicola caprae*	Cosmopolitan
	Bovicola crassipes	Cosmopolitan
	Bovicola limbata	Cosmopolitan
Domestic sheep	*Bovicola ovis*	Cosmopolitan
Bighorn sheep, Dall's sheep	*Bovicola jellisoni*	Western N. America
Mountain goat	*Bovicola oreamnidis*	Western N. America
Peccary	*Macrogyropus dicotylis*	Southwestern USA to S. America
Pocket gophers	*Geomydoecus* spp.	N. and Central America
	Thomomydoecus spp.	N. and Central America
Nutria	*Pitrufquenia coypus*	New World; introduced elsewhere
Porcupine	*Eutrichophilus setosus*	Canada to Northern Mexico

[a]Where extralimital distributions are indicated, the louse parasitizes the same or closely related host species in other regions.

louse, *Microthoracius mazzai*, can cause host irritation; interruption of normal feeding and sleeping regimes; biting, kicking, and rubbing against posts and shrubs (sometimes resulting in self-inflicted wounds); fleece damage; and lowered weight gains in alpacas and llamas (Cicchino et al. 1998). Ronald and Wagner (1973) reported deaths of spider monkeys (*Ateles geoffroyi*) caused by anemia resulting from severe pediculosis due to *Pediculus mjobergi*. Large infestations of *Haematomyzus elephantis* (Fig. 1.2F) on elephants can cause severe dermatitis, pruritis, and dry, scaly skin (Raghavan et al. 1968). Rodents and lagomorphs can also be adversely affected by louse infestations. In the Netherlands, morbidity and mortality of European red squirrels (*Sciurus vulgaris*) have been attributed to massive populations (up to 80,000 per squirrel) of *Neohaematopinus sciuri* (Beaucournu 1966). Laboratory rats and mice that are heavily infested with *Hoplopleura* spp. (Fig. 1.1B) or *Polyplax* spp. (Fig. 1.1H) are unthrifty and restless. They scratch incessantly and can become anemic, with death resulting in extreme cases (Kim et al. 1973). Infestations of the rabbit louse, *Haemodipsus ventricosus*, cause acute pruritis that predisposes the host to rub and scratch away its fur. Young rabbits infested by large numbers of this louse are debilitated to the extent that their growth can be retarded (Kim et al. 1973).

The effect of louse infestations on host health has been studied in far greater detail for domesticated mammals than for wild mammals. However, because domesticated hosts often survive as feral populations, some of these studies have relevance to wild mammals. For example, severe infestations of cattle lice can cause anemia; feeding inefficiency; weight loss (or reduced weight gains compared to uninfested cattle); fur/hide damage from grooming responses; and behavioral modifications such as kicking, licking, and reduced feeding times (Peterson et al. 1953; Collins and Dewhirst 1965; Kettle 1974, Cummins and Graham 1982; Gibney et al. 1985). A study by DeVaney et al. (1992) demonstrated reduced weight gains and altered blood parameters in calves that were infested with relatively low numbers of lice. Heifers are typically affected more severely than mature cattle, but sometimes pathogenic effects are minimal even with heavy louse infestations (Collins and Dewhirst 1965; Cummins and Graham 1982). Similar effects have been documented for domestic sheep, goats, horses, and hogs with large infestations of lice. Severe hog louse, *Haematopinus suis* (Fig. 1.1F), infestations also cause decreased activity and altered blood cell parameters in weaner pigs relative to control (uninfested) hosts (Davis and Williams 1986). Overall there was no difference in average daily weight gains or feed efficiency between hog louse–infested and uninfested weaner pigs in the study by Davis and Williams (1986). However, in a similar study by Kamyszek and Gibasiewicz (1986), hog louse–infested suckling and fattener piglets showed retarded development and reduced weight gains when compared to uninfested (control) piglets. Based on these studies, it is reasonable to assume that some or all of the detrimental effects resulting from louse infestations of domesticated mammals also occur in wild mammals belonging to the same or related species.

LICE AS VECTORS OF PATHOGENS TO WILD MAMMALS. Apparently, relatively few pathogens of wild mammals are transmitted by lice. This impression probably exists because there has been insufficient study of this topic rather because it is a true reflection of the phenomenon. Because they are obligate hematophages, it is not surprising that more sucking lice than chewing lice have been implicated as vectors of pathogens. In some cases, it has not been definitively ascertained whether pathogen transmission by lice involves a developmental cycle of the organism inside the louse (i.e., biological transmission) or short-term survival of the pathogen on the louse mouthparts or other structures (i.e., mechanical transmission). Although the etiologic agents of several diseases have been detected in, or isolated from, lice (especially sucking lice), some of these agents may have been imbibed with the blood meal, and lice may not be effective vectors of these pathogens. The causative agents of borreliosis (including Lyme disease), bartonellosis, brucellosis, salmonellosis, several viral and rickettsial infections, and murine trypanosomiasis fall into this category. However, the causative agents of zoonoses such as Q fever and tularemia are readily transmitted by rodent and lagomorph sucking lice that appear to play a role in the enzootic maintenance of these pathogens in nature.

The hog louse, *H. suis* (Fig. 1.1F) is a vector of swinepox virus to hogs (Bruner 1963). Also, Lebombo virus has been isolated from sucking lice (*Scipio aulacodi*) recovered from African cane rats (*Thryonomys swinderianus*), suggesting that these lice could be enzootic vectors of this zoonotic pathogen between their rat hosts (Karabatsos 1985). The seal louse, *Echinophthirius horridus* (Fig. 1.1A), has been implicated as a possible vector of the highly pathogenic seal morbillivirus in northern Europe (Beder 1990), but definitive data pertaining to its vectorial capacity for this virus are lacking.

The cosmopolitan bacteria *Haemobartonella muris* and *Eperythrozoon coccoides* are both transmitted to their rodent hosts by sucking lice. *H. muris* is transmitted to *Rattus* spp. by the spined rat louse, *Polyplax spinulosa* (Fig. 1.1H) (Crystal 1959; Durden and Musser 1994b), whereas *E. coccoides* is transmitted to house mice by the mouse louse, *Polyplax serrata* (Berkencamp and Wescott 1988). Transmission of two related pathogens, *Eperythrozoon suis* and *Eperythrozoon parvum*, both of which cause swine eperythrozoonosis, has been reported for infected hog lice feeding on splenectomized hogs under experimental conditions (Prullage et al. 1993).

An intriguing zoonosis that is maintained in flying squirrels and their ectoparasites is enzootic in North America (McDade 1987). The agent involved causes sporadic epidemic typhus in humans but causes inapparent, transient infections in southern flying squirrels (*Glaucomys volans*). The pathogen has been identified as *Rickettsia prowazekii*, which causes epidemic (louse-borne) typhus in humans; flying squirrel isolates are almost identical to strains that cause this form of epidemic typhus in humans. Under laboratory conditions, flying squirrel sucking lice, *Neohaematopinus sciuropteri* (Fig. 1.1G), and fleas efficiently transmit this rickettsial agent to flying squirrels (McDade 1987).

Chewing and sucking lice of cattle are known to be mechanical vectors of the skin fungus *Trichophyton verrucosum*, which causes dermatomycosis (i.e., ringworm) (Durden and Musser 1994b). Very likely, other species of lice are mechanical vectors of skin fungi and other dermal pathogens of wild mammals.

At least two species of apicomplexan protozoan parasites of rodents, *Hepatozoon gerbilli* and *Hepatozoon pitymysi*, have been found in the sucking lice *Polyplax stephensi* and *Hoplopleura acanthopus*, respectively, which may act as vectors of these agents to their rodent hosts (Smith 1996).

The seal heartworm *Dipetalonema spirocauda* is an important cause of mortality and morbidity in harbor seals throughout the Holarctic region (Conlogue et al. 1980; Skirnisson and Olafsson 1990). This heartworm undergoes biological development in the seal sucking louse, *Echinophthirius horridus* (Fig. 1.1A), which then transmits infective microfilariae to seals as it feeds on them (Geraci et al. 1981). A related filarial nematode, *Dipetalonema reconditum*, has been recovered from the chewing louse *Heterodoxus spiniger*

(Fig. 1.2A) and from the dog sucking louse *Linognathus setosus,* both of which are believed to be vectors of the infective microfilariae to canids (Pennington and Phelps 1969).

LICE AS INTERMEDIATE HOSTS OF PARASITES. The dog chewing louse *Trichodectes canis* (Fig. 1.2D), which parasitizes several species of wild canids (Table 1.5), is an intermediate host of the double-pored tapeworm, *Dipylidium caninum,* which usually parasitizes canids (Kim et al. 1973). Lice become parasitized when they ingest viable *D. caninum* eggs from dried host feces. Inside the louse, the tapeworm develops into the cysticercoid stage and then remains quiescent until it is ingested by the definitive (canid) host, typically during host grooming activities. In the canid alimentary canal, the cysticercoid is liberated, attaches to the gut wall, and metamorphoses into the adult tapeworm. Reproducing tapeworms complete the life cycle by releasing proglottids containing eggs that are voided in the host feces.

DIAGNOSIS. Louse infestations of wild mammals are best diagnosed when the host is immobilized during either biopsy or necropsy examinations. When visually searching for lice on host skin, particular attention should be paid to areas adjacent to alopecia or skin discoloration and to body regions that are inaccessible by grooming. On live mammals, host fur should be parted in order to locate lice attached to hair bases next to the skin surface; on dead hosts, lice tend to gradually migrate to the hair tips. Hosts that have been dead for more than 1–2 days will most likely have lost their lice to scavenging or predatory animals, especially arthropods. If feasible, a low-power binocular microscope should be used to aid in locating lice. Lice can also be collected using laboratory techniques such as dissolving skin in potassium hydroxide (Kim et al. 1986; Welch and Samuel 1989), washing skin sections in detergent solution (Henry and McKeever 1971), skin scrubbing (van Dyk and McKenzie 1992), and skin combing or brushing (Ignoffo 1958). On large animals, a random sampling technique can be used to estimate louse densities (Welch and Samuel 1989).

Attached lice should be collected with fine jeweler's forceps by gently grasping each specimen anteriorly close to its attachment site. Lice to be identified should then be added to appropriately labeled vials containing 70% ethanol in which they can be stored indefinitely. Lice stored in ethanol can later be cleared in 10% potassium hydroxide, dehydrated in a series of alcohols of ascending strength, further cleared in xylene, and then slide-mounted in Canada balsam for identification (Kim et al. 1986). Useful identification guides for various groups of lice are listed in the preceding sections in this chapter on "Classification, Taxonomy, and Morphology" and "Host Associations." Lice stored in ethanol can often be screened for pathogens using the polymerase chain reaction with appropriate DNA primers for the pathogen(s) under consideration. However, if pathogen isolates are required, lice should be stored alive on dry ice or in a liquid nitrogen tank in the field, then transferred to an appropriate freezer in a laboratory, depending on the pathogen under study.

IMMUNITY. In many cases, the precise mode of developmemt of host immunity against lice is incompletely understood. As with immune responses to most hematophagous arthropods, immunity to lice is often expressed as a reduction in engorgement rates, fecundity of females, and survival of eggs deposited after the immune blood meal (Jones 1996). An intriguing situation exists in house mice whereby areas of host skin subjected to a certain number of bites from the mouse louse (*Polyplax serrata*) develop immunity which does not readily spread to other areas of skin unless a surgical graft is made (Nelson et al. 1979). However, systemic immunity to lice can develop in house mice (Ratzlaff and Wikel 1990), domestic rats (Volf 1991), cattle (Jones 1996), and probably also in other parasitized mammals. In house mice parasitized by *P. serrata*, several host cell types such as neutrophils, eosinophils, and lymphocytes proliferate at louse attachment sites (Nelson et al. 1977, 1979), while lymphoid cells proliferate systemically (Ratzlaff and Wikel 1990). These cellular responses are accompanied by vasoconstriction, a decrease in the number of blood vessels, and epidermal thickening at louse infestation sites after about 5 weeks. About 4 weeks after the initial infestation, total body populations of *P. serrata* start to decline on immunocompetent mice. Presumably, immune responses against lice on wild mammals operate in a similar fashion.

CONTROL AND TREATMENT. Several techniques have been used to rid animals of lice, with varying degrees of success. These can be divided into behavioral techniques and chemical techniques. The former involve maintaining animals in uncrowded conditions to prevent the rapid spread of lice, shearing wool from sheep, and host grooming responses such as scratching, biting, and licking.

Chemicals that kill lice are called pediculicides, and a wide array of products is currently available. Pediculicidal dusts, powders, sprays, dips, ear tags, tail tags, collars, pour-ons, shampoos, and topical lotions are widely used veterinary products. Infested mammals destined to be incorporated into established herds or colonies should be quarantined until their lice have been eradicated. Lousy animals should be treated weekly for 2–4 weeks, and their caging or bedding should be disinfected simultaneously. Treatment with insecticides such as carbaryl, cypermethrin, deltamethrin, diazinon, lindane, and malathion is usually efficacious. Resin strips impregnated with insecticides can be used as neck collars, ear tags, tail tags, or gut boluses, or can simply be added to cages to control lice. Similar strips, insecticidal dust bags, or 'back rubbers' can be used as self-dosing rubbing stations for cattle, deer, and other ungulates. Because louse populations on most temperate ungulates increase during the cooler months, pediculicides should ideally be administered to them in the late fall.

Several recently developed parasiticides have shown promise as pediculicides. Avermectins such as abamectin, doramectin, and ivermectin kill lice. Prescribed doses of these compounds can be administered orally, topically, or by injection. The bacterium *Bacillus thuringiensis* var. *israelensis,* which is an effective biological control agent against numerous nuisance arthropods, also has pediculicidal properties. Some juvenile hormone analogs and insect growth regulators similarly show promise as pediculicides. The attempts to develop vaccines and hosts genetically resistant to louse infestation are fields with a great deal of current interest.

PUBLIC HEALTH CONCERNS. Because lice are quite host specific, species associated with wild mammals present only minor public health concerns. Nevertheless, hungry lice will occasionally feed on unusual hosts, and some monkey lice will readily feed on humans (Ronald and Wagner 1973). Because little is known about the relationship of certain zoonotic pathogens and lice associated with wild mammals, care should be taken to avoid accidentally crushing lice on human skin. As a prudent precaution, at the least, latex gloves should be worn when lice are collected during host biopsies or necropsies.

At least one species of louse, the dog chewing louse *Trichodectes canis* (Fig. 1.2D), has proven zoonotic importance because it is an intermediate host of *Dipylidium caninum;* if infected lice are inadvertently ingested (by children playing with dogs, etc.), this helminth can parasitize humans.

Humans are parasitized by the following three host-specific lice, none of which characteristically parasitize any other host species: the body louse, *Pediculus humanus humanus;* the head louse, *Pediculus humanus capitis;* and the crab (i.e., pubic) louse, *Pthirus pubis* (Durden and Musser 1994a,b).

DOMESTIC ANIMAL HEALTH CONCERNS. Most species of domestic mammals are parasitized by lice (Tables 1.1–1.5). Some of these hosts, such as dogs, horses, cattle, goats, and sheep, can be infested by two or more species of lice. Therefore, louse infestations of domestic animals have considerable economic importance. The situation can be exacerbated because feral populations of most of these domestic mammals persist in nature where they may serve as reservoirs of lice. For example, the three species of lice that parasitize domestic dogs (*Linognathus setosus, Heterodoxus spiniger,* and *Trichodectes canis*), also parasitize coyotes, wolves, feral dogs, and some other canids. Feral horses, cattle, goats, and other ungulates can similarly maintain feral louse populations that have the potential to transfer to domesticated conspecific (or sometimes, closely related) hosts. A puzzling phenomenon, which apparently confirms the transfer of lice from domestic to feral ungulates, is that of the sheep and goat louse *Linognathus africanus* parasitizing wild deer in sufficiently large numbers to cause mortality in the latter hosts (Brunetti and Cribbs 1971; Foreyt et al. 1986). The importance of louse infestations of livestock and pets has spurred several pharmaceutical and veterinary companies to develop insecticides with pediculicidal activity.

MANAGEMENT IMPLICATIONS. Because lice typically infest healthy, immunocompetent, wild mammals in low numbers, they do not appear to be a health burden to their hosts in most instances, and management programs are not warranted. However, in those situations where lice have the potential to transmit pathogens to their hosts or where lice multiply to large populations, as seems to sometimes occur when atypical hosts are parasitized, intervention may be recommended. Although relatively few pathogens are known to be transmitted to wild mammals by lice, this field has received insufficient study, and it seems likely that, with further research, blood-feeding lice will be implicated as vectors of more pathogens in the future.

LITERATURE CITED

Adhikary, C.C., and A.K. Ghosh. 1994. *Anopluran fauna of India. The sucking lice infesting domestic and wild animals.* Records of the Zoological Survey of India, Occasional Paper No. 164, 213 pp.

Barker, S.C. 1991. Taxonomic review of the *Heterodoxus octoseriatus* group (Phthiraptera: Boopiidae) from rock wallabies with the description of three new species. *Systematic Parasitology* 19:1–16.

Beaucournu, J.-C. 1966. Hyperinfestation d'ecureuils (*Sciurus vulgaris*) par un anoploure, *Neohaematopinus sciuri* Jancke 1931. *Annales de Parasitologie Humaine et Comparée* 41:203.

———. 1968. Les anoploures de lagomorphes, rongeurs et insectivores dans la région paléarctique occidentale et en particulier en France. *Annales de Parasitologie Humaine et Comparée* 43:201–271.

Beder, G. 1990. Rasterelektronenmikroskopische studie der Robbenlaus *Echinophthirius horridus* (Olfers 1816). *Mitteilungen der Deutsche Gesellschaft Allgemeine Angewandte Entomologie* 7:512–516.

Berkencamp, S.D., and R.B. Wescott. 1988. Arthropod transmission of *Eperythrozoon coccoides* in mice. *Laboratory Animal Science* 38:398–401.

Bruner, D.W. 1963. The pox diseases of man and animals. In *Diseases transmitted from animals to man,* 5th ed. Ed. T.G. Hull. Springfield, IL: Charles C. Thomas, pp. 386–400.

Brunetti, O., and H. Cribbs. 1971. California deer deaths due to massive infestation by the louse (*Linognathus africanus*). *California Fish and Game* 57:138–153.

Chin, T.-H. 1998. A scanning electron microscope study of *Mirophthirus liae* Chin and confirmation of the family status of the Mirophthiridae (Phthiraptera: Anoplura). *Journal of Medical Entomology* 35:596–598.

Cicchino, A.C., M.E.M. Cobenas, G.M. Bulman, J.C. Diaz, and A. Laos. 1998. Identification of *Microthoracius mazzai* (Phthiraptera: Anoplura) as an economically important parasite of alpacas. *Journal of Medical Entomology* 35:922–930.

Collins, R.C., and L.W. Dewhirst. 1965. Some effects of the sucking louse, *Haematopinus eurysternus*, on cattle on unsupplemented range. *Journal of the American Veterinary Medical Association* 146:129–132.

Conlogue, G.J., J.A. Ogden, and W.J. Foreyt. 1980. Pediculosis and severe heartworm infection in a harbor seal. *Veterinary Medicine/Small Animal Clinician* 75:1184–1187.

Crystal, M. M. 1959. The infective index of the spined rat louse, *Polyplax spinulosa*, in the transmission of *Haemobartonella muris* (Mayer) of rats. *Journal of Economic Entomology* 52:543–544.

Cummins, L.J., and J.F. Graham. 1982. The effect of lice infestation on the growth of Hereford calves. *Australian Veterinary Journal* 58:194–196.

Davis, D.P., and R.E. Williams. 1986. Influence of hog lice, *Haematopinus suis*, on blood components, behavior, weight gain and feed efficiency of pigs. *Veterinary Parasitology* 22:307–314.

DeVaney, J.A., T.M. Craig, L.D. Rowe, C. Wade and D.K. Miller. 1992. Effects of low levels of lice and internal nematodes on weight gain and blood parameters in calves in central Texas. *Journal of Economic Entomology* 85:144–149.

Durden, L.A. 1983. Sucking louse (*Hoplopleura erratica*: Insecta, Anoplura) exchange between individuals of a wild population of eastern chipmunks, *Tamias striatus*, in central Tennessee, USA. *Journal of Zoology, London* 201:117–123.

———. 1990. Phoretic relationships between sucking lice (Anoplura) and flies (Diptera) associated with humans and livestock. *The Entomologist* 109:191–192.

———. 1991. A new species and an annotated world list of the sucking louse genus *Neohaematopinus* (Anoplura: Polyplacidae). *Journal of Medical Entomology* 28:694–700.

Durden, L.A., and G.G. Musser. 1994a. The sucking lice (Insecta, Anoplura) of the world: A taxonomic checklist with records of mammalian hosts and geographical distributions. *Bulletin of the American Museum of Natural History* 218:1–90.

———. 1994b. The mammalian hosts of the sucking lice (Anoplura) of the world: A host-parasite list. *Bulletin of the Society for Vector Ecology* 19:130–168.

Emerson, K.C. 1972. *Checklist of the Mallophaga of North America (north of Mexico)*. Parts I–IV. Dugway, UT: Deseret Test Center.

Emerson, K.C., and R.D. Price. 1975. Mallophaga of Venezuelan mammals. *Brigham Young University Science Bulletin, Biological Series* 20(3): 1–77.

———. 1981. A host-parasite list of the Mallophaga on mammals. *Miscellaneous Publications of the Entomological Society of America* 12:1–72.

———. 1985. Evolution of Mallophaga on mammals. In *Coevolution of parasitic arthropods and mammals*. Ed. K. C. Kim. New York: Wiley, pp. 233–255.

———. 1988. A new species of *Haematomyzus* (Mallophaga: Haematomyzidae) off the bush pig, *Potamochoerus porcus*, from Ethiopia, with comments on lice found on pigs. *Proceedings of the Entomological Society of Washington* 90:338–342.

Ferris, G.F. 1919–1935. Contributions toward a monograph of the sucking lice. Parts I–VIII. *Stanford University Publications University Series, Biological Sciences* 2:1–634.

———. 1951. The sucking lice. *Memoirs of the Pacific Coast Entomological Society* 1:1–320.

Foreyt, W.J., G.G. Long, and N.L. Gates. 1978. *Trichodectes canis:* Severe pediculosis in coyotes. *Veterinary Medicine/Small Animal Clinician* 73:503–505.

Foreyt, W.J., D.H. Rice, and K.C. Kim. 1986. Pediculosis of mule deer and white-tailed deer fawns in captivity. *Journal of the American Veterinary Medical Association* 189:1172–1173.

Geraci, J.R., J.F. Fortin, D.J. St. Aubin, and B.D. Hicks. 1981. The seal louse, *Echinophthirius horridus:* An intermediate host of the seal heartworm, *Dipetalonema spirocauda* (Nematoda). *Canadian Journal of Zoology* 59:1457–1459.

Gibney, V.J., J.B. Campbell, D.J. Boxler, D.C. Clanton, and G.H. Deutscher. 1985. Effects of various infestation levels of cattle lice (Mallophaga: Trichodectidae and Anoplura: Haematopinidae) on feed efficiency and weight gains of beef heifers. *Journal of Economic Entomology* 78:1304–1307.

Hafner, M.S., and S.A. Nadler. 1988. Phylogenetic trees support the coevolution of parasites and their hosts. *Nature, London* 332:258–259.

Hellenthal, R.D., and R.D. Price. 1991. Biosystematics of the chewing lice of pocket gophers. *Annual Review of Entomology* 36:185–203.

———. 1994. Two new subgenera of chewing lice (Phthiraptera: Trichodectidae) from pocket gophers (Rodentia: Geomyidae), with a key to all included taxa. *Journal of Medical Entomology* 31:450–466.

Henry, L.G., and S. McKeever. 1971. A modification of the washing technique for quantitative evaluation of the ectoparasite load of small mammals. *Journal of Medical Entomology* 8:504–505.

Hopkins, G.H.E. 1949. The host-associations of the lice of mammals. *Proceedings of the Zoological Society of London* 119:387–604.

Hopkins, G.H.E., and T. Clay. 1952. *A checklist of the genera and species of Mallophaga*. London: British Museum (Natural History), 362 pp.

Ignoffo, C.M. 1958. Evaluation of techniques for recovering ectoparasites. *Proceedings of the Iowa Academy of Science* 65:540–545.

Johnson, P.T. 1960. *The Anoplura of African rodents and insectivores*. United States Department of Agriculture Technical Bulletin No. 1211, 116 pp.

———. 1964. The hoplopleurid lice of the Indo-Malayan subregion (Anoplura: Hoplopleuridae). *Miscellaneous Publications of the Entomological Society of America* 4(3): 68–102.

———. 1972. Sucking lice of Venezuelan rodents, with remarks on related species (Anoplura). *Brigham Young University Science Bulletin, Biological Series* 17(5): 1–62.

Jones, C.J. 1996. Immune responses to fleas, bugs, and sucking lice. In *The immunology of host-ectoparasitic arthropod relationships*. Ed. S. K. Wikel. Wallingford, UK: CAB International, pp. 150–174.

Kamyszek, F., and W. Gibasiewicz. 1986. Pediculosis in pigs in the light of clinical and laboratory studies [In Polish]. *Wiadomosci Parazytologiczne* 32:190–198.

Karabatsos, N. (Ed.). 1985. *International catalogue of arboviruses including certain other viruses of vertebrates*, 3d ed. San Antonio: American Society of Tropical Medicine and Hygiene, 1147 pp.

Kéler, S. von. 1971. A revision of the Australasian Boopiidae (Insecta: Phthiraptera) with notes on the Trimenoponidae. *Australian Journal of Zoology, Supplementary Series* 6:1–126.

Kettle, P.R. 1974. The influence of cattle lice (*Damalinia bovis* and *Linognathus vituli*) on weight gain in beef animals. *New Zealand Veterinary Journal* 22:10–11.

Kim, K.C. 1985. Evolution and host associations in Anoplura. In *Coevolution of parasitic arthropods and mammals.* Ed. K. C. Kim. New York: Wiley, pp. 197–231.

———. 1987. Order Anoplura. In *Immature insects,* Vol. 1. Ed. F.W. Stehr. Dubuque, IA: Kendall/Hunt, pp. 224–245.

Kim, K.C., and H.W. Ludwig. 1978. The family classification of the Anoplura. *Systematic Entomology* 3:249–284.

Kim, K.C., K.C. Emerson, and R.D. Price. 1973. Lice. In *Parasites of laboratory animals.* Ed. R. J. Flynn. Ames: Iowa State University Press, pp. 376–397.

Kim, K.C., H.D. Pratt, and C.J. Stojanovich. 1986. *The sucking lice of North America. An illustrated manual for identification.* University Park: Pennsylvania State University Press, 241 pp.

Kühn, H.J., and H.W. Ludwig. 1967. Die Affenläuse der Gattung *Pedicinus. Zeitschrift für Zoologische Systematik und Evolutionsforschung* 5:144–297.

Ledger, J.A. 1980. *The arthropod parasites of vertebrates in Africa south of the Sahara.* Vol. 4, *Phthiraptera (Insecta).* Publications of the South African Institute for Medical Research, No. 56, 327 pp.

Lodha, K.R. 1964. Some observations on *Microthoracius cameli* (Linnaeus) infestation in camels in Rajasthan, India. *Ceylon Veterinary Journal* 12:18–20.

Lyal, C.H.C. 1985. Phylogeny and classification of the Psocodea, with particular reference to the lice (Psocodea: Phthiraptera). *Systematic Entomology* 10:145–165.

McDade, J.E. 1987. Flying squirrels and their ectoparasites: Disseminators of epidemic typhus. *Parasitology Today* 3:85–87.

Mech, L.D., R.P. Thiel, S.H. Fritts, and W.E. Berg. 1985. Presence and effects of the dog louse *Trichodectes canis* (Mallophaga, Trichodectidae) on wolves and coyotes from Minnesota and Wisconsin. *American Midland Naturalist* 114:404–405.

Méndez, E. 1990. Identificacion de los anopluros de Panama. Panama City, Panama: Editorial Universitaria, 42 pp.

Mishra, A.C. 1981. *The hoplopleurid lice of the Indian subcontinent (Anoplura: Hoplopleuridae).* Records of the Zoological Survey of India, Miscellaneous Publications, Occasional Paper No. 21, 128 pp.

Nelson, W.A., J.E. Keirans, J.F. Bell, and C.M. Clifford. 1975. Host-ectoparasite relationships. *Journal of Medical Entomology* 12:143–166.

Nelson, W.A., J.F. Bell, C.M. Clifford, and J.E. Keirans. 1977. Interaction of ectoparasites and their hosts. *Journal of Medical Entomology* 13:389–428.

Nelson, W.A, J.F. Bell, and S.J. Stewart. 1979. *Polyplax serrata:* Cutaneous cytologic reactions in mice that do (CFW strain) and do not (C57BL strain) develop resistance. *Experimental Parasitology* 48:259–264.

Pennington, N.E., and C.A. Phelps. 1969. Canine filariasis on Okinawa, Ryukyu Islands. *Journal of Medical Entomology* 6:59–67.

Peterson, H.O., I.H. Roberts, W.W. Becklund, and H.E. Kemper. 1953. Anemia in cattle caused by heavy infestations of the blood-sucking louse *Haematopinus eurysternus. Journal of the American Veterinary Medical Association* 122:373–376.

Price, R.D. 1987. Order Mallophaga. In *Immature insects,* vol. 1. Ed. F. W. Stehr. Dubuque, IA: Kendall/Hunt, pp. 215-223.

Price, R.D., and O.H. Graham. 1997. *Chewing and sucking lice as parasites of mammals and birds.* United States Department of Agriculture, Agricultural Research Service, Technical Bulletin No. 1849, 257 pp. plus appendices.

Prullage, J.B., R.E. Williams, and S.M. Gaafar. 1993. On the transmissibility of *Eperythrozoon suis* by *Stomoxys calcitrans* and *Aedes aegypti. Veterinary Parasitology* 50:125–135.

Raghavan, R.S., K.R. Reddy, and G.A. Khan. 1968. Dermatitis in elephants caused by the louse *Haematomyzus elephantis* (Piagot [sic.] 1869). *Indian Veterinary Journal* 45:700–701.

Ratzlaff, R.E., and S.K. Wikel. 1990. Murine immune responses and immunization against *Polyplax serrata* (Anoplura: Polyplacidae). *Journal of Medical Entomology* 27:1002–1007.

Rékási, J. 1994. Chewing lice parasitizing mammals in central Europe with notes on louse taxonomy and biogeography. *Parasitologia Hungarica* 27:57–67.

Ronald, N.C., and J.E. Wagner. 1973. Pediculosis of spider monkeys: A case report with zoonotic implications. *Laboratory Animal Science* 23:872–875.

Samuel, W.M., and D.O. Trainer. 1971. Seasonal fluctuations of *Tricholipeurus parallelus* (Osborn 1896) (Mallophaga: Trichodectidae) on white-tailed deer *Odocoileus virginianus* (Zimmermann 1780) from south Texas. *American Midland Naturalist* 85:507–513.

Scanlon, J.E. 1960. The Anoplura and Mallophaga of the mammals of New York. *Wildlife Diseases* 5:1–121.

Schwartz, C.C., R. Stephenson, and N. Wilson. 1983. *Trichodectes canis* on the gray wolf and coyote on Kenai Peninsula, Alaska. *Journal of Wildlife Diseases* 19:372–373.

Séguy, E. 1944. *Faune de France.* Vol. 43, *Insectes ectoparasites (Mallophages, Anoploures, Siphonaptères).* Paris: Librairie de la faculté des Sciences, 684 pp.

Skirnisson, K., and E. Olafsson. 1990. Parasites of seals in Icelandic waters, with special reference to the heartworm *Dipetalonema spirocauda* Leidy 1858 and the sucking louse *Echinopthirius* (sic.) *horridus* Olfers 1916 [In Icelandic]. *Natturufraedingurinn* 60:93–102.

Smith, T.G. 1996. The genus *Hepatozoon* (Apicomplexa: Adeleina). *The Journal of Parasitology* 82:565–585.

Timm, R.M., and R.D. Price. 2000. A new species of *Eutrichoophilus* (Phthiraptera: Trichodectidae) from the Brazilian black dwarf porcupine (Rodentia: Erethizontidae). *Journal of the Kansas Entomological Society* 72:28–31.

———. 1994a. *Revision of the chewing louse genus* Eutrichophilus *(Phthiraptera: Trichodectidae) from the New World porcupines (Rodentia: Erethizontidae).* Fieldiana, Zoology, New Series No. 76, 35 pp.

———. 1994b. A new species of *Felicola* (Phthiraptera: Trichodectidae) from a Costa Rican Jaguar, *Panthera onca* (Carnivora: Felidae). *Proceedings of the Biological Society of Washington* 107:114–118.

van Dyk, P.J., and A.A. McKenzie. 1992. An evaluation of the efficacy of the scrub technique in quantitative ectoparasite ecology. *Experimental and Applied Acarology* 15:271–283.

Volf, P. 1991. *Polyplax spinulosa* infestation and antibody response in various strains of laboratory rats. *Folia Parasitologica* 38:355–362.

Welch, D.A., and W.M. Samuel. 1989. Evaluation of random sampling for estimating density of winter ticks (*Dermacentor albipictus*) on moose (*Alces alces*) hides. *International Journal for Parasitology* 19: 691–693.

Werneck, F.L. 1948. *Os malofagos de mamiferos.* Parte I, *Amblycera e Ischnocera (Philopteridae e parte de Trichodectidae).* Rio de Janeiro: Revista Brasileira de Biologia, 243 pp.

Werneck, F.L. 1950. *Os malofagos de mamiferos.* Parte II, *Ischnocera (continuacao de Trichodectidae) e Rhyncophthirina.* Rio de Janeiro: Insituto Oswaldo Cruz, 207 pp.

Westrom, D.R., and J.R. Anderson. 1983. The population dynamics of *Solenopotes ferrisi* (Anoplura: Linognathidae) on the Columbian black-tailed deer *Odocoileus hemionus columbianus. Canadian Journal of Zoology* 61:2060–2063.

Westrom, D.R., B.C. Nelson, and G.E. Connolly. 1976. Transfer of *Bovicola tibialis* (Piaget) (Mallophaga: Trichodec-

tidae) from the introduced fallow deer to the Columbian black-tailed deer in California. *Journal of Medical Entomology* 13:169–173.

Whitaker, J.O., Jr. 1982. *Ectoparasites of mammals of Indiana.* Indiana Academy of Science Monograph No. 4, 240 pp.

2

BITING FLIES (CLASS INSECTA: ORDER DIPTERA)

SANDRA A. ALLAN

INTRODUCTION. Flies are often biting and serious pests of wild mammals that elicit a variety of defensive behaviors from hosts (Walker and Edman 1986). They belong to the order Diptera and are characterized by the presence of one pair of wings. In some flies such as the louse or bat flies, wings are lost once adults contact the host. Flies are holometabolous with four life stages: the egg, larva (often with four stadia), a non-feeding pupa, and an adult. Three suborders comprise the order: Nematocera, Brachycera and Cyclorrhapha. The Nematocera typically include small delicate flies usually with beaded antenna, palps of 4–5 segments, and aquatic or semi-aquatic larvae. Only females feed on blood. Biting flies in this suborder are mosquitoes, black flies, biting midges, and sand flies. Flies in Brachycera are stout-bodied with large eyes, short antennae, and larvae found in aquatic or semi-aquatic habitats. They include snipe flies, deer flies, and horse flies, the females of which feed on blood. In Cyclorrhapha, adults are stout-bodied, antennae have a hair or bristle-like structure on the third segment, and larvae tend to be found in decaying plant and animal tissues (i.e., vegetation, manure, carrion, wounds). This group includes louse and bat flies and muscoid flies (Superfamily Muscoidea) such as eye gnats, face flies, horn flies, stable flies, moose flies, and blow flies that produce larvae that feed on decaying or fresh vertebrate tissue (myiasis). Bot flies and warble flies also produce myiasis and are discussed in Chapter 3. Adults of most muscoid flies feed on blood or other secretions.

Reports on the direct effects of biting flies on wild mammals are few, probably because flies feed quickly and are only in contact with the host for a relatively short time, yet effects of feeding can be quite dramatic and include localized irritation, disease transmission, and death. Lankester (1987), in reviewing the biting insects of moose, felt that the many biting insects that harass wild cervids were little studied yet constituted an important stress factor for the host. Accordingly, this chapter reviews the interaction of wild mammals in North America with the most important of the biting flies, including mosquitoes, biting midges, sand flies, black flies, snipe flies, deer and horse flies, louse and bat flies, muscoid flies, and blow flies causing myiasis.

MOSQUITOES. Mosquitoes are small (3–9 mm), slender-bodied flies with a long proboscis, long anten-

nae, and wings with scales on the veins and margins. They belong to the family Culicidae. Worldwide there are more than 3500 species in three subfamilies: Anophelinae, Culicinae, and Toxorhynchitinae (Knight and Stone 1977). In North America, there are more than 167 species in 14 genera: *Aedes, Anopheles, Culex, Culiseta, Coquillettidia, Deinocerites, Haemagogus, Mansonia, Orthopodomyia, Psorophora, Sabethes, Toxorhynchites, Uranotaenia,* and *Wyeomyia* (Wood et al. 1979; Darsie and Ward 1981). Identifications can be made using Wood et al. (1979) and Darsie and Ward (1981).

Life History. Immature mosquitoes are aquatic, and eggs are laid either singly on vegetation near the edge of the water or in rafts on the surface of the water. Larvae emerge from the eggs and obtain food by filter feeding. The pupal stage is also aquatic and very active. Adults emerge from pupal skins at the surface of the water (Clements 1992). Nectar sources, visited by both sexes of adults, provide energy used for flight (Magnarelli 1979). Mating occurs within several days after emergence and may occur in swarms, depending on species. Only female mosquitoes feed on blood, which is subsequently used for egg production. Mosquitoes feed by inserting stylets in the proboscis into blood vessels or a hematoma produced by repeated probing. Mosquito species often differ in the times of feeding throughout the day; however, most mosquito species are active at dawn and dusk. After eggs are deposited, another blood meal may be obtained for further ovarian development. A few species are autogenous and produce the initial egg batch without a blood meal. Generation times for mosquitoes vary from several weeks to a year (Clements 1992).

Mosquitoes locate potential hosts through use of visual cues including color, intensity, and background contrast (Allan et al. 1987) and olfactory cues such as carbon dioxide, 1-octen-3-ol, phenols, and butanone (Kline et al. 1990). Olfactory cues also play a role in the location of nectar sources (Foster and Hancock 1994) and potential oviposition sites (Bentley and Day 1989; Allan and Kline 1995).

Epizootiology

DISTRIBUTION AND HOST RANGE. Mosquitoes are present throughout North America [for distribution maps of individual species see Darsie and Ward (1981) and Wood et al. (1979)]. Mosquitoes are generally considered as either fixed or opportunistic blood feeders (Edman et al. 1972). Fixed blood feeders such as *Culex territans* feed primarily from one group of hosts, in this case, amphibians, but most mosquitoes are opportunistic blood feeders that obtain blood from a wide variety of available hosts (Downe 1962). *Culex* spp. generally feed on birds rather than mammals, although a narrow host range is rare among mosquitoes (Edman 1974; Magnarelli 1977). *Culex nigropalpis* is opportunistic; hosts in Florida include cattle, rabbits, horses, egrets, ibis, passerine birds, quail, turkeys, terns, herons, dogs, opossums, cats, and armadillos (Nayar 1982). This species annually shifts its blood-feeding pattern from birds in the spring and summer to mammals in the summer and fall (Edman and Taylor 1968). In the western United States, *Culex tarsalis* also undergoes a similar host shift (Templis et al. 1967; Reeves et al. 1963).

The seasonal host shift in feeding by *Cx. nigropalpis* may be due to movement of the mosquitoes from wooded areas to open habitats during the summer and fall when afternoon rainfall is frequent (Bidlingmayer 1971). The propensity of some mosquito species to remain in local protected habitats such as woodlands versus open areas affects the availability of hosts for feeding and, alternatively, the choice of host species. If mosquitoes remain in certain areas/habitats, they will be restricted to local fauna.

As a group, female *Culiseta* spp. feed primarily on large mammals; however, some species such as *Culiseta melanura* (vector of eastern equine encephalitis) feed preferentially on birds (Hayes 1961; Magnarelli 1977). Various other mosquito species serve as bridge vectors and are capable of transmitting the virus from infected birds to mammals (Scott and Weaver 1989). Females of *Aedes* are often aggressive biters; they feed on small to large mammals. Blood meals of Arctic *Aedes* spp. include caribou, musk ox, voles, and waterfowl and other birds (Corbet and Downe 1966). In New Jersey *Aedes sollicitans* feed primarily on mammals (over 86%), the majority of which are large mammals (deer, humans, horses, cows, pigs) and the remainder small mammals (dogs, rabbits, rodents, raccoons) (Crans et al. 1990). Templis (1975) reported that some mosquito species fed two or more times on different hosts to complete a blood meal prior to oviposition. Magnarelli (1977) used precipitin tests to determine that over 91% of the blood-engorged *Aedes* collected in Connecticut fed on mammals. Of those mosquitoes tested, *Ae. abserratus, Ae. canator,* and *Ae. vexans* fed on cattle and horses, and *Ae. abserratus* fed on deer. Nasci (1985) reported that *Ae. vexans* was a moderately opportunistic species with a preference for larger mammals (horses, deer and cattle). Blackmore et al. (1998) presented data suggesting that *Anopheles quadrimaculatus* and *Coquillettidia perturbans* are involved in the Midwestern transmission of Cache Valley virus. Although the vertebrate reservoir for Cache Valley virus is unknown, high antibody

prevalence has been obtained in livestock and large ungulates in the Midwest (Blackmore et al. 1998). In North Carolina, Robertson et al. (1993) identified mosquito blood meals and determined that *An. quadrimaculatus* fed principally on white-tailed deer and horses, while *Culex erraticus* was opportunistic and fed on mammals (49%), reptiles and amphibians (20%), and birds (31%). *Ae. albopictus* is an opportunistic feeder (Sullivan et al. 1971). In a recent study, 21% of the blood meals were obtained from avian hosts and 79% from mammalian hosts including rabbits (24.5%), deer (13.6%), dogs (13.6%), humans (8.2%), squirrels (7.3%), opossums (4.5%), myomorph rodents other than *Rattus* (3.6%), raccoons (0.9%), and cattle (0.1%) (Savage et al. 1993). In a comparison in host choice between two sibling species of treehole-breeding mosquitoes in northern Indiana, Nasci (1982) reported that *Ae. triseriatus* fed predominately on chipmunks and deer and *Ae. hendersoni* fed on tree squirrels and raccoons. Blood meals identified from *Ae. triseriatus* in Indiana were primarily from chipmunks (61%) except in habitats where chipmunks were absent, and then gray squirrels were the primary hosts (65%) (Nasci 1985). In a comparison among urban, suburban, and rural sites, more *Ae. triseriatus* fed on deer in the rural site than in the urban and suburban sites (6% in each); however, the chipmunk remained a consistently preferred host in all sites (35%–50%) (Nasci 1985). In fact, Gauld et al. (1974) suggested that the level of circulating LaCrosse virus in Wisconsin was related to density of chipmunk and *Ae. triseriatus* populations. Pinger and Rowley (1975) analyzed blood meals from field-collected *Ae. trivittatus* in Iowa and reported that over 68% fed on eastern cottontail rabbits. In a similar study in Indiana, Nasci (1985) reported a very opportunistic feeding pattern for *Ae. trivittatus* in three different habitats. Blood meals from an urban site were identified from dogs (43%), rabbits (24%), and cats (14%); from a suburban site blood meals were identified from horses (37%), deer (29%), raccoons (12%), and rabbits (8%); and from a rural site, blood meals were identified from deer (57%) and raccoons (21%). Hosts vary in degree of defensive behavior, and chipmunks and tree squirrels appear to tolerate feeding by a moderate number of mosquitoes; however, nocturnal rodents such as cotton rats and cotton mice are highly intolerant of mosquito feeding (Edman and Spielman 1986).

The most severe pest species for man and wild mammals alike include *Ae. albopictus, Ae. dorsalis, Ae. aegypti, Ae. hexodontus, Ae. impiger, Ae. nigripes, Ae. sollicitans, Ae. stimulans, Ae. vexans, Cq. perturbans, Cx. tarsalis,* and *Psorophora columbiae* (Wood et al. 1979; Darsie and Ward 1981).

ENVIRONMENTAL LIMITATIONS. Preferred larval habitats vary between species; however, species can be generally categorized as those associated with permanent (marshes, streams, ponds) and temporary (snow melt pools, ditches, tree holes, containers) habitats of fresh water or with salt or brackish water. In general, the greatest densities of mosquitoes are adjacent to larval habitats. Adults of some species such as *Aedes sollicitans, Ae. vigilax,* and *Ae. vexans* disperse considerable distances from the larval habitat while other species such as *Ae. triseriatus* remain in close proximity (Service 1980). There are various reports of dispersal of mosquitoes by winds, and these have been recently reviewed by Service (1997). Piles of tires filled with water serve as habitat for container-breeding mosquitoes such as *Ae. triseriatus* and *Ae. albopictus. Ae. triseriatus* is an efficient vector of La Crosse virus, and the presence of tire piles or the natural larval habitats, tree holes, in proximity to human habitations are considered important risk factors in the epidemiology of La Crosse encephalitis (Hedberg et al. 1985). Management of mosquitoes is generally localized through aerial applications of insecticide and treatment, modifications, or removal of larval breeding sites. Often these procedures elicit concerns of environmental contamination or disturbance of environmentally sensitive areas. Dale et al. (1998) summarized the usefulness of geographic information systems combined with remote sensing analysis for mosquito management and disease risk assessment.

Clinical Signs. Clinical signs are few and range from localized reddened swelling at the bite site to mosquito avoidance behavior by the host [ear twitching, leg stomping, tail flicking (Walker and Edman 1986); muscle tremor (Sota et al. 1991)].

Pathology and Disease Transmission to Wild Mammals. Feeding by mosquitoes may range in intensity from very minor with slight local irritation and itching to severe effects such as exsanguination and death. Bites often cause whealing and delayed papules that appear within several hours after the bite and persist for several days. In delayed mosquito bite reactions, there is an early influx of eosinophils and neutrophils and a subsequent accumulation of CD4+ lymphocytes (Karppinen et al. 1996). With the increase in the number of feeding mosquitoes, host behavior can change to irritation and avoidance of the mosquitoes. The amount of blood lost through feeding is usually trivial; feeding by large numbers of mosquitoes, however, particularly *Aedes* and *Psorophora,* has been reported to cause animal distress or death [in cattle (Abbitt and Abbitt 1981)]. The gregarious behavior of reindeer and caribou has been interpreted as a response to severe infestations of mosquitoes in arctic and subarctic habitats (Calef and Heard 1980; Morschel and Klein 1997).

In addition to the direct effects of feeding, mosquitoes are effective vectors of a variety of agents, only some of which are pathogenic to wild mammals. Mosquitoes have been implicated in the transmission to wild mammals of viruses including arboviruses such as western equine encephalitis, eastern equine encephalitis, Venezuelan equine encephalitis, St. Louis encephalitis, and several viruses in the California group

(Calisher et al. 1986). Primary vectors of western equine encephalitis virus include *Culex tarsalis* in the western United States in irrigated areas as well as *Ae. melanimon* (California), *Ae. dorsalis* (Utah and New Mexico), and *Culiseta melanura* in the eastern United States; vectors of eastern encephalitis virus include *Cs. melanura, Culex nigripalpis, Coquillettidia perturbans, Ae. sollicitans,* and *Ae. vexans;* Venezuelan encephalitis virus includes a wide range of species such as *Ae. taeniorhynchus, Cq. perturbans, Psorophora,* and *Culex* spp.; and vectors of St. Louis encephalitis virus include various species of *Culex* such as *Cx. pipiens, Cx. quinquefasciatus* (Gulf coast, Ohio, and Mississippi River Valley), *Cx. nigropalpis* (Florida), and *Cx. tarsalis* (western states) (Sudia et al. 1975; Mitchell et al. 1980; Monath 1988).

The importance of California group viruses in causing disease in livestock and wild mammals is unknown, although infections of deer, elk, and other large mammals are well known (Eldridge et al. 1987). Of the California group viruses, Cache Valley virus is widespread in North America with white-tailed deer as the primary vertebrate host and with *Aedes taeniorhynchus* and *Ae. sollicitans* as vectors on the east coast (Yuill and Thompson 1970); *Anopheles quandrimaculatus* and *Coquillettidiaperturbans* have been implicated as possible vectors in the Midwest (Blackmore et al. 1998). Jamestown Canyon virus (associated with white-tailed deer) is exclusively associated with *Culiseta inornata* in the West; in the East primary vectors are *Aedes communis* group, *Ae. stimulans, Ae. triseriatus, Anopheles punctipennis, An. quadrimaculatus* (reviewed in Grimstad 1989), and *Ae. provocans* (Heard et al. 1990). Boromisa and Grimstad (1987) suggested that in northern Indiana, transmission of Jamestown Canyon virus is directly correlated with the size of spring *Ae. stimulans* populations. The primary vectors of Keystone virus (associated with white-tailed deer, cotton rats, and rabbits) are *Ae. atlanticus* along the Atlantic seaboard and *Ae. infirmatus* in Florida (LeDuc 1979). The primary vectors of LaCrosse virus (associated with gray squirrels, tree squirrels, and eastern chipmunks in eastern deciduous forest habitats) are *Ae. triseriatus* and *Ae. canadensis* (Grimstad 1989). In a laboratory study, Grimstad et al. (1980) reported that the frequency of probing on hosts was greater by arbovirus(La Crosse)-infected *Ae. triseriatus*. Snowshoe hare virus (associated with snowshoe hares) appears to involve two transmission cycles; one with *Culiseta inornata* and the other with univoltine spring *Aedes* species (including *Ae. implicatus, Ae. canadensis, Ae. communis, Ae. hexodontus* and *Ae. nigripes*) (Grimstad 1989). Trivattus virus (associated with cottontail rabbits) is primarily vectored by *Ae. trivittatus* except in Florida, where the vector is *Ae. infirmatus* (Grimstad 1989). Potosi virus cycles between various mammalophilic mosquitoes and deer (McLean et al. 1996; Mitchell et al. 1996, 1998).

Mosquitoes also act as vectors of nematodes such as *Pelecitus scapiceps,* filarid of the limb joints of lagomorphs (Bartlett 1983, 1984); *Dirofilaria immitis* in black bears, coyotes, gray foxes, and red foxes (Crum et al. 1978; Hubert et al. 1980; Simmons et al. 1980; King and Bohning 1984); *Setaria yehi* to deer (mule, white-tailed)(Becklund et al. 1969; Weinmann et al. 1973); and *Setaria labiatopalillosa* in antelope, bison, moose, mule deer, bighorn sheep, caribou, horses, and cattle (Becklund and Walker 1969). The prevalence of *D. immitis* in black bears was 8% (Crum et al. 1978). The prevalence of *D. immitis* in coyotes was reported as 66% in northeast Arkansas (King and Bohning 1984), 8.3%–27.3% in northern California (Acevedo and Theis 1982), 12.5% in Indiana (Kazacos and Edberg 1979), and 3.6% in Iowa (Franson et al. 1976). In gray foxes, prevalence was 16% in Alabama and Georgia (Simmons et al. 1980) and 3.7% in Indiana (Kazacos and Edberg 1979); in red foxes prevalence was 3.6% in Illinois (Hubert et al. 1980) and 2.7% in Indiana (Kazacos and Edberg 1979). The primary vectors of *Dirofilaria immitis* are *Aedes vexans, Anopheles punctipennis, An. quadrimaculatus, Ae. stricticus,* and *Ae. trivittatus* (Christensen and Andrew 1976; Todaro et al. 1977; Buxton and Mullen 1980; Tolbert and Johnson 1982).

Immunity. Mellanby (1946) first reported the repeated exposure of humans to mosquito bites resulted in a regular pattern of skin sensitivity, ultimately ending in a reactive state with repeated exposure; subsequent research was reviewed by Nelson (1987). Cutaneous reactions to mosquito bites in humans can be divided into five different stages ranging from immediate whealing and delayed bite papules to nonreactivity. Arthus-type local and systemic symptoms also can occur, but anaphylactic reactions are very rare (Reunala et al. 1990). The feeding of mosquitoes on sensitized hosts can result in reduced mosquito fecundity or other physiological effects (Sutherland and Ewen 1974; Ramasamy et al. 1992). The role of saliva in these responses was confirmed by Hudson et al. (1960); they severed salivary ducts of mosquitoes that failed to elicit hypersensitivity responses with subsequent feedings on sensitized hosts. Hypersensitivity to mosquito feeding has been reported in sheep (Jones and Lloyd 1987), guinea pigs (French and West 1971), rabbits (McKiel and West 1961), and cats (Power and Ihrke 1995). In cats, mosquito bite sensitivity ranges from multiple pinpoint papular crusts on the muzzle to severe reactions resulting in larger ulcerative areas. The latter, when healed, may remain alopecic (Power and Ihrke 1995). Kay and Kemp (1994) summarized several studies with various hosts on experimental vaccinations against mosquitoes. Effects of vaccination ranged from no change in feeding to higher mosquito mortality, reduced oviposition, and reduced infection rates with viruses and *Plasmodium* spp.

Control and Treatment. Control of adults is primarily by aerial application of insecticides (Mount et al. 1996). Larvae are controlled through habitat reduction

(removal of standing water, draining ditches and marshes, etc.) (Wolfe 1996), applications of insecticides or oil in the water, or biological control agents (pathogens such as *Bacillus thuringiensis* var. *israeliensis* or *Bacillus sphaericus* or predators such as *Gambusia*)(Legner 1995). Insect growth regulators are effective for mosquito control yet are relatively nontoxic to fish and wildlife (Mulla 1995), and it is anticipated that they will be utilized more in vector control programs. Personal protection from mosquitoes includes the use of insecticides, repellents or protective clothing (i.e., veils, hats), and insecticide-impregnated clothing.

Public Health Concerns. Mosquitoes are important as pests due to annoyance and blood loss caused by feeding and as vectors of diseases. In North America, mosquitoes are primarily important as vectors of eastern equine encephalitis, western equine encephalitis, Cache Valley virus, and St. Louis encephalitis (Yuill and Thompson 1970; Calisher et al. 1986; Scott and Weaver 1989; Sexton et al. 1997). Worldwide, mosquitoes are vectors of devastating diseases such as malaria, dengue, yellow fever, and filariasis (*Wuchereria, Brugia*). Malaria was present in various regions in North America and was eradicated locally; competent vectors are indigenous in North America, however, and occasionally locally acquired cases occur (Dawson et al. 1996; Barat et al. 1997).

Domestic Animal Concerns. Feeding by mosquitoes has considerable economic impact on livestock production and contributes significantly to a loss in cattle production through reduction in weight gain and milk production estimated at over $24 million in 1965 (USDA 1965). In addition to the severe annoyance caused by mosquito bites, mosquitoes are vectors of eastern equine encephalitis, western equine encephalitis, Venezuelan equine encephalitis, and St. Louis encephalitis to horses; *Dirofilaria immitis* to dogs, cats, and ferrets; and *Setaria yehi* (Calisher et al. 1986; Bowman 1995) and *Setaria equina* to horses, mules, burros, and cattle (Becklund and Walker 1969; Durden 1984; LeBrun and Dziem 1984). Several species including *Aedes vexans* and *Culex quinquefasciatus* serve as vectors of *D. immitis;* susceptibility of mosquito species to *D. immitis* differs, however, with geographic strain (Loftin et al. 1995). Sixteen species of mosquitoes in four genera have been implicated as vectors of dog heartworm in the United States (Scoles 1994). In addition, feeding by mosquitoes has been reported to reduce weight gain of cattle due to blood loss and reduced feeding by cattle (Steelman et al. 1972).

BITING MIDGES. Biting midges are tiny flies (0.6–5.0 mm) with long antennae (15 segments) and short mouthparts belonging to the Family Ceratogoponidae (i.e., Heleidae). They are known by a variety of common names including biting midges, punkies, no-see-ems, and sand flies. Wings are superimposed over the back at rest and often spotted. Flies in this family that blood-feed generally belong to the genera *Culicoides, Leptoconops,* or *Forcipomyia* (i.e., *Lasiohelea*). Biting midges are vectors of epizootic hemorrhagic disease and bluetongue viruses (Gibbs and Greiner 1989). Keys to North American biting midges are provided in Fox (1955), Wirth and Atchley (1973), and Downes and Wirth (1981).

Life History. Eggs are laid singly near damp habitats. The larvae of *Culicoides* spp., which are aquatic or semi-aquatic, are present in sand, mud, manure, decaying vegetation, water in tree-holes, and in debris in the intertidal zone along the coast. They are thought to be scavengers. The duration of the larval stage varies considerably as larvae overwinter in a variety of temperate zones. Larvae of *Leptoconops* are present in sandy or clay/silt soils and those of *Forcipomyia* are often in moist places such as under bark or moss (Downes and Wirth 1981).

Mating usually occurs in swarms just after emergence of adults. Adults of *Culicoides* spp. are crepuscular or nocturnal and are strong fliers, but they are generally found close to breeding sites. Adults of *Leptoconops* spp. generally bite throughout the day. In a recent study in Utah, *Leptoconops americanus'* greatest biting activity occurred when temperatures were above 15° C on calm, sunny days (Strickman et al. 1995). Adults of both sexes feed on nectar but only females possess biting mouthparts and feed on blood. Some species are autogenous for the first oviposition, but all species require blood meals for the second and subsequent ovipositions. Jamnback (1969) reported that adult *Culicoides* were highly sensitive to moisture loss and were inactive during the day except in wooded humid woodlands or on wet, humid, calm days in the open. Biting habits vary between species; for example some midges feed preferentially only on one body region (Schmidtmann et al. 1980). Females blood-fed at 3–4-day intervals on mammals, birds, reptiles, and other invertebrates. Adult flies are common in warm months throughout North America. Seasonal prevalence varies between species and geographic location.

Attraction of some *Culicoides* species to hosts and host-mimicking traps appears to be related to the presence of host-produced odors such as carbon dioxide and 1-octen-3-ol (Kline et al. 1994; Mullens and Gerry 1998).

Epizootiology

DISTRIBUTION. *Leptoconops* are primarily prevalent in arid western regions of the United States, *Culicoides* are found throughout North America, and *Lasiohelia* are reported from eastern North America. Details of the geographic distribution of individual species are presented in Battle and Turner (1971), Wirth and Atchley (1973) and Blanton and Wirth (1979).

HOST RANGE. Information on host range is limited because it is difficult to observe biting midges feeding on hosts. For this reason information on hosts on which midges feed is based on trapping studies with selected hosts or precipitin tests for blood-meal identification (Templis and Nelson 1971). Few biting midge species appear to be highly host specific (Kettle 1977), and most reports are from domestic livestock (cattle, sheep) (Zimmerman and Turner 1983; Anderson and Holloway 1993; Raich et al. 1997). Twelve species of *Culicoides* were collected in North Dakota in association with white-tailed deer habitat and livestock operations (Anderson and Holloway 1993). At a site enzootic for hemorrhagic disease in Georgia, Smith et al.(1996b) collected *C. lahillei* (73%), *C. stellifer* (16%), *C. biguttatus* (6%), *C. niger* (3%), *C. spinosus* (2%) and *C. paraensis* (0.2%) from white-tailed deer. In a similar study during epizootics of hemorrhagic disease, *C. variipennis* [confirmed vector of epizootic hemorrhagic disease (EHD)] was collected in low numbers along with *C. lahillei, C. paraensis,* and *C. stellifer,* which were abundant (Smith and Stallknecht 1996). Mullen et al. (1985) reported *C. debilipalpis, C. niger, C. obsoletus, C. paraensis, C. sanguisuga,* and *C. stellifer* from white-tailed deer in Alabama. *Culicoides debilipalpis* was the most predominant species, followed by *C. paraensis* and *C. stellifer* in late July and August. Mullens and Dada (1992) used drop traps and precipitin tests to confirm that *Culicoides brookmani, C. variipennis, C. copiosus* group, and the *Leptoconops kerteszi* group fed on bighorn sheep in California. Members of the *L. kerteszi* group also were collected from a trap baited with a domestic rabbit (Mullens and Dada 1992).

ENVIRONMENTAL LIMITATIONS. Biting midges are associated with moist habitats. Eggs and larvae are prone to desiccation and require moist habitats (dung, rotting vegetation, tree holes, and riverbeds), and adults require moist sites for resting (Jamnback 1969). Larvae of some species are tolerant of salt and are present in high numbers in salt marshes or saline lakes (Kettle 1977). Nuisance of biting midges to wild mammals is greatest for those in closest proximity to larval habitats.

Pathology and Disease Transmission to Wild Mammals. Direct effects of feeding by species such as *C. furens, C. robertsi* and *Leptoconops torrens* may be inapparent or severe as characterized by bulla formation, detached epidermis, serous fluid with neutrophils and perivascular infiltrations by lymphocytes, eosinophils, monocytes, and leucocytes (reviewed in Nelson 1987). Effects of *Culicoides* bites can also include allergic dermatitis, which is best characterized in livestock and horses (Riek 1953). Direct effects on wildlife species are undocumented but may be present. Allergic dermatitis (known as sweat itch or Queensland itch in horses) is due to development of hypersensitivity to feeding *Culicoides*. Initial lesions are papules and with development of hypersensitivity may eventually lead to pruritus (Riek 1953). Perez de Leon et al. (1997) reported a reddish halo surrounding a petechial hemorrhage at the site of bites in native sheep and rabbits and identified a salivary vasodilator from *C. variipennis* as likely responsible for this effect. Perez de Leon and Tabachnick (1996) also reported apyrase activity that might act in the development of the *Culicoides* hypersensitivity response.

In addition to direct effects of feeding, biting midges vector disease agents such as bluetongue virus (BT) to wild mammals including bighorn sheep, mule deer, black-tailed deer, white-tailed deer, pronghorn antelope, and other wild ruminants (Hourrigan and Klingsporn 1975; Pence 1991). The primary vector of both BT virus and EHD virus in North America is *C. variipennis* (Prestwood et al. 1974; Thomas 1981; Tabachnick 1996), which is comprised of three subspecies: *C. variipennis variipennis, C. v. sonorensis and C. v. occidentalis* (Tabachnick 1992). *Culicoides variipennis sonorensis* is an efficient vector of BT virus, and *C. v. variipennis* is a less efficient vector (Tabachnick and Holbrook 1992). *Culicoides variipennis sonorensis* is documented from several locations in Virginia and Maryland (Schmidtmann et al. 1998) and California (Holbrook and Tabachnick 1995) but is known to be absent in New England (Holbrook et al. 1996). *Culicoides insignus* is also a known vector of BT virus, and 11 other species are suspected vectors (Gibbs and Greiner 1989). Adult female *Culicoides* become infected with BT and EHD virus when feeding on a viremic ruminant host (Sohn and Yuill 1991). Most ruminant species appear to be susceptible to BT virus, and severe clinical disease may develop in the white-tailed deer, the pronghorn, and the desert bighorn sheep. Epizootic hemorrhagic disease (EHD) virus can cause a disease similar in severity to BT in white-tailed deer, mule deer, black-tailed deer, and bighorn sheep or a milder disease as in pronghorn antelope (Gibbs and Greiner 1989; Pence 1991). This virus has been isolated from field-collected *C. variipennis* and other species (*C. venustus* and *C. lahillei*) are incriminated as potential vectors through experimental studies (Jones et al. 1977, 1983; Smith et al. 1996a). Vesicular stomatitis virus is transmitted to white-tailed deer by several species of *Culicoides* (Davidson and Nettles 1997). Several species of *Culicoides* are also vectors of eastern equine encephalitis and several of the California group arboviruses such as Buttonwillow (Reeves et al. 1970; Hardy et al. 1970), Lokern, and Main Drain (Nelson and Scrivani 1972). *Culicoides arubae*, collected from horses, is a suspected vector of Venezuelan equine encephalitis virus in Texas (Jones et al. 1972).

Control and Treatment. These flies are associated with moist habitats. The flies generally do not travel far from the larval habitat and may often be avoided by moving further away from the habitat. Modification and reduction of larval habitats by draining for coastal species that breed in salt marsh habitats and mangrove swamps (reviewed in Blanton and Wirth 1979); however, these measures are often very expensive, and while they may provide effective control they may not be appropriate in environmentally sensitive areas. Control usually includes use of insecticides such as ultra-low-volume applications or application of pesticides to larval habitats (reviewed in Gibbs and Greiner 1989), use of repellents on hosts (Braverman and Chizov-Ginzburg 1997), and housing animals inside buildings (Blanton and Wirth 1979).

Public Health Concerns. *Culicoides* and *Leptoconops* are important as pests and can be extremely annoying; bites are painful. In some coastal areas of Florida the tremendous numbers of these flies "makes life almost unbearable" (Blanton and Wirth (1979). The small flies are difficult to see, hard to detect, and extremely persistent in biting. Often the flies have significantly negative effects on outdoor recreation (Linley and Davies 1971).

Domestic Animal Concerns. Feeding by several *Culicoides* species can elicit hypersensitive responses in horses known as sweat itch or Queensland itch (Fadok and Greiner 1990; Anderson et al. 1991). *Culicoides variipennis* is the vector of BT virus to cattle and sheep (Giggs and Greiner 1989; Wieser-Schimpf et al. 1993); this disease causes an estimated loss of $125 million a year due to lost trade with BT-free countries (Tabachnick 1996). *Culicoides variipennis* is the primary vector of *Onchocerca cervicalis* in horses and *Onchocerca gibsoni* in cattle (Bowman 1995; Foil et al. 1984).

PHLEBOTOMINE SAND FLIES. Phlebotomine sand flies are tiny flies (0.6–5 mm) with hairy bodies, erect wings, and long antennae and legs belonging to the subfamily Phlebotominae in the family Psychodidae. This family is largely tropical, with over 600 species. Blood-feeding species are known as phlebotomine sand flies or gnats. Females are blood-feeding with piercing mouthparts and usually require a blood meal for ovarian development; however, some species are autogenous. Sand flies of the greatest importance in the New World belong to the genus *Lutzomyia* (Young and Perkins 1984).

Life History. Adults are generally nocturnal and are most active from dawn to dusk. By day, adults rest in secluded sites such as dark corners in buildings, crevices, and caves, under vegetation, or in burrows. The flight range of sand flies is restricted to within a few hundred meters of their resting sites and flies are active only with little or no wind (Hall 1936). The cutting mouthparts lacerate the skin and flies feed from hemorrhages in surface capillaries. This feeding often produces distinct discomfort (Tesh and Guzman 1996). Flies tend to feed more readily on certain parts of the host body such as the belly and genital areas. Eggs are deposited in small batches in high humidity environments such as cracks, crevices, or burrows and incubate 6–17 days. Larvae feed on organic debris and occur in decaying vegetable matter, mud, moss, or water. Larvae and pupae develop slowly in soil, burrows, and leaf litter and around tree bases, with larval diapause occurring in temperate areas (Lewis 1974). The entire life cycle may occur in 7–10 weeks, but larval diapause may extend the life cycle of some species. Adult females lay eggs ~5–7 days after blood-feeding. Depending on species, females may feed again after oviposition, but flies are generally quite short-lived (Bram 1978). Adult activity is limited to the summer in warmer climates. Overwintering occurs as diapausing fourth-instar larvae in mammal burrows. Sand flies may be present year round in warm climates such as Texas, with some fluctuation throughout the year in areas with mild climates.

Epizootiology

DISTRIBUTION AND HOST RANGE. Young and Perkins (1984) summarized the known geographic distributions of sand flies north of Mexico with updates by McHugh (1991). Hosts include a range of small and large mammals as well as cold-blooded animals. Species in North America include *Lutzomyia anthophora,* which is found in Texas and feeds on small mammals including rabbits (Addis 1945; Young and Perkins 1984); *L. apache* from Arizona (Young and Perkins 1984); *L. aquilonia* from burrows of yellow-bellied marmots (*Marmota flaventris*) in Alberta, British Columbia, Colorado, and Washington (Shemanchuck et al. 1978); *L. californica* from California, Arizona, Texas, and Washington; *L. cruciata* from Florida and Georgia, an experimental vector of cutaneous leishmaniasis (*Leishmania mexicana*) (Young and Perkins 1984); *L. diabolica* from Texas (Hall 1936); *L. oppidana* from the western mountain regions of the United States and Canada; *L. shannoni,* which is from the southeastern United States (Delaware south to Argentina) and feeds on a variety of mammals (Young and Perkins 1984); *L. stewarti* from California; *L. tanyopsis* from Arizona (Young and Perkins 1984); *L. texana* from armadillo burrows in Texas (Young and Perkins 1984); *L. vexator* from across the United States and southern Ontario (Downes 1972); *L. vexator occidentis* from burrows of woodchucks (*Marmota monax*) in Montana (Chaniotis 1974); and *Lutzomyia xerophila* from California (Young and Perkins 1984). Several of these species have been collected from mammal nests (*L. californica, L. oppidana, L. stewarti, L. vexator, L. vexator occidentis*) but are believed to feed on cold-blooded animals in the nests (Harwood 1965; Chaniotis 1967). Identification of hosts of *L. shannoni* in Georgia by indirect ELISA of blood meals revealed that flies fed on white-tailed deer (81%), feral swine (16%), horses (1.5%), and raccoons (0.6%) and reflected opportunistic host selection (Comer et al. 1994). A recent study by Mead and Cupp (1995) reported on collections by vacuum aspiration and CDC

miniature light traps of *L. anthophora* from nests of the woodrat (*Neotoma albigula*) and rock squirrel (*Citellus variegatus*) in Arizona.

ENVIRONMENTAL LIMITATIONS. These flies are highly associated with high humidity habitats and generally are found in association with habitats such as burrows or nests. Tree holes are important diurnal resting sites for *Lutzomyia shannoni,* the presumed vector of vesicular stomatitis virus, and Comer et al. (1993) reported that treehole availability, sand fly abundance, and abundance of antibody to vesicular stomatitis virus were greater in mature live oak forests than in other forest types. The relative abundance of *L. shannoni* was influenced significantly by the availability of tree holes, and virus infection in wild swine was linked to forest type, with virus presence the greatest in areas with abundant populations of *L. shannoni* (Comer et al. 1993).

Pathology and Disease Transmission to Wild Mammals. Feeding by sand flies results in localized irritation. In addition, sand flies are vectors of several viruses. *Lutzomyia shannoni* is both a competent transstadial and transovarial vector of the New Jersey serotype of vesicular stomatitis virus (Comer et al. 1990) and serves as both the vector and the reservoir (Comer et al. 1991). Antibodies to the virus are present in both white-tailed deer (*O. virgininaus*) and wild swine (*Sus scrofa*) (Comer et al. 1993). *Lutzomyia anthopora* is a suspected vector of Rio Grande virus, which was isolated from *Neotoma* woodrats near Brownsville, Texas (Endris et al. 1983), as was a virus of the phlebotomine fever group (Calisher et al. 1977).

Control and Treatment. Location of breeding habitats is often difficult, and control is primarily targeted at adults through residual insecticide sprays on buildings and resting sites (Tesh and Guzman 1996) and in animal burrows (Robert and Perich 1995). Repellents significantly reduce biting of humans (Perich et al. 1995).

Public Health Concerns. In North America, the only species known to bite man is *Lutzomyia cruciata* in Texas (Lindquist 1936). Cutaneous leishmaniasis and antibodies in man and dogs have been reported from Texas (Shaw et al. 1976), and recently McHugh et al. (1993) reported the isolation of *Leishmania mexicana* from *Lutzomyia anthophora* collected from the nest of a southern plains woodrat (*Neotoma microplus*).

Management Implications. Deforestation and habitat destruction through urbanization is thought to reduce sand fly populations (Lewis 1974) or to cause some zoophilic and syvlatic species to adapt to feeding on man in domestic or peridomestic situations (Walsh et al. 1993). In a study on the distribution of seropositive wild swine or deer to vesicular stomatitis virus, maritime live oak forests with significantly more tree holes (larval habitat of *Lutzomyia shannoni*) had significantly higher levels of seropositive animals (Comer et al. 1993). The Holocene portions of Ossabaw Island had the highest prevalence of vesicular stomatitis virus antibodies in white-tailed deer, and the predominant forest in these areas is a near-climax maritime live oak forest. This part of the island has poor soil, was never cleared for agriculture, and had minimal selective timber removal. In the Pleistocene portion of the island, virus activity is lower; vegetation has been cleared for agriculture with well-drained soils, and the area is currently covered with pine forest that does not provide favored habitat (tree holes) for *L. shannoni* (Comer et al. 1993).

BLACK FLIES. Black flies constitute significant problems to wildlife and domestic animals as well to man due to their aggressive blood-feeding habits (Crosskey 1961; Steelman 1976; Fredeen 1977). Excessive feeding by black flies can result in death by exsanguination, toxic salivary secretions, or obstruction of nasal and bronchial passageways (Crosskey 1961; Fredeen 1973).

These dark, small, hump-backed flies (1–5.5 mm), often referred to as black flies, buffalo flies, turkey gnats, or buffalo gnats, are members of the Family Simuliidae. The wings of adults are short and veins are prominent toward the anterior margin. This group consists of ~23 genera and 1554 species worldwide with approximately 147 species in North America (Peterson 1981). The primary genera in North America include *Simulium, Prosimulium, Cnephia, Twinnia,* and *Gymnopais.* A key to genera of larvae and adults is provided by Petersen (1981). Keys to species in various regions are presented in references cited below for geographical distributions.

Life History. Eggs are laid in batchs on the water surface or on objects in moving water. Larvae filter feed while attached by silk to rocks and other objects in the swiftest portion of the water. Pupae are also attached to the substrate. Adult flies emerge, and female flies blood-feed several days after emergence; females use the short, stout proboscis to cut the skin and provide anchorage, then blood is drawn from a subdermal hematoma. Some species produce the first egg batch without a blood meal (Anderson 1987). Both sexes also feed on nectar, sap, or honeydew, which provide fuel for flight, ovarian development, and increased survival (Crosskey 1990). Many species of black flies are strong fliers and may be present at considerable distances from water. In fact, recaptures of marked flies of *Simulium euryadminiculum, Simulium venustum (s.l.),* and *Prosimulium mixtum/fuscum* were made up to 8 km (Algonquin Park, Ontario), 35 km (Chalk River, Ontario), and 5.2 km (Adirondack Mountains, New York), respectively, from the source of release (Bennett and Fallis 1971; Baldwin et al. 1975; White and Morris 1985). Females may feed and oviposit repeatedly.

Mammalophilic black flies blood-feed during daylight hours. In wooded areas, particularly on warm cloudy days, feeding may occur throughout the day; in open areas, however, feeding occurs primarily during dawn and dusk. Feeding may intensify just prior to a storm. Black flies are primarily univoltine in the north. Black flies often occur in large swarms in late spring and early summer near swiftly moving streams. Black flies readily disperse several kilometers from breeding sites, and some species have been reported to be transported by winds over 80 km away (Crosskey 1990).

Epizootiology

DISTRIBUTION. Black flies are found throughout North America but are particularly abundant in the north temperate and subarctic regions. Some of the more important pest species include *Prosimulium mixtum* (northeast), *Simulium venustum* (widespread), *Simulium jenningsi* complex (widespread), and *Simulium arcticum* (north). Regional distributions are provided by Pinkovsky and Butler (1978) (Florida), Bask and Harper (1979) (New York), Bruder and Crans (1979) (New Jersey), Lewis and Bennett (1979) (Canadian Maritimes), Fredeen (1981) (Canada), Westwood and Brust (1981) (Manitoba), Mohsen and Mulla (1982) (California), Stone (1964) and Cupp and Gordon (1983) (northeastern United States), Currie (1986) (Alberta), Adler and Kim (1986) and Adler and Mason (1997) (Saskatchewan), and Stone and Snoddy (1969) (Alabama).

The primary pest species of mammals in North America are *Simulium venustum* (widely distributed), *Prosimulium mixtum* (northeast), *Simulium jenningsi* complex (widely distributed), *Simulium arcticum* (northern), *Simulium vittatum* (western), *Simulium rugglesi* (eastern), and *Simulium meridionale* and *Cnephia pecuarum* (throughout the Mississippi Valley) (Fredeen 1973; Laird 1981).

HOST RANGE. In general, black flies are more host specific than mosquitoes and feed on a wide range of domestic and wild mammals and birds. Some species feed primarily on mammals and others are primarily ornithophilic. Black flies use both olfactory cues such as CO_2 and visual cues (color, shape, movement) and heat for location of hosts (Sutcliffe 1986; Allan et al. 1987). Many species have distinct feeding preferences for certain body regions of the host (Sutcliffe 1986; Yee and Anderson 1995).

In a study on adult black flies in Algonquin Park, Ontario, Canada, *Simulium venustum* was reported feeding most often on white-tailed deer (Davies and Petersen 1956). McCreadie et al. (1994) collected black flies on the Avalon Peninsula, Newfoundland, from humans and from traps baited with fox, snowshoe hare, lynx, rabbit, and caribou. Blood-fed females of the *Simulium rostratum/verecundum* complex were only collected from caribou. *Simulium truncatum/ venustum* complex fed on fox, lynx, rabbit, and caribou and were collected around humans. *Simulium tuberosum* also fed on rabbit and fox. McCreadie et al. (1985) reported on a variety of black fly species that fed on cattle in Newfoundland. Pledger et al. (1980) collected 15 species of black flies from trapped wild moose and a hand-reared tame moose in Alberta during a study of the vector of the filarid nematode, *Onchocerca cervipedis*. Six species fed on the lower legs, belly, and brisket and around the anus and areas with short, sparse hair.

ENVIRONMENTAL LIMITATIONS. Black flies are associated with sources of strong or swiftly moving water including both large rivers (such as the Athabasca River, Alberta) and small streams that are well aerated and support larval development. Immatures are sensitive to pollution, and populations have decreased in affected waterways (Jamnback 1969). Recently, with increased emphasis on restoration of clean water sources, black fly populations have increased.

Clinical Signs. Animals often scratch bite sites. Toxins injected during a severe attack can result in a general illness known as black fly fever (Fredeen 1973) and in more severely affected animals (cattle and humans), breathing may be jerky and heavy and muscles may tremble. Animals with these symptoms may die in 15 minutes to 2 hours or recover totally in 48 hours. Chronic exposure to large numbers of feeding black flies can result in loss of weight (Fredeen 1973).

Pathology and Disease Transmission to Wild Mammals. Lesions occur at feeding sites. A typical lesion consists of a round, pink swollen area with a droplet of dried blood at the feeding site (Fredeen 1973). Reaction to black fly saliva can be rapid with fluid-filled swellings. Hypersensitivity to feeding may also occur. Extreme annoyance and pruritus can result from flies feeding inside ears or on the head, chest, thighs and ventral abdomen. Feeding sites may become edematous. In cattle, trauma from fly feeding can interfere with feeding calves (Fredeen 1973).

Extensive feeding by black flies can result in mortality. Populations of *Simulium arcticum* from the Saskatchewan and Athabasca Rivers, Alberta, are large enough in 3 or 4 years in 10 to result in cattle mortality (Fredeen 1973). From 1944 to 1948 more than 1300 animals were killed in Saskatchewan by *S. arcticum* (Fredeen 1973). Postmortem examinations of the cattle indicate that death occurs from increased permeability of the capillaries and loss of fluid from the circulatory system in response to a toxic response (Rempel and Arnason 1947). Nelson (1987) reviewed effects of feeding of black flies on humans and cattle. In humans, the feeding lesion increases to an indurated papule followed by involutional vesicle formation, sometimes with cervical adenopathy, chills, and pyrexia. Cattle endemic to black fly areas are usually unaffected by black fly feeding whereas naive animals often display severe systemic effects and die. These animals exhibit

depression, anorexia, cariasthenia, edema of the neck, and death within 5 to 12 hours. In necropsy, serogleantinous edema of the neck and lower belly, extensive fluid in the pericardium, lymphadenopathy, and punctate and striate hemorrhages in the epicardium, myocardium, endocardium, and epithelium of the small intestine are observed. At the feeding lesion, there is extensive necrosis and separation of the epidermis, hyperemic corium, eosinophils, and a perivascular infiltration primarily of eosinophils (Nelson 1987).

Black flies vector several filarid nematodes of wildlife including *Onchocerca cervipedes* to Columbian black-tailed deer [*Prosimulium impostor* (Weinmann et al. 1973)] and moose [*Simulium decorum* and *S. venustum* (Pledger et al. 1980)] and *Dirofilaria ursi* to bears [*Simulium venustum s.l.* (Addison 1980)], and they are implicated as vectors of vesicular stomatitis viruses to deer in Colorado [*Simulium bivittatum, Simulium vittatum* (Francy et al. 1988; Cupp et al. 1992)].

Immunity. Humans and cattle appear to acquire immunity. People exposed repeatedly to black flies generally respond less severely than previously exposed individuals (Nelson 1987). Little is known of the mechanisms, but there is current research exploring the potential for desensitizing individuals to black fly bites (Cross et al. 1993).

Control and Treatment. Area-wide control of black flies is difficult due to the migration of adults and the presence of larvae in environmentally sensitive habitats. Current control methods and alternative biological control methods such as use of predators, parasites, and pathogens have been reviewed in Laird (1981) and Kim and Merritt (1986). Control is targeted primarily against the late stage larvae in localized areas through treatment of water with insecticides (Westwood and Brust 1981). Insect growth regulators and *Bacillus thuringiensis* var. *israeliensis* (Teknar, Vectobac) are promising effective control methods. Molloy (1992) demonstrated that use of *B. t. israeliensis* had relatively little adverse impact on aquatic nontarget organisms. Use of repellents, insecticides, and physical barriers (head nets, ear nets, etc.) provide protection from biting adults. Domestic or game-ranched animals can be housed in shelters.

Public Health Concerns. The incessant swarming and biting of black flies, at least in temperate North America, "can make spring and early summer outdoor activity an excruciating ordeal for man and beast alike" (Sutcliffe 1986). Feeding by black flies on man can produce effects ranging from temporary localized irritation as a result of localized hypersensitivity reactions to potentially fatal systemic responses (Frazier and Asheville 1973; Pinheiro et al. 1974). The movement and buzzing of flies around the head are intensely annoying, and secondary infection often results from scratching feeding lesions. Some individuals react more strongly than others to feeding and may present with black fly fever characterized by headache, fever, nausea, and swollen painful lymph glands.

In man, black flies serve as vectors for viruses, protozoa, and helminthics worldwide. Black flies in North America are not known to be important vectors of disease to man or animals, but they are vectors of onchocerciasis elsewhere. Gray et al. (1996) documented the severe economic impact of the presence of black flies in the *Simulium jenningsi* group on revenue from a private golf club in the South Carolina Piedmont.

Domestic Animal Concerns. Effects of black flies feeding on livestock range from local irritation as a result of a few bites, to severe dermatitis (Anderson and Minson 1985; Cupp 1996), to death due to reaction to injected saliva as documented from *Simulium arcticum* in Saskatchewan (Rempel and Arnason 1947; Charnetski and Haufe 1981). Feeding of black flies on domestic animals causes many indirect losses such as sterility and decreased milk production and weight gains (Charnetski and Haufe 1981). In some areas, the presence of black flies can render regions unfavorable for livestock production (Millar and Rempel 1944). Black flies are implicated as vectors of eastern equine encephalitis virus (Anderson et al. 1961) and are reported as vectors of vesicular stomatitis virus (Cupp et al. 1992) and *Setaria equina* in horses (Dalmat 1955) and of *Onchocerca lienalis* in cattle (Lok et al. 1983).

Management Implications. Control of black fly larvae through treatment of streams or rivers with pesticides has serious implications for nontarget organisms; thus, such approaches should be reserved for serious threats. Use of microbial insecticides such as *B. thuringiensis* var. *israeliensis* has fewer nontarget effects (Laird 1981).

TABANIDS AND SNIPE FLIES. Tabanids and snipe flies cause considerable pain and annoyance to man, livestock, and wild mammals due to their persistent circling flight and painful cutting mouthparts. Disease transmission by these flies usually occurs as a result of mechanical transmission. Heavy feeding by these flies causes livestock to bunch together and cease feeding (Jamnback 1969)

Horse flies and deer flies are stout-bodied flies with large eyes and heads and are in the family Tabanidae. Deer flies, *Chrysops* spp., are ~6–11 mm in length, yellow-orange with dark markings, and often with dark patterns on the wings. Horse flies, including the genera *Tabanus, Hybomitra, Atylotus, Haematopota, Silvius, Diachlorus, Chlorotabanus, Leucotabanus* and *Chloropus,* are large flies 9–33 mm in length that range in color from green to black. Deer flies in the genus *Chrysops* are smaller than horse flies and yellowish-brown and often with spotted wings. There are over 2000 species of tabanids worldwide, with 295 species in the Nearctic region in North America. Identification

of adult tabanids can be made to genus using Pechuman and Tesky (1981) and to species using Stone (1938) and Brennan (1935) along with regional keys (Tidwell 1973; Pechuman 1981; Pechuman et al. 1983). Snipe flies belong to the families Rhagionidae and Anthericidae and are gray-black and ~4–15 mm in length with a pointed abdomen and often with spotted wings. Legs are often elongated. Most blood-feeding snipe flies belong to the genera *Symphoromyia* (Rhagionidae) and *Suragina* (Anthericidae). Snipe flies can be identified using Cole (1969), Usinger (1973), James and Turner (1981), and Webb (1981).

Life History. Eggs are laid in masses on vegetation adjacent to or above aquatic or semi-aquatic habitats. Larvae hatch and develop in the mud. Larvae of most species inhabit wet soil [marshes, bogs, streams, and ponds (fresh or saline)], but some species are also present in dry soil (Pechuman and Tesky 1981). Larvae of deer flies feed on vegetation, while horse fly larvae are predaceous. Many species are associated with a specific larval habitat (Goodwin et al. 1985). Pupation occurs at the soil surface. Tabanids are generally univoltine, but generation times, depending on species, can range from 3 months to 2–3 years. Generally, different species emerge at specific times of the year and are present for a short period of time. Only female flies blood-feed and inflict a painful bite using blade-like mouthparts to cut the skin and sponging mouthparts to ingest the blood. After feeding, oogenesis is complete, the female oviposits, and 3–4 days later is ready for another blood meal. Many tabanid species only require a blood meal for the second and subsequent egg batches (Pechuman 1972). A life cycle may require 2 months to 2 years to complete, depending on species and location (Foil and Hogsette 1994). Because of the painful bite, feeding tabanids are often interrupted by host behavior, and the interruption of feeding and transfer from one host to another enhances the mechanical transmission of diseases by these flies (Jamnback 1969). Most adult tabanids are active during the warmer parts of the year, and activity occurs during the warmer hours of the day. Some species, however, are crepuscular. *Chrysops* fly repeatedly in circles around the head and shoulders and are very persistent in their attacks. Many tabanids are specific in their feeding sites on hosts (Mullens and Gerhardt 1979). Relatively little is known of the life history of snipe flies. Larvae are generally in damp soil rich in organic matter and *Symphoromyia* larvae have been collected from woodland/grass soils (Lane and Anderson 1982). Larvae are likely predaceous (James and Turner 1981).

Adult horse flies are present in the warmer months of the year, and intensity of attack is greatest adjacent to larval habitats (i.e., marshes, swamps). In a study in Louisiana, an estimate of 43,000 horse flies produced per acre has been made and landing rates of up to 1000 flies/hour on horses in southern Louisiana has been reported (Foil and Foil 1988). Using mark-recapture methods, Cooksey and Wright (1989) estimated the average number of host-seeking *Tabanus abactor* to be 1651 to 2225 females per hectare. Obviously these flies have a high potential impact on wild mammals.

Attraction of tabanids to potential hosts appears to involve various visual cues such as color, pattern, and background contrast (Allan and Stoffolano 1986a,b,c; Allan et al. 1987) and olfactory cues such as carbon dioxide, 1-octen-3-ol, and ammonia (Hayes et al. 1993; LePrince et al. 1994).

Epizootiology

DISTRIBUTION. Tabanids are found throughout North America, and geographic distributions of individual species are reported in Stone (1938), Brennan (1935), and Tesky (1990). The most common genera of tabanids are *Tabanus, Hybomitra,* and *Chrysops.* The most well known pests include *Tabanus atratus* (eastern states), *T. punctifer* (western states), *T. sulcifrons* (Midwest), *T. quinquevittatus, T. nigrovittatus, T. lineola, Chrysops atlanticus,* and *Hybomitra lasiopthalma* in the east. Distributions of snipe flies are presented in Cole (1969) and Webb (1977). The major pest species include *Symphoromyia atripes* (Alaska, Alberta, Montana, and California), *S. hirta* (eastern states and Alberta), *S. limata* (southern California), *S. sackeni* (California)(James and Turner 1981), and *Suragina concinna* (Webb 1981).

HOST RANGE. Tabanids are severe nuisances of a wide range of domestic and wild mammals. Tabanids are not host specific and have opportunistic feeding behaviors such as those in the genus *Tabanus* that have a very broad host range including reptiles. General preferences are observed for *Haematopota* that appear to feed preferentially on Bovidae (Oldroyd 1964) and the genus *Chrysops* that commonly feed on deer. Some tabanid species demonstrate clear preferences for landing and feeding on particular body regions of animals, as demonstrated with studies on cattle (Mullens and Gerhardt 1979). Deer and moose also are heavily attacked by deer flies and horse flies (Smith et al. 1970). White-tailed deer in Algonquin Park, Ontario, were hosts to 3 species of *Chrysops* (Davies 1959), 14 species each of *Chrysops* and *Hybomitra,* and 2 species of *Tabanus* (Smith et al. 1970). Smith et al. (1970) collected 32 species of tabanids from man, deer, and moose in Algonquin Park and concluded that one of the most important factors influencing the preference of a given host for feeding is the availability of the host in a given habitat (i.e., lakeshore, river, woodland). In general, deer flies fed on smaller hosts; horse flies (*Hybomitra*) fed on larger hosts. Moose were fed upon mostly by *Hybomitra* and a few *Chrysops. Hybomitra affinis* fed exclusively on moose but not on deer or man. Most deer flies were collected from man, compared to deer and moose. Lane and Anderson (1982) reported that the most common hosts of *Chrysops hirsuticallus* were cattle and Columbian black-tailed deer, but they also fed on black-tailed jackrabbits, Virginia

opossum, and raccoon. In Louisiana, deer are considered the major host of tabanids (Wilson and Richardson 1969). Reports of attacks by snipe flies usually involve man; however, Hoy and Anderson (1978) also reported attacks of Columbian black-tailed deer by large numbers of flies.

ENVIRONMENTAL LIMITATIONS. Larvae are present in aquatic and semi-aquatic habitats such as marshes or along rivers or lakes, and the numbers of adult tabanids are higher adjacent to these areas. Deer flies are usually present in woodlands or adjacent to woodlands while horse flies may be present in open areas. Snipe flies are generally present in wooded areas or areas of dense vegetation (Jamnback 1969; Pechuman 1981).

Clinical Signs. Feeding by tabanids is sharply painful and often produces a swollen red area with a central bleeding feeding lesion. Anaphylaxis in humans has been reported from tabanid bites (Hemmer et al. 1998).

Snipe flies are known to inflict painful bites in man, but there is little information on clinical signs in wildlife. Hoy and Anderson (1978) reported that deer attacked by swarms of snipe flies would become nervous and attempt to dislodge flies from their faces by brushing against inanimate objects or grooming with the hind foot. To avoid attack, deer also would assume a head-down, ears-flattened, legs-out, low-profile, resting posture ("reduced silhouette").

Pathology and Disease Transmission to Wild Mammals. Tabanids produce a painful bite, and feeding can result in considerable blood loss (up to 0.5 ml/fly). Flies stay on the host only long enough to feed. Wounds often ooze afterwards and other flies may feed from the wounds. These flies cause severe annoyance to animals as well as man.

The annoyance of feeding by biting flies and tabanids, in particular, often elicits avoidance behavior on the part of the host to reduce the feeding. Based on a study of captive animals, Sein (1985) (cited in Lankester and Samuel 1998) suggested that moose are less bothered by biting flies than are caribou. Moose may wallow or coat themselves in mud to protect their legs and belly from biting flies (Sein 1985). Duncan and Vigne (1979) observed that horses in large groups were attacked less by tabanids than horses in small groups. Hughes et al. (1981) noted that when horse flies were abundant and feeding, horses modified their behavior to move as a group from feeding areas to open windy areas. Different hosts vary in their tolerance to feeding; Smith et al. (1970) noted that moose appeared tolerant of severe attack by tabanids whereas deer were extremely restive and tried to dislodge flies.

Tabanids are also both mechanical and biological vectors of a range of disease agents, as is thoroughly reviewed by Krinsky (1976) and Foil (1989). Diseases associated with tabanids include equine infectious anemia (Foil et al. 1983), vesicular stomatitis, western equine encephalitis, hog cholera, anthrax (Krinsky

1976), tularemia (Jellison 1950), *Anaplasma* (Roberts et al. 1968), California encephalitis (Jamestown Canyon and LaCrosse) (Grimstad 1989), and try-panosomes (suspected vector of *Trypanosoma cervi* of deer) (Kistner and Hanson 1969) as well as nematodes such as *Elaeophora schneideri* (Pence 1991). *Elaeophora schneideri* naturally occurs in mule deer, elk, white-tailed deer, Sika deer, and moose (Chapter 12, this book). It is transmitted by many species of horseflies of the genera *Hybomitra* and *Tabanus* (summarized by Pence 1991; Chapter 12, this book) and all intermediate hosts of *E. scheideri* are reviewed by Anderson (Chapter 12, this book). In a study on South Island, South Carolina, the prevalence of infection of *Tabanus lineola hinellus* with *Elaeophora schneideri* was biphasic, with peaks in mid-May (1.23%) and mid-August (1.22%) (Couvillion et al. 1986). The intensity of infection with *E. schneideri* was highest in late summer. Clark and Hibler (1973) reported infective larvae of *Elaeophora schneideri* from *Hybomitra laticornis, H. tetricabrubilata,* and *Tabanus eurycerus* collected in the Gila National forest in New Mexico. About 90% of the larval nematodes were collected from *H. laticornis,* and ~16% of flies examined were infected. *Hybomitra tetricarubulata* and *T. eurycerus* contained 5.0% and 3.2% of the nematodes found, respectively. An average of 25 larval *E. schneideri* were found in each infected fly (Clark and Hibler 1973). Snipe flies are important primarily due to their painful bite.

Control and Treatment. Control of tabanids is very difficult due to the large numbers of species present in an area and their varied larval habitats, differing seasonal distributions, and the short contact time between flies and the host (Goodwin et al. 1985; Foil and Hogsette 1994). Repellents in the forms of wipe-ons or sprays provide short-lived relief for horses (Harris and Oehler 1977) and when applied as aerosols or impregnated in clothing provide temporary relief for humans (Catts 1968). Treatment with insecticides such as organophosphates or pyrethroids as spray, pour-on or ear-tag formulations provides short-term control for livestock (Goodwin et al. 1985; Foil et al. 1991). A moderate level of area-wide control through use of ultra-low-volume insecticide sprays can provide temporary relief if application timing is correct (Axtell and Dukes 1974). Use of traps such as box traps that attract and collect flies can be effective in reducing some local tabanid populations such as *Tabanus nigrovittatus* on eastern saltmarshes (Wall and Doane 1980). Because few tabanids enter buildings, housing animals can reduce fly feeding (Foil and Hogsette 1994). Control of larvae through water management or use of insecticides can be effective but is not feasible due to the diversity and size of habitats and environmental concerns (Goodwin et al. 1985). Proximity of livestock to wooded areas increases likelihood of problems with tabanids feeding (Foil and Hogsette 1994).

Public Health Concerns. The primary concern of public health is the annoyance caused by feeding, and this can have a significant negative effect on use of certain recreational areas. Anaphylaxis to tabanids, although rare, has been documented in man (Freye and Litwin 1996). Tabanids can serve as mechanical vectors of tularemia (Krinsky 1976). Snipe flies can inflict a "keen and painful bite" to humans and responses in humans vary from no effect to severe human allergic responses (Turner 1979). Pechuman (1972) reported on deer flies causing considerable irritation to fishermen, lumbermen, and other people outdoors in New York.

Domestic Animal Concerns. Tabanids are severe pests of domestic animals in some regions (Pechuman 1972). Pastured livestock may suffer intensely with normal grazing being interrupted, resulting in slower weight gain and lower milk production as reported in cattle (Goodwin et al. 1985; Granett and Hansens 1957). Effects of tabanids feeding on cattle can be devastating, and Tashiro and Schwardt (1949) estimated that 40 *Tabanus sulcifrons* feeding would result in a loss of 115 cc of blood in 1 hour. Similarly, Hollander and Wright (1980) estimated a total blood loss of 200 cc/day in Oklahoma with an average of 10% of tabanids feeding successfully. In addition, tabanids have been documented as mechanical transmitters of over 35 pathogenic agents of livestock (Foil 1989). In North America, the primary diseases vectored by tabanids include anaplasmosis of cattle in the Mississippi River area (Roberts et al. 1968) and equine infectious anemia virus of horses (Foil 1989). Snipe flies have been reported to feed and seriously annoy cattle in Alberta (*Symporomyia hirta;* Shemanchuk and Weintraub 1961) and horses and sheep in British Columbia (Hearle 1928).

Management Implications. Due to the difficulty in locating and treating larval habitats that are often environmentally sensitive areas, control is targeted towards reduction of annoyance of adults through use of repellents and insecticides.

LOUSE FLIES AND BAT FLIES. These bloodsucking flies are often present on cervids and bats, but there appear to be few documented ill effects to the hosts. This group consists of dorsoventrally flattened flies (sometimes wingless) with piercing mouthparts. Louse flies belong to the family Hippoboscidae, which includes flies that parasitize birds and mammals. In the United States, 31 species have been identified, of which 6 parasitize mammals. Louse flies are reddish brown and small (~6 mm) with a well-developed head. The families Nycteribiidae (spider-like bat flies) and Streblidae (bat flies) contain species that only parasitize bats. Streblids are small flies with a reduced head and long legs, and they somewhat resemble spiders. Nycteribiids are very small, spider-like flies with generally reduced wings and a small narrow head resting in a thoracic groove (Bequaert 1957; Cole 1969). Flies can be identified using Cole (1969), Peterson and Maa (1970), and Bequaert (1957).

Life History. All adult members of the Hippoboscidae are blood-feeding external parasites. The female produces one offspring at a time, eggs are retained and hatched, and the larvae develop in ~1 week within a uterine pouch. When ready to pupate, they are extruded by the female. Pupae are within a brown or black, oval, hard, seed-like pupal case that is sometimes glued to the hair or wool of the host (as in the sheep ked, *Melophagus ovinus*). Most often, however, larvae drop from the host or are deposited on the ground by the females and found in nests and bedding areas. The time of pupal development varies between species. The life cycle may last ~14–30 days, with females producing ~12 young in total. The frequency of feeding of females appears to be correlated to the 6- day gestation period. Wingless male and female *Lipoptena cervi* remain on hosts most of the year. In spring, larvae are deposited in the hair and pupae fall to the ground. Adults emerge in the fall. As soon as the ked finds a host, the wings detach and the ked begins to feed (Bequaert 1942). Both *Lipoptena depressa* and *L. cervi* appear to have one generation per year with young produced in the summer, overwintering as pupae, and emerging as adults the next spring or summer. Hippoboscids have one pair of wings that are retained by species of *Lipoptena* and *Neolipoptena* for only a day or two. Flies in *Melophagus* are wingless, and *Hippobosca* retain wings throughout their life. The life cycles of Nycteribiidae and Streblidae are similar.

Epizootiology

DISTRIBUTION AND HOST RANGE. There are four species of louse flies that feed on mammals (Bequaert 1957). *Lipoptena cervi,* an introduced louse fly from the Palearctic, is well established on white-tailed deer of northeastern North America. *Lipoptena mazamae* commonly occurs on white-tailed deer of the southern United States and Central and South America (Bequaert 1957); occurrence is also reported on black-buck antelope (Mertins et al. 1992), exotic deer (axis, fallow, Sika) (Richardson and Demarais 1992), and cattle (Drummond 1966). In the United States it is common on deer from South Carolina to Texas. Forrester (1992) reported *L. mazamae* on Florida panthers but concluded that it was a case of accidental parasitism as a result of predation. *Lipoptena depressa* and *Neolipoptena ferrisi* are common and often occur together, on mule and white-tailed deer of western North America (Bequaert 1957; Senger and Capelle 1959; Eads and Campos 1984; Kennedy et al. 1987; Mertins et al. 1992). *Lipoptena depressa* is generally found on mule deer.

Species of bat flies reported from bats include *Basilia antrozoi, Basilia corynorhini, Basilia forcipata,* and *Basilia boardmani* in the family Nycteribiidae and *Trichobius major* and *Trichobius corynorhini* in the family Streblidae.

PREVALENCE AND INTENSITY. Louse flies can be prevalent and abundant on deer; most published data is of *Lipoptena mazamae* on southern populations of white-tailed deer. Davis (1973) found *L. mazamae* on 90 of 94 white-tailed deer examined in east Texas; deer had up to 2300 keds. Samuel and Trainer (1972) and Forrester et al. (1996) reported *L. mazamae* on 64% and 82%, respectively, of white-tailed deer in southern Texas and southern Florida, respectively. Demarais et al. (1987) reported *L. mazamae* on 21 of 32 deer in central Mississippi but did not find them on 62 and 32 deer from northern and southern Mississippi, respectively. In a 3-year study on the distribution and seasonal abundance of deer keds on Columbian black-tailed deer in California, *L. depressa* was present on all 71 deer, and *Neolipoptena ferrisi* was present on 85% of deer examined (Westrom and Anderson 1992). Most *L. depressa* were present on the posterior regions of the deer (65%), and most *N. ferrisi* were present on the head (95%). Mean intensities were 424 (range 21–1563) (*L. depressa*) and 61 (range 1–481) (*N. ferrisi*). *Lipoptena depressa* was bivoltine with peaks of keds on deer in midsummer and early winter. There was no significant difference in prevalence of *L. depressa* on hosts of different ages or sexes or from different habitats. Winged forms of *L. depressa* were less abundant than the winter forms (63.4%), and winged forms were absent from December to late March and for 2 months in summer. Significantly fewer *N. ferrisi* were present on fawns (1–12 months) than on middle-aged (13–36 months) or old (> 37 months) deer. Cowan (1943) estimated that up to 2400 *L. depressa* occurred on black-tailed deer, while Dixon and Herman (1945) removed 1350 louse flies from a mule deer in California.

ENVIRONMENTAL LIMITATIONS. Moisture content in the substrate may affect ked populations. In a study on deer in south Florida, prevalence of *L. mazamae* was lower in October than in March, June, and August. Forrester et al. (1996) speculated that the lower prevalence could be due to greater rainfall in the fall that would decrease dry habitat available for successful pupation. In addition to a seasonal effect, deer from the sample site with high water levels had lower levels of *L. mazamae* than deer from sites with lower water levels. Samuel and Trainer (1972) reported similar findings.

Clinical Signs. Infestations of louse and bat flies are determined by the presence of the flies. Hippoboscidae are flat, dark brown insects, with or without wings. Nycteribiidae are small, spider-like wingless insects with a small head that folds back into the thorax. Streblidae are similar to the Nycteribiidae, but the head does not bend into the thorax; flies may be wingless or winged.

Pathology and Disease Transmission to Wild Mammals. There are no reports of negative impact of louse flies feeding on wildlife, although Strickland et al. (1981), in reference to *Lipoptena* and *Neolipoptena* on deer, suggests that one might expect heavy infestations to result in anemia and mechanical damage to the host. Strickland et al. (1981) proposed that since other species of keds are vectors of trypanosomes in domestic sheep and goats that *L. mazamae* could be a vector of the deer trypanosome, *Trypanosoma cervi*. Forrester et al. (1996) (see above discussion) indicated that high numbers of keds on deer could explain the high prevalence of *T. cervi* in deer of south Florida. The effects of bat fly infestations on bats is unknown (Forrester 1992).

Immunity. Domestic sheep acquire resistance to *Melophagus ovinus* with repeated exposure (Nelson and Kozub 1980). Sheep ked populations cycle annually due to the development of acquired resistance (Nelson 1962) as the skin becomes resistant to feeding keds. Acquired resistance in sheep is a local phenomenon in the infested area of skin (Nelson and Kozub 1980) and consists of a chronic inflammatory response combined with specific immune effector elements (Baron and Nelson 1985).

Control and Treatment. Control of keds on domestic sheep is achieved by use of insecticide dips and sprays (Khan et al. 1989; Bowman 1995).

Public Health Concerns. The bite of *Lipoptena cervi* is fairly painless but may be followed by a pruritic welt for several weeks (Bequaert 1942). Since sheep keds are known to annoy people handling sheep (Bequaert 1957), it is likely that keds from the occasional hunter-killed, heavily infested deer could be bothersome to hunters. The bat fly *(Trichobius major)* is known to bite humans (Constantine 1970).

Domestic Animal Concerns. While louse flies have been reported as vectors of agents in other parts of the world, they have not been reported as such in North America. The sheep ked, *Melophagus ovinus* is found on domestic sheep throughout North America and when present in high numbers can cause unthriftiness. *Melophagus ovinus* transmits *Typanosoma melophagium* to sheep, which appears to result in localized skin lesions (Nelson 1988). The prolonged presence of keds on sheep may result in reduction of wool growth (Nelson and Slen 1968) and production of skin nodules or cockles (Hanigan et al. 1976). *Lipoptena* may also attack cattle and horses (Bequeart 1942; Drummond 1966).

Management Implications. These flies appear to have no negative impact on populations of wild mammals.

MUSCOID FLIES. Flies in this group include biting and nonbiting flies in several families that are important for their nuisance status to wild mammals as well as being disease vectors or causing myiasis. Nonbiting flies in the genus *Hippelates* of the family Chloropidae are known as eye gnats and are small (1.0–2.5 cm), shiny black flies with aristate antennae. Flies in the family Muscidae are thick-bodied, gray-black in color with grayish stripes on the thorax, and ~4–9 mm in length. They include nonbiting flies such as the face fly, *Musca autumnalis,* and biting flies such as the horn fly, *Haematobia irritans,* stable fly, *Stomoxys calcitrans,* and moose fly, *Haematobosca alcis.* Both males and females of the horn, stable, and moose fly feed on blood. The common bluebottle and greenbottle flies in the family Calliphoridae and those in the family Sarcophagidae are important as they cause myiasis or tissue damage due to the feeding of larvae in wounds or tissues of domestic and wild mammals. These flies are medium to large, thick-bodied, and either metallic blue or green (Calliphoridae) or grey-brown with large distinct thoracic stripes and a checkered, striped, or spotted pattern on the abdomen (Sarcophagidae). Important species in Calliphoridae include *Cochliomyia hominivorax* (or *Callitroga americana* in older literature) (New World screwworm fly, primary screwworm fly), *Cochliomyia macellaria* (secondary screwworm fly), *Chrysomya rufifacies* (hairy maggot blow fly), *Phormia regina* (black blow fly)*, Phaenicia* (i.e., *Lucilia*) *sericata* (green bottle fly)*,* and *Protophormia terrae-nova*e. In the family Sarcophagidae six species have been implicated in myiasis in humans (James 1947). Most are secondary invaders of wounds and only *Wohlfahrtia* deposit larvae on healthy tissue (James 1948). These include *Wohlfahrtia vigil (W. opaca* in western North America is considered a subspecies by some) and *Wohlfahrtia meigeni* (Hall 1979; Wall and Shearer 1997).

Life History. Eye gnats *(Hippelates)* oviposit in moist friable soil and larvae burrow and feed on decomposing organic material. Pupation generally occurs in the top 3–4 cm of soil. Depending on food abundance and temperature, a generation may be completed in 2 weeks to several months. Adults have sponging mouthparts with sharp spines and feed on secretions from eyes, genitals, and wounds produced by other flies (Harwood and James 1979). Females require protein for egg development (Greenberg 1973).

Flies in the family Muscidae include those that feed only on secretions (face fly) and those that feed on blood (horn fly, stable fly, and moose fly). All feed on nectar. The face fly, *Musca autumnalis,* is found crawling over the faces of its hosts (usually cattle) and feeds with sponging mouthparts on ocular and nasal discharges and saliva as well as blood from wounds from biting flies and appear to stimulate tear production (Treece 1960; Krafsur and Moon 1997). Small spines on the mouthparts can cause irritation and mechanical damage to eye tissue. Males are seldom on cattle but rest on nearby surfaces (Treece 1960). Females deposit eggs only in fresh cow feces or, in their absence, feces of bison, swine, or humans (Bay et al. 1968; Burger and Anderson 1970). Larvae develop in 2–4 days and adults emerge from the whitish puparia ~14 days after eggs are deposited (Pickens and Miller 1980). The complete life cycle lasts 2–3 weeks. Adult horn flies, *Haematobia irritans,* maintain almost continuous contact (day and night) with hosts (usually cattle, sometimes horses), frequently biting with their piercing, sucking mouthparts and obtaining blood. Horn flies generally feed on the back and sides of the host. Under experimental conditions, female horn flies spend an average of 163 min/day feeding while males spend 96 min/day (Harris et al. 1974). Female flies require multiple blood meals for oviposition, which must occur in fresh bovine feces. In warm weather, larvae develop rapidly and adults may emerge within 2 weeks; in cold weather development may take several months (Thomas et al. 1987). Stable flies (*Stomoxys calcitrans*) oviposit in decaying moist vegetation (i.e., straw or hay, seaweed, lawn cuttings), sometimes combined with manure, and larvae develop in 6–26 days depending on temperature. Adults emerge from the brown pupae ~1 month after eggs are deposited. Both males and females blood-feed with stiletto-like piercing mouthparts, and a single blood meal supports development of an egg mass (Foil and Hogsette 1994). Flies feed within 3–4 minutes of landing on hosts; their feeding action is painful to the host (Harwood and James 1979). Stable flies generally feed below the knees and hocks of hosts but also may be found on the sides and back when populations are large (Foil and Hogsette 1994). Stable flies often disperse, making local control difficult (Greenberg 1973; Foil and Hogsette 1994). Adults of the moose fly, *Haematobosca alcis,* also maintain close contact with the host and are often visible on the rump or in swarms over the hind quarters. Females leave the host only to deposit eggs in very fresh moose feces, where larval development occurs (Burger and Anderson 1974).

Calliphorid flies are oviparous and lay eggs on wounded or infected skin or on skin soiled with feces. Larvae feed in wounds causing myiasis. They then drop to the ground and pupate and molt to adults (Greenberg 1973). *Cochliomyia hominivorax* is an obligate parasite of mammals that will infest almost any species of mammal. Eggs (200–400) are laid in rows overlapping like shingles at the edge of the wound. Sometimes, eggs are deposited on top of previously laid masses. In this species, larvae assume a characteristic position with head in the wound and spiracles positioned to obtain air. Larvae rarely leave the wound, but feed on the tissue in a pocket, enlarging the wound, which often attracts oviposition by other blow fly species. Larvae feed until fully developed (~100–200 hours) (Hall 1948). *Cochliomyia macellaria* is generally a carrion breeder but may be a secondary invader of wounds. Females oviposit in masses of 40–250 eggs in infected wounds or existing myiases. Sometimes several females oviposit together, resulting in a large mass of eggs. Larvae that feed in the wound often migrate out of the wound into wool or hair. They are mature in

~6 days. Pupation occurs on the ground. The average life cycle takes ~9–39 days depending on temperature (James 1948). Flies are most abundant in late summer and early fall and in southern Florida and Texas are present year round (Hall 1948). *Chrysomya rufifacies* is saprophagous but may also act as a facultative endoparasite (Wall and Shearer 1997). Eggs are deposited in masses of 50–200, and this is generally one of the first flies to oviposit on a fresh carcass. It is a secondary invader on wounds and acts as a scavenger in dead tissue. *Phormia, Protophormia* and *Phaenicia sericata* usually oviposit in carrion but also may act as secondary invaders and oviposit in wounds of livestock and wild mammals, causing myiasis. *Phormia regina* larvae are normally saprophagous but may be common in causing wound myiasis. This species is generally most abundant in early spring but is present year round in southern states. Eggs are laid in masses of 12–80, and the life cycle may take 10–15 days. *Protophormia terrae-novae* are common during the summer and very abundant in subarctic regions, where it has been known to kill reindeer (Hall 1948). Eggs are deposited in masses of 12–80 with a total development time of 15–16 days. *Phaenicia sericata* is a common carrion breeding fly and is one of the first to attack dead animals (Hall 1948). It occasionally oviposits in batches of 80–170 eggs in carrion but will also oviposit on blood and discharge from wounds or body openings and is most often the species associated with myiasis of vaginal canals and infected sores (Greenberg 1973). There can be up to eight generations per year in some southern states. Sarcophagid flies such as *Wohlfahrtia* are larviparous and deposit larvae into skin lesions (i.e., tick bites, scratches) or mucous membranes at natural orifices. *Wohlfahrtia vigil* is an obligate parasite, and larvae feed 5–7 days then drop to the ground and pupate. This species remains in the dermal tissue and causes furuncular myiasis that may contain up to five larvae (Wall and Shearer 1997).

Adult eye gnats are present during the warm months, with a long season in the south. Adults are highly mobile and are present considerable distances from the larval habitats (Dow 1959; Mulla and March 1959). Adult face flies, horn flies, and stable flies are present in the warm months and are diurnally active. Adults of these species are also strong fliers and are found considerable distances from the larval habitat. Adult blowflies are most abundant in midsummer to late summer (Hall 1948).

Eye gnats can be identified using Sabrosky (1941). Other muscoid flies can be identified using Cole (1969), Hall (1948, 1979) and Greenberg (1971).

Epizootiology

DISTRIBUTION. The most common eye gnats include *Hippelates bishoppi* (widespread), *H. collusor* (southwestern United States), *H. pallipes* (widespread), and *H. pusilio* (southeastern United States). Face flies are present in the western United States and north of South

Carolina. Stable flies and horn flies are widespread in North America (Cole 1969; Greenberg 1971). The distribution of the moose fly *Haematobosca alcis* overlaps that of its primary host, moose (Anderson and Lankester 1974). The New World screwworm fly, *Cochliomyia hominivorax*, has been eradicated north of Mexico through an on-going sterile male release program (Reichard et al. 1992), but prior to that was primarily in southeastern and south central states, with reports in northern states. The threat of reintroduction is a concern in the southern states. *Cochliomyia macellaria* is found throughout North America north to Quebec (Greenberg 1971). *Chrysomya rufifacies* is only present in some southern states (from Texas to California) and Hawaii (Shishido and Hardy 1969; Gagne et al. 1982). *Phormia regina* is present throughout North America (Hall 1948), and *Protophormia terrae-novae* is found in northern regions (Wall and Shearer 1997). *Phaenicia sericata* and *Wohlfahrtia* spp. are common throughout North America (Cole 1969; Greenberg 1971), and *P. sericata* is the most abundant blowfly species in the Midwest from late June to August (Greenberg 1973). *Wohlfahrtia vigil* is present in northern North America.

HOST RANGE. Adult *Hippelates* generally feed on large mammals including livestock, dogs, and humans. This group appears to be nonspecific in host range (Sabrowsky 1941; Greenberg 1973). Face flies feed primarily on cattle but also have been reported from horses, deer, antelope, and bison (Harwood and James 1979). Horn flies are generally only associated with cattle, although sometimes horses, sheep, and, rarely, dogs, swine, and humans are hosts (Treece 1960; Foil and Hogsette 1994). *Haematobosca alcis* feeds primarily on moose, and adult flies are closely associated with the host at all times (Lankester and Samuel 1998). Stable flies are not host-specific and feed on a wide range of hosts including livestock (Greenberg 1973), wild mammals (i.e., moose, see Lankester and Samuel 1998), bighorn sheep (Mullens and Dada 1992), man, and dogs (Foil and Hogsette 1994). Stable flies also can be a nuisance at zoos, particularly for big cats (Rugg 1982). Calliphorid flies causing myiasis are not host-specific, and larvae may feed on a wide range of species including domestic and wild mammals (Zumpt 1965). *Protophomia terrae-novae* can be a parasite of sheep, cattle, and reindeer, whereas *Phormia regina* is more commonly reported from livestock. *Phaenicia sericata* is found on a range of hosts throughout North America. *Wohlfartia vigil* is an obligate parasite reported from a wide range of wild mammals such as mink, fishers, foxes, nestling cottontail rabbits, adult Townsend voles, nestling *Microtus pennsylvanicus,* and rabbits and domestic mammals such as rabbits, cats, and dogs, and even man (Dong 1977, summarized in Craine and Boonstra 1986). *Wohlfartia meigeni* is an obligate parasite of mink and foxes, often in the farming industry. Wild mammalian hosts of blow flies and flesh flies that cause myiasis are summarized by Baum-

gartner and MacKey (1988) who report on 42 species of mammals parasitized by 30 species of myiasis-producing flies. Prior to its eradication, the primary screwworm was reported feeding on many wild mammals, and Hall (1948) reported that no North American mammals were exempt from myiasis caused by this species. Such reports included cottontail rabbits, jackrabbits, opossum, coyote, antelope (Capelle 1971), white-tailed deer (Capelle 1971; Forrester 1992), black bear, and wild hogs (Forrester 1992). In a summary of parasites reported from mammals in Florida, Forrester (1992) reported collections of blow fly larvae belonging to *Sarcophaga, Callipohora, Phaenicia,* and *Phormia regina* from white-tailed deer in Florida.

Pathology and Disease Transmission to Wild Mammals. Eye gnats are extremely annoying and persistent in feeding. Repeated feeding may cause localized irritation either from mechanical damage caused by the spines on the mouthparts or from infection. Eye gnats are incriminated as mechanical vectors of pinkeye (Payne et al. 1977) and are associated with transmission of yaws among humans in the West Indies (Greenberg 1973) and anaplasmosis among cattle (Roberts 1968). Infectious keratoconjunctivitis (pinkeye) can be mechanically transferred between animals by feeding flies. While the exact role of flies is unclear, several outbreaks of infectious keratoconjunctivitis have been reported from mule deer in Utah (Taylor et al. 1996), bighorn sheep in Montana (Meagher et al. 1992), and white-tailed deer, pronghorn antelope, and moose (Thorne 1982 cited in Taylor et al. 1996). Face flies cause significant irritation during feeding and are mechanical vectors of pinkeye in cattle (Hall 1984) and biological vectors of eyeworms (*Thelazia gulosa* in cattle; *T. skrjabini* in cattle and horses; *T. lacrymalis* in horses) (reviewed in Geden and Stoffolano 1982). *Thelazia skrjabini* has also been reported from white-tailed deer in Alberta (Kennedy et al. 1993). Kennedy (1993) examined prevalence of *Thelazia* eyeworms in beef cattle grazing on different pasture zones in Alberta. Prevalence was lower in short- and mid-grass pastures (0%–15%) than in transitional or aspen parklands (6.2%–7.4%) or rough fescue or woodland pastures (11.3%–18.4%), and the author suggested that pasture type may limit the number of face fly vectors. The horn fly is primarily a nuisance of cattle, but there is some confusion amongst reports on the number of feeding flies required before economic loss such as reduced weight gain occurs (Foil and Hogsette 1994). The horn fly is a biological vector of the nematode, *Stephanofilaria stilesi,* which causes a dermatological condition in cattle (Hibler 1966). Stable flies generally feed on cattle and horses; however, they have also been reported from wild mammals such as bighorn sheep (Mullens and Dada 1992). These nasty biters are easily disturbed, often flying from one host to another to feed. This behavior makes them excellent mechanical vectors of disease in man and livestock, and they have been incriminated as vectors of louse-borne relapsing fever, anthrax, brucellosis (summarized in Harwood and James 1979) and equine infectious anemia (Foil et al. 1985). The stable fly is the intermediate host of the nematode *Habronema microstoma* in horses (Stoffolano 1970). Cattle bunch together when stable fly populations are large, possibly to decrease fly attack (Weiman et al. 1992). Moose flies do not appear to be serious pests of moose, and it is unclear whether they are responsible for raw, wet lesions present just above the hock on the back legs of the moose (Lankester and Samuel 1998).

Untreated extensive myiasis may ultimately lead to death of a host, as indicated by the dramatic loss of livestock (cattle, sheep, goats) and wild mammals (Hall 1948; Zumpt 1965; Michener 1993). Losses can be extensive in the presence of the primary screwworm infestations (Reichard et al. 1992). Before eradication of the primary screwworm, it was considered the most important arthropod parasite of white-tailed deer in Florida and Texas, with an estimated 25%–80% of fawns lost annually in south Texas to myiasis (Scruggs 1979). After the eradication, deer populations increased in south Florida (Harlow and Jones 1965). Effects of myiasis include direct damage and secondary infection. Feeding by a few larvae is generally tolerated, although myiasis with as few as four larvae of *Wohlfahrtia vigil* has caused mortality in fox pups (Capelle 1971). Nestling *Microtus pennsylvanicus* with myiasis caused by *Wohlfahrtia vigil* were dead or moribund with an average of 10.8 larvae per vole (Craine and Boonstra 1986). A total of 4 of 43 nests had nestlings parasitized by *W. vigil;* in all cases all nestlings in the nest were parasitized with extensive affected tissue (up to 30%).

Immunity. Relatively little has been documented of immunity in this group. The horn fly and stable fly are susceptible to immune effector elements in a host blood meal as indicated in a study by Schlein and Lewis (1976). Antibody responses in cattle infested with horn flies peaked 4 weeks after fly abundance reached 150 flies per animal, but correlations between antibody response and fly abundance were extremely variable among animals (Baron and Lysyk 1995). When rabbits were immunized with extracts of various tissues from stable flies, horn flies that fed on the rabbits had greater mortality than those feeding on unvaccinated animals. Sandeman (1992) reviewed the potential for development of a vaccine against myiasis-producing flies such as *Lucilia cuprina,* and a recent study by Casu et al. (1997) reported larval growth inhibition and a candidate vaccine antigen purified from the peritrophic membrane of larvae. Acquired resistance has been documented for the Australian species, *Lucilia cuprina,* and the immunoglobulin fraction isolated from sera of previously infested sheep significantly slowed larval growth (Eisemann et al. 1990).

Control and Treatment. Control of muscoid flies on wild mammals is not feasible due to the highly interventive nature of the control methods (application of

insecticide to individual animals, etc.). For animals that are managed on farms or ranches, control methods used for domestic livestock may be appropriate. Eye gnats can be temporarily controlled by use of ultra-low-volume applications of insecticides (Axtell 1972), but eye gnats rapidly build resistance to insecticides and treatment of breeding habitats can be costly (Mulla 1962). Use of attractant baits in spot treatments with a toxicant in a removal trapping study demonstrated a rapid decrease in eye gnat populations (Mulla and Axelrod 1974). Face flies, horn flies, and stable flies are primarily controlled on livestock through the use of insecticide applied directly (sprays, dips), by self-application (dust bags, oilers) or by sustained-release (ear tags, boluses) (Harwood and James 1979; Drummond 1985; Derouen et al. 1995). Use of such methods for control of flies on wildlife is limited because direct and sustained-release methods require direct intervention. Self-application is more conducive for fly control on wild mammals; however, effective and equal treatments of individuals is difficult to achieve. Repellents are generally used for control of flies on horses (Foil and Hogsette 1994). Insecticide resistance in horn flies and stable flies to synthetic pyrethroid and organophosphate insecticides has been reported (Cilek et al. 1991; Cilek and Knapp 1993; Cilek and Greene 1994) and is widespread. On the other hand, ivermectin (as a pour-on) provides control of horn flies, and a single dose of pour-on reduced horn fly populations for ~6 weeks in Missouri (Marley et al. 1993).

Management of larval habitats through timely removal of manure, wet bedding, decaying organic matter, and accumulated seaweed effectively decreases local adult populations. The ability of these flies to fly moderate distances contributes to the reinfestation of some locations. Other methods of control also entail use of traps (sticky or pesticide treated) and electrocution grids. Use of naturally occurring biological control agents such as predators, parasites, and pathogens appear to have some potential for control of manure-breeding flies (Drummond 1985; Foil and Hogsette 1994).

Treatment of existing lesions and wounds could reduce incidence of myiasis in captive animals. Existing infestations are generally treated by surgical removal of the larvae or direct application of a wound dressing or smear containing insecticide. Control or prevention of blow fly myiasis in wild mammals is generally impractical. Use of methods effective for livestock may be useful for mammals managed on ranches. In a field study on calves in Australia, prophylactic use of ivermectin was successful against *Cochliomyia hominivorax* (Benitez Usher et al. 1994). Prevention of myiasis in sheep in Australia was obtained through use of insecticides by James et al. (1994), Levot et al. (1998), and Rugg et al. (1998), who used ear-tags, sprays, and ivermectin (intraruminal controlled-release bolus), respectively. Use of injectable ivermectin and moxidectin did not protect sheep from infestation with *Wolfahrtia magnifica* in

Hungary (Farkas et al. 1996). Topical, subcutaneous, and oral administration of ivermectin in reindeer has been evaluated for bot control and may also affect control of myiasis (Oksanen et al. 1993).

Public Health Concerns. Eye gnats and face flies can be annoying pests of humans. Stable flies are vicious biters and cause considerable human discomfort, often resulting in decreased use of recreational areas such as beaches (Newson 1977). Calliphorid flies are occasionally reported as causing human myiasis (Hall 1979; Wall and Shearer 1997). Reports of human myiasis include cases caused by *Phaenicia sericata* (Hall 1948; Greenberg 1984), *Phormia regina* (Hall et al. 1986; Miller et al. 1990), *Cochliomyia macellaria* (Smith and Clevenger 1986), *Sarcophaga* spp. (Arbit et al. 1986) and *Calliphora* spp. (Hall 1948).

Domestic Animal Concerns. Eye gnats are highly irritating pests of livestock when present in high numbers and are incriminated as vectors of pinkeye and bovine mastitis (Sanders 1940). Face flies cause considerable irritation while feeding and increase incidence of pinkeye in the northern states and Canada; costs of reduced weight gain and reduced milk production are estimated at over $50 million yearly (Steelman 1976). The primary pests of cattle production (beef and dairy) are stable flies and horn flies, both of which are responsible for significant economic loss each year. It is estimated that the economic impact of the horn fly alone on cattle production in North America approaches $1 billion (Cupp et al. 1998). In addition, stable flies can be mechanical vectors of a variety of diseases listed above. Beef cattle exposed to stable flies may gain less weight and utilize feed less efficiently than fly-free cattle (Campbell et al. 1987; Weinman et al. 1992). Derouen et al. (1995) indicated that there was 17% more weight gain on treated pastured cattle than on untreated cattle. Weiman et al. (1992) reported that cattle responded to stable flies by bunching together to protect their front legs, thereby increasing heat stress and causing reduction in weight gain.

The primary screwworm caused major economic impact on the livestock industry in the United States prior to its eradication, with estimated losses of over $100 million annually (Steelman 1976). The incidence of myiasis in domestic animals has decreased dramatically with this eradication, but it is still present due to the other species of Calliphorid flies present throughout North America. Dogs and cats are often hosts for myiasis-producing larvae (Hendrix 1991).

Management Implication. The presence of *Hippeletes* and stable, face, and horn flies can be reduced by effective management and timely removal of manure, soiled bedding, and decaying organic matter. The incidence of myiasis is more difficult to control other than by prompt treatment of wounds and lesions on animals.

LITERATURE CITED

Mosquitoes

Abbitt, B., and L.G. Abbitt. 1981. Fatal exsanguination of cattle attributed to an attack of salt marsh mosquitoes (*Aedes sollicitans*). *Journal of the American Veterinary Medical Association* 179:1397–1400.

Acevedo, R.A., and J.H. Theis. 1982. Prevalence of heartworm (*Dirofilaria immitis* Leidy) in coyotes from five northern California counties. *American Journal of Tropical Medicine and Hygiene* 31:968–972.

Allan, S.A., and D.L. Kline. 1995. Evaluation of organic infusions and synthetic compounds mediating oviposition in *Aedes albopictus* and *Aedes aegypti* (Diptera: Culicidae). *Journal of Chemical Ecology* 21:847–860.

Allan, S.A., J.D. Day, and J.D. Edman. 1987. Visual ecology of biting flies. *Annual Review of Entomology* 32:297–316.

Barat, L.M., J.R. Zucker, A.M. Barber, M.E. Parise, L.A. Paxton, J.M. Roberts, and C.C. Campbell. 1997. Malaria surveillance—United States, 1993. *Morbidity and Mortality Weekly Report* 46:27–47.

Bartlett, C.M. 1983. Zoogeography and taxonomy of *Dirofilaria scapiceps* (Leidy, 1886) and D. *uniformis* Price, 1957 (Nematoda: Filariodea) of lagomorphs in North America. *Canadian Journal of Zoology* 61:1011–1022.

Bartlett, C.M. 1984. Development of *Dirofilaria scapiceps* (Leidy, 1886) (Nematoda: Filarioidea) in *Aedes* spp. and *Mansonia perturbans* (Walker) and responses of mosquitoes to infection. *Canadian Journal of Zoology* 62:112–129.

Becklund, W.W., and M.L. Walker. 1969. Taxonomy, hosts and geographic distribution of the *Setaria* (Nematoda: Filaroidea) in the United States and Canada. *The Journal of Parasitology* 55:359–368.

Bentley, M.D., and J.F. Day. 1989. Chemical ecology and behavioral aspects of mosquito oviposition. *Annual Review of Entomology* 34:401–421.

Bidlingmayer, W.L. 1971. Mosquito flight paths in relation to environment. I. Illumination levels, orientation and resting areas. *Annals of the Entomological Society of America* 16:1121–1131.

Blackmore, C.G.M., M.S. Blackmore, and P.R. Grimstad. 1998. Role of *Anopheles quadrimaculatus* and *Coquillettidia perturbans* (Diptera: Culicidae) in the transmission cycle of Cache Valley virus (Bunyaviridae: Bunyavirus) in the Midwest, USA. *Journal of Medical Entomology* 35:660–664.

Boromisa, R.D., and P.R. Grimstad. 1987. Seroconversion rates to Jamestown Canyon virus among six populations of white-tailed deer (*Odocoileus virginianus*) in Indiana. *Journal of Wildlife Diseases* 23:23–33.

Bowman, D.D. 1995. *Georgis' Parasitology for Veterinarians*, 6th ed. Philadelphia, PA: W. B. Saunders Company.

Buxton, B.A., and G.R. Mullen. 1980. Field isolations of *Dirofilaria* from mosquitoes in Alabama. *The Journal of Parasitology* 66:140–144.

Calef, G., and D.C. Heard. 1980. The status of three tundra wintering herds in northeastern mainland Northwest territories. In *Proceedings 2nd reindeer/caribou symposium, Roros, Norway,* Part B. Ed. E. Reimers, E. Gaare, and S. Skjenneberg. Pp. 582–594.

Calisher, C.H., D.B. Francy, G.C. Smith, D.J. Murth, J.S. Lazuick, N. Karabatsos, W.L. Jakob, and R.E. McLean. 1986. Distribution of Bunyamwera serogroup viruses in North America 1956–84. *American Journal of Tropical Medicine and Hygiene* 35:429–443.

Christensen, B.M., and W.N. Andrew. 1976. Natural infection of *Aedes trivittatus* (Coq) with *Dirofilaria immitis* in central Iowa. *The Journal of Parasitology* 62:276–280.

Clements, A.N. 1992. *The Biology of Mosquitoes.* New York: Chapman and Hall.

Corbet, P.S., and A.E.R. Downe. 1966. Natural hosts of mosquitoes in northern Ellesmere Island. *Arctic* 19:153–161.

Crans, W.J., L.J. McCuiston, and D.A. Sprenger. 1990. The blood-feeding habits of *Aedes sollicitans* (Walker) in relation to eastern equine encephalitis virus in coastal areas of New Jersey I. Host selection in nature determined by precipitin tests on wild caught specimens. *Bulletin of the Society for Vector Ecology* 15:144–148.

Crum, J.M., V.F. Nettles, and W.R. Davidson. 1978. Studies on endoparasites of the black bear (*Ursus americanus*) in the southeastern United States. *Journal of Wildlife Diseases* 14:178–186.

Dale, P.E.R., S.A. Ritchie, B.M. Territo, C.D. Morris, A. Muhar, and B.H. Kay. 1998. An overview of remote sensing and GIS for surveillance of mosquito vector habitats and risk assessment. *Journal of Vector Ecology* 23:54–61.

Darsie, R.F. Jr., and R.A. Ward. 1981. Identification and geographical distribution of the mosquitoes of North America, north of Mexico. *Mosquito Systematics Supplement* 1:1–313.

Dawson, M., P.T. Johnson, L. Feldman, R. Glover, J. Koehler, P. Blake, and K.E. Toomey. 1996. Probable locally acquired mosquito-transmitted *Plasmodium vivax* infection—Georgia, 1996. *Morbidity and Mortality Weekly Report* 46:264–267.

Downe, A.E.R. 1962. Some aspects of host selection by *Mansonia perturbans* (Walk.)(Diptera: Culicidae). *Canadian Journal of Zoology* 40:725–732.

Durden, L.A. 1984. Natural incidence of *Setaria equina* (Nematoda: Filaroidea) from *Aedes canadensis* (Diptera: Culicidae) in North America. *Journal of Medical Entomology* 21:472–473.

Edman, J.D. 1974. Host-feeding patterns of Florida mosquitoes. III. *Culex (Culex)* and *Culex (Neoculex). Journal of Medical Entomology* 11:95–104.

Edman, J.D., and A. Spielman. 1986. Blood-feeding by vectors: Physiology, ecology, and vertebrate defense. In *The arboviruses: Epidemiology and ecology,* vol. 1. Ed. T.P. Monath. Boca Raton, FL: CRC Press, pp. 153–189.

Edman, J.D., and D.J. Taylor. 1968. *Culex nigropalpis:* Seasonal shift in the bird-mammal feeding ratio in a mosquito vector of human encephalitis. *Science* 161:67–68.

Edman, J.D., L.A. Webber, and H.W. Kale. 1972. Host-feeding patterns of Florida mosquitoes. II. *Culiseta. Journal of Medical Entomology* 9:29–434.

Eldridge, B.F., C.H. Calisher, J.L. Fryer, L. Bright, and D.J. Hobbs. 1987. Serological evidence of California serogroup virus activity in Oregon. *Journal of Wildlife Diseases* 23:199–204.

Foster, W.A., and R.G. Hancock. 1994. Nectar-related olfactory and visual attractants for mosquitoes. *Journal of the American Mosquito Control Association* 10:288–296.

Franson, J.C., R.D. Jorgensen, and E.K. Boggess. 1976. Dirofilariasis in Iowa coyotes. *Journal of Wildlife Diseases* 12:165–166.

French, F.E., and A.S. West. 1971. Skin reaction specificity of guinea pig immediate hypersensitivity to bites of four mosquito species. *The Journal of Parasitology* 57:396–400.

Gauld, L.W., R.P. Hanson, W.H. Thompson, and S.K. Sinha. 1974. Observations on a natural cycle of LaCrosse virus (California group) in southwestern Wisconsin. *American Journal of Tropical Medicine and Hygiene* 23:983–992.

Grimstad, P.R. 1989. California group virus disease. In *The arboviruses: Epidemiology and ecology,* vol. 2. Ed. T. P. Monath. Boca Raton, FL: CRC Press, pp. 99–136.

Grimstad, P.R, Q.E. Ross, and G.B. Craig, Jr. 1980. *Aedes triseriatus* (Diptera: Culicidae) and LaCrosse virus II. Modifications of mosquito feeding behavior by virus infection. *Journal of Medical Entomology* 17:1–7.

Hayes, R.O. 1961. Host preferences of *Culiseta melanura* and allied mosquitoes. *Mosquito News* 21:179–187.

Heard, P.B., M.B. Zhang, and P.R. Grimstad. 1990. Isolation of Jamestown Canyon virus (California serotype) from *Aedes* mosquitoes in an enzootic focus in Michigan. *Journal of the American Mosquito Control Association* 6:461–468.

Hedberg, C.W., J.W. Washburn, and R.D. Sjogren. 1985. The association of artificial containers and La Crosse encephalitis cases in Minnesota, 1979. *Journal of the American Mosquito Control Association* 1:89–90.

Hubert, G.F., Jr., T.J. Kick, and R.D. Andrews. 1980. *Dirofilaria immitis* in red foxes in Illinois. *Journal of Wildlife Diseases* 16:229–232.

Hudson, A., L. Bowman, and C.W.M. Orr. 1960. Effects of absence of saliva on blood feeding by mosquitoes. *Science* 131:1730.

Jones, C.J., and J.E. Lloyd. 1987. Hypersensitivity reactions and hematolytic changes in sheep exposed to mosquito (Diptera: Culicidae) feeding. *Journal of Medical Entomology* 24:71–76.

Karppinen, A., I. Pantala, A. Vaalasti, T. Palosuo, and T. Reunala. 1996. Effect of cetirizine on the inflammatory cells in mosquito bites. *Annals of Experimental Allergy* 26:703–709.

Kay, B.H., and D.H. Kemp. 1994. Vaccines against arthropods. *American Journal of Tropical Medicine and Hygiene* 50(s): 87–96.

Kazacos, K.R., and E.O. Edberg. 1979. *Dirofilaria immitis* infection in foxes and coyotes in Indiana. *Journal of the American Veterinary Medical Association* 175:909–910.

King, A.W., and A.M. Bohning. 1984. The incidence of heartworm *Dirofilaria immitis* (Filaroidea) in the wild canids of northeast Arkansas. *Southwestern Naturalist* 29:89–92.

Kline, D.L., W. Takken, J.R. Wood, and D.A. Carlson. 1990. Field studies on the potential of butanone, carbon dioxide, honey extract, 1-oct-3-ol, L-lactic acid and phenols as attractants for mosquitoes. *Medical and Veterinary Entomology* 4:383–391.

Knight, K.L., and A. Stone. 1977. *A catalog of the mosquitoes of the world (Diptera: Culicidae),* 2d ed. College Park, MD: Thomas Say Foundation, Entomological Society of America.

Lankester, M. W. 1987. Pests, parasites, and diseases of moose (*Alces alces*) in North America. *Swedish Wildlife Research Supplement* 1(Part 2): 461–490.

LeBrun, R.A., and G.M. Dziem. 1984. Natural incidence of *Setaria equina* (Nematoda: Filarioidea) from *Aedes canadensis* (Diptera: Culicidae) in North America. *Journal of Medical Entomology* 21:472–473.

LeDuc, J.W. 1979. The ecology of California group viruses. *Journal of Medical Entomology* 16:1–17.

Legner, E.F. 1995. Biological control of Diptera of medical and veterinary importance. *Journal of Vector Ecology* 20:59–120.

Loftin, K.M., R.L. Byford, M.J. Loftin, and M.E. Craig. 1995. Potential mosquito vectors of *Dirofilaria immitis* in Bernalillo Co., New Mexico. *Journal of the American Mosquito Control Association* 11:90–93.

Magnarelli, L.A. 1977. Host feeding patterns of Connecticut mosquitoes (Diptera: Culicidae). *American Journal of Tropical Medicine and Hygiene* 26:547–551.

———. 1979. Diurnal nectar-feeding of *Aedes canator* and *Ae. sollicitans* (Diptera: Culicidae). *Environmental Entomology* 8:949–945.

McKiel, J.A., and A.S. West. 1961. Effects of repeated exposures of hypersensitive humans and laboratory rabbits to mosquito antigens. *Canadian Journal of Zoology* 39:597–603.

McLean, R.G., L.J. Kirk, R.B. Shriner, P.D. Cook, E.E. Myers, J.S. Gill, and E.G. Campos. 1996. The role of deer as a possible reservoir host of Potosi virus, a newly recognized arbovirus in the United States. *Journal of Wildlife Diseases* 32:444–452.

Mellanby, K. 1946. Man's reaction to mosquito bites. *Nature* 158:554.

Mitchell, C.J., D.B. Francy, and C.T. Monath. 1980. Arthropod vectors. In *St. Louis Encephalitis.* Ed. T.P. Monath. Washington, DC: American Public Health Association, pp. 1313–1379.

Mitchell, C.J., G.C. Smith, N. Karabatsos, C.G. Moore, D.B. Francy, and R.S. Nasci. 1996. Isolation of Potosi virus from mosquitoes collected in the United States, 1989–94. *Journal of the American Mosquito Control Association* 12:1–7.

Mitchell, C.J., L.D. Haramis, N. Karabatsos, G.C. Smith, and V.J. Starwalt. 1998. Isolation of La Crosse, Cache Valley, and Potosi viruses from *Aedes* mosquitoes (Diptera: Culicidae) collected at used-tire sites in Illinois during 1994–1995. *Journal of Medical Entomology* 35:573–577.

Monath, T.P. (Ed.) 1988. *The arboviruses. Epidemiology and ecology,* vols. 1–5. Boca Raton, FL: CRC Press.

Morschel, F.H. and D.R. Klein. 1997. Effects of weather and parasitic insects on behavior and group dynamics of caribou of the Delta Herd, Alberta. *Canadian Journal of Zoology* 75:1659–1670.

Mount, G.A., T.L. Biery, and D.G. Haile. 1996. A review of ultra-low-volume aerial sprays of insecticide for mosquito control. *Journal of the American Mosquito Control Association* 12:601–618.

Mulla, M. 1995. The future in insect growth regulators in vector control. *Journal of the American Veterinary Medical Association* 11:269–273.

Nasci, R.S. 1982. Differences in host choice between the sibling species of treehole mosquitoes, *Aedes triseriatus* and *Aedes hendersoni. American Journal of Tropical Medicine and Hygiene* 31:411–415.

Nasci, R.S. 1985. Behavioral ecology of variation in blood-feeding and its effect on mosquito-borne diseases. In *Ecology of mosquitoes: Proceedings of a workshop.* Ed. L.P. Lounibos, J.R. Rey, and J.H. Frank. Vero Beach: Florida Medical Entomology Laboratory, pp. 293–303.

Nayar, J.K. 1982. *Bionomics and physiology of* Culex nigropalpis *(Diptera: Culicidae) of Florida: An important vector of disease.* Florida Agricultural Experiment Station Bulletin 827.

Nelson, W.A. 1987. Other blood sucking and myiasis-producing flies. In *Immune responses in parasitic infections: Immunology, immunopathology and immunoprophylaxis.* Ed. E.J.L. Soulsby. Vol. 4, *Protozoa, arthropods and invertebrates.* Boca Raton, FL: CRC Press, pp. 293–303.

Pinger, R.R. and W.A. Rowley. 1975. Host preferences of *Aedes trivittatus* (Diptera: Culicidae) in central Iowa. *American Journal of Tropical Medicine and Hygiene* 24:889–893.

Power, H.T., and P.J. Ihrke. 1995. Selected feline eosinophilic skin diseases. *Veterinary Clinics of North America: Small Animal Practice* 25:833–850.

Ramasamy, M.S., K.A. Srikinshnaraj, S. Wijekoone, L.S. Jesuthason, and R. Ramasamy. 1992. Host immunity to mosquitoes: Effect of antimosquito antibodies on *Anopheles tesselatus* and *Culex quinquefasciatus* (Diptera: Culicidae). *Journal of Medical Entomology* 29:934–938.

Reeves, W.C., C.H. Templis, R.E. Bellamy, and M.F. Lofy. 1963. Observations on the feeding habits of *Culex tarsalis* in Kern county, California, using precipitating sera produced in birds. *American Journal of Tropical Medicine and Hygiene* 12:929–935.

Reunala, T., H. Brummer-Korrenkontio, P. Lappalainer, L. Rasanen, and T. Palosuo. 1990. Immunology and treatment of mosquito bites. *Clinical and Experimental Allergy* 20(Supplement 4): 19–24.

Robertson, L.C., S. Prior, C.S. Apperson, and W.S. Irby. 1993. Bionomics of *Anopheles quadrimaculatus* and *Culex erraticus* (Diptera: Culicidae) in the Falls Lake basin, North Carolina: Seasonal changes in abundance and gonotrophic status and host feeding patterns. *Journal of Medical Entomology* 30:689–698.

Savage, H.M., M.L. Nielylski, G.C. Smith, C.J. Mitchell, and G.B. Craig, Jr. 1993. Host-feeding patterns of *Aedes albopictus* (Diptera: Culicidae) at a temperate North American site. *Journal of Medical Entomology* 30:27–34.

Scoles, G.A. 1994. Surveying for vectors of dog heartworm. *Vector Control Bulletin of the North Central States* 3:59–67.

Scott, T.W., and S.C. Weaver. 1989. Eastern equine encephalitis virus: Epidemiology and evolution of mosquito transmission. *Advances in Virus Research* 37:277–328.

Service, M.W. 1980. Effects of wind on the behavior and distribution of mosquitoes and black flies. *International Journal of Biometeorology* 24:347–353.

———. 1997. Mosquito (Diptera: Culicidae) dispersal—the long and short of it. *Journal of Medical Entomology* 34:579–588.

Sexton, D.J., P.E. Rollin, E.B. Breitschwerdt, G.R. Corey, S.A. Meyers, M.R. Dumais, M.D. Bowen, C.S. Goldsmith, S.R. Zain, S.T. Nichol, C.J. Peters, and T.G. Ksiazek. 1997. Life-threatening Cache Valley virus infection. *New England Journal of Medicine* 336:547–549.

Simmons, J.M., W.S. Nicholson, E.P. Hill, and D.B. Briggs. 1980. Occurrence of *Dirofilaria immitis* in gray fox (*Urocyon cinereargenteus*) in Alabama and Georgia. *Journal of Wildlife Diseases* 16:225–228.

Sota, T., E. Hayamizu, and M. Mogi. 1991. Distribution of biting *Culex tritaeniorynchus* (Diptera: Culicidae) among pigs: Effects of host size and behavior. *Journal of Medical Entomology* 28:428–433.

Steelman, C.D., T.W. White, and P.E. Schilling. 1972. Effects of mosquitoes on the average daily gain of feedlot steers in southern Louisiana. *Journal of Economic Entomology* 65:462–466.

Sudia, W.D., V.F. Newhouse, L.D. Beadle, D.L. Miller, J.G. Johnston, Jr., R. Young, C.H. Calisher, and K. Maness. 1975. Epidemic Venezuelan equine encephalitis in North America in 1971. Vector studies. *American Journal of Epidemiology* 101:17–35.

Sullivan, M.F., D.J. Gould, and S. Maneechai. 1971. Observation on the host range and feeding preferences of *Aedes albopictus* (Skuse). *Journal of Medical Entomology* 8:713–716.

Sutherland, G.B., and A.B. Ewen. 1974. Fecundity decrease in mosquitoes ingesting blood from specifically sensitized mammals. *Journal of Insect Physiology* 20:655–666.

Templis, C.H. 1975. Host feeding patterns of mosquitoes, with a review of arboviruses and analysis of blood meals by serology. *Journal of Medical Entomology* 11:635–653.

Templis, C.H., D.B. Francy, R.O. Hayes, and M.F. Lofy. 1967. Variations in patterns of seven culicine mosquitoes on vertebrate hosts in Weld and Larimer Counties, Colorado. *American Journal of Tropical Medicine and Hygiene* 16:111–119.

Todaro, W.S., C.D. Morris, and N.A. Heacock. 1977. *Dirofilaria immitis* and its potential mosquito vectors in central New York State. *American Journal of Veterinary Research* 38:1197–1200.

Tolbert, R.H., and W.E. Johnson, Jr. 1982. Potential vectors of *Dirofilaria immitis* in Macon county, Alabama. *American Journal of Veterinary Research* 43:2054–2056.

Walker, E.D., and J.D. Edman. 1986. Influence of defensive behavior of eastern chipmunks and gray squirrels (Rodentia: Sciuridae) on feeding success of *Aedes triseriatus* (Diptera: Culicidae). *Journal of Medical Entomology* 23:1–10.

Weinmann, C.J., J.R. Anderson, W.M. Longhurst, and G. Connolly. 1973. Filarial worms of Columbian black-tailed deer in California. I. Observations in the vertebrate hosts. *Journal of Wildlife Diseases* 9:213–220.

Wolfe, R.J. 1996. Effects of open water management on selected total marsh resources: A review. *Journal of the American Mosquito Control Association* 12:701–712.

Wood, D.M., P.T. Danks, and R.A. Ellis. 1979. *The Insects and Arachnids of Canada.* Part 6, *The Mosquitoes of Canada. Diptera: Culicidae.* Ottawa, Ontario: Agriculture Canada Publication 1686.

United States Department of Agriculture. 1965. Livestock and poultry losses. In *Losses in Agriculture.* Washington, DC: U.S. Department of Agriculture Handbook No. 29, pp. 72–84.

Yuill, T.M., and P.H. Thompson. 1970. Cache Valley virus in the Del Mar Va peninsula. IV. Biological transmission of the virus by *Aedes sollicitans* and *Aedes taeneorynchus. American Journal of Tropical Medicine and Hygiene* 19:513–519.

Biting Midges

Anderson, G.S., P. Belton, and N. Kleider. 1991. *Culicoides obseletus* (Diptera: Ceratopogonidae) as a causal agent of *Culicoides* hypersensitivity (sweet itch) in British Columbia. *Journal of Medical Entomology* 28:685–693.

Anderson, R.R., and H.L. Holloway. 1993. *Culicoides* (Diptera: Ceratopogonidae) associated with white-tailed deer habitat and livestock operations in the northern Great Plains. *Journal of Medical Entomology* 30:625–627.

Battle, F.V., and E.C. Turner. 1971. *A systematic review of the genus* Culicoides *(Diptera: Ceratopogonidae) in Virginia with a geographic catalog of the species occurring in the eastern United States north of Florida.* Virginia Polytechnical Institute and State University Research Division Bulletin No. 44, 129 pp.

Blanton, F.S., and W.W. Wirth. 1979. *The sand flies of Florida (Diptera: Ceratopogonidae).* Vol. 10, *Arthropods of Florida and neighboring land areas.* Gainesville: Florida Department of Agriculture and Consumer Services.

Braverman, Y., and A. Chizov-Ginzburg. 1997. Repellency of synthetic and plant derived preparations for *Culicoides imicola. Medical and Veterinary Entomology* 11:355–360.

Bowman, D.D. 1995. *Georgis' parasitology for veterinarians,* 6th ed. Philadelphia, PA: W. B. Saunders Company.

Davidson, W.R., and V.F. Nettles. 1997. *Field manual of wildlife diseases in the southeastern United States,* 2nd. ed. Athens, GA: Southeastern Cooperative Wildlife Disease Survey, University of Georgia.

Downes, J.A. , and W.W. Wirth. 1981. Ceratopogonidae. In *Manual of Nearctic Diptera,* vol. 1. Hull, Quebec: Agriculture Canada Monograph No. 27, pp. 293–303.

Fadok, V.A., and E.C. Greiner. 1990. Equine insect hypersensitivity: Skin test and biopsy results correlated with clinical data. *Equine Veterinary Journal* 22:236–240.

Foil, L., D. Stage, and T.R. Klein. 1984. Assessment of wild-caught *Culicoides* (Ceratopogonidae) species as natural vectors of *Onchocerca cervicalis* in Louisiana. *Mosquito News* 44:204–206.

Fox, I. 1955. A catalogue of the bloodsucking midges of the Americas (*Culicoides, Leptoconops* and *Lasiohelia*) with keys to the subgenera and Nearctic species, a geographic index and bibliography. *Journal of Agriculture of the University of Puerto Rico* 39:214–285.

Gibbs, E.P.J., and E.C. Greiner. 1989. Bluetongue and epizootic hemorrhagic disease. In *The arboviruses: Epidemiology and ecology,* vol. 2. Ed. T.P. Monath. Boca Raton, FL: CRC Press, pp. 39–70.

Hardy, J.L., R.P. Scrivani, R.N. Lyness, R.L. Nelson, and D.R. Roberts. 1970. Ecologic studies on buttonwillow virus in Kern County, California 1961–1968. *American Journal of Tropical Medicine and Hygiene* 19:552–563.

Holbrook, F.R., and W.J. Tabachnick. 1995. (Diptera: Ceratopogonidae) *Culicoides variipennis* complex in California. *Journal of Medical Entomology* 32:413–419.

Holbrook, F.R., W.J. Tabachnick, and R. Brady. 1996. Genetic variation in populations of *Culicoides variipennis* complex in the six New England states, USA. *Medical and Veterinary Entomology* 10:173–180.

Hourrigan, J.L., and A.L. Klingsporn. 1975. Epizootiology of bluetongue: The situation in the United States of America. *Australian Veterinary Journal* 51:203–208.

Jamnback, H. 1969. *Bloodsucking flies and other outdoor nuisance arthropods of New York state.* New York State Museum and Science Series Memoirs 19.

Jones, R.H., H.W. Potter, Jr., and H.A. Rhodes. 1972. Ceratopogonidae attacking horses in south Texas during the 1971 VEE epidemic. *Mosquito News* 32:507–509.

Jones, R.H., R.D. Roughton, N.M. Foster, and B.M. Bando. 1977. *Culicoides,* the vector of epizootic hemorrhagic disease in white-tailed deer in Kentucky in 1971. *Journal of Wildlife Diseases* 13:2–8.

Jones, R.H., E.T. Schmidtmann, and N.M. Foster. 1983. Vector-competence studies for bluetongue and epizootic hemorrhagic disease viruses with *Culicoides venustus. Mosquito News* 43:184–186.

Kettle, D.S. 1977. Biology and bionomics of bloodsucking ceratopogonids. *Annual Review of Entomology* 22:33–51.

Kline, D.L., D.V. Hagan, and R. Wood. 1994. *Culicoides* responses to 1-octen-3-ol and carbon dioxide in salt marshes near Sea Island, Georgia, USA. *Medical and Veterinary Entomology* 8:25–30.

Linley, J.R., and J.B. Davies. 1971. Sandflies and tourism in Florida and the Bahamas and the Caribbean area. *Journal of Economic Entomology* 64:262–278.

Mullen, G.R., M.E. Hayes, and K.E. Nusbaum. 1985. Potential vectors of bluetongue and epizootic hemorrhagic disease viruses in cattle and white-tailed deer in Alabama. In *Bluetongue and Related Orbiviruses.* Ed. T. L. Barber, M. M. Johnson, and B. I. Osburn. New York: Alan Liss, Inc., pp. 201–206.

Mullens, B.A., and C.E. Dada. 1992. Insects feeding on desert bighorn sheep, domestic rabbits and Japanese quail in the Santa Rosa mountains of southern California. *Journal of Wildlife Diseases* 28:476–480.

Mullens, B.A., and A.C. Gerry. 1998. Comparison of bait cattle and carbon dioxide-baited suction traps for collecting *Culicoides variipennis sonorensis* (Diptera: Ceratopogonidae) and *Culex quinquefasciatus* (Diptera: Culicidae). *Journal of Medical Entomology* 35:245–250.

Nelson, R.L., and R.P. Scrivani. 1972. Isolations of arboviruses from parous midges of the *Culicoides variipennis* complex and parous rates in biting populations. *Journal of Medical Entomology* 9:277–281.

Nelson, W.A. 1987. Other blood-sucking and myiasis-producing flies. In *Immune responses in parasitic infections: Immunology, immunopathology and immunoprophylaxis.* Ed. E.J.L. Soulsby. Vol. 4, *Protozoa, arthropods and invertebrates.* Boca Raton, FL: CRC Press, pp. 175–209.

Pence, D.B. 1991. Elaeophorosis in wild ruminants. *Bulletin of the Society for Vector Ecology* 16:149–160.

Perez de Leon, A.A., and W.J. Tabachnick. 1996. Apyrase activity and adenosine diphosphate induced platelet aggregation inhibition by the salivary gland proteins of *Culicoides variipennis,* the North American vector of bluetongue viruses. *Veterinary Parasitology* 61: 327–328

Perez de Leon, A.A., J.M. Ribeiro, W.J. Tabachnick, and J.G. Valenzuela. 1997. Identification of a salivary vasodilator in the primary North American vector of bluetongue viruses, *Culicoides variipennis. American Journal of Tropical Medicine and Hygiene* 57: 375–381.

Prestwood, A.K., T.P. Kistner, F.E. Kellogg, and F.A. Hayes. 1974. The 1971 outbreak of hemorrhagic disease among white-tailed deer of the southeastern United States. *Journal of Wildlife Diseases* 10:217–224.

Raich, T., M. Jacobson, F. Holbrook, R. Babion, C. Blair, and B. Beaty. 1997. *Culicoides variipennis* (Diptera: Ceratopogonidae) host selection in Colorado. *Journal of Medical Entomology* 34:247–249.

Riek, R.F. 1953. Studies on allergic dermatitis (Queensland itch) of the horse. 1. Description, distribution, symptoms and pathology. *Australian Veterinarian Journal* 29:177–184.

Reeves, W.C., R.P. Scrivani, J.L. Hardy, D.R. Roberts, and R.L. Nelson. 1970. Buttonwillow virus, a new arbovirus isolated from mammals and *Culicoides* midges in Kern County, California. *American Journal of Tropical Medicine and Hygiene* 19:544–551.

Schmidtmann, E.T., C.J. Jones, and B. Gollands. 1980. Comparative host-seeking activity of *Culicoides* (Diptera: Ceratopogonidae) attracted to pastured livestock in central New York state, USA. *Journal of Medical Entomology* 17:221.

Schmidtmann, E.T., F.R. Holbrook, E. Day, T. Taylor, and W.J. Tabachnick. 1998. *Culicoides variipennis* (Diptera: Ceratopogonidae) complex in Virginia. *Journal of Medical Entomology* 35:18–824.

Smith, K.E., and D.E. Stallknecht. 1996. *Culicoides* (Diptera: Ceratopogonidae) collected during epizootics of hemorrhagic disease among captive white-tailed decr. *Journal of Medical Entomology* 33:507–510.

Smith, K.E., D.E. Stalknecht, and V.F. Nettles. 1996a. Experimental infection of *Culicoides lahillei* (Diptera: Ceratopogonidae) with epizootic hemorrhagic disease virus serotype 2 (Orbivirus: Reoviridae). *Journal of Medical Entomology* 33:117–122.

Smith, K.E., D.E. Stallknecht, C.T. Sewell, E.A. Rollor, G.R. Mullen, and R.R. Anderson. 1996b. Monitoring of *Culicoides* spp. at a site enzootic for hemorrhagic disease in white-tailed deer in Georgia, USA. *Journal of Wildlife Diseases* 32:627–642.

Sohn, R. and T.M. Yuill. 1991. Bluetongue and epizootic hemorrhagic disease in wild ruminants. *Bulletin of the Society of Vector Ecology* 16:17–24.

Strickman, D., R. Wirtz, P. Lawyer, J. Glick, S. Stockwell, and M. Perich. 1995. Meteorological effects on the biting activity of *Leptoconops americanus* (Diptera: Ceratopogonidae). *Journal of the American Mosquito Control Association* 11:15–20.

Tabachnick, W.J. 1992. Genetic differentiation among populations of *Culicoides variipennis* (Diptera: Ceratopogonidae), the North American vector of bluetongue virus. *Annals of the Entomological Society of America* 85:140–147.

———. 1996. *Culicoides variipennis* and bluetongue-virus epidemiology in the United States. *Annual Review of Entomology* 41:23–43.

Tabachnick, W.J., and R.J. Holbrook. 1992. The *Culicoides variipennis* complex and the distribution of bluetongue viruses in the United States. *Proceedings of the U.S. Animal Health Association* 96:207–212.

Templis, C.H., and R.L. Nelson. 1971. Blood feeding pattern of midges in *Culicoides variipennis* complex in Kern County, California. *Journal of Medical Entomology* 8:532–534.

Thomas, F.C. 1981. Hemorrhagic disease and parasites of the white-tailed deer. *Publications of the Tall Timbers Research Station* 7:87–96.

Weiser-Schimpf, L., W.C. Wilson, D.D. French, A. Baham and L.D. Foil. 1993. Bluetongue virus in sheep and cattle and *Culicoides variipennis* and *C. stellifer* (Diptera: Ceratopogonidae) in Louisiana. *Journal of Medical Entomology* 30:719–724.

Wirth, W.W., and W.R. Atchley. 1973. *A Review of the North American* Leptoconops *(Diptera: Ceratopogonidae).* Graduate Studies, Texas Technical University, No. 5, 57 pp.

Zimmerman, R.H,. and E.C. Turner, Jr. 1983. Host-feeding patterns of *Culicoides* (Diptera: Ceratopogonidae) collected from livestock in Virginia, USA. *Journal of Medical Entomology* 20:514–519.

Phlebotomine Sand Flies

Addis, C.J. 1945. *Phlebotomus (Dampfomyia) anthophorus,* n. sp. and *Phlebotomus diabolicus* Hall from Texas (Diptera: Psychodidae). *The Journal of Parasitology* 31:119–127.

Bram, R.A. 1978. *Surveillance and collection of arthropods of veterinary importance.* Washington, DC: United States Department of Agriculture Handbook No. 518.

Calisher, C.H., R.G. McLain, G.C. Smith, D.M. Sanyd, D.J. Muth, and J.S. Lazuick. 1977. Rio Grande—a new phlebobomine fever group virus from south Texas. *American Journal of Tropical Medicine and Hygiene* 26:997–1002.

Chaniotis, B.N. 1967. The biology of California *Phlebotomus* (Diptera: Psychodidae) under laboratory conditions. *Journal of Medical Entomology* 4:221–33.

———. 1974. Phlebotomine sandflies in Montana: First report. *Mosquito News* 34: 334–335.

Comer, J.A., B.B. Tesh, G.B. Modi, J.L. Corn, and V.F. Nettles. 1990. Vesicular stomatitis virus, New Jersey serotype: Replication in and transmission by *Lutzomyia shannoni* (Diptera: Psychodidae). *American Journal of Tropical Medicine and Hygiene* 42:483–490.

Comer, J.A., D.E. Stallknecht, J.L. Corn, and V.F. Nettles. 1991. *Lutzomyia shannoni* (Diptera: Psychodidae): A biological vector of the New Jersey serotype of vesicular stomatitis virus on Ossabaw Island, Georgia. *Parassitologia* 33:151–158.

Comer , J.A., D.M. Kavanaugh, D.E. Stallknecht, G.O. Ware, J.L. Corn, and V.F. Nettles. 1993. Effect of forest type on the distribution of *Lutzomyia shannoni* (Diptera: Psychodidae) and vesicular stomatitis virus on Ossabaw Island, Georgia. *Journal of Medical Entomology* 30:555–560.

Comer, J.A., W.S. Irby, and D.M. Kavanaugh. 1994. Hosts of *Lutzomyia shannoni* (Diptera: Psychodidae) in relation to vesicular stomatitis virus on Ossabaw Island, Georgia, USA. *Medical and Veterinary Entomology* 8:325–336.

Downes, J.A. 1972. Canadian records of *Phlebotomus vexator,* *Trichomyia nuda,* and *Marunia lanceolata* (Diptera: Psychodidae). *Canadian Entomologist* 104:1135–1136.

Endris, R.G., R.B. Tesh, and D.G. Young. 1983. Transovarial transmission of Rio Grande virus (Bunyaviridae: Phlebotomus) by the sand fly, *Lutzomyia anthophora. Ameri-*

can *Journal of Tropical Medicine and Hygiene* 32:862–864.

Hall, D.G. 1936. *Phlebotomus (Brumptomyia) diabolicus,* a new biting gnat from Texas (Diptera: Psychodidae). *Proceedings of the Entomological Society of Washington* 38:27–29.

Harwood, R.F. 1965. Observations on distribution and biology of *Phlebotomus* sand flies from northwestern North America. *Pan Pacific Entomologist* 41:1–4.

Lewis, D.J. 1974. The biology of Phlebotomidae in relation to Leishmaniasis. *Annual Review of Entomology* 19:363–384.

Lindquist, A.W. 1936. Notes on the habits and biology of a sand fly, *P. diabolicus* Hall, in southwestern Texas. *Proceedings of the Entomological Society of Washington* 38:29–32.

McHugh, C.P. 1991. Distributional records for some North American sand flies, *Lutzomyia* (Diptera: Psychodidae). *Entomological News* 102:192–194.

McHugh, C.P., M. Grogl, and R.D. Kreutzer. 1993. Isolation of *Leishmania mexicana* (Kinetoplastida: Trypanosomatidae) from *Lutzomyia anthophora* (Diptera: Psychodidae) collected in Texas. *Journal of Medical Entomology* 30:631–633.

Mead, D.G., and E.W. Cupp. 1995. Occurrence of *Lutzomyia anthophora* (Diptera: Psychodidae) in Arizona. *Journal of Medical Entomology* 32:747–748.

Perrich, M.J., D. Strickman, R.A. Wirtz, S.A. Stockwell, J.I. Glick, R. Burge, G. Hunt, and P.G. Lauya. 1995. Field evaluation of four repellents against *Leptoconops americanus* (Diptera: Ceratopogonidae) biting midges. *Journal of Medical Entomology* 32:306–307.

Robert, L.L. and M.J. Perich. 1995. Phlebotomine sand fly (Diptera: Psychodidae) control using a residual pyrethroid insecticide. *Journal of American Mosquito Control Association* 11:195–199.

Shaw, P.K., T.Loren, and D. Juranek. 1976. Autochthonous dermal leishmaniasis in Texas. *American Journal of Tropical Medicine and Hygiene* 25:788–796.

Shemanchuck, J.A., R.H. Robertson, and K.R. Depner. 1978. Occurrence of two species of *Phlebotomus* sandflies in burrows of yellow-bellied, *Marmota flaviventris nosophora,* in southern Alberta. *Canadian Entomologist* 110:1355–1358

Tesh, R.B., and H. Guzman. 1996. Sand flies and the agents they transmit. In *The biology of disease vectors.* Ed. B. J. Beaty and W. C. Marquardt. Niwot: University Press of Colorado, pp. 117–127.

Walsh, J.F., D.H. Molyneux, and M.H. Birley. 1993. Deforestation: Effects on vector-borne disease. *Parasitology* 106(Supplement): s55–s75.

Young, D.G., and P.V. Perkins. 1984. Phlebotomine sand flies of North America (Diptera: Psycodidae). *Mosquito News* 44:263–304.

Black Flies

Addison, E.M. 1980. Transmission of *Dirofilaria ursi* Yamaguti, 1941 (Nematoda: Onchocercidae) of black bears (*Ursus americanus*) by blackflies (Simuliidae). *Canadian Journal of Zoology* 58:1913–1922.

Adler, P.H., and K.C. Kim. 1986. The black flies of Pennsylvania (Simuliidae: Diptera): Bionomics, taxonomy and distribution. *Pennsylvania State University Agriculture Experiment Station Bulletin* 856, 88 pp.

Adler, P.H., and P.G. Mason. 1997. Black flies (Diptera: Simuliidae) of east-central Saskatchewan, with descriptors of a new species and implications for pest management. *Canadian Entomologist* 129:81–91.

Allan, S.A., J.F. Day, and J.D. Edman. 1987. Visual ecology of biting flies. *Annual Review of Entomology* 32:297–316.

Anderson, J.R. 1987. Reproductive strategies and gonotrophic studies of blackflies. In *Blackflies: Ecology, population management and annotated world list.* Ed. K.C. Kim and R.W. Merritt. University Park: Pennsylvania State University, pp. 276–294.

Anderson, F.L., and K.L. Minson. 1985. Generalized equine dermatitis associated with black fly (Simuliidae) infestation. *Proceedings of the Annual Meeting of the Utah Mosquito Abatement Association 1985–86,* pp. 38–39.

Anderson, J., V. Leer, S. Vadlamudi, S. Hanson, and G. DeFoliart. 1961. Isolation of eastern equine encephalitis virus from Diptera in Wisconsin. *Mosquito News* 21:244–248.

Baldwin, W.F., A.S. West, and J. Gomery. 1975. Dispersal pattern of black flies (Diptera: Simuliidae) tagged with ^{32}P. *Canadian Entomologist* 107:113–118.

Bask, C., and P.P. Harper, 1979. Seasonal succession, emergence, voltinism and distribution of Laurentian black flies (Diptera: Simuliidae). *Canadian Journal of Zoology* 57:627–639.

Bennett, G.F., and A.M. Fallis. 1971. Flight range, longevity and habitat preference of female *Simulium eryadminiculum* Davies (Diptera: Simuliidae). *Canadian Journal of Zoology* 49:1203–1207.

Bruder, K.W., and W.J. Crans. 1979. *The black flies (Simuliidae: Diptera) of the Stony Brook watershed of New Jersey, with emphasis on parasitism by mermithid nematodes (Mermithidae: Nematoda).* Bulletin of the New Jersey Agriculture Experiment Station, No. 851, 21 pp.

Charnetski, W.A., and W.O. Haufe. 1981. Control of *Simulium arcticum* Malloch in Northern Alberta. In *Black flies: The future for biological methods in integrated control.* Ed. M. Laird. New York: Academic Press, pp. 117–132.

Cross, M.L., M.S. Cupp, E.W. Cupp, F.B. Ramberg, and F.J. Enriquez. 1993. Antibody responses of BALB/c mice to salivary antigens of hematophagous black flies (Diptera: Simuliidae). *Journal of Medical Entomology* 30:725–734.

Crosskey, R.W. 1961. The black flies—pests of man and animals. Part K. Biology and economic importance. *Pest Technology* 3:182–186.

———. 1990. *The natural history of blackflies.* Chichester, England: Wiley.

Cupp, E.W. 1996. Black flies and the diseases they transmit. In *The biology of disease vectors.* Ed. B.J. Beaty and W.C. Marquardt. Niwot: University Press of Colorado, pp. 98–109.

Cupp, E.W., and A.E. Gordon. 1983. *Notes on the systematics, distribution, and bionomics of black flies (Diptera: Simuliidae) in the northeastern United States.* Search Agriculture No. 25, Ithaca, NY: Cornell University Agricultural Experiment Station, 75 pp.

Cupp, E.W., C.J. Mare, M.S. Cupp, and F.B. Ramberg. 1992. Biological transmission of vesicular stomatitis virus (New Jersey) by *Simulium vittatum* (Diptera: Simuliidae). *Journal of Medical Entomology* 29:137–140.

Currie, D.C. 1986. *An annotated list of and keys to the immature black flies of Alberta (Diptera: Simuliidae).* Memoirs of the Entomological Society of Canada, No. 134.

Dalmat, H. 1955. *The black flies of Guatemala and their role as vectors of onchocerciasis.* Smithsonian Miscellaneous Collection No. 125.

Davies, D.M., and B.V. Peterson. 1956. Observations on the mating, feeding, ovarian development and oviposition of adult black flies. *Canadian Journal of Zoology* 34:615–655.

Francy, D.B., C.G. Moore, G.C. Smith, W.L. Jakob, S.A. Taylor, and C.H. Calisher. 1988. Epizootic vesicular stomatitis in Colorado, 1982: Isolation of virus from insects collected along the northern Colorado Rocky Mountain front range. *Journal of Medical Entomology* 24:343–347.

Frazier, C.A., and N.C. Asheville. 1973. Biting insects. *Archives of Dermatology* 107:400–402.

Fredeen, F.J.H. 1973. *Black flies*. Ottawa, Ontario: Canada Department of Agriculture Publication 940.

———. 1977. A review of the economic importance of black flies (Simuliidae) in Canada. *Quaestiones Entomologica* 13:219–229.

———. 1981. Keys to the black flies (Simuliidae) of the Saskatchewan River in Saskatchewan. *Quaestiones Entomologica* 17:189–210.

Gray, E.W., P.H. Adler, and R. Noblet. 1996. Economic impact of black flies (Diptera: Simuliidae) in South Carolina and development of a localized suppression program. *Journal of the American Mosquito Control Association* 12:676–678.

Jamnback, H. 1969. *Bloodsucking flies and other outdoor nuisance arthropods of New York state*. Albany, NY: State Museum and Science Service Memoir 19.

Kim, K.C., and R.W. Merritt. 1986. *Black flies: Ecology, population management, and annotated word list*. University Park: The Pennsylvania State University.

Laird, M. 1981. *Blackflies: The Future for biological methods in integrated control*. New York: Academic Press.

Lewis, D.J., and G.F. Bennett. 1979. An annotated list of the black flies (Diptera: Simuliidae) of the Maritime Provinces of Canada. *Canadian Entomologist* 111:1227–1230.

Lok, J.B., E.W. Cupp, and M.J. Bernard. 1983. *Simulium jenningsi* (Diptera: Simuliidae): A vector of *Onchocerca lienalis* Stiles (Nematoda: Filarioidea) in New York. *American Journal of Veterinary Research* 44:2355–2358.

McCreadie, J.W., M.H. Colbo, and G.F. Bennett. 1985. The seasonal activity of hematophagous Diptera attaching cattle in insular Newfoundland. *Canadian Entomologist* 117:995–1006.

McCreadie, J.W., M.H. Colbo, and F.F. Hunter. 1994. Notes on sugar feeding and selected wild mammalian hosts of black flies (Diptera: Culicidae) in Newfoundland. *Journal of Medical Entomology* 31:566–570.

Millar, J.L., and J.G. Rempel. 1944. Livestock losses in Saskatchewan due to black flies. *Canadian Journal of Comparative Medicine* 8:334–337.

Mohsen, Z.H. and M.S. Mulla. 1982. The ecology of black flies (Diptera: Simuliidae) in some southern California streams. *Journal of Medical Entomology* 19:72–85.

Molloy, D.P. 1992. Impact of black fly (Diptera: Simuliidae) control agent *Bacillus thuringiensis israeliensis* (Diptera: Chironomidae) and other nontarget insects: Results of field trials. *Journal of the American Mosquito Control Association* 8:24–31.

Nelson, W.A. 1987. Other blood sucking and myiasis-producing flies. In *Immune responses in parasitic infections: Immunology, immunopathology and immunoprophylaxis*. Vol. 4, *Protozoa, arthropods and invertebrates*. Ed. E.J.L. Soulsby. Boca Raton, FL: CRC Press, pp. 175–209.

Petersen, B.V. 1981. Simuliidae. In *Manual of Nearctic Diptera*, vol. 1. Hull, Quebec: Agriculture Canada Monograph No. 27, pp. 355–391.

Pinherio, F.P., G. Bensebath, D. Costa, O.M. Maroa, Z.C. Lins, and A.H.P. Andrade. 1974. Haemorrhagic syndrome of Altamire. *Lancet* 1:639–642.

Pinkovsky, D.D., and J.F. Butler. 1978. Black flies of Florida. I. Geographic and seasonal distribution. *Florida Entomologist* 61:257–267.

Pledger, D.J., W.M. Samuel, and D.A. Craig. 1980. Black flies (Diptera: Simuliidae) as possible vectors of legworm (*Onchocerca cervipedes*) in moose of central Alberta. *Proceedings of the North American Moose Conference and Workshop* 16:171–202.

Rempel, J.G., and A.P. Arnason. 1947. An account of three successive outbreaks of the black fly, *Simulium arcticum*. *Science and Agriculture* 27:428–445.

Steelman, C.D. 1976. Effects of external and internal arthropods parasites on domestic livestock production. *Annual Review of Entomology* 21:155–178.

Stone, A. 1964. Simuliidae and Thaumaleidae. *Guide to the insects of Connecticut*. State Geological and Natural History Survey of Connecticut Bulletin No. 47.

Stone, A., and E.L. Snoddy. 1969. The black flies of Alabama (Diptera: Simuliidae). *Bulletin of the Alabama Agricultural Experiment Station* 390:1–93.

Sutcliffe, J.F. 1986. Black fly host location: A review. *Canadian Journal of Zoology* 64:1041–1053.

Weinmann, C.J., J.R. Anderson, W.M. Longhurst, and G. Connolly. 1973. Filarial worms of Columbian black-tailed deer in California. 1. Observations in the vertebrate hosts. *Journal of Wildlife Disease* 9:213–220.

Westwood, A.R., and R.A. Brust. 1981. Ecology of black flies (Diptera: Simuliidae) of the Souris River, Manitoba, as a basis for control strategy. *Canadian Entomologist* 113:223–234.

White, D.J., and C.D. Morris. 1985. Bionomics of anthropophilic Simuliidae (Diptera) from the Adirondack mountains of New York state, USA. 1. Adult dispersal and longevity. *Journal of Medical Entomology* 22:190–199.

Yee, W.L., and J.R. Anderson. 1995. Trapping black flies (Diptera: Simuliidae) in northern California. II. Testing visual cues used in attraction to CO_2-based animal head models. *Journal of Vector Ecology* 20:26–39.

Tabanids and Snipe Flies

Allan, S.A. and J.G. Stoffolano, Jr. 1986a. The effects of hue and intensity on visual attraction of adult *Tabanus nigrovittatus* (Diptera: Tabanidae). *Journal of Medical Entomology* 23:83–91.

———. 1986b. Effects of background contrast on visual attraction and orientation of *Tabanus nigrovittatus* Macquart (Diptera: Tabanidae). *Environmental Entomology* 15:689–694.

———. 1986c. The importance of pattern in visual attraction of *Tabanus nigrovittatus* (Diptera: Tabanidae). *Canadian Journal of Zoology* 64:2273–2280.

Allan, S.A., J.D. Day, and J.D. Edman. 1987. Visual ecology of biting flies. *Annual Review of Entomology* 32:297–316.

Axtell, R.C., and J.C. Dukes. 1974. ULV chemical control of mosquitoes, *Culicoides* and tabanids in coastal North Carolina. *Proceedings of the California Mosquito Control Association* 42:99–101.

Brennan, J.M. 1935. The Pangoniinae of Nearctic America, Diptera: Tabanidae. *University of Kansas Science Bulletin* 22:249–402.

Catts, E.P. 1968. DEET-impregnated net shirt repels biting flies. *Journal of Economic Entomology* 61:472–474.

Clark, G.G., and C.P. Hibler. 1973. Horse flies and *Elaeophora schneideri* in the Gila National Forest, New Mexico. *Journal of Wildlife Diseases* 8:21–25.

Cole, F.R. 1969. *The flies of western North America*. Berkeley: University of California Press.

Cooksey, L.M., and R.E. Wright. 1989. Population estimation of the horse fly, *Tabanus abactor* (Diptera: Tabanidae) in north central Oklahoma. *Journal of Medical Entomology* 26:167–172.

Couvillion, C.E., V.F. Nettles, D.C. Sheppard, R.L. Joyner, and O.M. Bannaga. 1986. Temporal occurrence of third-stage larvae of *Elaeophora schneideri* in *Tabanus lineola hinellus* on South Island, South Carolina. *Journal of Wildlife Diseases* 22:196–200.

Davies, D.M. 1959. Seasonal variation of tabanids (Diptera) in Algonquin Park, Ontario. *Canadian Entomologist* 91:548–553.

Duncan, P., and N. Vigne. 1979. The effect of group size in horses on the rate of attacks by blood-sucking flies. *Animal Behavior* 27:623–625.

Freye, H.B., and G. Litwin. 1996. Coexistent anaphylaxis to Diptera and Hymenoptera. *Annals of Allergy, Asthma and Immunology* 76:270–272.

Foil, L. 1989. Tabanids as disease agents. *Parasitology Today* 5:88–96.

Foil, L., and C. Foil. 1988. Dipteran parasites of horses. *Equine Practice.* 10:21–39.

Foil, L.D., and J.A. Hogsette. 1994. Biology and control of tabanids, stable flies and horn flies. *Revue du Scientifique et Technologie* 13:1125–1158.

Foil, L.D., C.L. Meek, W.V. Adams, and C.J. Issel. 1983. Mechanical transmission of equine infectious anemia virus by deer flies (*Chrysops flavidus*) and stable flies (*Stomoxys calcitrans*). *American Journal of Veterinary Research* 44:155–156.

Foil, L.D., D.J. LePrince, and R.L. Byford. 1991. Survival and dispersal of horse flies (Diptera: Tabanidae) feeding on cattle sprayed with a sublethal dose of fenvalerate. *Journal of Medical Entomology* 28:663–667.

Grimstad, P.R. 1989. California group virus disease. In *The arboviruses: Epidemiology and ecology,* vol. 2. Ed. T.R. Monath. Boca Raton, FL: CRC Press, pp. 99–136.

Goodwin, J.T., B.A. Mullens, and R.R. Gerhardt. 1985. *The tabanidae of Tennessee.* The University of Tennessee Agricultural Experiment Station Bulletin 642.

Granett, P. and E.J. Hansens. 1957. Further observations on the effect of biting fly control on milk production in cattle. *Journal of Economic Entomology* 50:332–336.

Harris, R.L., and P.P. Oehler. 1977. Control of tabanids on horses. *Southwestern Entomologist* 1:194–197.

Hayes, R.O., O.W. Doane, Jr., E. Sakolsky, and S. Berick. 1993. Evaluation of attractants in traps for greenhead fly (Diptera: Tabanidae) collections on a Cape Cod, Massachusetts, salt marsh. *Journal of American Mosquito Control Association* 9:436–440.

Hearle, E. 1928. *Insects of the season 1928 in British Columbia. Insects affecting livestock and man.* 59th Annual Report of the Entomological Society of Ontario, 35 pp.

Hemmer, W.M., D. Focke, D. Vieluf, B. Berg-Drewniok, M. Gotz, and R. Jarisch. 1998. Anaphylaxis induced by horsefly bites: Identification of a 69 Kd IdE-binding salivary gland protein from *Chrysops* spp. (Diptera: Tabanidae) by western blot analysis. *Journal of Allergy and Clinical Immunology* 101:134–136.

Hollander, A.L., and R.E. Wright. 1980. Impact of tabanids on cattle: Blood meal size and preferred feeding sites. *Journal of Economic Entomology* 73:431–433.

Hoy, J.B., and J.R. Anderson. 1978. Behavior and reproductive physiology of blood-sucking snipe flies (Diptera: Rhagionidae: *Symphoromyia*) attacking deer in northern California. *Hilgardia* 46:113–168.

Hughes, R.D., P. Duncan, and J. Dawson. 1981. Interactions between Carmague horses and horseflies (Diptera: Tabanidae). *Bulletin of Entomological Research* 71:227–242.

James, M.T., and W.J. Turner. 1981. Rhagionidae. In *Manual of Nearctic Diptera,* vol. 1. Hull, Quebec: Agriculture Canada Monograph No. 27, pp. 483–488.

Jamnback, H. 1969. *Bloodsucking flies and other outdoor nuisance arthropods of New York state.* Albany, NY: State Museum and Science Service Memoir 19.

Jellison, D.W. 1950. Tularemia, geographical distribution of deer fly fever and the biting fly, *Chrysops discalis* Williston. *United States Public Health Reports* 65:1321–1329.

Kistner, T.P., and W.L. Hanson. 1969. Trypanosomiasis in white-tailed deer. *Bulletin of Wildlife Diseases* 6:437–440.

Krinsky, W.L. 1976. Animal disease agents transmitted by horse flies and deer flies (Diptera: Tabanidae). *Journal of Medical Entomology* 13:225–275.

Lane, R.S., and J.R. Anderson. 1982. Breeding sites for snipe flies (Rhagionidae) and other diptera in woodland grass soils. *Journal of Medical Entomology* 19:104–108.

Lankester, M.W., and W.M. Samuel. 1998. Pests, parasites and diseases. In *Ecology and management of the North American moose,* a Wildlife Management Institute Book. Ed. A.W. Franzmann and C.C. Schwartz. Washington and London: Smithsonian Institution Press, pp. 479–517.

LePrince, D.J., L.J. Hribar, and L.D. Foil. 1994. Responses of horseflies (Diptera: Tabanidae) to Jersey bullocks and canopy traps baited with ammonia, octenol and carbon dioxide. *Journal of Medical Entomology* 31:729–731.

Mullens, B.A., and R.R. Gerhardt. 1979. Feeding behavior of some Tennessee tabanids. *Environmental Entomology* 8:1047–1051.

Oldroyd, H. 1964. *The natural history of flies.* New York: W.W. Norton and Co.

Pechuman, L.L. 1972. *The horse flies and deer flies of New York (Diptera: Tabanidae).* Search Agriculture No. 2. Ithaca, NY: Cornell University Agricultural Experiment Station.

———. 1981. *The horse flies of New York (Diptera: Tabanidae).* Search Agriculture No. 18. Ithaca, NY: Cornell University Agricultural Experiment Station.

Pechuman, L.L., and H.J. Teskey. 1981. Tabanidae. In *Manual of Nearctic Diptera,* vol. 1. Hull, Quebec: Agriculture Canada Monograph No. 27, pp. 463–478.

Pechuman, L.L., D.W Webb, and H.J. Teskey. 1983. The Diptera, or the flies, of Illinois. 1. Tabanidae. *Bulletin of the Illinois Natural History Survey* 33:1–22.

Pence, D.B. 1991. Elaeophorosis in wild ruminants. *Bulletin of the Society for Vector Ecology* 16:149–160.

Roberts, R.H., W.A. Pund, H.F. McCory, J.W. Scales, and J.C. Collins. 1968. The relative roles of the Culicidae and Tabanidae as vectors of anaplasmosis. *Proceedings of the National Anaplasmosis Conference* 5:183–190.

Sein, R. 1985. Biting flies (Diptera) attracted to, and their effect on the behaviour of captive moose (*Alces alces*) and captive woodland caribou (*Rangifer tarandus caribou*) in northwestern Ontario. Honours Thesis, Lakehead University, Thunder Bay, Ontario, 98 pp

Shemanchuk, J.A., and J. Weintraub. 1961. Observations on the biting and swarming of snipe flies (Diptera: *Symphoromyia*) in the foothills of southern Alberta. *Mosquito News* 21:238–243.

Smith, S.M., D.M. Davies, and V.I. Golini. 1970. A contribution to the bionomics of the Tabanidae (Diptera) of Algonquin Park, Ontario: Seasonal distribution, habitat preferences and biting records. *Canadian Entomologist* 102:1461–1473.

Stone, A. 1938. *The Horseflies of the subfamily Tabanids of the Nearctic region.* Washington, DC: United States Department of Agriculture Miscellaneous Publication 305.

Tashiro, H. and H.H. Schwardt. 1949. Biology of the major species of horse flies in central New York. *Journal of Economic Entomology* 42:269–272.

Tesky, H.J. 1990. *The Insects and Arachnids of Canada.* Part 16, *The Horse Flies and Deer Flies of Canada and Alaska (Diptera: Tabanidae).* Ottawa, Ontario: Ministry of Supply and Services.

Tidwell, M.A. 1973. The Tabanidae (Diptera) of Louisiana. *Tulane Studies in Zoology* 18:1–93.

Turner, W.I. 1979. A case of severe human allergic response to bites of *Symphoromyia* (Diptera: Rhagionidae). *Journal of Medical Entomology* 15:138–139.

Usinger, R.L. 1973. *Aquatic insects of California.* Berkeley: University of California Press.

Wall, W., Jr., and O.W. Doane, Jr. 1980. Large scale use of box traps to study and control saltmarsh greenhead flies (Diptera: Tabanidae) on Cape Cod, Massachusetts. *Environmental Entomology* 9:371–375.

Webb, D.W. 1977. The Nearctic Anthericidae (Insecta: Diptera). *Journal of Kansas Entomological Society* 50:473–495.

———. 1981. Anthericidae. In *Manual of Nearctic Diptera,* vol. 1. Hull, Quebec: Agriculture Canada Monograph No. 27, pp. 479–482

Wilson, B.H., and C.G. Richardson. 1969. Tabanid hosts in estuarine and alluvial areas of Louisiana. *Annals of the Entomological Society of America* 62:1043–1046.

Louse and Bat Flies

Baron, R.W., and W.A. Nelson. 1985. Aspects of the humoral and cell-mediated immune responses of sheep to the ked *Melophagus ovinus* (Diptera: Hippoboscidae). *Journal of Medical Entomology* 22:544–549.

Bequaert, J.C. 1942. A monograph for the Melophaginae, or ked flies, of sheep, goats, deer and antelopes (Diptera, Hippoboscidae). *Entomologist America* 22:1–220.

Bequaert, J.C. 1957. The Hippoboscidae or louse flies (Diptera) of mammals and birds. II. Taxonomy, evolution and revision of American genera and species. *Entomologist America* 36:417–611.

Bowman, D.D. 1995. *Georgis' parasitology for veterinarians.* Philadelphia, PA: W.B. Saunders Company.

Cole, F. R. 1969. *The flies of western North America.* Berkeley, CA: University of California Press.

Constantine, D.G. 1970. Bats in relation to the health, welfare, and economy of man. In: *Biology of bats.* Ed. W.A. Wimsath. New York: Academic Press, pp. 319–449.

Cowan, I.M. 1943. Notes on the life history and morphology of *Cephenemyia jellisoni* Townsend and *Lipoptena depressa* Say, two dipterous parasites of the Columbian black-tailed deer (*Odocoileus hemionus columbianus* (Richardson). *Canadian Journal of Research (D)* 21:171–187.

Craine, I.T., and R. Boonstra. 1986. Myiasis in *Wohlfahrtia vigil* in nestling *Microtus pennsylvanicus. Journal of Wildlife Diseases* 22:587–589.

Davis, J.W. 1973. Deer ked infestation on southern populations of white-tailed deer in east Texas. *The Journal of Wildlife Management* 37:183–186.

Demarais, S., H.A. Jacobson, and D.C. Guynn. 1987. Effects of season and area on ectoparasites of white-tailed deer (*Odocoileus virginianus*) in Mississippi. *Journal of Wildlife Diseases* 23:261–266.

Dixon, J.S., and C.M. Herman. 1945. Studies on the condition of California mule deer at Sequoia National Park. *California Fish and Game* 31:3–11.

Drummond, R.O. 1966. *Lipoptena mazamae* Rondani (Diptera: Hippoboscidae), a louse fly of deer, on cattle in southwestern Texas. *The Journal of Parasitology* 52:825.

Eads, R.B., and Campos, E.G. 1984. Notes on the deer keds, *Neolipoptena ferrisis* and *Liptoptena depressa* (Diptera: Hippoboscidae) from Colorado, USA. *Journal of Medical Entomology* 21:245.

Forrester, D.J. 1992. *Parasites and diseases of wild mammals in Florida.* Gainesville: University Press of Florida.

Forrester, D.J., G.S. McLaughlin, S.R. Telford, Jr., G.W. Foster, and J.W. McCown. 1996. Ectoparasites (Acari, Mallophaga, Anoplura, Diptera) of white-tailed deer, *Odocoileus virginianus,* from southern Florida. *Journal of Medical Entomology* 33:96–101.

Hannigan, M.V., A.L. Everett, L.H. Roberts, and J. Naghski. 1976. Microscopic study of leather defects and histological and other physical changes in sheep skins due to ked-produced cockle. *Journal of the American Leather Chemistry Association* 71:411.

Kennedy, M.J., R.A Newman, and G.A. Chalmers. 1987. First record of *Lipoptena depressa* (Diptera: Hippoboscidae) from Alberta, Canada. *Journal of Wildlife Diseases* 23:506–507.

Khan, B.A., W.T. Whitmore, and L.A. Goonewardene. 1989. Permethrin pour-on for sheep ked (*Melophagus ovinus*) control in Alberta. *Journal of Animal Science* 67:172.

Mertins, J.W., J.L. Schlater, and J.L. Corn. 1992. Ectoparasites of the blackbucked antelope (*Antelope cervicapra*). *Journal of Wildlife Diseases* 28:481–484.

Nelson, W.A. 1962. Development in sheep of resistance to the ked, *Melophagus ovinus* (L.) 1. Effects of seasonal manipulations of infestations. *Experimental Parasitology* 12:41–44.

———. 1988. Skin eruptions in ked infected sheep. *Veterinarian Record* 122:472.

Nelson, W.A., and G.C. Kozub. 1980. *Melophagus ovinus* (Diptera: Hippoboscidae): Evidence of local mediation of acquired resistance of sheep to keds. *Journal of Medical Entomology* 17:291–297.

Nelson, W.A., and S.B. Slen. 1968. Weight gains and wool growth in sheep infested with the sheep ked, *Melophagus ovinus. Experimental Parasitology* 22:223.

Peterson. B.V. and T.C. Maa. 1970. A new *Lipoptena* from Chile with a key to the New World species (Diptera: Hippoboscidae). *Canadian Entomologist* 102:1117–1122.

Richardson, M.L., and S. Demarais. 1992. Parasites and condition of co-existing populations of white-tailed and exotic deer in south-central Texas. *Journal of Wildlife Diseases* 28:485–489.

Samuel, W.M., and D.O Trainer. 1972. *Lipoptena mazamae* Rondini, 1878 (Diptera: Hippoboscidae) on white-tailed deer in southern Texas. *Journal of Medical Entomology* 9:104–106.

Senger, C.M., and K.J. Capelle. 1959. Louse flies from mule and white-tailed deer in western Montana. *The Journal of Parasitology* 45:32.

Strickland, R.K., R.R. Gerish, and J.S. Smith. 1981. Arthropods. In *Diseases and parasites of white-tailed deer.* Ed. W.R. Davidson, F.A. Hayes, V.F. Nettles, and F.F. Kellogg. Tallahassee, FL: Tall Timbers Research Station, pp. 363–389.

Westrom, D.R., and J R. Anderson 1992. The distribution and seasonal abundance of deer keds (Diptera: Hippoboscidae) on Columbian black-tailed deer (*Odocoileus hemionus columbianus*) in northern California. *Bulletin of the Society for Vector Ecology* 17:57–69.

Muscoid Flies

Anderson, R.C., and M.W. Lankester. 1974. Infectious and parasitic diseases and arthropod pests of moose in North America. *Le Naturaliste Canadien* 101:23–50.

Arbit, E., R.E. Varon, and S.S. Brem. 1986. Myiatic scalp and skull infection with diptera *Sarcophaga:* Case report. *Neurosurgery* 18:361–362.

Axtell, R.C. 1972. Fly control in caged-poultry houses: Comparison of larviciding and integrated control programs. *Journal of Economic Entomology* 63: 1734–1737.

Baron, R.W., and T.J. Lysyk. 1995. Antibody responses in cattle infested with *Haematobia irritans irritans* (Diptera: Muscidae). *Journal of Medical Entomology* 32:630–635.

Baumgartner, D.L., and D. MacKey. 1988. Review of myiasis (Insecta: Diptera: Calliphoridae, Sarcophagidae) of Nearctic wildlife. Seventh Annual Symposium of the National Wildlife Rehabilitators Association, Denver, Colorado. *Wildlife Rehabitiation* 7:3–46.

Bay, D.E., C.W. Pitts, and G.M. Ward. 1968. Oviposition and development of the face fly in feces of six species of animals. *Journal of Economic Entomology* 61:1733–1736.

Benitez Usher, C., J. Cruz, L. Carvalho, A. Bridi, D. Farrington, R.A. Barrick, and J. Eagleson. 1997. Prophylactic use of ivermectin against cattle myiasis caused by *Cochliomyia hominovorax* (Coquerel, 1858). *Veterinary Parasitology* 72:215–220.

Burger, J.F., and J.R. Anderson. 1970. Association of the face fly, *Musca autumnalis,* with bison in North America. *Annals of the Entomological Society of America* 63:655–659.

———. 1974. Taxonomy and life history of the moose fly *Haematobosca alcis,* and its association with the moose, *Alces alces shirasi* in Yellowstone National Park. *Annals of the Entomological Society of America* 67:204–214.

Campbell, J.B., I.L. Berry, D.J. Boxler, R.L. Davis, D.C. Clanton, and G.H. Deutscher. 1987. Effects of stable flies (Diptera: Muscidae) on weight gain and feed efficiency of feedlot cattle. *Journal of Economic Entomology* 80:117–119.

Capelle, K.J. 1971. Myiasis. In *Parasitic diseases of wild mammals.* Ed. J.W. Davis, and R.C. Anderson. Ames: Iowa State University Press, pp. 279–305.

Casu, R., C. Eisemann, R. Pearson, G. Riding, I. East, A. Donaldson, L. Cadogan, and R. Tellam. 1997. Antibody-mediated inhibition of the growth of larvae from an insect causing cutaneous myiasis in a mammalian host. *Proceedings of the National Academy of Science, USA* 94:8939–8944.

Cilek, J.E., and G.L. Greene. 1994. Stable fly (Diptera: Muscidae) insecticide resistance in Kansas cattle feedlots. *Journal of Economic Entomology* 87:275–279.

Cilek, J.E., and F.W. Knapp. 1993. Enhanced diazinon susceptibility in pyrethroid-resistant horn flies (Diptera: Muscidae): Potential for insecticide resistance management. *Journal of Economic Entomology* 86:1303–1307.

Cilek, J.E., C.D. Steelman, and F.W. Knapp. 1991. Horn fly (Diptera: Muscidae) insecticide resistance in Kentucky and Arkansas. *Journal of Economic Entomology* 84:756–762.

Cole, F.R. 1969. *The flies of western North America.* Berkeley: University of California Press.

Craine, I.T.M., and R. Boonstra. 1986. Myiasis by *Wohlfahrtia vigil* in nestling *Microtus pennsylvanicus. Journal of Wildlife Diseases* 22:587–589.

Cupp, E.W., M.S. Cupp, J.M.C. Ribeiro, and S.E. Kunz. 1998. Blood-feeding strategy of *Haematobia irritans* (Diptera: Muscidae). *Journal of Medical Entomology* 35:591–595.

Derouen, S.M., L.D. Foil, J.W. Know, and J.M. Turpin. 1995. Horn fly (Diptera: Muscidae) control and weight gains of yearling beef cattle. *Journal of Economic Entomology* 88:666–668.

Dong, L. 1977. First report of human myiasis due to *Wohlfahrtia vigil opaca* in California and a review of the distribution of the subspecies in the state. *California Vector Views* 24:3–4, 13–17.

Dow, R.P. 1959. A dispersal of adult *Hippelates pusio,* the eye gnat. *Annals of the Entomological Society of America* 52:372–281.

Drummond, R.O. 1985. New methods for applying drugs for the control of ectoparasites. *Veterinary Parasitology* 18:111–119.

Eisemann, C.H., L.A. Johnston, M. Broadmeadow, B.M. O'Sullivan, R.A. Donaldson, R.D. Pearson, T. Vuocolot, and J.T. Kerr. 1990. Acquired resistance of sheep to larvae of *Lucilia cuprina* assessed in vivo and in vitro. *International Journal for Parasitology* 20:99–305.

Farkas, R., H.J. Hall, M. Daniels and L. Borzsonyi. 1996. Efficacy of ivermectin and moxidectin injection against lar-

vae of *Wohlfahrtia magnifica* (Diptera: Sarcophagidae) in sheep. *Parasitology Research* 82:82–86.

Foil, L.D., and J.A. Hogsette. 1994. Biology and control of tabanids, stable flies and horn flies. [6] *Revue du Scientifique et Technologie.* (Paris: Office International des Epizooties.) 13:1125–1158.

Foil, L.D., C.L. Meek, W.V. Adams, and C.J. Issel. 1985. Mechanical transmission of equine infectious anemia virus by deer flies (*Chrysops flavidus*) and stable flies (*Stomoxys calcitrans*). *American Journal of Veterinary Research* 44:155–156.

Forrester, D.J. 1992. *Parasites and diseases of wild mammals in Florida.* Gainesville: University Press of Florida.

Gagne, R.J., R.R. Gerrish, and K.D. Richard. 1982. Correspondence. *Entomological Society of America Newsletter* 5:9.

Geden, C.J., and J.G. Stoffolano, Jr. 1982. Nematode parasites of other dipterans. In *Plant and insect nematodes.* Ed. W.J. Nickle. New York: Marcel Dekker, pp. 849–898.

Greenberg, B. 1971. *Flies and disease.* Vol. 1, *Ecology, classification, and biotic associations.* Princeton, NJ: Princeton University Press.

———. 1973. *Flies and disease.* Vol. 2, *Biology and disease transmission.* Princeton, NJ: Princeton University Press.

———. 1984. Two cases of human myiasis caused by *Phaenicia sericata* (Diptera: Calliphoridae) in Chicago area hospitals. *Journal of Medical Entomology* 21:615.

Hall, D.G. 1948. *The blowflies of North America.* College Park, MD: The Thomas Say Foundation, Entomological Society of America.

Hall, R.D. 1979. The blow flies of Missouri: An annotated checklist (Diptera: Calliphoridae) *Transactions of the Mississippi Academy of Science* 13:33–36.

———. 1984. Relationship of the face fly (Diptera: Muscidae) to pinkeye in cattle: A review and synthesis of the relevant literature. *Journal of Medical Entomology* 21:361–365.

Hall, R.D., P.C. Anderson, and D.P. Clark. 1986. A case of human myiasis caused by *Phormia regina* (Diptera: Calliphoridae) in Missouri, USA. *Journal of Medical Entomology* 23:578–579.

Harlow, R.F., and F.K. Jones. 1965. *The white-tailed deer in Florida.* Florida Game and Fresh Water Fish Commission, Technical Bulletin No. 9.

Harris, R.L., J.A. Miller, and E.D. Frazer. 1974. Horn flies and stable flies: Feeding activity. *Annals of the Entomological Society of America* 67:891–894.

Harwood, R.F., and M.T. James. 1979. *Entomology in human and animal health,* 7th ed. New York: Macmillan.

Hendrix, C.M. 1991. Facultative myiasis in dogs and cats. *Compendium for Continuing Education for the Practicing Veterinarian* 13:86–93.

Hibler, C.P. 1966. Development of *Stephanofilaria stilesi* in the horn fly. *The Journal of Parasitology* 52:890–898.

James, M.T. 1948. The flies that cause myiasis in man. *United States Department of Agriculture Miscellaneous Publication* 631, 175 pp.

James, P.J., H.K. Mitchell, K.S. Cockrum, and P.M. Ancell. 1994. Controlled release insecticide devices for protection of sheep against head strike caused by *Lucilia cuprina. Veterinary Parasitology* 52:113–128.

Kennedy, M.J. 1993. Prevalence of eyeworms (Nematoda: Thelazioidea) in beef-cattle grazing on different range pasture zones in Alberta, Canada. *The Journal of Parasitology* 79:866–869.

Kennedy, M.J., D.T. Moraiko, and B. Treichel. 1993. First report of immature *Thalazia skrjabini* (Nematoda: Thelazioidea) from the eyes of a white-tailed deer, *Odocoileus virginianus. Journal of Wildlife Diseases* 29:159–160.

Krafsur, E.S., and R.D. Moon. 1997. Bionomics of the face fly, *Musca autumnalis. Annual Review of Entomology* 42:503–523.

Lankester, M.W., and W.M. Samuel. 1998. Pests, parasites and diseases. In *Ecology and management of the North American moose,* a Wildlife Management Institute Book. Ed. A.W. Franzmann and C.C. Schwartz. Washington and London: Smithsonian Institution Press, pp. 479–517.

Levot, G.W., and N. Sales. 1998. Effectiveness of a mixture of cyromasine and diazinon for controlling flystrike on sheep. *Australian Veterinary Journal* 76:343–344.

Meagher, M., W.J. Quinn and L. Stackhouse. 1992. Chlamydial-caused infectious keratoconjunctivitis in bighorn sheep of Yellowstone National Park. *Journal of Wildlife Diseases* 28:171–176.

Marley, S.E., R.D. Hall, and R.M. Corwin. 1993. Ivermectin cattle pour-on: Duration of a single late spring treatment against horn flies, *Haematobia irritans* (L.)(Diptera: Muscidae) in Missouri, USA. *Veterinary Parasitology* 51:176–172.

Michener, G.R. 1993. Lethal myiasis of Richardson's ground squirrels by the sarcophagid fly, *Neobellieria citellivora. Journal of Mammalogy* 74:148–155.

Miller, K.B., L.J. Hribar, and L.J. Saunders. 1990. Human myiasis caused by *Phormia regina* in Pennsylvania. *Journal of the American Podiatrist Medical Association* 80:600–602.

Mulla, M.S. 1962. The breeding niches of *Hippelates* gnats. *Annals of the Entomological Society of America* 55:389–393.

Mulla, M.S., and H. Axelrod. 1974. Attractants for synanthropic flies: Attractant-toxicant formulations, their potency against a *Hippelates* eye gnat. *Journal of Economic Entomoogy* 67:13–16.

Mulla, M.S., and R.B. March. 1959. Flight range, dispersal patterns and population density of the eye gnat *Hippelates collusor* (Townsend). *Annals of the Entomological Society of America* 52:641–646.

Mullens, B.A., and C.E. Dada. 1992. Insects feeding on desert bighorn sheep, domestic rabbits and Japanese quail in the Santa Rosa mountains of southern California. *Journal of Wildlife Diseases* 28:476–480.

Newson, H.D. 1977. Arthropod problems in recreation areas. *Annual Review of Entomology* 22:333–353.

Oksanen, A., M. Nieminen, and T. Soveri. 1993. A comparison of topical, subcutaneous and oral administrations of ivermectin to reindeer. *Veterianrian's Record* 133:312–314.

Payne, W.J., Jr., J.R. Cole, E.L. Snoddy, and H.R. Seiboldt. 1977. The eye gnat *Hippelates pusilis* as a vector of bacterial conjunctivitis using rabbits as an animal model. *Journal of Medical Entomology* 13:599–603.

Pickens, L.G., and R.W. Miller. 1980. Biology and control of the face fly, *Musca autumnalis* (Diptera: Muscidae). *Journal of Medical Entomology* 17:195–210.

Reichard, R.E., T.M. Vargas, and M. AbuSowa. 1992. Myiasis: The battle continues against screwworm infestation. *World Health Forum* 13:130–138.

Roberts, R.H. 1968. A feeding association between *Hippelates* and Tabanidae on cattle: Its role in transmission of anaplasmosis. *Mosquito News* 28:236–237.

Rugg, D. 1982. Effectiveness of Williams traps in reducing the numbers of stable flies (Diptera: Muscidae). *Journal of Economic Entomology* 75:857–859.

Rugg, D., D. Thompson, R.P. Gogoloweski, G.R. Allerton, R.A. Barrick, and J.S. Eagleson. 1998. Efficacy of ivermectin in a controlled-release capsule for the control of breech strike in sheep. *Australian Veterinary Journal* 76:350–354.

Sabrosky, C.W. 1941. The *Hippelates* flies or eye gnats: Preliminary notes. *Canadian Entomologist* 73:23–27.

Sandeman, R.M. 1992. Biotechnology and the control of myisais diseases. In *Animal parasite control utilizing biotechnology.* Ed. W. K. Yong. Boca Raton, FL: CRC Press, pp. 275–301.

Sanders, D.A. 1940. A *Musca domestica* and *Hippelates* flies, vectors of bovine mastitis. *Science* 92:286.

Schlein, Y., and C.T. Lewis. 1976. Lesions in hematophagous flies after feeding on rabbits immunized with fly tissues. *Physiological Entomology* 1:55–59.

Scruggs, C.G. 1979. The origin of the screwworm control program. In *The screwworm problem.* Ed. R. H. Richardson. Austin: University of Texas Press, pp. 11–18.

Shishido, W.H., and D.E. Hardy. 1969. Myiasis in newborn calves in Hawaii. *Proceedings of the Hawaiian Entomological Society* 20:435–438.

Smith, D.R., and R.R. Clevenger. 1986. Nosocomial nasal myiasis. *Archives of Pathology and Laboratory Medicine* 110:439–440.

Steelman, C.D. 1976. Effects of external and internal arthropod parasites on domestic livestock production. *Annual Review of Entomology* 21:155–178.

Stoffolano, J.G. Jr. 1970. Nematodes associated with the genus *Musca. Bulletin of the Entomological Society of America* 16:194–203.

Taylor, S.K., V.G. Viera, E.S. Williams, R. Pilkington, S.L. Fedorchak, K.W. Mills, J.L. Cavender, A.M. Boerger-Fields, and R.E. Moore. 1996. Infectious keratoconjunctivitis in free-ranging mule deer (*Odocoileus hemionus*) from Zion National Park, Utah. *Journal of Wildlife Diseases* 32:326–330.

Thomas, G.L., R.D. Hall, and I.L. Berry. 1987. Diapause of the horn fly (Diptera: Muscidae) in the field. *Environmental Entomology* 60:1092–1097.

Thorne, E.T. 1982. Infectious keratoconjunctivitis. In *Diseases of wildlife in Wyoming.* Ed. E.T. Thorne, N. Kingston, W.R. Jolley, and R.C. Bergstrom. Cheyenne: Wyoming Game and Fish Department, pp. 81–84.

Treece, R.E. 1960. Distribution, life-history and control of the face fly in Ohio. *Proceedings of the North Central Branch of the Entomological Society of America* 15:107.

Wall, R., and D. Shearer. 1997. *Veterinary entomology.* New York: Chapman and Hall.

Weiman, G.A., J.B. Campbell, J.A. Deshazer, and I.L. Berry. 1992. Effects of stable flies (Diptera: Muscidae) and heat stress on weight gain and feed efficiency of feeder cattle. *Journal of Economic Entomology* 85:1835–1842.

Zumpt, F. 1965. *Myiasis in man and animals in the Old World.* London: Butterworth and Co.

3

BOT FLIES AND WARBLE FLIES (ORDER DIPTERA: FAMILY OESTRIDAE)

DOUGLAS D. COLWELL

INTRODUCTION. Bot fly and warble fly larvae are obligate parasites of mammals, living within host tissues or body cavities. Larvae resident in body cavities feed on cellular debris and mucosal secretions. Tissue–invading larvae feed on digested connective tissue, serum, and white blood cells. The condition of being parasitized by fly maggots is commonly known as myiasis.

Several dipteran families, the Calliphoridae (blow flies), Sarcophagidae (flesh flies) and Oestridae (bot and warble flies), have representatives that cause myiasis. The nature of the association between the maggots and the host varies across these groups. In some the relationship is facultative; that is, maggots are capable of developing in decaying organic matter, but can develop within and consume necrotic host tissues (e.g., Calliphoridae and Sarcophagidae). In others the relationship is obligatory and maggots require living hosts and their tissues/secretions for successful development [e.g., Oestridae (bot/warble flies)].

All members of the Oestridae have larval stages that are obligate parasites of mammals. Wood (1987) has placed all bot and warble flies into a single family, the Oestridae. This has reduced previous familial designations, Hypodermatidae, Oestridae, Gasterophilidae, Cuterebridae, to subfamily status. Wood's (1987) revision suggests that the group is monophyletic, a contention later supported by Pape (1992).

This chapter considers the life history, diagnosis, immunity, and pathology of oestrid parasites in the subfamilies Oestrinae (nose and pharyngeal bots), Hypodermatinae (warbles), and Cuterebrinae (cuterebrid or rodent bots). Distinctive oviposition behaviors, larval morphology, and developmental sites within the host differentiate the members of these three groups (see Fig. 3.1).

Female Oestrinae (nasal/pharyngeal bots) are viviparous and deposit or forcibly eject packets of larvae onto the muzzle or eyes of the host, often without landing. The newly deposited larvae migrate quickly into the eyes, nose, or mouth before migrating into the nasal cavities of the host where first instar development is completed. Second and third instars of the Oestrinae develop within the sinus cavities or pharyngeal regions of their hosts.

Female Hypodermatinae (warble) are oviparous, landing on the host, sometimes only briefly, to attach eggs directly onto the hair. First instars penetrate the host's skin and migrate within connective tissue.

Female Cuterebrinae (bots) are oviparous, depositing eggs on vegetation or on the ground at sites frequented by the potential hosts. Eggs hatch when warmed by the approach of a potential host. Newly hatched larvae locate the host and enter the body through moist openings such as the nares or eyes. Included in the Cuterebrinae is the human or tropical bot fly, *Dermatobia hominis,* which uses mammophilic transporter flies to carry its eggs to the host.

Second and third instars of the subfamilies Hypodermatinae and Cuterebrinae develop within subdermal, granulomatous cysts. The host reaction provides a rich resource, and the larvae are able to acquire sufficient nutrients to allow completion of the adult phase without feeding.

This chapter updates and extends the reviews of Zumpt (1957), Capelle (1971), Sabrosky (1986), and Guimares (1989). This will include new information on identification, life history, pathology, immunity, impact of the parasites on their hosts, and control. Table 3.1 summarizes the genera selected for discussion. Little new information has emerged on the remaining genera (see Table 3.2), and readers are encouraged to consult the reviews of Zumpt (1965) and Papavero (1977) for discussion of these genera. If there is no information on certain topics (e.g., Clinical Signs) under the various genera reviewed, that subsection is deleted.

GENERAL MORPHOLOGY. Adult oestrids have a broad head, usually flattened (front to back), with relatively small eyes (see Wood 1987). Small, three-segmented antennae are sunken into a pit on the face. The third antennal segment is globular and fits into the cup-like second segment that is attached to the head by a short first segment. The arista, on the terminal (third) segment, is slender and is either bare (Oestrinae and Hypodermatinae) or plumose (Cuterebrinae). Mouthparts are small and inconspicuous or completely absent. The thorax is covered with occasional hairs (pilose) or it is densely longhaired throughout. Legs are short, robust, and hairy. The abdomen is globular with a shiny integument that is often overlain by long, colored hairs.

First instars are small (1–2 mm), white, have a general muscomorph body form (Teskey 1981), and usually have one or two bands of spines per segment. The cephalic segment has a variable number of sensory

46

Nose & pharyngeal bots (Oestrinae)

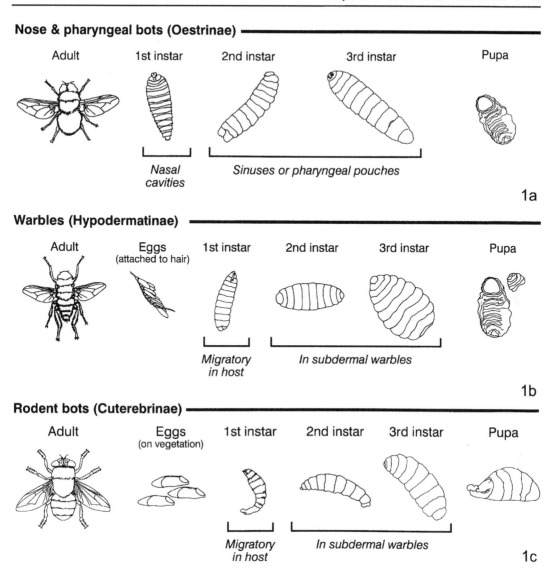

FIG. 3.1—Life cycle diagrams of representatives of three subfamilies in the family Oestridae: (**a**) Oestrinae (nose and pharyngeal bots)—adult flies are larviparous, depositing first instar larvae onto eyes or nares of hosts; development of later instars taking place in nasal sinuses or pharyngeal pouches. (**b**) Hypodermatinae (warbles)—oviparous adults attach eggs to host hair; first instars penetrate the skin and undergo migration within the host; later instars develop within host produced granulomas (warbles). (**c**) Cuterebrinae (rodent bots)—oviparous adults attach eggs to a substrate in the vicinity of host activity; first instars locate host and enter through natural openings; short migration is followed by development in host granulomas (warbles). (**Note:** Images are not to scale.)

structures that are used to locate the host and locate suitable sites of entry into the host's body. The mandibles are well developed and conspicuous. Posterior spiracles are small or absent, and anterior spiracles are absent.

Second instars are medium–sized (12–20 mm), white or cream, and have spines distributed in a variety of patterns. The posterior spiracles of second instars are present as a circular plate with numerous pores (< 100).

Third instars are large (20–35 mm), robust, and have variable numbers of spines with variable distributions. Some larvae are completely covered with flat, plate-like spines (e.g., Cuterebrinae) while others have very few spines (e.g., *Oestrus*). New third instars are white or cream colored, and the spines have little or no melanin. Mature third instars are either very dark in color (completely black in many cases) or are cream with distinctive bands of highly melanized spines. The

Table 3.1. Host, parasite, and distribution list of warble and bot fly species in selected genera from three sub-families of the family Oestridae

Subfamily/ Genera/ Species	Hosts	Distribution
Oestrinae		
Pharyngomyia:		
picta	*Cervus elaphus, C. nippon,*	Europe, central Asia
	Dama dama, Capreolus capreolus	
dzerenae	'mongolian gazelle'	Central Asia
Cephenemyia:		
apicata	*Odocoileus hemionus*	Nearctic (western)
auribarbis	*C. elaphus, D. dama*	Europe
jellisoni	*O. hemionus, O. virginianus, Alces alces americanus,*	Nearctic (western)
	C. elaphus canadensis	
phobifera	*O. hemionus, A. alces americanus*	Nearctic (eastern)
pratti	*O. hemionus, O. virginianus*	Nearctic (southwest)
stimulator	*C. capreolus*	Palearctic
trompe	*Rangifer rangifer, O. hemionus*	Holarctic
ulrichii	*A. alces*	Central & eastern Europe
Kirkioestrus:		
blanchardi	*Alcelaphus buselaphus, A. lichtensteini*	Central & southern Africa
minutus	*A. buselaphus, A. lichtensteini, Connoachaetes taurinus,*	Central Africa
	Damaliscus korrigum	
Rhinoestrus:		
antidorcitis	*Antidorcas marsupialis*	Southern Africa
giraffae	*Giraffa camelopardalis*	"Tanganika"
hippopotami	*Hippopotamus amphibius*	Central Africa
nivarleti	*Potamochoerus porcus*	Central Africa
phacochoeri	*Phacochoerus aethiopicus*	Central Africa
steyni	*Equus burchelli, E. zebra*	Southern Africa
tshernyshevi	*Ovis ammon*	Central Asia
usbekistanicus	*E. burchelli*	Africa, central Asia
Oestrus:		
aureoargentatus	*Hippotragus niger, H. equinus,*	Sub-Saharan Africa
	D. korrigum, D. lunatus, A. buselaphus,	
	A. lichtensteini, C. taurinus	
bassoni	*A. buselaphus*	Southwest Africa
caucasicus	*Capra caucasica, C. ibex,*	Central Asia, Europe
	C. pyrenaica, C. sibirica	
ovis	*O. ovis, C. ibex, O. canadensis, O. virginianus,* and	Worldwide
	many others	
variolosus	*D. korrigum, D. dorcas, D. lunatus,*	Sub-Saharan Africa
	A. buselaphus, A. lichtensteini, H. niger, O. gazella,	
	C. taurinus	
Gedoelstia:		
cristata	*C. gnou, C. taurinus, A. buselaphus,*	Throughout host range
	A. lichtensteini, D. korrigum	
Hypodermatinae		
Hassleri	*C. gnou, C. taurinus, A. buselaphus*	Throughout host range
	A. lichtensteini, D. borrigum, D. dorcas,	
	D. lunatus	
Oestromyia:		
leporina	*Microtis arvalis, M. agrestis,*	Palearctic
	Pitymus subterraneus, Arvicola terrestris, Ondatra	
	zibethicus, Ochotona alpina, O. daurica,	
	M. oeconomis, M. gregalis, Citellus undulatus	
marmotae	*Marmota caudata*	Central Asia
prodigiosa	*O. daurica, O. pallas*	Central Asia
Hypoderma:		
actaeon	*C. elaphus*	Palearctic
diana	*C. elaphus, C. capreolus, O. orientalis*	Palearctic
tarandi	*R. rangifer*	Holarctic
Cuterebrinae		
Cuterebra	See Sabrosky (1986)	
Alouattamyia:		
baeri	*Alouatta palliata*	Neotropics
Metacuterebra:		
almeidai	Host unknown	Brazil
apicalis	*Oryzomys subflavus, Bolomys*	Neotropics
	lasiurus, Thalpomys cerradensis, Holochilus sciureus	
cayennensis	*Didelphys* sp.*, Sciurus aestuans, Caluromys philander*	Neotropics
detrudator	*Proechimys semispinosus, Oryzomys* spp.*, Marmosa*	Neotropics
	murina	
funebris	Host unknown	Neotropics
megastoma	Host unknown	Brazil
patagonia	Host unknown	Argentina
pessoai	Host unknown	Trinidad, Brazil
rufiventris	Host unknown	Peru, Ecuador, Brazil
infulata	Host unknown	Brazil
simulans	*Didelphys* sp.*, C. philander*	Surinam
townsendi	*M. murina*	Brazil

Table 3.2. Host and parasite list of genera not selected for inclusion because of the paucity of new information on development and host relationships

Subfamily/Genus	No. of Species	Hosts
Oestrinae		
Pharyngobolus	1	African elephant
Tracheomyia	1	Kangaroo
Cephalopina	1	Camels
Hypodermatinae		
Oestroderma	1	Pikas
Portschinskia	1	Mice, pikas
Strobiloestrus	3	*Kobus* spp.
Pavlovskiata	1	Goitered antelope
Pallasiomyia	1	Saiga antelope
Przhevalskiana	6	Gazelles, goats
Cuterebrinae		
Rogenhofera	4	Rodents
Dermatobia	1	Various mammals
Pseudogametes	1	Rodents and marsupials

cephalic segment is relatively small, and the mandibles are prominent and curved. Posterior spiracles in Oestrinae and Hypodermatinae are present as a pair of disc-shaped plates with numerous slit-like openings (usually > 100/plate); each plate encloses a prominent remnant of the second instar spiracle, known as the ecdysal scar. In the Cuterebrinae the posterior spiracles are composed of two sets of three serpentine slits each with numerous openings (see Wood 1987).

Nasal/Pharyngeal Bots (Oestrinae). Nasal/pharyngeal bot flies are medium to large, heavy-bodied flies. Generally, adults are sparsely pilose (e.g., *Oestrus*); however, some genera are densely haired (e.g., *Cephenemyia*). Body coloration is brown to grey with an overall mottled appearance. In those species with dense hair, the body coloration is obscured. Mouthparts are small and compact or are completely atrophied; the antennae are small and sunken into a pit. Sexual dimorphism is evident in the difference between male and female interocular distance, the females having a larger space between the eyes than the males.

Nasal/pharyngeal bot flies are viviparous; eggs have thin translucent shells and develop within the body of the females. First instars are muscomorph in form, but are distinctly dorsoventrally flattened, with large, prominent mouth hooks, well-developed and numerous lateral spines, and a set of posterior crochets or hooks (see Colwell and Scholl 1995). These features aid the newly deposited larvae in the migration from the external surfaces into the host nasal cavities. Cuticular sensilla on the larvae are usually well developed and are present in higher numbers than in the Hypodermatinae (see Colwell 1986; Colwell and Scholl 1995). This is a consequence of the need to locate suitable entry sites and to find appropriate development sites within the host.

Second and third instar larvae are large, robust, and usually cylindrical, although in the later instar there is

often a distinct flattening of the ventral surface. Bands of well-developed spines are present on most body segments, and mouth hooks are prominent. Posterior spiracles are present on the terminal abdominal segments as prominent spiracular plates. These plates are pierced by more than 100 pores that open into sieve-like felt chambers. Pigmentation of third instar spines becomes darker as the third instar larvae reach maturity. Larvae do not become completely black, as do third instars of the Hypodermatinae and Cuterebrinae.

Warble Flies (Hypodermatinae). Warble flies are medium to large, heavy-bodied flies with a dense covering of hairs over most of the body. The hairs are golden and black in color, which gives adults a bee-like appearance. Mouthparts are usually completely atrophied. Small antennae are sunken into the facial pit and have a bare arista. Sexual dimorphism is evident in the increased interocular separation of the females. Eggs are smooth surfaced and have a unique terminal attachment organ that completely surrounds the hair shaft (Cogley et al. 1981), keeping the egg well anchored and somewhat resistant to removal through grooming. First instars have a delicate musciform body with small, sparsely distributed spines (Colwell 1986). Larval cuticular sensilla are generally fewer in number than on the larval Oestrinae or Cuterebrinae. This reflects the limited amount of searching and migration by the larvae on the host surface; they move directly to the skin and penetrate prior to embarking on internal migrations. Second and third instars are large, cylindrical, and robust. Simple spines are distributed in bands on both dorsal and ventral surfaces. Both spines and mouth hooks are less prominent than in the Oestrinae. The posterior segments have well-defined posterior spiracles composed of two terminal spiracular plates. Each plate is pierced by > 100 pores that open into sieve-like felt chambers (Colwell 1989a) Mature third instars are completely black in color. Spine and spiracular plate structure can be used to identify the species (Colwell et al. 1998; see Figs. 3.8 and 3.9, below, in section on *Hypoderma*).

Bots (Cuterebrinae). Cuterebrid bot flies are very large, robust flies with prominent eyes and a fine covering of hairs that are often in contrasting colors. This feature gives the flies a mottled appearance. Sexual dimorphism occurs in the coloration of several species, male and female flies of the same species having distinctly different color patterns on the body (Sabrosky 1986). Vestigial mouthparts are present but are hidden beneath dense facial hairs. The eyes are large, with the interocular space being greater in the females than in the males. When alive, males of those species that parasitize lagomorphs are often distinguished by the presence of red spots or bands on the eyes. Small antennae, concealed within the facial pit, have plumose arista.

Cuterebrid eggs have a thick, highly sculptured outer chorion and may be flattened on the ventral surface (see Colwell et al. 1999). They are usually firmly attached to the substrate by the ovipositing female. First instars are muscomorph in form, with well-developed bands of stout spines, and characteristically have an adhesive sac at their posterior end that aids in attachment of the larvae to surfaces and host hair. The larvae are well endowed with cuticular sensilla used to locate the host and find a suitable opening through which they can enter the host. Mouth hooks are large.

Second instars, in all but the monospecific genus *Dermatobia,* have well-developed and widely distributed spines. The posterior spiracles appear as paired, convoluted bars with numerous slit-like openings in each bar.

Third instars are large, cylindrical, and robust, some weighing more than 3 g. Broad, spade-like spines cover the entire body. Cephalic segments are relatively small, and the mouth hooks are usually small. Posterior spiracles are present as paired sets of three prominent serpentine bars, each having a large number of slit-like openings. Mature larvae are completely black. During pupation the anterior spiracles are everted, giving a distinctive appearance to these pupae.

GENERAL LIFE HISTORY
AND DEVELOPMENT

Nasal/Pharyngeal Bots (Oestrinae) (Fig. 3.1a). Males gather at aggregation sites with highly species-specific ecological characteristics (Catts 1964, 1994). Sites are usually prominent hilltops that are further partitioned by species-specific preferences (Catts 1994). Man-made structures, such as wooden fire-observation towers, have been used as aggregation sites for members of the genus *Cephenemyia*. Males await passing females and capture them in flight. Mating, which usually takes place on the ground, may last 20 minutes.

Females have a completely developed complement of eggs at the time of eclosion. Single eggs develop in each ovariol during the pupal period and no additional eggs are formed posteclosion (Cepeda-Palacios and Scholl 1999). The number of eggs per female varies from 108 to 590 (*Oestrus ovis:* D.D. Colwell, unpublished).

Females are vivparous, and several days are required for the inseminated eggs to embryonate. Embryonation occurs in a specialized feature of the common oviduct referred to as a uterus. The developmental period can range from 12 to 16 days and is temperature dependent (P.J. Scholl and D.D. Colwell, unpublished).

Gravid females are attracted to increased concentrations of CO_2 (Anderson and Nilssen 1990, 1996a,b) associated with potential hosts. Few other details regarding host selection are clearly established, although recent electro-antennogram studies have indicated that *Cephenemyia trompe* responds to dimethyl disulphide, a compound found in extracts of interdigital glands of reindeer (Tømmerås et al. 1993). Fly responses to traps baited with CO_2 and dimethyl sulphide did not confirm the laboratory findings (Nilssen et al. 1996). Females have a small number of tarsal sensilla, suggesting that they do not require sensory information from contact with the host in order to initiate larviposition (D.D. Colwell, unpublished).

Larvipositing females discharge packets of first instars toward the nose/mouth region or toward the eye of the host. The packets contain 3–35 larvae (Cogley and Anderson 1981) surrounded by a viscous uterine fluid that provides moisture and aids larval adherence to the host. The uterine fluid dissolves rapidly when exposed to mucous secretions or water and questing larvae quickly search for and move toward the oral opening. Larvae are positively thermotactic, negatively phototactic, and negatively geotactic.

First instars migrate quickly into the nasal cavities of the host. The development period of first instars varies widely, ranging from several days to several months. Individuals from the same fly may not all develop at the same rate. Factors affecting first instar development are not clearly understood, although there are indications that larval crowding and host immunity are components in the regulatory process. Second and third instar development usually takes place at a second site (e.g., the nasal sinuses or the pharyngeal pouch) and can be quite variable in length.

Warble Flies (Hypodermatinae) (Fig. 3.1b). Males gather at distinctive aggregation sites, but in contrast to Oestrinae or Cuterebrinae these flies do not seek high points. Instead the flies gather along dry stream beds or roadways in small valleys. Males will perch on tall grass or shrubs waiting for passing females. *Hypoderma tarandi* are unique in having two distinct types of aggregation sites depending on the biome in which they are found (Anderson et al. 1994). In the treeless tundra they gather at rocky areas along dry riverbeds; in wooded valleys, flies gather at sites along roads or tracks. Use of mating sites allows males, who are incapable of sustained flights, to maximize their reproductive efforts and allows females to waste less energy searching for males and thus conserve energy for host–searching.

Following mating, the oviparous females depart in search of hosts. Distances traveled can be amazing, particularly when in pursuit of migrating species such as reindeer (Nilssen and Anderson 1995) or wildebeest. Nilssen and Anderson (1995), in a series of laboratory studies, estimated the maximum postmating flight range of female *H. tarandi* to be in the range of 600–900 km.

Mated female flies are attracted to increased concentrations of CO_2 (Anderson and Nilssen 1990) as evidenced by the success of trapping schemes that used CO_2–baited traps. Tømmerås et al. (1993) showed that, in the laboratory, female *H. tarandi* respond to dimethyl trisulphide, a component extracted from the interdigital glands of reindeer. However, no increases in trap catches were noted when this compound was used as bait (Nilssen et al. 1996). The role of thermal or visual characteristics of hosts has not been evaluated. Host acceptance criteria are also poorly understood in these flies; however, indirect evidence suggests that tarsal chemosensilla play some role in the final stages of host acceptance. This observation is supported by studies of warble flies of domestic livestock showing that the numbers of tarsal chemosensilla are co-related with the type of oviposition behavior (Colwell and Berry 1993). Increasing requirement for sensory acuity is correlated with increased numbers of tarsal chemosensilla.

Female warble flies emerge from the puparium with eggs fully developed (Scholl and Weintraub 1988). As in the Oestrinae, only two eggs develop, almost simultaneously, in each ovariole. The total egg complement ranges from 400 to 850 eggs/female (Scholl and Weintraub 1988; Anderson and Nilssen 1996a,b).

Ovipositing females attach eggs individually or in groups to the base of host hair shafts, which protect them from being removed by host grooming activity and from variations in temperature and humidity. Females apparently are selective in their choice of hairs, preferentially placing eggs on hairs with a small diameter. Most data are available for warble flies of domestic livestock, but recent research with *H. tarandi* has broadened the understanding of developmental requirements of eggs (Karter et al. 1992). Eggs of this species are capable of development over a relatively broad range of temperatures (20° C–37° C), but exhibit the optimum, in terms of developmental rate and survival, in the temperature ranges found in the microenvironment of the reindeer pelage.

Newly hatched larvae show positive thermotaxis, but show no phototaxis or geotaxis (Karter et al. 1992). They move quickly to the skin and penetrate using regurgitated enzymes that dissolve the tissue. *Hypoderma tarandi* use a collagenase similar to that known from *H. bovis* and *H. lineatum,* the cattle parasites (Boulard et al. 1996). *Hypoderma bovis* and *H. lineatum* secrete two serine proteinases that have not been reported from *H. tarandi*. Migration within the host is also accomplished with these enzyme(s). At least one of the major secretory enzymes is known to cleave the C3 component of the complement cascade (Baron 1990; Boulard 1989); this gives it the ability to down-regulate the development of host immunity.

First instars complete their development when they reach sites beneath the skin on the dorsal region of the host. Here they digest small holes in the skin and molt to the second instar. During this development they are encapsulated in a host granuloma, known as a warble. Second and third instar development is completed within the granuloma with the larvae feeding on serum and abundant white blood cells.

Mature third instars emerge from the host and fall to the ground, where they actively burrow into grass and leaf litter. Within a short period of time larvae form a puparium and begin the metamorphosis to adult. This development is temperature-dependent and has been modeled for *H. tarandi* (Nilssen 1997a). Variation in environmental conditions influences the emergence of

adult flies and thus will affect the timing of the other parasitic life stages.

Bots (Cuterebrinae) (Fig. 3.1c). Male cuterebrids also gather at aggregation sites to await passing females (Catts 1982, 1994). Mating site specificity is not known for many species. Females are oviparous, but unlike other oestrids, they require several days after eclosion for egg development to be completed (Scholl 1991). They are refractory to mating during this process. Egg numbers range from 1200 to 4000/female. Oviposition sites are highly specific and are usually located where host activity brings them into close proximity (e.g., rodent burrows by *Cuterebra polita*). Females use the large number of tarsal sensilla (e.g., 5000/tarsus) to select oviposition sites. These sensilla presumably aid detection of low-intensity chemical cues indicative of the preferred host.

Eggs require 5–7 days to fully embryonate, after which larvae emerge in response to sudden increases in temperature and CO_2 concentration associated with the presence of a potential host. Eggs in an individual cluster will not hatch simultaneously, presumably an adaptation that reduces larval mortality if the emergence is in response to an inappropriate host.

First instars have numerous cuticular sensilla used to find hosts and a site for entry into the body. Entry is through a moist opening (e.g., eyes, nares) or a fresh skin lesion. Moisture is presumably an attractant (Hunter et al. 1972). Newly hatched larvae can live several hours after emerging from the egg. They appear to be positively thermotactic. Within the host the larvae move to the nasal passages or esophagus and trachea, usually within 2–3 days. From these locations the larvae penetrate the host and undergo a migration through the thoracic and abdominal cavities to the final subdermal site of development (Gingrich 1981). The migration within the host typically lasts 3–6 days, with the route terminating at a subdermal site. Larvae tend migrate to species-specific locations on the host's body.

At the subdermal tissue sites, larvae open a small hole in the host's skin and complete the second and third instars. Larvae at subdermal sites are quickly surrounded by a host granuloma, forming the characteristic 'warble' (Cogley 1991). The location of these sites is often species specific (e.g., 70% of the larvae of *Alouattamyia baeri* are found on the throat/neck region of infested howler monkeys). These instars require 25–30 days to complete development. Mature third instars leave the warble, often at a time coincident with the period of highest activity by the host. The mature larvae will burrow quickly into the soil or beneath the surface litter. Mature third instars of tropical species will rapidly burrow to depths of 15 cm. Pupation occurs within 2 days. A pupal diapause allows the species that occur in temperate regions to overwinter.

Second and third instars feed on sera and white blood cells (Colwell and Milton 1998), a rich nutrient source that allows dramatic and rapid growth. It has been estimated that overall increase in mass from the first instar to the mature third instar is in the order of 100,000-fold (Catts 1982)

IMPORTANCE OF BOTS AND WARBLES TO MAMMALS.

The impact of oestrid myiasis on the health and productivity of wild mammals is, with rare exceptions, not particularly well defined. Traumatic and lethal effects seen as a result of myiasis caused by *Cochliomyia hominovorax* (the screwworm), *Neobellieria citellivora* (a parasite of Richardson's ground squirrel) (see Michener 1993) or *Wohlfahrtia* spp. is not common with the oestrids. Conventional wisdom suggests that oestrid parasites have evolved with their hosts over long periods and the relationship has thus developed towards a more benign state.

Impact on the host can be categorized into (1) impacts resulting from oviposition/larviposition activities of adult females and (2) impacts resulting from migration and development of larvae and subsequent host response.

Impacts Relating to Adult Flies. The impact of oviposition/larviposition activity of nose bot and warble flies has been examined in detail for several important species. Reindeer exposed to the combined attacks of blood-feeding flies and oestrids show a dramatic reduction in food intake as they leave preferred grazing sites to take refuge on windswept slopes or snow patches (Downes et al. 1986; Russel and Dixon 1990; Mörschel and Klein 1997). Reduction in intake will have an effect on both gain and milk production. The latter effect will presumably reduce gain in suckling calves. It has also been postulated that the extensive postcalving migration of reindeer is a strategy developed for parasite avoidance (Folstad et al. 1991). Dudley and Milton (1990) found that the energy expenditure associated with fly-deterrence behavior in howler monkeys represented a significant proportion of the daily energy budget.

Host responses to the larviposition behavior of nose bots can be dramatic. Peculiar and specific evasive responses of deer to larviposition flights of *Cephenemyia* spp. have been described thoroughly (Anderson 1975). Deer quickly learn to associate the activity of the large flies with irritating activities of larvae as they enter the nasal passages or eyes. Despite dramatic evasive behavior, the impact on the host remains in question. However, fly attack can be viewed as a stressor that initiates changes in neurochemical systems regulating several behavioral and physiological systems. These changes may reduce host fitness (see Colwell and Kavaliers 1992; Colwell et al. 1997).

Subtle consequences of bot fly oviposition/larviposition behavior may be postulated from research that has demonstrated activation of opioid peptides in rodents parasitized by nematodes and coccidia as well as in rodents under biting fly attack (Kavaliers and Colwell 1992; Colwell and Kavaliers 1993). Altered opioid peptide mechanisms in parasitized animals can have far reaching consequences as this group of neurochemicals influences a wide number of physiological and behavioral systems. For example, opioid peptide activation in parasitized hosts and in animals under fly attack mediates changes in activity patterns, mate selection, and learning. Similarly, opioid activation influences the function of various components of the immune system that may affect the impact of parasitism. There is no need for direct damage to the host as it has been shown that hosts previously exposed to biting fly attack exhibit anxiety and opioid activation when exposed to subsequent fly attack without biting (Colwell et al. 1997).

Cuterebrid flies do not interact directly with their hosts during oviposition. As a result they are not known to have any impact on host fitness.

Impacts Relating to Larval Stages. Impact of early larval stages (i.e., first instars) on the host may be relatively minor and transient. For example, hosts that have been infested previously with warble larvae often exhibit a characteristic "rash" where the larvae have penetrated the skin (Wolf 1959). Colwell (1989b) demonstrated the movement of eosinophils and mast cells into the skin areas through which larvae are migrating. There was significant degranulation of these cells, which contributed to the rash-like conditions described in cattle and reindeer following penetration of first instars. Presumably similar reactions occur during penetration of other warble larvae. These changes are of relatively short duration and may be of little significance to the host. However, the lesions may serve as a site for entry of other pathogens.

Subsequent interactions between larvae and the host may be of more importance to host fitness. *Hypoderma* spp. from cattle secrete or regurgitate a serine proteinase, Hypodermin A, that has immunosuppressive effects (Chabaudie and Boulard 1992). The consequences of the immunosuppression have not been quantified, but during times of stress in cattle (i.e., weaning) this may contribute to the development of other disease states. Similarly, the effect of the general immunosuppression in infested deer may be reflected in a predisposition of the infested animals to other diseases. Similar proteinases have not been described from *Hypoderma* spp. infesting wild mammals. However, immunoreactive Hypodermin C, a potent collagenase, is known from two species of *Hypoderma* that infest wildlife (*H. tarandi* and *H. actaeon*: D.D. Colwell et al., unpublished) (*H. diana*: Boulard et al. 1996).

Warbles have an impact on the weight gain of domestic livestock, but the effect has not been universal and may relate to the level of dietary intake and the level of parasitism. In wildlife, the research has suggested that there is little impact. Arneberg et al. (1996) found that infestations with *Hypoderma* and *Cephenemyia* did not influence feed intake in reindeer, and similarly Oksanen et al. (1992, 1993) found that weight gains were not influenced by the presence of these parasites or by removal of parasites with macrocyclic lactone parasiticides (Oksanen et al. 1998). Postcalving migrations that characterize most reindeer populations have been hypothesized to be a behavioral adaptation reducing overall parasite burdens (Folstad et al. 1991). Those herds with shorter migratory routes tend to have increased prevalence and intensities of *H. tarandi,* although any movement away from calving grounds will reduce gastrointestinal and lungworm nematode transmission.

Controversy exists about the impact of cuterebrid parasitism on hosts. Negative effects have been reported on the growth, survival, and reproduction of *Microtus townsendi* parasitized by *C. fontinella* (Boonstra et al. 1980). In contrast, other research has reported no impact (Hunter et al. 1972; Catts 1982). Estimates have been made that the growing maggots take up 1%–3.5% of the rodent's nutrient budget (Smith 1975; Munger and Karasov 1994). This has been coupled with an indication that there may also be an increase in the basal metabolism (Munger and Karasov 1994). Despite these observations, the general conclusion of these studies was that the impact was of little consequence. A contrasting study (Gummer et al. 1997) has suggested that parasite-induced reallocation of physiological resources can be of significance in the survival of host species under highly limiting conditions. Infested hosts expend resources on developing one or more large granulomas (i.e., the warble surrounding the maggot) and on maintaining humoral and cellular immune responses and must also support the increase in mass of the larvae (an increase in the order of 10^5). Thus, when nutrient is limiting, parasitism may be a factor in host survival. Milton (1996) supports this with observations on reduced survival of juvenile howler monkeys heavily parasitized by *Alouattamyia baeri*. A further impact of cuterebrid parasitism in howler monkeys has been the predilection of the screwworm (*C. hominovorax*) to oviposit on or near the openings of the warble in howler monkeys infested with *A. baeri* (K. Milton, unpublished). This observation is in contrast to those made by Ruiz-Martinez et al. (1996), who did not observe any association between *Dermatobia hominis* lesions and fly strike in a variety of domestic and wild mammals in Central America.

CONTROL. Control of oestrid myiasis is achieved through the application of classical systemic insecticides and parasiticides that kill the larval stages within the host. With the advent of the broad-spectrum macrocyclic lactone parasiticides, the practice has become relatively easy; application difficulties commonly encountered with the application of organophosphates can be alleviated through the use of baits dosed with an orally effective formulation. This approach has been used to control helminths in deer and, while not free of problems, it could work well if applied to intensively managed game populations. The major concern with this group of compounds is the off-target impacts and reduction of dung degradation.

Use of the sterile insect technique, coupled with chemical suppression, has not been attempted with any species of oestrid affecting wildlife. The technique has, however, been successfully applied to the control of cattle grubs (Kunz et al. 1990) Production of large numbers of insects for sterilization and release was the major factor limiting the control of cattle grubs.

Vaccines for the protection of cattle against *Hypoderma* spp. have been developed and have shown promise. The approach utilized recombinant secretory proteins that are also found in the species of *Hypoderma* infesting deer and reindeer. Reduction of populations of oestrid flies attacking reindeer could be achieved if a suitable delivery system were developed.

GENUS *PHARYNGOMYIA*

Description. Flies are moderately large with a black and white pattern on the abdomen and thorax. The color is partially obscured by a dense covering of whitish hairs. Two species parasitize cervids and a "mongolian" gazelle in the Palearctic region. Little is known of the species reported from the gazelle and the remaining observations refer to *P. picta.*

Newly deposited first instars have distinctive swellings on each of the second through fifth anterior segments. As first instars grow, the posterior of each segment enlarges, giving the larvae a lobulated appearance. Third instars are slightly dorsoventrally flattened with well-defined rows of spines on all segments except for the posterior two. Distinct brown or black spots are evident on posterior segments of nearly mature third instars. Antennal lobes of third instars are widely separated at the base. This characteristic can be used to separate these larvae from those of *Cephenemyia* spp. that may co-occur in the same hosts. Anterior spiracles are clearly evident at this stage. Broad, flat spiracular plates, with features that allow distinction of these larvae from those of *Cephenemyia* (Zumpt 1965), are evident on the terminal abdominal segment, as are the terminal spines.

Life History. Limited information is available on the biology and behavior of the adult flies of this genus, although they are likely similar to other Oestrinae. Zumpt (1965) indicates a period of fly activity between June and August in southern and central Africa.

Sugar (1976b) reported the presence of first instars in the nasal cavities of red deer (*Cervus elaphus*) in most months, with large numbers being recorded in collections made during November and February. However, the first appearance each year was in early May. Ruiz-Martinez and Palomares (1993), examining red deer between November and March in southern Spain, found first instars in three sites, nasal, oral, and pharyngeal. This suggests that larvae had begun to mature and had moved from nasal sites to pharyngeal sites, which indicates that in Spain the period of adult activity is earlier than that proposed by Zumpt (1965).

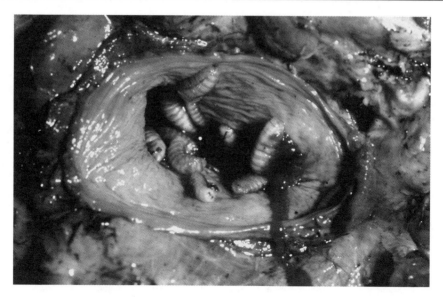

FIG. 3.2—Third instar *Pharyngomyia picta* within the retropharyngeal pouch of a red deer (*Cervus elaphus*). (Photograph by J. Martinez-Moreno, University of Cordoba, Spain.)

Zumpt reported that most second and third instars were recovered from pharyngeal sites in February through April, although some were recorded as late as June and July. In southcentral Spain, Ruiz-Martinez and Palomares (1993) reported the lowest prevalence and intensity of this species in red deer in March, which suggests an earlier period of activity for adults in this warmer region. High summer temperatures of southern Spain probably preclude adult fly activity. At higher elevations, in central Spain, the prevalence and intensities in red deer reached maximum values in January, while the lowest values were noted in June (De la Fuente et al. 1999). These authors reported evidence for two generations of *P. picta* per year.

Mature larvae exit through the nasal openings to pupate on the ground. Pupal development is short, ranging from 26 to 32 days under laboratory conditions (Sugar 1976b).

Distribution and Host Range. *Pharyngomyia picta* has a Holarctic distribution and is reported from a variety of cervids in Europe and central Asia (Table 3.1). The overall distribution appears to match that of the principal hosts.

Prevalence and Intensity. In southern Spain, prevalence in red deer varied from 80% to 100% from November to February then declined to ~30% by March (Ruiz-Martinez and Palomares 1993). Intensity in this study ranged from 25 to 30 larvae in November and December, but declined to less than 10 in March. All fallow deer (*Dama dama*) examined between February and April in southern Spain were infested with the intensity of infestation ranging from 14 to 34 larvae (Ruiz et al. 1993). De la Fuente et al. (2000) reported prevalence in red deer as high as 60% in January with a second peak of the same magnitude in August. The mean intensity was much higher in January than in August (35 vs. 7).

Clinical Signs. External symptoms of infestation with *Pharyngomyia* are few, although some nasal discharge may be evident in heavily infested hosts.

Pathology/Diagnosis/Immunity. Larvae developing in pharyngeal pouches likely induce responses similar to that known for *Cephenemyia* (Cogley 1987). A group of third instar larvae is shown, in situ, within a pharyngeal pouch of a red deer collected in Spain (Fig. 3.2).

There is little evidence that hosts develop protective immunity. Ruiz-Martinez and Palomares (1993) reported small variation between age classes of red deer in Spain, but differences were not suggestive of acquired immunity. No differences in the prevalence or intensity of infestation were reported in different age classes of red deer in central Spain (de la Fuente et al. 2000).

Diagnosis requires recovery of larvae from the nasal cavities or pharyngeal pouches of infected hosts. Recovered third instars can be identified to species; however, if possible, mature specimens should be allowed to pupate and adults reared for definitive identification. Earlier instars are difficult to identify to species, and there are no known methods for culturing these stages to maturity.

Control and Treatment. Broad-spectrum, macro-cyclic lactone endectocides are likely effective, and there is the possibility for management of these parasites through the use of treated baits or untreated baits that attract animals to wick-based applicators.

Public Health Concerns. There are no documented cases of human infestation.

Domestic Animal Concerns. There are no reports of infestation of domestic species. The high host specificity of this genus suggests that there is little likelihood of a problem developing.

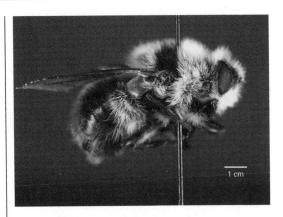

FIG. 3.3—Lateral view of female *Cephenemyia* sp. Note the dense covering of hairs on the head and body.

GENUS *CEPHENEMYIA*

Description. Flies are bumblebee-like in appearance with long yellow and black hairs covering a shining black body. A distinct band of black hairs crosses the thorax and the abdomen and legs are covered with predominantly black hairs (Fig. 3.3). The face is completely covered with dense hairs that obscure the absence of mouthparts. First instars are dorsoventrally flattened with well-developed ventral spines and a cluster of hooks on the terminal abdominal segment. Third instars may be as small as 12 mm long, but grow to over 25 mm. This stage becomes gradually dark and opaque as they mature. Mature or nearly mature third instars have well-developed spines, usually tipped in black, on dorsal and ventral surfaces. Bases of the antennal lobes on the third instar cephalic segment are set close together, a feature that can be used to distinguish larvae from those of *Pharyngomyia* (Zumpt 1965).

Larval stages are difficult to identify to species. Bennett and Sabrosky (1962) provide a key for separating four of the Nearctic species, although its utility is in doubt (see Samuel and Trainer 1971).

Life History. Adults are not often seen by the casual observer, but a substantial amount of research has been conducted on their mating (Catts 1964) and larviposition behavior (Anderson 1975). Larviposition is delayed until the fertilized eggs can embryonate. There is no information on the activities of the females during embryonation, but Anderson (1975) reported collecting females at CO_2-baited traps that had full ovaries or partially developed larvae in the uterus. This suggests that females move into the vicinity of potential hosts prior to completion of embryogenesis. Gravid females are attracted to elevated concentrations of CO_2. Other olfactory and visual cues are probably involved in host selection and acceptance, although the responsiveness to deer or reindeer (*Rangifer* spp.) models varies between species (Breev 1950; Dudzinski 1970a,b; Anderson 1975). Larviposition behavior also varies between species and may be more or less variable within a species. Anderson (1975) has detailed descriptions of larvipostion behavior of *C. jellisoni* and *C. apicata,* and others may be found in Hadwen (1926).

Distribution and Host Range. Eight species parasitize a variety of cervids throughout the Holarctic (Table 3.1). Of these, one (*C. trompe*) parasitizes members of the genus *Rangifer* throughout its Holarctic distribution (Table 3.1). Four species are exclusively Nearctic, and three are exclusively Palearctic. Host specificity is high and appears to be influenced by the female flies' ability to select appropriate targets for larviposition.

Prevalence and Intensity. Prevalence of *C. phobifera* in white-tailed deer (*Odocoileus virginianus*) was 62% over a 12-year period (Bennett 1962). Deer < 6 months of age had lower prevalence and intensities than deer > 6 months. McMahon and Bunch (1989) reported 100% of road-killed mule deer (*Odocoileus hemionus*) were infested with *Cephenemyia* spp. in Utah. Percent prevalence of *C. stimulator* in roe deer (*Capreolus capreolus*) from Poland ranged from 4 to 87 (Dudzinski 1970b). Samuel and Trainer (1971) found that percent prevalence of *Cephenemyia* spp. was higher in deer from areas with more dense canopy cover, suggesting that flies exhibit a preference for more heavily treed areas. These authors also noted higher prevalence in older deer, an observation that raises questions about the effectiveness of learned responses to fly attacks.

Percent prevalence of *C. auribarbis* in sympatric red deer (*Cervus elaphus*) and fallow deer (*Dama dama*) was 81% and 59%, respectively (Ruiz *et al.* 1993). *Cephenemyia auribarbis* co-occurred with *Pharyngomyia picta* in 23% of the cases studied (Ruiz et al. 1993). Prevalence of *Cephenemyia* spp. tends to be highest in young (< 1 year) and older (> 5 years) deer. In a recent survey of *C. auribarbis* in red deer in a high plain area of central Spain (de la Fuente et al. 2000), highest prevalence (50%) occurred in February.

Numbers of larvae per host are: 1–55 (*C. phobifera,* whitetails), 5–35 (*C. stimulator,* roe deer), 22–65 (*Cephenemyia* spp., mule deer: McMahon and Bunch

1989), 4.5–5.6 (*C. auribarbis,* red deer: Ruiz et al. 1993), and 3.3–6.7 (*C. auribarbis,* fallow deer: Ruiz et al. 1993). Maximal mean intensity of *C. auribarbis* in red deer from central Spain was seen in December (8 larvae/host: de la Fuente et al. 2000).

Clinical Signs Occasional deaths, resulting from penetration of the cranial cavity (Johnson et al. 1983) and weight loss (Dudzinski 1970b), have been attributed to infestation with *Cephenemyia* spp. However, in general there are few symptoms that have been reported in association with the infestation.

Pathology/Diagnosis/Immunity. First instars are found primarily in the recesses of the ethmoid bone, although some have been reported associated with the turbinate bones (Bennett 1962; Dudzinski 1970a; Cogley 1987). Second and third instars are exclusively located in the retropharyngeal pouches.

Infected deer have the retropharyngeal recess enlarged to form a pouch, the size of which varies with the number and size of the infesting larvae (Cogley 1987). Pathological changes include a reduced epithelial layer with a loss of cilia, reduction of the number of mucous glands, fibrous tissue invasion with increased vascularization, and eosinophil infiltration into pouch wall. These changes are accompanied by a mucopurulent discharge. Other authors have reported that the keratitis is often associated with *C. trompe* infestations in semidomestic reindeer (Rehbinder 1970).

Prevalence and intensity decline with increasing host age (Bennett 1962; Samuel and Trainer 1971; Anderson 1975); this decline may be the result of acquired immunity. However, there have been no studies of the host immune response to these parasites and some studies have found that animals > 5 years of age have a higher prevalence and intensity than younger animals.

Larvae have been reported in a variety of unusual locations, but these reports are often discounted as being the result of postmortem migration. Reports of severe neurological symptoms (Foreyt et al. 1994) and death (e.g., Johnson et al. 1983) following larval penetration of the cranial cavity and auditory regions are considered unusual, and there is little evidence that these parasites are major mortality factors in host populations (McMahon and Bunch 1989).

Comments on diagnosis of *Pharyngomyia* (above) apply here. Keys are available for some third instars.

Control and Treatment. Macrocyclic lactone parasiticides effectively control these larvae (Oksanen and Nieminen 1996).

Public Health Concerns. There are no documented cases in humans.

Domestic Animal Concerns. Physical features of the host nasal region probably prevent establishment of first instars in hosts other than the primary ones (Cog-

ley and Anderson 1981). Misguided larviposition attempts, where larvae land on inappropriate sites such as the eye, have been implicated in the development of keratitis (Rehbinder 1970).

Management Implications. Larvae can cause problems for host individuals (see above), but they apparently cause no problems for host populations.

GENUS *KIRKIOESTRUS*

Description. Flies are moderate in size, reddish brown to dark brown in color, usually with a black pattern on the abdomen. Thorax and abdomen are covered with dense fine hairs of variable color. Legs are also densely haired and usually black. Adults of the two species, *K. minutus* and *K. blanchardi,* are separated by differences in wing venation and leg color (Zumpt 1965).

First instar *K. minutus,* described by Horak et al. (1980), have a distinctive, rounded anterior and blunt posterior. Single bands of spines are present ventrally and laterally at the posterior edge of each segment. Second instars are nearly cylindrical with single rows of spines on all thoracic and abdominal segments, mostly on the ventral surface. A prominent cluster of spines is located terminally, on the postanal bulge. Spine numbers on the postanal bulge are diagnostic; *K. blanchardi* has 12–20, and *K. minutus* has 5–9. Third instars are yellowish brown in color. The body is cylindrical, with some flattening of the ventral surface and a gentle narrowing toward the anterior segments. Spine patterns are similar to the second instar and are diagnostic, as previously mentioned.

Life History. No information is available on the life history and behavior of the adults. Presumably they exhibit characteristics that reflect the trends evident for other members of this subfamily. Larval stages are known from studies of naturally infested wild hosts. In the blue wildebeest (*Connochaetes taurinus*) first instars of *K. minutus* are found within nasal passages and nasal septa, usually during April through August (Horak et al. 1980). Second and third instars are found in the frontal sinuses and around the entrance to these structures. The later stages are found throughout the year except for November and December. From May through August larvae of all three stages are found in some hosts. The total development time within the host has been estimated as short as 30 days. Pupal development is temperature-dependent and varies from 31–32 days in March to 53–58 days in July.

Distribution and Host Range. *Kirkioestrus* is restricted to central and southern Africa (Table 3.1). Members parasitize antelope and wildebeest throughout these regions. *Kirkioestrus minutus* appears to have low host specificity, infesting hosts in three genera (*Alcelaphus, Connochaetes,* and *Damaliscus*). *Kirkioestrus blanchardi* is more specific, infesting only *Alcelaphus* spp.

Prevalence and Intensity. In Kruger National Park all host animals older than 3 months were infested with larvae of *K. minutus.* Up to 145 larvae were found in individual hosts. Variation between months was significant, with peak intensities being recorded in November and January. Between-year variation in intensity is high and is presumably influenced by abiotic factors that regulate pupal and adult survival.

Clinical Signs. Clinical symptoms of infestation are rarely evident, although a nasal discharge may be present.

Diagnosis. Comments on diagnosis of *Pharyngomyia* (above) apply here.

Control and Treatment. There are no recommendations for control, although it is likely that they are susceptible to macrocyclic lactone parasiticides.

Public Health Concerns. There are no documented cases of human infestation.

Management Implications. Howard (1977) suggested that there is little impact of this parasite at the host population level.

GENUS *RHINOESTRUS*

Description. Flies range from medium (11 mm) to large (20 mm) in size. They are characterized by the presence of tubercles, of variable size, on most body regions. Setae are often present on each tubercle. The thorax usually bears several large wheals on the pronotum and mesonotum, and these also have setae present. There are 11 species described in this genus.

First instars are dorsoventrally flattened, with three to seven rows of small spines at the anterior edge of each segment. The cephalic segment has prominent antennal lobes, and the mouth hooks are long and well developed (Guitton et al. 1996). At this stage the posterior stigmal plates have few openings. Second instar cephalic segments are large with prominent antennal lobes. The mouth hooks have become relatively smaller, in comparison to those in first instars. Spines on the thoracic and abdominal segments are slightly larger, but distribution remains similar to that of the first instar. The stigmal plates are relatively small with large pore-like openings.

Third instar cephalic segments are proportionally smaller than in the other instars. The antennal lobes are less distinct. Mouth hooks are prominent and of similar relative size to the second instar. Stigmal plates are large, with the central ecdysal scar clearly evident.

Life History. Knowledge of the behavior and life history of adults is limited to those species attacking domestic equids. Females of *R. purpureus* produce 700–800 larvae. The developmental rate of first instars is variable, resembling that of *Oestrus ovis.* In warmer climates there may be two generations per year. First instars migrate to the pharyngeal area just prior to molting to the second instar. Second and third instar development takes place in the same location.

Distribution and Host Range. Two of the known species, *R. latifrons* and *R. purpureus,* are exclusively parasites of domestic horses and donkeys; two other species (*R. steyni* and *R. usbekistanicus*) are reported from zebras (*Equus burchellii, Equus zebra*), of which the latter is also occasionally reported from domestic horses (Table 3.1). Two species with South African distribution are known from Springbuck (*Antidorcas marsupialis*). In central Africa one species is known from each of the giraffe, bushpig, warthog, and hippopotamus. A single species is reported from the "Argali" (*Ovis ammon*) in central Asia. Host specificity is generally high, although no experimental data support this observation.

Clinical Signs. Clinical symptoms of infestation are rarely evident, although a nasal discharge may be present.

Diagnosis. Comments for *Pharyngomyia* (above) apply here.

Control and Treatment. Several organophosphate systemic insecticides and the macrocyclic lactone parasiticides are effective.

Public Health Concerns. There are no documented cases of human infestation.

Domestic Animal Concerns. Except for those species known to have low host specificity, there are few concerns regarding domestic animals.

GENUS *OESTRUS*

Description. Flies are moderate in size with variable appearance. Abdomens have a light pilosity overlying a general black or grey color (Fig. 3.4). Heads are characterized by the presence of randomly distributed glossy black pits, and the thorax has a number of black tubercles (Fig. 3.5). *Oestrus aureoargentatus* has a dense yellow pilosity on the thorax, but the black tubercles are still clearly evident. *Oestrus ovis* and *O. caucasicus* are very similar except for the presence of distinctive black wing veins in the latter. Both species are sparsely pilose with a highly mottled yellow-brown to grey coloration. Adult *O. variolosus* are reddish brown with yellow, moderately dense pilosity and have a distinctive discal cross-vein.

Adult mouthparts are vestigial, although observations suggest that flies can imbibe water, as has been demonstrated for some other oestrids (Catts and Garcia 1963). Both sexes are active and aggressive fliers. Sexual dimorphism is evidenced in the greater interocular distance seen in the female flies.

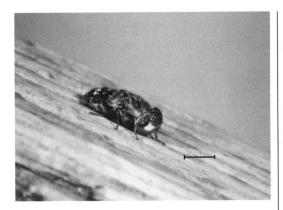

FIG. 3.4—Adult *Oestrus ovis,* habitus view. Hairs are absent on the thorax and abdomen. (Bar = 0.5 cm) (Photograph by P. J. Scholl, Fort Dodge Animal Health, New Jersey.)

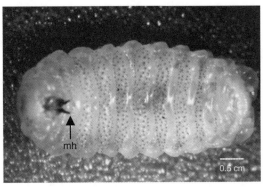

FIG. 3.6—Dorsal view of third instar *Oestrus ovis,* recovered from naturally infested sheep (*Ovis aries*). Note the prominent mouth hooks (**mh**). (Photograph by P. J. Scholl, Fort Dodge Animal Health, New Jersey.)

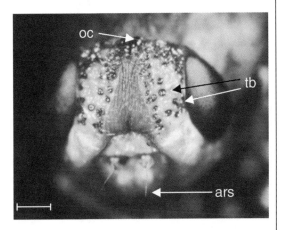

FIG. 3.5—Close-up view of the head of *Oestrus ovis.* Note the prominent tubercles (tb), as well as the ocelli (oc) and arista (ars) on the antenna. (Bar = 0.5 cm) (Photograph by P. J. Scholl, Fort Dodge Animal Health, New Jersey.)

First instars are somewhat dorsoventrally flattened (see Colwell and Scholl 1995) with well-developed spines on the ventral and lateral surfaces. Mouth hooks are prominent, and a group of strong hooks is present on the last abdominal segment. Posterior spiracles are difficult to see at this stage. Second instars are highly variable in size and are usually white. Spines and mouth hooks are well developed. Characteristic spiracular plates are visible on the terminal segments. Third instars are robust and moderate in size (Fig. 3.6). They move about aggressively when expelled from the host. Prominent mouth hooks (Fig. 3.6) are highly sclerotized, as are the bands of spines present on the ventral surfaces of thoracic and abdominal segments. Third

instars of *O. caucasicus* have strong dorsal spines. Spiracular plates are conspicuous on the terminal abdominal segment and are completely black on mature specimens.

Life History. Life cycle information comes primarily from work done on *O. ovis* in domestic sheep. Porchinski (1913) gives a detailed account, based on work conducted in Russia. The developmental period of the first instars, ejected from passing females onto the host nose, is highly variable, lasting 1–9 months. Factors that influence the length of development are not established, although host immunity and crowding may be two (D.D. Colwell, unpublished). Prior to molting, first instars move into the frontal sinuses where the remainder of their development takes place. Mature third instars migrate from the sinuses, fall to the ground, and pupate under the surface litter. Pupal development is highly dependent on environmental conditions, but averages ~6 weeks. Egg development occurs during the pupal stage, and oogenesis is complete prior to adult eclosion. Newly emerged flies mate quickly, after which eggs move from the ovary to begin embryonation in the uterus. Developmental rate of infective larvae is temperature dependent (12–17 days at 16°C–20°C: D.D. Colwell, unpublished).

Distribution and Host Range. *Oestrus ovis* has a worldwide distribution, largely coincident with man's movement of domestic sheep and goats (Table 3.1). Larvae have low host specificity; a variety of wildlife species host this parasite. Three species, *O. aureoargentatus, O. bassoni,* and *O. variolosus,* infest hosts in the tribes Alcelaphini and Hippotragini throughout sub-Saharan Africa (Table 3.1). One species (*O. caucasicus*) appears to have a relatively narrow host range, being found only in some members of the Caprini, such as the Siberian ibex (*Capra ibex*) (Grunin 1957). Larvae have also been reported from *Capra sibirica* in

Mongolia (Minar et al. 1985). Recently the range has been extended to include Europe with descriptions of infestations in the Spanish ibex (*Capra pyrenaica*), and there are suggestions that this parasite is widely distributed in the Palearctic region (Perez et al. 1996).

Prevalence and Intensity. *Oestrus caucasicus* was reported to have a mean prevalence of 74% with significantly more female Spanish ibex being parasitized than males (Perez et al. 1996). Prevalence also increased with host age, with fewer animals ≤ 1 year being parasitized than those > 5 years of age. Intensity ranged from 1 to 142, with a mean intensity of 25.4 ± 27.3 larvae. Older hosts had higher intensities than younger ones.

Clinical Signs. Clinical symptoms are rarely evident, although a nasal discharge may be present. Levels of circulating eosinophils may be elevated during some phases of the infestation (Nguyen et al. 1996).

Diagnosis. Comments for *Pharyngomyia* (above) apply here. Detection of circulating antibodies, through the use of ELISA or other related techniques has been used for diagnosis of infestation in sheep. These approaches have not been applied to diagnosis in wildlife although potentially then could be (Bautista-Garfias et al. 1988; Innocenti et al. 1995). Elevation of mast cells and eosinophils in infested animals may increase susceptibility to respiratory diseases (Nguyen et al. 1996).

Control and Treatment. Larvae are controlled by application of systemic organophosphate insecticides and the macrocyclic lactone parasiticides.

Public Health Concerns. Female flies are not particularly selective in their choice of hosts, and numerous examples of human ophthalmomyiasis are reported worldwide (e.g., Rakusin 1970; Reingold et al. 1984; Repkeny 1985; Amr et al. 1993).

Domestic Animal Concerns. Domestic animals are probably the major source of infestation of wildlife. However, with the advent of highly effective macrocyclic lactone endectocides and their growing usage in domestic sheep, the potential for transmission of *O. ovis* to wildlife is greatly reduced. At present, wildlife species are more likely to act as reservoirs for reinfestation of domestic sheep with *O. ovis*.

Management Implications. Movement of *O. ovis* infested sheep can pose a threat to related wildlife species. In North America, however, the ease of treatment has reduced the danger of this occurrence.

GENUS *GEDOELSTIA*

Description. Flies are moderately sized, generally brown in color with the thorax covered by dense brown hairs and with black patches on the abdomen. Abdominal segments have large laterally located tubercles that terminate in sharp spines. The two species can be separated on the basis of the presence of black glossy weals on the dorsal thorax of *G. cristata*. In addition, abdominal tubercles on *G. hässleri* are smaller than the ones found on *G. cristata*.

First instars have large mouth hooks and a characteristic pattern of spines on the anterior thoracic segments. The species can be differentiated on the basis of differences in spine patterns on the dorsal surface: the anterior margin of each segment has a two short bands on *G. hässleri*, whereas on *G. cristata* the bands are long, almost extending across the width of the specimen. Posterior spiracles are bell shaped and are subterminal. Second and third instars are without spines dorsally and have only a few spines on the ventral surface. Large third instars have typical spiracular plates with a characteristic suture running vertically down from the ecdysal scar. This feature allows easy identification of third instars of this genus.

Life History. Females larviposit on or near the eyes, and first instars begin an unusual migration. Larvae apparently move from the eye into the vascular system or travel along the optic nerve and migrate to the subdural cavity and dura mater. Larvae move to the nasal cavities via the foramina of the cribriform plate and ethmoid bones. The last two instars complete development at that site (Basson 1966; Horak and Butt 1977). Mature third instars migrate from the host's nasal cavities, fall to the ground, and burrow into the soil to pupate. Pupal development period ranges from 21 to 66 days (Basson 1966).

Fly activity and oviposition occur from October to May. This coincides with the recovery of the highest number of first instars. Second and third instars are recovered from hosts throughout the year, with peak infestations recorded in the spring. Larvae appear to mature at different rates and exit the host throughout the year. Horak and Butt (1977) suggest that larvae maturing during the winter months do not survive to produce flies.

Distribution and Host Range. This genus is restricted to the central and southern regions of Africa and are parasites of Alcelaphine antelopes (blue wildebeest, black wildebeest—*C. gnou*), common and Lichtenstein's hartebeest (*Alcelaphus buselaphus* and *A. lichtensteini*), blesbok (*Damaliscus dorcas phillipsi*), tsessebe (*Damaliscus lunatus*), and koorigum (*Damaliscus korrigum*) (Table 3.1).

Prevalence and Intensity. Prevalence in blesbok is reported to be 100% with intensities ranging from 93 to 248 larvae (Horak and Butt 1977).

Clinical Signs. No clinical signs are associated with infestations.

Pathology and Diagnosis. Pathologic changes have been noted in a variety of tissues in natural hosts. Small petechial hemorrhages were noted in ocular conjunctiva; small lesions were found in the cardiovascular system and in the meninges. None of the changes appeared to have serious consequences.

Regarding diagnosis, comments for *Pharyngomyia* (above) apply here.

Control and Treatment. There are no recommendations for treatment of animals infested with these nose bots. However, it is likely that application of macrocyclic lactone parasiticides would be effective.

Domestic Animal Concerns. Infestations of domestic livestock, including sheep, cattle, goats, and horses, produce a severe disease condition referred to as "utipeuloog" (Basson 1962a,b,c). This disease is manifested in three forms, ophthalmic, encephalitic, and cardiac, coinciding with the three major organ systems affected by the migrating larvae. Outbreaks associated with the movement of wildebeest through livestock-producing regions have resulted in up to 75% morbidity in the livestock.

GENUS *OESTROMYIA*

Description. Flies are small with an orange and yellow head and a distinctive black ocellar triangle. Mouthparts of *O. leporina* are severely reduced (Rietschel, 1981). The thorax and abdomen are black with dark hairs on the thorax, while the abdomen is naked. The legs are black. Five species are described, but little is known about two.

Eggs have an attachment organ similar to that described for *Hypoderma*. First instars are hyaline with large mouth hooks and sparsely distributed rows of spines. They resemble *H. lineatum* (Colwell 1986). Second instars are yellowish with distinct anterior thoracic spiracles. Bands of small, posteriorly directed spines are present on each segment. Third instars are cream colored, but darken to a dark greyish green as they mature. Third instar *O. leporina* are very similar in overall appearance to *Hypoderma* spp. (see Colwell et al. 1998).

Life History. Adult *O. leporina* have been shown to be capable of imbibing water, which may extend their survival in the wild. The majority of information on development has been obtained for *O. leporina* in both natural and laboratory hosts. Females produce ~500 eggs.

First instars penetrate the skin and undergo migration in the loose connective tissues (Reitschel 1975). Following a brief migration (3–4 days), larvae appear beneath the skin in posterior regions. A hole is digested in the skin, and a typical warble is formed.

Second instars develop for 16–25 days. Third instars complete their development within ~10 days. The mature third instars exit the host and quickly burrow into the soil to pupate. Pupae enter a diapause that lasts 4–5 months.

Distribution and Host Range. *Oestromyia* spp. are restricted to the Palearctic region, where they are parasites of rodents and lagomorphs of the family Ochotonidae (pikas) and Marmotidae (Table 3.1). Species infesting pikas and marmots tend to be host specific. In contrast, *O. leporina* has been described from a range of hosts, including voles, muskrats, and squirrels (Golubev 1960; Sugar 1976a). Laboratory rodents have also been successfully infested (Reitschel 1975).

Prevalence and Intensity. Volf et al. (1990) reported that prevalence was variable between years (range: 0.1–12). Rarely will the prevalence be > 50%. Hosts usually have one larva, but occasionally there may be as many as seven. Golubev (1960) reported lower prevalences of *O. leporina* in younger voles than in older animals. This is in contrast to *O. marmotae* in which older animals have dramatically lower prevalences than the young.

Pathology/Diagnosis/Immunity. The only pathological changes reported are those associated with the development of the furuncle surrounding the developing second and third instar larvae. Reitschel (1975) found that laboratory rodents acquire a protective immunity following primary infestation, although conflicting evidence from field studies does not support the development of solid immunity.

Comments on diagnosis of *Pharyngomyia* (above) apply here.

GENUS *HYPODERMA*

Description. Flies are medium sized with a dense covering of yellow/gold hairs. They have a striking resemblance to bumble bees. Legs are lightly haired. The facial region of the head is covered with long, dense hairs that obscure the absence of functional mouthparts.

The eggs are smooth surfaced and cream colored and are attached to the hairs of the host by the ovipositing females. A special attachment organ on the basal portion aids in holding the eggs firmly on the hair shaft (Cogley et al. 1981). Newly hatched first instars are white with a sparse covering of small spines (see Colwell 1986). No features are known to distinguish larvae of the various species, although the cattle-infesting species can be distinguished by the structure of the cephalopharyngeal skeleton. Second instars are stouter and broader than first instars and have small bands of spines on each segment. Third instars are robust and have distinctive bands of spines on both ventral and dorsal surfaces. These larvae are a light cream colored at first, but gradually darken until they are completely black at maturity.

Several characteristics can be used to distinguish between third instars of this genus. Distribution of spines on the anterior segments (Fig 3.7.) are distinct for each species. In addition, the spiracular plates of the

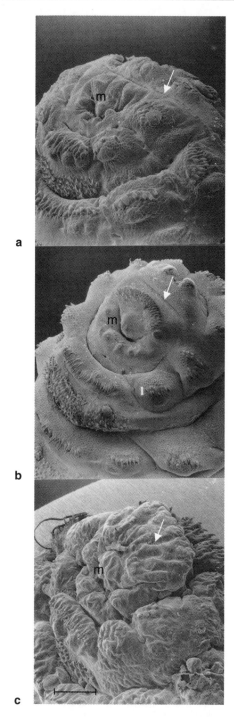

a

b

c

FIG. 3.7—Scanning electron micrographs of the cephalic and thoracic segments of third instar *Hypoderma actaeon, H. diana,* and *H. tarandi.* (**a**) *H. actaeon:* note the absence of spines between the opercular suture (arrow) and the mouth (m), as well as the small band of heavy spines ventral to the mouth. (**b**) *H. diana:* note the band of spines between the opercular suture (arrow) and the mouth (m), the spines ventral to the mouth are light and are more numerous than in the other species. (**c**) *H. tarandi:* note the few large spines between the opercular suture (arrow) and the mouth (m) and the band of robust spines ventral to the mouth. (Bar = 0.5 cm)

various species have characteristics that allow identification of species (Fig. 3.8), and there are differences in spine morphology (Figs. 3.9, 3.10; also see Colwell et al. 1998).

Life History. Much data are derived from studies on species from cattle, although new data have recently been reported for *H. tarandi* from reindeer. Mated females immediately engage in host-finding behavior, often flying immense distances in pursuit of migrating hosts such as reindeer (Nilssen and Anderson 1995). Environmental conditions necessary for flight are stringent, temperatures between 18° C and 22° C, with wind speeds less than 6 km/hour. Little is known of the oviposition behavior of the species parasitizing deer in Europe, but the extensive investigations on the reindeer fly provide good indications. Female *H. tarandi* have a complement of ~600 eggs [range: 354–824 (Nilssen 1997b)], not unlike that of the cattle-infesting species.

First instars move rapidly to the skin surface where they penetrate. *Hypoderma tarandi* first instars are known to move through connective tissue toward the back and rump of infested reindeer. Occasionally, larvae will enter muscle tissue, but this is not usual and may be deleterious. First instars increase in size approximately tenfold before molting. Little is known about migratory paths of first instar *H. diana* and *H. actaeon.*

Second and third instar development takes place within the granulomatous warble (Fig. 3.11). The granuloma increases in size as the larva grows and becomes quite evident in later stages. Larvae acquire all the nutrients required to complete development, pupate, produce eggs, and have fat body reserves to support extensive postmating flights in search of hosts.

Mature third instars exit the host and pupate within a short period of time. Pupal development is influenced by temperature and can take several weeks to complete.

Distribution and Host Range. Two species (*H. actaeon* and *H. tarandi*) appear to be host specific, although *H. tarandi* seems less so, being reported from red deer (Nilssen and Gjershaug 1988), roe deer (Skjenneberg and Slagsvold 1968), and muskox (*Ovibos moschatus*) (Jansen 1970). It is unclear if these larvae would be able to complete development in other than the primary host. *Hypderma diana* has a broader host range, having been reported from several deer species and mouflon (*Ovis ammon*). The cattle species are occasionally reported from wildlife; for example, *H. bovis* in North American bison (*Bison* spp.) and musk ox (Jansen 1970).

Hypoderma tarandi occurs throughout the range of its host, *Rangifer tarandus,* thus having a Holarctic distribution. The remaining species, *H. diana* and *H. actaeon,* are Palearctic in distribution.

Prevalence and Intensity. The prevalence of *H. tarandi* in Europe varies between herds, depending on host behavior during the postlarval period (Folstad et

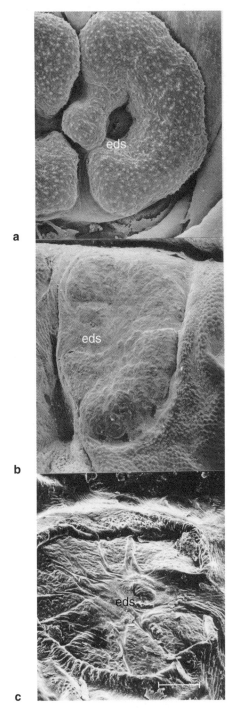

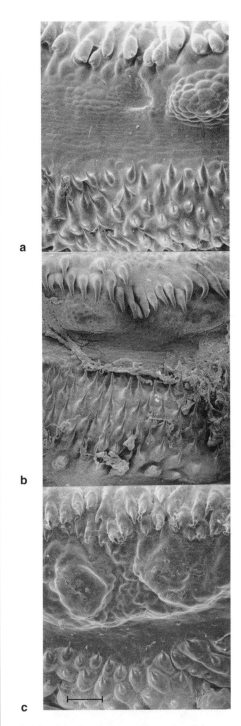

FIG. 3.8—Scanning electron micrographs of one posterior spiracular plate of third instar *Hypoderma actaeon, H. diana,* and *H. tarandi.* (**a**) *H. actaeon:* note the ecdysal scar (eds) completely surrounded by the plate, and the deep indentation of the plate around the ecdysal scar and note the spine on each spiracular opening. (**b**) *H. diana:* note the flat plate with the ecdysal scar incompletely surrounded and the absence of spines at the openings. (**c**) *H. tarandi:* note the flat plate completely surrounding the ecdysal scar, note also the absence of spines and the cuticular ridges subdividing the plate (arrows). (Bar = 0.3 mm)

FIG. 3.9—Scanning electron micrographs of the post-oral, ventral spines on the first thoracic segment of third instar *Hypoderma actaeon, H. diana,* and *H. tarandi.* A cluster of posterior directed spines (upper) is shown with the accompanying cluster of anterior directed spines (lower). (**a**) *H. actaeon:* note the posteriorly directed spines are robust, with broad bases and blunt tips; anteriorly directed spines have narrow bases and sharp tips. (**b**) *H. diana:* note the posteriorly directed spines have narrow bases and rounded tips; anteriorly directed spines have narrow bases and sharp tips. (**c**) *H. tarandi:* note the posteriorly directed spines have broad bases and rounded tips; anteriorly directed spines have broad bases and sharp tips. (Bar = 0.1 mm)

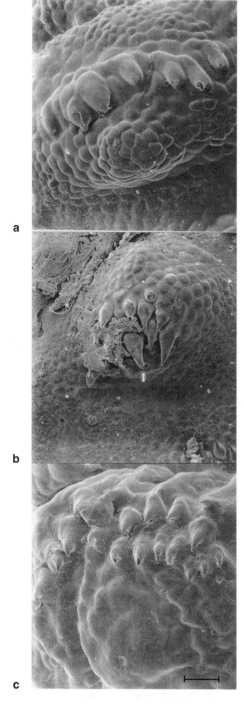

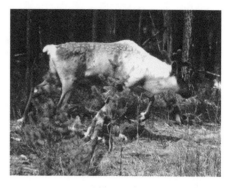

FIG. 3.11—Caribou (*Rangifer tarandus*) heavily infested with *Hypoderma tarandi*. Warbles containing second and third instars are present along the entire dorsal surface. Photograph was taken near Grande Cache, Alberta, May 1998. (By Michael Gray, Lethbridge, Alberta.)

al. 1991). Prevalence and intensity tend to be lower in herds that migrate from their calving grounds, the site where most larval stages emerge and drop from hosts, than in herds that remain near calving areas. Prevalence in males is higher than in females (Kelsal 1972; Folstad et al. 1991; Thomas and Kiliaan 1990). In North America, prevalence declines with increasing latitude, but postcalving migration tends to influence the prevalence in much the same way as in Europe (Thomas and Kiliaan 1990).

Intensities tend to range from 15 to 450 larvae. Younger animals have higher intensities than older animals, which may reflect acquired immunity similar to that seen in cattle (Folstad et al. 1991)

Prevalence of infestation with *H. diana* and *H. actaeon* in red deer and roe deer from central Europe and in red deer from Spain is 65%–98% (Sugar 1976a; Martinez-Gomez et al. 1990). Intensities range from 1 to 220 larvae.

Clinical Signs. There are no described clinical symptoms of warble infestation prior to the appearance of the granulomatous, subdermal furuncles (Fig. 3.11) occupied by the developing second and third instar larvae.

Diagnosis and Immunity. Hypodermosis is usually diagnosed by detection of larvae in furuncles on the back. Recovered third instars can be identified to species; however, mature specimens should be allowed to pupate and adults reared for definitive identification. Earlier instars are difficult to identify to species, and there are no known methods for culturing these stages to maturity.

Early diagnosis of infestations is possible through detection of specific antibodies, usually to secretory/excretory antigens, in serum. The techniques, which are classical approaches to detection of antibodies in serum (e.g., ELISA, complement fixation, indirect hemagglutination) have been developed for the cattle

FIG. 3.10—Scanning electron micrographs of the ventrolateral spines on the first throracic segment of third instar *Hypoderma actaeon, H. diana,* and *H. tarandi.* These spines are associated with a small pit sensillum, located below each spine cluster. (**a**) *H. actaeon:* note the robust spines, with broad bases and blunt tips. (**b**) *H. diana:* note the delicate spines with sharp tips, usually clustered close to the sensillum. (**c**) *H. tarandi:* note the broad based spines with sharp tips, not clustered near sensillum. (Bar = 100 μm)

species but are transferable to wildlife (Monfray and Boulard 1990).

Reindeer acquire protective immunity to *H. tarandi* (Folstad et al. 1989) as evidenced by the reduced larval intensities in older females. Male reindeer have increased intensities of infestation until their fifth year. This suggests the impairment of acquired immunity occurs in these males as a result of the presence of high levels of testosterone and stress-induced corticosteroids (Folstad et al. 1989). This trend is not evident in male castrates.

Control and Treatment. Systemic insecticides and/or macrocyclic lactone parasiticides are effective. The latter drugs are effective against larvae at all stages. Baits treated with macrocyclic lactone parasiticides offer an excellent option for controlling these parasites in wild ungulates.

Public Health Concerns. There are numerous reports of human ophthalmomyiasis resulting from larvae of *H. tarandi* (Kearney et al. 1991). Most reports come from Europe, where the reindeer hosts are semidomesticated and there is a close association between the hosts and herders. However, a recent report of ophthalmomyiasis in a Canadian Inuit suggests that the phenomenon may be underreported (Safneck et al. 1998). There is also the possibility that as the reindeer herds of northern Canada become more intensively managed, there will be an increased likelihood of accidental infestations.

Domestic Animal Concerns. Host specificity is generally considered to be high, and there are no known reports of transmission from wildlife to domestic livestock.

Management Implications. In some studies, weight gain of semidomesticated reindeer infested with *H. tarandi* is reduced (Oksanen and Nieminen 1996), but Arneberg et al. (1996) found no correlation between the presence of *H. tarandi* and reduced intake or weight gains. Intensity of infestation in the latter study was low.

Larvae present in warbles on the back reduce the aesthetic quality of affected animals (Fig. 3.11). Hides from animals harvested during that time are not usable. In addition, the carcass becomes unsightly, and substantial trim loss results from removal of affected areas. These factors combine to reduce the value of affected animals to hunters and thus present a concern for wildlife managers.

GENUS *CUTEREBRA*

Description. Flies are large and robust with a shining black or blue abdomen. The face, thorax, and abdomen are covered with patches of short hairs that give a mottled appearance. Several species exhibit a sexual

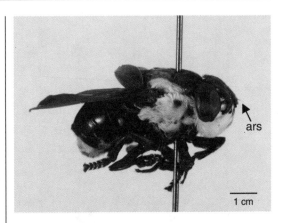

FIG. 3.12—Lateral view of a female *Cuterebra fontinella* reared from a larva collected from *Peromyscus maniculatus*. Note the long hairs on the thorax, the color pattern of the hairs and the bare abdomen (ars = arista). (Photograph by F. Brouwers, Taber, Alberta.)

dimorphism, with females being solid colors while the males have distinct white patches (e.g., *C. fontinella*) (Fig. 3.12). Males of several species that parasitize lagomorphs have characteristic red eyespots or bands that run vertically down the eye. These markings fade quickly after death. Legs are covered with dense hairs.

Eggs are dark in color and have a prominent operculum. Outer surfaces of the eggs are highly sculptured. Eggs of most species have the ventral surface distinctly flattened (see Colwell et al. 1999). There are numerous species for which the eggs remain undescribed.

Newly hatched first instars are white with 2–3 rows of large, recurved spines at the posterior edge of the thoracic and abdominal segments. Similar spines are also on the cephalic segment. These larvae have a large number of cuticular sensilla on the cephalic segment as well as on the body (see Colwell 1986). These presumably enable larvae to find the host and locate suitable sites to enter the host's body. Mouth hooks are well developed and prominent. The posterior "adhesive sack" aids the larvae in moving and in attaching to the host hair. The small posterior spiracles are located subterminally on the last abdominal segment. The second instars, living within the subdermal furuncle, are white to cream colored. Spine patterns vary between species, although they are generally simpler in shape than those of the first instar and are more generally distributed. The relative size of the cephalic segment is reduced in comparison to first instars. Spiracular plates with convoluted openings are located on the posterior abdominal segment.

Large third instars range in color from creamy white to black. They become darker as they mature. Spines are more numerous and larger than on the second instars, often covering the entire body. Terminal spirac-

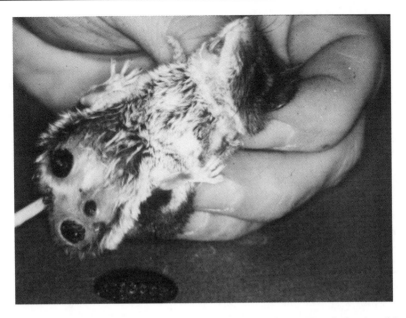

FIG. 3.13—Ventral view of a deer mouse (*Peromyscus* sp.) infested with *Cuterebra* sp. Note the location of the warbles containing the larvae. (Photograph by C. R. Baird, University of Idaho, Moscow, Idaho.)

ular plates are prominent and bear three highly convoluted spiracular openings.

Life History. Females emerge from puparia with the eggs partially developed and require several days for completion of egg development (Scholl 1991). Males generally emerge before the females and gather at aggregation sites. Mated females are oviparous and search for highly specific oviposition sites. Selection and acceptance of these oviposition sites is probably regulated by the detection of host chemicals.

Embryonation requires several days, after which eggs are capable of hatching in response to enviromental changes associated with the proximity of a potential host. Not all larvae from a single batch will hatch at the same time.

Newly hatched first instars are aggressive in their host-finding and in their search for openings through which to enter the host. Once inside, internal migration requires only a few days, after which the larvae move to subdermal sites and are enclosed within the host-derived warble. Warbles with developing second and third instars are found at specific locations on the host (Fig. 3.13), although some variation in location is evident.

Second and third instar development occurs within the warble, and increases in size are large and rapid. Mature third instars leave the host and burrow beneath surface debris and soil to pupate. In temperate species pupae will overwinter in a diapause state.

Distribution and Host Range. *Cuterebra* are found throughout the New World as parasites of rodents and lagomorphs. Sabrosky (1986) provides an excellent summary of the hosts and distribution of the known species. Some species have strict host specificity while others have a broad host range. *Cuterebra polita* is an example of the latter which has usually been reported from *Thomomys* but recently has been described from a population of Ord's kangaroo rats (*Dipodomys ordii*) in southeastern Alberta (Gummer et al. 1997). There are also numerous reports of larvae developing in what may be termed aberrant hosts (Sabrosky 1986), including humans (Baird et al. 1989) and domestic livestock.

Prevalence and Intensity. Prevalence of bot infestation is highly variable, with reports ranging from < 2% to > 30%. Seasonal variation in prevalence is usual, particularly in the northern range where the insects overwinter as diapausing pupae.

Clinical Signs. Few clinical signs of infestation have been described prior to the development of the furuncle containing the developing second and third instar larvae. Occasional reports of coughing and wheezing have been noted in experimental hosts (Baird 1971) and there are also reports of unilateral paralysis and death from aberrant movement of larvae (Catts 1982). The most evident clinical manifestation is the granulomatous furuncle within which the larvae complete development (Fig. 3.13).

Diagnosis and Immunity. Diagnosis of cuterebrid infestations is based on presence of the larva within the furuncle. Recovered third instars can usually be identified to species, however mature specimens should be allowed to pupate and adults reared for definitive identification. Specimens from temperate regions will usually enter a pupal diapause and will require a period of culture at low temperature before development will proceed following culture at warmer temperatures. Earlier instars are difficult to identify to species, and there are no known methods for culturing these stages to maturity.

Infested hosts develop circulating antibodies to larval antigens that can be detected prior to the appearance of larvae in the furuncle. Standard techniques such as ELISA have been used for detection of antibodies, but their usefulness as a diagnostic tool in wildlife has not been examined.

Control and Treatment. Cuterebrid larvae are sensitive to the macrocyclic lactone parasiticides. These compounds are extremely effective against bots at all stages. Treatment of baits offers a potential option for controlling these parasites in wildlife populations.

Public Health Concerns. There are occasional reports of human infestation (Baird et al. 1989). These cases tend to occur during late summer when adult flies are most numerous. Human infestations have resulted from incidental hatching of eggs that occur when the ovipositional environment is encountered during outdoor activities.

Domestic Animal Concerns. Domestic animals are occasionally accidental hosts of *Cuterebra* spp. (Catts 1982). Their impact is generally of little concern.

Management Implications. Assessment of the impact of cuterebrid infestations on host populations has produced equivocal results. Gummer et al. (1997) suggest that the cost of cuterebrid parasitism to hosts whose nutiriton is limited may be sufficient to reduce reproductive success and survival. Similar observations have been made for other genera of cuterebids (see Milton 1996).

GENUS *ALOUATTAMYIA*

Description. Only one species, *A. baeri,* is known (Table 3.1). Flies are large and completely black and have a dense covering of black hairs. Males have a characteristic vertical red stripe running across their eyes, a feature that quickly fades after death (Colwell and Miton 1998).

Eggs are laid in long rows and are firmly attached to the substrate. The outer surface is highly sculptured, and a prominent dorsal operculum is present (see Colwell et al. 1999). Newly hatched first instars are white, highly active maggots with well-developed mouth hooks and rows of recurved spines on the posterior edge of each thoracic and abdominal segment. These larvae have numerous, diverse cuticular sensilla on the

cephalic segment and on the thoracic and abdominal segments. Second instars are white, with prominent mouth hooks and rows of spines on all segments. Spines have a simple shape and are uniformly distributed. Third instars, initially cream colored after the molt become black at maturity. The entire body of this stage has a dense covering of broad, flat spines.

Pupae are black with a prominent operculum through which the adult fly will emerge. At pupariation the anterior spiracles are extruded. They are white and stand out prominently at the anterior end of the pupa.

Life History. There is no information on adult behavior although it is suspected that they have habits similar to those of other cuterebrids. There is one anecdotal report of males aggregating high in the tropical rain forest (Catts 1982). Laboratory studies suggest the females deposit eggs on leaf or tree surfaces. Development of the larvae within the eggs takes ~5 days at 26° C. Proximity of the host, which results in a rapid warming of the eggs and an increase in CO_2 concentration, will trigger hatching.

Laboratory studies suggest that larvae enter the host through moist body openings and go through a short migration within the host prior to reaching subdermal sites, usually around the neck (Colwell and Milton 1998). The migratory period within a laboratory host (*Oryctolagus cuniculus*) is 5–6 days.

Second and third instars develop within furuncles, feeding on host serum and white blood cells. Development in *Oryctolagus cuniculus* requires 32–37 days, after which the larvae exit the furuncle, fall to the ground, and rapidly bury themselves in the leaf litter and soil. Mature third instars pupate within 1–2 days. Development of adults takes 35–48 days at 26° C, with the males developing more quickly than the females (36 vs. 39 days).

Distribution and Host Range. *A. baeri* is thought to be highly host specific, parasitizing hosts of the howler monkey genus, *Alouatta*. The primary host is the mantled howler monkey, *A. palliata*. There are only occasional reports from other hosts, including another monkey *Aotus trivirgatus* and man (Catts 1982). In addition, artificial infestations have been established in laboratory rabbits (Colwell and Milton 1998). Reports of infestations occur throughout the range of the host: Central America and the tropical rain forest regions of South America.

Prevalence and Intensity. Milton (1996) described the seasonal changes in prevalence and intensity in an isolated population of howler monkeys. Although there is substantial between-year variation, prevalence tends to fall during the dry season. Intensities also vary between years, but differences between age groups are not evident.

Clinical Signs. Hosts develop large furuncles that are clearly evident (Fig. 3.14).

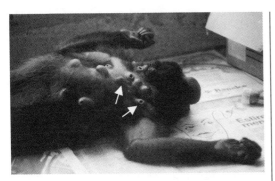

FIG. 3.14—View of a Howler monkey (*Alouatta palliata*) from Barro Colorado Island, Panama, infested with *Alouattamyia baeri*. Furuncles or warbles containing larvae are evident around the throat and on the chest (arrows). Larvae are predominantly third instar as evidenced by the large size of the warbles and the large openings.

Diagnosis and Immunity. Infested monkeys develop antibodies to a range of second and third instar proteins (Baron et al. 1996). However, there appears to be little indication that protective immunity is acquired by the host as prevalence and intensity of infestation in older animals is not different from that of younger monkeys (Milton 1996). K. Milton and N. Lerchka (unpublished) found no significant alterations in white blood cell populations in monkeys with a wide range of infestation intensities.

Diagnosis of infestations is based on presence of the larva within the furuncle. Recovered third instars can be identified; however, mature specimens should be allowed to pupate, and adults should be reared for definitive identification. Earlier instars are difficult to identify, and there are no known methods for culturing these stages to maturity.

Control and Treatment. No control methods have been developed for the larvae of this genus. The sensitivity of many other oestrid larvae to macrocyclic lactone parasiticides suggests that they may be effective; however, application may be difficult. The use of treated baits would not likely be useful given the specialized diet of the howler monkey.

Public Health Concerns. There is only one case report of human infestation; larvae were recovered from the scalp of two indigenous people in the Amazon basin (Guimaraes and Coimbra 1982).

Domestic Animal Concerns. Host specificity of this genus appears to be high, and there are no reports of accidental infestations other than the one human case. It appears that the host specificity is the result of the ecological requirements of the ovipositing flies and not barriers to development in unusual hosts. This contention is supported by development of larvae in experimental hosts (rabbits) (Colwell and Milton 1998).

Management Implications. A long-term study of howler monkey populations on Barro Colorado island in Panama (Milton 1996) suggested that these maggots are a major factor restricting the growth of the monkey populations at this site.

GENUS *METACUTEREBRA*

Description. Flies are large and have a dense covering of fine hairs. Both abdomen and thorax are light colored with patches of dark hairs in either bands (abdomen) or speckles (thorax). Males may have large dark patches on the dorsal surface of the thorax. Legs are dark with a dense covering of hairs. Males have a characteristic vertical red eye band that disappears shortly after death.

The brown eggs are elongate, cylindrical and slightly pointed at both ends and have a distinct flattening of the ventral surface. They have a highly sculptured outer surface and a prominent, dorsal operculum (Leite and Williams 1989). Newly hatched first instars are whitish, with prominent bands of large, recurved spines at the posterior edge of the cephalic, thoracic, and abdominal segments. The mouth hooks are large and prominent. Cephalic sensilla are large and numerous. The larvae use a terminal adhesive sac both to attach to the substrate and as an aid in locomotion.

Second and third instars have not been described.

Life History. *Metacuterebra* larvae are generally parasites of rodents (Table 3.1). Life cycle observations in this genus have been made on *M. apicalis* (Leite and Williams 1988, 1989) in natural hosts that include a number of neotropical rodents and in laboratory hosts.

Female *M. apicalis* have a large reproductive capacity (2500–2900 eggs/female). Under experimental conditions the eggs are attached to a filter paper substrate in rows (Leite and Williams 1988). The natural oviposition sites and substrates have not been determined. Eggs of *M. apicalis* require 7–10 days to develop at ~26° C. As with other cuterebrids, eggs of this species hatch in response to warming and an increase in CO_2 concentration. The newly hatched first instars enter the host via a moist body opening, the nares or eye. Development within the host, including the period of time in the subdermal warble, ranges from 21–26 days in the usual host *Oryzomys subflavus* to 22 –31 days in the laboratory rat (*Rattus norvegicus*). Mature third instars are large (1.32g ♂; 1.49g ♀) and quickly form puparia following exit from the host. Pupal development was similar for males and females (~32 days). The sex ratio appears skewed in favor of females, but data are limited. Under laboratory conditions the flies are extremely short lived (~6 days), although there are reports of the flies living up to 15 days.

Distribution and Host Range. All described species are Neotropical, ranging from Mexico to northern Argentina. The host range appears to be broad; there are reports of this genus parasitizing several species of cricetid rodents as well as marsupials (*Metachirus nudicaudatus, Didelphis* sp.). Rats (*Rattus norvegicus*) have been reported as hosts in artificial infestations.

Prevalence and Intensity. Recent research by Vieira (1993) on several rodent species from the cerrado of central Brazil showed that prevalence varied between the species of host (range: 3%–11%). Prevalence was much higher in the rodents of a tropical rainforest (range: 12%–50%) (Bossi and Bergallo 1992) than on the dry cerrado. The mean intensities in the two biomes were similar at ~1.0. Everard and Aitken (1972) and Twigg (1965) report similar prevalences in tropical rain forests.

Clinical Signs. Development of large subcutaneous furuncles is the most evident clinical sign. There is a likelihood that some respiratory symptoms may be observed since the life cycle resembles that of *Cuterebra.*

Diagnosis. Diagnosis of infestations is based on presence of the larva within the furuncle. No keys are available for larval stages. Recovered third instars should be allowed to pupate, and should be adults for definitive identification. Earlier instars are difficult to identify, and there are no known methods for culturing these stages to maturity.

LITERATURE CITED

Amr, Z.S., B.A. Amr, and M.N. Abo-Shehada. 1993. Ophthalmomyiasis externa caused by *Oestrus ovis* L. in the Ajloun area of northern Jordan. *Annals of Tropical Medicine and Parasitology* 87:259–262.

Anderson, J.R. 1975. The behavior of nose bot flies (*Cephenemyia apicata* and *C. jellisoni*) when attacking black-tailed deer (*Odocoileus hemionus columbianus*) and the resulting reactions of the deer. *Canadian Journal of Zoology* 53:977–992.

Anderson, J.R., and A.C. Nilssen. 1990. The method by which *Cephenemyia trompe* (Modeer) larvae invade reindeer (*Rangifer tarandus*). *Rangifer, Special Issue* 3:291–297.

Anderson, J.R., and A.C. Nilssen. 1996a. Trapping oestrid parasites of reindeer: The response of *Cephenemyia trompe* and *Hypoderma tarandi* to baited traps. *Medical and Veterinary Entomology* 10:337–346.

———. 1996b. Trapping oestrid parasites of reindeer: The relative age, fat body content and gonotrophic conditions of *Cephenemyia trompe* and *Hypoderma tarandi* females caught in baited traps. *Medical and Veterinary Entomology* 10:347–353.

Anderson, J.R., A.C. Nilssen, and I. Folstad. 1994. Mating behavior and thermoregulation of the reindeer warble fly, *Hypoderma tarandi* L. (Diptera: Oestridae). *Journal of Insect Behavior* 7:679–706.

Arneberg, P., I. Folstad, and A.J. Karter. 1996. Gastrointestinal nematodes depress food intake in naturally infected reindeer. *Parasitology* 112:213–219.

Baird, C.R. 1971. Development of *Cuterebra jellisoni* (Diptera: Cuterbridae) in six species of rabbits and rodents. *Journal of Medical Entomology* 8:615–622.

Baird, J.K., C.R. Baird, and C.W. Sabrosky. 1989. North American cuterebrid myiasis. *Journal of the American Academy of Dermatology* 21:763–772.

Baron R.W. 1990. Cleavage of purified bovine complement component C3 in larval *Hypoderma lineatum* (Diptera: Oestridae) hypodermins. *Journal of Medical Entomology* 27:899–904.

Baron, R.W., D.D. Colwell, and K. Milton. 1996. Antibody immunoglobulin G (IgG) response to bot fly (*Alouattamyia baeri*) parasitism in a howler monkey (*Alouatta palliata*) population in Panama. *Medical Entomology* 33:946–951.

Basson, P.A. 1962a. Studies on specific oculo-vascular myiasis of domestic animals (utipeuloog). I. Historical review. *Onderstepoort Journal of Veterinary Research* 29:81–87.

———. 1962b. Studies on specific oculo-vascular myiasis of domestic animals (utipeuloog). II. Experimental transmission *Onderstepoort Journal of Veterinary Research* 29:203–209.

———. 1962c. Studies on specific oculo-vascular myiasis of domestic animals (utipeuloog). III. Symptomatology, pathology, aetiology and epizootiology. *Onderstepoort Journal of Veterinary Research* 29:211–240.

———. 1966. Gedoelstial myiasis in antelopes of Southern Africa. *Onderstepoort Journal of Veterinary Research* 33:77–92.

Bautista-Garfias, C.R., R.M. Angulo-Contreras, and E. Garay-Garzon. 1988. Serologic diagnosis of *Oestrus ovis* (Diptera: Oestridae) in naturally infested sheep. *Medical and Veterinary Entomology* 2:351–355.

Bennett, G.F. 1962. On the biology of *Cephenemyia phobifera* (Diptera: Oestridae), the pharyngeal bot of the white-tailed deer, *Odocoileus virginianus*. *Canadian Journal of Zoology* 40:1195–1210.

Bennett, G.F., and C.W. Sabrosky. 1962. The nearctic species of the genus *Cephenemyia* (Diptera: Oestridae). *Canadian Journal of Zoology* 40:431–448.

Boonstra, R., C.J. Krebs, and T.D. Beecham. 1980. Impact of bot fly parasitism on *Microtus townsendii* populations. *Canadian Journal of Zoology* 58:1683–1692.

Bossi, D.E.P., and H. de G. Bergallo. 1992. Parasitism by cuterebrid botflies (*Metacuterebra apicalis*) in *Orzomys nitidus* (Rodentia: Cricetidae) and *Metachirus nudicaudatus* (Marsupialia: Didelphidae) in a southeastern Brazilian rain forest. *The Journal of Parasitology* 78:142–145.

Boulard C. 1989. Degradation of bovine C3 by serine proteases from parasites *Hypoderma lineatum* (Diptera: Oestridae). *Veterinary Immunology and Immunopathology* 20:387–398.

Boulard, C., C. Villejoubert, and N. Moire. 1996. Cross-reactive stage-specific antigens in the Oestridae family. *Veterinary Research* 27:535–544.

Breev, K. A. 1950. The behaviour of blood sucking insects and bot flies and the reaction of the reindeer to the attack [In Russian]. *Sbornik Trudov Naucho-Issledovatel'skogo Institua Meditsinskoi Parazitologii I Tropicheskoi Meditsing Gruzinskoi SSR* 12:167–198.

Capelle K.J. 1971. Myiasis. In *Parasitic diseases of wild mammals*. Ed. J.W. Davis and R.C. Anderson. Ames: The Iowa State University Press, pp. 279–305.

Catts, E.P. 1964. Field behaviour of adult *Cephenemyia* (Diptera: Oestridae). *The Canadian Entomologist* 96:579–585.

———. 1982. Biology of New World bot flies: Cuterebridae. *Annual Review of Entomology* 27:313–338.

———. 1994. Sex and the bachelor bot (Diptera: Oestridae). *American Entomologist* Fall 1994: 153–160.

Catts, E.P., and R. Garcia. 1963. Drinking by adult *Cephenemyia* (Diptera: Oestridae). *Annals of the Entomological Society of America* 56:660–663.

Cepeda-Palacios, R., and P.J. Scholl. 1999. Gonotrophic development in *Oestrus ovis* (Diptera: Oestridae). *Journal of Medical Entomology* 36:435–440.

Chaboudie, N., and C. Boulard. 1992. Effect of hypodermin A, an enzyme secreted by *Hypoderma lineatum* (Insect Oestridae), on the bovine immune system. *Veterinary Immunology and Immunopathology* 31:167–177.

Cogley, T.P. 1987. Effects of *Cephenemyia* spp. (Diptera: Oestridae) on the nasopharynx of black-tailed deer (*Odocoileus hemionus columbianus*). *Journal of Wildlife Diseases* 23:596–605.

———. 1991. Warble development by the rodent bot *Cuterebra fontinella* (Diptera: Cuterebridae) in the deer mouse. *Veterinary Parasitology* 38:275–288.

Cogley, T.P., and J.R. Anderson. 1981. Invasion of black-tailed deer by nose bot fly larvae (Diptera: Oestridae: Oestrinae). *International Journal for Parasitology* 11:281–286.

Cogley, T.P., J.R. Anderson, and J. Weintraub. 1981. Ultrastructure and function of the attachment organ of warble fly eggs (Diptera: Oestridae: Hypodermatinae). *International Journal of Insect Morphology and Embryology* 10:7–18.

Colwell, D.D. 1986. Cuticular sensilla on newly hatched larvae of *Cuterebra fontinella* Clark (Diptera: Cuterebridae) and *Hypoderma* spp. (Diptera: Oestridae). *International Journal of Insect Morphology and Embryology* 75:385–392.

———. 1989a. Scanning electron microscopy of the posterior spiracles of cattle grubs. *Medical and Veterinary Entomology* 3:391–398.

———. 1989b. Host-parasite relationships and adaptations to parasitism of first instar cattle grubs, *Hypoderma bovis* (L.) and *H. lineatum* (Vill.). Ph.D. thesis, Department of Environmental Biology, University of Guelph, Guelph, Ontario, 226 pp.

Colwell, D.D., and N.M. Berry. 1993. Tarsal sensilla of warble flies [*Hypoderma bovis* and *H. lineatum* (Diptera: Oestridae)]. *Annals of the Entomological Society of America* 86:756–765.

Colwell, D.D., and M. Kavaliers. 1992. Evidence for activation of endogenous opioid systems in mice following short exposure to stable flies. *Medical and Veterinary Entomology* 6:159–164.

———. 1993. Evidence for involvement of endogenous opioid peptides in altered nociceptive responses of mice infected with *Eimeria vermiformis*. *The Journal of Parasitology* 79:751–756.

Colwell, D.D., and E.G. Kokko. 1986. Preparation of dipteran larvae for scanning electron microscopy using a freeze substitution technique. *Canadian Journal of Zoology* 64:797–799.

Colwell, D.D., and K. Milton. 1998. Development of *Alouattamyia baeri* (Diptera: Oestridae) from howler monkeys (*Alouatta palliata*) on Barro Colorado Island, Panama. *Journal of Medical Entomology* 35:674–680.

Colwell, D.D., and P.J. Scholl. 1995. Cuticular sensilla on newly hatched larvae of *Gasterophilus intestinalis* (deGeer) and *Oestrus ovis* (L.). *Medical and Veterinary Entomology* 9:85–93.

Colwell, D.D., M. Kavaliers, and T.J. Lysyk. 1997. Stable fly mouthpart removal influences stress and anticipatory responses in mice. *Medical and Veterinary Entomology* 11:310–314.

Colwell, D.D., F.J. Martinez-Moreno, A. Martinez-Moreno, S. Hernandez-Rodriquez, C. De la Fuente-Lopez, J.M. Alunda, and M.J.R. Hall. 1998. Comparative scanning electron microscopy of third instar *Hypoderma* spp. (Diptera: Oestridae). *Medical and Veterinary Entomology* 12:181–186.

Colwell, D.D., C.R. Baird, B. Lee, and K. Milton. 1999. Scanning electron microscopy and comparative morphometrics of eggs from six bot fly species (Diptera: Oestridae). *Journal of Medical Entomology* 36(6): 803–810.

de la Fuente, C. de la, J.M. San Miguel, M. Santin, J.M. Alunda, I. Dominquez, A. Lopez, M. Carballo, and A. Gonzalez. 2000. Pharyngeal bot flies in *Cervus elaphus* in central Spain: Prevalence and population dynamics. *The Journal of Parasitology* (in press).

Downes, C.M., J.B. Theberge, and S.M. Smith. 1986. The influence of insects on the distribution, microhabitat choice, and behaviour of the Burwash caribou herd. *Canadian Journal of Zoology* 64:622–629.

Dudley, R., and K. Milton. 1990. Parasite deterrence and the energetic costs of slapping in howler monkeys. *Journal of Mammology* 71:463–465.

Dudzinski, W. 1970a. Studies on *Cephenemyia stimulator* (Clark) (Diptera, Oestridae), the parasite of the European roe deer, *Capreolus capreolus* (L.) I. Biology. *Acta Parasitologica Polonica* 18:555–572.

———. 1970b. Studies on *Cephenemyia stimulator* (Clark) (Diptera, Oestridae), the parasite of the European roe deer, *Capreolus capreolus* (L.) II. Invasiology. *Acta Parasitologica Polonica* 18:573–592.

Everard, C.O.R., and T.H. Aitken. 1972. Cuterebrid flies from small mammals in Trinidad. *The Journal of Parasitology* 58:189–190.

Folstad, I., A.C. Nilssen, O. Halvorsen, and J. Andersen. 1989. Why do male reindeer *Rangifer t. tarandus*) have higher abundance of second and third instar larvae of *Hypoderma tarandi* than females? *Oikos* 55:87–92.

———. 1991. Parasite avoidance: The cause of post-calving migrations in Rangifer. *Canadian Journal of Zoology* 69:2423–2429.

Foreyt W.J., C.W. Leathers, and G. Hattan. 1994. Bot fly larvae (*Cephenemyia jellisoni*) as a cause of neurologic signs in elk. *Journal of Wildlife Diseases* 30:470–471.

Gingrich, R.E. 1981. Migratory kinetics of *Cuterebra fontinella* (Diptera: Cuterebridae) in the white-footed mouse, *Peromyscus leucopus*. *The Journal of Parasitology* 67:398–402.

Golubev, P.D. 1960. The water vole (*Arvicola terrestris* L.)— A new host of the warble fly, *Oestromyia leporina* Pall [in Russian]. (Diptera, Hypodermatidae). *Entomologicheskoe Obozrenie* 39:316–363.

Grunin, K.Y. 1957. Botflies (oestridae)[in Russian]. *Fauna USSR, Insecta, Diptera* 19:1–146.

Guimaraes, J.H. 1971. Notes on the hosts of Neotropical Cuterebini (Diptera, Cuterebridae), with new records from Brazil [in Portuguese]. *Papeis Aulsos de Zoologia (Sao Paulo)* 25:89–94.

———. 1989. Revisao das especies sul-americana da familia Cuterebridae (Diptera, Cyclorhapha). Ph.D. thesis, Universidade de Sao Paulo, Sao Paulo, 188pp.

Guimaraes, J.H., and C.E.A. Coimbra. 1982. Miase humana por *Alouattamyia baeri* (Shannon and Greene) (Diptera: Cuterebridae). *Revista Brasileira Zoologica* 1:35–39.

Guitton C., P. Dorchies, and S. Morand. 1996. Scanning electron microscopy of larval instars and imago of *Rhinoestrus usbekistanicus* Gan, 1947 (Oestridae). *Parasite* 3:155–159.

Gummer, D.L., M.R. Forbes, D.J. Bender, and R.M.R. Barclay. 1997. Botfly (Diptera: Oestridae) parasitism of Ord's kangaroo rats (*Dipodomys ordii*) at Suffield National Wildlife Area, Alberta, Canada. *The Journal of Parasitology* 83:601–604.

Hadwen, S. 1926. Notes on the life history of *Oedemagena tarandi* L. and *Cephenemyia trompe* Modeer. *The Journal of Parasitology* 13:56–65.

Horak, I.G., and M.J. Butt. 1977. Parasites of domestic and wild animals in South Africa. III. *Oestrus* spp. and *Gedoelstia hässleri* in the blesbok. *Onderstepoort Journal of Veterinary Research* 44:113–118.

Horak, I.G., J. Boomaker, and V. DeVos. 1980. A description of the immature stages of *Kirkoestrus minutus* (Rodhain and Bequaert, 1915) (Diptera: Oestridae), and the life cycle and seasonl prevalence of this fly in blue wildebeest. *Onderstepoort Journal of Veterinary Research* 47:23–30.

Howard, G.W. 1977. Prevalence of nasal bots (Diptera: Oestridae) in some Zambian hartebeest. *Journal of Wildlife Diseases* 13:400–404.

Hunter, D.M., R.F.M.S. Sadleir, and J.M. Webster. 1972. Studies on the ecology of cuterebrid parasitism in deer mice. *Canadian Journal of Zoology* 50:25–29.

Innocenti, L., M. Masetti, G. Macchioni, and F. Giorgi. 1995. Larval salivary gland proteins of the sheep nasal bot fly (*Oestrus ovis* L.) are major immunogens in infested sheep. *Veterinary Parasitology* 60:273–282.

Jansen, J., Jr. 1970. Hypodermatid larvae (Diptera: Hypodermatidae) from the muskox, *Ovibos moschatus. Entomologische Berichten (Amsterdam)* 30:222–224.

Johnson J.L., J.B. Campbell, A.R. Doster, G. Nason, and R.J. Cagne. 1983. Cerebral abscess and *Cephenemyia phobifera* in a mule deer in central Nebraska. *Journal of Wildlife Diseases* 19:279–280.

Karter, A.J., I. Fostad, and J. Anderson. 1992. Abiotic factors influencing embryonic development, egg hatching, and larval orientation in the reindeer warble fly, *Hypoderma tarandi. Medical and Veterinary Entomology* 6:355–362.

Kavaliers, M., and D.D. Colwell. 1992. Parasitism, opioid systems and host behavior. *Advances in Neuroimmunology* 2:287–295.

Kearney, M.S., A.C. Nilssen, A. Lyslo, P. Syrdalen, and L. Dannevig. 1991. Ophthalmomyiasis caused by the reindeer warble fly larva. *Journal of Clinical Pathology* 44:276–284.

Kelsall, J.P. 1972. Warble fly distribution among some Canadian caribou. In *Proceedings of the 1st International Reindeer and Caribou Symposium*, pp. 509–517.

Kunz, S.E., P.J. Scholl, D.D. Colwell, and J. Weintraub. 1990. Use of sterile insect releases in an IPM program for control of *Hypoderma lineatum* and *H. bovis* (Diptera: Oestridae): A pilot test. *Journal of Medical Entomology* 27:523–529.

Leite, A.C.R., and P. Williams. 1988. The life cycle of *Metacuterebra apicalis* (Diptera: Cuterebridae). *Memorias de Instituto Oswaldo Crus* 83:485–491.

———. 1989. Morphological observations on the egg and first instar larva of *Metacuterebra apicalis* (Diptera: Cuterebridae). *Memoires Instituto des Oswaldo Crus* 84:123–130.

Martinez Gomez, F., S. Hernandez Rodriguez, P. Ruiz Sanchez, R. Molina Rodero, and A. Martinez Moreno. 1990. Hypodermosis in the red deer *Cervus elaphus* in Cordoba, Spain. *Medical and Veterinary Entomology* 4:311–314.

McMahon, D.C., and T.D. Bunch. 1989. Bot fly larvae (*Cephenemyia* spp., Oestridae) in mule deer (*Odocoileus hemionus*) from Utah. *Journal of Wildlife Diseases* 25:636–638.

Michener, G.R. 1993. Lethal myiasis of Richardson's ground squirrels by the sarcophagid fly *Neobellieria citellivora. Journal of Mammalogy* 74:148–155.

Milton, K. 1996. Effects of bot fly (*Alouattamyia baeri*) parasitism on a free-ranging howler monkey (*Alouatta palliata*) population in Panama. *Journal of Zoology* 239:39–63.

Minar, J.S., S. Lobachev, M. Kiefer, and D. Bazardorzh. 1985. New findings of warble flies (Hypodermatidae, Oestridae) of wild animals in Mongolia. *Folia Parasitologia* 32:89–91.

Monfray K., and C. Boulard. 1990. Preliminary evaluation of four immunological tests for the early diagnosis of *Hypoderma tarandi* causing hypodermosis in reindeer. *Medical and Veterinary Entomology* 4:297–302.

Mörschel, F.M., and D.R. Klein. 1997. Effects of weather and parasitic insects on behavior and group dynamics of caribou of the Delta Herd, Alaska. *Canadian Journal of Zoology* 75:1659–1670.

Munger J.C., and W.H. Karasov. 1994. Costs of bot fly infection in white-footed mice: Energy and mass flow. *Canadian Journal of Zoology* 72:166–173.

Murphy S.M., and J.A. Curatolo. 1987. Activity budgets and movement rates of caribou encountering pipelines, roads and traffic in northern Alaska. *Canadian Journal of Zoology* 65:2483–2490.

Nilssen, A.C. 1997a. Effect of temperature on pupal development and eclosion dates in the reindeer oestrids *Hypoderma tarandi* and *Cephenemyia trompe* (Diptera: Oestridae). *Environmental Entomology* 26:296–306.

———. 1997b. Factors affecting size, longevity and fecundity in the reindeer oestrid flies *Hypoderma tarandi* (L.) and *Cephenemyia trompe* (Modeer). *Ecological Entomology* 22:294–303.

Nilssen, A.C., and J.R. Anderson. 1995. Flight capacity of the reindeer warble fly, *Hypoderma tarandi* L., and the reindeer nose bot fly, *Cephenemyia trompe* (Modeer) (Diptera: Oestridae). *Canadian Journal of Zoology* 73:1228–1238.

Nilssen, A.C., and J.O. Gjershaug. 1988. Reindeer warble fly larvae found in red deer. *Rangifer* 8:35–37.

Nilssen, A.C., B.A. Tømmerås, R. Schmid, and S.B. Evensen. 1996. Dimethyl sulphide is a strong attractant for some calliphorids and a muscid but not for the reindeer oestrids *Hypoderma tarandi* and *Cephenemyia trompe. Entomologia Experimentalis et Applicata* 79:211–218.

Nguyen, V.K., N. Bourges, D. Condorcet, and P. Dorchie. 1996. Mast cells and eosinophils in upper respiratory mucosa of sheep infected with *Oestrus ovis* (Lynne, 1761) larvae. *Parasite* 3:217–221.

Oksanen, A., and M. Nieminen. 1996. Larvicidal effectiveness of doramectin against natural warble (*Hypoderma tarandi*) and throat bot (*Cephenemyia trompe*) infections in reindeer. *Medical and Veterinary Entomology* 10:395–396.

Oksanen, A., H. Norberg, and M. Nieminen. 1998. Ivermectin treatment did not increase slaughter weight of first-year reindeer calves. *Preventive Veterinary Medicine* 35:209–217.

Oksanen, A., M. Nieminen, T. Soveri, and K. Kumpula. 1992. Oral and parenteral administration of ivermectin to reindeer. *Veterinary Parasitology* 41:241–247.

Oksanen, A., M. Nieminen, and T. Soveri. 1993. A comparison of topical, subcutaneous and oral administration of ivermectin to reindeer. *The Veterinary Record* 133:312–314.

Papavero, N. 1977. *The world Oestridae (Diptera), mammals and continental drift*. The Hague: W. Junk, 240pp.

Pape, T. 1992. Phylogeny of the Tachinidae family-group (Diptera: Calyptratae). *Tijdschrift voor Entomologie* 135:43–86.

Perez, J.M., J.E. Granados, R.C. Soriguer, and I. Ruiz-Martinez. 1996. Prevalence and seasonality of *Oestrus causcasicus* Grunin, 1948 (Diptera: Oestridae) parasitizing the Spanish ibex, *Capra pyrenaica* (Mammalia: Artiodactyla). *The Journal of Parasitology* 82:233–236.

Porchinskii, I.A. 1913. The sheep nose bot (*Oestrus ovis* L.): Its biology, characteristics, methods of control and relation to man [In Russian]. *Trudy Biuro Po Entomolgii* 10:1–65.

Rakusin, W. 1970. Ocular myiasis interna caused by the sheep nasal bot fly (*Oestrus ovis* L.). *South African Medical Journal* 44:1155–1157.

Rehbinder, C. 1970. Observations of first instar larvae of nostril fly (*Cephenemyia trompe* L.) in the eye of reindeer and their relation to keratitis in this animal. *Acta Veterinaria Scandinavia* 11:338–339.

Reingold, W.J., J.B. Robin, D. Leipa, D.J. Schanzlin, and R. E. Smith. 1984. *Oestrus ovis* ophthalmomyiasis externa. *American Journal of Ophthalmology* 97:7–10.

Reitschel, G. 1975. Die laborzucht der dasselfliege *Oestromyia leporina* Pall. (Diptera, Hypodermatidae) und ihre biologischen voraussetzungen. *Zietschrift fur Parasitenkunde* 47:299–306.

———. 1981. Bau und Funktion der imaginalen Mundwekzeuge der Dasselfliege *Oestromyia leporina* (Diptera: Hypodermatidae). *Entomologia Generalis* 7:161–165.

Repkeny, I. 1985. Oestrida Legylarva a szemben. (Sheep-nose bot-flies in human eyes.) *Parasitologia Hungarica* 18:99–102.

Ruiz, I., R.C. Soriguer, and J.M. Perez. 1993. Pharyngeal bot flies (Oestridae) from sympatric wild cervids in southern Spain. *The Journal of Parasitology* 79:623–626.

Ruiz-Martinez I., and F. Palomares. 1993. Occurrence and overlapping of pharyngeal bot flies *Pharyngomyia picta* and *Cephenemyia auribarbis* (Oestridae) in red deer of southern Spain. *Veterinary Parasitology* 47:119–127.

Ruiz-Martinez, I., F. Gomez, J.M. Perez, and F.A. Poudevigne. 1996. The role of botfly myiasis due to *Dermatobia hominis* L. (Diptera: Cuterebridae) as a predisposing factor to New World screwworm myiasis (*Cochliomyia hominivorax* Coquerel) (Diptera: Calliphoridae). *Annals of the New York Academy of Sciences* 791:434–442.

Russell, D.E., and W.A. Dixon. 1990. Activity budgets, food habits and habitat selection of the Porcupine Caribou herd during the summer insect season. *Rangifer, Special Issue* 3:255.

Sabrosky, C.W. 1986. North American species of *Cuterebra*, the rabbit and rodent bot flies (Diptera: Cuterebridae). College Park, MD: Entomological Society of America, 240 pp.

Safneck, J.R., R. Leicht, T. Galloway, and D.D. Colwell. 1998. Fly in the eye: Ophthalmomyiasis due to *Hypoderma tarandi*. Abstract, Canadian Ophthalmic Pathologists Society Meeting, Calgary, June 26.

Samuel, W.M., and D.O. Trainer. 1971. Pharyngeal botfly larvae in white-tailed deer. *Journal of Wildlife Diseases* 7:142–146.

Scholl, P.J. 1991. Gonotrophic development in the rodent bot fly *Cuterebra fontinella* (Diptera: Oestridae). *Journal of Medical Entomology* 28:474–476.

Scholl, P.J., and J. Weintraub. 1988. Gonotrophic development in *Hypoderma lineatum* and *H. bovis* (Diptera: Oestri-dae), with notes on reproductive capacity. *Annals of the Entomological Society of America* 81:318–324.

Skjenneberg, S., and L. Slagsvold. 1968. *Reindfiften og dens naturgrunnlag*. Oslo: Scandanavian University Books, 332 pp.

Smith, D.H. 1975. An ecological analysis of a host-parasite association: *Cuterebra approximata* (Diptera: Cuterebridae) in *Peromyscus maniculatus* (Rodentia: Cricetidae). Ph.D. Dissertation, University of Montana, Missoula, 175 pp.

Sugar, I. 1976a. On the incidence of larvae of Hypodermatidae in the games and wild rodents of Hungary. *Parasitologia Hungarica* 9: 85–96.

———. 1976b. Seasonal incidence of larvae of *Pharyngomyia picta* (Meigen) 1824 and *Cephenemyia auribarbis* (Meigen) 1824 (Oestridae) in red deer (*Cervus elaphus hippelaphus*) in Hungary. *Parasitologia Hungarica* 9:73–84.

Teskey, H.J. 1981. *Manual of Nearctic Diptera*. Vol. 1, *Morphology and terminology—Larvae*. Agriculture Canada Research Branch Monograph No. 27, pp. 65–88.

Thomas, D.C., and H.P.L. Kiliaan. 1990. Warble infestations in some Canadian caribou and their significance. *Rangifer, Special Issue* 3:409–417.

Tømmerås, B.A., A. Wibe, A.C. Nilssen, and J.R. Anderson. 1993. The olfactory response of the reindeer nose bot fly, *Cephenemyia trompe* (Oestridae), to components in interdigital pheromone gland and urine from the host reindeer, *Rangifer tarandus. Chemoecology* 4:115–119.

Twigg, G.I. 1965. Warbles on Holochilus sciureus from the coast of British Guiana. *Journal of Mammalogy* 46:98–100.

Vieira, E.M. 1993. Occurrence and prevalence of bot flies, *Metacuterebra apicalis* (Diptera: Cuterebridae), in rodents of cerrado from central Brazil. *The Journal of Parasitology* 79:792–795.

Volf, P., J. Lukes, and V. Srp. 1990. Study on the population of the warble fly, *Oestromyia leporina* (Pallas 1778) (Diptera, Hypodermatidae) in Bohemia. *Folia Parasitologica* 37:187–190.

Wolf, L.S. 1959. Observations on the histopathological changes caused by the larvae of *Hypoderma bovis* (L.) and *Hypoderma lineatum* (DeVill.) (Diptera: Oestridae). *Canadian Journal of Animal Science* 39:145–157.

Wood, D.M. 1987. Oestridae. In *Manual of Nearctic Diptera*, vol. 2. Ed. J. F. McApline. Ottawa: Agriculture Canada Monograph No. 28, pp. 1147–1158.

Zumpt, F. 1965. *Myiasis in man and animals in the Old World*. London: Butterworths, 267 pp.

4

TICKS (CLASS ARACHNIDA: ORDER ACARINA)

SANDRA A. ALLAN

INTRODUCTION. Ticks are the most important group of ectoparasites of wild mammals, primarily because they feed on blood and tissue fluids in order to develop and because of the wide range of pathogenic agents that they transmit. In addition, they cause local irritation at the site of feeding, blood loss from severe infestations, wounds as sites for secondary infection, and tick paralysis.

Ticks are obligate ectoparasites belonging to the order Acarina and are readily distinguished from insects by the leathery appearance of the body and the fused head, thorax, and abdomen. Antennae are absent. The mouthparts are fused, with palps, chelicerae, hypostome, and basis capitulum to form a capitulum. Ticks are divided into two families: Argasidae (soft-bodied ticks), a relatively small group comprising ~170 species, and Ixodidae (hard ticks), a larger group comprising over 650 species (Oliver 1989). They undergo four life stages: egg, larva (3 pairs of legs), nymph (4 pairs of legs and no genital pore), and adult (4 pairs of legs and a genital pore).

This chapter reviews the association of soft and hard ticks with wild mammals in North America north of Mexico.

SOFT TICKS. Soft ticks (family Argaside) lack a hardened dorsal scutum. The body shape is roughly oval with leathery wrinkled cuticle. The capitulum of nymphs and adults is situated on the ventral surface and is not readily obvious from above. Adult mouthparts project anteriorly. Males and females are not readily distinguished. Argasid ticks can be identified using Cooley and Kohls (1944). Because argasid ticks feed rapidly (several minutes to hours), they are rarely collected on hosts. Most species are nidicoles (i.e., nest dwellers), and all species feed multiple times as nymphs and adults.

Four genera (*Argas, Ornithodoros, Otobius* and *Antricola*) are present in North America. Adult *Argas* spp. are flattened with a yellowish brown leathery cuticle and a sharp lateral margin that can be seen even when ticks are engorged. This genus will not be mentioned further because most members preferentially feed on birds, although there are occasional reports of some species (*Argas persicus, Argas miniatus, Argas sanchezi, Argas radiata*) feeding on man and livestock (Bishopp and Trembley 1945). Adult *Ornithodoros* spp. are globular in shape, while adult *Otobius* spp. have a granulated integument. Adult *Antricola* spp. are flattened and marginated with a leathery semitransparent skin (Sonenshine 1991). Ticks in the genus *Antricola* feed on bats, generally in South and Central America and only one species has been reported from North America.

Life History. Almost all argasid ticks have a multi-host feeding pattern with each on different individuals in the same species or different species (Hoogstraal and Aeschlimann 1982). The acquisition of several blood meals for nymphs and adults is facilitated by their presence in nest and shelters to which the vertebrate hosts repeatedly return. The general life cycle of argasid ticks may range from several months to years with female argasids feeding and ovipositing several times (Hoskins and Cupp 1988). Length of life cycle varies by species from 3 to 4 months for *Ornithodoros hermsi, Ornithodoros puertoricensis,* and *Ornithodoros turicata* to 14 months for *Ornithodoros coriaceus* (reviewed in Adeyeye 1982). Eggs, which are generally deposited in small batches in crevices, vary in number from 200 to 1500 eggs/female/lifetime, depending on species. Once on a mammalian host, larvae of most species feed quickly, often in 12–15 minutes. Some species on birds or bats feed slowly (7–10 days) (Oliver 1989). Larvae detach, hide in cracks, crevices, or under debris and molt to nymphs. The number of nymphal instars varies between species and often within a species (Oliver 1989); in general each stage requires a blood meal. For instance, *Ornithodoros hermsi* and *O. coriaceus* have three and up to seven nymphal instars, respectively, with each feeding on a host. Adult males of some species, such as *Ornithodoros parkeri,* develop with one fewer nymphal instar than females (Oliver 1989). The number of nymphal instars is not consistent even in the same species and may vary based on nutrition (Sonenshine 1991). Feeding by nymphs and adults may range from 30 minutes to several hours (Oliver 1989). Excess fluid is excreted by the coxal glands during tick feeding; this excess fluid excretion is unique to soft ticks (Laviopierre and Riek 1955). Adult ticks emerge and mate off the host. Both males and females blood-feed. Females use the blood meals for egg development. In general, *Ornithodoros* spp. lay eggs in batches of 10–150 eggs, with variation due to factors such as size of blood meal and temperature (summarized in Adeyeye 1982; Endris et al. 1991a). For *Ornithodoros puertoricensis,* females completed 7–11 gonotrophic cycles per year depending on temperature (Endris et al. 1991b).

Departures from this general pattern occur. Larvae in the subgenus *Ornithodoros* do not feed; this behavior is possibly related to the fact that these ticks inhabit burrows that may house hosts irregularly (Hoogstraal and Aeschlimann 1982). First-instar nymphs of the subgenus *Alectorobius* (North American species include *Ornithodoros dyeri, Ornithodoros kelleyi, Ornithodoros puertoricensis, Ornithodoros talaje* and *Ornithodoros yunatensis*) do not feed, and adults of *Otobius megnini, Otobius lagophilus,* and *Antricola* sp. have poorly developed mouthparts and also are nonfeeding (Hoogstraal 1985b).

The life cycles of the spinose ear tick, *Otobius megnini* (the common name refers to spines on the cuticle of the nymph), and *O. lagophilus* are specialized, and each uses one host on which the larvae and two nymphal instars feed (Oliver 1989). Larvae of *O. megnini* enter ears of hosts, feed, and form a bladder-like grub. This stage molts to the first-stage nymph, which feeds and molts, and the engorged second-stage nymph drops to the ground and molts to an adult. Mating and oviposition occur on the ground, and in *O. megnini* ~1500 eggs are deposited (Hoogstraal 1985a). Drummond (1967) reported that *O. megnini* on cattle in southern Texas had poorly defined seasonal activity with an inconsistent peak of activity in late summer and fall. The life cycles of *O. megnini* and *O. lagophilus* can be completed in 2–4 months (Hoogstraal 1985a).

In general, argasid ticks are nidicolous and are present in the nests, burrows, buildings, and sleeping areas of their hosts. Survival of nonfeeding ticks is dependent on humidity. Most argasids can resist long periods of starvation during their development, thus extending their life span (Sonenshine 1991). Soft ticks can survive many years, even in arid or semiarid environments, if they can obtain frequent blood meals and appropriate shelter (e.g., in crevices) (Sonenshine 1991). Diapause also regulates many species and may coordinate development with return of hosts to nests or burrows (Sonenshine 1991). *Ornithodoros kelleyi* feed on bats in roosting sites, but not in hibernation sites (Sonenshine 1991).

Most argasids (*Argas, Ornithodoros*) are nocturnal and feed at night and thus are seldom found on hosts collected and examined during the day.

Epizootiology

DISTRIBUTION AND HOST RANGE. Numerous argasid ticks infest shelters used by bats, and many of these are host specific. Soft ticks primarily associated with bats with distribution limited to the south include *Ornithodoros concanensis, O. dugesi, O. dyeri, O. rossi, O. stageri, O. yumatensis,* and *Antricola coprophilus* (Table 4.1). Several of these species are more frequently collected in bat retreats than on the hosts themselves, making identification of host species difficult. *Ornithodoros kelleyi* has a widespread distribution throughout North America and feeds on insectivorous bats as nymphs and adults (Sonenshine 1993).

Ornithodoros coriaceus has been collected primarily from rodents in hot and temperate regions along the Pacific (Cooley and Kohls 1944). Distribution of *O. hermsi* is often collected in association with nests of chipmunks in hollow trees and logs and in cabins frequented by small rodents (Kohls et al. 1965). In western states, *O. parkeri* inhabits burrows and nests of various small mammals (Kohls et al. 1965). *Ornithodoros sparnus* has been reported mostly from the nests of woodrats in Arizona and Utah (Kohls et al. 1965). In the Caribbean, *O. puertoricensis* feeds primarily on rats, and there are occasional reports from other mammals. *Ornithodoros talaje* is generally reported from South and Central America but is established in the southern United States. *Ornithodoros turicata* is primarily associated with burrow-inhabiting species but is also reported from domestic animals and man (Cooley and Kohls 1944; Kohls et al. 1965).

In general, *Otobius megnini* is associated with arid and semiarid plateau regions in southern and Pacific coastal regions (Cooley and Kohls 1944), although some populations are established in Florida and Louisiana (Kierans and Litwak 1989). It is widely distributed in western and southwestern states and British Columbia and is mainly reported from domestic livestock with some reports from white-tailed deer (Cooley and Kohls 1944; Bishopp and Trembley 1945; Rich 1957), mountain sheep (Rich and Gregson 1968), and lions in zoos (Munas Diniz et al. 1987). This tick is native to North America but has been accidentally introduced to other continents.

There are few prevalence and intensity data published for soft ticks on wild mammals.

ENVIRONMENTAL LIMITATIONS. Argasid ticks are highly specialized in being able to maintain favorable water balance; they tolerate lower humidities and higher temperatures than hard ticks (Oliver 1989). Most species live in arid or semiarid hot environments, usually in nests, burrows, or shelters of their vertebrate hosts (Sonenshine 1993). Such sites are used either seasonally or for short periods of time by hosts. Thus, the rapid feeding time of nymphs and adults and the ability of these ticks to survive long periods in the absence of hosts enhance tick survival. *Otobius megnini* is an exception to the nidicolous habit and parasitizes wide-ranging ungulates in dry habitats (Oliver 1989). It is often associated with livestock stables and shelters, as females lay eggs in cracks and crevices and larvae emerge and crawl onto hosts (Parrish 1949). Ticks can persist unfed at least 2 years in empty corrals or stables. The bat tick, *O. kelleyi,* exhibits an ovipositional diapause (i.e., oviposition delayed 100+ days) when fed on hibernating bats, but oviposits normally on posthibernating bats (Sonenshine and Anastos

TABLE 4.1—Hosts, geographic distribution, and diseases vectored by North American Argasid ticks that feed on mammals

Species (Common Name)	Location	Diseases	Mammalian Hosts[a]
Antricola coprophilus	Arizona, Texas, Mexico	—	Bats (suspected)
Ornithodoros concanensis	Arizona, Colorado, Montana, Texas, Wyoming	—	Bats (*Eptesicus fuscus, Myotis velifer, Pipistrellus subflavus, Tadarida brasiliensis*)
Ornithodoros coriaceus (pajaroello tick)	California, Mexico	Relapsing fever, epizootic bovine abortion, bluetongue, African swine fever	Rodents (*Sciurus, Eutamias, Peromyscus*), Deer (*Odocoileus*), Domestic (cattle, sheep), Man (rarely)
Ornithodoros dugesi	Mexico, Texas	—	Bats, Man (rarely)
Ornithodoros dyeri	Arizona, California, Mexico	—	Bats (*Pizonyx vivesi, Balantiopteryx plicata*)
Ornithodoros eremicus	Utah	—	Deer mouse (*Peromyscus maniculatus*)
Ornithodoros hermsi	California, Colorado, Florida, Idaho, Nevada New Mexico, Oregon, Washington, British Columbia	Relapsing fever	Chipmunk (*Eutamias*), Deer mouse (*Peromyscus*), Woodrat (*Neotoma*), Bat, Man (rarely)
Ornithodoros kelleyi	Widespread	—	Bats (*Eptesicus fuscus, Antrozous pallidus, Pipistrellus hesperus, Pipistrellus subflavus, Myotis subulatus subulatus* [this species now split as *Myotis leibii* (in eastern N. America) and *M. ciliolabrum* (in western N. America)], *Myotis lucifugus lucifugus, Myotis californicus pallidus*), Man (rarely)
Ornithodoros parkeri	California, Colorado, Idaho, Montana, Nevada, Oregon, Utah, Washington, Wyoming	Relapsing fever, spotted fever	Rodents (*Citellus, Dipodomys, Cynomys, Peromyscus, Marmota*), Rabbit (*Sylvilagus, Lepus*), Weasel (*Mustela*), Man (rarely)
Ornithodoros puertoricensis	Puerto Rico, Virgin Islands, Haiti, Dominican Republic	African swine fever	Rat (*Rattus, Proechimys, Neotomys*), Rabbit (*Sylvilagus*), Domestic (cat), Man (rarely)
Ornithodoros rossi	Arizona	—	Bat (*Eptesicus fuscus, Macrotus californicus, Leptonycteris nivalis*)
Ornithodoros sparnus	Arizona, Utah	—	Woodrat (*Neotoma*), Deer mouse (*Peromyscus*), Deer (*Odocoileus*)
Ornithodoros stageri	Arizona, California, Oklahoma, Texas	—	Bat (*Myotis velifer, Tadarida mexicana, Antrozous pallidus*), Man (rarely)
Ornithodoros talaje	Arizona, California, Colorado, Florida, Kansas, New Mexico, Oklahoma, Texas, Utah, Mexico	Mexican-American relapsing fever	Rodent (*Citellus, Dipodomys*), Woodrat (*Neotoma*), Domestic (dog, cat), Man (rarely)
Ornithodoros turicata (relapsing fever tick)	Arizona, California, Colorado, Florida, Kansas, New Mexico, Oklahoma, Texas, Utah, Mexico	Relapsing fever, Rocky Mountain spotted fever, tularemia, Mexican-American relapsing fever, African swine fever (not in North America)	Ground squirrel (*Citellus beecheyi, C. fisheri*), Prairie dog (*Cynomys*), Woodrat (*Neotoma*), Kangaroo rat (*Dipodomys*), Rabbit (*Syvilagus*), Domestic (pig, cattle, horse), Man (rarely)
Ornithodoros yumatensis	Arizona, California, Florida, Georgia, Texas	—	Bats [*Myotis velifer, Plecotus (= Corynorhinus) townsendii, Plecotus rafinesquii, Desmodus rotundus, Pipistrellus subflavus, Myotis ausroriparius*], Man (rarely)
Otobius lagophilus	Alberta, California, Colorado, Idaho, Montana, Nevada, Oregon, Wyoming	Colorado tick fever	Cottontail rabbit (*Sylvilagus*), Jackrabbit (*Lepus*), Pika (*Ochotona*), Domestic cat (rarely)
Otobius megnini (spinose ear tick)	Arizona, California, Colorado, Florida, Georgia, Idaho, Kansas, Louisiana, Mississippi, Missouri, Montana, Nebraska, Nevada, New Mexico, North Carolina, Oregon, South Dakota, Wyoming, British Columbia, Mexico	Otoacariasis, tick paralysis, suspected Q fever	White-tailed deer (*Odocoileus virginianus*), Mule deer (*Odocoileus hemionus hemionus*), Rabbit (*Sylvilagus, Lepus*), Coyote (*Canis latrans*), Elk (*Cervus elaphus*), Mountain goat (*Oreamnos americanus*), Mountain sheep (*Ovis canadensis*), Domestic (cat, dog, horse, cattle, goat, sheep, pig, mule), Man (rarely)

[a] Names as from sources.

Sources: Cooley and Kohls (1944), Bishopp and Trembley (1945), Kohls and Clifford (1963), Kohls et al. (1965), Wilson and Baker (1972), Cook (1972), Williams et al. (1976), Fox (1977), Pfaffenberger and Valencia (1988).

1960). *Ornithodoros kelleyi* live in cracks and crevices of roosts and emerge during the day to feed on roosting bats. This species can become established in human habitations with the presence of roosting bats (Cilek and Knapp 1992). When bats migrate to caves and caverns for hibernation, the ticks remain in the roosting sites (Sonenshine 1993).

Clinical Signs. Clinical signs include painful bites, in some species, and lesions. Symptoms of *Otobius megnini* infestation include shaking of the head, ear scratching, trauma of the external ear, secondary infection, convulsions, and deafness (Gregson 1973; Strickland et al. 1976). Infested animals show increasing signs of nervous and digestive disorders. Infested cattle assume a head-heavy stance, followed by lack of muscle coordination, collapse, and death (Rich 1957).

Pathology and Disease Transmission. Direct effects of feeding include trauma, pruritus, local inflammation, and subcutaneous nodules. Del Cacho et al. (1994) evaluated the sequential histological development of feeding sites of the tropical bat tick, *Argas vespertillonis* on *Eptesicus serotinus*. Initially, neutrophils and Langerhans' cells were the major components of cellular infiltrate. Skin had hyperkeratosis with superficial crusting, and this was restricted to the area immediately around the feeding site. *Ornithodoros coriaceus* is the vector of relapsing fever (*Borrelia hermsi*) and epizootic bovine abortion (Schmidtmann et al. 1976) and an experimental vector of African swine fever (Groocock et al. 1980) (Table 4.1). *Ornithodoros hermsi, O. parkeri,* and *O. talaje* are vectors of relapsing fevers caused by *Borrelia hermsi, B. parkeri,* and *B. mazzotti,* respectively (Sonenshine 1993). Spirochetes of Mexican-American relapsing fever are transmitted to hosts in coxal gland fluid (Hoskins and Cupp 1988). Feeding by *Ornithodoros turicata* causes irritation and edema. This species is a vector of relapsing fever (*Borrelia turicata*) (Butler and Gibbs 1984), *B. parkeri* (Davis and Burgdorfer 1955), tularemia, and possibly, *Leptospira ballum* and *L. pomona* (Burgdorfer 1956). Potential vectors of African swine fever in the Caribbean region include *Ornithodoros coriaceus, O. turicata, O. puertoricensis, O. tajale,* and *O. dugesi* (Butler and Gibbs, 1984; Endris et al. 1991b). The painful and irritating effects of feeding by *Otobius megnini,* deep in the ears of hosts, include ulceration and damage to the ear drums and auricular nerves (Rich 1957). In addition these ticks can serve as vectors for a number of pathogens (Table 4.1) that are transmitted in saliva or coxal gland secretions while feeding or by infected feces or ingestion of an infected tick (Hoskins and Cupp 1988). This species is also incriminated as a possible vector of Q fever (*Coxiella burnetti*) (Marrie 1990) and a cause of tick paralysis (Gregson 1973).

Immunity. There has been little documentation of immune responses to many of the soft ticks (Allen 1987), although there is some evidence of development of host resistance (Johnston and Brown 1985). Johnston and Brown (1985) demonstrated intense cutaneous basophilia and eosinophilia in sensitized guinea pigs in response to feeding by *Ornithodoros parkeri*. Repeated feeding by *Argas polonicus* adults and nymphs on pigeons did not elicit resistance in pigeons, but repeated exposure to larvae in the laboratory resulted in low resistance (Dusbabek et al. 1989). Dusbabek et al. (1989) suggested that low resistance might develop because *A. polonicus* feed rapidly. Immune response to tick antigens has been documented in infested hosts with no significant development of resistance to tick-feeding. Details of the immunopathology are presented in Allen (1987), who indicated that reactions to argasid bites by guinea pigs included very marked involvement of basophil leucocytes in reactions to secondary and subsequent infestations. In bite sites from secondary infestations, basophils were involved with a vesicular degranulation mechanism, anaphylactic degranulation, and disintegration of cells caused by cytotoxic mechanisms. Feeding ticks completed blood meals before arrival and degranulation of basophils at the feeding site, possibly contributing to the lack of resistance effects seen (Allen 1987). Need and Bulter (1991) reported reduced survival of *Ornithodoros tajale* (a relatively long-feeding species) fed on CD1 mice immunized with tick extracts compared to no effect on *O. turicata* (a relatively rapid feeder). Del Cacho (1994) proposed that the bat *E. serotinus* developed immunity to *Argas vespertilionis* infestations by producing a new layer of epidermis that interfered with tick-feeding.

Control and Treatment. Control of soft ticks on captive animals is through sanitation and destruction of breeding sites (nests, deer and cattle bedding, etc.) and use of acaricides, generally in spray, pour-on, and ear-tag formulations. Spinose ear ticks can be controlled through removal of ticks in ears followed by application of treatments (insecticides) in the ears or use of insecticide-impregnated ear tags (Lancaster 1984).

Public Health Concerns. Soft ticks are occasional pests of man due to irritation from feeding and to transmission of diseases to man (Table 4.1). Direct effects from feeding on man have been reported for *Ornithodoros coriaceus* in the western United States (painful bite and severe toxic reaction) (Furman and Loomis 1984), *O. talaje* (painful bite), *Argus persicus* (painful bite), and *Otobius megnini* (painful bite) (Stickland et al. 1976; Harrison et al. 1997). In contrast, Eads and Campos (1984) reported that bites by *Otobius megnini* were painless. Bites by *Ornithodoros turicata* were reported by Cooley and Kohls (1944) to be painless, but were followed in a few days by intense local irritation and swelling. Subcutaneous nodules often developed and persisted several months. In North America, agents causing relapsing fever have been isolated from *Ornithodoros hermsi (Borrelia hermsi), O. turicata (B. turicatae)* and *O. parkeri (B. parkeri)* (Sonenshine 1993). Additionally, *O. hermsi* also has been implicated as a vector of Q fever (Sonenshine 1993) and *O. talaje* as a vector of Mexican-American relapsing fever (*B. mazzottii*) (Davis 1956).

Domestic Animal Concerns. Feeding *Otobius megnini* can cause otoacariasis, which entails extreme irritation, edema, muscle spasms, hemorrhage, pain, and death in livestock (Stickland et al. 1976; Madigan et al. 1995). Cattle and horses can host up to 35 nymphs per ear on average (Drummond 1967). In western states, *Ornithodoros coriaceus* serves as a vector of bovine epizootic abortion caused by *Borrelia coriaceae* (Lane and Manweiler 1988), and bluetongue (Stott et al. 1985.

HARD TICKS. Hard ticks are some of the more common ectoparasites of wild mammals in North America, in part because of their widespread distribution and prolonged association with the host while blood-feeding. The most common ticks on wild mammals of North America belong to the genera, *Ixodes, Amblyomma, and Dermacentor.* Ticks in the genera *Haemaphysalis* are less common, and those in *Rhipicephalus* and *Boophilus* are rare due to difficulty in establishing in temperate climates and a concerted effort to eradication, respectively.

Ixodid ticks (i.e., hard ticks) have a hardened dorsal plate or scutum. Sexual dimorphism is marked in adults with the scutum covering the entire dorsal surface of males and only the anterior portion of the body of females as well as nymphs and larvae. Ixodid ticks are generally teardrop shaped with an anterior capitulum that is obvious from a dorsal view.

Hard ticks require three blood meals for development and to complete the life cycle. Each stage blood-feeds once, detaches from the host, and molts to the subsequent life stage on the ground. Often the larva, nymph, and adult feed on different hosts (i.e., three-host ticks). Some species such as *Dermacentor albipictus* (=nigrolineatus) are one-host ticks (all stages feed on the same individual host). Most of the life cycle of one-host ticks occurs on the host with only gravid females, egg masses, and host-seeking larvae present on the ground. Females and immature hard ticks become greatly distended when blood-fed; females, for instance, often ingest more than 100 times their body weight (Sonenshine 1991). Blood meals are used for molting to the next stage or production of eggs. Eggs are laid in a mass of ~100–10,000 in ~3–30 days (depending on species and temperature); they are deposited on the soil, in a crevice, or beneath leaves. Males generally obtain small blood meals and expand little in size. Hard ticks feed relatively slowly and remain on the host ~3–14 days before detaching. For instance, *Dermacentor variabilis* feed 3–6 days as larvae, 4–7 days as nymphs, and 7–10 days as adult females (Atwood and Sonenshine 1967). After feeding as immatures, molting occurs after an interval that varies between species and with temperature. For *D.*

variabilis, molting of fed larvae and nymphs requires ~8 and 17 days, respectively (Sonenshine 1991). There are ~650 species of Ixodidae (Cupp 1991) of which ~54 are established in North America. While some of these feed exclusively on birds or reptiles, most feed on wild mammals.

Ixodes. This is the largest genus of hard ticks worldwide. Of the 34 indigenous species of *Ixodes* in North America, most feed on mammals. In general *Ixodes* spp. have a wide host range, with immatures feeding on a variety of rodents; however, some species such as *I. dentatus, I. muris,* and *I. spinipalpis* are very host specific. Members of *Ixodes* are nidicolous (and often closely associated with the nests or shelters of their hosts) and are very host specific (Sonenshine 1991).

Ixodes are inornate ticks (2–4 mm) without eyes or festoons and with long mouthparts. Males have seven ventral plates. An anal groove (inverted U-shaped) anterior to the anus separates this genus from other hard ticks. Species can be identified using keys of Clifford et al. (1961) (larvae), Durden and Keirans (1996) (nymphs), Keirans and Clifford (1978), and Keirans and Litwak (1989) (adults). Detailed distributions of species are in Bishopp and Trembley (1945) and Durden and Keirans (1996).

LIFE HISTORY. All *Ixodes* are three-host ticks with life cycles requiring at least 1 year to complete. Some species such as *I. scapularis* (= *dammini*) and *I. pacificus* require at least 2 years (Spielman et al. 1985; Peavey and Lane 1996). Egg masses are deposited on the ground. Numbers of eggs include up to 3000 (*I. scapularis*) (Fish 1993), 1600 (*I. minor*) (Banks et al. 1998), and 1280 (*I. cookei*) (Farkas and Surgeoner 1991). Larvae emerge and attach to hosts (small mammals or birds) and feed. After engorgement, larvae detach and molt to nymphs on the ground. Nymphs seek and attach to hosts (usually small to midsized rodents or birds), detach from the host when replete, and molt to adults on the ground. Adults attach to hosts (usually midsized or large mammals); females feed, detach, and oviposit. Males blood-feed very little if at all. Mating occurs prior to host-finding or on the host.

Patterns of seasonal abundance differ between species. Adult *I. angustus* are present year round in nests of mammalian hosts, with immatures present after October (Bishop and Trembley 1945). Allred et al. (1960) reported larvae in May, nymphs from May to September, and adults from May to August. Adult *I. cookei* were most abundant in February, with larvae and nymphs present during the winter in Virginia (Sonenshine and Stout 1971). All stages were most abundant in fall and winter in Arkansas with few collected in midsummer (Tugwell and Lancaster 1962). Ko (1972) reported most larvae present in August and nymphs and adults in May to July in southern Ontario. Larvae of *I. dentatus* were most active in fall, with an additional small peak of activity in spring (Tugwell and Lancaster 1962; Sonenshine 1979). Nymphs were active in fall and winter, and adult density on rabbits was greatest in the fall and winter (Tugwell and Lancaster 1962; Sonenshine 1979). All stages of *I. kingi* were present on hosts throughout the year, but were most abundant during spring and summer (Bishopp and Trembley 1945). *Ixodes muris* has been collected on hosts from April to October, with adults present from spring to early fall (Bishopp and Trembley 1945; Lacombe et al. 1999). Adult *I. neotomae* were collected from black-tailed jackrabbits in California in fall and winter (Lane and Burgdorfer 1988). Adult *I. pacificus* were collected in winter and spring, with females feeding from December to March and immatures present in May and June. In California, *I. pacificus* was the most abundant tick on deer in fall (35.1 ticks/deer) and least abundant in summer (0.2 ticks/deer) (Westrom et al. 1985). Immatures are usually present in spring and summer (Peavey and Lane 1996). All stages of *I. texanus* were collected on mammals throughout the year (Bishopp and Trembley 1945). In South Carolina and Georgia, adults of *I. minor* were present from midsummer to October, larvae in November, and nymphs in November, May, and June (summarized in Banks et al. 1998). All stages of *I. scapularis* were most abundant in October and November in Arkansas (Tugwell and Lancaster 1963). In general, adult *I. scapularis* are collected from October to April (Rogers 1953; Watson and Anderson 1976; Spielman et al. 1985; Fish and Dowler 1989; Goddard 1992). In the northeast and Midwest, nymphs are present in spring and summer, with a peak in June; larvae are present in summer, with a peak in August (Watson and Anderson 1976; Spielman et al. 1985; Fish and Dowler 1989). In Florida, larvae were present from May to August, with a peak in May; and nymphs were present from May to September, with a peak in June (Rogers 1953). Less is known of the life history of other species of *Ixodes*.

Predeliction sites often vary between species. On deer, *I. scapularis* attach primarily on dorsal regions with 87% of adults found on the head, neck, and brisket. In general, bucks were more heavily infested than does in the fall (Schmidtmann et al. 1998). Watson and Anderson (1976) reported adults attached mostly to the neck and shoulders of white-tailed deer; larvae to belly, legs, and groin; and nymphs to head, forelegs, brisket, and shoulders. Westrom et al. (1985) reported that 80% of all *I. pacificus* attached to the venter of black-tailed deer.

EPIZOOTIOLOGY

DISTRIBUTION AND HOST RANGE. Details of the geographic distribution and host records of *Ixodes* spp. established in North America are presented in Table 4.2. Robbins and Keirans (1992) presented an overview of hosts of *Ixodes*. Most species have relatively narrow host ranges (e.g., *I. banks,* mostly beaver; *I. eastoni,* arvicolid and cricetid rodents; and *I. soricis,* shrews and shrew-moles). Some *Ixodes* feed on a wide range of host species, as immatures feeding on small mammals or birds and as adults on mid- to large-sized mammals. For example, immature *I. affinis* parasitize rodents, deer, and sometimes, birds; adults feed on deer, bobcat, and dogs. *Ixodes angustus* is a parasite of a wide range of arvicolid and cricetid rodents, soricid insectivores, and their predators, and adults are often collected in nests of hosts. Immature *I. tovari* are found on birds and rodents; adults are often on large mammals and rabbits. Primary hosts of *I. kingi* include carnivores, ground squirrels, and prairie dogs east of the Rocky Mountains and pocket gophers, kangaroo rats, and sigmodontine mice west of the Rockies (Durden and Keirans 1996).

Adult *I. pacificus* parasitize mid-to-large vertebrates (primarily deer as well as other hosts such as dogs and rabbits); they quest (host-seek) on vegetation 50 cm or more above the soil surface (Loye and Lane 1988). Nymphal *I. pacificus* infest diurnally active lizards and rodents but are rare on nocturnally active rodents (Lane 1990b). Lane et al. (1995) concluded that lizards were selected because they most frequented areas where *I. pacificus* quested. Studies by James and Oliver (1990), however, did not indicate a preference between lizards or white laboratory mice. The behavior of the immature *I. pacificus* seeking hosts in shaded environments apparently resulted in the selection of lizards as hosts. The diurnal questing of nymphs under the leaf litter resulted in increased contact with day-active lizards and the California ground squirrel as potential hosts rather than with nocturnal rodents (Furman and Loomis 1984; Lane et al. 1995).

Ixodes scapularis has been reported from 41 species of mammals, 57 species of birds, and 14 species of lizards (Keirans et al. 1996b) and now occurs in 32 eastern and central states of the United States (Dennis et al. 1998). Its distribution has expanded steadily over time in the northeastern United States (White et al. 1991), perhaps due to expanding populations of white-tailed deer (see Dennis et al. 1998). Adults feed on 27 species of mammals. White-footed mice serve as the most important hosts for immatures (in the north) and also serve as a reservoir of Lyme disease in endemic areas (Wilson et al. 1985). Large mammals are preferred host of adults. White-tailed deer are the most important hosts of adults and often are examined for surveillance (Spielman et al. 1985).

PREVALENCE AND INTENSITY. There are many recent reports of *I. scapularis* on wild mammals, especially white-tailed deer, because of its involvement in transmission of Lyme disease. In some studies, this species is the only or the most common tick present on deer (Watson and Anderson 1976; Durden et al. 1991). Reported percent prevalences on deer vary (e.g., 13–50 in Mississippi: Demararis et al. 1987; 54 in North Carolina: Apperson et al. 1990; 21–81 in Alabama: Durden et al. 1991; 10 in Minnesota: Gill et al. 1993). Smith (1977) reported the following percent prevalences on deer from Alabama (75%), Arkansas (98%), Florida (54%), Georgia (76%), Louisiana (99%), Mississippi

TABLE 4.2—Hosts, geographic distribution, and diseases vectored by North American Ixodes that feed on mammals

Species	Distribution	Diseases	Mammalian Hosts[a]
Ixodes affinis	Florida, Georgia, South Carolina	—	White-tailed deer (*Odocoileus virginianus*), Bobcat (*Felis rufus*), Raccoon (*Procyon lotor*), Virginia opossum (*Didelphis marsupialis*), Southern short-tailed shrew (*Blarina carolinensis*), Cotton mouse (*Peromyscus gossypinus*), Cotton rat (*Sigmodon hispidus*), Woodrat (*Neotoma*), Eastern gray squirrel (*Sciurus carolinensis*), Florida panther (*Felis concolor coryi*), Domestic (dog), Man (rarely)
Ixodes angustus	Northern U.S. and Canada (scattered)	Implicated Lyme disease[b]	Ground squirrel (*Citellus, Spermophilus*), Chipmunk (*Eutamias*), Townsend chipmunk (*Eutamias townsendi*), Squirrel (*Tamiasciurus, Sciurus, Glaucomys*), Antelope squirrel (*Ammospermophilus*), Lemming (*Synaptomys*), Woodrat (*Neotoma*), Mouse and Vole (*Clethrionomys, Peromyscus, Mus, Mictrous, Zapus, Perorognathus, Napaeozapus*), Mole (*Parascalops, Neurotrichus*), Pocket gopher (*Thomomys*), Heather vole (*Phenacomys*), Rabbit (*Sylvilagus, Lepus*), Pika (*Ochotona*), Mountain beaver (*Aplodontia*), Raccoon (*Procyon lotor*), Ringtail (*Bassariscus astutus*), Opossum (*Didelphis marsupialis*), Roof rat (*Rattus rattus*), Shrew (*Sorex, Blarina*), Little brown bat (*Myotis lucifugus*), Domestic (cat, dog), Man
Ixodes banksi	Alabama, Arkansas, Connecticut, Michigan, Missouri, New York, Wisconsin, Ontario	Implicated tularemia	Beaver (*Castor canadensis*), Muskrat (*Ondatra zibethicus*), Man (rarely)
Ixodes conepati	New Mexico, Texas	—	Skunk (*Conepatus, Mephitis*), Rock squirrel (*Spermophilus variegatus*), Ringtail (*Bassariscus astutus*)
Ixodes cookei	East of the Mississippi and eastern Canada	Powassan virus, tularemia, spotted fever group rickettsia, *Ackertia marmotae* (nematode)	Woodchuck, Marmot (*Marmota*), Raccoon (*Procyon lotor*), Skunk (*Mephitis, Spilogale*), Ground squirrel (*Citellus*), Otter (*Lutra canadensis*), Fox (*Vulpes vulpes, Urocyon cinereargenteus*), Weasel, Ferret, Mink (*Mustela*), Opossum (*Didelphis marsupialis*), Porcupine (*Erethizon dorsatum*), Prairie dog (*Cynomys*), Badger (*Taxidea taxus*), Coyote (*Canis latrans*), Ringtail (*Bassariscus astutus*), Mouse (*Peromyscus*), Squirrel (*Sciurus*), Marten, Fisher (*Martes*), Cougar (*Felis concolor*), Domestic (cat, cattle, dog), Man
Ixodes dentatus	East of the Mississippi	Lyme disease, Connecticut virus, implicated Rocky Mountain spotted fever, tularemia	Rabbit (*Sylvilagus, Lepus*), Mouse and Vole (*Peromyscus, Microtus*), Muskrat (*Ondatra zibethicus*), Domestic (sheep), Man
Ixodes eadsi	Texas	—	Mouse (*Peromyscus, Reithrodontomys, Mus, Liomys*), Shrew (*Sorex*), Chipmunk (*Eutamias*), Cotton rat (*Sigmodon hispidus*)
Ixodes eastoni	South Dakota, Wyoming	—	Mouse (*Peromuscus, Zapus*), Vole (*Clethrionomys, Microtus*), Shrew (*Sorex*), Chipmunk (*Tamias*)
Ixodes hearli	California, Montana, Oklahoma, Oregon, Texas, British Columbia	—	Raccoon (*Procyon lotor*), Squirrel (*Tamiasciurus*)
Ixodes jellisoni	California, Utah	Implicated Lyme disease	Kangaroo rat (*Dipodomys*), Pocket mouse (*Perognathus*), Pocket gopher (*Thomomys*), Man (rarely)
Ixodes kingi	Midwestern and western U.S., Alberta, Saskatchewan	Implicated tularemia	Ground squirrel (*Citellus*), Prairie dog (*Cynomys*), Woodchuck (*Marmota*), Badger (*Taxidea taxus*), Pocket gopher (*Thomomys*), Rabbit (*Sylvilagus*), Pocket mouse (*Perognathus*), Kangaroo rat (*Dipodomys*), Woodrat (*Neotoma*), Mink, Ferret (*Mustela*), Wolf (*Canis lupus*), Skunk (*Mephitis, Spilogale*), Raccoon (*Procyon lotor*), Red fox (*Vulpes vulpes*), Domestic (cat, dog)

TABLE 4.2 *(continued)*

Species	Distribution	Diseases	Mammalian Hosts[a]
Ixodes marxi	East of Mississippi, Nova Scotia, Ontario	Implicated Powassan virus[b]	Squirrel (*Sciurus, Tamiasciurius, Glaucomys*), Chipmunk (*Eutamias*), Fox (*Vulpes*), Raccoon (*Procyon lotor*), Rabbit (*Lepus*), Domestic (cat, dog), Man (rarely)
Ixodes marmotae	Colorado, Idaho, Montana, Oregon, Utah, Washington, Wyoming, British Columbia	—	Porcupine (*Erethizon dorsatum*), Woodchuck (*Marmota*), Ground squirrel (*Spermophilus*), Woodrat (*Neotoma*)
Ixodes minor	Florida, Georgia, South Carolina	Implicated Lyme disease[b]	Eastern rice rat (*Oryzmys*), Woodrat (*Neotoma*), Cotton rat (*Sigmodon hispidus*), Rat (*Rattus*), Mice (*Peromyscus, Mus*), Woodchuck (*Marmota monax*), Eastern gray squirrel (*Sciurus carolinensis*), Eastern spotted skunk (*Spilogale putorius*), Cottontail rabbit (*Sylvilagus floridanus*)
Ixodes muris	Northeastern U.S. south to South Carolina, Newfoundland, Nova Scotia, Ontario	Implicated human babesiosis	Mouse (*Peromyscus, Zapus, Napaeozapus*), Shrew (*Blarina, Sorex*), Rabbit (*Sylvilagus*), Rat (*Rattus*), Vole (*Microtus*), Muskrat (*Ondatra zibethicus*), Domestic (cat, dog), Man (rarely)
Ixodes neotomae	California, New Mexico, Utah	Lyme disease	Woodrat (*Neotoma*), Mice (*Peromyscus*), Rabbit (*Lepus, Sylvilagus*), Muskrat (*Ondatra zibethicus*), Kangaroo rat (*Dipodomys*), Gray fox (*Urocyon cinereoargenteus*), Domestic (dog)
Ixodes ochotonae	California Colorado, Idaho, Montana, Nevada, South Dakota, Utah, Washington, Wyoming, British Columbia, Saskatchewan	—	Pika (*Ochotona princeps*), Woodrat (*Neotoma*), Mouse and Vole (*Peromyscus, Microtus, Clethrionomys*), Chipmunk (*Tamias*), Pocket gopher (*Thomomys*), Squirrel (*Tamiasciurus*), Ground squirrel (*Spermophilus*), Heather vole (*Phenacomys*), Fox (*Urocyon cinereoargentatus*)
Ixodes pacificus (western black-legged tick)	Arizona, California, Nevada, Oregon, Utah, Washington, British Columbia	Lyme disease, tularemia, tick paralysis, ehrlichiosis, implicated anaplasmosis, spotted fever group rickettsia, equine ehrlichiosis	Columbian black-tailed deer (*Odocoileus hemionus columbianus*), Mouse (*Peromyscus, Perognathus, Zapus*), Woodrat (*Neotoma*), Ground squirrel (*Citellus*),Wolf (*Canis lupus*), Cougar (*Felis concolor*), Bobcat (*Felis rufus*), Coyote (*Canis latrans*), Rabbit (*Sylvilagus, Lepus*), Chipmunk (*Eutamias*), Shrew (*Sorex*), Mole (*Scapanus*), Mink (*Mustela*), Squirrel (*Tamiasciurus*), Domestic (burro, cat, cattle, dog, goat, horse, mule), Man
Ixodes peromysci	California	—	Deer mouse (*Peromyscus maniculatus*)
Ixodes rugosus	California, Oregon, Washington, British Columbia	—	Skunk (*Spilogale, Mephitis*), Fox (*Vulpes*), Weasel (*Mustela*), Coyote (*Canis latrans*), Domestic (Dog)
Ixodes scapularis (=*dammini*) (black-legged tick)	Eastern U.S. and Canada	Lyme disease, human babesiosis, human granulytic erhlichiosis, tularemia, spotted fever group rickettsia, anaplamosis, Powassan virus	White-tailed deer (*Odocoileus virginianus*), Mouse and Vole (*Peromyscus, Blarina, Microtus, Mus, Cleithrodontomys*), Squirrel (*Sciurus, Tamiasciurus*), Raccoon (*Procyon lotor*), Opossum (*Didelphis marsupialis*), Fox (*Vulpes vulpes, Urocyon cinereargentatus*), Cotton rat (*Sigmodon hispidus*), Rice rat (*Oryzomys palustris*), Rat (*Rattus*), Chipmunk (*Eutamias, Tamias*), Rabbit (*Sylvilagus, Lepus*), Feral swine (*Sus scrofa*), Coyote (*Canis latrans*), Wolf (*Canis lupus*), Bobcat (*Felis rufus*), Skunk (*Mephitis*), Florida panther (*Felis concolor coryi*), Bobcat (*Felis rufus floridana*), Domestic (cat, cattle, dog, goat, horse, mule, pig, sheep), Man
Ixodes sculptus	Western states, British Columbia, Alberta, Saskatchewan	—	Ground squirrel (*Citellus*), Chipmunk (*Eutamias*), Mouse (*Peromyscus*), Weasel (*Mustela*), Woodrat (*Neotoma*), Skunk (*Mephitis*), Rabbit (*Lepus*), Raccoon (*Procyon lotor*), Red fox, Badger (*Taxidea taxus*), Pocket gopher (*Geomys*), Prairie dog (*Cynomys*), Domestic (cat, goat), Man (rarely)
Ixodes soricis	Pacific Northwest states, British Columbia	—	Shrew (*Sorex*), Shrew-mole (*Neurotrichus*), Pocket gopher (*Thomomys*), Man (rarely)

(continued)

TABLE 4.2 (*continued*)

Species	Distribution	Diseases	Mammalian Hosts[a]
Ixodes spinipalpis	Pacific Northwest states, Colorado, Alberta, British Columbia	Lyme disease, Powassan virus	Woodrat (*Neotoma*), Mouse (*Peromyscus, Reithrodontomys*), Chipmunk (*Eutamias*), Ground squirrel (*Citellus*), Squirrel (*Tamiasciurus*), Shrew (*Sorex*), Weasel (*Mustela*), Pika (*Ochotona princeps*), Rabbit (*Lepus, Sylvilagus*)
Ixodes texanus	Widespread	Implicated raccoon babesiosis (*Babesi lotori*), implicated Rocky Mountain spotted fever	Raccoon (*Procyon lotor*), Badger (*Taxidea taxus*), Skunk (*Spilogale, Mephitis*), Opossum (*Didelphis marsupialis*), Rabbit (*Sylvilagus, Lepus*), Squirrel (*Sciurus*), Weasel, Mink (*Mustela*), Marten (*Martes*), Woodchuck (*Marmota*), Bobcat (*Lynx rufus*), Domestic (dog), Man
Ixodes tovari	Texas	—	Rabbit (*Sylvilagus, Lepus*), Domestic (cattle, goats)
Ixodes woodi	Alabama, Arizona, California, Colorado, Idaho, Indiana, Kansas, Nevada, New Mexico, North Carolina, Oklahoma, Oregon, Texas, Washington, Wyoming	—	Woodrat (*Neotoma*), Mouse (*Peromyscus*), Pocket gopher (*Pappogeomys*), Raccoon (*Procyon lotor*), Kangaroo rat (*Dipodomys*), Shrew (*Notiosorex*), Cotton rat (*Sigmodon hispidus*), Skunk (*Spilogale, Mephitis*), Man (rarely)

[a]Names as from sources.
[b]Agent isolated from field-collected ticks, but no documented evidence of vector status.
Sources: Bishopp and Trembley (1945), Cooley and Kohls (1945), Gregson (1956), Wilson and Baker (1972), Keirans and Clifford (1978), Spielman et al. (1979), Lane and Burgdorfer (1988), Hall et al. (1991), Robbins and Keirans (1992), Durden and Keirans (1996), Keirans et al. (1996a,b).

(94%), North Carolina (99%), Oklahoma (91%), South Carolina (69%), Tennessee (7%), and Virginia (56%). Annual prevalence of *I. scapularis* on deer in south Florida ranged from 11% to 48% from 1984 to 1990, while prevalence between sites varied from 6%–49% (Forrester et al. 1996). Numbers of *I. scapularis* on deer are usually fairly low [e.g., 2.9–10.7 ticks/deer in Alabama (Durden et al. 1991); 4.0 ticks/deer in Minnesota (Gill et al. 1993)]. For information on adult *I. scapularis* on other mammals see Table 4.1, Greiner et al. 1984 (feral swine in Florida), Fish and Dowler 1989 (opossum, raccoon, and skunk in New York), and Wehinger et al. 1995 (Florida panther and bobcat).

Immature *I. scapularis* are reported from a wide range of hosts; prevalence and intensity vary considerably between studies. Mean numbers of larvae and nymphs on white-footed mice were 36/host and 6.3/host, respectively, in Massachusetts (Wilson and Spielman 1985) and 3.4/host and 1.3/host, respectively, in Connecticut (Stafford et al. 1995). Short-tailed shrews along coastal Massachusetts were infested with an average of 1.1 larvae/host and 0.01 nymph/host (Telford et al. 1990). In New York, *I. scapularis* larvae were present on *Peromyscus leucopus* (94%, 8 ticks/host), *Procyon lotor* (94%, 136 ticks/host) and *Didelphis marsupialis* (100%, 54 ticks/host) (Fish and Daniels 1990). In collections of larval *I. scapularis* in Alabama, over 88% were from cotton mice, 9% from golden mice, and 2% from cotton rats (Luckhardt et al.

1991). Apperson et al. (1993) reported that lizards were more heavily infested as hosts of *I. scapularis* than rodents.

Prevalence of *I. cookei* on groundhogs includes 29% and 38% in Ontario (Ko 1972; Farkas and Surgeoner 1991; respectively), and 25% in New York state (Cohn et al. 1986). Mean intensities were 8.4 (larvae), 2.3 (nymphs), and 0.8 (adults) (Farkas and Surgeoner 1991). Ouellette et al. (1997) reported average infestations in North Carolina of less than one tick per raccoon of larvae, nymphs, and adults of *I. scapularis* and 1.3 larvae, 1.3 nymphs, and 0.8 females of *I. texanus*. In Georgia, prevalence and intensity of *I. scapularis* were 2% and 1.0 (raccoon) and 19% and 3.4 (opossum); similar data for *I. texanus* were 24% and 3.4 (raccoon), and 0 (opossum) (Pung et al. 1994). In Alberta, *Clethrionomys gapperi* was the major small mammal host of *I. angustus* despite the abundance of *Peromyscus maniculatus* (Sorensen and Moses 1998). Prevalence and intensity of *I. dentatus* on cottontail rabbits from Massachusetts were 85% and 11.6 (adult ticks, peak in April), 62% and 5.4 (nymphs, peak in October), and 85% and 54.7 (larvae, peak in September) (Telford and Spielman 1989). *Ixodes minor* was the most common ectoparasite of eastern woodrats in coastal South Carolina (prevalence 70%, intensity 14.7) (Durden et al. 1997). Maupin et al. (1994) reported intensities of *I. spinipalpis* from 0.13 to 14.8 ticks/host on *Neotoma mexicana* from three sites in Colorado.

ENVIRONMENTAL LIMITATIONS. All stages of *Ixodes* are highly prone to desiccation, and microhabitat contributes greatly to off-host survival of these ticks. Environmental factors limiting survival have been thoroughly examined for *I. scapularis* because of its role as a vector of Lyme disease. Kitron et al. (1991, 1992) used a geographic information system (GIS) in Illinois to compare the spatial distribution of tick-infested and uninfested white-tailed deer and studied the spatial distribution of deer around sites where *I. scapularis* were present and where Lyme disease transmission occurred. Tick-infested deer were concentrated around known enzootic foci, indicating that these foci were the only important sources of tick infestations. Tick presence was associated with deer, sandy soil, hardwoods, and proximity to major rivers (Kitron et al. 1991). The spatial distribution of ticks and Lyme disease cases was analyzed by county in Wisconsin (Kitron and Kazmierczak 1997) and was significantly correlated with spatial distribution of human cases. Degree of forest cover was also clustered in the same area. Kitron and Kazmierczak (1997) showed positive spatial autocorrelation (clusters) of ticks, Lyme disease, and forests in Wisconsin. Using data from Landsat thermatic mappers, Glass et al. (1995) associated forest cover and location of residences with Lyme disease cases to identify risk categories for Lyme disease. Dister et al. (1997) used similar data and GIS to integrate it with canine seroprevalence to Lyme disease and found a high correlation with seroprevalence and proportions of deciduous forest and densely vegetated residential areas adjacent to woods.

Adult female *I. scapularis* feed mostly on white-tailed deer, and deer density strongly influences reproduction and abundance of this tick (Wilson et al. 1988; Deblinger et al. 1992). Increased abundance of deer over time is a proposed explanation for increasing regional abundance of *I. scapularis* (Spielman et al. 1985). Immature *I. scapularis* feed on a wide range of small and medium-sized mammals as well as on birds and reptiles (Keirans et al. 1996b). The availability of hosts does not appear to limit the presence of *I. scapularis* (Wilson 1998). Wilson (1998) presents a discussion of conditions influencing the distribution and abundance of *I. scapularis*. Tick abundance in Maryland was positively correlated with well-drained sandy soils with low water levels and negatively correlated with urban land use patterns, wetlands, and amount of privately owned lands and soils saturated with water (Glass et al. 1994).

Ixodes pacificus is most common along the temperate west coast, with some disjunct populations inland (Table 4.1). An isolated population in Arizona is present in a region where snowmelt provides sufficient moisture and vegetation to support the population (Dennis et al. 1998). In Utah, *I. pacificus* is found in narrow bands of riverine habitat (Dennis et al. 1998). *Ixodes angustus* is often associated with cool moist habitats such as forest and riparian areas and is thought to be associated with nests of hosts (Robbins and Keirans 1992). In Colorado, *I. spinipalpis* is present in the semiarid foothills, but off-host stages are exclusively associated with woodrat nests that provide high humidity and moderate temperatures appropriate for survival (Maupin et al. 1994).

PATHOLOGY AND DISEASE TRANSMISION. The bites of *Ixodes* ticks can cause irritation, trauma, and sometimes paralysis (Nelson 1973; Strickland et al. 1976; Lane et al. 1984). Occasionally, bites of some species such as *I. angustus* and *I. scapularis* have been reported as causing inflamed lesions (Durden and Keirans 1996). Ko (1972) reported strong local tissue reactions by groundhog to feeding *I. cookei;* after 2 days of feeding, attachment sites were red, and by 3 days, fluid-filled swellings were present. The swellings were hard and consisted mainly of fibrous tissue. Seven days after attachment, extensive areas were heavily infiltrated with neutrophils, lymphocytes, and plasma cells. A case of tick paralysis in a western harvest mouse *(Reithrodontomys megalotis)* has been associated with *I. pacificus* (Botzler et al. 1980).

Ixodes spp. are effective vectors of a wide range of diseases (Table 4.2). While Lyme disease causes little to no pathology in wild mammals, mammals are reservoirs of the disease, and the causal agent, *Borrelia burgdorferi*, has been isolated from a wide range of species (Spielman et al. 1985; Moody et al. 1994; summarized in Ginsberg 1994). The primary vectors of Lyme disease in North America include *I. scapularis* (Oliver et al. 1993; Spielman et al. 1985) and *I. pacificus* (Brown and Lane 1992). Other less important vectors include *I. angustus* (Damrow et al. 1989; Banerjee et al. 1994), *I. cookei* (Levine et al. 1991), *I. dentatus* (Telford and Spielman 1989), *I. jellisoni* (Keirans et al. 1996a), *I. minor* (Durden and Keirans 1996), *I. neotomae* (Brown and Lane 1992), and *I. spinipalpis* (Maupin et al. 1994). Since *I. dentatus, I. neotomae,* and *I. spinipalpis* rarely feed on man, they maintain the disease in enzootic cycles among the mammalian reservoir hosts and the ticks that feed on them (e.g., between *I. spinipalpis* and the Mexican woodrat, *Neotoma mexicana:* Maupin et al. 1994; between *I. neotomae* and dusky-footed woodrats, jackrabbits, cottontails, California kangaroo rats, and deer mice: Brown and Lane 1996). Spirochetes have been isolated from *I. angustus, I. jellisoni,* and *I. minor,* but at most, they may only serve as minor vectors.

Along the Pacific coast, *I. pacificus* feed as immatures on deer mouse *(Peromyscus maniculatus)*, dusky-footed woodrat *(Neotoma fuscipes)*, and California kangaroo rat *(Dipodomys californicus)*, which are implicated as reservoirs *of Borrelia burgdorferi* (Lane 1990a; Brown and Lane 1992). *Ixodes pacificus* is also considered a bridge vector of *B. burgdorferi* to humans from the enzootic cycle maintained between *I. spinipalpis* and *Neotoma* (Brown and Lane 1992). The apparent reluctance of *I. pacificus* to feed on deer mice contributes to the low prevalence of infection in this species (Richter et al. 1996). In northeastern and upper

Midwestern states, the white-footed mouse (*Peromyscus leucopus*) is the primary reservoir for *B. burgdorferi* and the most important host for immature *I. scapularis* (Spielman et al. 1985). In southern states, cotton *rats (Sigmodon hispidus),* cotton mice (*Peromyscus gossypinus*), eastern woodrats (*Neotoma floridanus*), and rice rats (*Oryzomys palustris*) may also be involved as reservoirs (Oliver et al. 1993, 1995; Levin et al. 1995). Both *I. scapularis* and *I. pacificus* feed readily on man as infected nymphs and adults.

Ixodes scapularis is also considered the primary vector of human granulocytic ehrlichiosis (Pancholi et al. 1995) as well as human babesiosis (caused by *Babesia microti*) (Spielman et al. 1985), which is also vectored by *I. pacificus* (Oliveira and Kreier 1979) and *I. muris* (Spielman et al. 1984). The white-footed deer mouse is also the primary reservoir of human granulocytic ehrlichiosis (Telford et al. 1996) and babesiosis (Spielman et al. 1985). *Ixodes scapularis* is an efficient laboratory vector of deer babesiosis caused by *Babesia odocoilei* (Kocan and Kocan 1991). *Ixodes texanus* is a vector of *Babesia lotori* (Anderson et al. 1981).

Vectors implicated in the transmission of Powassan virus include *I. cookei* (Farkas and Surgeoner 1991), *I. marxi* (McLean and Larke 1963), *I. spinipalpis* (Keirans and Clifford 1983), and *I. scapularis* (Costero and Grayson 1993). This virus appears to be maintained in raccoons, foxes, weasels, skunks, and possibly groundhogs, squirrels, and lagomorphs (Durden and Keirans 1996). Rocky Mountain spotted fever also is reported to be transmitted by *I. dentatus* (Clifford et al. 1969) and spotted fever group rickettsia have been isolated from both *I. scapularis* and *I. texanus* (Anderson et al. 1986; Sonenshine 1991). Vectors of tularemia include *I. banksi, I. cookei, I. dentatus, I. kingi,* and *I. pacificus* (Lawrence et al. 1965; Thorpe et al. 1965; Stickland et al. 1976; Artsob et al. 1984; Westrom et al. 1985). The vector of Connecticut virus in eastern cottontails is *I. dentatus* (Main and Carey 1980). A splenopathogenic piroplasm is transmitted to tundra redback voles in Alaska by *I. angustus* (Fay and Rausch 1969). *Ixodes scapularis* has been implicated in the transmission of anaplasmosis (Strickland et al. 1976). The filarioid nematode *Ackertia marmotae* was transmitted in the laboratory to groundhogs by *I. cookei* (Ko 1972).

IMMUNITY. Various species of hard ticks induce host resistance that is immunologically mediated (Wikel 1996). The expression of this immunological response varies with different hosts and tick species (reviewed by Brown 1985; Wikel 1996; and Wikel and Bergman 1997). Effects of acquired resistance include decreases in engorgement weights, engorgement success, egg deposition, and hatching rates; longer feeding periods; and increases in preoviposition periods and egg and tick mortality (Wikel 1996). Most research has been conducted with cattle or laboratory animals with only a few reports of acquired resistance in wild mammals. Resistant hosts often develop cutaneous reactions at the feeding site that differ greatly from nonresistant sites.

Often an influx of basophils and eosinophils surround the attached mouthparts, indicative of cutaneous basophil hypersensitivity. Degranulation occurs, and histamine inhibits tick salivation and engorgement (reviewed in Wikel and Bergman 1997).

Acquired resistance to *I. scapularis* is considered not to be elicited in *Peromyscus leucopus, P. gossypinus,* or *Mus musculus,* but it has been reported in the guinea pig (Davidar et al. 1989; Galbe and Oliver 1992). Allan and Appel (1992), however, did report mild evidence of acquired resistance in both white mice and *P. leucopus* with repeated exposure to *I. scapularis.* Raccoons developed immune resistance to infestation by larval *I. scapularis* after repeated applications of nymphs and larvae (Craig et al. 1996). Production of anti-tick salivary gland extract antibodies correlated to development of resistance to infestation that prevented nearly 90% of larvae from feeding. It has been suggested that host resistance does not develop in natural or preferred hosts (Galbe and Oliver 1992), and Ribeiro (1989) suggested that substances in saliva of some ticks inhibit cell-mediated immunity. To enhance survival and successful blood-feeding, ticks have evolved a mechanism to develop host immunosuppression (Wikel and Bergman 1997). Wikel et al. (1997) exposed BALB/C mice to pathogen-free *I. scapularis* nymphs four times and observed decreased infection with *B. burgdorferi* during the fifth exposure. Only 17% of the multiply infested mice became infected compared to 100% of the control mice (single exposure). The basis for this resistance to infection and its implications in the epidemiology of tick-borne diseases is unknown.

CONTROL AND TREATMENT. Immense effort has been expended towards the control of *I. scapularis* and *I. pacificus* because of their roles as major vectors of Lyme disease. Most research on the control of these ticks has focused on the use of insecticides, host management, vegetation management, biological control, and personal protection measures (Wilson and Deblinger 1993; summarized in Schmidtmann 1994; Ginsberg 1994). While most *I. scapularis* are associated with woods, wooded suburban sites, and ecotone areas, ticks on lawns and ornamental plantings pose significant risks (Fish 1995). Tick control efforts by licensed operators in these locations in Connecticut primarily used cyfluthrin, chlorpyrifos, and carbaryl to target control of these ticks in peridomestic locations (Ginsberg 1994; Stafford 1997). Prescribed burning of forests (especially pine-dominated) is a management method that is effective in decreasing populations of *I. scapularis* (Wilson 1986; Mather et al. 1993), as well as *Dermacentor albipictus* (Drew et al. 1985), *D. variabilis* (Smith et al. 1946), *Amblyomma maculatum* (Scifres et al. 1988), and *A. americanum* (Davidson et al. 1994). Recent efforts have been made toward host-targeted control with passive-application acaricide on the host by use of a feeding device or application of acaricides to materials used as nesting materials (summarized in Schmidtmann 1994).

PUBLIC HEALTH CONCERNS. Man can be affected directly by the discomfort and irritation of bites from *Ixodes* or by the transmission of diseases by the ticks (Table 4.2). Man is commonly fed upon by *I. scapularis* and *I. pacificus,* less commonly by *I. cookei,* and rarely by several other species (Lane 1994; Campbell and Bowles 1994; Felz et al. 1996; Walker et al. 1998). Feeding *I. pacificus* elicit strong responses that often result in edema, chronic sores, ulcer, fever, mild rashes, and headaches (Lane 1994).

The most common tick-borne disease in North America is Lyme disease. The vectors of this and other diseases, and the enzootic cycles involved, have been discussed previously. Further information on human Lyme disease, ehrlichiosis, and babesiosis are provided by Spielman et al. (1985), Lastavica (1992), Oliver et al. (1993), and Pancholi et al. (1995).

DOMESTIC ANIMAL CONCERNS. Feeding by *Ixodes* can cause irritation and blood loss. *Ixodes scapularis* can reach pest proportions on livestock (Strickland et al. 1976). Tick paralysis has been reported from feeding by *I. pacificus* on dogs, humans, and other animals (Nelson 1973; Lane et al. 1984) and rarely from *I. scapularis* on dogs (Gregson 1973). Dogs are the most common and best-documented domestic animal to be infected with Lyme disease (Appel et al. 1993). Clinical effects of Lyme disease on dogs, cats, horses, and cows are summarized by Parker and White (1992) and Ginsberg (1994). While many species are occasional vectors of disease (Table 4.2), *Ixodes* are rarely associated with other diseases of domestic animals. Recently, *I. pacificus* has been implicated in the transmission of *Ehrlichia equi* to horses (Richter et al. 1996).

MANAGEMENT IMPLICATIONS. Although *Ixodes* are commonly found on wild rodents and other wild mammals, infestations seldom cause severe effects such as unthriftiness or death. White-tailed deer are a characteristic species of subclimax forests and are becoming increasingly common in the urban environment. They have been linked to the presence and abundance of *I. scapularis* (Main et al. 1981; Lastavica 1992). Numbers of larval *I. scapularis* have been correlated with the abundance of deer on various Massachusetts islands (Wilson et al. 1985). However, the correlation of deer presence with *I. scapularis* populations is not absolute: populations of *I. scapularis* have been reported from locations where deer are not present (Main et al. 1981; Duffy et al. 1994), and in these cases other midsized mammals serve to maintain tick populations. Lastavica et al. (1989) reported a high correlation between the presence of deer and the frequency of households with Lyme disease around a Massachusetts nature preserve. Management efforts have been focused on removal or containment of deer to reduce tick populations (Stafford 1993). While successful in reducing tick numbers, these methods are not feasible for prolonged and widespread control. Recent efforts include experimental treatment of deer (as the primary host of adults) or small rodents (as primary hosts of immatures) with acaricide (reviewed in Schmidtmann 1994). These host-targeted treatments appear to be promising, but efficacy has been variable with host-targeted control based on *Peromyscus* (Stafford 1992). Maupin et al. (1991) studied the landscape ecology of *I. scapularis* in Westchester Co., New York, and demonstrated that the presence of *I. scapularis* is critically associated with the presence of forested habitats in developed suburban neighborhoods.

Amblyomma. Ticks of the genus *Amblyomma* feed on a wide range of species of wild mammals. Effects of feeding may be innocuous or result in irritation around the feeding sites, anemia, paralysis, transmission of a disease agent, or death of the host. Several species are important from a public health standpoint, because they vector several important diseases in man and other animals.

Adult *Amblyomma* are moderate to large ticks (4–8 mm), often with highly ornate patterns on the dorsal scutum. This genus is generally tropical or subtropical with eight species established in North America; six species feed at least occasionally on mammals (Keirans and Durden 1998). They are *A. americanum* (lone star tick), *A. cajennense* (Cayenne tick), *A. imitator, A. inornatum, A. maculatum* (Gulf Coast tick) and *A. tuberculatum.* The lone star tick, *A. americanum,* is the best known of the North American species because of its importance as pest and vector species of man, domestic livestock, and wildlife. Of the others, *A. cajennense* and *A. imitator* are only known from southern Texas, being more abundant in Mexico and South America (Strickland et al. 1976; Strey et al. 1996). The two non–mammal-feeding species are *A. dissimile,* which feed entirely on snakes, and *A. rotundatum,* which feed primarily on amphibians and reptiles. All species use three hosts, with adult ticks feeding, in general, on large hosts (mainly cattle and white-tailed deer) and immatures feeding on small mammals or birds.

Amblyomma spp. are characterized by long mouthparts and palps (second segment) as well as eyes and festoons. Species can be distinguished using keys in Jones et al. (1972) and Keirans and Litwak (1989) (adults), Keirans and Durden (1998) (nymphs), and Clifford et al. (1961) (larvae).

LIFE HISTORY. Because *Amblyomma* is a "southern" genus of tick, with development retarded by cooler temperatures (Semtner et al. 1973) and low relative humidity (Koch and Dunn 1980b), one can find ticks in all stages of development on or off hosts throughout the year. There is usually one generation per year. The general life cycle typically involves three hosts: Gravid females drop from hosts and oviposit on the ground or under debris. Egg masses contain large numbers of eggs with up to 8300 eggs for *A. americanum,* 18,000 eggs for *A. maculatum,* and 7700 eggs for *A. cajennense* (Strickland et al. 1976). Eggs hatch, and larvae attach to small mammals and ground-frequenting birds.

After dropping from the host and molting, nymphs attach to another host (small mammal or ground-frequenting bird). After feeding, nymphs detach and molt, and adults emerge and attach to hosts (mammals) on which they mate and feed. Males often remain on the host but blood-fed females leave the host.

In general, all stages of *A. americanum* are most abundant on hosts in spring and summer, with some variation from one region to the next. Samuel and Trainer (1970) reported that adult *A. americanum,* though present year round on white-tailed deer in south Texas, were most prevalent in spring. On white-tailed deer in Oklahoma, the greatest infestations of larvae occurred in late July and August, nymphs peaked from April to October, and adults peaked from late May to July (Patrick and Hair 1977). In Virginia, most larvae were present in August or September, most nymphs in August and September, and most adults in May to June (Sonenshine and Levy 1971). In Georgia, peak larval activity occurred from July to September, nymphal activity from April to June, and adult activity from March through May (Davidson et al. 1994). Koch (1982) recovered most *A. americanum* immatures from dogs in southeastern Oklahoma and northwestern Arkansas in August. Semtner et al. (1973) recovered most larvae of *A. americanum* from vegetation in August and September in Oklahoma and September in Mississippi, respectively; nymphs predominated in June and August to September (Oklahoma) and May and August (Mississippi).

Feeding by adult *A. maculatum* was greatest on cattle in Texas in September, with feeding by immatures on birds in January and February (Teel et al. 1988). Presumably, feeding by immatures on mammals occurs at the same time. Most adult *A. maculatum* were collected during summer from deer in south Texas (Samuel and Trainer 1970). Adult *A. maculatum* were collected from vegetation from May to September in South Carolina (Clark et al. 1998). Larval and nymphal *A. maculatum* peaked in abundance on birds in coastal Texas in December and February to March, respectively (Teel et al. 1998). In northern Oklahoma, the peak abundance of larvae and nymphs occurred in July and August (Williams and Hair 1976). Larvae of *A. maculatum* were only collected from trapped rodents in South Carolina in July to October, and nymphs were collected March, April, and July to September.

All stages of *A. cajennense* can be collected throughout the year (Strickland et al. 1976). Seasonal peaks for larvae have been reported in midsummer to fall (Teel et al. 1998). Adult *A. tuberculatum* have been collected year round (Bishopp and Trembley 1945), with larvae present during late fall and winter (Rogers 1953; Wilson and Baker 1972).

Feeding site preferences often vary with species of host, species of tick, and life stage. Adult *A. americanum* attach to livestock on thin-skinned areas such as ears (outside surface), dewlap, escutcheon, and axillary and inguinal region. In severe infestations, adults attach all over the body (Strickland et al. 1976). On deer, pre-ferred attachment sites for lone star ticks are around the eyes and on the ears (Bolte et al. 1970; Bloemer et al. 1988). Most adult *A. americanum* were on the front and underside of coyotes and on the legs and tail of gray foxes; most immatures were on the legs, tail, and ventral regions (Bloemer and Zimmerman 1988). Larvae and nymphs of *A. americanum* were found over the body of raccoons in North Carolina but were concentrated on the head (larvae 49%, nymphs 61%) (Ouellette et al. 1997).

Adult *A. maculatum* attach almost exclusively inside the pinna of the ear of large mammals such as cattle, horses, deer, and feral swine (Strickland et al. 1976; Greiner et al. 1984). Most adult *A. inornatum* (72%) attached to the medial surface of the hind leg of deer (fawns preferred), while adult *A. maculatum* attached to antlers in velvet (32%) and ears (29%) (Samuel and Trainer 1970). Most immature *Amblyomma* spp. (55%) were attached to ears. Adult *A. cajennense* frequently attach to ears, flanks, wither, tail, and mane of horses and all over the body of cattle (Strickland et al. 1976).

EPIZOOTIOLOGY

DISTRIBUTION AND HOST RANGE. In North America, *Amblyomma* is generally limited to the southern states, with the greatest occurrence in the southeast (Table 4.3). All six mammalian species have been reported from white-tailed deer; four (*A. americanum, A. cajennense, A. inornatum* and *A. maculatum*) commonly infest livestock (Strickland et al. 1976). The two primary North American species, *A. americanum* and *A. maculatum,* use small-to-large mammals as hosts. White-tailed deer are the prominent wild mammalian host of adult *A. americanum* (Demarais et al. 1987; Bloemer et al. 1988). Deer also serve as hosts for immatures. Adults are found on a wide range of large mammals that include cattle, horses, and dogs, while immatures feed on small to medium-sized mammals as well as birds (Wilson and Baker 1972). Gray foxes and coyotes are considered important hosts, as they become heavily infested with all stages of lone star ticks (Bloemer and Zimmerman 1988). They, along with other small and medium-sized wild mammals, such as red fox and raccoons, are the most commonly reported hosts (Sonenshine and Stout 1971; and Koch and Dunn 1980a). Ouellette et al. (1997) reported that *A. americanum* was the most abundant tick on raccoon in North Carolina, with all stages present. Conflicting reports exist about the role of small rodents as hosts for immatures. Schulze et al. (1984) reported that *Peromyscus leucopus* was the primary host of immature *A. americanum* in New Jersey. In other studies, immatures were rarely found on small rodents (Wilson and Baker 1972; Zimmerman et al. 1987; Clark et al. 1998).

The Gulf Coast tick, *A. maculatum,* is generally concentrated along areas bordering the Gulf of Mexico and the Atlantic Coast (Bishopp and Trembley 1944), although Clark et al. (1998) noted abundant popula-

TABLE 4.3—Hosts, geographic distribution, and diseases vectored by North American *Amblyomma* that feed on mammals

Species (Common Name)	Distribution	Diseases	Mammalian Hosts[a]
Amblyomma americanum (lone star tick)	Southeastern and south-central U.S. (north to New Jersey)	Rocky Mountain spotted fever tularemia, ehrlichiosis, tick paralysis, Q fever, babesiosis (*Babesia cervi*)	White-tailed deer (*Odocoileus virginianus*), Cotton rat (*Sigmodon hispidus*), Rice rat (*Oryzomys palustris*), Squirrels (*Sciurus, Tamiasciurus*), Norway rat (*Rattus norvegicus*), Southern pocket gopher (*Geomys pinetis*), Florida mink (*Mustela vison*), Coyote (*Canis latrans*), Fox (*Vulpes vulpes, Urocyon cinereoargenteus*), Mountain lion (*Felis concolor*), Bobcat (*Lynx rufus*), Wolf (*Canis lupus, Canis rufus*), Skunk (*Mephetis mephitis*), Raccoon (*Procyon lotor*), Rabbit (*Sylvilagus, Lepus*), Bear (*Ursus americanus*), Woodchuck (*Marmota flaviventris, Marmota monax*), Badger (*Taxidea taxus*), Mouse (*Mus*), Florida panther (*Felis concolor coryi*), Otter (*Lutra canadensis*), Feral swine (*Sus scrofa*), Blackbuck antelope (*Antilope cericapra*), Opossum (*Didelphis marsulialis*), Sambar deer (*Cervus unicolor*), Domestic (cat, cattle, dog, horse, sheep, pig, mule, goat), Man
Amblyomma cajennense (cayenne tick)	Southern Texas	Spotted fever group rickettsia	White-tailed deer (*Odocoileus virginianus*), Coyote (*Canis latrans*), Raccoon (*Procyon lotor*), Peccary (*Pecari angulatus*), Feral swine (*Sus scrofa*), Domestic (cattle, dog, donkey, goat, horse, sheep), Man (rarely)
Amblyomma imitator	Southern Texas	—	Deer (*Odocoileus virginianus*), Peccary (*Pecari angulatus*), Domestic (cattle, goat, horse), Man (rarely)
Amblyomma inornatum	Southern Texas	—	White-tailed deer (*Odocoileus virginianus*), Coyote (*Canis latrans*), Rabbit (*Sylvilagus, Lepus*), Ground squirrel (*Citellus*), Armadillo (*Dasypus novemcinctus*), Peccary (*Pecari angulatus*), Cotton rat (*Sigmodon hispidus*), Domestic (cattle, dog, goat), Man (rarely)
Amblyomma maculatum (Gulf Coast tick)	Southeastern U.S. (up to Oklahoma)	Tick paralysis, predisposes for myiasis	White-tailed deer (*Odocoileus virginianus*) Rabbit (*Sylvilagus, Lepus*), Feral swine (*Sus scrofa*), Coyote (*Canis latrans*), Raccoon (*Procyon lotor*), Wolf (*Canis lupus*)[b], Skunk (*Mephitis*), Squirrel (*Sciurus*), Cotton rat (*Sigmodon hispidus*), Rice rat (*Oryzomys palustris*), Roof rat (*Rattus rattus*), Fox (*Vulpes vulpes, Uroyon cinereoargenteus*), Bear (*Ursus*), Bobcat (*Felis rufus*), Florida panther (*Felis concolor coryi*), Sambar deer (*Cervus unicolor*), Domestic (cat, cattle, dog, goat, pig, horse, sheep, mule), Man (rarely)
Amblyomma tuberculatum (gopher tortoise tick)	Southeastern U.S. (north to S. Carolina)	—	Rabbit (*Sylvilagus*), Fox (*Vulpes vulpes, Uroyon cinereoargenteus*), Fox Squirrel (*Sciurus niger*), Gray squirrel (*Sciurus carolinensis*), White-tailed deer (*Odocoileus virginianus*), Domestic (cattle, dog)

[a] Names as from sources.
[b] Must be *Canis rufus* (editors).
Sources: Cooley and Kohls (1944), Bishopp and Trembley (1945), Wilson and Baker (1972), Coombs and Springer (1974), Strickland et al. (1976), Forrester (1992), Mertins et al. (1992), Keirans and Durden (1998).

tions > 160 km inland. A wide range of species serve as hosts for *A. maculatum* (Table 4.3*)*, with immatures feeding primarily on birds and occasionally small to medium-sized mammals, and adults on larger mammals. Feral swine and white-tailed deer, in that order, appear to be the preferred wild hosts in North America.

Amblyomma cajennense is fairly indiscriminate in host range and is reported from a wide range of mammals (Table 4.3). All stages readily feed on large mammals such as livestock (Stickland et al 1976). Adult *A.*

tuberculatum feeds exclusively on tortoises, and the geographic range of this species coincides with that of its primary host, the gopher tortoise (Cooley and Kohls 1944). Immatures, however, may be present on a range of mammals as well as reptiles and ground-frequenting birds (Keirans and Durden 1998). Adult *A. inornatum* feed on a range of large mammals, while immatures feed on ground-dwelling birds and small mammals such as ground squirrels, armadillo, and coyotes (Keirans and Durden 1998). In addition, there has been a report of one larva of *A. dissimile,* a snake-feeding species in Florida, collected from a cotton mouse in Florida (Durden et al. 1993).

PREVALENCE AND INTENSITY. Lone star ticks are commonly found on deer throughout their range. Abundance of *A. americanum* can be very high, and Sonenshine and Levy (1971) reported densities of 1334–4212/ha (adults), 2145–3857/ha (nymphs) and 16 958/ha (larvae) on vegetation in Virginia. Lone star ticks were less common in exposed habitats such as old fields or pastures than in dense woodlands. In a comparison of seven forest types, more ticks (up to 5.5-fold more) were present in a relatively undisturbed subclimax forest compared to a mixed, old-wood-lot community (Sonenshine and Levy 1971). Prevalences vary on white-tailed deer (e.g., 10% in south Texas: Samuel and Trainer 1970; 24% in Alabama: Durden et al. 1991; 44% in North Carolina: Apperson et al. 1990). Smith (1977) reported the following percent prevalences on deer from Alabama (33%), Arkansas (17%), Florida (26%), Georgia (31%), Mississippi (22%), North Carolina (32%), Oklahoma (23%), South Carolina (44%), and Virginia (52%). Prevalence and mean intensity on fawns in Illinois were 80% and 21.6 ticks/fawn, respectively (Nelson et al. 1984).

Infestations on individual animals can reach high numbers, and Bishopp and Trembley (1945) reported 4800 ticks, mostly *A. americanum* nymphs, on ears of a deer in North Carolina. Infestations of *A. americanum* larvae on deer in Oklahoma averaged 3175/deer in July 1993 and 700/deer in August 1974 (Patrick and Hair 1977). Infestations of nymphs reached 565/deer in 1973 and 360/deer in 1974. Demarais et al. (1987) reported that *A. americanum* was the predominant tick species collected from white-tailed deer in Mississippi, with all stages present throughout the year.

Other species serve as hosts for *A. americanum* and are important for disseminating the species. In Tennessee, percent prevalences of *A. americanum* were 100% (striped skunk, woodchuck, gray fox), 72% (raccoon), 46% (opossum), 44% (eastern cottontail rabbit), and 50% (feral cats) (Zimmerman et al. 1988). Mean intensities of larvae, nymphs, and adults were 573, 65, and 0.4 (striped skunk); 383, 80, and 1.5 (raccoon); 49, 9, and 1 (woodchuck); 8.7, 0.8, and 0.2 (opossum); and 8.4 larvae and 2.6 nymphs on rabbit, 3.2 nymphs and 3.1 larvae on squirrel, and 156 larvae on fox. Average infestations of *A. americanum* on raccoon in North Carolina were 45.2 larvae, 78.6 nymphs, and 0.5 adults/host, with highest populations from July to September (Ouellette et al. 1997). In Georgia, prevalence and intensity of *A. americanum* on raccoon and opossum were 69% and 14%, respectively, and 181 and 32, respectively (Pung et al. 1994). The highest mean intensities on half-body counts on coyotes in Tennessee were 103 adults in May, 137 nymphs in June, and 5075 larvae in September (Bloemer and Zimmerman 1988). Mean numbers were lower on gray foxes (30 adults, 103 nymphs, and 2480 larvae). In south Florida < 1%

of feral swine were infested with *A. americanum* in comparison to 86% infested with *A. maculatum* (Greiner et al. 1984).

Prevalence of *A. maculatum* varies by host and location. Greiner et al. (1984) reported the tick from 86% of feral swine in south Florida. Reports from white-tailed deer include the following: 18% (south Texas: Samuel and Trainer 1970), 10% (south Florida: Forrester et al. 1996), 5% (southeastern states: Smith 1977), and 1% (Alabama: Durden et al. 1991). Prevalences on Florida panther and bobcat were 14% and 1%, respectively (Wehinger et al. 1995).

Amblyomma cajennense and *A. inornatum* have been reported from collared peccaries in Texas (98% and 5%, respectively) (Samuel and Low 1970). Most adult *A. inornatum* (76%) on deer occurred on young fawns (Samuel and Trainer 1970). Larval *A. tuberculatum* have been reported from deer (Smith 1977).

ENVIRONMENTAL LIMITATIONS. Temperature and relative humidity are two primary factors limiting tick distribution abundance and survival (Semtner et al. 1971a). Most ixodid ticks lose water when exposed to low relative humidity (< 80%), and a humid microhabitat is essential for off-host survival (Sonenshine 1993). Sauer and Hair (1971) demonstrated that the critical equilibrium humidity for adult lone star ticks is ~85%, below which survival is decreased. Hair and Bowman (1986) concluded that two factors related to abundance of lone star ticks are the presence of suitable hosts and an area that provides protection for the hosts and conservation of moisture with the presence of a forest canopy and vegetative ground cover.

The lone star tick is particularly common in secondary growth forest habitat with a dense understory. In the southeastern states, it is usually associated with habitat that is primarily oak-hickory, post-oak, blackjack oak, and persimmon-sassafras-elm forests (Semtner et al. 1971b; Hair and Bowman 1986). *A. americanum* is abundant in brushy pastures and wooded areas, especially those with dense underbrush (Semter et al. 1971a), and less frequently in exposed habitats such as old fields or pastures (Sonenshine and Levy 1971). Tick numbers decrease in taller woody vegetation, while adults and nymphs are more numerous in taller grassy vegetation. In Oklahoma, survival of adults was significantly higher in bottomland oak-hickory habitats, with lowest day temperatures and highest humidities, than in upland woods or meadows (Semter et al. 1973a). Larval survival of *A. americanum* was shortest in meadow habitat (10–19 days) and longest in bottomland oak-hickory habitat (33–106 days) (Patrick and Hair 1975). Under optimal conditions, unfed ticks can survive > 250 days (Strickland et al. 1976).

Habitats that support large numbers of white-tailed deer are likely to develop large lone star tick populations (Bolte et al. 1970), as deer are the most important hosts of adults and also serves as hosts for immatures. Deer use of various habitats influence distribution of ticks in these habitats, but ultimately climatic factors control the ability of the tick to survive (Patrick and Hair 1977).

Similar environmental requirements hold for other *Amblyomma.* Prevalence of *A. maculatum* and *A. inornatum* was significantly greater on young fawns captured in dense vegetation than on fawns from moderate or sparse vegetation (Samuel and Trainer 1970). Survival of *A. maculatum* during summer months was greater in canopied habitats than in meadows (Fleetwood 1985). The coastal prairie of Texas was found to support higher densities of adult *A. maculatum* than do the Rio Grande Plains (Teel et al. 1988).

Amblyomma cajennense is a tropical/subtropical species found consistently in drier regions in Texas. These ticks are more resilient to water loss and less tolerant of cold than are *A. maculatum* and *A. americanum* (Strey et al. 1996).

CLINICAL SIGNS. Feeding by ticks on cattle and deer, particularly by *A. americanum* on ears, produces thickened skin, scaliness, and partial denuding of hair (Bishopp and Trembley 1945). Davidson et al. (1985) reported mild focal cutaneous and subcutaneous inflammation associated with attachment sites of *A. americanum* on deer. Feeding by *A. maculatum* on ears of cattle can cause inflammation, production of yellowish exudate, edema, and deformation of the ear due to destruction of the cartilage (Strickland et al. 1976; Drummond 1987). Descriptions of the histology of feeding sites of all stages of *A. americanum* on guinea pigs are described by Brown and Knapp (1980a,b).

PATHOLOGY AND DISEASE TRANSMISSION TO WILD MAMMALS. Feeding by *Amblyomma* is particularly annoying to hosts, because this genus has long mouthparts. Effects of feeding are well documented in livestock and deer. Bites often form erythemous areas that may develop into suppurating lesions (Strickland et al. 1976). Kellogg et al. (1971) reported intradermal hemorrhage, small abscesses at attachment sites, hair loss, and moderate and infrequent hematomas as a result of feeding. In livestock, feeding sites can lead to secondary infection or myiasis (Strickland et al. 1976).

Effects of lone star ticks on whitetails include pruritis, hematoma, intradermal hemorrhage, blood loss, thickened skin, infection with pathogenic agents, and death (Bolte et al. 1970; Kellogg et al. 1971; Strickland et al. 1976). Demarais et al. (1987) indicated that the direct pathogenic effect of tick-feeding on deer was difficult to assess, but could partially contribute to leucocytosis and decreased packed-cell volumes. Fawns are particularly vulnerable (Bolte et al. 1970). Infestations, particularly on the head and around the eyes of newborn fawns, resulted in erosion of all hide, flesh, and connective tissue and ligaments around eyes of 6 of 18 fawns (Bolte et al. 1970). The sequence of events after tick attachment around eyes included initial swelling and development of a lesion in 3–7 days with an

increased eye secretion, necrosis in 5–7 more days with rupturing of blood vessels and free-flowing blood, possible host reaction, and secondary infection. All tissue within 5 cm was disintegrated, and mucus, lymph, and blood flowed from the wound. In eastern Oklahoma 17% of fawns < 6 weeks old were blinded by damage from tick-feeding around the head; 5% died (Bolte et al. 1970). Emerson (1969) suggested that blood loss caused by lone star ticks could kill fawns in Texas. Barker et al. (1973) produced anemia in fawns infested experimentally with *Theileria*-infected lone star ticks.

Feeding by *A. maculatum* and *A. americanum* (less so) also may result in tick paralysis in humans and large mammals (Stickland et al. 1976). *Amblyomma maculatum* feeding on whitetails can lead to suppurating wounds and destruction of the ear cartilage (Strickland et al. 1976). Severe infestations can be debilitating for hosts and can cause death.

The lone star tick, *A. americanum,* is a vector or suspected vector of several diseases involving wild mammals (Table 4.3). Forty-two percent of ticks collected in Arkansas were positive for the rickettsia causing Rocky Mountain spotted fever (Burgdorfer 1975). The lone star tick is implicated in causing tick paralysis (Arthur 1961) and vectoring Q fever, tularemia, deer babesiosis and theileriasis (Samuel and Trainer 1970; Kellogg et al. 1971; Barker et al. 1973; Strickland et al. 1976). Recently, it has been implicated as a vector of human monocytic ehrlichiosis (*Ehrlichia chaffeensis*) (Dumler and Bakken 1998). The role of wild mammals in this disease cycle is currently under investigation. Deer infected with *E. chaffeensis* do not show clinical evidence of disease, but mild histological changes may be present (Ewing et al. 1995). Lockhardt et al. (1998) studied the seroreactivity of wild rodents (cotton mouse, gray squirrel, fox squirrel, Norway rat, house mouse, white-footed mouse, eastern harvest mouse, rice rat, and cotton mouse) in Georgia and South Carolina to *Erhlichia chaffeensis*. Despite the presence of both *A. americanum* and *E. chaffeensis,* these mammals were seronegative. Lockhardt et al. (1998) concluded that this reflected the rare feeding of infected nymphs on these rodents and that wild rodents were at low risk of exposure with limited, if any, involvement in the epidemiology of *E. chaffeensis.*

IMMUNITY. The literature on immunity to ticks has been extensively reviewed by Allen (1987), George (1992), and Wikel (1996). Most studies on immunity have been conducted with laboratory animals or cattle. Acquired resistance to *A. maculatum* (Strother et al. 1974) and *A. americanum* (George et al. 1985) has been reported in cattle. Stronger acquired resistance and heightened in vivo lymphocyte responses to salivary gland extracts were expressed in purebred cattle with experimental infestations of *A. americanum* (George et al. 1985). After exposure of cattle to *A. americanum,* cutaneous cellular responses occur; these responses are consistent with cutaneous basophil hypersensitivity (George 1992). The responses occurred ~24 hours after attachment and were characterized by epidermal vesiculation and cellular infiltrates of neutrophils, eosinophils, and basophils. Repeated feeding of *A. americanum* larvae on guinea pigs resulted in induced immunity. After 24 hours, there was a dominance of basophils (69% of total cells) at the feeding site, and about 75% tick rejection occurred. Immune sera recipients had increased presence of mononuclear cells (69% of infiltrate) and a weak cutaneous basophil response (24% of infiltrate). Rejection of hosts was generally associated with both responses (Brown and Askenase 1981).

CONTROL AND TREATMENT. Control of *Amblyomma* can be achieved on livestock through use of insecticides as dusts, sprays, pour-ons, and ear-tag formulations and in recreation areas through acaricide applications; vegetation management or reduction, including use of herbicides and controlled burning; and host exclusion (reviewed in Barnard et al. 1988). Some formulations of ivermectin may also provide control (Miller et al. 1989; Pound et al. 1996; Miller et al. 1997). Nonchemical control of *A. americanum* by habitat modification (i.e., clearing and establishing a permanent pasture) was very effective, and excluding animals from a wooded area was moderately effective at controlling ticks (Meyer et al. 1982).

PUBLIC HEALTH CONCERNS. Tick bites can be a nuisance for people living in regions where tick populations are high. The lone star tick was the most common tick removed from humans in Georgia and South Carolina (Felz et al. 1996) and comprised 34% of ticks removed from U.S. Air Force personnel across the United States (Campbell and Bowles 1994). All three tick life stages feed on people, causing irritation (due to the painful bite) and, possibly, subsequent infection. Adult *A. maculatum* feed infrequently on man, and this species comprised only 1% of ticks biting humans in Georgia and South Carolina (Felz et al. 1996).

The lone star tick is an efficient vector of human monocytic ehrlichiosis (*Ehrlichia chaffeensis*) in the south central and eastern United States. The geographic distribution of human ehrlichiosis caused by *E. chaffeensis* and the geographic range of *A. americanum* are similar (Eng et al. 1990). All of the 30 sites with antibodies of *E. chaffeensis* from white-tailed deer in the southeastern United States contained populations of *A. americanum* (Lockhardt et al. 1996). *Amblyomma americanum* may also be the vector of *Borrelia lonestari,* which causes a Lyme disease–like illness (Barbour et al. 1996). Other diseases such as Rocky Mountain spotted fever, tularemia, and Q fever are associated with this species (Table 4.3). A spotted fever group rickettsia, possibly related to human cases of rickettsiosis, was recently isolated from *A. cajennense* in south Texas (Billings et al. 1998), and this species is a vector of Rocky Mountain spotted fever in Brazil and Columbia (Billings et al. 1998). Transmission of

human disease is not associated with *A. maculatum,* although tick paralysis may be (Strickland et al. 1976).

DOMESTIC ANIMAL CONCERNS. Three species of *Amblyomma, A. americanum, A. maculatum,* and *A. cajennense,* may infest livestock in such large numbers as to produce irritability, low weight gain, anemia, and death (Drummond 1987). Attachment of adult *A. maculatum* onto ears produces inflammation, edema, and deformation of the ears, and feeding lesions may predispose animals to myiasis and secondary bacterial infection (Drummond 1987). Intense infestations may also lead to hide damage. *Amblyomma maculatum* is a potential vector of heartwater, a deadly African ruminant disease also present in the Caribbean (Uilenberg 1982).

MANAGEMENT IMPLICATIONS. The reliance of ticks on high relative humidity in favorable habitats such as dense brush and woodlands is important for potential management strategies. Vegetation alteration of wooded areas results in dramatic reduction of lone star tick populations due to changes in temperature, relative humidity, and soil moisture (Clymer et al. 1970). At a campground area in Kentucky, treatment with acaricide and mowing resulted in a significant decrease in numbers of *A. americanum* larvae and nymphs collected on opossums and rabbits (Zimmerman et al. 1988). Haile and Mount (1987) developed a computer model of the life cycle of *A. americanum* that simulates the effects of major environmental variables on population dynamics. Variables include weather (temperature, relative humidity), habitat type, host density, day length, and host-finding rate. The growth rate of tick population per generation is increasingly sensitive to changes in parameters.

Dermacentor. These are large ticks that feed primarily on large mammals. Most species are three-host ticks with adults parasitizing large mammals and immatures feeding on small mammals including rodents, insectivores, and lagomorphs. Two species are one-host ticks; these infest large ungulates.

Ticks in the genus *Dermacentor* have short mouthparts and palps, rectangular basis capitulum, and festoons and eyes. They are moderate-sized ticks (2–6 mm long), usually with ornate markings on the scutum. Males do not have ventral plates or shields. Ticks can be identified using keys of Brinton et al. (1965), Furman and Loomis (1984), Yunker et al. (1986), and Keirans and Litwak (1989).

LIFE HISTORY. The two species of one-host ticks, *Dermacentor* (=*Anocentor*) *nitens* and *D. albipictus,* feed on equids and members of Cervidae, respectively. In both species, blood-feeding, molting, and mating all occur on the same host. Only gravid females detach from the host. In three-host ticks, eggs that are deposited on the ground hatch, and larvae emerge to seek and attach to hosts (generally a small mammal).

Once blood-fed, larvae detach and seek refuge under leaf litter before molting to nymphs. Nymphs emerge and seek and attach to hosts (generally a small mammal). After blood-feeding, nymphs detach and molt to adults. Adults seek and attach to a host (often a larger mammal), feed, and mate on the host; once fully blood-fed, the female drops from the host to oviposit on the ground. Egg masses vary in size between species and with the amount of blood ingested. Egg masses may include as many as 3400 (*D. nitens*), 4400 (*D. albipictus*), 7400 (*D. andersoni*), 4500 (*D. occidentalis*), or 6500 eggs (*D. variabilis*) (Strickland et al. 1976). Eggs hatch in ~4 weeks. Blood-feeding is completed in 4–14 days, depending on stage, and the subsequent molting requires ~2–4 weeks. Most species complete a life cycle in 1–2 years, depending on host availability and environmental conditions. Under laboratory conditions, *D. variabilis* can complete a generation in 3 months (Sonenshine 1979, 1991).

All stages of *D. albipictus* are present on hosts between fall and spring (Drew and Samuel 1989). In northern regions, larvae ascend vegetation and aggregate in clumps on tips of vegetation in September and October (Drew and Samuel 1985). Once on the host (usually moose, elk, or deer), larvae feed, and nymphs are produced about 3 weeks later. Nymphs do not blood-feed until January to March (Drew and Samuel 1989). The long-lasting nymphal stage is only typical for *D. albipictus* in the northern part of its range (Addison et al. 1979; Samuel and Barker 1979). Adults are most common in March and April, and engorged females detach in late March through April, with oviposition occurring in June (Drew and Samuel 1989). This seasonal pattern of detachment of gravid females may be influenced by photoperiod. In southern regions the life cycle can be completed in as little as a month (Ernst and Gladney 1975).

The life cycle of *D. andersoni* can take 1–2 years, with 3 years required at high altitudes. Larvae of *D. andersoni* are most numerous in July; nymphs are generally present in summer. Adults are active from March to July, with peak abundance in April and May (Wilkinson 1968; Gregson 1973). Immature *D. paumapertus* are found on rabbits in cool weather, and adults may be found year round (Bishopp and Trembley 1945). All stages of *D. nitens* are present throughout the year (Despins 1992). Larvae and nymphs of *D. occidentalis* are most abundant on hosts in spring and summer; adults are present throughout the year, with a peak in April and May (Strickland et al. 1976). Adult *D. hunteri* are active from July to December (Bishopp and Trembley 1945). In Arkansas, larvae of *D. variabilis* were present year round, with nymphs present from April to September and adults from May to July (Tugwell and Lancaster 1962). In Virginia unfed larval *D. variabilis* emerge from a winter diapause, with peak activity in April; nymphs become abundant in May or June; and adults are active from April to August. Adults consists of overwintering survivors (active earlier) and young adults that emerge that year (later peak) (Sonen-shine 1979). In South Carolina, larval activity occurs from November to April, nymphs are most abundant in April, and adults are most abundant in June (Clark et al. 1998).

All stages of *D. nitens* are commonly found in the ears of equines (Despins 1992). In dense infestations, ticks also may be present in the mane or nose or under the tail. Infestations of *D. variabilis* often occur on the head, ears, and back of dogs and in the tail brush and mane of horses (in Schmidtmann et al. 1998). Preferred attachment sites of *D. andersoni* differ between montane and prairie regions; ticks from montane regions attach to the upper body, and those from prairie regions attach to the lower body (Wilkinson and Lawson 1965). In British Columbia, *D. andersoni* attaches to the anterior part of the backline, often near the ears and the poll, of livestock and near or on the head of man (Gregson 1973).

EPIZOOTIOLOGY

DISTRIBUTION AND HOST RANGE. An overview of geographic and host ranges of *Dermacentor* is presented in Table 4.4. The winter tick, *D. albipictus* is a widespread species with several color variants, one of which (*D. nigrolineatus*) is present in the southeastern United States. These species are synonymized. Variation within *D. albipictis* is widespread (Crosbie et al. 1998). *Dermacentor albipictus* is the northernmost member of the genus, occurring to 62°N in western Canada (Samuel 1989). The primary host of this tick is moose (Addison et al. 1979), although moose may have acquired *D. albipictus* from deer (Mooring and Samuel 1998a). It readily feeds on other cervids and is infrequently present on other mammals.

Dermacentor andersoni is present in many of the northwestern states and western Canada. It is generally not considered host specific and feeds on a wide variety of mammals, primarily at high elevations (Wilkinson 1967). Adult ticks generally feed on larger mammals, and immatures feed on small mammals. Carey et al. (1980) reported that larvae were most abundant on smaller mammals, deer mice, and chipmunks; nymphs on larger sciurids; and adults on porcupines. In Rocky Mountain National Park, Colorado, deer mice (*Peromyscus maniculatus*), least chipmunks (*Eutamias minimus*), and golden mantled ground squirrels (*Spermophilus lateralis*) were principal hosts of larvae; golden-mantled ground squirrels and least chipmunks were principal hosts of nymphs; and porcupines were principle hosts of adults (Carey et al. 1980).

Dermacentor occidentalis is present along the Pacific coast and infests a wide range of mammals. Adults occur on large mammals (i.e., deer, cattle) and immatures on mammals of all sizes. Nymphs feed mostly on nocturnal rodents (Lane 1990b), and the preference of nymphs to quest about 4–10 cm above the ground is possibly why nymphs are primarily found on rodents and lagomorphs (Lane et al. 1995). The distribution of *D. nitens* is tropical, with established

TABLE 4.4—Hosts, geographic distribution, and diseases vectored by *Dermacentor*, *Rhipicephalus*, *Haemaphysalis*, and *Boophilus* that feed on mammals

Species (Common Name)	Distribution	Diseases	Mammalian Hosts[a]
Dermacentor albipictus (=*nigrolineatus*) (winter tick)	Northern, eastern, western U.S. and Canada (not Alaska)	Tick paralysis, bovine anaplasmosis (implicated)	Moose (*Alces alces*), Elk (*Cervus elaphus*), White-tailed deer (*Odocoileus virginianus*), Mule deer (*Odocoileus hemionus hemionus*), Columbian black-tailed deer (*Odocoileus hemionus columbianus*), Woodland caribou (*Rangifer tarandus*), Pronghorn (*Antilocapra americana*), Mountain goat (*Oreamnos americanus*), Bighorn sheep (*Ovis canadensis*), Coyote (*Canis latrans*), Black bear (*Ursus americanus*), Mouse (*Peromyscus*), Bison (*Bison bison*), Peccary (*Tayassu tajacu*), Domestic (cat, cattle, horse, mule), Man (rarely)
Dermacentor andersoni (Rocky Mountain wood tick)	Northwestern U.S. and Canada	Rocky Mountain spotted fever, tick paralysis, tularemia, bovine anaplasmosis, Q fever, Colorado tick fever, Powasson encephalitis	Mule deer (*Odocoileus hemionus hemionus*), Elk (*Cervus elaphus*), Mountain goat (*Oreamnos americanus*), Pronghorn (*Antilocapra americana*), Ground squirrel (*Citellus, Spermophilus*), Chipmunk (*Eutamias*), Squirrel (*Tamiasciurus*), Pocket gopher (*Thomomys*), Prairie dog (*Cynomys*), Coyote (*Canis latrans*), Rabbit (*Sylvilagus, Lepus*), Badger (*Taxidea taxus*), Woodrat (*Neotoma*), Woodchuck (*Marmota flaviventris*), Bighorn sheep (*Ovis c. canadensis*), Porcupine (*Erethizon dorsatum*), Mouse and Vole (*Zapus, Microtus, Peromyscus, Lemmiscus, Clethrionomys*), Pika (*Ochotona princeps*), Weasel (*Mustela*), Bison (*Bison bison*), Bobcat (*Lynx rufus*), Bear (*Ursus*), Domestic (cat, cattle, dog, goat, horse, mule, pig, sheep), Man (rarely)
Dermacentor halli	Texas	—	Peccary (*Pecari angulatus*)
Dermacentor hunteri	Arizona, California	Bovine anaplasmosis	Desert bighorn sheep (*Ovis canadensis*)
Dermacentor (=*Anocenter*) *nitens* (Tropical horse tick)	South Florida, south Texas	Equine babesiosis	White-tailed deer (*Odocoileus virginianus*), Florida panther (*Felis concolor coryi*), Domestic (horse, cattle, goat, mule)
Dermacentor occidentalis (Pacific coast tick)	California, Oregon	Tick paralysis, bovine anaplasmosis, Q fever, Colorado tick fever, tularemia	Mule deer (*Odocoileus hemionus hemionus*), Ground squirrel (*Citellus*), White-footed mouse (*Peromyscus*), Woodrat (*Neotoma*), Rabbit (*Sylvilagus, Lepus*), Pocket mouse (*Perognathus*), Chipmunk (*Eutamias*), Domestic (cattle, dog, horse, mule, sheep), Man (rarely)
Dermacentor parumapertus (the rabbit *Dermacentor*)	Southwestern states	Tick paralysis, Rocky Mountain spotted fever, tularemia	Rabbit (*Lepus, Sylvilagus*), Pocket mouse (*Perognathus*), Kangaroo rat (*Dipodomys*), Coyote (*Canis latrans*), Deer (*Odocoileus*), Domestic (cattle)
Dermacentor variabilis (American dog tick)	Eastern U.S. and Canada, Pacific coast, Idaho, Montana	Rocky Mountain spotted fever, babesiosis, tick paralysis, anaplasmosis, Q fever, tularemia, cytauxzoonosis	White-tailed deer (*Odocoileus virginianus*), Mouse (*Peromyscus, Mus, Zapus, Reithrodontomys, Ochrotomys*), Vole (*Mictrotus, Pitymys*), Cotton rat (*Sigmodon hispidus*), Rice rat (*Orzomys palustris*), Rabbit (*Sylvilagus, Lepus*), Raccoon (*Procyon lotor*), Badger (*Taxidea taxus*), Coyote (*Canis latrans*), Fox (*Vulpes vulpes, Urocyon cinereoargenteus*), Muskrat (*Ondatra zibethicus*), Opossum (*Didelphis marsupialis*), Peccary (*Pecari angulatus*), Squirrel (*Sciurus, Tamiaciurus, Glaucomys*), Shrew (*Blarina, Sorex*), Rat (*Rattus*), Southern pocket gopher (*Geomys*), Woodrat (*Neotoma*), Feral swine (*Sus scrofa*), Porcupine (*Erithizon dorsatum*), Woodchuck (*Marmota monax*), Wolf (*Canis lupus*), Bear (*Ursus americanus*), Mountain lion (*Felis concolor*), Florida panther (*Felis concolor coryi*), Bobcat (*Lynx rufus*), Weasel (*Mustela*), Skunk (*Mephitis, Spilogale*), Otter (*Lutra canadensis*), Sambar deer (*Cervus unicolor*), Domestic (cat, cattle, dog, goat, horse, mule, pig, sheep), Man

TABLE 4.4 (*continued*)

Species (Common Name)	Distribution	Diseases	Mammalian Hosts[a]
Rhipicephalus sanguineus (brown dog tick)	Widespread	Canine ehrlichiosis, canine babesiosis, Rocky Mountain spotted fever, tularemia, bovine anaplasmosis, Q fever, tick paralysis, haemobartonellosis	Coyote (*Canis latrans*), Rabbit (*Sylvilagus*), White-tailed deer (*Odocoileus virginianus*), Domestic (cattle, dog), Man (rarely)
Haemaphysalis chordeilis	Southeastern and eastern U.S. into Canada	—	Rabbit (*Sylvilagus, Lepus*), Squirrel (*Tamiasciurus*), Woodchuck (*Marmota flaviventris*), Domestic (cat, cattle, horse, sheep), Man (rarely)
Haemaphysalis leporispalustris	Widespread	Rocky Mountain spotted fever, Q fever, tularemia	Rabbit (*Sylvilagus, Lepus*), Mouse (*Peromyscus*), Ground squirrel (*Citellus*), Fox (*Vulpes vulpes, Urocyon cinereoargenteus*), Squirrel (*Sciurus, Tamaisciurus*), Woodrat (*Neotoma*), Roof rat (*Rattus rattus*), Chipmunk (*Eutamias*), Cotton rat (*Sigmodon hispidus*), Bobcat (*Lynx rufus*), Peccary (*Pecari angulatus*), Raccoon (*Procyon lotor*), Woodchuck (*Marmota*), Blackbuck antelope (*Antilope cervicapra*), White-tailed deer (*Odocoileus virginianus*), Domestic (cat, goat)
Boophilus annulatus (cattle fever tick)	Mexico and south (eradicated from U.S.)	Bovine babesiosis, anaplasmosis	White-tailed deer (*Odocoileus virginianus*), Domestic (buffalo, cattle, horse, goat, mule, sheep)
Boophilus microplus (tropical cattle tick)	Mexico and south (eradicated from U.S.)	Bovine babesiosis, anaplasmosis	White-tailed deer (*Odocoileus virginianus*), Domestic (cattle, horse, goat, sheep)

[a] Names as from sources.

Sources: Bishopp and Trembley (1945), Gregson (1956), Kellogg et al. (1971), Wilson and Baker (1972), Meleney 1975, Sonenshine (1979, 1993), Strickland et al. (1976), Forrester (1992), Mertins et al. (1992), Crosbie et al. (1998), Keirans and Durden (1998).

populations in south Texas and south Florida. Most collections are from horses, with rare reports from wild and domestic mammals. *Dermacentor* spp. that have limited geographic and host ranges include *D. halli,* which feed primarily on peccaries in Texas; *D. hunteri,* which feed on bighorn sheep in Arizona and California; and *D. parumapterus,* which feed on lagomorphs, chiefly black-tailed jackrabbits, as adults and immatures, and occasionally on other mammals as immatures, in arid regions of the southwestern states (Bishopp and Trembley 1945). *Dermacentor variabilis* is present in eastern North America and has a wide host range, with immatures feeding on small mammals and adults feeding on larger mammals (Campbell and Mackay 1979; Zimmerman et al. 1988; Fish and Dowler 1989).

PREVALENCE AND INTENSITY. The winter tick does well on moose. In western Canada all moose (222) and elk (52), 8 of 10 white-tailed deer, and 7 of 8 bison examined from 1977 to 1996 were infested with *D. albipictus* (Mooring and Samuel 1999). Mean densities are low on deer (0.53/cm²), but high (> 1.00/cm²) on moose (Samuel and Welch 1991; Welch et al. 1991). Numbers on individual moose often exceed 50,000

(Samuel and Welch 1991). Highest densities on elk occurred on the top of the shoulder, at the dorsal base of the neck, and between the rear legs, with the maximum number of ticks reported on an elk as 9000 (Samuel et al. 1991). Welch et al. (1991) experimentally infested hosts with larvae of *D. albipictus* and obtained the highest yield of engorged females from moose (8% of initial infestation), followed by elk (0.23%), mule deer (0.6%), and white-tailed deer (0%), suggesting that moose are highly suitable hosts for this species. Bison do not appear to support high numbers of *D. albipictus* (133 ticks/animal or 0.009/cm²) (Mooring and Samuel 1998b). Mooring and Samuel (1998b) suggest that this is the result of highly effective grooming, possibly in combination with the presence of a physical barrier (tightly packed mat of hair at skin surface).

Rogers (1975) and Manville (1978) report *D. albipictus* from black bear; numbers were few and prevalence was low. In Alabama, prevalence of *D. albipictus* on white-tailed deer was 15%; some deer were infested with more than 200 ticks (Durden et al. 1991). Luckhardt et al. (1992) reported that 27% of the ticks collected from hunter-killed deer in Alabama were *D. albipictus.* Smith (1977) reported *D. albipictus* on < 1% of deer and *D. nigrolineatus* (now considered *albipictus*) on 13% of 4024 tick-infested deer examined from the southeastern states.

Numerous studies document the interactions between the American dog tick, *D. variabilis,* and the wide variety of hosts on which it feeds. Most (99.6%) of 645 feral swine in southern Florida were infested (Greiner et al. 1984); *D. variabilis* constituted 86% of the ticks collected. Ticks were present year round, with the lowest prevalence in winter. Other records include prevalences of 30% on feral swine in the southern Appalachians (Henry and Conley 1970); 78% on collared peccary in south Texas (Samuel and Low 1970); 91% (adult ticks) and 4% (nymphs) on opossum on Merritt Island, Florida (Durden et al. 1993); 14% and 69% on opossum and raccoon, respectively, in Georgia, with average infestations of 32 and 181 ticks, respectively (Pung et al. 1994); 92% and 66% on panther and bobcat, respectively, in Florida (Wehinger et al. 1995); 56% on black bears in the Lake Superior region, with numbers ranging from 1 to 165 per bear (Robers 1975); and 73% on bears from northern Wisconsin, with an average of 117 ticks per bear (Manville 1978).

One of the important hosts for immature *D. variabilis* is *Peromyscus leucopus.* Prevalence and mean intensity of infestations have been reported as 21% and 2.2 in West Virginia (Joy and Briscoe 1994), 19% and 1.2 in Maryland (Durden 1992), 27% and 3.2 in Ontario (Lindsay et al. 1991), 37% and 3.8 in Tennessee (Zimmerman et al. 1987), 58% and 5.2 in Maryland (Carroll et al. 1989), 45% and 1.8 larvae and 4.3 nymphs in Connecticut (Stafford et al. 1995), and 57% and 12.8 in Tennessee (Durden and Wilson 1991). In Virginia, 58% of all immature *D. variabilis* from small mammals were collected in the field-forest ecotone, with 16% collected in an open area, 17% in a low deciduous habitat, and 10% in a deciduous medium-height habitat (Sonenshine and Levy 1971). In Kansas, *D. variabilis* was collected from 16 species of mammals, and all life stages were reported from *Sciurus niger* (Brillhart et al. 1994).

In Colorado, mean numbers of larval and nymphal *D. andersoni,* by host, were *Peromyscus maniculatus* (0.59 larvae, 0.09 nymphs), *Spermophilus lateralis* (0.64 larvae, 4.47 nymphs), *Spermophilus richardsoni* (0.11 larvae, 0.51 nymphs), *Eutamias minimus* (2.05 larvae, 0.96 nymphs), and *Eutamias umbrinus* (2.20 larvae, 0.29 nymphs) (Carey et al. 1980).

ENVIRONMENTAL LIMITATIONS. The distribution of *D. albipictus* is widespread, with greater abundance in mountain or upland habitats. In southeastern Missouri, intensity of infestation on hunter-killed white-tailed deer was higher on deer from upland, rather than lowland, habitats (Kollars et al. 1997). Larvae, which are the only host-seeking stage on vegetation, are highly tolerant of cold and snow (Gregson 1956; Samuel and Welch 1991). Even so, fewer engorged females of *D. albipictus* survived, fewer eggs were produced, and

fewer larvae survived in aspen forest habitats of Alberta, compared to grasslands or bogs, possibly because temperatures were lower in the aspen habitat (Drew and Samuel 1986). Patrick and Hair (1975) reported higher survival of engorged females in forested habitats than in meadows, which were too hot and dry for survival. These studies, while representing some of the extremes in conditions for survival of this species, indicate the importance of suitable microhabitats for survival of the off-host stages of this tick.

The Rocky Mountain wood tick, *D. andersoni,* is generally present in areas of low shrubs in cool to moderate latitudes at altitudes between 300 and 2175 m (Wilkinson 1967). High abundance of *D. andersoni* adults was associated with shallow soils, steep slopes, moderate shrub cover, relatively abundant pine, abundant log litter, exposed rocks, and rock interstices (Carey et al. 1980). South-facing slopes in the upper montane region contained many of these attributes, and free-ranging adult ticks appeared confined to these regions.

The American dog tick occurs in damp, grassy, brush-covered areas of the eastern, central, and Pacific United States in association with low deciduous shrubs (Bishopp and Trembley 1945; Wilkinson 1967). Sonenshine and Levy (1971) concluded that the old field-forest ecotone was the most important for adults of this tick in Virginia, but that this habitat was not as satisfactory for survival of immature stages. Adult *D. variabilis* are collected most often on grassy paths (Newhouse 1983; Micher and Rockett 1993) and edges of trails, roads, meadows, and clearings (Sonenshine 1991). The abundance of these ticks along paths may be related to host scent (Smith et al. 1946), and experimental results indicate greater attraction of nymphs to rabbit and dog hair than to cotton (Dukes and Rodriguez 1976). The distribution of *D. variabilis* and its mammalian hosts in relation to vegetation type in Nova Scotia was studied by Campbell and MacKay (1979). Nymphs of *D. variabilis* occurred most frequently in old field and ecotone areas with *Microtus pennsylvanicus* and *Zapus hudsonicus.* Nymphs were often collected from *Microtus pennsylvanicus,* but also from *Peromyscus leucopus,* in ecotone and woodland areas. Over half the larvae collected were from *Clethrionomys gapperi* and *Peromyscus* in ecotone-powerline, shrubs-trees, and mixed wood areas, with many fewer collected from open habitats. These host associations were likely related to the preference of *Clethrionomys* for wetter areas and the higher survival of larvae in these moist habitats. *Peromyscus* have wider ranges than the other species and may disperse blood-fed larvae that subsequently molt to nymphs in a wider range of habitats. The shift in relative numbers of each life stage from one vegetation type to another was due to differences in environmental factors (i.e., humidity) that affect tick survival and interspecific differences in the timing of seasonal activity and the density of mammalian hosts (Campbell and MacKay 1979). Carroll and Nichols (1986) reported that numbers of host-seeking adult *D. variabilis* in a sweet gum field in Maryland reflected changes in the population density of *Microtus pennsylvanicus,* a preferred host species. In Massachusetts, Smith et al. (1946) reported a decrease in numbers of *D. variabilis* adults after *M. pennsylvanicus* populations were poisoned.

Environmental conditions in habitats also influence behavior and distribution of other tick species. Host-seeking by *D. occidentalis* nymphs is reported to be reversibly related to soil temperature and positively related to ambient relative humidity (Lane et al. 1995). Nymphs of *D. occidentalis* climb low vegetation and seek hosts at ~4 to 10 cm above the soil surface. This was proposed by Lane et al. (1995) to partly explain why 18 of the 23 reported nymphal hosts of this species are rodents and lagomorphs instead of larger vertebrates such as deer.

Ambient temperature and relative humidity significantly increased oviposition and egg hatch of *D. nitens,* and experimental conditions characteristic of the tropical/subtropical habitat of *D. nitens* increased survival of this species (Despins 1992). The geographic distribution of this species is limited to areas (Texas and southern Florida) where optimal conditions exist (Despins 1992). *Dermacentor parumapertus* is a "desert" species (Bishopp and Trembley 1945) and is present in arid regions in southwestern states in association with its lagomorph hosts.

PATHOLOGY AND DISEASE TRANSMISSION TO WILD MAMMALS. Feeding by *Dermacentor* can result in local inflammation, edema, hemorrhage, irritation, and even tick paralysis. Tick paralysis is a flaccid, ascending paralysis that occurs in a wide range of vertebrates after attachment of one or more ticks. Although it has been associated with 43 species in 10 genera worldwide, only *D. andersoni, D. variabilis,* and *D. occidentalis* commonly cause the condition in North America (Gregson 1973). Tick paralysis has been reported from mule deer, bison, black-tailed deer, black bear, gray fox, striped skunk, coyote, western harvest mouse, and the red wolf (Kohls and Kramis 1952; Brunetti 1965; Loomis and Bushnell 1968; Wilkinson 1970; Gregson 1973; Jessup 1979; Botzler et al. 1980; Lane 1984; Beyer and Grossman 1997). Wilkinson (1985) reported that *D. andersoni* collected from Kamloops, British Columbia, were significantly more effective in inducing paralysis or ataxia in lambs than ticks collected from Alberta and proposed that a population difference existed in induction of tick paralysis. A paralyzed gray fox regained full use of the rear legs within 48 hours after 117 adult *D. variabilis* were removed (Jessup 1979).

Effects of feeding by *D. albipictus* are well documented and may be severe enough to include death of moose. Heavily infested moose groom extensively (Samuel 1991) and suffer from alopecia (McLaughlin and Addison 1986; Samuel et al. 1986), loss of visceral fat stores (McLaughlin and Addison 1986), anemia, and death (Glines and Samuel 1989). Tick-related

moose die-offs are reported often (e.g., Berg 1975; Samuel and Barker 1979; Addison and Smith 1981). Elk, mule deer, and white-tailed deer groom in response to ticks, but suffer only mild alopecia, often around the base of the neck in elk (Murie 1951; Welch et al. 1991). Elk become infested (Kistner 1982), though rarely with large infestations; however, mortality associated with ticks has been reported (Murie 1951).

Dermacentor are effective vectors of a variety of pathogenic agents (Table 4.4). Enzootic cycles of Rocky Mountain spotted fever and tularemia are maintained between mammalian reservoirs by the vectors *D. variabilis, D. andersoni,* and *D. parumapertus* (Bishopp and Trembley 1945). A moose disease caused by *Klebsiella paralytica* is vectored by *D. albipictus,* which has also been implicated as a vector of bovine anaplasmosis and Rocky Mountain spotted fever (Stickland et al. 1976; Sonenshine 1993). *Dermacentor hunteri* has been associated with bovine anaplasmosis in desert bighorn sheep (Crosbie et al. 1997). *Dermacentor occidentalis* also may serve as a vector of bovine anaplasmosis in wild cervids (see Kuttler 1984). An enzootic cycle of *Cytauxzoon felis* is maintained between *D. variabilis* and the reservoir host, bobcat. This disease is highly fatal to domestic cats (Blouin et al. 1984).

IMMUNITY. Various species of *Dermacentor* are capable of inducing high levels of resistance in hosts with repeated exposure to feeding ticks. These responses are best documented in livestock (cattle) and laboratory animals (rabbits, guinea pigs, white mice) and are characterized by responses such as reductions in survival of ticks, weight of fed ticks, molting, and oviposition (Trager 1939; den Hollander and Allen 1985; Wikel 1979, 1996). Allen and Humphreys (1979) reported significant reduction in weight of adult *D. variabilis* fed on calves immunized with extracts of partially fed ticks. Trager (1939) repeatedly exposed guinea pigs or laboratory rabbits to feeding *D. variabilis* larvae and induced high resistance. When the experiment was repeated using natural hosts, deer mice, low resistance was evident. C-4 deficient guinea pigs repeatedly exposed to *D. andersoni* larvae developed resistance with engorgement of larvae during subsequent infestations (Wikel 1979). At attachment sites, resistant guinea pigs developed cutaneous reactions characterized by intradermal vesicles filled with numerous basophils. Acquired resistance was elicited in BALB/c mice with repeated exposures to *D. variabilis* larvae (den Hollander and Allen 1985). Fewer engorged larvae and reduced weights of fed larvae were obtained with subsequent exposures. Histological examination of feeding sites revealed slight reactions to primary infestations and increasingly severe reactions to subsequent infestations, with numerous mast cells and eosinophils present.

These responses may interfere with pathogen transmission by the vector. Bell et al. (1979) reported that induction of acquired resistance of rabbits to

D. andersoni reduced experimental transmission of tularemia. Salivary gland extracts of *D. andersoni* can prolong clotting of whole blood (Gregson 1960) and contain materials effective against intrinsic and extrinsic coagulation systems, but lack fibrinolytic activity (Gordon and Allen 1991). Ramachandra and Wikel (1992) found that salivary gland extracts of engorging female *D. andersoni* suppressed various host immune responses including normal lymphocytes to the T-cell mitogen; concanavalin A; elaboration of the macrophage cytokines interleukin-1, IL-1, and tumor necrosis factor alpha, TNF; and the lymphocyte cytokines interleukin -2, LL-2, and gamma interferon. Acquired resistance to *D. variabilis* in guinea pigs is associated with basophil-rich skin reactions; however, in mice with few basophils, acquired resistance was associated with increased numbers of dermal mast cells (Steeves and Allen 1990).

The degree of grooming by moose induced by infestations of *D. albipictus* may be a result of developing resistance of the host to the ticks (Glines and Samuel 1989). Moose infested with equal numbers of ticks varied in the intensity of grooming response.

CONTROL AND TREATMENT. Control can be obtained through habitat modification, clearing vegetation (including herbicide application), burning vegetation (grass, woodlots), area application of acaricide, host-targeted application of acaricide, host removal or exclusion, or the introduction of parasites or predators (summarized in Schmidtmann 1994). Sonenshine and Haines (1985) used a tube baited with food and acaricide to treat voles and mice; tick infestations were reduced 81%–100% on small mammals. A similar bait tube was used successfully by Lane et al. (1998). *Dermacentor* on livestock can be controlled through use of topical or systemic insecticides (Sonenshine 1993). Haile et al. (1990) developed a computer-simulation model for reduction of *D. variabilis* populations and Rocky Mountain spotted fever. Integrated pest management was the most effective management method indicated by the model.

PUBLIC HEALTH CONCERNS. Adults of *D. variabilis* and, less commonly, *D. occidentalis* and *D. andersoni,* are frequently reported feeding on man, often resulting in irritation (Strickland et al. 1976; Furman and Loomis 1984). Tick paralysis in man is usually associated with *D. occidentalis,* with infrequent cases involving *D. variabilis* (Gregson 1973). Felz et al. (1996) reported that 11% of ticks feeding on humans in Georgia and South Carolina were *D. variabilis.* Walker et al. (1998) reported that 51% of ticks identified from humans were *D. variabilis* and 8% were *D. albipictus.* Campbell and Bowles (1994) reported 34% of ticks collected from Air Force personnel were *D. variabilis.* Both *D. variabilis* and *D. andersoni* readily feed on man and often transmit Rocky Mountain spotted fever, tularemia, Q fever, and Colorado tick fever to man (Sonenshine 1993; Schreifer and Azad 1994). Also, *D. variabilis*

and *D. andersoni* have been implicated as vectors of Powassan virus (Artsob 1989). Other *Dermacentor* species serve as vectors of these diseases to other hosts but rarely feed on man (Table 4.4).

DOMESTIC ANIMAL CONCERNS. Feeding by *Dermacentor* ticks can directly result in irritation, local inflammation, edema, hemorrhage, and tick paralysis (Gregson 1973; Strickland et al. 1976). Tick paralysis in livestock is generally limited to the northwestern region of North America and is usually associated with *D. andersoni* or *D. occidentalis* (Gregson 1966, 1973; Wilkinson 1982). Tick paralysis in dogs is also a serious problem and is associated with *D. occidentalis* and *D. variabilis* (Gregson 1973; Strickland et al. 1976; Lane et al. 1984). In dense infestations, feeding by *D. nitens* on horses can result in skin that is thickened, swollen, and encrusted with blood (Despins 1992). In heavy infestations ticks are found in the ears, where skin becomes thickened and inflamed, and in the nasal diverticulum, the mane, the perineal region, and the ventral midline.

In addition to direct effects of feeding, *Dermacentor* vectors diseases to domestic animals (Table 4.4). The primary vector of bovine anaplamosis is *D. andersoni* (Kuttler 1984); other vectors are *D. occidentalis* and *D. variabilis* (Kuttler 1984). Cytauxzoonosis, a fatal disease of domestic cats, is vectored by *D. variabilis* (Blouin et al. 1984). Equine piroplasmosis, caused by *Babesia caballi,* is transmitted by *D. nitens* (Stiller and Frerichs 1979).

Rhipicephalus, Haemaphysalis,* and *Boophilus. Several other species of hard ticks are present in the following genera: *Rhipicephalus sanguineus; Haemaphysalis leporispalustris, H. chordeilis, and Boophilus.* Two species of *Boophilus, annulatus* and *microplus,* were originally present in the United States, but due to their roles as vectors of Texas cattle fever, they were eradicated and are currently only present in Mexico and south (as well as on other continents). They are included here because of their potential reintroduction.

Rhipicephalus are small (3–4.5 mm), inornate, red-brown ticks with short mouthparts, eyes, festoons, and a hexagonal basis capitulum. Males have ventral plates. *Haemaphysalis* are small (2–3 mm), eyeless, inornate ticks with festoons and short, conical palps, the second segment of which projects beyond the lateral margin of the basis capitulum. There are no ventral plates in males. *Boophilus* are small (3–5 mm), inornate ticks, with very short, ridged, compressed palps, a hexagonal basis capitulum, eyes, no festoons, and ventral shields in males. Adults can be identified using the keys in Keirans and Litwak (1989).

LIFE HISTORY. *Rhipicephalus sanguineus* is a three-host tick, and often all three stages will feed on the same species of host. Eggs masses of up to 4000 are deposited in crevices or cracks (often in kennels), and larvae hatch and attach to a host. All stages may feed on the same species of host, but each will detach, molt on the ground, and reattach to another individual host. The life cycle may occur in as short as 2 months, and several generations may occur each year in warm climates (Strickland et al. 1976). Ticks are found on hosts year round in semitropical/tropical climates and from spring to fall in cooler climates. Immature *R. sanguineus* usually attach on the neck, and adults attach all over the body and often between toes of the host.

Haemaphysalis are three-host ticks; immatures feed on small mammals and birds, and adults feed on larger mammals. The life cycle is completed in 90–400 days (depending on temperature). *Haemaphysalis chordeilis* is more often collected from fall to early spring in southern states and from spring to fall in northern states (Bishopp and Trembley 1945). *Haemaphysalis leporispalustris* is active throughout the year in the southern part of its range, with activity ceasing during winter in the north (Tugwell and Lancaster 1963; Sonenshine and Stout 1970; Lane and Burgdorfer 1988). Larvae are most active July to December, nymphs most active August to September, and adults are present in all months, with a peak in May (Sonenshine and Stout 1970). Immatures have been collected from hosts year round (Tugwell and Lancaster 1963; Lane and Burgdorfer 1988). All three stages may be present on a host at one time (Gregson 1956). Most blood-fed stages of *H. leporispalustris* drop from the host (rabbit) during the 6-hour period before dusk, when the host is in its resting place (George 1971). This synchronization of detachment concentrates the ticks and enhances host-finding for the next stage. In general, ticks of this species attach to the head of the hosts; on rabbits, many are attached on the head, especially around the eye and ears (Bishopp and Trembley 1945; Gregson 1956).

Cattle are the primary hosts of the one-host ticks, *Boophilus annulatus* and *B. microplus*. Egg masses consisting of 2000–4000 eggs are laid on the ground. After hatching in ~19–40 days (depending on time of year), larvae seek and attach to hosts. Larvae blood-feed and molt on the host, as do the subsequent nymphal and adult stages. Gravid females detach and oviposit on the ground. Under favorable conditions, the life cycle may be completed in 40 days, and several generations can be completed in a year in semitropical/tropical climates (Strickland et al. 1976).

EPIZOOTIOLOGY

DISTRIBUTION AND HOST RANGE. The geographic distribution and host ranges for these species are summarized in Table 4.4. The brown dog tick, *Rhipicephalus sanguineus,* is widely distributed throughout the world and is found throughout North America, particularly in protected habitats such as kennels. Collections of *R. sanguineus* are primarily from dogs in North America, occasionally from man (Rhodes and Norment 1979; Harrison et al. 1997), and rarely from wild mammals such as white-tailed deer

(Kellogg et al. 1971). In Africa, where the species is indigenous, adults feed on a wide variety of carnivores and large mammals, and immatures feed on smaller mammals (Hoogstraal and Aeschlimann 1982).

Haemaphysalis chordeilis is present in eastern North America, where adults feed on birds and immatures feed primarily on birds, with infrequent collections from mammals (Bishopp and Trembley 1945; Sonenshine 1979). Lagomorphs are the primary hosts of *H. leporispalustris,* which is a common species with a widespread distribution across North America. Adults feed almost exclusively on lagomorphs; immatures, however, also feed on a variety of small mammals and birds (Sonenshine and Stout 1970; Stafford et al. 1995). In a ten-state survey, 78% of 339 Eastern cottontail rabbits were infested (Harrison et al. 1997). Lane and Burgdorfer (1988) reported *H. leporispalustris* on 24 of 26 black-tailed jackrabbits in California. Although this species is rarely reported from deer (Kellogg et al. 1971), all blackbuck antelopes on a ranch in Texas were infested with *H. leporispalustris* immatures, leading to the speculation that a local population had adapted to feeding on antelope (Mertins et al. 1992).

Boophilus were reported from 17 states prior to being eradicated from North America north of Mexico. While *B. annulatus* is primarily considered a pest of cattle, deer can serve as at least a short-term host and disperse ticks along the Mexican-Texas border (Cooksey et al. 1989). The primary hosts of *B. microplus* are cattle, with collections from deer as well as other species of livestock (Strickland et al. 1976, 1981).

ENVIRONMENTAL LIMITATIONS. *Rhipicephalus sanguineus* is primarily associated with kennels and dwellings in temperate regions and is only able to survive year round outdoors in tropical and semitropical regions. It does not survive temperatures < 5° C (Enigk and Grittner 1953). In semitropical and tropical climates, it may be established in unprotected sites (Stickland et al. 1976).

PATHOLOGY AND DISEASE TRANSMISSION TO WILD MAMMALS. Feeding by *R. sanguineus* can cause inflammation, edema, hyperemia, hemorrhage, and thickened skin. Details of the histopathological interactions between the tick and dogs are detailed in Theis and Budwiser (1974) and Theis et al. (1976). Ticks in this group are vectors of several diseases to wild mammals, humans, and domestic animals (Table 4.4). Canine ehrlichiosis (*Erhlichia canis*) associated with a massive infestation of *R. sanguineus* was diagnosed in wolves, dogs, and wolf-dog crosses in a zoo in north-central Florida (Harvey et al. 1979). Rocky Mountain spotted fever may be maintained in enzootic cycle among wildlife species by *H. leporispalustris* with movement of infected rabbit ticks between locations by migratory birds (Sonenshine 1993). In addition, this tick is the primary vector of tularemia among rabbits (Sonenshine 1993). Infestations of 4000 to 5000 *H.*

leporispalustris/rabbit were reported by Bishopp and Trembley (1945), who proposed that such infestations are likely to weaken the hosts.

IMMUNITY. Guinea pigs have been used as a model to study acquired immunity in ticks, and an immune response was observed with repeated exposure of nymphs/adults of *R. sanguineus* (Brown and Askenase 1981). This cell-mediated immune response was characterized by infiltration of eosinophils in the guinea pig. Dogs generally do not appear to develop immunity to repeated feeding by *R. sanguineus* (Theis and Budwiser 1974; Szabo et al. 1995a). However, Inokuma et al. (1997) reported that fewer adult female ticks were recovered on the second exposure than on the initial exposure; differences in engorgement size, duration, egg production, or hatch times were also reported. The local inflammatory response in dogs consists primarily of neutrophil infiltration (Theis and Budwiser 1974). In guinea pigs, however, a very strong resistance is developed (Szabo et al. 1995a), with a local inflammatory response consisting of mononuclear cells and basophils (Brown and Askenase 1981). An immediate type hypersensitivity reaction in dogs and guinea pigs was induced by Szabo et al. (1995b) using subcutaneous injection of tick extracts. The lack of this type of response in nature is likely due to mediation by salivary components.

Cottontail rabbit, *Sylvilagus floridanus,* acquired resistance to repeated infestation by *Haemaphysalis leporispalustris* (McGowan et al. 1979, 1982). Acquired resistance decreased feeding success of *Dermacentor variabilis* and may play a role in regulating tick populations and maintaining a balance between the parasite and host populations. There was no evidence of tick resistance in the snowshoe hare (*Lepus americanus*) (McGowan et al. 1982).

The immunity of hosts to ticks is probably best characterized for the one-host tick *Boophilus microplus,* where host immunity has long been documented. Naturally acquired immunity in cattle to larval *B. microplus* results in decreased numbers of engorged ticks with little effect on viability. Immunity induced against adult antigens has a more damaging effect on viability, engorgement, and oviposition (Willadsen et al. 1988). *Boophilus microplus* suffered extensive damage, including damaged or killed midgut cells, ruptured midgut caeca, and tissue damage due to escaped host leucocytes, when fed on cattle that were vaccinated with tick-midgut extracts (Agbede and Kemp 1986). This type of damage is unusual and is not typical of that observed with most natural infestations (Sonenshine 1993). A vaccine based on synthetic midgut antigen has been developed for control of *Boophilus microplus* on cattle and is available in Australia and Cuba (Sonenshine 1993).

CONTROL AND TREATMENT. Control of *R. sanguineus* includes insecticide treatment of kennel areas or buildings, reduction of cracks and crevices ticks can hide in, and insecticide treatment of dogs. Little effort is made to control *Haemaphysalis* because they rarely feed on domestic animals. Control of *Boophilus* includes use of chemical control, use of cattle or animal breeds naturally resistant to ticks, and pasture spelling or rotation (Sonenshine 1993).

PUBLIC HEALTH CONCERNS. *Rhipicephalus sanguineus* has been reported feeding on man (Harrison et al. 1997) and is a vector of tularemia and Q fever (Soneshine 1993) (Table 4.4). In surveys of ticks from human patients, *R. sanguineus* represented 0.7% in Georgia and South Carolina (Felz et al. 1996) and 7% from Air Force personnel across the United States (Campbell and Bowles 1994). Rickettsia of the spotted fever group have been isolated from *R. sanguineus;* however, the role of this species in the ecology of Rocky Mountain spotted fever is unknown (Schreifer and Azad 1994). Although incriminated as a vector of Rocky Mountain spotted fever (Schreifer and Azad 1994) and tularemia (Sonenshine 1993)*, H. leporispalustris* contributes little to human disease because it rarely feeds on man.

DOMESTIC ANIMAL CONCERNS. *Rhipicephalus sanguineus* is primarily a pest of dogs, and heavy infestation can result in irritation, unthriftiness, blood loss, and in some instances, disease transmission (Strickland et al. 1976) and tick paralysis (Gregson 1973) (Table 4.4). Numbers of *R. sanguineus* can build up around homes and dog quarters, and populations of several hundred adults per dog have been reported in southeastern Oklahoma (Koch 1982). In North America, *R. sanguineus* is the primary vector of several diseases in canines including canine babesiosis (*Babesia canis*) (Shortt 1972; Breitschwerdt 1984), canine ehrlichiosis (*Ehrlichia canis*) (Harvey et al. 1979; Greene and Harvey 1984; Mathew et al. 1996), canine hepatozoonsis (Panciera et al. 1997), and haemobartonellosis (Harvey 1984). It is also implicated in the transmission of *Babesia gibsoni* to dogs in California (Yamane et al. 1993) (Table 4.4).

Both *Boophilus annulatus* and *B. microplus* are effective vectors of bovine babesiosis (*Babesia bigemina*), a devastating disease of livestock (cattle, sheep, goats, horses) (Strickland et al. 1976). Prior to eradication, mortality resulting from this disease reached 90% in some susceptible cattle herds (Sonenshine 1993), and estimates of annual losses from ticks and babesiosis in the United States in 1906 reached $130.5 million (Harwood and James 1979).

LITERATURE CITED

Soft Ticks

Adeyeye, O.A. 1982. Field studies on *Ornithodoros turicata* Duges in the gopher tortoise (*Gopherus polyphemus* Daudin) habitat in north central Florida. M.S. Thesis, Department of Entomology, University of Florida, Gainesville, FL.

Allen, J.R. 1987. Immunology, immunopathology and immunopropylaxis of tick and mite infestations. In *Immune responses in parasitic infections: Immunology, immunopathology and immunoprophylaxis.* Vol., IV, *Protozoa, arthropods and invertebrates.* Ed. E.J.L. Soulsby,. Boca Raton, FL: CRC Press, pp. 141–174.

Bishopp, F.C., and H.L. Trembley. 1945. Distribution and hosts of certain North American ticks. *The Journal of Parasitology* 31:1–54.

Burgdorfer, W. 1956. The possible role of ticks as vectors of *Leptospira.* Transmission of *Leptospira pomona* by the argasid tick *Ornithodoros turicata* and the persistence of this organism in its tissues. *Experimental Parasitology* 5:571–579.

Butler, J.F., and E.P.J. Gibbs. 1984. Distribution of potential soft tick vectors of African swine fever in the Caribbean region (Acari: Argasidae). *Preventative Medicine* 2:63–70.

Cilek, J.E., and FW. Knapp. 1992. Occurrence of *Ornithodoros kelleyi* (Acari: Argasidae) in Kentucky. *Journal of Medical Entomology* 29:349–351.

Cook, B. 1972. Hosts of *Argas cooleyi* and *Ornithodoros concanensis* (Acarina: Argasidae) in a cliff-face habitat. *Journal of Medical Entomology* 9:315–317.

Cooley, R.A., and G.M. Kohls. 1944. *The Argasidae of North America, Central America and Cuba.* American Midland Naturalist Monographs 1, 152 pp.

Davis, G.E. 1956. A relapsing fever spirochete, *Borrelia mazzottii* (sp. nov.), from *Ornithodoros talaje* from Mexico. *American Journal of Hygiene* 63:13–17.

Davis, G.E., and W. Burgdorfer. 1955. Relapsing fever spirochetes: An aberrant strain of *Borrelia parkeri* from Oregon. *Experimental Parasitology* 4:100–106.

Del Cacho, E., A. Estrada-Pena, A. Sanchez, and J. Serra. 1994. Histological response of *Epticus serotinus* (Mammalia: Chiroptera) to *Argas vespertilionis* (Acari: Argasidae). *Journal of Wildlife Diseases* 30:340–345.

Drummond, R.O. 1967. Seasonal activity of ticks (Acarina: Metastigmata) on cattle in southwestern Texas. *Annals of the Entomological Society of America* 60:439–447.

Dusbabek, F., S. Lukes, V. Matha, and L. Grubhoffer. 1989. Antibody-mediated response of pigeons to *Argas polonicus* larval feeding and characterization of larval antigen. *Folia Parasitologia* 36:89–92.

Eads, R.B., and E.G. Campos. 1984. Human parasitism by *Otobius megnini* (Acari: Argasidae) in New Mexico, USA. *Journal of Medical Entomology* 21:224.

Endris, R.G., T.M. Haslett, M.J. Monahan, and J.G. Phillips. 1991a. Laboratory biology of *Ornithodoros (Alectorobius) puertoricensis* (Acari: Argasidae). *Journal of Medical Entomology* 28:49–62.

Endris, R.G., T.M. Haslett, and W.R. Hess. 1991b. Experimental transmission of African swine fever virus by the tick *Ornithodoros (Alectorobius) puertoricensis* (Acari: Argasidae). *Journal of Medical Entomology* 28:854–858.

Fox, I. 1977. The domestic cat, *Felis cattus,* a new host record for the tick, *Ornithodoros puertoricensis. Journal of Agriculture of the University of Puerto Rico* 61:509.

Furman, D.P., and E.C. Loomis. 1984. The ticks of California (Acari: Ixodida). *Bulletin of the California Insect Survey* 25:1–239.

Gregson, J.D. 1973. *Tick paralysis: An appraisal of natural and experimental data.* Canada Department of Agriculture Monograph No. 9, 109 pp.

Groocock, C.M., W.R. Hess, and W.J. Gladney. 1980. Experimental transmission of African swine fever virus by *Ornithodoros coriaceus* an Argasid tick indigenous to the USA. *American Journal of Veterinary Research* 421:591–594.

Harrison, B.A., B.R. Engbor, and C.S. Apperson. 1997. Ticks (Acari: Ixodidae) uncommonly found biting humans in North Carolina. *Journal of Vector Ecology* 22:6–12.

Hoogstraal, H. 1985a. Ticks. In *Parasites, pests and predators.* Ed. S.M. Gaafar, W.E. Howard, and R.E. Marsh. Amsterdam: Elsevier, pp. 347–370.

———. 1985b. Argasid and Nuttalliellid ticks as parasites and vectors. *Advances in Parasitology* 24:135–238.

Hoogstraal, H., and A. Aeschlimann. 1982. Tick-host specificity. *Bulletin de Societie Entomologique Suisse.* 55:5–32.

Hoskins, J.D., and E.W. Cupp. 1988. Ticks of Veterinary importance. Part II. The Argasidae family: Identification, behavior and associated diseases. *Compendium of Continuing Education for the Practicing Veterinarian* 10:699–708.

Johnston, C.M., and S.J. Brown. 1985. Cutaneous and systemic cellular responses induced by feeding of the argasid tick, *Ornithodoros parkeri. International Journal of Parasitology* 15: 621–628.

Kohls, G.M., and C.M. Clifford. 1963. *Ornithodoros sparnus* sp. n. a parasite of wood rats, *Neotoma* spp. and deer mice, *Peromyscus* spp. in Utah and Arizona (Acarina: Argasidae*). The Journal of Parasitology* 49:857–861.

Kohls, G.M., D.E. Sonenshine, and C.M. Clifford. 1965. The systematics of the subfamily Ornithodorinae (Acarina: Argasidae) II. Identification of the larvae of the Western Hemisphere and descriptions of three new species. *Annals of the Entomological Society of America* 58: 331–364.

Lancaster, J.L., Jr. 1984. Ear tags provide spinose ear tick control. *Arkansas Farm Research* 33:8.

Lane, R.S., and S.A. Manweiler. 1988. *Borrelia coriaceae* in its tick vector, *Ornithodoros coriaceus* (Acari: Argasidae), with emphasis on transtadial and transovarial infection. *Journal of Medical Entomology* 25:172–177.

Laviopierre, M.M.J., and R.F. Riek. 1955. Observations on the feeding habits or argasid ticks and on the effect of their bites on laboratory animals, together with a note on the production of coxal fluid by several of the species studied. *Annals of Tropical Medicine and Parasitology* 49:96–113.

Madigan, J.E., S.J. Valberg, C. Ragle, and J.L. Moody. 1995. Muscle spasms associated with ear tick (*Otobius megnini*) infestations in five horses. *Journal of the Veterinary Medical Association of America* 207:74–76.

Marrie, T.J. 1990. *Q-Fever.* Vol. 1, *The Disease.* Boca Raton, FL: CRC Press, Inc.

Munas Diniz, L.S., H.E. Belluomini, L.P. Travassas Filho, and M.B. Da Koche. 1987. Presence of the ear mite, *Otobius megnini* in the external ear canal of lions (*Panthera leo*). *The Journal of Zoo Animal Medicine* 18:154–155.

Need, J.T., and J.F. Butler. 1991. Possible application of the immune response of laboratory mice to the feeding of argasid ticks. *Journal of Medical Entomology* 28:250–253.

Oliver, J.H., Jr. 1989. Biology and systematics of ticks (Acari: Ixodida). *Annual Review of Ecology and Systematics* 20:397–430.

Parrish, H.E. 1949. Recent studies on the life history and habits of the ear tick. *Journal of Economic Entomology* 42:416–419.

Pfaffenberger, G.S., and V.B. Valencia. 1988. Ectoparasites of sympatric cottontails *(Sylvilagus audubonii* Nelson) and jackrabbits (*Lepus californicus* Means) from the high plains of New Mexico. *The Journal of Parasitology* 74:842–846.

Rich, G.B. 1957. The eartick, *Otobius megnini* (Duges)(Acarina: Argasidae), and its record in British Columbia.

Canadian Journal of Comparative Medicine 21:416–418.

Rich, G.B., and J.D. Gregson. 1968. The first discovery of free-living larvae of the ear tick, *Otobius megnini* (Duges), in British Columbia. *Journal of the Entomological Society of British Columbia* 65:22–23.

Schmidtmann, E.T., R.B. Bushnell, E.C. Loomis, M.N. Oliver, and J.H. Theis. 1976. Experimental and epizootiological evidence associating *Ornithodoros coriaceus* Koch with the exposure of cattle to epizootic bovine abortion in California. *Journal of Medical Entomology* 13:292–299.

Sonenshine, D.E. 1991. *Biology of ticks,* Vol. 1. New York: Oxford University Press.

———. 1993. *Biology of ticks.* Vol. 2. New York: Oxford University Press.

Sonenshine, D.E., and G. Anastos. 1960. Observations on the life history of the bat tick, *Ornithodoros kelleyi* (Acarina: Argasidae). *The Journal of Parasitology* 46:449–454.

Strickland, R.K., R.R. Gerrish, J.L. Hourrigan, and G.O. Schubert. 1976. *Ticks of veterinary importance.* Washington, DC: APHIS, U.S. Department of Agriculture Handbook 485, 122 pp.

Stott, J.L., B.I. Osburn, and L. Alexander. 1985. *Ornithodoros coriaceus* (pajaroello tick) as a vector of bluetongue virus. *American Journal of Veterinary Research* 46:1197–1199.

Williams, J.E., I. Somsak, F.H. Tap, D.C. Cavanaugh, and P.K. Russell. 1976. Kaeng Khoi virus from natural infected bed bugs and immature free tailed bats. *Bulletin of the World Health Organization* 53:365–369.

Wilson, N., and W.W. Baker. 1972. Ticks of Georgia (Acarina: Metastigmata). *Bulletin of the Tall Timbers Research Station.* 10:1–29.

Hard Ticks

Addison, E.M., and L.M. Smith. 1981. Productivity of winter ticks (*Dermacentor albopictus*) collected from moose killed on Ontario roads. *Alces* 17:136–146.

Addison, E.M., F.J. Johnson, and A. Fyvie. 1979. *Dermacentor albipictus* of moose (*Alces alces*) in Ontario. *Journal of Wildlife Diseases* 15:281–284.

Agbede, R.I.S., and Kemp, D.H. 1986. Immunization of cattle against *Boophilus microplus* extracts derived from adult female ticks: Histopathology of ticks feeding on vaccinated cattle. *International Journal of Parasitology* 16:35–41.

Allan, S.A., and M.J. Appel. 1992. Acquired resistance to *Ixodes dammini:* Comparison of hosts. In *Host-regulated developmental mechanisms in vector arthropods.* Ed. D. Borovsky and A. Spielman. Proceeding of the Third Symposium. Vero Beach: University of Florida-IFAS, pp. 255–262.

Allen, J.R. 1987. Immunology, immunopathology and immunopropylaxis of tick and mite infestations. In *Immune responses in parasitic infections: Immunology, immunopathology and immunoprophylaxis.* Vol. IV, Protozoa, arthropods and invertebrates. Ed. E.J.L. Soulsby. Boca Raton, FL: CRC Press, pp. 141–174.

Allen, J.R., and S. Humphreys. 1979. Immunization of guinea pigs and cattle against ticks. *Nature* 280:491–493.

Allred, D., D. Eldenback, and L.D. Ahite. 1960. Ticks of the genus Ixodes in Utah. *Brigham Young University Bulletins of Biology Series* 1:1–42.

Anderson, J.F., L.A. Magnarelli, and A.J. Sulzer. 1981. Raccoon babesiosis in Connecticut, USA: *Babesia lotori* sp. N. *The Journal of Parasitology* 67:417–425.

Anderson, J.F., L.A. Magnarelli, R.N. Phillip, and W. Burgdorfer. 1986. *Rickettsia rickettsii* and *Rickettsia montana* from ixodid ticks in Connecticut. *American Journal of Tropical Medicine and Hygiene* 35:187–191.

Appel, M.J., S.A. Allan, R.H. Jacobsen, T.L. Lauderdale, Y.F. Chang, S.J. Shin, T.W. Thomford, R.J. Rodhunter, and B.A. Summers. 1993. Experimental Lyme disease in dogs. *Journal of Infectious Diseases* 167:651–664.

Apperson, C.S., J.F. Levine, and W.L. Nicholson. 1990. Geographic occurrence of *Ixodes scapularis* and *Amblyomma americanum* (Acari: Ixodidae) infesting white-tailed deer in North Carolina. *Journal of Wildlife Diseases* 26:550–553.

Apperson, C.S., J.F. Levine, T.L. Evans, A. Braswell, and J. Heller. 1993. Relative utilization of reptiles and rodents as hosts by immature *Ixodes scapularis* (Acari: Ixodidae) in the coastal plain of North Carolina. *Experimental and Applied Acarology* 7: 719–731.

Artsob, H. 1989. Powassan encephalitis. In *The Arboviruses: Epidemiology and ecology,* vol. 4. Ed. T. P. Monath. Boca Raton, FL: CRC Press, pp. 29–49.

Artsob, H., L. Sence, G. Surgeoner, J. McCreadie, J. Thorsen, C. Th'ng, and V. Lampotang. 1984. Isolation of *Francisella tularensis* and Powassan virus from ticks (Acari: Ixodidae) in Ontario, Canada. *Journal of Medical Entomology* 21:165–168.

Arthur, D.R. 1961. *Ticks and disease.* Evanston, IL: Row, Peterson and Co., 445 pp.

Banerjee, S.N., M. Banjeree, J.A. Smith, and K. Fernando. 1994. Lyme disease in British Columbia—An update. *British Columbia Medical Journal* 36:540–541.

Banks, C.W., J.H. Oliver, Jr., J.B. Phillips, and K.L. Clark. 1998. The life cycle of *Ixodes minor* (Acari: Ixodidae) in the laboratory. *Journal of Medical Entomology* 35:496–499.

Barbour, A.G., G.O. Maupin, G.J. Teltow, C.J. Carter, and J. Piesman. 1996. Identification of an uncultivable *Borrelia* species in the hard tick *Amblyomma americanum*—Possible agent of a Lyme-like illness. *Journal of Infectious Diseases* 173:403–409.

Barker, R.W., A.L. Hoch, R.G. Buckner, and J.A. Hair. 1973. Hematologic changes in white-tailed deer fawns (*Odocoileus virginianus*) infested with *Theileria*-infected lone star tick. *The Journal of Parasitology* 59:1091–1098.

Barnard, D.R., G.S. Mount, H.G. Koch, D.G. Haile, and G.I. Garris. 1988. *Management of the lone star tick in recreation areas.* Washington, DC: U.S. Department of Agriculture Agricultural Handbook 682, 33 pp.

Bell, J.F., S.J. Stewart, and S.K. Wikel. 1979. Resistance to tick-borne *Francisella tularensis* by tick-sensitized rabbits: Allergic klendusity. *American Journal of Tropical Medicine and Hygiene* 28:876–880.

Berg, W.E. 1975. *Management implications of natural mortality of moose in northwestern Minnesota.* Proceedings of the 11th North American Moose Conference and Workshop, Winnipeg, 24–28 March 1975. Thunder Bay, Ontario: Lakehead University School of Forestry, pp. 332–342.

Beyer, A.B., and M. Grossman. 1997. Tick paralysis in a red wolf. *Journal of Wildlife Diseases* 33:900–902.

Bishopp, F.C., and Trembley, H.L. 1945. Distribution and hosts of certain North American ticks. *The Journal of Parasitology* 31:1–54.

Billings, A.N., Y. Xue-jie, P.D. Teel, and D.H. Walker. 1998. Detection of a spotted fever group rickettsia in *Amblyomma cajennense* (Acari: Ixodidae) in south Texas. *Journal of Medical Entomology* 35:474–478.

Bloemer, S.R., and R.H. Zimmerman. 1988. Ixodid ticks on the coyote and gray fox at Land between the Lakes, Kentucky-Tennessee, and importance for tick dispersal. *Journal of Medical Entomology* 85:5–8.

Bloemer, S.R., R.H. Zimmerman, and K. Fairbanks. 1988. Abundance, attachment sites, and density estimators of lone star ticks (Acari: Ixodidae) infesting white-tailed deer. *Journal of Medical Entomology* 25:295–300.

Blouin, E.F., A.A. Kocan, B.L. Glen, K.M. Kocan, and J.A. Hair. 1984. Transmission of *Cytauxzoon felis,* 1979 from bobcats, *Felis rufus* (Schreber), to domestic cats by *Dermacentor variabilis* (Say). *Journal of Wildlife Disease* 20:241–242.

Bolte, J.R., J.A. Hair, and J. Fletcher. 1970. White-tailed deer mortality following tissue destruction induced by lone star ticks. *The Journal of Wildlife Management* 34:546–552.

Botzler, R.G., J. Albrecht, and T. Schaefer 1980. Tick paralysis in a western harvest mouse (*Reithrodontomys megalotis*). *Journal of Wildlife Diseases* 16:223–224.

Breitchwerdt, E.B. 1984. Babesiosis. In *Clinical microbiology and infectious diseases of the dog and cat.* Ed. C.E. Greene. New York: W. B. Saunders, pp. 796–805.

Brinton, E.P., D.E. Beck, and D.M. Allred. 1965. Identification of the adults, nymphs and larvae of ticks of the genus *Dermacentor* Koch (Ixodidae) in the western United States. *Brigham Young University Science Bulletin Biology Series* 5:1–44.

Brown, S.J. 1985. Immunology of acquired resistance to ticks. *Parasitology Today* 1:166–171.

Brown, S.J., and P.W. Askenase. 1981. Cutaneous basophil responses and immune resistance of guinea pigs to ticks: Passive transfer with peritoneal exudate cells or serum. *The Journal for Parasitology* 127:2163–2167.

Brown, S.J., and F.W. Knapp. 1980a. *Amblyomma americanum:* Sequential histological analysis of larval and nymphal feeding sites on guinea pigs. *Experimental Parasitology* 49:188–205.

———. 1980b. *Amblyomma americanum:* Sequential histological analysis of adult feeding sites on guinea pigs. *Experimental Parasitology* 49:303–318.

Brown, R.N., and R.S. Lane. 1992. Lyme disease in California: A novel enzootic transmission cycle of *Borrelia burgdorferi. Science* 256:1439–1442.

———. 1996. Reservoir competence of four chaparral-dwelling rodents for *Borrelia burgdorferi* in California. *American Journal of Tropical Medicine and Hygiene* 54:84–91.

Brunetti, O. 1965. Tick paralysis in California deer. *California Fish and Game* 51:208–210.

Burgdorfer, W. 1975. A review of Rocky Mountain spotted Fever (Tick-borne typhus), its agent and its tick vectors in the United States. *Journal of Medical Entomology* 12:269–278.

Campbell, A., and P.R. MacKay. 1979. Distribution of the American dog tick, *Dermacentor variabilis* (Say), and its small-mammal hosts in relation to vegetation types in a study area of Nova Scotia. *Canadian Journal of Zoology* 57:1950–1959.

Campbell, B.S., and D.E. Bowles. 1994. Human bite records in a United States Air Force population, 1989–1993: Implications for tick-borne disease risk. *Journal of Wilderness Medicine* 5:405–412.

Carey, A.B., R.G. Mclean, and G.O. Maupin. 1980b. The structure of a Colorado tick fever ecosystem. *Ecological Monographs* 50:131–151.

Carroll, J.F., and J.D. Nichols. 1986. Parasitism of meadow voles, *Microtus pennsylvanicus* (Ord), by American dog ticks, *Dermacentor variabilis* (Say) and adult tick movement during high host density. *Journal of Entomological Science* 21:102–113.

Carroll, J.F., E.T. Schmidtmann, and R.M. Rice. 1989. White-footed mice: Tick burdens and role in the epizootiology of Potomac horse fever in Maryland. *Journal of Wildlife Diseases* 25:397–400.

Clark, K.L. , J.H. Oliver, Jr. D.B. McKechnie, and D.C. Williams. 1998. Distribution, abundance and seasonal

activities of ticks collected from rodents and vegetation in south Florida. *Journal of Vector Ecology* 23:89–105.

Clifford, C.M., M.G. Anastos, and A. Elbl. 1961. The larval ixodid ticks of the eastern United States (Acarina: Ixodidae). *Miscellaneous Publications of the Entomological Society of America* 2:215–237.

Clifford, C.M., D.E. Sonenshine, E.L. Atwood, C.S. Robins, and L.E. Hughes. 1969. Tests on ticks from wild birds collected in the eastern United States for rickettsiae and viruses. *American Journal of Tropical Medicine and Hygiene* 18:1057–1061.

Clymer, B.D., D.E. Howell, and J.A. Hair. 1970. Environmental alteration in recreation areas by mechanical and chemical treatment as a means of lone star tick control. *Journal of Economic Entomology* 63:504–509.

Cohn, D.L., H.N. Erb, J.R. Georgi, and B.C. Tennant. 1986. Parasites of the laboratory woodchuck (*Marmota monax*). *Laboratory Animal Science* 36:298–302.

Cooksey, L.M., R.B. Davey, E.H. Ahrens, and J.E. George. 1989. Suitability of white-tailed deer as hosts for cattle fever ticks (Acari: Ixodidae). *Journal of Medical Entomology* 26:155–158.

Cooley, R.A., and G.M. Kohls. 1944. The genus *Amblyomma* (Ixodidae) in the United States. *The Journal of Parasitology* 30:77–111.

———. 1945. *The genus* Ixodes *in North America.* Washington, DC: National Institute of Health Bulletin No. 184, 246pp.

Coombs, D.W., and M.D. Springer. 1974. Parasites of feral pig x European wild boar hybrids in southern Texas. *Journal of Wildlife Diseases* 10:436–441.

Costero, A., and M.A. Grayson. 1993. Experimental transmission of Powassan virus by *Ixodes dammini* ticks. *American Journal of Tropical Medicine and Hygiene* 49:22.

Craig, L.E., D.E. Norris, M.L. Sanders, G.E. Glass, and B.S. Schwartz. 1996. Acquired resistance and antibody response of raccoons (*Procyon lotor*) to sequential feedings of *Ixodes scapularis* (Acari: Ixodidae). *Veterinary Parasitology* 63:291–301.

Crosbie, P.R., W.L. Goff, D. Stiller, D.A. Jessup, and W.M. Boyce. 1997. The distribution of *Dermacentor hunteri* and *Anaplasma* sp. in desert bighorn sheep (*Ovis canadensis*). *The Journal of Parasitology* 83:31–37.

Crosbie, P.R., W.M. Boyce, and T.C. Rodwell. 1998. DNA sequence variation in *Dermacentor hunteri* and estimated phylogenies of *Dermacentor* spp. (Acari: Ixodidae) in the New World. *Journal of Medical Entomology* 35:277–288.

Cupp, E.W. 1991. Biology of ticks. *Veterinary Clinics of North America: Small Animal Practice* 21:1–24.

Damrow, T., H. Freedman, R.S. Lane, and K.L. Preston. 1989. Is *Ixodes* (*Ixodiopsis*) *angustus* a vector of Lyme disease in Washington State? *Western Journal of Medicine* 150:580–582.

Davidar, P., M. Wilson, and J.M.C. Ribeiro. 1989. Differential distribution of immature *Ixodes dammini* (Acari: Ixodidae) on rodent hosts. *The Journal of Parasitology* 75:898–904.

Davidson, W.R., J.M. Crum, J.L. Blue, D.W. Sharp, and J.H. Phillips. 1985. Parasites, diseases, and health status of sympatric populations of fallow deer and white-tailed deer in Kentucky. *Journal of Wildlife Diseases* 21:153–159.

Davidson, W.R., D.A. Siefken, and L.H. Creekmore. 1994. Influence of annual and bienniel prescribed burning during March on the abundance of *Amblyomma americanum* (Acari: Ixodidae) in central Georgia. *Journal of Medical Entomology* 31:72–81.

Deblinger, R.D., M.L. Wilson, and A. Spielman. 1992. Reduced abundance of immature *Ixodes dammini* (Acari: Ixodidae) following gradual reduction of deer density. *Journal of Medical Entomology* 31:875–877.

Demarais, S., H.A. Jacobson, and D.C. Guynn. 1987. Effects of seasons on ectoparasites of white-tailed deer (*Odocoileus virginianus*) in Mississippi. *Journal of Wildlife Diseases* 23:261–266.

den Hollander, N., and J.R. Allen. 1985. *Dermacentor variabilis:* Acquired resistance to ticks in BALB/c mice. *Experimental Parasitology* 59:118–129.

Dennis, D.T., T.S. Nekomoto, J.C. Victor, W.S. Paul, and J. Piesman. 1998. Reported distribution of *Ixodes scapularis* and *Ixodes pacificus* (Acari: Ixodidae) in the United States. *Journal of Medical Entomology* 35:629–638.

Despins, J.L. 1992. Effects of temperature and humidity on ovipositional biology and egg development of the tropical horse tick, *Dermacentor (Anocentor) nitens. Journal of Medical Entomology* 29:332–337.

Dister, S.W., D. Fish, S.M. Bros, D.H. Frank, and B.L. Wood. 1997. Landscape characterization of peridomestic risk for Lyme disease using satellite imagery. *American Journal of Tropical Medicine and Hygiene* 57:687–692.

Drew, M.L., and W.M. Samuel. 1985. Factors affecting transmission of larval winter ticks, *Dermacentor albopictus* (Packard), to moose, *Alces alces* L., in Alberta, Canada. *Journal of Wildlife Disease* 21:274–282.

———. 1986. Reproduction of the winter tick, *Dermacentor albipictus,* under field conditions in Alberta, Canada. *Canadian Journal of Zoology* 64:714–721.

———. 1989. Instar development and disengagement rate of engorged female winter ticks, *Dermacentor albipictis* (Acari: Ixodidae) following single- and trickle-exposure of moose (*Alces alces*). *Experimental and Applied Acarology* 6:189–196.

Drew, M.L., W.M. Samuel, G.M. Lukiwski, and J.N. Willman. 1985. An evaluation of burning for control of winter ticks, *Dermacentor albipictus,* in central Alberta. *Journal of Wildlife Diseases* 21:313–315.

Drummond, R.O. 1987. Economic aspects of ectoparasites of cattle in North America. In *Proceedings XXIII World Veterinary Congress Symposium, The Economic Impact of Parasitism of Cattle.* Lawrenceville, NJ: Veterinary Learning Systems.

Duffy, D.C., S.R. Campbell, D. Clark, C. DiMotta, and S. Gurney. 1994. *Ixodes scapularis* (Acari: Ixodidae) deer tick mesoscale populations in natural areas: Effects of deer, area and location. *Journal of Medical Entomology* 31:152–158.

Dukes, J.C., and J.H. Rodriguez. 1976. A bioassay for host-seeking responses of tick nymphs. *Journal of the Kansas Entomological Society* 49:562–566.

Dumler, J.S., and J.S. Bakken. 1998. Human ehrlichioses: Newly recognized infections transmitted by ticks. *Annual Review of Medicine* 49:201–213.

Durden, L.A. 1992. Parasitic arthropods of sympatric meadow voles and white-footed mice at Fort Detrick, Maryland. *Journal of Medical Entomology* 29:761–766.

Durden, L.A., and J.E. Keirans. 1996. *Nymphs of the Genus* Ixodes *(Acari: Ixodidae) of the United States: Taxonomy, identification key, distribution, hosts, and medical/veterinary importance.* Monograph of the Thomas Say Publications in Entomology. Lanham, MD: Entomological Society of America.

Durden, L.A., and N. Wilson. 1991. Parasitic and phoretic arthropods of sylvatic and commensal white-footed mice (*Peromyscus leucopus*) in Central Tennessee, with notes on Lyme disease. *The Journal of Parasitology* 77:219–223.

Durden, L.A., S. Luckhardt, G.R. Mullen, and S. Smith. 1991. Tick infestations of white-tailed deer in Alabama. *Journal of Wildlife Diseases* 27:606–614.

Durden, L.A., J.S. H. Klompen, and J.E. Keirans. 1993. Parasitic arthropods of sympatric opossums, cotton rats, and cotton mice from Merritt Island, Florida. *The Journal of Parasitology* 79:283–286.

Durden, L.A., C.W. Banks, K.L. Clark, B.V. Bebey, and J.H. Oliver, Jr. 1997. Ectoparasite fauna of the eastern woodrat, *Neotoma floridana:* Composition, origin and comparison with ectoparasite faunas of western woodrat species. *The Journal of Parasitology* 83:374–381.

Emerson, H.R. 1969. A comparison of parasitic infestations of white-tailed deer (*Odocoileus virginianus*) from central and east Texas. *Bulletin of the Wildlife Disease Association* 5:137–139.

Enigk, K., and I. Grittner. 1953. Zur Zucht und Biologie der Zecken. *Zeitschrift für Parasitenkunde* 16:56–83.

Eng, T.R., J.R. Harkess, D.B. Fishbain, J.E. Dawson, C.N. Greene, M.A. Redus, and F.T. Satalowich. 1990. Epidemiological, clinical and laboratory findings of human ehrlichiosis in the United States, 1988. *Journal of the American Medical Association* 264:2251–2258.

Ernst, S.E., and W.J. Gladney. 1975. *Dermacentor albipictus:* Hybridization of the two forms of the winter tick. *Annals of the Entomological Society of America* 68:63–67.

Ewing, S.A., J.E. Dawson, A.A. Kocan, R.W. Barker, C.K. Warner, R. J. Panciera, J.C. Fox, K.M. Kocan, and E.F. Blouin. 1995. Experimental transmission of *Ehrlichia chaffeensis*(Rickettsiales: Ehrlichieae) among white-tailed deer by *Amblyomma americanum*(Acari: Ixodidae*). Journal of Medical Entomology* 32:368–374.

Farkas, M.J., and G.A. Surgeoner. 1991. Developmental times and fecundity of *Ixodes cookei* Packard under laboratory conditions. *Canadian Entomologist* 123:1–12.

Fay, F.H., and R.L. Rausch. 1969. Parasitic organisms in the blood of arvicoline rodents in Alaska. *The Journal of Parasitology* 55:1258–1265.

Felz, M.W., L.A. Durden, and J.H. Oliver, Jr. 1996. Ticks parasitizing humans in Georgia and South Carolina. *The Journal of Parasitology* 82:505–508.

Fish, D. 1993. Population ecology of *I. dammini.* In *Ecology and environmental management of Lyme disease.* H.S. Ginsberg (ed.). Rutgers University Press, New Brunswick, New Jersey, pp. 25–42.

———. 1995. Environmental risk and prevention of Lyme disease. *American Journal of Medicine* 98(Supplement 4A): 2S–9S.

Fish, D., and T.J. Daniels. 1990. The role of medium-sized mammals as reservoirs of *Borrelia burgdorferi* in southern New York. *Journal of Wildlife Diseases* 26:339–345.

Fish, D., and D.C. Dowler. 1989. Host associations of ticks (Acari: Ixodidae) parasitizing medium-sized mammals in a Lyme disease endemic area of southern New York. *Journal of Medical Entomology* 26:200–209.

Fleetwood, S.C. 1985. The environmental influence of selected vegetation microhabitats on the various life stages of *Amblyomma maculatum* Koch (Acari: Ixodidae). Ph.D. thesis, Texas A & M University, College Station, Texas.

Forrester, D.J. 1992. *Parasites and diseases of wild mammals in Florida.* Gainesville: University Press of Florida.

Forrester, D.J., G.S. McLaughlin, S.R. Telford Jr., G.W. Foster, and J.W. McCown. 1996. Ectoparasites (Acari, Mallophaga, Anoplura, Diptera) of white-tailed deer, *Odocoileus virginianus,* from southern Florida. *Journal of Medical Entomology* 33:96–101.

Furman, D.P., and E.C. Loomis. 1984. *The ticks of California.* Bulletin of the California Insect Survey, No. 25. Berkeley: University of California Press.

Galbe, J., and J.H. Oliver, Jr. 1992. Immune response of lizards and rodents to larval *Ixodes scapularis* (Acari: Ixodidae). *Journal of Medical Entomology* 29:774–783.

George, J.E. 1971. Drop-off rhythms of engorged rabbit ticks, *Haemaphysalis leporispalustris* (Packard 1896) (Acari: Ixodidae). *Journal of Medical Entomology* 18:129–133.

———. 1992. Naturally acquired immunity as an element in strategies for the control of ticks on livestock. *Insect Science and its Application* 13:515–524.

George, J.E., R.L. Osburn, and S.K. Wikel. 1985. Acquisition and expression of resistance by *Bos indicus* and *Bos indicus* x *Bos taurus* calves to *Amblyomma americaunum* infestations. *The Journal of Parasitology* 71:174–182.

Gill, J.S., R.C. Johnson, M.K. Sinclair, and A.R. Wesbrod. 1993. Prevalence of the Lyme disease spirochete, *Borrelia burgdorferi*, in deer ticks (*Ixodes dammini*) collected from white-tailed deer (*Odocoileus virginianus*) in Saint Croix State Park, Minnesota. *Journal of Wildlife Diseases* 29:64–72.

Ginsberg, H.S. 1994. Lyme disease and conservation. *Conservation Biology* 8:343–353.

Glass, G.E., F.P. Amerasinghe, J.M. Morgan, III, and T.W. Scott. 1994. Predicting *Ixodes scapularis* abundance on white-tailed deer using geographic information systems. *American Journal of Tropical Medicine and Hygiene* 51:538–544.

Glass, G.E., B.S. Schwartz, J.M.I. Morgan, D.T. Johnson, P.M. Noy, and E. Israel. 1995. Environmental risk factors for Lyme disease identified with geographic information systems. *American Journal of Public Health* 85:944–948.

Glines, M.V., and W.M. Samuel. 1989. Effect of *Dermacentor albipictus* (Acari: Ixodidae) on blood composition, weight gain and hair coat of moose, *Alces alces*. *Experimental and Applied Acarology* 6:197–213.

Goddard, J. 1992. Ecological studies of adult *Ixodes scapularis* in central Mississippi: Questing activity in relation to time of year, vegetation type and meteorological conditions. *Journal of Medical Entomology* 29:501–506.

Gordon, J.R., and J.R. Allen. 1991. Factors V and VII anticoagulant activities in the salivary glands of feeding *Dermacentor andersoni* ticks. *The Journal of Parasitology* 77:167–170.

Greene, C.E., and J.W. Harvey. 1984. Canine ehrlichiosis. In *Clinical microbiology and infectious diseases of the dog and cat*. Ed. C.E. Greene. New York: W. B. Saunders, pp. 545–561

Gregson, J.D. 1956. *The Ixodoidea of Canada*. Scientific Services, Entomological Division, Canadian Department of Agricultural Publications, No. 930:1–92.

———. 1960. Morphology and functioning of the mouthparts of *Dermacentor andersoni*. *Parasitology* 57:1–8.

———. 1966. Records of tick paralysis in British Columbia. *Journal of the Entomological Society of British Columbia* 63:13–18.

———. 1973. *Tick paralysis. An appraisal of natural and experimental data*. Ottawa: Canadian Department of Agriculture Monograph No. 9.

Greiner, E.C., P.P. Humphrey, R.C. Belden, W.B. Frankenberger, D.H. Austin, and E.P.J. Gibbs. 1984. Ixodid ticks on feral swine in Florida. *Journal of Wildlife Diseases* 20:114–119.

Haile, D.G., and G.A. Mount. 1987. Computer simulation of population dynamics of the lone star tick, *Amblyomma americanum* (Acari: Ixodidae). *Journal of Medical Entomology* 27:750–755.

Haile, D.G., G.A. Mount, and L.M. Cooksey. 1990. Computer simulation of management strategies for American dog ticks (Acari: Ixodidae) and Rocky Mountain spotted fever. *Journal of Medical Entomology* 27:686–696.

Hair, J.A., and J.L. Bowman. 1986. Behavioral ecology of *Amblyomma americanum* (L.). In *Morphology, physiology and behavioral biology of ticks*. Ed. J.R. Sauer and J.A. Hair. Chichester, UK: Ellis Horwood, pp. 406–427.

Hall, J.E., J.W. Armine, Jr., R.D. Gais, V.P. Kolanko, B.E. Hagenbush, V.F. Gerenscen, and S.M. Clark. 1991. Para-

sitism of humans in West Virginia by *Ixodes cookei* (Acari: Ixodidae), a potential vector of Lyme borreliosis. *Journal of Medical Entomology* 28:186–189.

Harrison, B.A., B.R. Engbor, and C.S. Apperson. 1997. Ticks (Acari: Ixodidae) uncommonly found biting humans in North Carolina. *Journal of Vector Ecology* 22:6–12.

Harvey, J.W. 1984. Hemobartonellosis. In *Clinical microbiology and infectious diseases of the dog and cat*. Ed. C.E. Greene. New York: W. B. Saunders, pp. 545–561.

Harvey, J.W., C.F. Simpson, J.M. Gaskin, and J.H. Sameck. 1979. Erhlichiosis in wolves, dogs and wolf-dog crosses. Journal of the American Veterinary Medical Association 9:901–905.

Harwood, R.F., and M.T. James. 1979. *Entomology in human and animal health*, 7th ed. New York: MacMillan Publishing Co., Inc.

Henry, V.G., and R.H. Conley. 1970. Some parasites of European wild hogs in the southern Appalachians. *The Journal of Wildlife Management* 34:913–917.

Hoogstraal, H., and A. Aeschlimann. 1982. Tick-host specificity. *Bulletin de Sociétié Entomologique Suisse* 55:5–32.

Inokuma, H., K. Tamura, and T. Onishi. 1997. Dogs develop resistance to *Rhipicephalus sanguineus*. *Veterinary Parasitology* 68:295–297.

James, A.M., and J.H. Oliver, Jr. 1990. Feeding and host preference of immature *Ixodes dammini, I. scapularis* and *I. pacificus* (Acari: Ixodidae). *Journal of Medical Entomology* 27:324–332.

Jessup, D.A. 1979. Tick paralysis in a grey fox. *Journal of Wildlife Diseases* 15:271–272.

Jones, E.K., C.M. Clifford, J.E. Keirans, and G.M. Kohls. 1972. Ticks of Venezuela (Acarina: Ixodoidea) with a key to the species of *Amblyomma* in the Western Hemisphere. *Brigham Young University Science Bulletin* 17:1–40.

Joy, J.E., and N.J. Briscoe. 1994. Parasitic arthropods of white-footed mice at McClintock Wildlife Station, West Virginia. *Journal of the American Mosquito Control Association* 10:108–111.

Keirans, J.E., and C.M. Clifford. 1978. The genus *Ixodes* in the United States: A scanning electron microscope study and keys to the adults. *Journal of Medical Entomology* 15(Supplement 2).

———. 1983. *Ixodes (Pholeoixodes) eastoni* n. sp. (Acari: Ixodidae), a parasite of rodents and insectivores in the Black Hills of South Dakota, USA. *Journal of Medical Entomology* 20:90–98.

Keirans, J.E., and L.A. Durden. 1998. Illustrated key to nymphs of the tick genus *Amblyomma* (Acari: Ixodidae) found in the United States. *Journal of Medical Entomology* 35:489–495.

Keirans, J.E., and T.R. Litwak. 1989. Pictorial key to the adults of hard ticks, family Ixodidae (Ixodida: Ixodoidea), east of the Mississippi River. *Journal of Medical Entomology* 26:435–448.

Keirans, J.E., R.N. Brown, and R.S. Lane. 1996a. *Ixodes (Ixodes) jellisoni* Cooley & Kohls, and *Ixodes (Ixodes) neotomae* Cooley (Acari: Ixodidae): Descriptions of the immature stages from California. *Journal of Medical Entomology* 33:319–327.

Keirans, J.E., H.J. Hutcheson, L.A. Durden, and J.S.H. Klompen. 1996b. *Ixodes (Ixodes) scapularis* (Acari: Ixodidae): Redescription of all active stages, distribution, hosts, geographic variation and medical and veterinary importance. *Journal of Medical Entomology* 33:297–318.

Kellogg, F.E., T.P. Kistner, R.K. Strickland, and R.R. Gerrish. 1971. Arthropod parasites collected from white-tailed deer. *Journal of Medical Entomology* 8:495–498.

Kistner, T.P. 1982. Diseases and parasites. In *Elk of North America: Ecology and management*. Ed. J.W. Thomas and D.E. Toweill. Harrisburg, PA: Stackpole Books, pp. 181–217.

Kitron, U., and J.J. Kazmierczak. 1997. Spatial analysis of the distribution of Lyme disease in Wisconsin. *American Journal of Epidemiology* 145:558–566.

Kitron, U., J.K. Bouseman, J.A. Neilson, and C.J. Jones. 1991. Use of the ARC/INFO GIS to study the distribution of Lyme disease ticks in Illinois. *Preventative Veterinary Medicine* 11:243–248.

Kitron, U., C.J. Jones, J.K. Bouseman, J.A. Nelson, and D.L. Baumgartner. 1992. Spatial analysis of the distribution of *Ixodes dammini* (Acari: Ixodidae) on white-tailed deer in Ogle County, Illinois. *Journal of Medical Entomology* 29:259–266.

Ko, R.C. 1972. The transmission of *Ackertia marmotae* Webster, 1967 (Nematoda: Onchocercidae) of groundhogs (*Marmota monax*) by *Ixodes cookei*. *Canadian Journal of Zoology* 50:437–450.

Kocan, A.A., and K.M. Kocan. 1991. Tick-transmitted protozoan diseases of wildlife in North America. *Bulletin of the Society Vector Ecology* 16:94–108.

Koch, H.G. 1982. Seasonal incidence and attachment sites of ticks (Acari: Ixodidae) on domestic dogs in southeastern Oklahoma and northwestern Arkansas. *Journal of Medical Entomology* 19:293–298.

Koch, H.G., and J.C. Dunn. 1980a. Ticks collected from small and medium-sized wildlife hosts in LeFlore County, Oklahoma. *Southwestern Entomology* 5:214–221.

———. 1980b. Oviposition, egg hatch and larval survival of lone star ticks held at different temperatures. *Southwestern Entomologist* 5:169–174.

Kohls, G.M., and N.J. Kramis. 1952. Tick paralysis in the American buffalo, *Bison bison* (Linn.). *Northwestern Scientist* 26:61–64.

Kollars, T.M., L.A. Durden, E.J. Masters, and J.H. Oliver, Jr. 1997. Some factors affecting infestation of white-tailed deer by blacklegged ticks (Acari: Ixodidae) in southeastern Missouri. *Journal of Medical Entomology* 34:372–375.

Kuttler, K.L. 1984. *Anaplasma* infections in wild and domestic ruminants: A review. *Journal of Wildlife Diseases* 20:12–20.

Lacombe, E.H., P.W. Rand, and R.P. Smith. Jr. 1999. Severe reaction in domestic animals following the bite of *Ixodes muris* (Acari: Ixodidae). *Journal of Medical Entomology* 36:27–232.

Lane, R.S. 1984. New host records of ticks (Acari: Argasidae and Ixodidae) parasitizing wildlife in California and a case of tick paralysis in a deer. *California Fish and Game* 70:11–17.

———. 1990a. Susceptibility of the western fence lizard (*Sceloporus occidentalis*) to the Lyme borreliosis spirochete (*Borrelia burgdorferi*). *American Journal of Tropical Medicine and Hygiene* 42:75–82.

———. 1990b. Infection of deer mice and pinyon mice (*Peromyscus* spp.) with spirochetes at a focus of Lyme borreliosis in northern California, USA. *Bulletin of the Society of Vector Ecology* 15:25–32.

———. 1994. Tick paralysis: An underreported disease of dogs in California. *California Veterinarian* 38:14–16.

Lane, R.S., and W. Burgdorfer. 1988. Spirochetes in mammals and ticks (Acari: Ixodidae) from a focus of Lyme borreliosis in California. *Journal of Wildlife Diseases* 24:1–9.

Lane, R.S., J. Peek, and P.J. Donaghey. 1984. Tick (Acari: Ixodidae) paralysis in dogs from northern California: Acarological and clinical findings. *Journal of Medical Entomology* 21:321–326.

Lane, R.S., J.E. Kleinjan, and G.B. Schoeler. 1995. Diel activity of nymphal *Dermacentor occidentalis* and *Ixodes pacificus* (Acari: Ixodidae) in relation to meteorological

factors and host activity periods. *Journal of Medical Entomology* 32:290–299.

Lane, R.S., L.E. Casher, C.A. Peavey, and J. Piesman. 1998. Modified bait tube controls disease-carrying ticks and fleas. *California Agriculture* 52:43–47.

Lastavica, C.C. 1992. Deer, ticks, and Lyme disease. *New York State Journal of Medicine* 92:3.

Lastavica, C.C., M.L. Wilson, V.P. Bernardi, A. Spielman, and R. D. Deblinger. 1989. Rapid emergence of a focal epidemic of Lyme disease in coastal Massachusetts. *New England Journal of Medicine* 320:133–137.

Lawrence, W.H., K.L. Hays, and S.A. Graham. 1965. *Arthropodous ectoparasites from some northern Michigan mammals*. Occasional Papers of the Museum of Zoology of University of Michigan, No. 639.

Levin, M., J.F. Levine, C.S. Apperson, D.E. Norris, and P.B. Howard. 1995. Reservoir competence of the rice rat (Rodentia: Cricetidae) for *Borrelia burgdorferi*. *Journal of Medical Entomology* 32:135–142.

Levine, J.F., D.E. Sonenshine, W.L. Nicholson, and R.T. Turner. 1991. *Borrelia burgdorferi* in ticks (Acari: Ixodidae) from coastal Virginia. *Journal of Medical Entomology* 28:668–674.

Lindsay, L.R., I.K. Barker, G.A. Surgeoner, S.A. McEwen, L.A. Elliot, and J. Kolar. 1991. Apparent incompetence of *Dermacentor variabilis* (Acari: Ixodidae) and fleas (Insects: Siphonaptera) as vectors of *Borrelia burgdorferi* in an *Ixodes dammini* endemic area of Ontario, Canada. *Journal of Medical Entomology* 28:750–753.

Lockhardt, J.M., W.R. Davidson, D.E. Stallknecht and J.E. Dawson. 1996. Site-specific geographic association between *Amblyomma americanum* (Acari: Ixodidae) infestations and *Ehrlichia chaffeensis* (Rickettsiales: Ehrlichiae) antibodies in white-tailed deer. *Journal of Medical Entomology* 33:153–158.

———. 1998. Lack of seroreactivity to *Ehrlichia chaffeensis* among rodent populations. *Journal of Wildlife Diseases* 34:392–396.

Loomis, E.C., and R.B. Bushnell. 1968. Tick paralysis in California livestock. *Journal of Veterinary Research* 29:1089–1093.

Loye, J.E., and R.S. Lane. 1988. Questing behavior of *Ixodes pacificus* (Acari: Ixodidae) in relation to meteorological and seasonal factors. *Journal of Medical Entomology* 25:391–398.

Luckhardt, S., G.R. Mullen, and J.C. Wright. 1991. Etiologic agent of Lyme disease of Lyme disease, *Borrelia burgdorferi*, detected in ticks (Acari: Ixodidae) collected at a focus in Alabama. *Journal of Medical Entomology* 28:652–657.

Luckhardt, S., G.R. Mullen, L.A. Durden, and J.C. Wright. 1992. *Borrelia* sp. in ticks recovered from white-tailed deer in Alabama. *Journal of Wildlife Diseases* 28:449–452.

Main, A.J., and A.B. Carey. 1980. Connecticut virus: A new sawgrass group virus from *Ixodes dentatus* (Acari: Ixodidae). *Journal of Medical Entomology* 17:473–476.

Main, A.J., H.E. Sprance, K.O. Kloter, and S.E. Brown. 1981. *Ixodes dammini* (Acari: Ixodidae) on white-tailed deer (*Odocoileus virginianus*) in Connecticut. *Journal of Medical Entomology* 18:487–492.

Manville, A.M. 1978. Ecto- and endoparasites of the black bear in northern Wisconsin. *Journal of Wildlife Diseases* 14:97–101.

Mather, T.N., D.C. Duffy, and S.R. Campbell. 1993. An unexpected result from burning vegetation to reduce Lyme disease transmission risks. *Journal of Medical Entomology* 30:642–645.

Mathew, J.S., S.A. Ewing, R.W. Barker, J.C. Fox, J.E. Dawson, C.K. Warner, G.L. Murphy, and K.M. Kocan. 1996.

Attempted transmission of *Ehrlichia canis* by *Rhipicephalus sanguineus* after passage in cell culture. *American Journal of Veterinary Research* 57:1594–1598.

Maupin, G.O., D. Fish, J. Zultowsky, E.C.G. Campos, and J. Piesman. 1991. Landscape ecology of Lyme disease in a residential area of Westchester County, New York. *American Journal of Epidemiology* 133:1105–1113.

Maupin, G.O., K.L. Gage, J. Piesman, J. Montenieri, S.L. Sviat, L. VanderZanden, C.M. Happ, M. Dolan, and B.J.B. Johnson. 1994. Discovery of an enzootic cycle of *Borrelia burgdorferi* in *Neotoma mexicana* and *Ixodes spinipalpis* from northern Colorado, an area where Lyme disease in nonendemic. *Journal of Infectious Diseases* 170:636–643.

McGowan, M.J., J.H Camin, and R.W. McNew. 1979. Field study of the relationship between skin-sensitizing antibody production in the cottontail rabbit, *Sylvilagus floridanus,* and infestation by the rabbit tick, *Haemaphysalis leporispalustris* (Acari: Ixodidae). *The Journal of Parasitology* 65:692–699.

McGowan, M.J., R.W. McNew, J.T. Homer, and J.H. Camin. 1982. Relationship between skin-sensitizing antibody production in the eastern cottontail, *Sylvilagus floridanus,* and infestations by the rabbit tick, *Haemaphysalis leporispalustris,* and the American dog tick, *Dermacentor variabilis* (Acari: Ixodidae). *Journal of Medical Entomology* 19:198–203.

McLaughlin, R.F., and E.M. Addison. 1986. Tick (*Dermacentor albipictus*)-induced winter hair-loss in captive moose (*Alces alces*). *Journal of Wildlife Diseases* 22:502–510.

McLean, D.M., and R.P.B. Larke. 1963. Powassan and Stillwater viruses: Ecology of two Ontario arboviruses. *Canadian Medical Association Journal* 88:182–185.

Meleney, W.P. 1975. Arthropod parasites of the collared peccary, *Tayassu tajacu (Artiodactyla tayassuidae),* from New Mexico. *Journal of Parasitology* 61:530–534.

Mertins, J.W., J.L. Schlater, and J.L. Corn. 1992. Ectoparasites of the blackbuck antelope (*Antilope cervicapra*). *Journal of Wildlife Diseases* 28:481–484.

Meyer, J.A., J.L. Lancaster, Jr., and J.S. Simco. 1982. Comparison of habitat modification, animal control, and standard spraying for control of the lone star tick. *Journal of Economic Entomology* 75:524–529.

Micher, K.M., and C.L. Rockett. 1993. Field investigations on the American dog tick *Dermacentor variabilis,* in northeast Ohio (Acari: Ixodidae). *The Great Lakes Entomologist* 26:61–70.

Miller, J.A., G.I. Garris, J.E. George, and D.D. Oehler. 1989. Control of lone star ticks (Acari: Ixodidae) on Spanish goats and white-tailed deer with orally administered ivermectin. *Journal of Economic Entomology* 22:1650–1656.

Miller, J.A., G.I. Garris, and D.D. Oehler. 1997. Control of lone star ticks on cattle with ivermectin. *Journal of Agricultural Entomology* 14:199–204.

Moody, K.D., G.A. Terwilliger, G.M. Mansen, and S.W. Barthold. 1994. Experimental *Borrelia burgdorferi* infection in *Peromyscus leucopus*. *Journal of Wildlife Disease* 30:155–161.

Mooring, M.S., and W.M. Samuel. 1998a. The biological basis of grooming in moose: Programmed versus stimulus-driven grooming. *Animal Behaviour* 56:1561–1570.

———. 1998b. Tick defense strategies in bison: The role of grooming and hair coat. *Behavior* 135:693–718.

———. 1999. Premature winter hair loss in free-ranging moose (*Alces alces*) infested with winter ticks (*Dermacentor albipictus*) is correlated with grooming rate. *Canadian Journal of Zoology* 77:148–156.

Murie, O.J. 1951. *The elk of North America.* Stackpole Company, Harrisburg, PA; The Wildlife Management Institute, Washington, DC. Reprinted 1979. Jackson, WY: Teton Bookshop, 376 pp.

Nelson, B.C. 1973. Tick paralysis in a dog caused by *Ixodes pacificus* Cooley and Kohls (Acarina: Ixodidae). *California Vector Views* 20:80–82.

Nelson, T.A., K.Y. Grubb, and A. Woolf. 1984. Ticks on white-tailed deer fawns from southern Illinois. *Journal of Wildlife Diseases* 20:300–302.

Newhouse, V.F. 1983. Variations in population density and rickettsial infection rates in a local population of *Dermacentor variabilis* (Acarina: Ixodidae) ticks in the Piedmont of Georgia. *Environmental Entomology* 12:1737–1746.

Oliveira, M.R., and J.P. Kreier. 1979. Transmission of *Babesia microti* using various species of ticks as vectors. *The Journal of Parasitology* 816–817.

Oliver, J.H., Jr., F.W. Chandler, Jr., M.P. Lutrell, A.M. James, D.E. Stallknecht, B.S. McGuire, H.J. Hutcheson, G.A. Cummins, and R.S. Lane. 1993. Isolation and transmission of the Lyme disease spirochete from the southeastern United States. *Proceedings of the National Academy of Sciences, USA* 90:7371–7375.

Oliver, J.H., Jr., F.W. Chandler, Jr., A.M. James, F.H. Sanders, Jr., H.J. Hutcheson, L.O. Huey, B.S. McGuire, and R.S. Lane. 1995. Natural occurrence and characterization of the Lyme disease spirochete *Borrelia burgdorferi,* in cotton rats (*Sigmodon hispidus*) from Georgia and Florida. *The Journal of Parasitology* 81:30–36.

Ouellette, J., C.S. Apperson, P. Howard, T.L. Evans, and J.F. Levine. 1997. Tick-raccoon associations and the potential for Lyme disease spirochete transmission in the coastal plain of North Carolina. *Journal of Wildlife Diseases* 33:28–39.

Pancholi, P., C.P. Kolbert, P.D. Mitchell, K.D. Reed, J.S. Dumler, J.S. Bakken, S.R. Telford, III, and D.H. Persing. 1995. *Ixodes dammini* as a potential vector of human granulocytic ehrlichiosis. *Journal of Infectious Diseases* 172:1007–1012.

Panciera, R.J., N.T. Gatto, M.A. Crystal, R.G. Helman, and R.W. Ely. 1997. Canine hepatozoonosis in Oklahoma. *Journal of the American Animal Hospital Association* 33:221–225.

Parker, J.L., and K.W. White. 1992. Lyme borreliosis in cattle and horses: A review of the literature. *Cornell Veterinarian* 3:253–274.

Patrick, C.D., and J.A. Hair. 1975. Ecological observations on *Dermacentor albipictus* (Packard) in eastern Oklahoma (Acari: Ixodidae). *Journal of Medical Entomology* 12:393–394.

———. 1977. Seasonal abundance of lone star ticks on white-tailed deer. *Environmental Entomology* 6:263–269.

Peavey, C.A., and R.S. Lane. 1996. Field and laboratory studies on the timing of oviposition and hatching of the western black-legged tick, *Ixodes pacificus* (Acari: Ixodidae). *Experimental and Applied Acarology* 20:695–671.

Pound, J.M., J.A. Miller, J.E. George, D.D. Oehler, and D.E. Harmel. 1996. Systemic treatment of white-tailed deer with ivermectin-medicated bait for control to control free-living populations of lone star ticks (Acari: Ixodidae). *Journal of Medical Entomology* 33:385–394.

Pung, O.J., L.A. Durden, C.W. Banks, and D.N. Jones. 1994. Ectoparasites of opossums and raccoons in southeastern Georgia. *Journal of Medical Entomology* 31:915–919.

Ramachandra, R.N., and S.K. Wikel. 1992. Modulation of the host immune response by ticks (Acari: Ixodidae): Impact of salivary gland extracts on host macrophage and lymphocyte cytokine production. *Journal of Medical Entomology* 29:818–826.

Rhodes, A.R., and E. Norment. 1979. Hosts of *Rhipicephalus sanguineus* (Acari: Ixodidae) in northern Mississippi, USA. *Journal of Medical Entomology* 16:488–492.

Ribeiro, J.M.C. 1989. Role of saliva in tick/host interactions. *Experimental and Applied Acarology* 7:15–20.

Richter, P.J., Jr., R.B. Kimsey, J.E. Madigan, and D.L. Brooks. 1996. Compatibility of two species of *Ixodes* ticks with murid hosts and its effect on transmission of Lyme disease spirochetes. *Medical and Veterinary Entomology* 10:291–294.

Robbins, R.G., and J.E. Keirans. 1992. *Systematics and ecology of the subgenus Ixodiopsis* (Acari: Ixodidae: Ixodes). Entomological Society of America Thomas Say Foundation 14:1–159.

Rogers, A.J. 1953. A study of the ixodid ticks of southern Florida, including the biology and life history of *Ixodes scapularis* Say (Ixodidae: Acarina). Ph.D. Thesis, University of Maryland, College Park, MD.

Rogers, L.L. 1975. Parasites of black bears of the Lake Superior region. *Journal of Wildlife Diseases* 11:189–192.

Samuel, W.M. 1989. Locations of moose in northwestern Canada with hair loss probably caused by the winter tick, *Dermacentor albipictus* (Acari: Ixodidae). *Journal of Wildlife Diseases* 25:436–439.

Samuel, W.M. 1991. Grooming by moose (*Alces alces*) infested with the winter tick (*Dermacentor albipictus*) (Acari): Mechanism for premature loss of winter hair. *Canadian Journal of Zoology* 69:1255–1260.

Samuel, W.M., and M.J. Barker. 1979. The winter tick, *Dermacentor albipictus* (Packard, 1869) on moose, *Alces alces* L., of central Alberta. *Proceedings of the North American Moose Conference Workshop* 15:303–348.

Samuel, W.M., and W.A. Low. 1970. Parasites of the collared peccary from Texas. *Journal of Wildlife Diseases* 6:16–28.

Samuel, W.M., and D.O. Trainer. 1970. *Amblyomma* (Acarina: Ixodidae) on white-tailed deer, *Odocoileus virginianus* (Zimmermann), from south Texas with implications for theileriasis. *Journal of Medical Entomology* 7:567–574.

Samuel, W.M., and D.A. Welch. 1991. Winter ticks on moose and other ungulates: Factors influencing their population size. Alces 27:169–182.

Samuel, W.M., D.A. Welch, and M.L. Drew. 1986. Shedding of the juvenile and winter hair coats of moose (*Alces alces*) with emphasis on the influence of the winter tick, *Dermacentor albipictus*. Alces 22:345–360.

Samuel, W.M., D.A. Welch, and B.L. Smith. 1991. Ectoparasites from elk (*Cervus elaphus nelsoni*) from Wyoming. *Journal of Wildlife Diseases* 27:446–451.

Sauer, J.R., and J.A. Hair. 1971. Water balance in the lone star tick (Acarina: Ixodidae): The effects of relative humidity and temperature on weight changes and total water content. *Journal of Medical Entomology* 8:479–485.

Schreifer, M.E., and A.F. Azad. 1994. Changing ecology of Rocky Mountain spotted fever. In *Ecological dynamics of tick-borne zoonoses.* Ed. D.E. Sonenshine and T.N. Mather. New York: Oxford University Press, pp. 314–326.

Schulze, T.L., G.S. Bowen, E.M. Bosler, M.F. Lakat, W.E. Parkin, R. Altman, B.G. Ormiston, and J.K. Shisler. 1984. *Amblyomma americanum*: A potential vector of Lyme disease in New Jersey. *Science* 224:601–603.

Scifres, C.J., T.W. Oldham, P.D. Teel, and D.L. Drawe. 1988. Gulf Coast tick (*Amblyomma maculatum*) populations and responses to burning of coastal prairie habitats. *Southwestern Naturalist* 33:55–64.

Schmidtmann, E.T. 1994. Ecologically based strategies for controlling ticks. In *Ecological dynamics of tick-borne zoonoses.* Ed. D.E. Sonenshine and T.N. Mather. New York: Oxford University Press, pp. 240–271.

Schmidtmann, E.T., J.F. Carroll, and D.W. Watson. 1998. Attachment-site patterns of adult black-legged ticks (Acari: Ixodidae) on white-tailed deer and horse. *Journal of Medical Entomology* 35:59–63.

Semtner, P.J., R.W. Barker, and J.A. Hair. 1971a. The ecology and behavior of the lone star tick (Acarina: Ixodidae). II.

Activity and survival in different ecological habitats. *Journal of Economic Entomology* 8:719–725.

Semtner, P.J., D.E. Howell, and J.A. Hair. 1971b. Ecology and behavior of the lone star tick (Acarina: Ixodidae). I. The relationship between vegetative habitat type and tick abundance and distribution in Cherokee Co., Oklahoma. *Journal of Medical Entomology* 8:329–335.

Semtner, P.J., J.R. Sauer, and J.A. Hair. 1973. The ecology and behavior of the lone star tick (Acarina: Ixodidae). IV. Abundance and seasonal distribution in different habitat types. *Journal of Medical Entomology* 10:618–628.

Shortt, H.E. 1972. *Babesia canis:* The life cycle and laboratory maintenance in its arthropod and mammalian hosts. *International Journal for Parasitology* 3:119.

Smith, J.S. 1977. A survey of ticks infesting white-tailed deer in 12 southeastern states. M.S. thesis, University of Georgia, Athens.

Smith, C.N., Cole, M.M., and H.K. Gouck. 1946. *Biology and control of the American dog tick.* U.S. Department of Agriculture Technical Bulletin 95.

Solberg, V.B., K. Neidhardt, M.R. Sardelis, F.J. Hoffman, R. Stevenson, L.R. Boobar, and H.J. Harlan. 1992. Field evaluation of two formulations of cyfluthrin for control of *Ixodes dammini* and *Amblyomma americanum* (Acari: Ixodidae). *Journal of Medical Entomology* 29:634–638.

Sonenshine, D.E. 1979. *Ticks of Virginia* (Acari: Metastigmata). The Insects of Virginia, No. 13. Virginia Polytechnic Institute and State University Research Bulletin 139.

———. 1991. *Biology of ticks,* vol. 1. New York: Oxford University Press.

———. 1993. *Biology of ticks,* vol. 2. New York: Oxford University Press.

Sonenshine, D.E., and G. Haines. 1985. A convenient methods for controlling populations of the American dog tick, *Dermacentor variabilis* (Acari: Ixodidae) in the natural environment. *Journal of Medical Entomology* 22:577–585.

Sonenshine, D.E., and G.J. Levy. 1971. The ecology of the lone star tick *Amblyomma americanum* (L.) in two contrasting habitats in Virginia (Acarina: Ixodidae). *Journal of Medical Entomology* 8:623–635.

Sonenshine, D.E., and I.J. Stout. 1970. A contribution to the ecology of ticks infesting wild birds and rabbits in the Virginia-North Carolina Piedmont (Acarina: Ixodidae). *Journal of Medical Entomology* 7:645–654.

———. 1971. Ticks infesting medium-sized wild mammals in two forest localities in Virginia (Acarina: Ixodidae). *Journal of Medical Entomology* 8:217–227.

Sorensen, T.C., and R.A. Moses. 1998. Host preferences and temporal tends of the tick, *Ixodes angustus* in North-Central Alberta. *The Journal of Parasitology* 84:902–906.

Spielman, A., C.M. Clifford, J. Piesman, and M.D. Corwin. 1979. Human babesiosis on Nantucket Island, USA: Description of the vector, *Ixodes (Ixodes) dammini,* n. sp. (Acarina: Ixodidae). *Journal of Medical Entomology* 15:218–234.

Spielman, A., J.F. Levine, and M.L. Wilson. 1984. Vectorial capacity of North American *Ixodes* ticks. *Yale Journal of Biology and Medicine* 57:507–513.

Spielman, A., M.L. Wilson, J.F. Levine, and J. Piesman. 1985. Ecology of *Ixodes dammini*-borne human babesiosis and Lyme disease. *Annual Review of Entomology* 30:439–460.

Stafford, K.C. III. 1992. Reduced abundance of host-targeted permethrin for the control of *Ixodes dammini* (Acari: Ixodidae) in southeastern Connecticut. *Journal of Medical Entomology* 25:717–720.

———. 1993. Reduced abundance of *Ixodes scapularis* (Acari: Ixodidae) with the exclusion of deer by electric fencing. *Journal of Medical Entomology* 30:986–996.

————. 1997. Pesticide use by licensed applicators for the control of *Ixodes scapularis* (Acari: Ixodidae) in Connecticut. *Journal of Medical Entomology* 34:552–558.

Stafford, K.C. III, V.C. Bladen, and Magnarelli, L.A. 1995. Ticks (Acari: Ixodidae) infesting wild birds (Aves) and white-footed mice in Lyme, CT. *Journal of Medical Entomology* 32:453–466.

Steeves, E.B.T., and J.R. Allen. 1990. Basophils in skin reactions of mast cell–deficient mice infested with *Dermacentor variabilis*. *International Journal for Parasitology* 20:655–667.

Stiller, D., and W.M. Frerichs. 1979. Experimental transmission of *Babesia caballi* to equines by different stages of the tropical horse tick. Record of Advances in Acarology 2:263.

Strey, O.F., P.D. Teel, M.T. Longnecker, and G.R. Needham. 1996. Survival and water-balance characteristics of unfed adult *Amblyomma cajennense* (Acari: Ixodidae). *Journal of Medical Entomology* 33:63–73.

Strickland, R.K., R.R. Gerrish, J.L. Hourrigan, and G.O. Schubert. 1976. *Ticks of veterinary importance.* Washington DC: APHIS, U.S. Department of Agriculture Handbook 485, 122 pp.

Strickland, R.K., R.R. Gerrish, and J.S. Smith. 1981. Arthropods. In *Diseases and parasites of white-tailed deer.* Ed. W.R. Davidson et al. Tallahassee, FL: Tall Timbers Research Station, pp. 363–389.

Strother, G.R., E.C. Burns, and L.I. Smart. 1974. Resistance of purebred Brahman, Hereford, and Brahman x Hereford crossbred cattle to the lone star tick, *Amblyomma americanum* (Acarina: Ixodidae). *Journal of Medical Entomology* 11:559–563.

Szabo, M.P.J., L.S. Mukai, P.C.S. Rosa, and G.H. Bechara. 1995a. Differences in the acquired resistance of dogs, hamsters, and guinea pigs to repeated infestations with adult ticks *Rhipicephalus sanguineus* (Acari: Ixodidae). *Brazilian Journal of Research in Animal Science* 32:43–50.

Szabo, M.P.J., J. Morelli, Jr., and G.H. Bechara. 1995b. Cutaneous hypersensitivity induced in dogs and guinea pigs by extracts of the tick *Rhipicephalus sanguineus* (Acari: Ixodidae). *Experimental and Applied Acarology* 11:723–730.

Teel, P.D., S.C. Fleetwood, S.W. Hopkins, and B. Cruz. 1988. Ectoparasites of eastern and western meadowlarks in the Rio Grande plains of south Texas. *Journal of Medical Entomology* 25:32–38.

Teel, P.D., S.W. Hopkins, W.A. Donahue, and O.F. Strey. 1998. Population dynamics of immature *Amblyomma maculatum* (Acari: Ixodidae) and other ectoparasites on meadowlarks and northern bobwhite quail resident to the coastal prairie of Texas. *Journal of Medical Entomology* 35:483–488.

Telford, S.R. III, and A. Spielman. 1989. Enzootic transmission of the agent of Lyme disease in rabbits. *American Journal of Tropical Medicine and Hygiene* 41:482–490.

Telford, S.R. III, T.N. Mather, G.H. Adler, and A. Spielman. 1990. Short-tailed shrews as reservoirs of the agents of Lyme disease and human babesiosis. *The Journal of Parasitology* 76:681–683.

Telford, S.R. III, J.E. Dawson, P. Katarobos, C.K. Werner, C.P. Kolbert, and D.H. Persing. 1996. Perpetuation of the agent of human granulocytic ehrlichiosis in a deer tick-rodent cycle. *Proceedings of the National Academy of Sciences* 93:6209–6214.

Theis, J.H., and P.D. Budwiser. 1974. *Rhipicephalus sanguineus:* sequential histopathology at the host-arthropod interface. *Experimental Parasitology* 36:77–105.

Theis, J.H., C.E. Franti, E. Engel, and J.R. Littrell. 1976. Changes in lymphatic fluid draining an area of inflammation induced by feeding *Rhipicephalus sanguineus*

(Acarina: Ixodidae) on the dog. *Journal of Medical Entomology* 13:2–39.

Thorpe, B.D., R.W. Sidwell, D.E. Johnson, K.L. Smart, and D.D. Parker. 1965. Tularemia in the wildlife and livestock of the Great Salt Lake Desert region, 1951 through 1964. *American Journal of Tropical Medicine and Hygiene* 14:622–637.

Trager, W. 1939. Acquired immunity to ticks. *The Journal of Parasitology* 25:57–81.

Tugwell, P., and J.L. Lancaster, Jr. 1962. Results of a tick-host study in northeast Arkansas. *Journal of the Kansas Entomological Society* 35:202–211.

————. 1963. Notes on the seasonal abundance of six tick species in Northwest Arkansas. *Journal of the Kansas Entomological Society* 36:167–171.

Uilenberg, G. 1982. Experimental transmission of *Cowdria ruminantium* by the Gulf coast tick, *Amblyomma maculatum:* danger of introducing heartwater and benign African theileriosis onto the American mainland. *American Journal of Veterinary Research* 43:1279–128.

Walker, E.D., M.G. Stobierski, M.L. Poplar, T.W. Smith, A.J. Murphy, P.C. Smith, S.M. Schmitt, T.M. Cooley, and C.M. Kramer. 1998. Geographic distribution of ticks (Acari: Ixodidae) in Michigan, with emphasis on *Ixodes scapularis* and *Borrelia burgdorferi*. *Journal of Medical Entomology* 35:872–882.

Watson, T.G., and Anderson, R.C. 1976. *Ixodes scapularis* Say on white-tailed deer (*Odocoileus virginianus*) from Long Point, Ontario. *Journal Wildlife Diseases* 12:66–71.

Wehinger, K.A., M.E. Roelke, and E.C. Greiner. 1995. Ixodid ticks from panthers and bobcats in Florida. *Journal of Wildlife Diseases* 3:480–485.

Welch, D.A., W.M. Samuel, and C.J. Wilke. 1991. Suitability of moose, elk, mule deer, and white-tailed deer as hosts for winter ticks (*Dermacentor albopictus*). *Canadian Journal of Zoology* 69:2300–2305.

Westrom, D.R., R.S. Lane, and J.R. Anderson. 1985. *Ixodes pacificus* (Acari: Ixodidae): Population dynamics and distribution on Columbian black-tailed deer (*Odocoileus hemionus columbianus*). *Journal of Medical Entomology* 22:507–511.

White, D.J., H.G. Chang, J.L. Benach, E.M. Bosler, S.C. Meldrum, R.G. Means, J.G. Debbie, G.S. Birkhead, and D.L. Morse. 1991. The geographic spread and temporal increase of the Lyme disease epidemic. *Journal of the American Medical Association* 266:1230–1236.

Wikel, S.K. 1979. Acquired resistance to ticks. *American Journal of Tropical Medicine and Hygiene* 28:586–590.

————. 1996. Host immunity to ticks. *Annual Review of Entomology* 41:1–22.

Wikel, S.K., and D. Bergman. 1997. Tick-host immunology: significant advances and challenging opportunities. *Parasitology Today* 13:383–389.

Wikel, S.K., R.N. Ramachandra, D.K. Bergman, T.R. Burkot, and J. Piesman. 1997. Infestation of pathogen-free nymphs of the tick *Ixodes scapularis* induces host resistance to transmission of *Borrelia burgdorferi* by ticks. *Infection and Immunology* 65:335–338.

Wilkinson, P.R. 1967. The distribution of *Dermacentor* ticks in Canada in relation to bioclimatic zones. *Canadian Journal of Zoology* 45:517–537.

————. 1968. Phenology, behavior and host-relations of *Dermacentor andersoni* Stiles in outdoor rodentaria and in nature. *Canadian Journal of Zoology* 46:677–689.

————. 1970. *Dermacentor* ticks on wildlife and new records of paralysis. *Proceedings of the Entomological Society of British Columbia* 67:24–29.

————. 1982. Paralysis by Rocky Mountain Wood ticks (Acari: Ixodidae) of cattle breeds other than Hereford. *Journal of Medical Entomology* 19:215–216.

———. 1985. Difference in parasitizing ability and sites of attachment to cattle of Rocky Mountain wood ticks (Acarina: Ixodidae) from three regions of western Canada. *Journal of Medical Entomology* 22:28–31.

Wilkinson, P.R., and J.E. Lawson. 1965. Differences of sites of attachment *of Dermacentor andersoni* Stiles to cattle in southeastern Alberta and in south central British Columbia, in relation to possible existence of genetically different strains of ticks. *Canadian Journal of Zoology* 43:408–411.

Willadsen, P., R.V. McKenna, and G.A. Riding. 1988. Isolation from the cattle tick*, Boophilus microplus,* of antigenic material capable of eliciting a protective immunological response in the bovine host. *International Journal of Parasitology* 18:183–189.

Williams, R.E., and J.A. Hair. 1976. Influence of Gulf Coast ticks on blood composition and weights of Eastern meadowlarks in Alabama. *Annals of the Entomological Society of America* 69:403–404.

Wilson, M.L. 1986. Reduced abundance of adult *Ixodes dammini* (Acari: Ixodidae) following destruction of vegetation. *Journal of Economic Entomology* 79:693–696.

———. 1998. Distribution and abundance of *Ixodes scapularis* (Acari: Ixodidae) in North America: Ecological process and spatial analysis. *Journal of Medical Entomology* 35:446–457.

Wilson, M.L., and R.D. Deblinger. 1993. Vector management to reduce the risk of Lyme disease. In *Ecology and environmental management of Lyme disease.* Ed. H.S. Ginsberg. New Brunswick, NJ: Rutgers University Press, pp. 126–156.

Wilson, M. L., and A. Spielman. 1985. Seasonal activity of immature *Ixodes dammini* (Acari: Ixodidae). *Journal of Medical Entomology* 22:408–414.

Wilson, M.L., G.H. Adler, and A. Spielman. 1985. Correlation between abundance of deer and that of the deer tick, *Ixodes dammini* (Acari: Ixodidae*). Annals of the Entomological Society of America* 78:172–176.

Wilson, M.L., S.R. Telford III, J. Piesman, and A. Spielman. 1988. Reduced abundance of immature *Ixodes dammini* (Acari: Ixodidae) following elimination of deer. *Journal ofMedical Entomology* 25:224–228.

Wilson, N., and W.W. Baker. 1972. Ticks of Georgia. *Bulletin of the Tall Timbers Research Station.* 10:1–29.

Yamane, I., I.A. Gardner, S.R. Telford III, T. Elward, J.A. Hair, and P.A. Conrad. 1993. Vector competence of *Rhipicephalus sanguineus* and *Dermacentor variabilis* for American isolates of *Babesia gibsoni. Experimental and Applied Acarology* 17:913–919.

Yunker, C.E., J.E. Keirans, C.M. Clifford, and E.R. Easton. 1986. *Dermacentor* ticks (Acari: Ixodoidea: Ixodidae) of the New World: A scanning electron microscope atlas. *Proceedings of the Entomological Society of Washington* 88:609–627.

Zimmerman, R.H., G.R. McWherter, and S.R. Bloemer. 1987. Role of small mammals in population dynamics and dissemination of *Amblyomma americanum* and *Dermacentor variabilis* (Acari: Ixodidae) at Land between the Lakes, Tennessee. *Journal of Medical Entomology* 24:370–375.

———. 1988. Medium-sized mammal host of *Amblyomma americanum* and *Dermacentor variabilis* (Acari: Ixodidae) at Land between the Lakes, Tennessee, and effects of integrated tick management on host infestations. *Journal of Medical Entomology* 25:461–466.

5

SARCOPTES SCABIEI AND SARCOPTIC MANGE

SET BORNSTEIN, TORSTEN MÖRNER, AND WILLIAM M. SAMUEL

INTRODUCTION. Sarcoptic mange, called scabies in man and mange in animals, is a common, widespread, highly contagious, mite-caused, skin disease of mammals. The etiologic agent is *Sarcoptes scabiei.* Clinical signs of acute sarcoptic mange include intense pruritus, erythematous eruptions, papule formation, seborrhoea and alopecia. Morbidity and mortality may be high. Many species of mammals, including man, may be infected. In this chapter we review some aspects of the epidemiology of this mite with emphasis on morphology, pathology, diagnosis, control and treatment, public health concerns and zoonotic aspects.

THE MITE. The itch mite, *Sarcoptes scabiei* (L. 1758) Latreille 1802 (Acaridida: Sarcoptidae) is a member of the suborder Sarcoptiformes, family Sarcoptidae (Fain 1968). Sarcoptidae include most of the "burrowing mites," that is, the genera *Sarcoptes, Notoedres,* and *Knemidocoptes. Sarcoptes scabiei* produces disease in many species of wild (free-ranging and captive) and domestic animals worldwide (Arlian 1989). As summarized by Arlian (1989), "Surprisingly for a disease that has afflicted humans since antiquity, little is directly known about the basic biology of the parasite, the host-parasite interactions, the host immune response, and host susceptibility."

Sarcoptes scabiei has a characteristic oval, ventrally flattened and dorsally convex, tortoise-like body. The body (idiosoma) surface is covered with fine striations; the dorsal idiosoma has fields of several stout setae, and the adult female has fields of numerous cuticular spines, which are taxonomically important features (Fig. 5.1) (Fain 1968; Pence et al. 1975). The male (213–285 µm long by 162–210 µm wide) is approximately two-thirds the size of the female (300–504 µm long by 230–420 µm wide) (Fain 1968). The short anterior first and second pair of legs, but not the third and fourth pair, extend beyond the anterior-lateral margins of the body. There are bell-shaped suckers (caruncles) on the long, unsegmented pedicels (pedicel plus caruncle equal pretarsus) on the tarsi of all legs of males and the anterior two pairs of females. Legs 3 and 4 of females and leg 3 of males each terminate in a long seta. The tarsi have two blade-like claws. The anus is terminal in both sexes. Close relatives of *Sarcoptes* have the following diagnostic morphological characters: *Notoedres* spp. have a dorsal anus; *Psoroptes* spp.

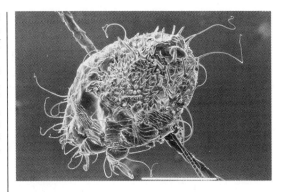

FIG. 5.1—Dorsal idiosoma of an adult female *Sarcoptes scabiei* from a red fox, *Vulpes vulpes.* (Bar = 100 µm).

have a smooth body, with long unsegmented pedicels; and *Chorioptes* spp. have short pedicels. Fain (1968) presents more detail on the morphology of larval, nymphal, and adult stages of *S. scabiei*

Sarcoptes from different hosts tend to be morphologically indistinguishable (Fain 1968), which raises the question of the systematic status of the genus. Do different isolates represent different species or should they be classified as different varieties of the same species (Arlian 1989)? There are two schools of thought. One is that different isolates (strains) should be designated distinct species (e.g., Kutzer 1970). In contrast, Fain (1968, 1978) concluded that different isolates represent one highly variable species. Pence et al. (1975) agree, based on a study of variation in chaetotaxy and denticulation of *Sarcoptes* on North American wild canids. Fain (1968) further proposed that humans were the original or primary hosts and that animals had acquired the mites from them.

Most of the morphological variations among isolates of *S. scabiei* from different hosts relate to the size, configuration, and number of the cuticular triangular spines (scales) on the dorsum of the females and to the presence or absence of the few ventrolaterally placed spines. Four morphological variations (types) are described (Fain 1968; Pence et al. 1975). Usually one species of host has a higher proportion of specimens of one type than of other types. Comprehensive systematic studies of host specificity of different *S. scabiei* variants (i.e., isolates from different mammal hosts)

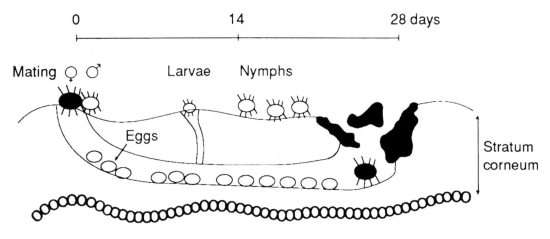

FIG. 5.2—Life cycle of *Sarcoptes scabiei.* (Illustration by R. Isaksson.)

have not been done. Crossbreeding studies of different isolates have not been done. However, molecular genetic analyses of 23 isolates of *S. scabiei* from nine host species (cattle, chamois, dog, red and silver fox, dromedary camel, raccoon dog, lynx, pig, and wombat) from four continents strongly support the view that the genus *Sarcoptes* consists of one heterogenous species (Zahler et al. 1999). Thus, we designate various isolates as variants (var.) of the particular host species from which they were isolated (examples, *S. scabiei* var. *canis, S. scabiei* var. *vulpes, S. scabiei* var. *suis,* etc.).

There is evidence indicating the existence of physiological differences between mites isolated from different hosts (Arlian 1989; Arlian et al. 1996a). From experimental transfer trials and from observations of natural infections, there are indications that host specificity occurs in some variants but not in others, and in some where it does occur, there is only partial specificity (Stone et al. 1972; Samuel 1981; Arlian et al. 1984a; Arlian et al. 1988a; Arlian 1989; Mörner 1992*).* Attempts to establish permanent *S. scabiei* infections in mice, rats, guinea-pigs, swine, cattle, cats, goats, and sheep isolated from dogs (*S. scabiei* var. *canis*) were unsuccessful (Arlian 1989). However, transient infestations lasted up to 13 weeks in some experimental hosts, some of which (e.g., cattle, goats, sheep, and swine) are known "natural" hosts of *S. scabiei.*

Sarcoptes scabiei was successfully transferred from dogs to (and passaged in) New Zealand white rabbits (Arlian et al. 1984a,b; Arlian et al. 1988a), but *S. scabiei* from humans and swine failed to infect New Zealand white rabbits (Arlian et al. 1988a). Mites were successfully transferred from sheep to goats and vice versa (Abu-Samra et al. 1984; Ibrahim and Abu-Samra 1987), to dromedary camels (Nayel and Abu-Samra 1986), and from goats to donkeys (Abu-Samra et al. 1985). Mange occurred in the recipients. Recent concern that scabies, prevalent in some Aborigine communities of Australia, originated from dingos, which host

S. scabiei var. *canis,* was tentatively disproved by molecular analyses (Walton et al. 1998).

LIFE HISTORY. All *S. scabiei* go through egg, larval, protonymphal, and tritonymphal life stages (Fain 1968; Arlian and Vyszenski-Moher 1988; Davis and Moon 1990a). *Sarcoptes scabiei* differ from many other mange mites in that they inhabit the epidermis of the skin, where tunnels are excavated in the outer layers (Fig. 5.2). All life stages can penetrate the skin surface (Heilesen 1946; Mellanby 1972; Van Neste 1988). Penetration is achieved by a combination of chewing movements with the chelicerae and a side to side movement of the gnathosoma. Mites burrow through the stratum corneum to the stratum granulosum and stratum spinosum, where they consume live cells or tissue fluid oozing into the burrows (Van Neste 1986, 1988; Arlian et al. 1988b). Because of continual outgrowth of the epidermis, much of the burrow, with contents such as eggs and feces, is located in the cornified layers of the epithelium.

Fertilized females, with a life expectancy of 4–6 weeks, lay eggs in these tunnels (Fig. 5.2). The eggs, which are oval and measure 150–200 μm by 175–250 μm, are laid at a rate of 3–4/day. They hatch within 3 days, and larvae, which have three pairs of legs, emerge. Some larvae migrate from the breeding tunnels made by the females and move in the skin. Others are found migrating on the skin or remain in the original tunnels or their extensions, which are sometimes referred to as molting pockets. There they develop into a first nymphal stage (protonymphs) in 3 to 4 days and into a second nymphal stage (tritonymph) ~3 days later. These nymphal stages remain in tunnels and molting pockets, wander on the skin surface, or form new tunnels and pockets. Nymphal stages have four pairs of legs. Another 2 to 4 days are required before the tritonymphs molt into adults. Thus, development from egg to adult takes ~2 weeks.

DISTRIBUTION, EPIDEMIOLOGY, AND TRANSMISSION.

Sarcoptes scabiei has been reported from more than 100 species of mammals and marsupials (Bak et al. 1997) (Table 5.1). Sarcoptic mange also has been reported from many species of wild mammals worldwide. Some of the most notable hosts include (1) canids in North America (Pence et al. 1983; Little et al. 1998b); (2) red foxes and other canids in Europe (Mörner 1992; Ippen et al. 1995; Gortazar et al. 1998); (3) red foxes and dingos in Australia (Gray 1937; McCarthy 1960; Hoyte and Mason 1961); (4) chamois, *Rupicapra* spp., and a variety of other ungulates in Europe (Ippen et al. 1995; Rossi et al. 1995; Fernández Morán et al. 1997); (5) felids in Europe (Mörner 1992,) and Africa (Young 1975); (6) wild boar in Europe (Ippen et al. 1995); (7) marsupials, especially wombats (*Vombatus ursinus*), in Australia (Arundel et al. 1977; Martin et al. 1998; Skerratt et al. 1998); and (8) a range of ungulates, primates, and canids in Africa (Zumpt and Ledger 1973; Young 1975; Kalema et al. 1998).

The epidemiology of sarcoptic mange in wildlife populations is not well understood and seems to differ between different areas of the world and animals species. In North America most literature (see review of Pence and Custer 1981) deals with epizootics in wild canids, mainly red foxes and coyotes (Todd et al. 1981; Pence et al. 1983; Pence and Windberg 1994), but also gray and red wolves, *Canis lupus* and *Canis rufus* (Pence et al. 1981; Todd et al. 1981). In Europe most recent literature deals with an epizootic of mange in red foxes of Fennoscandia (Mörner 1992) and in chamois in the Alps of southern Europe (Rossi et al. 1995; Fernandez Moran et al. 1997).

Prevalence of mange in trapped or hunter-killed coyotes in Alberta was ~20%, 1972–1975; prevalence in gray wolves poisoned during wolf reduction programs, 1972–1978, was 11% (Todd et al. 1981). Differences in body condition of mangy and non-mangy hosts were greatest for pups. Although little direct information is available on survival of mangy canids in the North, trappers and agricultural field personnel in Alberta see many mangy coyotes before, but not after, winter becomes severely cold (-30° C to 40° C) (W.M. Samuel, personal observation). Mangy coyotes rely more on carrion than do non-mangy coyotes, and they remain 50% closer to carrion sources than non-mangy coyotes (Todd et al. 1981).

In southern North America, Pence and Windberg (1994) evaluated the effect of an epizootic, 1975–1991, on coyotes in south Texas. They examined 1489 coyotes and found that 80% were infected during the peak (1980). Reduced ovulation and pregnancy rates were associated with severity of mange in adult females. Coyotes with severe mange tended to have less internal fat. Pence and Windberg (1994) suggested that the epizootic was caused by the appearance of a virulent strain of *S. scabiei* and enhanced by high densities of coyotes, but moderated by the social organization of the animals. They also concluded that the coyote population declined as a result of selection for mange-resistant individuals in the host population. They showed that the epizootic had little long-term effect on the coyote population in spite of coyotes experiencing ~70% mortality.

An epizootic of *S. scabiei* occurred in the wild red fox population of Finland in the mid-1960s, very likely the result of foxes crossing the Gulf of Finland from Estonia (Henriksson 1972). The disease spread to Sweden and Norway about 10 years later (Mörner 1992). The first case recorded in Sweden was in 1972 (Christensson 1972); a second case was reported in 1975 (Borg et al. 1976). Within 8 years, sarcoptic mange had spread throughout the mainland of the country killing over 50% of the red fox population (Danell and Hörnfeldt 1987; Lindström and Mörner 1985). In certain regions, mortalities (Fig. 5.3) of ~90% were reported (Mörner 1992). Substantial numbers of lynx (*Lynx lynx*) and marten (*Martes martes*) were also infected and died during the epizootic (Mörner 1992). Infected Arctic foxes (*Alopex lagopus*), first noticed in the mountains of northern Sweden in 1986, were caught, treated successfully, and released in 1987 (Mörner et al. 1988).

Prior to the epizootic, Swedish wildlife, including foxes and dogs, were naive to *S. scabiei;* in fact, the only recorded case of *S. scabiei* on any wildlife species earlier was a red fox found dead on the southern shore of Sweden in 1955 (S. Bornstein, unpublished). Dogs were very susceptible to sarcoptic mites from red foxes (Svensson 1983). The fox population began to recover during the late 1980s (Lindström et al. 1994).

The occurrence of sarcoptic mange in isolated populations can be a severe problem. For example, sarcoptic mange is thought to be the main cause of extinction of red foxes on the island of Bornholm, Denmark (Henriksen et al. 1993). Also, sarcoptic mange is the most common cause of death of chamois (see Fig. 1.37 in Sweatman 1971) and ibex, *Capra ibex*, in European mountain regions (Rossi et al. 1995; Fernández Morán et al. 1997). It is considered a threat to these endangered animals. Several waves of sarcoptic mange, with intervals between > 10–15 years, have been seen with a mortality of > 80%. Sarcoptic mange also occurs in Spanish ibex *(Capra pyrenaica)* and, less frequently, in roe deer *(Capreolus capreolus)* and red deer *(Cervus elaphus)* in parts of central and southern Europe (Ippen et al. 1995; Fernández Morán et al., 1997). In Australia *S. scabiei* var. *wombati* causes sporatic epizootics in wombats (see Fig. 1.38 in Sweatman 1971); such outbreaks "have the potential to threaten the long-term survival of small, remnant populations" (Martin et al. 1998).

Transmission of *S. scabiei* among wildlife occurs both by direct and indirect contact. Larvae and nymphs of *S. scabiei* frequently leave their burrows and wander on the skin (Arlian and Vyszenski-Moher 1988), which may harbor hundreds to several thousands of mites/cm^2 (W.M.Samuel, unpublished; Zeh 1974; Arlian et al. 1988c). Some may become dislodged from the host and

TABLE 5.1—List of reported species infected with *Sarcoptes scabiei*

Order/Family	Species	Scientific Name	Locality	Selected References
PRIMATES				
Cercopithecidae	Java-macac	*Macaca fascicularis*	Denmark[a]	Leerhøy and Jensen 1967
Hominidae	Man	*Homo sapiens*	Global	Fain 1978
Pongidae	Chimpanzee	*Pan troglodytes*	Africa	Zumpt and Ledger 1973
	Pygmy chimpanzee	*Pan paniscus*	Africa	Zumpt and Ledger 1973
	Orangutang	*Pongo pygmaeus*	The Netherlands[a]	Fain 1968
	Gibbon	*Hylobates leuciscus*	USA[a]	Fain 1968
CARNIVORA				
Canidae	Arctic fox	*Alopex lagopus*	Europe	Mörner et al. 1988
	Dog	*Canis familiaris*	Global[a]	Muller et al. 1989
	Dingo	*Canis familiaris dingo*	Australia	Gray 1937, McCarthy 1960
	Coyote	*Canis latrans*	America	Samuel 1981, Todd et al. 1981, Pence and Windberg 1994
	Gray wolf	*Canis lupus*	North America	Todd et al. 1981, Mörner, 1992
	Jackal	*Canis mesomelas*	Africa	Zumpt and Ledger 1973
	Red wolf	*Canis rufus*	North America	Pence et al. 1981
	Crab-eating fox	*Cerdocyon thous*	South America	Fain 1968
	Wild dog	*Lycaon pictus*	Africa	Mwanzia et al. 1995
	Racoon dog	*Nyctereutes procynoides*	Europe	Henriksson 1972
	Gray fox	*Urocyon cinereoargenteus*	North America	Stone et al. 1982
	Red fox	*Vulpes vulpes*	Australia, Holarctic	Gray 1937, Trainer and Hale 1969, Mörner 1981
Felidae	Cheetah	*Acinonyx jubatus*	Africa	Mwanzia et al. 1995
	Cat	*Felis catus*	Global[a]	Kershaw 1989
	Cougar	*Felis concolor*	USA[a]	Blair 1922
	Serval	*Felis serval*	Africa	Zumpt and Ledger 1973
	Lynx	*Lynx lynx*	Europe	Holt and Berg 1990, Mörner 1992
	Lion	*Panthera leo*	Africa	Young 1975
	Jaguar	*Panthera onca*	USA[a]	Blair 1922
	Leopard	*Panthera pardus*	Germany[a], USA[a]	Blair 1922
	Tiger	*Panthera tigris*	Vietnam[a]	Houdemer 1938
	Snow leopard	*Uncia uncia*	The Netherlands[a]	Peters and Zwart 1973
Mustelidae	Stone marten	*Martes foina*	Europe	Wetzel and Rieck 1962
	Pine marten	*Martes martes*	Europe	Holt and Berg 1990, Mörner 1992
	Fischer	*Martes pennanti*	North America	O'Meara et al. 1960
	Badger	*Mele meles*	Europe	Holt and Berg 1990
	Siberian polecat	*Mustela putorius*	Europe	Wetzel and Rieck 1962
	Stoat	*Mustela putorius furo*	Global[a]	Ryland and Gorham 1978
Procyonidae	Red panda	*Ailurus fulgens*	Sweden[a]	Bornstein 1992
	Coati	*Nasua nasua*	England[a]	Fain 1968
Protelidae	Aardwolf	*Proteles cirstatus*	Africa	Zumpt and Ledger 1973
Ursidae	Polar bear	*Thalarctos maritimus*	Czech Republic[a]	Jedlicka and Hojocova 1972
	Black bear	*Ursus americanus*	North America	Schmitt et al. 1987
	Brown bear	*Ursus arctos*	Czech Republic[a]	Jedlicka and Hojocova 1972
ARTIODACTYLA				
Bovidae	Impala	*Aepyceros melampus*	Africa	Zumpt and Ledger 1973
	Hartebeest	*Alcelaphus buselaphus*	Africa	Zumpt and Ledger 1973
	Barbary sheep	*Ammontragus lervia*	Israel[a]	Yeruham et al. 1996
	Springbok	*Antidorcas marsupialis*	Africa	Zumpt and Ledger 1973
	Pronghorn	*Antilope cervicapra*	Czech Republic[a]	Frolka and Rostinska 1984
	Cattle	*Bos taurus*	Global[a]	Fain 1968, Chakrabarti and Chaudhury 1984
	Water buffalo	*Bubalus bubalis*	Asia[a]	Chakrabarti et al. 1981
	Goat	*Capra hircus*	Europe[a], Africa[a], Asia[a]	Fain 1968, Garg 1973, Ibrahim and Abu-Samra 1985
	Ibex	*Capra ibex*	Europe	Rossi et al. 1995
	Nubian ibex	*Capra rubiana*	Israel[a]	Yeruham et al. 1996
	Iberian ibex	*Capra pyrenaica*	Europe	Palomares and Ruíz-Martìnez 1993
	Siberian ibex	*Capra sibirica*	Asia	Jakunin 1958, Vyrypaev 1985
	Oryx	*Connochaetes taurinus*	Africa	Zumpt and Ledger 1973

TABLE 5.1 *(continued)*

Order/Family	Species	Scientific Name	Locality	Selected References
	Mountain gazelle	*Gazella gazella*	Israel[a]	Yeruham et al. 1996
	Grants gazelle	*Gazella granti*	Africa	Wetzel 1984
	Thomson's gazelle	*Gazellea thomsoni*	Africa	Sachs and Sachs 1968
	Sable antelope	*Hippotragus niger*	Africa	Young 1975
	Waterbuck	*Kobus ellipsiprymnus*	Czech Republic[a]	Frolka and Rostinska 1984
	Arabian oryx	*Oryx leucoryx*	Israel[a]	Yeruham et al. 1996
	Sheep	*Ovis aries*	Europe[a], Africa[a], Asia[a]	Fain 1968, Okoh and Gadzama 1982, Chakrabarti and Chaudhury 1984
	Mouflon	*Ovis musimon*	Europe	Kerschlagl 1938, Kutzer 1970
	Steenbok	*Raphicerus campestris*	Africa	Zumpt and Ledger 1973
	Chamois	*Rupicapra rupicapra*	Europe	Onderscheka et al. 1968, Rossi et al. 1995
	African buffalo	*Syncerus caffer*	Africa	Zumpt and Ledger 1973
	Eland antelope	*Taurotragus oryx*	Israel[a]	Yeruham et al. 1996
	Kodu	*Tragelaphus strepsiceros*	Africa	Zumpt and Ledger 1973
Camelidae	Bactrian camel	*Camelus bactrianus*	England[a]	Fain 1968
	Dromedary	*Camelus dromedarius*	Asia[a], Arabia[a], Africa[a]	Lodha 1966, Higgins et al. 1984, Nayel and Abu-Samra 1986
	Lama	*Lama glama*	-	Kutzer 1970
	Guanaco	*Lama guanicoe*	-	Kutzer 1970
	Alpaca	*Lama pacos*	-	Kutzer 1970
	Vicuna	*Lama vicugna*	-	Kutzer 1970
Cervidae	Moose	*Alces alces*	Germany[a]	Ullrich 1938
	Roe deer	*Capreolus capreolus*	-	Kutzer 1970
	Red deer	*Cervus elaphus*	Europe	Kutzer 1970
	Sambar	*Cervus unicolor*	Africa	Fain 1968
	Reindeer	*Rangifer tarandus*	Russia[a]	Lange and Sokolova 1992
Giraffidae	Giraffe	*Giraffa camolopardalis*	France[a]	Mégnin 1877
	Warthog	*Phacochoerus aethiopicus*	Africa	Fain 1968
	Wild boar	*Sus scrofa*	Europe, North America	Wetzer and Rieck 1962, Smith et al. 1982
	Swine	*Sus scrofa domestica*	Global[a]	Chakrabarti 1990, Davis and Moon 1990b
Tayassuidae	White-lipped peccary	*Tayassu pecari*	America	Fain 1968
	Collared peccary	*Tayassu tajacu*	USA[a]	Meierhenry and Clausen 1977
PINNIPEDIA				
Phocidae	Harbour seal	*Phoca vitulina*	Europe	Jacobsen 1966
HYRACOIDEA				
Procaviidae	Gray hyrax	*Heterohyrax syriacus*	Africa	Wetzel 1984
	Rock dassie	*Procavia johnstoni*	Africa	Wetzel 1984
PERISSODACTYLA				
Equidae	Ass	*Equus asinus*	Arabia[a]	Abu Yaman 1978
	Horse	*Equus caballus*	Global[a]	Fain 1968, Abu Yaman 1978, Chakrabarti and Chaudhury 1984
Tapiridae	Tapir	*Tapirus terrestris*	Europe[a], USA[a]	Kutzer and Grünberg 1967, Fain 1968, Frolka and Rostinska 1984
RODENTIA				
Caviidae	Guinea pig	*Cavia porcellus*	France[a]	Fain 1968
	Capybara	*Hydrochaeris hydrochaeris*	Europe[a]	Fiebeger 1913, Fain 1968
Erethizontidae	Porcupine	*Erethizon dorsatum*	North America	Payne and O'Meara 1958
Muridae	African giant pouched rat	*Cricetomys gambianus*	Africa	Fain 1968
	House mouse	*Mus musculus*	USA[a]	Meierhenry and Clausen 1977
Sciuridae	Fox squirrel	*Sciurus niger*	North America	Allen 1942

(continued)

TABLE 5.1 *(continued)*

Order/Family	Species	Scientific Name	Locality	Selected References
LAGOMORPHA				
Leporidae	Brown hare	*Lepus europaeus*	Europe	Restani et al. 1985
	Mountain hare	*Lepus timidus*	Europe	Bornstein 1985
	Rabbit	*Oryctolagus cuniculus*	Europe, USA[a],	Fain 1968, Arlian et al. 1984a
	Marsh rabbit	*Sylvilagus palustris*	USA	Stringer et al. 1969
MARSUPIALIA				
Phascolarctidae	Koala	*Phascolarctos cinereus*	Australia	Barker 1974, Brown et al. 1981
Vombatidae	Wombat	*Lasiorhinus latifrons*	Australia	Fain 1968, Wells 1971
	Wombat	*Vombatus ursinus*	Australia	Gray 1937
INSECTIVORA				
Erinaceidae	African hedgehog	*Atelerix albiventris*	Africa	Okaeme and Osakawe 1985
	Hedgehog	*Erinaceus europaeus*	Israel, Germany	Kuttin et al. 1977, Saupe 1988
	Long-eared hedgehog	*Hemiechinus auritus*	Israel[a]	Yeruham et al. 1996

[a]Indicates that the infection has occurred in mammals in captivity.

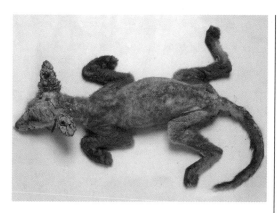

FIG. 5.3—Red fox with sarcoptic mange, including alopecia and crusted skin. (Photograph by B. Ekberg.)

fall off (Arlian and Vyszenski-Moher 1988). Mites may survive in the environment several weeks if conditions (microclimate) are optimal; that is, high relative humidity (RH) and low temperature prolongs their survival time (Arlian et al. 1989). Mites survived 8–19 days at 10°C–25° C at 97% RH, but died after a few hours when the ambient temperature was increased to 25°C–45° C and the RH was decreased to 45%. All life stages of *S. scabiei* var. *canis* survived 1–9 days at 15°–25° C and 25%–97% RH. How long mites retain the ability to penetrate host skin after being off the host is of great significance to the transmission of the disease. The time needed for *S. scabiei* var. *hominis,* immediately transferred from one host to another, to initiate penetration into the stratum corneum was ~10 minutes (Arlian et al. 1984b), and it took the mites ~35 minutes to become completely submerged. The time required for complete penetration into the stratum

corneum increased as a function of the time the mites had been off their host.

Experiments indicate that mites remain infective at least one-half to two-thirds of their survival time when dislodged from their host (Arlian 1989). Gerasimov (1958) showed that *S. scabiei* var. *vulpes* could be transmitted to uninfected red foxes occupying dens used previously by mangy animals. He also observed larval mites on the ovipositors of flies for ~24 hours after contact between the flies and a dead mangy carcass, suggesting the possibility of phoresy as a mechanism of transmission (Zeh 1974).

CLINICAL SIGNS. In many animal species, domestic and wild, acute sarcoptic mange is often characterized by intense pruritus accompanied by erythematous eruptions, papule formation, seborrhoea, and alopecia (Figs. 5.3, 5.4) (Sweatman 1971). These signs are not always observed because thick fur covers the lesions in many animals (Thomsett 1968). In chronic cases, crusting, hyperkeratosis, lichenification, and thickening of the skin are seen, and animals develop a foul aromatic odor. In severe cases lymphadenopathy occurs. Subcutaneous edema is often present, often seen on the face as squinting eyes shortly before death (Bornstein et al. 1995).

In wildlife, clinical signs reported are often of a generalized nature, obviously describing severely affected individuals. For example, Trainer and Hale (1969) describe the following clinical signs of sarcoptic mange in red foxes and coyotes: listlessness; emaciation; loss of fear of man; and hairless areas including muzzle, neck, shoulders, back, and sometimes the head and tail. Mangy wild canids are often easily approached and are seen in farmyards and in barns and dog houses, at base of farmed hay stacks, etc. Clinical signs in other species such as lynx and chamois are

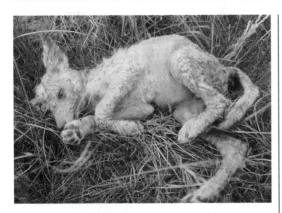

FIG. 5.4—Coyote, *Canis latrans,* found dead with severe sarcoptic mange.

similar to those described above (Pence et al. 1983; Mörner 1992; Ippen et al. 1995; Rossi et al. 1995; Fernández Morán et al. 1997).

PATHOGENESIS AND PATHOLOGY. The acute signs of sarcoptic mange are thought to be a manifestation of a hypersensitivity reaction to the mites. Both delayed (type IV) and immediate (type I) hypersensitivity reactions have been verified by skin tests in experimentally infected dogs (S. Bornstein, unpublished) and pigs (Davies and Moon 1990b). Little et al. (1998a) were not able to demonstrate any delayed (type IV) response in experimentally infected red foxes. Experimentally infected red foxes developed pronounced mast cell hyperplasia and infiltration with eosinophils as the earliest inflammatory cell response to infection (Little et al. 1998a), and elevated white blood cell counts were recorded. These results show that red foxes develop strong immediate hypersensitivity reactions to *S. scabiei* similar to those found in pigs (Davis and Moon 1990a), but contrary to some findings in other hosts (dogs, rabbits), red foxes were not resistant to reinfection.

Incubation periods of canids experimentally infected with *S. scabiei* vary from approximately 10 to 30 days (Stone et al. 1972; Samuel 1981; Mörner and Christensson 1984; Bornstein et al. 1995), depending on the infective dose. Stone et al. (1972) and Samuel (1981) observed that experimentally infected red foxes, dog-coyote hybrids, dogs, and coyotes developed papules ~2–3 weeks after exposure. Crusted lesions appeared ~4–5 weeks postexposure. Pelage became matted, hair was common in feces, and animals developed a foul aromatic odor, became restless, and spent much time licking and scratching infested areas ~1–2 months after exposure. By about day 50, lesions were encrusted and had coalesced, covering most of the body; serous exudate was extensive. Appetite remained fairly normal until 1 week before death, 2–3 months after infection.

Time of death likely depends on number of mites in the infection dose and individual resistance to infection.

One of three experimentally infected red foxes developed a well-demarcated hyperkeratotic lesion (Bornstein et al. 1995), a chronic localized mange without any systemic involvement, quite different from the deadly mange of the other two infected foxes. This could indicate that some naturally infected animals may develop local and long-lasting chronic infections. Such animals could act as carriers of the infection. Some necropsied red foxes with healed skin wounds suspected of having been primarily caused by *S. scabiei* infections, although no mites were present, had elevated serum levels of antibodies against *S. scabiei* (S. Bornstein, unpublished).

Progression of lesions among wild canids is similar (Fig. 5.5) (Pence et al. 1983; Mörner and Christensson 1984; Bornstein et al. 1995). Lesions in red foxes usually begin on the elbows and hocks and on the base of the tail (Mörner 1981) and spread anteriorly to the back and distally to the tail. The expression 'rat-tailed coyote' or 'rat-tailed wolf' is commonly heard in Alberta (W.M. Samuel, person observation). Skin lesions may be localized or generalized, covering more or less the whole body (Figs. 5.3, 5.4). Generalized alopecia is not always present in severely affected foxes. Although pruritus is not always a significant feature in infected red foxes (Stone et al. 1972; Mörner and Christensson 1984), it has been observed in wild, naturally infected red foxes (Borg et al. 1976). It is thought to increase the animal's difficulty in catching their natural prey. Also, as the disease progresses, animals become emaciated and debilitated; eventually, animals succumb to emaciation and dehydration.

Experimentally infected red foxes developed pronounced mast cell hyperplasia and infiltration with eosinophils as the earliest inflammatory cell response to infection (Little et al. 1998a). White blood cell counts, but not red blood cell parameters, differed significantly between infected and uninfected foxes. These results and unremarkable serum biochemistry values are similar to findings of Arlian et al. (1995) for dogs infected with *S. scabiei*. Wild infected coyotes displayed significant decreases in alpha-globulin and albumin and significant increases in gamma-globulin (Pence et al. 1983).

The most common macroscopic lesions found in animals with a thick haircoat (e.g., foxes) are exudation of body fluids, matted haircoat, and a thickened, hyperkeratotic and hyperpigmented skin. In severe cases, animals lose more or less all hair (Figs. 5.3, 5.4). Pence et al. (1983) described coyotes with severe mange as having "partial to almost total alopecia over the legs, flanks, shoulders, tail (rat-tail), ears, and face." Skin was "thickened, wrinkled, slate-gray in color, and with numerous suppurative encrustations." Histologically, lesions were pronouncedly hyperkeratotic with extensive accumulations of serum exudate and extravasated erythrocytes in the stratum corneum, pronounced acanthosis, some parakeratosis, hyperplastic stratum

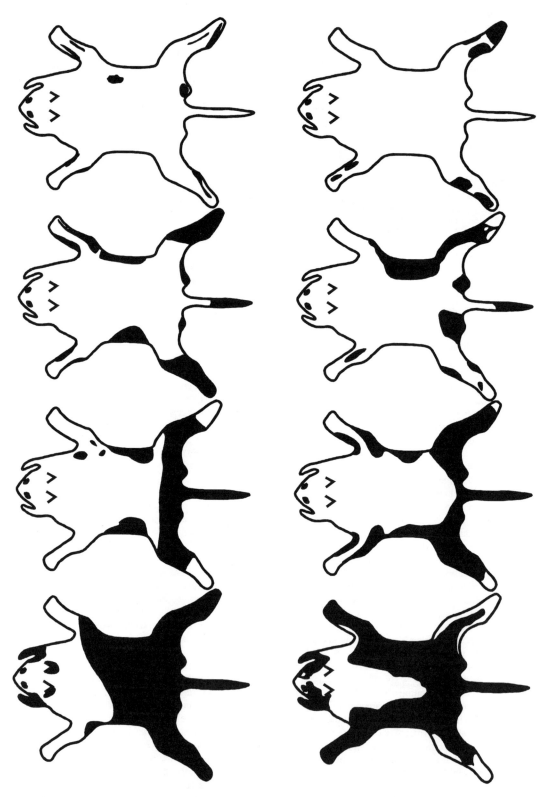

FIG. 5.5—Progression of skin damage (encrustation, alopecia) on 4 coyotes (left column) and 4 gray wolves (right) from Alberta. Percent of animal surface with skin damage is (top to bottom) 4%, 21%, 29%, and 67% for the coyotes and 6%, 20%, 39%, and 71% for the wolves. Distribution of skin damage was determined for 18 coyotes and 12 wolves (W.M. Samuel, unpublished).

germinativum, and a primary infiltration of neutrophils, lymphocytes, and plasma cells. Hair follicles and sebaceous glands were plugged at the surface and generally hyperplastic with a mild inflammatory response.

The inflammatory reaction varies among different species and different individuals. Varying degrees of superficial dermatitis, vasodilation, dermal edema, perivascular lymphocytic infiltration, epidermal spongiosis, hyperplasia, and para- and hyperkeratosis may be revealed at histological examinations. Eosinophils and mast cells are sometimes seen intermingled with neutrophils and macrophages. Neutrophils and plasma cells may be abundant in specimens taken from sites with epidermal erosions and crustings, which are often due to self-trauma (Muller et al. 1989; Jubb et al. 1993; Gross and Ihrke 1992). In the crusty, chronic, hyperkeratotic type of sarcoptic mange, massive numbers of the mites may be found (Pirilää et al. 1967; Dobson and Davies 1992; Arlian et al. 1988c).

DIAGNOSIS. Although most any pruritic skin condition can be caused by *S. scabiei* (Orkin and Maibach 1991), mange mimics a variety of skin disorders. Although distribution and spread of mange-induced lesions may provide a clue to diagnosis of the infection (Fig. 5.5), lesions can also vary from host to host, meaning that recovery and identification of mites are required for diagnosis by skin scrapings or skin biopsy. In addition, the demonstration of specific antibodies in sera of suspected infected animals strongly confirm the tentative diagnosis. Deep skin scrapings, even those including encrusted epidermis, can be negative (Hill and Steinberg 1993). Often, biopsies are not helpful, the one exception being wildlife with severe and chronic infestation (this is in contrast to acute sarcoptic mange in domestic animals).

Recovery techniques vary, but the following techniques are successful in recovering the parasite from live or dead hosts, respectively. On the living host, deep skin scrapings are made with a scalpel or similar blade-like tool to the point of oozing blood. Direct microscopic examination of scrapings is often not worth the effort. However, if the scrapings are heated gently, mites become active and more observable. If the host is dead, pieces of mangy skin are removed and placed in a petri dish. Heat from the light source of a stereomicroscope (~1 hour) stimulates mites to migrate from the skin. Failing this, scrapings are put in 10%–20% aqueous potassium hydroxide (KOH) solution. The material may be boiled in 20% KOH for a few minutes or put in a water bath (37° C) for a few hours using 10% KOH, until the material has become digested. Then the material is centrifuged (3 minutes at 3000 rpm) and the supernatant decanted. A few drops of glycerine are added to the sediment, which is then examined microscopically.

Serodiagnostic tests (ELISA) can support the diagnosis. This assay, which demonstrates specific antibodies to *S. scabiei*, has been developed for dogs and red foxes (Bornstein et al. 1995, 1996), pigs (Bornstein and Zakrisson 1993; Bornstein and Wallgren 1997), camels, lynx, and domestic cats (Bornstein et al. 1997a,b). This technique is used to verify whether an animal with skin lesions has been infected with *S. scabiei* or not. It is useful in diagnosing mange in animals with atypical or minute skin lesions and in conducting seroepidemiological surveys.

IMMUNOLOGY. The immune response to *S. scabiei* infection is not well understood. The question of whether or not an infection of *S. scabiei* induces protection to subsequent infections is controversial. Mites may induce relative protection against subsequent infections in some hosts, including humans, rabbits, and dogs (Arlian et al. 1994, 1996a,b), but not in others such as experimentally infected red foxes (Little et al. 1998a) and naturally infected dogs (S. Bornstein, unpublished). Mellanby (1977) associated the cyclical nature (15–30–year cycles) of scabies epidemics in humans, the spontaneous waning of the disease in reinfected patients, and in particular, the decrease in the mite burden in these patients (Mellanby 1944), to protective immunity.

The relative resistance to reinfection is thought to be associated with cell-mediated immune responses (Arlian et al. 1994). Cell-mediated reactions have been described in pigs (Davies and Moon 1990a). Both delayed and immediate hypersensitivity reactions were verified by skin tests in *S. scabiei* var. *suis*–infected swine (Sheehan 1975; Davies and Moon 1994b), in *S. scabiei* var. *vulpes*-infected dogs (S. Bornstein, unpublished) and in *S. scabiei* var. *vulpes*–infected guinea pigs (S. Bornstein, unpublished). Cell-mediated immune response is thought to be more important than humoral antibody response as regards protective immunity (Arlian et al. 1994). Studies suggest that Langerhans cells (CDI4$^+$) in the epidermis of dogs are involved in early immune responses in both primary infections and reinfections (Arlian et al. 1996b; Stemmer et al. 1996). In addition, it is suggested that T-lymphocytes (CD3e$^+$), CDLLc$^+$, MHC Class II$^+$ and CDIa$^+$ cells in the dermis (Stemmer et al. 1996), and CD4$^+$ cells (Arlian et al. 1997) play a significant role in the immune response to the mite.

Humoral antibodies to *S. scabiei* have been demonstrated in several hosts following infection (Bornstein 1995). Dogs and red fox seroconverted 2–5 and 5 weeks, respectively, after exposure to *S. scabiei* var. *vulpes* (Bornstein and Zakrisson 1993; Bornstein et al. 1995). Differences were partly explained by differences in infection methods, numbers of mites given, and individual responses. Naturally infected dogs seroconvert ~1–2 weeks after clinical signs appear (S. Bornstein, unpublished). Pigs experimentally infected with *S. scabiei* var. *suis* seroconverted 5–7 weeks following infection, depending on infective dose given (Bornstein and Zakrisson 1993).

CONTROL AND TREATMENT. Sarcoptic mange occurs normally in animal populations as a widespread and common disease. Controlling the disease by reducing infected animals through hunting may be counterproductive and result in more cases of mange because of high movement of animals into "animal-free" areas (Lindström and Mörner 1985). Treatment of single infected wild animals is usually of little value in wild populations. However, where mange is having an impact on small, isolated, and threatened populations (e.g., arctic fox or ibex), it may be worthwhile to capture, treat, and release such animals. This has been done successfully with arctic foxes in northern Sweden (Mörner et al. 1988).

Sarcoptic mange can occur in hosts in wildlife enclosures, game farms, or zoos. There are several effective drugs against sarcoptic mange available to be used topically, perorally, or parenterally. However, despite the use of effective acaricides (e.g., in modern pig breeding enterprises), many attempts to eradicate the infection have failed due to badly managed treatment procedures. Inadequate use of acaricides may keep the infection at a subclinical level. All in-contact animals should be treated, all at the same time. It is probably not necessary to treat, clean, or disinfect premises such as pens or stables (Jacobson et al. 1999). Avermectins are effective acaricides, having a systemic and prolonged effect. In addition, they work well against other parasites such as nematodes. Avermectins protect against *S. scabiei* between 9 and 18 days, during which time no reinfection occurs (Arendts et al. 1999). Quarantine and biosecurity measures should be enforced to prevent animals from becoming reinfected.

PUBLIC HEALTH CONCERNS. Humans are occasionally infected with *S. scabiei* of animal origin (Arlian 1989). This includes human infection from camel, cat, chamois, coyote, dog, ferret, fox, goat, horse, llama, pig, sheep, and water buffalo (Kutzer 1970; Fain 1978; Chakrabarti et al. 1981; Samuel 1981; Folz 1984; Chakrabarti 1990). Those infected include pig herders and slaughterers, researchers, wildlife biologists, trappers, animal care personnel, and pet owners. Most human infection from animal sources (and cross-infections between other species of hosts) is short-lived and self-limiting, lasting from a few days to several months (Arlian 1989). Scabies contracted from animals usually has a pattern of distribution different from that seen in classical human scabies. Lesions are frequently seen on the trunk, arms, and abdomen and rarely on the fingerwebs and genitalia. In addition the incubation period is markedly shortened, and mite burrows are not regularly seen (Orkin and Maibach 1991). Pruritus may be as intensive as in classical scabies, but symptoms usually wane within a few weeks. The nonhuman strain of the mite that infects man most frequently (30%–50% of cases) is that from dogs (Thomsett 1968; Folz 1984).

LITERATURE CITED

Abu-Samra, M.T., K.E.E. Ibrahim, and M.A. Aziz. 1984. Experimental infection of goats with *Sarcoptes scabiei* var. *ovis. Annals of Tropical Medicine and Parasitology* 78:55–61.

Abu-Samra, M.T., B.H. Ali, B.E. Musa, and K.E.E. Ibrahim. 1985. Experimental infection of the domestic donkey (*Equus asinus asinus*) with a goat strain of *Sarcoptes scabiei,* and treatment with ivermectin. *Acta Tropica* 42:217–224.

Abu Yaman, I.K. 1978. Insects and other pests affecting man and animals in Saudi Arabia. *Angewandte Parasitologie* 19:31–33.

Allen, D.L. 1942. Populations and habits of the fox squirrel in Allegen County, Michigan. *The American Midland Naturalist* 27:338–379.

Arendts, J.J., T. Skogerboe, and L.K. Ritzhaupt. 1999. Persistent efficacy of doramectin and ivermectin against experimental infestations of *Sarcoptes scabiei* var. *suis* in swine. *Veterinary Parasitology* 82:71–79.

Arlian, L.G. 1989. Biology, host relations, and epidemiology of *Sarcoptes scabiei. Annual Review of Entomology* 34:139–161.

Arlian, L.G., and D.L. Vyszenski-Moher. 1988. Life cycle of *Sarcoptes scabiei* var. c*anis. The Journal of Parasitology* 74:427–430.

Arlian, L.G., R.A. Runyan, and S.A. Estes. 1984a. Cross infestivity of *Sarcoptes scabiei. Journal of the American Academy of Dermatology* 10:979–986.

Arlian, L.G., R.A. Runyan, R.A. Achar, and S.A. Estes. 1984b. Survival and infestivity of *Sarcoptes scabiei* var. *canis* and var. h*ominis. Journal of the American Academy of Dermatolgy* 11:210–215.

Arlian, L.G., D.L. Vyszenski-Moher, and D. Cordova. 1988a. Host specificity of *S. scabiei* var. *canis* (Acari: Sarcoptidae) and the role of host odor. *Journal of Medical Entomology* 25:52–56.

Arlian, L.G., R.A. Runyan, and D.L. Vyszenski-Moher. 1988b. Water balance and nutritient procurement of *Sarcoptes scabiei* var. *canis* (Acari: Sarcoptidae). *Journal of Medical Entomology* 25:64–68.

Arlian, L.G., M. Ahmed, D.L. Vyszenski-Moher, S.A. Estes, and S. Achar. 1988c. Energetic relationship of *Sarcoptes scabiei* var. *canis* (Acari: Sarcoptidae) with the laboratory rabbit. *Journal of Medical Entomology* 25:57–63.

Arlian, L.G., D.L., Vyszenski-Moher, and M.J. Pole. 1989. Survival of adults and developmental stages of *Sarcoptes scabiei* var. *canis* when off the host. *Experimental and Applied Acarology* 6:181–187.

Arlian, L.G., M.S. Morgan, D.L. Vyszenski-Moher, and B.L. Stemmer. 1994. *Sarcoptes scabiei:* The circulating antibody response and induced immunity to scabies. *Experimental Parasitology* 78:37–50.

Arlian, L.G., M.S. Morgan, C.M. Rapp, and D.L. Vyszenski-Moher. 1995. Some effects of sarcoptic mange on dogs. *The Journal of Parasitology* 8:698–702.

Arlian, L.G., M.S. Morgan, and J.J. Arends. 1996a. Immunologic cross-reactivity among various strains of *Sarcoptes scabiei. The Journal of Parasitology* 82:66–72.

Arlian, L.G., M.S. Morgan, C.M. Rapp, and D.L. Vyszenski-Moher. 1996b. The development of protective immunity in canine scabies. *Veterinary Parasitology* 62:133–142.

Arlian, L.G., C.M. Rapp, B.T. Stemmer, M.S. Morgan, and P.F. Moore. 1997. Characterization of lymphocyte subtypes in scabietic skin lesions of naive sensitized dogs. *Veterinary Parasitology* 68:347–358.

Arundel, J.H., I.K. Barker, and I. Beveridge. 1977. Diseases of marsupials. In *The Biology of Marsupials.* Ed. B. Stonehouse and D. Gilmore. Baltimore, MD: University Park Press, pp. 148–149.

Bak, U., K. Hessellund, and J. Lykkegaard. 1997. Sarcoptic mange in red fox [In Danish]. Report Department of Zoology, University of Aarhus, Denmark, pp. 15–17.

Barker, I.K. 1974. *Sarcoptes scabiei* infestation of a koala (*Phascolarctos cinerus*), with probable human involvment. *Australian Veterinary Journal* 50:528.

Blair, W.R. 1922. *Report of the veterinarian.* 27th Annual Report of the New York Zoological Society, pp. 53–56.

Borg, K., D. Christensson, E. Fabiansson, T. Kronevi, P.O. Nilsson, and A. Uggla. 1976. Sarcoptic mange of red fox in Sweden [In Swedish]. *Svensk Jakt* 8:504–506.

Bornstein, P., and P. Wallgren. 1997. Serodiagnosis of sarcoptic mange in pigs. *Veterinary Record* 141:8–12.

Bornstein, S. 1985. The epidemiology of *Sarcoptes scabiei* in wild red foxes (*Vulpes vulpes*) in Sweden. *Proceedings 5th International Conference of Wildlife Disease Association,* Uppsala, Sweden, p. 10.

———. 1992. Sarcoptic mange in red fox [In Swedish]. *SVAvet* (The National Veterinary Institute, Uppsala, Sweden) 4:36–42.

———. 1995. *Sarcoptes scabiei* infections of the domestic dog, red fox and pig: Clinical and serodiagnostic studies. Dissertation, Swedish University of Agricultural Sciences and the National Veterinary Institute, Uppsala, Sweden, 131 pp.

Bornstein, S., and G. Zakrisson. 1993. Clinical picture and antibody response in pigs infected by *Sarcoptes scabiei* var. *suis. Veterinary Dermatology* 4:123–131.

Bornstein, S., G. Zakrisson, and P. Thebo. 1995. Clinical picture and antibody response to experimental *Sarcoptes scabiei* var. *vulpes* infection in red foxes (*Vulpes vulpes*). *Acta Veterinaria Scandinavica* 36:509–519.

Bornstein, S., P. Thebo, and. G. Zakrisson. 1996. Evaluation of an enzyme-linked immunosorbent assay (ELISA) for the serological diagnosis of canine sarcoptic mange. *Veterinary Dermatology* 7:21–28.

Bornstein, S., P. Thebo, G. Zakrisson, M.T. Abu-Samra, and G.E. Muhammed. 1997a. Demonstration of serum antibody to *Sarcoptes scabiei* in naturally infected camels: A pilot study. *Journal of Camel Practice and Research* 4:183–185.

Bornstein, S., B. Röken, and R. Lindberg. 1997b. An experimental infection of a lynx (*Felis lynx*) with *Sarcoptes scabiei* var. *vulpes.* 16th International Conference of the World Association for Advancement of Veterinary Parasitology, 10–15 August, Sun City, South Africa, p. 11.

Brown, A.S., A.A. Seawright, and G.T. Wilkinson. 1981. An outbreak of sarcoptic mange in a colony of koalas. In *Proceedings 4th International Conference Wildlife Disease Association,* Sydney, Australia, p. 111.

Chakrabarti, A. 1990. Pig handler's itch. *International Journal of Dermatology* 29:205–206.

Chakrabarti, A.N., and M.N. Chaudhury. 1984. Survey of incidence of mange in domestic animals in West Bengal (India). *Indian Veterinary Medical Journal* 8:39–48.

Chakrabarti, A.N., A.A. Chatterjee, K. Chakrabarti, and D.N. Sengupta. 1981. Human scabies from contact with water buffaloes infested with *Sarcoptes scabiei* var. *bubalis. Annals of Tropical Medicine and Parasitology* 75:353–357.

Christensson, D. 1972. Sarcoptic mange in a wild red fox [In Swedish]. *Svensk Veterinärtidning* 24:470–471.

Danell, K., and B. Hörnfeldt. 1987. Numerical responses by populations of red fox and mountain hare during an outbreak of sarcoptic mange. *Oecologia* 73:533–536.

Davis, D.P., and R.D. Moon. 1990a. Density of itch mite, *Sarcoptes scabiei* (Acari: Sarcoptidae) and temporal devel-

opment of cutaneous hypersensitivity in swine mange. *Veterinary Parasitology* 36:285–293.

Davis, D.P., and R.D. Moon. 1990b. Dynamics of swine mange: A critical review of the literature. *Journal of Medical Entomology* 27:727–737.

Dobson, K.J., and P.R. Davies. 1982. External parasites. In *Diseases of swine,* 7th ed. Ed. A.D. Leman, B. Straw, R.G. Clock, W.L. Mengeling, S. D'Allaire, and D.J. Taylor. Ames, Iowa: Wolfe Publishing Ltd., pp. 668–679.

Fain, A. 1968. Étude de la variabilité de *Sarcoptes scabiei* avec une révision des Sarcoptidae. *Acta Zoologica et Pathologica Antverpiensia* 47:1–196.

———. 1978. Epidemiological problems of scabieis. *International Journal of Dermatology* 17:20–30.

Fernández Morán, J., S. Gómez, F. Ballesteros, P. Quirós, J.L. Benito, C. Feliu, and J.M. Nieto. 1997. Epizootiology of sarcoptic mange in a population of cantabrian chamois (*Rupicapra pyrenaica parva*) in northwestern Spain. *Veterinary Parasitology* 73:163–171.

Fieberger, J. 1913. Untersuchungen über die Räude und ihre Erreger mit besonderer Berucksichtigung der Gemsenraude. Zeitschrift für Infektionskrankheiten. *Parasitäre Krankheiten und Hygiene der Haustiere* 14:341–365.

Folz, S.D. 1984. Canine scabies (*Sarcoptes scabiei*) infestation. *Compendium on Continuing Education for the Practising Veterinarian* 6:176–180.

Frolka, J., and J. Rostinska. 1984. Über die Wirksamkeit von Ivermectin MSD (IvomecR, EqvalanR) gegen Sarcoptesräude und Nematodenbefall bei Zootieren. *Erkrankungen der Zootiere* 26:455–462.

Garg, R.K. 1973. Studies on some important ectoparasites of goats. *Agra University Journal of Research (Science)* 22:69–70.

Gerasimov, Y. 1958. *Mange in wild foxes.* Translation of Russian game reports. Ottawa: Canadian Department of Northern Affairs National Resources.

Gortazar, C., R. Villafuerte, J.C. Blanco, and D. Fernadez-de-Luco. 1998. Enzootic sarcoptic mange in red foxes in Spain. *Zeitschrift fur Jagdwissenschaft* 44:251–256.

Gray, D.F. 1937. Sarcoptic mange affecting wild fauna in New South Wales. *Australian Veterinary Journal* 13:154–155.

Gross, T.L., and P.J. Ihrke. 1992. Perivascular diseases of the dermis. In *Veterinary dermatology.* Ed. T.L. Gross, P.J. Ihrke, and E.J. Walder. St. Louis, MO: Mosby Year Book, pp. 112–134.

Heilesen, B. 1946. Studies on *Acarus scabiei* and scabies. *Acta Dermatovenerologica* 26:1–370.

Henriksen, P., H.H. Dietz, S.A. Henriksen, and P. Gjelstrup. 1993. Sarcoptic mange in red fox in Denmark. A short report [In Danish]. *Dansk Veterinärtidskrift* 76:12–13.

Henriksson, K. 1972. Sarcoptic mange in wild red fox in Finland [In Finnish]. *Suomen Riista* 23:127–135.

Higgins, A.J., S.A. Al Mezani, and A.M. Abukhamseen. 1984. Observations on the incidence and control of *Sarcoptes scabiei* var. *camelii* in the Arabian camel. *Veterinary Record* 115:15–16.

Hill, P.B., and H. Steinberg. 1993. Difficult dermatological diagnosis. *Journal of the American Veterinary Medical Association* 202:873–874.

Holt, G., and C. Berg. 1990. Sarcoptic mange in red fox and other wild mammals in Norway [In Norwegian]. *Norsk Veterinärtidskrift* 102:427–432.

Houdemer, E.F. 1938. *Recherches de parasitologie comparée Indochinoise.* Paris: E. le Francois, 235 pp.

Ibrahim, K.E.E., and M.T. Abu-Samra. 1985. A severe outbreak of sarcoptic mange among goats naturally infected with a sheep strain of *Sarcoptes scabiei. Revue d'Elevage et de Médicine Vétérinaire des Pays Tropicaux* 38:258–265.

————. 1987. Experimental transmission of a goat strain of *Sarcoptes scabiei* to desert sheep and its treatment with ivermectin. *Veterinary Parasitology* 26:157–164.

Ippen, R., S. Nickel, and H-D. Schröder. 1995. *Krankheiten des Jagdbaren Wildes.* Berlin: Deutscher Landwirtschaftverlag, pp. 189–195.

Jacobsen, B. 1966. Eine durch Räudenmilbentfall verseuchte Hauterkrankung bei in freier Wildbahn lebenden Seehunden (*Phoca vitulina*). *Deutsche Tierärztliche Rundschau* 73:349–350.

Jacobson, M., S. Bornstein, and P. Wallgren. 1999. The efficacy of simplified eradication strategies against sarcoptic mange mite infections in swine herds monitored by an ELISA. *Veterinary Parasitology.* 81:249–258.

Jakunin, M.P. 1958. The occurrence of sarcoptic mange in ibex [In Russian]. *Trudy Instituta Zoologii. Akademia nauk Kazakhskoi SSR* 9:241.

Jedlicka, J., and M. Hojovcova. 1972. Sarcoptesräude bei Bären im Zoologischen Garten Brno. *Erkrankungen der Zootiere* 14:257–260.

Jubb, K.V.F., P.C. Kennedy, and N. Palmer. 1993. *Pathology of domestic animals,* 4th ed., vol. 1. St. Louis, MO: Academic Press, Inc.

Kalema, G., R.A. Koch, and E. Macfie. 1998. An outbreak of sarcoptic mange in free-ranging mountain gorillas (*Gorilla gorilla berengei*) in Bwindi Impenetrable National Park, South Western Uganda. *Proceedings AAZV and AAWV Joint Conference,* Omaha, Nebraska, USA, p. 438.

Kerschagl, W. 1938. Gamsräude und ihre Übertragung auf andere Wiltarten. *Der Deutsche Jä Illustrierte Süddeutsche Jagdzeitung* 59:711–712.

Kershaw, A. 1989. *Sarcoptes scabiei* in a cat. *Veterinary Record* 124:537–538.

Kuttin, E.S., A.M. Beemer, and U. Gerson. 1977. A dermatitis in a hedgehog associated with *Sarcoptes scabiei* and fungi. *Mykosen* 20:51–53.

Kutzer, E. 1970. Sarcoptes-Milben und Sarcoptesräude der Haustiere. Merkblätter Über angewandte Parasitenkunde und Schädlingsbekämpfung. *Angewandte Parasitologie* 11:1–22..

Kutzer, E., and W. Gruenberg. 1967. Sarcoptersräude (*Sarcoptes tapiri* nov. spec.) bei Tapiren (*Tapirus terrestris* L.). *Zeitschrift für Parasitenkunde* 29:46–60.

Lange, A.B., and T.V. Sokolova. 1992. Parasitism of the itch mite *Sarcoptes scabiei* (Acariformes: Sarcoptidae). *Parazitologiya* 26:281–295.

Leerhøy, J., and H.S. Jensen. 1967. Sarcoptic mange in a shipment of Cynomolgus monkeys. *Nordisk Veterinärmedicin* 19:128–130.

Lindström, E., and T. Mörner. 1985. The spreading of Sarcoptic mange among Swedish red foxes (*Vulpes vulpes L*) in relation to fox population dynamics. *Review Ecologie (Terre Vie)* 40:211–216.

Lindström, E.R., H. Andrén, P. Angelstam, G. Cederlund, B. Hörnfeldt, L. Jäderberg, P-A. Lemnell, B. Martinsson, K. Sköld, and J.E. Swensson. 1994. Disease reveals the predator: Sarcoptic mange, red fox predation, and prey populations. *Ecology* 75:1042–1049.

Little, S.E., W.R. Davidson, P.M. Rakich, T.L. Nixon, D.I. Bounous, and V.F. Nettles. 1998a. Responses of red foxes to first and second infection with *Sarcoptes scabiei*. *Journal of Wildlife Diseases* 34:600–611.

Little, S.E., W.R. Davidson, E.W. Howerth, P.M. Rakich, and V.F. Nettles. 1998b. Diseases diagnosed in red foxes from Southeastern United States. *Journal of Wildlife Diseases* 34:620–624.

Lodha, K.R. 1966. Studies on sarcoptic mange in camels (*Camelus dromedarius*). *Veterinary Record* 79:41–43.

Martin, R.W., K.A. Handasyde, and L.F. Skerratt. 1998. Current distribution of sarcoptic mange in wombats. *Australian Veterinary Journal* 76:411–414.

McCarthy, P.H. 1960. The presence of sarcoptic mange in the wild fox (*Vulpes vulpes*) in Central Queensland. *Australian Veterinary Journal* 36:359–360.

Mégnin, J.-P. 1877. *Monographie de la tribu des sarcoptes psoriques.* Paris: Librairie de E. Deyrolle Fils. 189 pp.

Meierhenry, E.F., and L.W. Clausen. 1977. Sarcoptic mange in collared peccaries. *Journal of the American Veterinary Medical Association* 171:983–984.

Mellanby, K. 1944. The development of symptoms, parasitic infection and immunity in human scabies. *Parasitology* 35:197–206.

————. 1972. *Scabies,* 2d ed. Middlesex, UK: E.W. Classey Ltd.

————. 1977. Biology of the parasite. In *Scabies and pediculosis.* Ed. M. Orkin, H.I. Maibach, L.C. Parish, and R.M. Schwartzman. Philadelphia, PA: J.B. Lippincott Co., pp. 8–16.

Mörner, T. 1981. The epizootic outbreak of sarcoptic mange in Swedish red foxes (*Vulpes vulpes*). In *Proceedings 4th International Conference Wildlife Disease Association,* Sydney, Australia, pp. 124–130.

————. 1992. Sarcoptic mange in Swedish wildlife. *Revue Scientifique et Technique Office International des Epizooties* 11:1115–1121.

Mörner, T., and D. Christensson. 1984. Experimental infection of red foxes (*Vulpes vulpes*) with *Sarcoptes scabiei* var. *vulpes*. *Veterinary Parasitology* 15:159–164.

Mörner, T., S. Bornstein, and G. Eriksson. 1988. Successful treatment of wild Arctic Foxes (*Alopex lagopus*) infested with *Sarcoptes scabiei* var. *vulpes*. Abstract, 37th WDA Annual Conference, Athens, GA.

Muller, G.H., R.W. Kirk and D.W. Scott. 1989. *Small animal dermatology,* 4th ed. Philadelphia, PA: W.B. Saunders Co.

Mwanzia, J.M., R. Kock, J.M. Wambua, N.D. Kock, and O. Jarret. 1995. An outbreak of sarcoptic mange in the free living cheetah (*Acinonyx jubatus*) in the Mara region of Kenya. In *Proceedings Joint Conference American Association of Zoo Veterinarians, Wildlife Disease Association and American Association of Wildlife Veterinarians,* East Lansing, MI, pp. 105–112.

Nayel, N.M., and Abu-Samra, M.T. 1986. Experimental infection of the one-humped camel (Camelus dromedarius) with *Sarcoptes scabiei* var. *camelii* and *S. scabiei* var. *ovis. Annals of Tropical Medicine and Parasitology* 80:553–561.

Okaeme, A.N., and M.E. Osakawe. 1985. Ectoparasites of the African hedgehog (*Atelerix albiventris,* Wagner) in the Kainji Lake area of Nigeria. *African Journal of Ecology* 23:167–169.

Okoh, A.E.J., and J.N. Gadzama. 1982. Sarcoptic mange of sheep in the Plateau State, Nigeria. *Bulletin of Animal Health and Production in Africa* 30:61–63.

O'Meara, D.C., D.D. Payne, and J.F. Witter. 1960. *Sarcoptes* infestation of a fisher. *The Journal of Wildlife Management* 24:339.

Onderscheka, K., E. Kutzer, and H.E. Richter. 1968. Die Räude der Gemse und ihre Bekämpfung. *Zeitschrift für Jagdwissenschaft* 14:12–27.

Orkin, M., and H.I. Maibach. 1991. Ectoparasitic diseases. In *Dermatology,* vol. 3. Ed. M. Orkin, H. Maibach, and M. V. Dahl Norwalk, VA: Appleton and Lange, pp. 205–214.

Palomares, F., and I. Ruíz-Martínez. 1993. Status und Aussichten für den Schutz der Population des Spanischen Steinbocks (*Capra pyrenaica* Schinz, 1938) im Sierra Mágina Naturpark in Spanien. *Zeitschrift für Jagdwissenschaft* 38:87–94.

Payne, D.D., and D.C. O'Meara. 1958. *Sarcoptes scabiei* infestation of a porcupine. *The Journal of Wildlife Management* 22:321–322.

Pence, D.B., and J.W. Custer. 1981. Host-parasite relationships in the wild Canidae of North America. II. Pathology of infectious diseases in the genus *Canis.* In *World-wide Furbearer Conference Proceedings,* 3–11 August 1980, Frostburg, MD. Ed. J.A. Chapman and D. Pursley. Pp. 760–845.

Pence, D.B., and L.A. Windberg. 1994. Impact of a sarcoptic mange epizootic on a coyote population. *The Journal of Wildlife Management* 58:624–63.

Pence, D.B., S.D. Casto, and W.M. Samuel. 1975. Variation in the chaetotaxy and denticulation of *Sarcoptes scabiei* (Acarina: Sarcoptidae) from wild canids. *Acarologia* 17:160–165.

Pence, D.B., J.W. Custer, and C.J. Carley. 1981. Ectoparasites of wild canids from the Gulf Coastal Prairies of Texas and Louisiana. *Journal of Medical Entomology* 18:409–412.

Pence, D.B., L.A. Windberg, B.C. Pence, and R. Sprowls. 1983. The epizootiology and pathology of sarcoptic mange in coyotes, *Canis latrans,* from South Texas. *The Journal of Parasitology* 69:1100–1115.

Peters, J.C., and P. Zwart. 1973. Sarcoptesräude bei Schneeleoparden. *Erkrankungen der Zootiere* 15:333–334.

Pirilää, V., P. Nourteva, and K. Kallela. 1967. The aetiologic agent of Norwegian scabies. *Transactions St. Johns Hospital Dermatological Society* 53:80–81.

Restani, R., M.P. Tampieri, C.G. Prati, and G. Vecchi. 1985. Sarcoptic mange in a hare [In Italian]. *Obietti e Documenti Veterinari* 6:53–57.

Rossi, L., P.G. Meneguz, P. de Martin, and M. Rodolfi. 1995. The epizootiology of sarcoptic mange in chamois, *Rupicapra rupicapra,* from the Italian Eastern Alps. *Parassitologia (Roma)* 37:233–240.

Ryland, L.M., and J.R. Gorham. 1978. The ferret and its diseases. *Journal of the American Veterinary Medical Association* 173:1154–1158.

Sachs, R., and C. Sachs. 1968. A survey of parasitic infestation of wild herbivores in the Serengeti region in northern Tanzania and the Lake Rukwa region in southern Tanzania. *Bulletin of Epizootic Diseases of Africa* 16:455–472.

Samuel, W.M. 1981. Attempted experimental transfer of sarcoptic mange (*Sarcoptes scabiei,* Acarina: Sarcoptidae) among red fox, coyote, wolf and dog. *Journal of Wildlife Diseases* 17:343–347.

Saupe, E. 1988. Die Parasitosen des Igels und ihre Behandlung [In German]. *Der Praktische Tierarzt* 69:49–54.

Schmitt, S.M., T.M. Cooley, P.D. Friedrich, and T.W.S. Van Veen. 1987. Clinical mange of the Black Bear (*Ursus americanus*) caused by *Sarcoptes scabiei. Journal of Wildlife Diseases* 23:162–165.

Sheehan, B.J. 1975. Pathology of *Sarcoptes scabiei* infection in pigs. *Veterinary Record* 94:202–209.

Skerratt, L.F., R.W. Martin, and K.A. Handasyde. 1998. Sarcoptic mange in wombats. *Australian Veterinary Journal* 76:408–410.

Smith, H.M., W.R. Davidson, V.F. Nettles, and R.R. Gerrish. 1982. Parasitisms among wild swine in southeastern United States. *Journal of the American Medical Veterinary Association* 181:1281–1284.

Stemmer, B.L., L.G. Arlian, M.S. Morgan, C.M. Rapp, and P.F. Moore. 1996. Characterization of antigen presenting cells and T-cells in progressing scabietic skin lesions. *Veterinary Parasitology* 67:247–258.

Stone, W.M., E. Parks, B.L. Weber, and F.J. Parks. 1972. Experimental transfer of sarcoptic mange from red foxes and wild canids to captive wildlife and domestic animals. *New York Fish and Game Journal* 19:1–11.

Stone, W.M., I.F. Salkin, and A. Martel. 1982. Sarcoptic mange in a gray fox. *New York Fish and Game Journal* 29:102–103.

Stringer, R.P., R. Harkema, and G.C. Miller. 1969. Parasites of rabbits in North Carolina. *The Journal of Parasitology* 55:328.

Svensson, T. 1983. Sarcoptic mange in red fox and dogs [In Swedish]. *Jagt och Jägare* 2:9–10.

Sweatman, G.K. 1971. Mites and pentastomes. In *Parasitic diseases of wild mammals.* Ed. J.W. Davis and R.C. Anderson. Ames: Iowa State University Press, pp. 3–64.

Thomsett, L.R. 1968. Mite infestation of man contracted from dogs and cats. *British Medical Journal* 3:93–95.

Todd, A.W., J.R. Gunson, and W.M. Samuel. 1981. Sarcoptic mange: An important disease of coyotes and wolves of Alberta, Canada. In *Worldwide Furbearer Conference Proceedings,* 3–11 August 1980, Frostburg, MD. Ed. J.A. Chapman D. and Pursley. Pp. 706–729.

Trainer D.O., and J.B. Hale. 1969. Sarcoptic mange in red foxes and coyotes in Wisconsin. *Bulletin of Wildlife Disease Association* 5:387–391.

Ullrich, H. 1938. Über einige neue Schmarotzermilben bei Elch, Biber und Schneehase. *Zeitschrift für Parasitenkunde* 10:553–558.

Van Neste, D.J. 1986. Immunology of scabies. *Parasitology Today* 2:194–196.

———. 1988. Human scabies in perspective. *International Journal of Dermatology* 27:10–15.

Vyrypaev, V.A. 1985. The influence of epizootics of *Sarcoptes* infection on the population of central asiatic mountain ibex in Tien-Shan. *Parazytologiya* 19:190–194.

Walton, S.F., A. Vale, J. McBroom, D. Taplin, L. Arlian, J.D. Mathews, B. Currie, and D.J. Kemp. 1998. Sympatric populations of dog-derived and human-derived *Sarcoptes scabiei* are genetically distinct in scabies-endemic communities in northern Australia. *Australian Society for Parasitology, Melbourne,* p. 48.

Wells, R.T. 1971. Maintenance of the hairy-nosed wombat (*Lasiorhinus latifrons*) in captivity. *International Zoo Yearbook* 11:30–31.

Wetzel, H. 1984. Vergleichende Untersuchungen an *Sarcoptes*-Milben von Wildtieren. *Zeitschrift für angewandte Zoologie* 71:233–243.

Wetzel, R., and W. Rieck. 1962. *Krankheiten des Wildes.* Hamburg: Verlag Paul Parey, 223 pp.

Yeruham, I., S. Rosen, A. Hadani, and A. Nyska. 1996. Sarcoptic mange in wild ruminants in zoological gardens in Israel. *Journal of Wildlife Diseases* 32:57–61

Young, E. 1975. Some important parasitic and other diseases of lion, *Panthera leo,* in the Kruger National Park. *Journal of the South African Veterinary Association* 46:181–183.

Zahler, M., A. Essig, R. Gothe, and H. Rinder. 1999. Molecular analyses suggests monospecificity of the genus *Sarcoptes* (Acari: Sarcoptidae). *International Journal of Parasitology* 29:759–766.

Zeh, J.B. 1974. Infestation of sarcoptic mange on red fox in New York. *New York Fish and Game Journal* 21:182–183.

Zumpt, F., and J.A. Ledger. 1973. Present epidemiological problems of sarcoptic mange in wild and domestic animals. *Journal of the Southern African Wildlife Management Association* 3:119–120.

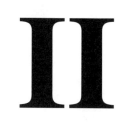

PART II

ENDOPARASITES

6

LIVER FLUKES

MARGO J. PYBUS

INTRODUCTION. Trematodes, along with Eucestodes, Monogeneans, and other minor groups, belong to the phylum Platyhelminthes, more commonly known as flatworms. All trematodes are parasitic and are classified in the subclass Digenea (species undergo multiplication within intermediate hosts and occur as endoparasites of many vertebrates and invertebrates) or the subclass Aspidobothrea (no multiplication in intermediates, primarily endoparasites of fish, reptiles, and molluscs) (Brooks 1989a,b; Rhode 1990). Trematodes are characterized by a one-way gut, external cuticle, protonephridia, and one or more external holdfast organs. Most are monoecious, and complete male and female reproductive systems occur in each individual. The life cycle of many trematodes is heteroxenous and may include one or more intermediate hosts (usually an invertebrate) and a final host (usually a vertebrate).

A wide range of digenetic trematodes (= flukes) occur in wild mammals. However, the majority of these species are not associated with significant disease conditions. This chapter focuses on a few species that have potential to be detrimental to the host and thus are of some concern to wildlife managers. Although adult digeneans can occur in numerous locations within the final host, this chapter is limited to those that occur within the liver as an example of the information, issues, and concerns associated with significant disease-causing trematodes in wild mammals.

FASCIOLOIDES MAGNA (BASSI, 1875) WARD, 1917.

Synonyms: (As in Swales 1935.) *Distomum magnum* Bassi, 1875; *Distomum hepaticum* Curtice, 1882; *Fasciola hepatica* Dinwiddie, 1889 (nec. Linnaeus, 1758); *Fasciola carnosa* Hassall, 1891; *Fasciola americana* Hassall, 1891; *Distomum texanicum* Francis, 1891; *Cladocoelium giganteum* Stossich, 1892; *Fasciola magna* (Bassi, 1875) Stiles, 1894

Common Names: giant liver fluke, large American liver fluke, deer fluke.

Life History. Adult *Fascioloides magna* occur in pairs or groups within fibrous capsules in the liver of infected ruminants. Mature flukes (up to 8 cm long) may release up to 4000 thick-walled operculate eggs per day (Swales 1935). Eggs are swept into the bile collecting system, enter the small intestine, and leave the host along with the feces (Fig. 6.1). Although embryonation can occur in moist feces (Swales 1935), eggs

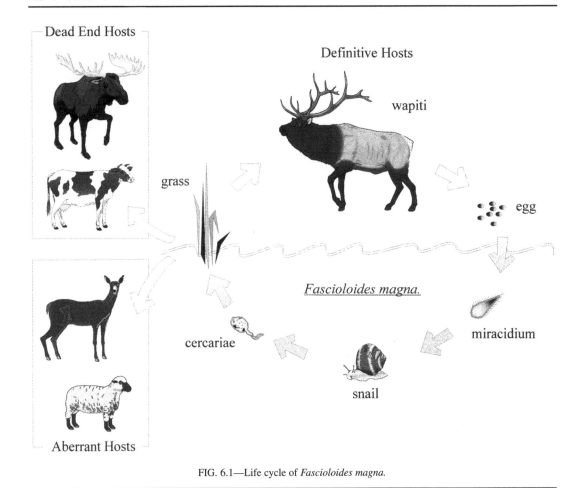

Dead End Hosts

Definitive Hosts

wapiti

grass

egg

Fascioloides magna.

miracidium

cercariae

snail

Aberrant Hosts

FIG. 6.1—Life cycle of *Fascioloides magna.*

hatch only in aerated water (Swales 1935; Campbell 1961). Fully developed miracidia produce proteolytic enzymes that release the operculum and allow hatching to occur. Low ambient temperature (< 20° C) retards development, and high temperature (34°C) results in abnormal embryonation and inability to hatch (Campbell 1961). Under summer field conditions, complete embryonation takes approximately 35 days (Swales 1935), but varies considerably with changes in temperature and moisture.

Free-swimming miracidia are very active but soon expend their energy and die if they do not find a suitable intermediate host in 1–2 days. They display positive phototaxis and strong chemotaxis for mucous produced by suitable intermediate hosts (Campbell 1961; Erhardová-Kotrlá 1971). Miracidia penetrate the tissues of suitable snail species, where they begin the multiplication phase of the cycle. Swales (1935) and Erhardová-Kotrlá (1971) provide detailed accounts of development within the snail. Each successful miracidium in the pulmonary sac of the snail develops into a sporocyst, which subsequently gives rise to up to 14 rediae. The rediae migrate to the snail's liver, and each gives rise to up to 9 daughter rediae. In turn, each daughter redia may produce 9 or 10 cercariae. Thus one miracidium may result in over 1000 free-swimming forms that emerge from the snail (usually at night) and encyst as metacercariae on aquatic vegetation. The inherent increase in numbers may compensate for a short life span and the inability of many miracidia to locate a suitable snail host. Time to complete development within the snail is 40–58 days (Swales 1935; Erhardová 1961) and is dependent on temperature and species of snail. In addition, development can be delayed, and *F. magna* may overwinter in various stages within infected snails (Erhardová-Kotrlá 1971).

Metacercariae remain viable on submerged or emergent vegetation for prolonged periods, particularly in cold water (Záhoř et al. 1966; Griffiths and Christensen 1972, 1974). There appear to be two primary periods of transmission to a final host. In the late summer and fall, large numbers of recently encysted metacercariae are available for ingestion by grazing herbivores, particularly young of the year. In the spring, cervids seek fresh green vegetation associated with wetlands at a time when a high proportion of encysted metacercariae are capable of invading host tissue (Erhardová-Kotrlá 1971).

Metacercariae are activated within the gut of a suitable ruminant. Activated larvae penetrate the intestinal wall, migrate along the ventral aspect of the peritoneal cavity, and then penetrate the liver, where they slowly grow and develop into adults. Rarely or in aberrant hosts, flukes may wander within the abdominal or thoracic cavities and penetrate other tissues within the final host, most often the lungs. However, such flukes generally do not survive or mature and thus do not contribute further to the parasite population.

Young flukes migrate within the liver tissue, apparently in search of another fluke (Foreyt and Todd 1976a; Foreyt et al. 1977), before becoming encapsulated in the hepatic parenchyma. Maturation and subsequent egg-laying occurs within the capsules. Thus, full-sized, gravid adults are found most often in groups of two or more individuals. Young flukes may remain immature for prolonged periods, perhaps years, if another fluke is not found. Adult flukes also have prolonged longevity and may live at least 5 years (Erhardová-Kotrlá 1971). Prepatent period in ruminant hosts can be as short as 3 months (Erhardova-Kotrla 1971) or as long as 7 months (Foreyt and Todd 1976a). Vitality or age of metacercariae may affect rate of establishment within the final host (Foreyt 1992).

Epizootiology

DISTRIBUTION. Giant liver fluke occurs in the liver of a variety of wild and domestic ruminants, primarily in North America (Table 6.1). Currently, *F. magna* is enzootic in five major areas: (1) the Great Lakes region; (2) the Gulf coast, lower Mississippi, and southern Atlantic seaboard; (3) northern Pacific coast; (4) the Rocky Mountain trench; and (5) northern Quebec and Labrador (Fig. 6.2). However, within these broad ranges, actual presence of giant liver flukes varies from locally abundant to locally absent. In addition, outlier populations exist as a result of translocation. Some early records of *Fasciola hepatica* may be misidentification of *F. magna* (e.g., Butler 1932).

Giant liver fluke was introduced into Italy in 1865 (Bassi 1875). Until recently, subsequent reports in Europe were sporadic and disjunct, with giant liver fluke reported in Germany (Salomon 1932), Poland (Slusarski 1955, 1956), the former Czechoslovakia (southern Bohemia) (Erhardová-Kotrlá 1971; Bojovic and Halls 1984), Austria (Pfeiffer 1983), Slovakia (Rajský et al. 1994), and Hungary (Majoros and Sztojkov 1994; Sztojkov et al. 1995). The apparently limited distribution of *F. magna* in Europe (Fig. 6.3) may be a result of translocation of infected wapiti (*Cervus elaphus nelsoni*) and white-tailed deer (*Odocoileus virginianus*) either directly from North America in the late nineteenth century or secondarily from enzootic areas

established in European game parks and reserves (Slusarski 1955; Erhardová-Kotrlá 1971). The parasite was slow to expand its range in Europe, perhaps due to the necessity of adapting to new molluscan and cervid hosts as well as to the differences in climate and vegetation in Europe (Kotrly and Kotrlá 1980). Recent reports suggest that *F. magna* may have become well established in red deer (*Cervus elaphus elaphus*) populations, and natural dispersal may be occurring within the upper Danube watershed.

Boomker and Dale-Kuys (1977) found giant liver fluke in the liver of a Brahman heifer in South Africa. The heifer had been imported recently from the United States. Similarly, Arundel and Hamir (1982) reported probable infection of *F. magna* (based on pathognomic hepatic lesions and the presence of eggs in hepatic parenchyma) in an imported ox in Australia. Although fluke eggs were found within the tissues of each animal, it is unlikely that giant liver flukes would establish a population in these instances. Recently, mature *F. magna* were found in a wapiti translocated from Canada to Cuba (Lorenzo et al. 1989). Suitable intermediate hosts appear to occur in the vicinity, but it is unknown if the fluke established a population.

HOST RANGE. Natural infections of *F. magna* occur primarily in cervids and bovids (Table 6.1). Experimental infections have been described in mule deer (*Odocoileus hemionus hemionus*) (Foreyt 1992, 1996a), bighorn sheep (*Ovis canadensis*) (Foreyt 1996b), wapiti (Foreyt 1996a), domestic sheep (Swales 1935; Foreyt 1989), domestic goats (Foreyt and Leathers 1980), chamois (*Rupicapra rupicapra*) and fallow deer (*Dama dama*) (Erhardová-Kotrlá and Blažek 1970), cattle (Swales 1936; Erhardová-Kotrlá and Blažek 1970), llama (Foreyt and Parish 1990), rabbits (Swales 1935; Griffiths 1962), and guinea pigs (Swales 1935; Griffiths 1962). Although many species are susceptible to infection, only a few cervids [wapiti, white-tailed deer, and caribou (*Rangifer tarandus*)] in North America and red deer/wapiti, white-tailed deer, and fallow deer in Europe, contribute significantly to maintaining populations of the fluke (see Pathology, this chapter). *Fascioloides magna* was first described from the liver of a wapiti stag (Bassi 1875). The earliest North American record involves flukes in a "deer" liver collected in ~1875 (Stewart 1882, as noted in Hall 1912). Early North American literature documents infections of *F. magna* in domestic species, primarily in states along the Gulf Coast (Francis 1891; Stiles and Hassall 1894; Hall 1912). However, since *F. magna* rarely matures in domestic species, these data probably reflect spillover of flukes from infected wild cervids.

All cervids and bovids do not contribute equally to the propagation of giant liver fluke. Following the suggestions of Swales (1935) and Foreyt (1996b), three primary types of final hosts occur (Table 6.2). *Definitive hosts* are those in which *F. magna* mature in thin-walled fibrous capsules within the liver, eggs are voided into the small intestine via the bile system, and

TABLE 6.1—Natural definitive hosts for *F. magna* (limited to early or first time reports)

Country	Host	Scientific Name	Locality	References
NORTH AMERICA				
Canada	Black-tailed deer	*Odocoileus h. columbianus*	British Columbia	Hadwen 1916
	Cattle	*Bos taurus*	British Columbia	Bruce 1930, Hilton 1930
	Wapiti	*Cervus elaphus*	Alberta	Swales 1935
	White-tailed deer	*O. virginianus*	Alberta	Swales 1935
	Mule deer	*O. h. hemionus*	Alberta	Swales 1935
	Yak	*B. grunniens*	Alberta	Swales 1935
	Cattalo	*B. taurus* χ *Bison bison*	Alberta	Swales 1935
	Cattle	*B. taurus*	Alberta	Swales 1935
	Caribou	*Rangifer tarandus*	Quebec	Choquette et al. 1971
	Moose	*Alces alces*	Ontario	Kingscote 1950
			British Columbia	Hilton 1930, Cowan 1951
	Bison	*Bison bison*	Alberta	Cameron 1923
United States	Wapiti	*C. elaphus*	Montana	Butler 1932, 1938
			Washington	Schwartz and Mitchell 1945
			Oregon	Dutson et al. 1967
	White-tailed deer	*O. virginianus*	New York	Stiles and Hassall 1894
			Florida, S. Carolina	Dinaburg 1939
			Montana	Aiton 1938
			Minnesota	Fenstermacher et al. 1943
			Texas	Olsen 1949
	Mule deer	*O. h. hemionus*	Montana	Senger 1963
	Black-tailed deer	*O. h. columbianus*	Washington	Schwartz and Mitchell 1945
	Moose	*A. alces*	Minnesota	Fenstermacher 1934
	Cattle	*B. taurus*	Texas	Francis 1891
	Sheep	*Ovis aries*	Michigan[a]	1906 - as reported in Hall 1912
			Montana	Hall 1914
			Texas	Olsen 1949
	Goat	*Capra hircus*	Texas	Olsen 1949
	Horse	*Equus caballus*	na[b]	listed in Swales 1935
	Pig	*Sus scrofa* f. dom.	na	Migaki et al. 1971
			Texas	Foreyt and Todd 1972
	Collared peccary	*Dicotyles tajacu*	Texas	Samuel and Low 1970
	Llama	*Lama glama*	Minnesota	Conboy et al. 1988
Cuba	Wapiti	*Cervus elaphus*		Lorenzo et al. 1989
EUROPE				
Austria	Fallow deer	*Dama dama*	Lower Austria	Pfeiffer 1983
Czech Republic	Red deer	*C. elaphus*	Southern Bohemia	Erhardova-Kotrla and Kotrly 1968
	Fallow deer	*D. dama*	Southern Bohemia	Ullrich 1930
	Roe deer	*Capreolus capreolus*	Southern Bohemia	Záhoř 1965
	White-tailed deer	*O. virginianus*	Southern Bohemia	Erhardová-Kotrlá 1971
	Sika deer	*Sika nippon*	Southern Bohemia	Erhardová-Kotrlá 1971
	Cattle	*B. taurus*	Southern Bohemia	Záhoř et al. 1966
Slovak Republic	Red deer	*Cervus e. elaphus*	Dunajska Streda	Rajský et al. 1994
Italy	Wapiti	*C. e. nelsoni*	Turin	Bassi 1875
	Fallow deer	*D. dama*	Turin	Bassi 1875
	Sambar	*Cervus unicolor*	Turin	Bassi 1875
	Blue bull	*Bosephalus tragocamelus*	Turin	Bassi 1875
	Goat	*Capra hircus*	Turin	Bassi 1875
	Sheep	*Ovis aries*	Turin	Bassi 1875
	Red deer	*C. e. elaphus*	Turin	Bassi 1875, Balbo et al. 1987
	Cattle	*B. taurus*	Turin	Balbo et al. 1987
	Horse	*E. callabus*	Turin	Balbo et al. 1987
	Wild boar	*Sus scrofa*	Turin	Balbo et al. 1987
Germany	Red deer	*C. e. elaphus*	Silesia	Salomon 1932
Hungary	Red deer	*C. e. elaphus*	Szigetkoz	Majoros and Sztojkov 1994
Poland	Red deer	*C. e. elaphus*	Silesia	Slusarski 1955, 1956

[a]Sheep came from the state of Washington.
[b]Not available.

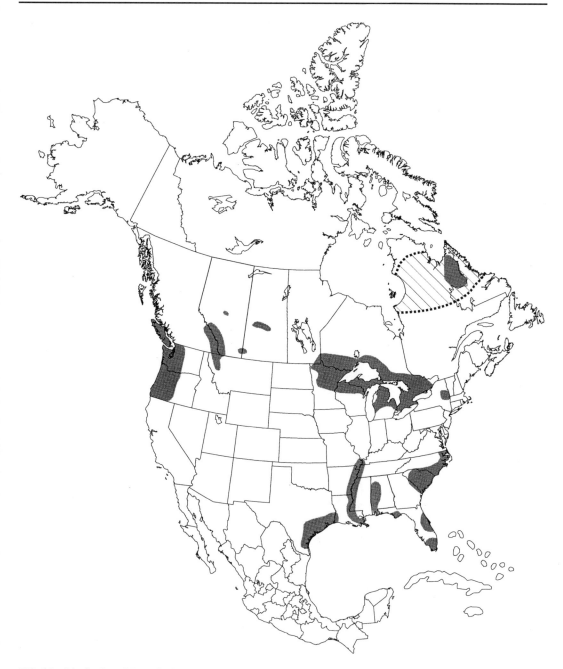

FIG. 6.2—Distribution of *Fascioloides magna* in North America. Region in northeastern Canada within dotted line indicates estimated distribution.

patent infections are established. Definitive hosts are primarily New World cervids. *Aberrant hosts* are those in which the parasite cannot successfully complete migration within the host. Such hosts often die acutely due to tissue damage associated with migrating immature flukes. Ovine species are the predominant hosts in this category. *Dead-end hosts* are those in which the flukes successfully reach the liver but rarely mature, and the few eggs produced usually do not reach the small intestine. Bovids, suids, llamas, and some Old World cervids generally are dead-end hosts for *F. magna*. Infections in humans have not been reported.

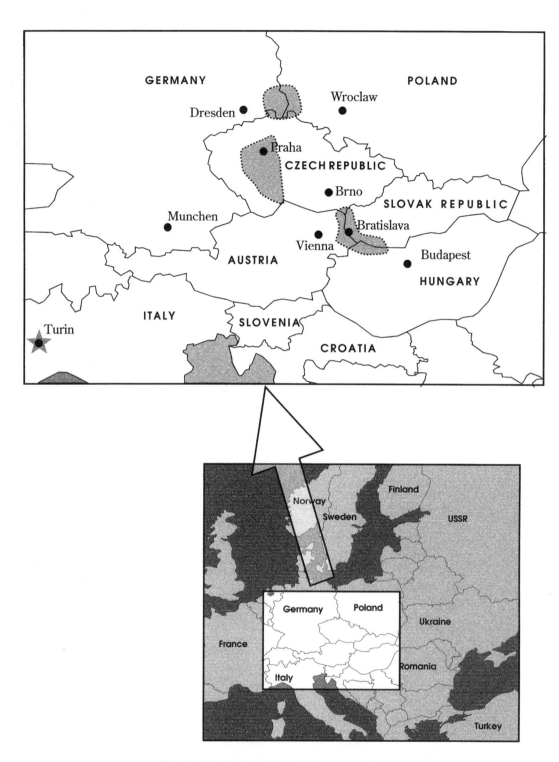

FIG. 6.3—Distribution of *Fascioloides magna* in Europe.

TABLE 6.2—Potential for final hosts to contribute to *F. magna* population[a]

Definitive Hosts	Dead-End Hosts	Aberrant Hosts
White-tailed deer	Moose	Domestic sheep
Wapiti	Sika deer	Domestic goat
Caribou	Sambar[b]	Chamois
Black-tailed deer		Bighorn sheep
Mule deer	Cattle	Mouflon
Red deer	Bison	
Fallow deer	Yak	Roe deer
	Horse	
	Domestic pig	
	Feral hog	
	Peccary	
	Llama	

[a]Assumes natural exposure occurs.
[b]Limited information; only one infected animal reported.

Only definitive hosts provide suitable conditions for maintaining a population of flukes in enzootic areas. Although some species (e.g., mule deer, bighorn sheep, horses) are susceptible to infection, inherent ecological barriers may preclude natural infection.

A variety of aquatic snails, generally *Lymnaea* spp., are reported as suitable intermediate hosts for *F. magna* in North America (reviewed in Foreyt 1981). Erhardová-Kotrlá (1971) exposed various snails collected in Czechoslovakia to giant liver flukes and documented a range of patterns in response. Miracidia did not penetrate into *Succinea oblonga, S. putris, Physa acuta,* or *L. palustris*. Only 2 of 507 *L. stagnalis* became infected, but both snails died before cercariae were present. Development of *F. magna* was arrested in *Radix peregra* subspp. prior to development of cercariae. Larval development was completed only in *L. truncatula*. The latter species was the only naturally infected intermediate host found in the study areas. Chroustová (1979) was able to infect and recover viable cercariae from *L. palustris* and suggested this species should be considered a potential intermediate host for *F. magna* in Czechoslovakia. Although the cumulative list of potential intermediate hosts is quite long, transmission on a local scale often involves only one or two species.

PREVALENCE AND INTENSITY. Prevalence in both intermediate and final hosts differs widely and reflects local conditions of wetland habitats, ungulate use and movements, and seasonal variations in moisture and temperature. Prevalence increases in areas where infected cervids congregate or spend prolonged periods. For example, prevalence of larval stages as high as 80% was recorded in snails in Czechoslovakia in an area used as a supplemental feeding ground for red deer (Erhardová-Kotrlá 1971). Similarly, prevalence of adult flukes as high as 86% was recorded in wapiti in the lower Bow valley in Alberta where wapiti occur year-round (Pybus 1990). Balbo et al. (1987) reported flukes in 100% of the red deer kept within a walled game park in Italy.

Shallow (1–35 cm depth), slightly alkaline (pH 7.9–8.2), warm water lowland areas with minimal canopy cover tend to have a higher abundance of suitable snails. Such areas also are attractive to various cervid species. Prevalence of *F. magna* in free-ranging hosts tends to be higher in river/swamp habitats than in dry uplands (Trainer 1969; Mulvey et al. 1991).

Prevalence of *F. magna* in definitive hosts increases with age; young of the year rarely are infected, and prevalence tends to increase among young age classes, then stabilize in older age classes (Flook and Stenton 1969; Foreyt et al. 1977; Addison et al. 1988; Lankester and Luttich 1988; Mulvey and Aho 1993; Pybus and Butterworth, forthcoming.). Prevalence of adult flukes is similar in male and female white-tailed deer (Behrend et al. 1973; Foreyt et al. 1977; Addison et al. 1988), caribou (Lankester and Luttich 1988), and wapiti (M.J. Pybus, unpublished). However, mean intensity generally is similar within infected age classes and both sexes. These data may indicate immunologic resistance in definitive hosts; however, this has not been investigated. Alternatively, the data may reflect differences in individual behavior that result in a proportion of the population that does not use emergent vegetation as a significant portion of the diet. Increased prevalence and intensity in high density situations may argue in favor of the opportunity for transmission as a primary factor in determining the dynamics of *F. magna* within the final host population. Superinfections can occur in both intermediate and final hosts. Over 600 cercariae may occur in a single *L. parva* (Swales 1935), and wapiti with 500–650 adult flukes have been observed (M.J. Pybus, unpublished). However, stunted growth, castration, and mortality can occur in snails heavily infected with developing *F. magna* (Erhardová-Kotrlá 1971), and excessive numbers of flukes may lead to mortality even in definitive hosts.

It is not clear whether final hosts continue to add to established infections (Addison et al. 1988; Mulvey et al. 1991) or not (Foreyt et al. 1977; Lankester and Luttich 1988; Majoros and Sztojkov 1994). Regardless, *F. magna* has an aggregated distribution in definitive host populations (Addison et al. 1988; Mulvey and Aho 1993). Most hosts have a few flukes, while the majority of the fluke population is carried in a few heavily infected individuals. For example, mean intensity in naturally infected white-tailed deer usually is less than 10 flukes (Olsen 1949; Foreyt et al. 1977; Addison et al. 1988; Forrester 1992); however, infections of 20–125 flukes are recorded (Olsen 1949; Pursglove et al. 1977; Forrester 1992; Mulvey and Aho 1993). A similar situation occurs in wapiti (Pybus and Butterworth, forthcoming), caribou (Huot and Beaulieu 1985; Lankester and Luttich 1988), and red deer (Balbo et al. 1987).

Although overall intensity was similar, white-tailed deer in Ontario had a higher proportion of capsules containing three or more flukes (30%) (Addison et al. 1988) than did more southern populations of white-tailed deer (15%) (Foreyt et al. 1977). The former authors suggest that the limited transmission period in northern climes may result in more synchronous invasion of the liver and a greater potential for flukes to be encapsulated in groups. They also suggest that the increasing proportion of capsules with three or more flukes in older deer may indicate that immature flukes can invade existing capsules. These interesting aspects of the epizootiology of *F. magna* warrant further study.

Prevalence and intensity in aberrant and dead-end hosts often reflect infections in sympatric definitive host populations, although the actual values generally are lower.

ENVIRONMENTAL LIMITATIONS. Seasonal conditions of moisture and temperature affect abundance and activity of the intermediate hosts as well as embryonation and subsequent development of the parasite. For example, prolonged snowcover in spring may delay emergence of snails from overwintering sites as well as extend the development time of miracidia within eggs. Seasonal drawdown or drought also limits the availability of intermediate hosts. Freezing temperatures kill eggs that are in advanced stages of development (Swales 1935); however, losses may be somewhat mitigated by protective snowcover (Erhardová-Kotrlá 1971). Regardless, overwintered eggs develop more slowly than those deposited in spring and summer (Erhardová-Kotrlá 1971). There must also be overlap of suitable intermediate and definitive hosts. Land use patterns that improve habitats for snails (e.g., dam-building, creation of ponds) or ungulates (e.g., prescribed burning, selective timber harvest, or agricultural land clearing: Yoakum et al. 1980) may increase the opportunities to establish populations of *F. magna*. Thus the complexity of the life cycle and the finite requirements of various developmental stages contribute to the limited populations of *F. magna*.

Additional limitations act at the interface between larval stages and the snail intermediate hosts. Snails in shallow warm water are more easily invaded by miracidia than those in cold-water streams (Erhardová-Kotrlá 1971). This may relate to the level of activity of the snail and the abundance or activation of chemical cues that facilitate targeting and penetration by the miracidia. This may also account for the lack of infection in snails from high-altitude mountains (850–1050 m) despite the presence of suitable intermediate and definitive hosts (Erhardová-Kotrlá 1971). Further limitations apparently relate to nutrition of the snails. Well-fed snails contain more mature rediae and cercariae than stunted snails (Kendall 1949). North American snails appear to withstand a greater intensity of infection than those in Europe; this ability may reflect the longer period of coadaptation within suitable intermediate hosts in North America (Erhardová-Kotrlá 1971).

Behavioral patterns of the final hosts may preclude infection in some species or individuals. For example, the lower Bow Valley in Banff National Park (Alberta) is heavily contaminated with *F. magna*. Most wapiti ≤ 2 years old are infected, yet mule deer and bighorn

sheep using the same general habitats are not infected (Butterworth and Pybus 1993). It is assumed that the latter two species minimize the amount of emergent vegetation consumed. Similarly, prevalence in white-tailed deer populations appears to be limited and rarely exceeds 65%–70%. Foreyt (1981) suggests that a proportion of white-tailed deer populations may not be susceptible to infection. The lack of infection could relate to immunologic protection or ecologic separation from infective metacercariae.

Old World cervids may provide suboptimal conditions for growth of the adult flukes. Morphology and morphometrics of adult giant liver flukes found in Europe differ slightly from those found in North America (Kotrlá and Kotrly 1980; Majoros and Sztojkov 1994).

Clinical Signs. Most infections of *F. magna* are subclinical. Occasionally lethargy, anorexia, depression, and weight loss occur shortly before death in aberrant hosts (Fenstermacher and Olsen 1942; Foreyt and Hunter 1980; Foreyt and Leathers 1980; Foreyt 1992; Foreyt 1996b). Dropsy (distended abdomen) was associated with liver fluke infection in wapiti (Hadwen 1939). Loss of condition has not been detected in definitive hosts (Flook and Stenton 1969; Huot and Beaulieu 1985; Addison et al. 1988).

Pathology and Pathogenesis. Pathologic changes within the final host differ among definitive, dead-end, and aberrant hosts. However, the primary lesions usually occur in the liver and are associated with mechanical damage due to migrating immature flukes or fibrous encapsulation of sedentary adult flukes. Infected livers often are enlarged, with rounded margins and fibrinous tags on the serosa. In some cases the fibrin tags extend as fibrous adhesions to the overlying diaphragm and adjacent peritoneum. Streaks of black pigment, pathognomic for *F. magna* infection, may be visible on the serosal surface or throughout the hepatic parenchyma. The hematin pigment is produced in the intestine of immature and adult flukes and consists of iron porphyrin (Campbell 1960; Blažek and Gilka 1970), a byproduct of feeding on blood. Pigment within tissues is a result of migration of immature flukes or filtration of hematin within the lymphatic system (Campbell 1960). It accumulates within hepatic cells and cannot be scraped away or separated from the tissue. Thin black fluid may leak from cut surfaces of infected livers. Pigmentation may occur in other tissues, including hepatic lymph nodes, omentum, mesenteries, lungs, and pulmonary lymph nodes, particularly in dead-end hosts or in severe infections.

On palpation, the texture of the liver may include soft flaccid areas (usually capsules containing adult flukes) or distended firm areas (usually thick-walled resolving capsules containing dead adults or masses of retained eggs). Tracks of tissue damage and hemorrhage may occur throughout the liver, wherever immature flukes have recently migrated. White fibrous cap-

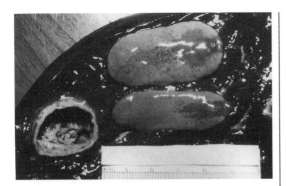

FIG. 6.4—*Fascioloides magna* in the liver of a naturally infected wapiti.

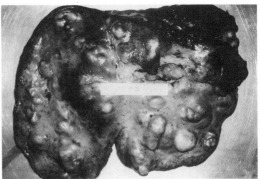

FIG. 6.5—Extensive liver damage associated with severe infection of *Fascioloides magna* in a wapiti.

sules distinctly demarcated from the adjacent hepatic parenchyma usually occur where adult flukes are found together. Histologically, changes progress from mechanical trauma to necrosis and chronic granulation tissue in infected livers.

DEFINITIVE HOSTS. Infections in definitive hosts are characterized by limited migration of immature flukes and by thin-walled fibrous capsules containing two or more adult flukes (Swales 1935; Foreyt et al. 1977; Addison et al. 1988) (Fig. 6.4). The initial migration pathways of immature flukes are replaced by fibrous tracks with no apparent relation to the architectural structure of the liver (Swales 1935). Capsules are of host origin and are an apparent attempt to prevent further migration of flukes within hepatic parenchyma. Swales (1935, 1936) provides a detailed description of the capsules. They consist of loose layers of vascularized collagen with patent afferent and efferent bile ducts. Older, denser tissue occurs on the periphery of the capsule, with the inner lining consisting of fine collagen fibrils and fibroblasts. Over time, efferent ducts may become blocked with fibrous tissue or eggs and detritus. This results in accumulation of pigmented fluids and fluke eggs within the capsule. As the capsule develops around the flukes, adjacent hepatic parenchyma is destroyed by pressure atrophy. The size of the capsule depends on the size and number of flukes enclosed as well as the amount of accumulated fluid and detritus.

More extensive changes are associated with increasing intensity of flukes and age of infection (Fig. 6.5). Emaciation and severe hepatic destruction were associated with 125 *F. magna* collected from a white-tailed deer in South Carolina (Pursglove et al. 1977). Acute peritonitis and exsanguination associated with rupture of the hepatic capsule and hepatic portal vein, respectively, were seen in wapiti naturally infected with extremely high numbers of flukes (> 500 flukes) in Alberta (Butterworth and Pybus 1993). Similarly, a wapiti calf given 2000 metacercariae died of acute fibrinous peritonitis

following rupture of the jejunum (Foreyt 1996a). Indeed, the original description of *F. magna* was a result of investigating mortality associated with severe infections in red deer and wapiti (Bassi 1875).

Chronic infections are associated with increased fibrosis throughout affected livers. This is particularly seen in wapiti, red deer, fallow deer, and caribou. Occlusion of bile ducts disrupts the patterned architecture of the liver and interferes with the flow of bile and blood. This may lead to further damage, including infarction, atrophy, and necrosis. Subsequent generation of functional liver tissue may result in extensive hypertrophy of the liver up to four or five times normal size (M.J. Pybus, unpublished). Despite the extensive changes in the liver, such individuals exhibit few, if any, clinical signs and do not have apparent loss of body condition as measured using fat depots. However, significant loss of body protein in cervids may occur without changes in fat indices (Reimers et al. 1982; Torbit et al. 1985; Huot 1989).

Fatal infections can occur in definitive hosts with severe infections. Mortality of naturally infected white-tailed deer (Pursglove et al. 1977), black-tailed deer (*Odocoileus hemionus columbianus*) (Cowan 1946), wapiti (Bassi 1875; M.J. Pybus, unpublished), and red deer (Balbo et al. 1987) as well as experimentally infected fallow deer (Erhardová-Kotrlá and Blažek 1970), wapiti (Foreyt 1996a), and mule deer (Foreyt 1992) has been reported.

Study of serologic changes in *F. magna* infections is limited. A decline in serum hemoglobin and packed-cell volume and an increase in serum gamma-globulin occurred in experimentally infected white-tailed deer fawns given 50 or 500 metacercariae (Foreyt and Todd 1979). Mild transitory anemia was noted early in infection (Foreyt and Todd 1979; Presidente et al. 1980); however, this did not result in clinical disease. No difference in serum chemistry values (calcium, magnesium, phosphorus) or weight gain of infected and uninfected fawns was detected. Serologic changes in naturally infected hosts have not been investigated.

ABERRANT HOSTS. Infections in aberrant hosts are characterized by excessive wandering of immature flukes, a lack of encapsulation, and death of the host. Damage is focused in the liver, although perforation of the hepatic capsule and penetration into various abdominal and pleural organs also may occur (Swales 1935; Foreyt and Todd 1976a; Foreyt and Leathers 1980; Stromberg et al. 1985). Acute hemorrhagic tracks and associated trauma and necrosis occur throughout the liver. Lesions are associated with acute and chronic inflammatory response involving plasma cells, eosinophils, and pigment-laden macrophages. Thickened vascular walls and thrombophlebitis often occur in hepatic veins. Diffuse fibrosis throughout the liver occurred in experimentally infected domestic goats (Foreyt and Leathers 1980). In cases of pulmonary involvement, hemorrhagic cavitations and generalized alveolar and interlobular edema may lead to atelectasis and fibrotic septae (Stromberg et al. 1985). Mortality usually occurs within 4–6 months (Swales 1935; Erhardová-Kotrlá and Blažek 1970; Erhardová-Kotrlá 1971; Foreyt and Todd 1976a; Foreyt and Leathers 1980) and may be associated with acute peritonitis before or after migrating larvae reach the liver. Rarely, mature flukes may occur, but few eggs are released prior to death of the host (Swales 1935; Campbell and Todd 1954; Erhardová-Kotrlá 1971).

Persistent eosinophilia in infected sheep was the only documented change from normal hematology and blood chemistry (Stromberg et al. 1985), although this aspect of infections has not been studied extensively. Prominent germinal centers in hepatic lymph nodes may indicate an active humoral immune response in infected domestic sheep (Stromberg et al. 1985).

Bighorn sheep appear particularly susceptible to fatal infection with *F. magna*. Foreyt (1996b) reported multifocal pyogranulomatous hepatitis, necrotizing hemorrhagic pneumonia, and hematin pigmentation in various organs of experimentally infected bighorn sheep. The liver was swollen to twice normal size, with coagulative hepatic necrosis and extensive migration pathways within the parenchyma. Up to 50%–75% of the liver was infiltrated with organizing fibroblasts and collagen deposition. Serosal surfaces of most abdominal organs and tissues were coated with a thick layer of fibrin and inflammatory cells. Extensive pulmonary involvement included serosanguinous fluid in the pleural cavity, fibrin tags over much of the pulmonary serosa, and occasional fluke migration tracks in the lung parenchyma. One bighorn sheep died with only a single immature *F. magna* recovered. However, there are no documented cases of natural infection in bighorn sheep despite their occurrence within highly contaminated environments (Butterworth and Pybus 1993).

DEAD-END HOSTS. Infections in dead-end hosts are characterized by excessive fibrosis, thick-walled encapsulation of flukes within hepatic parenchyma, and black pigmentation of various tissues. This is particularly evident in infections in cattle (Swales 1935;

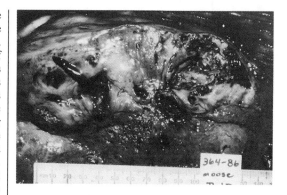

FIG. 6.6—*Fascioloides magna* in the liver of a naturally infected moose.

Záhoř et al. 1966; Erhardová-Kotrlá and Blažek 1970; Foreyt and Todd 1976a), although it also occurs in moose (*Alces alces*) (Lankester 1974), bison (*Bison bison*), yak, and bison χ cattle hybrids (Swales 1936). Migrating larvae successfully reach the liver but are then surrounded by dense fibrous tissue that may occlude the bile collection system and prevent eggs from escaping into the intestine. Foreyt and Todd (1974) suggest eggs may be found only in the feces of cattle with severe infections. In some cases, chronic calcification of capsules in the liver may occur.

Infections in moose tend to show increased fibrosis throughout the liver; however, flukes seldom are paired and remain as migrating immatures for extended periods (M.J. Pybus, unpublished). This results in extensive trauma and acute inflammation associated with hemorrhagic tracks through the hepatic parenchyma (Fig. 6.6). In chronic infections, large capsules (up to 10 cm in diameter) filled with material of variable consistency and color are common (Fenstermacher and Olsen 1942; Lankester 1974; M.J. Pybus, unpublished). Capsule walls 1–10 mm thick occur, although the margins often are indistinct and extend into adjacent tissue (Lankester 1974). In some cases, capsules are incomplete and do not surround migrating flukes. Damage to 50%–90% of the liver is not uncommon (Karns 1972; Lankester 1974; M.J. Pybus, unpublished). Severe damage, including significant hepatic hypertrophy, abdominal adhesions, and pulmonary involvement, often occurs even in light infections (< 20 flukes) (Butterworth and Pybus 1993). Loss of condition and mortality of infected individual moose have been reported (Fenstermacher and Olsen 1942; Karns 1972; Lankester 1974; Aho and Hendricks 1989).

Increased eosinophilia was documented in an experimentally infected domestic calf (Swales 1936), and low blood urea nitrogen and serum albumin/globulin ratio were detected in naturally infected moose (Karns 1973). Infections in swine are associated with extensive fibrosis of interlobular hepatic septae and black pigmentation in the abdominal cavity (Migaki et al.

1971; Foreyt et al. 1975). The interlobular septae in porcine liver may physically disrupt the migration of immature flukes. Occasionally *F. magna* matures in swine but eggs seldom occur in feces (Migaki et al. 1971; Foreyt et al. 1975). A similar situation may occur in collared peccary (*Dicotyles tajacu*) that occur in enzootic areas (Samuel and Low 1970).

Diagnosis. There are very few trematodes that occur within the liver of wild ruminants. Fully mature *F. magna* (up to 8 cm long by 3 cm wide) is by far the most conspicuous and is the only fluke that occurs within the hepatic parenchyma. *Fasciola hepatica, Fasciola gigantica,* and *Dicrocoelium dendriticum,* occasionally found in wild cervids and bovids that are sympatric with infected domestic species, occur in the bile ducts of the liver. In addition, *F. magna* can be distinguished by its rounded anterior and, unlike *F. hepatica* and *F. gigantica,* the oral and ventral suckers do not occur on an anterior cone. In *F. magna* the vitellaria occur only on the ventral side of the intestinal ceca. The robust *F. magna* is easily differentiated from *D. dendriticum,* a tiny (1–2 mm), slender fluke sharply tapered at each end and shaped like a lancet.

Infections in intermediate hosts generally are detected by identification of gymnocephalous cercariae released from captive snails or in crushed snails. A recent study using reverse transcriptase-polymerase chain reaction techniques could not differentiate snails infected with *F. hepatica* from those with *F. magna* infections (Rognlie et al. 1994). However, the test was considered specific to within the Fasciolidae.

Infections in the final host usually are detected at postmortem. Infections in live definitive hosts may be detected by searching for eggs in feces. Eggs of *F. magna* generally are larger (~160 x 96 µm; range 114–168 µm long x 94–96 µm wide) than those of *F. hepatica* (~135 x 75 µm; range 128–142 µm x 68–82 µm) but smaller than eggs of *F. gigantica* (156–197 µm x 90–104 µm). Fasciolid eggs have a high specific gravity, and Wobeser et al. (1985) recommend a 2 M Sheather's sugar solution as most suitable for floating eggs of *F. magna.* Foreyt (1981, 1992) recommends use of a modified sedimentation technique. Reliable diagnosis of infections in aberrant and dead-end hosts requires postmortem examination.

Serum enzymes (e.g., glutamate dehydrogenase and gamma-glutamyl transferase) are effective indicators of acute liver cell damage and chronic hepatofibrosis, respectively. These enzymes have been used to diagnose *F. hepatica* infections in cattle and sheep (Boray 1982). Similar studies of *F. magna* in wild and domestic species have not been conducted. However, given the type of liver damage, particularly in domestic species, these enzymes may be useful in diagnosing giant liver fluke infections. Extrapolating from other host-parasite relationships, serologic tests used to diagnose infections in domestic species should be thoroughly validated before they are used to assess infections in wildlife species (Gardner et al. 1996).

Antigens associated with the tegument (Trudgett et al. 1988) or from metabolic products (Sinclair and Wassall 1988) of *F. hepatica* can be used successfully to detect infections in domestic species. Antigenic differences between *F. magna* and *F. hepatica* have been described (Qureshi et al. 1995).

Immunity. There is little evidence to suggest an effective immune response to infection with *F. magna* in most hosts. Although the cellular reaction differs among hosts, it reflects a general response to the type and extent of tissue damage rather than a direct response to the parasites. Occasionally, dead flukes are found within capsules in chronic infections; however, it is not known whether the flukes were killed by a host response or "died of natural causes."

Control and Treatment. An interesting, if not unique, approach to control of liver flukes is presented by Hall (1934). The author provides the outline of a military campaign against *F. hepatica* (the "deadliest of the enemy forces in the army of parasites of sheep, also an enemy of cattle") and its allies ("certain snails [used] as lines of communication from invaded definitive host areas to uninvaded areas"). The campaign is built on a rigorous review of the parasite life cycle and where it is most vulnerable, the same basic approach used in more modern (and less military) times. Many aspects of the campaign are applicable to controlling *F. magna.*

Early control recommendations focused on separation of livestock and cervids, removal of cervid definitive hosts, or fencing of livestock away from natural wetlands in enzootic areas. In addition, a variety of physical (i.e., drainage) or chemical (copper sulphate) treatments of wetlands were encouraged in order to limit or eliminate snail populations. The combined effects of removal of cervids, removal of snails, and burning of emergent vegetation successfully eradicated *F. magna* from a park in Alberta (Swales 1935; Pybus 1990). However, most of the wetland treatments are associated with significant environmental impacts to other species, including fish. In addition, some herbicides may decrease embryonation time in snails and result in increased numbers available to act as intermediate hosts (Christian and Thompson 1990).

More recent investigations of treatment and control focus on prophylactic treatment of infected hosts (Table 6.3). Infections are difficult to treat because the flukes are not directly within the bile ducts, and sufficient amounts of chemical cannot get into the capsules in the liver. As a result, most anthelminthics effective against *F. hepatica* do not work well against *F. magna* (Foreyt and Todd 1976b). Similarly, some treatments are most successful against immature flukes (e.g., rafoxanide), while others are more effective against adult flukes (e.g., oxyclozanide). This diminishes the efficacy of their control. Triclabendazole appears to have broad-spectrum efficacy against adult and immature *F. magna* in a variety of hosts.

TABLE 6.3—Treatment and control of *F. magna* in natural (N) or experimental (E) infections in various hosts

Host		Agent	Dose (mg/kg)	Efficacy (%)	Effective Against	Reference
Wild						
White-tailed deer	N	Oxyclozanide	13–29	100	Adults	Foreyt and Todd 1973
	N	Albendazole	11–54	38	Adults and immatures	Foreyt and Drawe 1978
	N	Albendazole	5–17	82–84	Adults	Qureshi et al. 1990
	N	Clorsulon	12–30	80	Immatures	Foreyt and Drawe 1985
				92	Adults	
	N	Albendazole	17–46	67	Immatures	Foreyt and Drawe 1985
				89	Adults	
	N	Triclabendazole	10	100	Adults and immatures	Qureshi et al. 1989
	N	Triclabendazole	11	63[a]	Adults and immatures	Qureshi et al. 1994
	N	Hexachlorophene	12–26	0	Immatures	Foreyt and Todd 1976b
				50	Adults	
	N	Nitroxynil	11–24	50	Immatures	Foreyt and Todd 1976b
				0	Adults	
	N	Rafoxanide	12–25	75	Immatures	Foreyt and Todd 1976b
				0	Adults	
	N	Clioxanide	16–38	0	Adults and immatures	Foreyt and Todd 1976b
	N	Diamphenethide	255–280	0	Adults and immatures	Foreyt and Todd 1976b
	N	Hexachloroethane	463–629	0	Adults and immatures	Foreyt and Todd 1976b
Wapiti	N	Triclabendazole	50–60	90	Immatures	Pybus et al. 1991
				98	Adults	
Red deer	N	Diamphenethide	140	'high'	Adults and immatures	Balbo et al. 1987
Domestic						
Cattle	N	Albendazole	15–45	94–99	na[b]	Ronald et al. 1979
	E	Clorsulon	21	75–100	Immatures	Foreyt 1988
	N	Rafoxanide	10–15	100	Adults and immatures	Foreyt and Todd 1974
	N	Oxyclozanide	7–15	27	Live adults and immature flukes remained	Foreyt and Todd 1974
	N	Triclabendazole	6–12	77–88	Study incomplete	Craig and Huey 1984
Sheep	N	Albendazole	7.5		Approved by USDA	Stromberg et al. 1983
	E	Clorsulon	21	92	Immatures	Foreyt 1988
Goats	E	Albendazole	15	99	Prevented fatal infection	Foreyt and Foreyt 1980
	E	Triclabendazole	20	99	Immatures	Foreyt 1989

[a]Reduction in herd prevalence following access to treated bait.
[b]Not available.

Direct treatment of infected hosts is applicable only in situations of translocation of wild cervids from enzootic areas or husbandry of captive and farmed cervids. In addition, treatment of domestic species is feasible as part of on-going individual herd health management programs. Currently, treatment of natural populations of cervids is largely unfeasible. However, feed (Qureshi et al. 1990) and bait (Qureshi et al. 1994) treated with triclabendazole was effective against *F. magna* in naturally infected captive and free-ranging white-tailed deer, respectively. Similarly, diamphenathide (but not rafoxanide) fed in medicated pellets effectively controlled giant liver fluke infections in captive red deer (Balbo et al. 1987). In the latter situation, successful treatment was associated with improved body condition and calving rate. This approach may be useful where wild deer or wapiti occur in captive situations or in high density on limited range. In addition, the efficacy of burning emergent vegetation as a means of limiting transmission to domestic and wild species in enzootic areas by reducing the number of metacercariae seems worthy of study.

Domestic Animal Health Concerns. Natural infections of *F. magna* occur in a variety of domestic livestock in North America and Europe. Infections in aberrant hosts are of primary concern. In enzootic areas, wild definitive hosts act as reservoirs of infection for domestic species. High prevalence in wild species may preclude husbandry of domestic sheep (Stromberg et al. 1983) or goats (Foreyt and Leathers 1980) in some areas of the United States. Although mortality of naturally infected bovine calves has been reported (Stromberg et al. 1983), impacts on dead-end hosts generally are not so direct. Most infections are subclinical and go untreated or undetected until postmortem in a slaughterhouse. Condemnation of livers, loss of weight, loss of milk production, and unthrifty offspring have been associated with infections of *F. magna* in cattle (Foreyt and Todd 1976c; Schillhorn van Veen 1987). Undoubtedly millions of dollars in revenues to cattle producers are lost in enzootic areas throughout North America. Similar concerns have been expressed in Europe (Balbo et al. 1987), but the magnitude of impact is not so great due to the restricted distribution and abundance of the fluke.

Most infections in domestic species occur as individuals graze in contaminated wetlands. However, ingestion of viable metacercariae on dry grass and hay also can establish infections (Záhoř et al. 1966). Erhardová-Kotrlá (1971) recommended leaving wetland hay at least 3 months before feeding it to cattle, although viable metacercariae of *F. hepatica* were found on stored hay after 8 (Marek 1927) and 17 months (Rajcevic 1929). Infective stages of *F. hepatica* and *F. gigantica* can be killed in silage (Alicata 1938; Wikerhauser and Brglez 1961). A similar situation may occur with *F. magna.*

There is minimal concern associated with giant liver fluke infections in domestic pigs or feral swine. However, these species may increase snail abundance by creating wallows that collect water and in which suitable snail intermediate hosts can be found (Foreyt et al. 1975). In enzootic areas, this could increase the risk of infection in other domestic or in wild species. The few reports of infection in horses (Swales 1935; Balbo et al. 1987) and llama (Conboy et al. 1988) suggest that *F. magna* is not a significant risk for these species even in enzootic areas. There are no recent reports of *F. magna* in wild bison herds; however, infections occur in some captive herds (M.J. Pybus, unpublished).

Origin of *Fascioloides magna.* The current disjunct populations in North America imply that giant liver fluke was not widely distributed in early white-tailed deer populations (the only indigenous primary definitive host in North America) or that the flukes disappeared over much of their former range in eastern North America. Similarly, European colonization of North America occurred from east to west, yet all early records of *F. magna* occur in the west (mainly as spillover into cattle). During the period of commercial hunting and overexploitation of wild game in the late 1800s, there were no records or concerns expressed about fluke infections in white-tailed deer in eastern North America.

It is generally accepted that *F. magna* is of North American origin (Bassi 1875). The fluke may have evolved with ancestral *Odocoileus* spp., as evidenced by the apparent coadaptation and relatively benign infections in white-tailed deer and black-tailed deer. Mule deer, a more recent form of the genus, are not so well adapted and have an increased potential for tissue damage and fatal infections. As a contemporary of ancestral *Odocoileus* spp., giant liver fluke may have been widespread in ancient *Odocoileus* spp. in major wetland habitats throughout North America. However, white-tailed deer populations are considered to have declined steadily since 1500 (Fig.6.7) and were extirpated from large portions of their former range, particularly in eastern portions of the continent by 1900 (McCabe and McCabe 1984). A widespread translocation program was used to restore deer populations throughout their former range (McCabe and McCabe 1984).

Cervus elaphus is of Eurasian origin and entered North America during the Pleistocene epoch ~11,000–

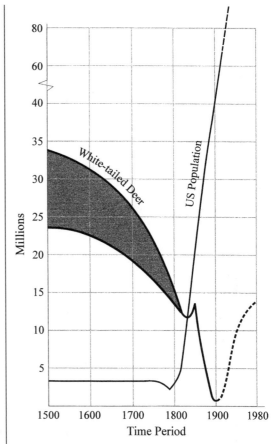

FIG. 6.7—Estimated white-tailed deer populations in North America relative to human populations in the United States [After McCabe and McCabe (1984); used with the permission of the Wildlife Management Institute.].

70,000 years ago (Bryant and Maser 1982). The species dispersed south and east across the continent, giving rise to eastern and western forms of wapiti. These forms overlapped with white-tailed deer throughout the cordilleran and mixed hardwood biomes, where they could have encountered *F. magna* in contaminated wetlands. Eastern populations of caribou, *Rangifer tarandus,* ranged as far south as Alabama in eastern North America (Churcher et al. 1989) and would have overlapped with white-tailed deer as well as the now extinct eastern wapiti (*C. elaphus canadensis*) in the Great Lakes and eastern boreal areas (Banfield 1974; Bryant and Maser 1982).

How does this relate to the current populations of *F. magna*, which are disjunct and isolated into relatively small pockets across North America? It is suggested that the widespread steady decline of white-tailed deer since the sixteenth century, followed by extirpation of big game across much of North America, resulted in the disappearance of giant liver fluke over much of its former range. However, populations may have remained in three primary refuge areas: (1) where wapiti persisted in the western slopes of the Rocky Mountains in British Columbia and Montana, as well as in the coastal islands and remote areas of British Columbia and Washington; (2) where white-tailed deer persisted in the inaccessible swamps of the Mississippi and Gulf coast; and (3) where caribou remained unavailable for harvest in the boreal forests of northern Quebec and Labrador. This suggestion is based on early written records of giant liver fluke in "deer" and wapiti in the west and along the Gulf Coast (Stiles and Hassall 1894; Hall 1912; Hadwen 1916; Swales 1933), and current foci of apparently natural populations of flukes.

Natural dispersal from these isolated remnants has been limited. White-tailed deer do not appear to spread *F. magna* despite availability of appropriate intermediate and definitive host populations (e.g., Florida, Alberta). The relationship between giant liver fluke and white-tailed deer appears to be finely tuned to allow the parasite to maintain populations but not to overwhelm the host. Prevalence in local populations of white-tailed deer rarely exceeds 60%–70%, and mean intensity is 5–10 flukes per infected deer. The flukes occur in thin-walled capsules that allow unhindered release of eggs; however, the egg output is moderated by the reduced number of mature flukes. This situation appears to maintain the fluke in core areas of its distribution but does not allow for dispersal beyond those foci. The critical limiting factors in the life cycle of *F. magna* may be the limited longevity of miracidia in the environment and the limited rate of establishment of metacercariae in the final host. Thus, infected deer moving away from enzootic foci may not carry enough mature flukes to ensure sufficient eggs and miracidia for the fluke to establish a new population.

Although one or two dispersing white-tailed deer cannot provide the threshold of parasite productivity needed to establish new populations, this threshold can be attained when deer are translocated as a group or kept in confined areas (e.g., Dobris forest enclosure in the former Czechoslovakia). Upon release, translocated animals often stay within a relatively small range, increasing the probability that the threshold for maintaining *F. magna* will be established in new wetland areas.

In contrast, the relationship between *F. magna* and wapiti/red deer is not so finely tuned. Prevalence and intensity are considerably higher than in white-tailed deer and so is the potential for damage to the liver. Although there have been no studies of egg output from infected wapiti, there appears to be an increased potential for egg production and subsequent release into the environment. This potential may increase the success of translocating liver flukes in infected wapiti or red deer and provide the basis for the current distribution of *F. magna* in much of western North America and Europe.

As in white-tailed deer, natural dispersal among wapiti populations appears to be slow. The current distribution in North America is largely restricted to Roosevelt wapiti in western Oregon, Washington, and British Columbia (Vancouver Island) and Rocky Mountain wapiti on the west slopes of the Rockies from the headwaters of the Columbia River in southeastern British Columbia to the Flathead area of western Montana. It is documented on the eastern slopes of the Rockies only in the vicinity of Waterton National Park, Alberta (Flook and Stenton 1969; Kingscote et al. 1987), and Banff National Park, Alberta (Flook and Stenton 1969; Pybus 1990), where it appears to have spilled over through mountain passes from enzootic areas in Montana and British Columbia, respectively. Movement into the Banff area probably occurred as recently as the early 1960s (Flook and Stenton 1969), but *F. magna* is now well established in the vicinity of Banff townsite (Butterworth and Pybus 1993). Similarly, natural dispersal of giant liver fluke in red deer in Europe has only recently occurred (Majoros and Sztojkov 1994; Spakulová et al. 1997).

Management Implications. Infections of *F. magna* have management implications in three broad areas: translocation in wild cervids, population impacts within free-ranging and farmed cervids, and reservoir hosts for spillover into domestic species.

TRANSLOCATION. It is well established that *F. magna* may be translocated along with infected cervids, primarily wapiti. The original description of *F. magna* followed its translocation in infected wapiti from North America to a game park near Turin, Italy (Bassi 1875). Introductions of *F. magna* into the former Czechoslovakia may have occurred in infected white-tailed deer (Kotrlá and Kotrly 1977; Bojovic and Halls 1984) and wapiti/red deer (Erhardová-Kotrlá and Kotrly 1968). The fluke established populations and remains a serious management concern in these areas (Bojovic and Halls 1984; Balbo et al. 1987; P. Lanfranchi, personal communication). Occurrence of *F. magna* in Austria was related to translocation of infected fallow deer (Pfeiffer 1983). The most recent range extension of giant liver fluke may have involved movement of infected red deer across the Danube River along the Hungary/Slovak border (Majoros and Sztojkov 1994). Indeed, the entire present-day distribution of *F. magna* throughout Europe reflects the purposeful movement of undetected infections in definitive hosts and the subsequent management in small, often fenced, reserves or game parks.

Translocations also have occurred within North America. Although there were early recommendations against translocation of infected white-tailed deer from enzootic areas to non-enzootic areas (Olsen 1949), the disjunct distribution of *F. magna* in white-tailed deer in the southeastern United States probably resulted from previous translocations of infected deer (Holland 1959; Pursglove et al. 1977; Christian et al. 1984). In Canada, liver flukes were translocated in infected wapiti from Wainwright, Alberta, to Burwash, Ontario (Kingscote

1950). However, widespread foci of liver flukes in white-tailed deer throughout southern Ontario (Kingscote 1950) and some Great Lakes states (Fenstermacher et al. 1943; Cheatum 1951) suggest *F. magna* was already present in the region. Its presence in Ontario was largely unnoticed until fatal infections in cattle and sheep adjacent to the introduced wapiti were detected (Kingscote 1950).

Wainwright, Alberta, is a particularly interesting example of translocation and localized distribution of giant liver fluke. Buffalo National Park was established at Wainwright, Alberta in 1909 to receive 661 plains bison transferred from Montana (Lothian 1981). In addition, six wapiti translocated from Banff National Park in 1910 (where giant liver flukes were not known to occur) and seven from the Flathead River region (Pablo herd) of Montana in 1911 (Lloyd 1927) became the foundation of a herd of wapiti within the park at Wainwright. *Fascioloides magna* was first detected in bison in the Wainwright herd in 1923 (Cameron 1923). Liver fluke became well established in the park until it was eradicated in the late 1930s (Swales 1935; Pybus 1990). There is no record of giant liver fluke occurrence outside the park or in eastern or central Alberta during or since that time. How did *F. magna* get to Wainwright? Since patent *F. magna* infections in bison are rare and the fluke apparently did not establish in other locations where bison from Montana were translocated, this appears to be yet another case of translocation of giant liver fluke along with infected wapiti, this time from Montana.

Other pockets of *F. magna* in Western Canada are associated with translocation of infected wapiti. Although there is no direct evidence of introduction of *F. magna* into Elk Island National Park (EINP) in Alberta, its occurrence there and no where else in central Alberta implies that it was introduced at some time. The park is enclosed by an 8-foot (~3-m) game fence, and ungulate densities, primarily wapiti, moose, and bison, are some of the highest on record (Blythe and Hudson 1987). Cowan (1951) provides a "record of occurrence" of *F. magna* in bison from EINP but gives no further details. The fluke was not reported in 500 bison from EINP in 1959-60 (Choquette et al. 1961), nor has it been found in bison since that time (Canadian Parks Service, unpublished data). In 1987 *F. magna* was detected in a moose from EINP (M.J. Pybus, unpublished). Since that time, surveys indicate infection in approximately 80%–90% of the adult wapiti in the northern portion of the park (M.J. Pybus, unpublished). In central Alberta, *F. magna* was translocated with infected wapiti from EINP to a game farm in east central Alberta (Pybus 1990) and probably central Saskatchewan (see Wobeser et al. 1985). White-tailed deer in the vicinity of these foci apparently are not infected (Wobeser et al. 1985; M.J. Pybus, unpublished). Thus, local populations of *F. magna* persist as isolated foci despite the presence of white-tailed deer and wetland habitats in adjacent areas.

Translocation of giant liver fluke in captive cervids is of increasing concern. The report of mature *F. magna* in an imported wapiti in Cuba (Lorenzo et al. 1989), despite pre-import diagnostic evaluation, is an example of the risk to non-enzootic areas. In particular, the extensive commercial movement of wapiti in North America increases the risk to domestic and wild hosts, and has the potential to completely alter the current distribution and range of *F. magna*. Translocation of liver flukes in captive wapiti into eastern Montana (Hood et al. 1997) and its occurrence on game farms in non-enzootic areas of Alberta (M.J. Pybus, unpublished) have already occurred.

POPULATION IMPACTS. The impact of *F. magna* on wild populations is not well documented. Although death of individuals may occur, there is little evidence of population control as a result of infection. Decreased moose calf survival (Karns 1972) and lower blood urea nitrogen and serum albumin/globulin ratio (Karns 1973) were documented in northwest Minnesota where *F. magna* was more prevalent. More commonly, *F. magna* may be a factor predisposing infected moose to increased predation or loss of condition/productivity (Lankester 1974; Berg 1975). Roe deer (*Capreolus capreolus*) appear to be particularly susceptible to infections, and population declines in enzootic areas have been documented (Záhoř 1965; Erhardová-Kotrlá 1971).

Subtle impacts were documented in infected white-tailed deer populations. Mulvey and Aho (1993) reported significantly lower body weights and number of antler points in infected yearling male deer. Similarly, infected males 2.5–3.5 years old lost significantly more weight during the rut than uninfected deer of the same age. In most age classes, male deer with the largest intensities (> 25 flukes) consistently had lower body weights than others in their age class. The differences were not reflected in kidney fat index. The authors suggest there may be a threshold intensity above which detrimental effects are observed. The actual threshold may differ with host age, ecological and physiological conditions, and perhaps host genetic characteristics. Effects were more pronounced in young deer than in old, perhaps relating to damage during the migration of young flukes within the liver. Reduced growth in early years may limit the ability of an individual male deer to attain full growth potential and thus reduces the chance of reproductive success, particularly in northern areas where the effects may be added to stress associated with weather and food limitation (Mulvey and Aho 1993). The potential for decreased trophy value of infected red deer, roe deer, and fallow deer is a management concern in enzootic areas in Europe (Majoros and Sztojkov 1994).

A number of authors suggest that potential adverse effects in definitive hosts are most likely to occur in conjunction with other stressors and should be evaluated when seasonal components of nutrition or reproduction are limiting (e.g., late winter). Increased winter mortality in infected white-tailed deer (Cheatum 1951) and perhaps moose (Fenstermacher and Olsen 1942) has been suggested. Adult males may be at greatest risk, following depletion of energies during the rut and increased energy demands during the winter. These comments also may pertain to other free-ranging definitive hosts (wapiti, caribou, red deer, fallow deer). Liver fluke can have direct impact on populations of aberrant hosts (as discussed earlier).

Numbers and prevalence of infection can build in captive animals in game parks, reserves, or game farms with resulting population impacts. Old World cervids may be at particular risk. Increased density of farmed cervids and repeated use of wetland areas can increase opportunities for transmission of *F. magna*. In addition, irrigation of marginal pastures can increase snail abundance. These features of intensive husbandry increase the potential risks to game farm cervids and to adjacent or sympatric domestic livestock. Use of marginal lands also may increase the potential for dissemination to wild cervids. The concerns are exacerbated by the difficulty in diagnosis of infections in live animals. Often there are no clinical signs and animals remain in good body condition. For example, *F. magna* was an incidental finding in a herd of 344 farmed wapiti slaughtered during a bovine tuberculosis eradication program, yet 80% of the herd was infected (Whiting and Tessaro 1994). Giant liver fluke is an increasing concern for game farm producers and agricultural managers in western North America. Significant mortality also has been documented in Europe in captive wapiti (Bassi 1875), red deer (Balbo et al. 1987), and roe deer (Záhoř 1965). Following anthelmintic treatment, captive red deer showed significantly improved condition and productivity (Balbo et al. 1987).

RESERVOIRS FOR INFECTION OF DOMESTIC SPECIES. As indicated earlier, domestic species cannot maintain populations of giant liver fluke in the absence of infected wild hosts. Given the potential damage to primary livestock species, wildlife managers should be aware of the situation with *F. magna* in local cervid populations and consider the potential impacts associated with increasing or relocating herds of definitive hosts relative to known enzootic areas.

Management Recommendations.
1. Wapiti, red deer, white-tailed deer, and fallow deer should not be translocated from enzootic to non-enzootic areas without appropriate anthelmintic treatment.
2. Husbandry of captive or game farm cervids in enzootic areas and in infected herds should include regular treatment with an effective fascioloidicide.
3. Husbandry of susceptible domestic species in enzootic areas should include pasture management to exclude access by infected definitive hosts, limitation of access to contaminated wetlands, or regular anthelmintic treatment with an effective fascioloidicide.
4. Additional anthelminthics effective against *F. magna* should be investigated in order to avoid resistance to repeated application of the same drug.

FASCIOLA HEPATICA LINNÉ, 1758.
Synonyms: As in (Stiles and Hassall 1894, 1895.)
Planaria latiuscula Goeze, 1782; *Distoma hepaticum* Abildg, 1786; *Fasciola humana* Gmelin, 1789; *F. lanceolata* Rudolphi, 1803; *Distoma hepaticum* Dujardin, 1845; *Distomata hominis* Taylor 1884; *Distomum hepaticum* Leuckart, 1889; *D. cavias* Sons, 1890; *Cladocoelium hepaticum* Stossich, 1892.
Common Names: common liver fluke, sheep liver fluke.

Fasciola hepatica has the potential to infect many domestic species, but is found primarily in domestic sheep, goats, and cattle. It has a cosmopolitan distribution, and occasionally infections in wild ungulates are reported. There is no evidence that wild species can maintain populations of common liver fluke in the absence of suitable domestic hosts. Fascioliasis is an important disease of domestic ruminants in all countries where suitable conditions for successful intermediate hosts occur (Radostits et al. 1994). However, it will receive minimal discussion in this chapter, as it is not of significant concern as a disease in wild mammals. For more information, the reader should consult the extensive literature regarding this species in domestic hosts.

Fasciola hepatica is a trematode of the family Fasciolidae in the subclass Digenea. Adult flukes are up to 30 mm long, dorsoventrally flattened, with an oral and ventral sucker. The oral sucker occurs on an anterior cone [although this may be difficult to ascertain in some individuals (Slusarski 1955)].

Life History. The life history of *F. hepatica* is essentially the same as that of *F. magna*. Eggs hatch in aerated water, and the free-swimming miracidium seeks a lymnaeid snail intermediate host. Some snail species can be suitable intermediate hosts for both *F. hepatica* and *F. magna* (Dunkel et al. 1996), and the distributions of the two species overlap in local areas in Europe (Erhardová-Kotrlá 1971) and North America (Francis 1891; Foreyt and Todd 1972; Knapp et al. 1992). There is polyembryony within the snails, and eventually numerous cercariae are released into the water. The cercariae encyst on aquatic vegetation, where they can withstand a wide range of environmental conditions prior to being ingested by a suitable final host.

In the final host, adult *F. hepatica* occur in the bile ducts of the liver, where they are associated with enlargement and calcification of the ducts. As with *F. magna,* there can be an extended length of time as immature flukes in the liver. Operculate eggs released from mature flukes directly enter the bile collecting system and then the small intestine. Mean egg size is 135 μm ± 7 μm × 75 μm ± 7 μm (Kendall and Parfitt 1959). Patent infections generally occur 8–10 weeks after infection.

Epizootiology. Wild hosts naturally infected with *F. hepatica* include black-tailed deer (Kermode 1916, questioned in Cowan 1946; Longhurst and Douglas 1953; Browning and Lauppe 1964), "deer" (Herman 1945; confirmed by Olsen 1949), white-tailed deer (Lang 1977), moose (Wetzel and Enigh 1936; Nilsson 1971), mule deer (Lang 1977), sika deer (Drózdz 1963), fallow deer, red deer, roe deer (Nilsson 1971; Barth and Schaich 1973), bison (Locker 1953; Bergstrom 1967), and beaver (*Castor canadensis*) (Lang 1977). In addition, there is a long history of common liver fluke infections in various lagomorph species, including jack rabbits (*Lepus californicus*), cottontail rabbits (*Sylvilagus* sp.), European hare (*Lepus europaeus*), and mountain hare (*Lepus timidus*) as reviewed in Olsen (1948). Lang (1977) reported infection in snowshoe hare (*Lepus americanus*). In general, infected hares and rabbits are common in enzootic areas and may contribute to maintaining or spreading the fluke population.

Common liver fluke often is absent in cervids despite infection in domestic species and despite *F. magna* infections in cervids (Price 1953; Foreyt and Todd 1972; Prestwood et al. 1975). Infections in cervids generally are incidental cases in a few individuals, although prevalence and intensity appear higher in Europe than in North America. Experimental infection of black-tailed deer (Kistner and Koller 1975), white-tailed deer (Presidente et al. 1974, 1975; Foreyt and Todd 1976d), roe deer, and red deer (Barth and Schaich 1973) are reported. Field and experimental studies indicate that wild cervids are not significant reservoirs of *F. hepatica*. The limited infections may be mediated by ecological barriers that limit exposure and/or inherent resistance to infection.

Pathology. Natural infections in cervids generally are not associated with clinical signs or significant pathology (Price 1953; Lang 1977). However, there is an indication of increased mortality in infected roe deer in the Netherlands (Jansen 1965), and experimental infection indicated *F. hepatica* is more pathogenic in roe deer than in red deer (Barth and Schaich 1973). Similarly, black-tailed deer are readily infected with *F. hepatica*, while white-tailed deer are relatively resistant (Presidente et al. 1974; Kistner and Koller 1975). Acute fascioliasis associated with migrating immature flukes occurs in black-tailed deer (Kistner and Koller 1975). In white-tailed deer, migrating larvae are destroyed prior to causing extensive damage (Presidente et al. 1974, 1975).

Infections in hares and rabbits are associated with limited enlargement and fibrosis of bile duct walls and distortion of the general hepatic surface (Olsen 1948).

Control and Treatment. There is extensive literature regarding the control and treatment of *F. hepatica* in domestic species (Boray 1982; Shah et al. 1984; Roberts and Suhardono 1996). In wild species, rafoxanide was effective in removing *F. hepatica* from captive and free-ranging roe and red deer (Barth and Schaich 1973). Efficacy was 92%–99% against adult

flukes and 66% against immature flukes. In addition, egg output of *F. hepatica* was reduced significantly following treatment with rafoxanide at 5–15 mg/kg (Barth and Schaich 1973). These authors also noted a safety range up to 45 mg/kg in roe deer and 75 mg/kg in red deer and no tissue residues after 14 days in treated red deer. However, in most cases treatment of free-ranging cervids is not feasible and, generally, not warranted. Treatment may be appropriate for captive cervids held in close proximity to or sympatric with infected sheep and cattle in enzootic areas. Efficacy of treatment in domestic species may be reduced in areas where infected lagomorphs occur (Olsen 1948).

Public Health Concerns. Hepatic fascioliasis in humans is occasionally documented in enzootic areas. The following information is taken from a review by Facey and Marsden (1960). Most cases are individual and are detected at autopsy or during surgery. However, local outbreaks of acute clinical disease have been reported in Argentina, Britain, Cuba, France, Germany, and Uruguay. In some cases, infection with one or two flukes may result in severe reactions and may be difficult to treat. Clinical signs can occur during the acute phase while larvae are migrating to and within the liver. They include recurrent bouts of epigastric pain, prolonged fever, enlarged liver, pyrexia, and weight loss. Infections may become patent in approximately 4 months, at which time diagnosis can be confirmed by finding eggs in feces. Treatment with chloroquine sulphate was successful in relieving clinical signs; however, unwanted side effects occurred and viable eggs remained in the feces. Emetine hydrochloride is more successful at removing flukes. Infection may occur when people consume emergent vegetation, often species of watercress that are contaminated with viable metacercariae.

Domestic Health Concerns. There are considerable health and management concerns regarding *F. hepatica* infections in domestic species (Wilson et al. 1982; Roberts and Suhardono 1996). Infections generally are subclinical; however, acute mortality and chronic production losses may occur in domestic species, particularly sheep and cattle (Sinclair 1967). Bovine and ovine livers containing liver flukes are condemned. Fatal infections occur most often in young sheep during their first summer (Wilson et al. 1982). Cattle are more resistant to infection than sheep. Concentration of livestock in riparian habitats, irrigation of pastures, and repeated use of contaminated wetlands increase the risks to a variety of domestic species. Infections in wild cervids are unlikely to contribute to the risks to livestock; however, infections in lagomorphs may be a reservoir for supplementing infections in domestic species.

Management Implications. In North America, there are no management concerns associated with *F. hepatica* infections in wild cervids. However, in Europe infections may be associated with reduced productivity in captive and semicaptive cervids. Similarly, liver flukes are not known to impact lagomorph populations but may have management implications for sympatric domestic species.

FASCIOLA GIGANTICA COBBOLD, 1855.

Synonoms: *Fasciola gigantea* Cobbold, 1856; *Distomum giganteum* Diesing, 1958; *Distomua hepaticum* ex. p. Gervais and van Beneden, 1858; *Fasciola gigantea* Cobbold, 1859; *Cladocoelium giganteum* ex. p. Stossich, 1892; *Fasciola hepatica angusta* Railliet, 1895; *Distomum hepaticum aegyptica* Looss, 1896.
Common name: liver fluke.

Fasciola gigantica was found originally in a captive Nubian giraffe (*Giraffa camelopardalis*) in a travelling menagerie in Britain (Cobbold 1855). However, it is primarily a parasite of domestic species in Africa, Asia, and India. Similar to *F. hepatica,* this fluke is reported infrequently in wild mammals. Infections in wild species occur most often where the fluke is enzootic in domestic species (Bindernagel 1972); however, in some cases, wild hosts may maintain a population of flukes without involvement of domestic species (Cheruiyot 1987). There is considerable literature associated with *F. gigantica* infections in domestic species, particularly in Africa. Fabiyi (1987) provides a general overview of infections in cattle, sheep, and goats. Pertinent information relative to infections in wild mammals is summarized herein.

Fasciola gigantica is a large fluke in the family Fasciolidae. Adult flukes are up to 75 mm long x 3–12 mm wide. The general body outline is elongate and straight-sided (Kendall and Parfitt 1959). The anterior end extends as a narrow cone that bears the oral and ventral suckers. It can be differentiated from *F. hepatica* by the larger size of the egg (156–197 µm x 90–104 µm in *F. gigantica*) (Alicata 1938) and the restricted distribution of the testes in *F. gigantica* (Kendall and Parfitt 1959). *Fascioloides magna* lacks the anterior cone, has the vitellaria restricted ventral to the intestinal ceca, and generally has a smaller egg (114–168 µm x 94–96 µm). Both *Fasciola gigantica* and *F. hepatica* occur within the bile ducts of the liver; whereas, *F. magna* occurs in the hepatic parenchyma. In general, *F. magna* occurs in North America and parts of central Europe, *F. hepatica* occurs worldwide in temperate regions, and *F. gigantica* is widespread in tropical regions.

Life History. Similar to the previous two species in this chapter, *F. gigantica* has a heteroxenous life cycle involving herbivorous vertebrates as final hosts and aquatic snails as intermediate hosts. Transmission is focused around fresh water areas where suitable lymnaeid snails are abundant.

Adult flukes occur in the bile ducts of the liver, and eggs are passed in feces. They develop rapidly at room temperature and hatch as early as 14 days (Alicata 1938). The active miracidia are strongly phototropic but short-lived. Development within the snail is completed within 39 days in Hawaii (Alicata 1938). Free-swimming cercariae encyst on aquatic vegetation and maintain viability for at least 3 months (Bitakaramire 1968). The cycle is completed when suitable final hosts ingest contaminated vegetation. Patent infections occur 75–85 days later.

Epizootiology

DISTRIBUTION. *Fasciola gigantica* occurs in a variety of domestic and wild mammals in the order Artiodactyla over a wide geographic distribution, including eastern, western, and southern Africa, southeast Asia, India, Indochina, Nepal, Europe (Spain), and the United States (Hawaii). Given the wide geographic and host range of *F. gigantica,* there may be physiological races of both the fluke and its intermediate hosts (Kendall and Parfitt 1959).

HOST RANGE, PREVALENCE, AND INTENSITY. Principal hosts of *F. gigantica* are cattle, sheep, and goats; however, infections in giraffe, hippopotamus (*Hippopotamus amphibius*), African buffalo (*Syncerus caffer*), blue wildebeest (*Connochaetes taurinus*), sassaby (*Damaliscus korrigum*), waterbuck (*Kobus ellipsiprymnus*), Uganda kob (*Adenota kob*), puku (*Kobus varondi*), and Jackson's hartebeest (*Alcelaphus buselaphus*) are reported (Cobbold 1855; Round 1968; Bindernagel 1972). Bindernagel (1972) reported prevalence of 47%–58% in buffalo, kob, and hartebeest in Uganda, but oribi (*Ourebia ourebi*) were not infected. Prevalence was similar in males and females and generally did not differ among age classes. Mean intensity in infected wild hosts was low (< 10), and maximum intensity in an individual was 66 flukes. Prevalence in adjacent cattle herds was 80%. The role of cattle in maintaining infections in wild hosts was considered possible but undetermined (Bindernagel 1972).

ENVIRONMENTAL LIMITATIONS. Cheruiyot (1987) reviewed the epizootiology of *F. gigantica* and described the following factors as important in maintaining enzootic foci: (1) a wide range of susceptible hosts ensures dispersion of eggs, increased transmission, and increased fluke population; (2) extended longevity of eggs, metacercariae, and adults helps maintain flukes in the absence of transmission; (3) polyembryony within intermediate hosts and high egg output of adult flukes, particularly in domestic species, increases fluke productivity; (4) increased susceptibility of young cattle and sheep provides access to a large population of naive final hosts; and (5) agricultural areas increase the potential for transmission due to presence of standing water, suitable habitats for snails, and abundant and sedentary final hosts (especially cattle). In addition, hibernation and estivation of snails allows for survival of snails and fluke larvae in harsh conditions. Local floods may aid in dispersal of snails and fluke larvae. Snails are difficult to control due to hermaphroditic reproduction (enhances reproductive potential in small populations) and to the lack of control measures that are effective against snail eggs. In concert, these factors increase the opportunities for *F. gigantica* to establish and maintain populations.

Pathology. As with the common liver fluke, *F. gigantica* is associated with significant damage to the liver in domestic hosts. Severe anemia, acute verminous hepatitis, and bile duct degeneration may occur during the migration phase as immature flukes wander through tissues in the abdominal cavity. Proliferation of periductal and perivascular connective tissue as well as granulomatous nodules containing dead adult flukes, eggs, or cellular debris occur in chronic infections. Acute infections may be associated with mortality in young animals. Chronic infections are associated with debilitation and production losses in various domestic hosts.

In wild hosts, pathologic changes may be limited. Cirrhosis and calcification of bile ducts occurred in severe infections in buffalo and kob (Bindernagel 1972); however, lesions generally were not significant. In a number of cases, flukes occurred only in the gall bladder, and investigators are cautioned against looking only in the bile ducts (Bindernagel 1972).

Diagnosis. Morel (1987) compared various techniques for diagnosing infections of *F. gigantica* and concluded that the differential flotation technique (a two-stage process using saturated salt and zinc sulphate of specific gravity 1.3, Sewell and Hammond 1972) was more sensitive than a standard flotation technique (one step, zinc sulphate at specific gravity 1.5). There was no difference between results from sedimentation and differential flotation, but sedimentation was more laborious.

Considerable research effort has been directed towards serologic tests for *F. gigantica* in domestic species; however, results are variable and of limited use in field situations, largely due to cross-reaction with other species of parasites (Schillhorn van Veen 1980).

Control and Treatment. Recommended methods to limit infections of *F. gigantica* in domestic species include simultaneous anthelminthic treatment, removal of stock from infected pastures by fencing or seasonal rotation, drainage of wetlands, and chemical or mechanical destruction of snails (Roberts and Suhardono 1996). Use of natural herbal molluscicide may be effective against intermediate hosts of *F. hepatica* and *F. gigantica* and less toxic to nontarget species (Singh and Singh 1994). However, control of snails generally is not recommended due to the large number of water sources, the reproductive potential of the snails, and the labour-intensive activities needed to ensure good coverage of snail populations.

A wide range of anthelminthics have been used to try to control *F. gigantica* infections, but efficacy differs among anthelminthics depending on stage of development (adult versus immature flukes), species of host, and local epizootiology (Fabiyi 1987). As with other liver flukes, triclabendazole is reported to have high efficacy against adult and immature *F. gigantica* in a variety of hosts (Mahato et al. 1994; Waruiru et al. 1994). Efficacy is diminished after 6–8 weeks if reinfection occurs on contaminated pasture subsequent to treatment. Attempts to use irradiated metacercariae as a protective vaccine to prevent infection with *F. hepatica* or *F. gigantica* in domestic species have shown potential, but results are inconsistent (Nansen 1975; A/gadir et al. 1987; Haroun et al. 1988). Similarly, investigations of immunologic resistance and control of infections are making progress but further work is needed (Haroun and Hillyer 1986). Control methods in wild populations are not reported and may not be warranted.

DICROCOELIUM DENDRITICUM (RUDOLPHI, 1819) LOOSS, 1899.

Synonoms: (after Mapes 1951): *Fasciola lanceolata* Rudolphi, 1803; *Distoma dendriticum* Rudoplhi, 1819; *Distoma lanceolatum* (Rudolphi, 1803) Mehlis, 1825; *Distomum dendriticum* (Rudolphi, 1803) Diesing, 1850; *Dicrocoelium lanceolatum* (Rudolphi, 1803) Weinland, 1858; *Dicrocoelium lanceatum* Stiles and Hassall, 1896; *Dicrocoelium dendriticum* (Rudolphi, 1819) Looss, 1899; *Distoma lanceolato* Baldi, 1900; *Distomum lanceatum* (Stiles and Hassall, 1896) Anglas and de Ribaucourt, 1902; *Fasciola dendriticum* (Rudolphi, 1819) Brumpt, 1913; *Dicrocoelium macaci* Kobayashi, 1915; *Dicrocoelium vitrinus* (v. Lonstow, 1887) Adam and LeLoup, 1934.

Common Names: lancet fluke, lanceolate fluke, little liver fluke.

Members of the family Dicrocoeliidae generally are characterized as medium to small endoparasitic distomes producing xiphidiocercariae having a stylet but no eyespots. They occur in the bile ducts, pancreas, and gall bladder of non-piscine vertebrates. *Dicrocoelium dendriticum* occurs in the bile ducts of a wide range of domestic and wild mammals including species of ovids, bovids, suids, equids, cervids, rodents, lagomorphs, primates, and camelids (Mapes 1951). It has a wide distribution in Europe and Asia but is limited in North America. Apparently *D. dendriticum* is of Eurasian origin and was introduced to eastern North America (Mapes 1951). The early North American records include infections in domestic sheep and mink (*Mustela vison*) in Canada (Nova Scotia and Prince Edward Island, respectively) (Conklin and Baker 1930) and cattle in the United States (New York) (Price and Kinchelow 1941). Subsequent distribution may have increased in conjunction with movements of infected domestic livestock. Lancet fluke has been found in localized areas of British Columbia (Lewis 1974) and southeastern Alberta (Pybus 1990).

Life History. The lancet fluke has a terrestrial life cycle involving two intermediate hosts: various species of terrestrial snails (e.g., *Cionella lubrica* and *Zebrina detrita*) and ants (*Formica* spp.). Mature eggs occur in the feces of infected definitive hosts. They are resistant to environmental conditions and remain viable for long periods. The miracidia hatch only after the eggs are ingested by a suitable molluscan host (Mattes 1936; Neuhaus 1936, 1938) in which they migrate to the snail's liver and undergo normal trematode polyembryony. Large numbers of cercariae eventually migrate to the pulmonary chamber within the snail, where they secrete a thin cyst wall and are then coated with snail mucus (a "slime ball"). Apparently, slime balls are produced in response to decreased environmental temperature (Krull and Mapes 1952) and are expelled during respiration of the snail. Development within the snail may take 4–5 months.

In order to continue the life cycle, the slime balls must be eaten by ants. In the ant, most cercariae form encysted metacercariae in the abdomen, but a few migrate to the subesophageal ganglion, where they encyst. These latter metacercariae are associated with altered behavior of infected ants. As air temperature drops in the evening, infected ants climb up vegetation, clamp onto the grass tips with their mandibles, and become torpid (Hohorst and Graefe 1961; Anokin 1966). The ants remain attached until air temperature increases (usually the next morning). Paralyzed ants were not found at temperatures > 20°C (Schuster and Neumann 1988). The altered behavior appears to increase the chances that infected ants will be ingested by grazing herbivores during peak foraging times at dusk and dawn. Once ingested by a suitable final host, the metacercariae from the ants excyst in the gut, move up the common bile duct, and disperse throughout the biliary system of the liver (Krull 1958). Migration is rapid, and invasion of the liver occurs within hours of infection. Patent infections in final hosts occur 8–10 weeks after ingestion of infected ants (Krull 1958).

Host Range. *Dicrocoelium dendriticum* is primarily a parasite of domestic species, particularly sheep and mouflon. However, spillover into wild species can occur. Lancet fluke has been found in sheep, goats, cattle, mouflon, chamois, red deer, fallow deer, moose, roe deer, sika deer, Japanese serow (*Capricornis crispus*), wild boars (*Sus scrofa*), European hare, jackrabbits (*Oryctolagus cuniculus*), mountain hare, pika (*Ochotona hyperborea*), woodchuck (*Marmota monax*), European marmot (*Marmota marmota*), and foxes (*Vulpes fulva*) (Mapes 1951; Erhardová-Kotrlá 1971; Nilsson 1971; Sugár 1978; Sakamoto et al. 1982; Nakamura et al. 1984). In Sweden, *D. dendriticum* was present in 22% of 462 roe deer, 16% of 19 moose, 3% of 353 European hares, and 11% of 407 mountain hares (Nilsson 1971). Infections were more common in animals older than 1 year. Wild cervids, lagomorphs, and marmots have been implicated as reservoirs of infection of lancet fluke in domestic species (Mapes 1951;

Nilsson 1971). Reports from wild mammals in North America are limited to incidental infections in woodchuck, white-tailed deer, mule deer, and wapiti (Mapes and Baker 1950; Mapes 1951; Schulte et al. 1976; Pybus 1990).

Pathology. There appears to be little immunologic resistance to infection with *D. dendriticum,* and high intensities can result in domestic species. In addition, infections frequently are concurrent with infections of *F. hepatica.* In such cases, clinical signs of loss of condition and anemia may occur in domestic species. Acute fatal infections also can occur, particularly in sheep. Increasing fibrosis within the liver is the primary feature of the pathologic changes associated with lancet fluke infection. Damage occurs initially at hepatic portal triads and then extends along connecting bile ducts throughout the liver parenchyma. The severity and extent of the lesions increase with increasing duration of infection. In chronic cases, there may be extensive bile duct hyperplasia with proliferation of tubulomucous glands. The external appearance of the liver may be distorted with protrusions and scars. Extensive cirrhosis, cholangitis, and disruption of the architecture and drainage patterns within the liver may occur. Secondary bacterial invasions are rare.

Intensities of infection in cervids and other wild hosts appear to remain low, and damage tends to be limited or inapparent. Infections are characterized by an accumulation of brightly coloured viscid exudate in the bile ducts. There was cholangitis and extensive accumulation of thick yellow/brown exudate in the biliary system throughout the liver of one mule deer in Alberta (Pybus 1990). Infections may persist in fallow deer and white-tailed deer for at least 3 years (Erhardová-Kotrlá and Kotrly 1970).

Diagnosis. Infections in live hosts may be detected by isolation of characteristic eggs in feces. Eggs of *D. dendriticum* are asymmetrically oval (flattened on one side), with an indistinct operculum and thick yellow-brown shell. Eggs (36–45 µm x 22–30 µm) are embryonated when laid and contain a miracidium with two prominent round vesicles (Mapes 1951). Mapes (1951) recommended a sugar solution with specific gravity of 1.347 as best for separating *D. dendriticum* eggs from fecal debris.

The majority of infections are identified at postmortem. Adult worms are tiny (8 mm long x 2 mm wide) and strongly tapered at each end and are readily differentiated from other trematodes that may inhabit the liver.

Control and Treatment. Drug treatment is available for use in domestic species, but often high doses are required in order to be effective (Mustafović 1983). Benzimidazoles and praziquantel can be used effectively; however, control is difficult due to widespread abundance of suitable snails and ants. Drug treatment in conjunction with rotational pasture management may limit infections in domestics. Treatment of wild hosts generally is unfeasible and unwarranted.

Public Health Concerns. A few cases of verminous hepatitis due to infection with lancet fluke in humans have been reported (Mapes 1951; Meunier et al. 1984; Drabick et al. 1988). Zoonotic potential exists from ingestion of infected ants or water contaminated with ants. In addition, eggs of *D. dendriticum* may occur in human feces for a few days after ingestion of infected liver. However these individuals are not infected. Eggs ingested in liver tissue pass through the human gut and are eliminated. Treatment with praziquantel can be effective (Drabick et al. 1988).

Management Implications. Management of *D. dendriticum* in wild populations generally is not warranted. In situations of acute outbreaks of dicrocoeliasis in domestic species, the role of wild species as possible reservoirs should be assessed. A survey of infection in wild species, particularly cervids and lagomorphs, may elucidate their role in the local epizootiology of the fluke. Appropriate management actions could then be tailored to the specific situation. Removal or reduction of local populations, in conjunction with rigorous domestic herd health management, may be helpful in reducing losses of domestic species.

METORCHIS CONJUNCTUS (COBBOLD, 1860) LOOSS, 1899.

Synonyms: (As in Cameron 1944.) *Distoma conjunctum* Cobbold, 1860 (not *D. conjunctum* of Lewis and Cunningham, 1872 or McConnell, 1876); *Metorchis conjunctum* Looss, 1899; *Parametorchis noveboracensis* Hung, 1926; *Parametorchis intermedius* Price, 1929; *Parametorchis canadensis* Price, 1929; *Parametorchis manitobensis* Allen and Wardle, 1934.

Common Name: Canadian liver fluke.

Metorchis conjunctus is a moderate-sized opisthorchiid trematode (1–6.6 mm long x 1–2.6 mm wide) that occurs in the bile ducts and gall bladder in a variety of fish-eating mammals. It was originally described from a red fox that died in the London Zoological Gardens (Cobbold 1860). Natural hosts include red fox, gray fox (*Urocyon cinereoargenteus*), mink, fisher (*Martes pennanti*), raccoon (*Procyon lotor*), wolf (*Canis lupus*), dog, and cat (Cameron 1944; Holmes and Podesta 1968; Mills and Hirth 1968; Dick and Leonard 1979). Experimental infections have been established in dog, cat, red fox, silver fox, mink, ferret (*Mustela putorius*), and cotton rat (*Sigmondon hispidus*) (Cameron 1944; Watson 1981a). A few cases in humans have been reported (Cameron 1944; Unruh et al. 1973).

Life History. Canadian liver fluke has a heteroxenous life cycle including two intermediate hosts (suitable aquatic snails and fishes) and a definitive host (fish-eating mammals) (Fig. 6.8). Embryonated eggs produced by adult females are released into the biliary system and occur in the feces of definitive hosts. The eggs are ingested by snails, *Amnicola limosa* (Cameron 1944), or related species (Holmes and Podesta 1968). Within the snail, miracidia migrate to the liver and develop through the usual sporocyst, rediae, and cercariae stages. Pleurolophocercous cercariae, complete with a long tail with dorsoventral fin folds as well as anterior spines and hair-like processes, leave the snails and may occur in clouds in warm shallow waters (Watson 1981b). Cercariae actively penetrate the body surfaces of various fishes, particularly white suckers (*Catostomus commersonii*) (Cameron 1944) and fallfish (*Semotilus corporalis*) (Watson 1981b), where they encyst in lateral muscles along the length of the fish. Only calcified cysts were found in brook trout (*Salvelinus fontinalis*), suggesting they may be an unsuitable intermediate host. In white sucker, live metacercariae can persist for at least 14 months (Watson 1981b). When ingested by a carnivore, metacercariae are digested from the fish tissue, migrate up the bile duct, and enter the biliary system within the liver. Patent infections occur approximately 1 month later, and adult flukes can survive at least 7 years in cats (Cameron 1945). Mink (Cameron 1944) and raccoon (Meyer 1949) may be the primary definitive hosts.

Distribution. Distribution of *M. conjunctus* is restricted to North America. It generally reflects the range of *A. limosa* within the Hudson Bay watershed. In Canada it is present south of Hudson's Bay and the southern Nunavut Territory border, east of the height of land in Saskatchewan and east central Alberta (Cameron et al. 1940; Holmes and Podesta 1968; Unruh et al. 1973), and north of the St. Lawrence River drainage (Fig. 6.9). Occasional reports from the Canadian maritime provinces (Smith 1978), northeastern United States (Dikmans 1945; Meyer 1949; Mills and Hirth 1968), and the Great Lakes region (Sweatman 1952) suggest that the fluke may be present throughout the St. Lawrence region. E.M. Addison (personal communication) examined large numbers of mink (> 3000) from Ontario and found *M. conjunctus* in 5%–6% (Hudson Bay watershed, northern Ontario) and 1%–3% in mink from southwestern Ontario. Local distribution was patchy except that liver flukes were not found in mink from eastern Ontario or west of Thunder Bay. Jordan and Ashby (1957) report infection in a dog that had apparently not left South Carolina. The fluke is relatively common in sled dogs fed uncooked fish in northcentral Canada (Cameron et al. 1940; Mongeau 1961; Unruh et al. 1973). Infections in captive, ranched furbearers (see Mills and Hirth 1968) do not necessarily reflect natural distribution of the fluke.

Pathology. Lesions caused by *M. conjunctus* are characterized by proliferation of biliary epithelium and progressive thickening of the bile ducts. Extent of damage

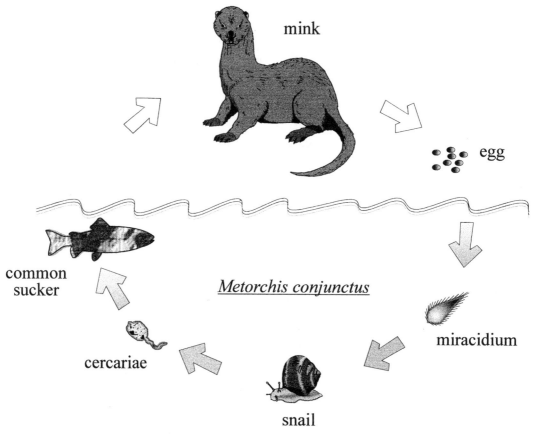

mink

egg

Metorchis conjunctus

common
sucker

miracidium

cercariae

snail

FIG. 6.8—Life cycle of *Metorchis conjunctus*.

may be related to the number of flukes present, the duration of infection, and the species of definitive host. Emaciation and mortality of heavily infected cats, ferrets, and mink has been recorded (Cameron 1945). Severe infections in northern dogs may be complicated by concurrent infection with infectious canine hepatitis (Mongeau 1961). Two of 7 infected wolves in Saskatchewan were emaciated (Wobeser et al. 1983). These wolves had flukes in the bile and pancreatic ducts, with marked fibrosis and dilatation of the liver and pancreas. Lesions were considered sufficient to cause potential disruption of the endocrine/exocrine functions of the pancreas. Pancreatic involvement appears to occur as an overflow of flukes from the liver in high intensity infections. In the 5 wolves with only hepatic infections, lesions were limited to nodular or cord-like swellings within the hepatic parenchyma that reflected greatly dilated bile ducts and accumulation of viscid yellow-green fluid (Wobeser et al. 1983). One of 98 wolves and 4 of 75 coyotes in Alberta were infected (Holmes and Podesta 1968); however, no significant lesions were noted. Verminous granulomas in the liver were a

common feature of infection in raccoons (Mills and Hirth 1968).

Diagnosis. Adult flukes are 1–6 mm in length, are linguiform in shape, and have a spiny cuticle. Size differs among different hosts. The distinctive eggs of *M. conjunctus* can be used to identify patent infections. The yellowish brown eggs are 22–32 μm x 11–18 μm. They have a distinct operculum and are fully embryonated when laid (Cameron 1944). However, most infections in wild mammals are detected during postmortem examination of the liver.

Public Health. Infection of Canadian liver fluke in humans is rare and is associated with eating raw or lightly smoked fish. The metacercariae are not killed at temperatures below 71° C (Cameron 1945). Cysts are not visible to the naked eye, increasing the risk of accidental human infection. Most human infections are associated with eating white sucker from the enzootic regions of northcentral Canada (Unruh et al. 1973). Public health officials in the enzootic area should be

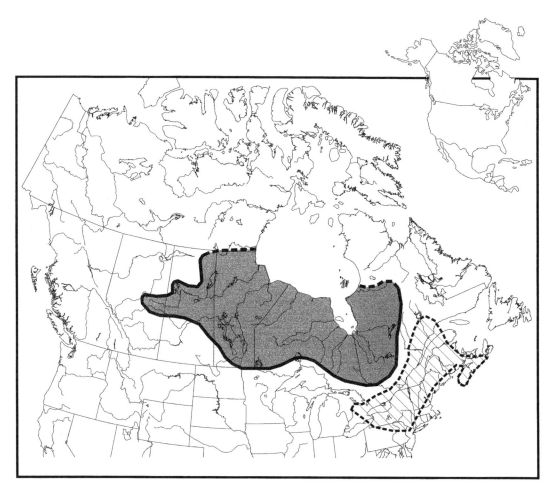

FIG. 6.9—Distribution of *Metorchis conjunctus* in naturally infected hosts. Shaded area = documented limits; area within dotted line = estimated limits.

aware of the potential for infection in cases of unexplained biliary/hepatic dysfunction.

Management Implications. Canadian liver fluke is unlikely to be a concern in the management of free-ranging wildlife. Fish-eating mammals within the Hudson Bay, and perhaps the St. Lawrence, watershed are likely to be infected, but the impacts appear to be minimal. Infection could cause individual mortality in free-ranging wildlife where there is local heavy reliance on infected fish or in captive canids fed raw infected fish. Ingestion of raw fish by humans, particularly white sucker from the enzootic area, should be discouraged.

LITERATURE CITED

Addison, E.M., J. Hoeve, D.G. Joachim, and D.J. McLachlin. 1988. *Fascioloides magna* (Trematoda) and *Taenia hydatigena* (Cestoda) from white-tailed deer. *Canadian Journal of Zoology* 66:1359–1364.

A/gadir, H., E.M. Haroun, and A.A. Gameel. 1987. The protective effect of irradited metacercariae of *Fasciola gigantica* against homologous challenge in sheep. *Journal of Helminthology* 61:137–142.

Aho, R.W., and J. Hendrickson. 1989. Reproduction and mortality of moose translocated from Ontario to Michigan. *Alces* 25:75–80.

Aiton, J.F. 1938. Enlarged spleen in whitetail deer at Glacier National Park. *Transactions of the North American Wildlife Conference* 3:890–892.

Alicata, J.E. 1938. *Observations on the life history of* Fasciola gigantica, *the common liver fluke of cattle in Hawaii, and the intermediate hosts,* Fossaria ollula. Hawaii Agricultural Experiment Station, University of Hawaii, Bulletin No. 80, 22 pp.

Anokin, I.A. 1966. Daily rhythm in ants infected with metacercariae of *Dicrocoelium dendriticum* [In Russian]. *Dokladȳ Akademii Nauk SSSR* 166:757–759.

Arundel, J.H., and A.N. Hamir. 1982. *Fascioloides magna* in cattle. *Australian Veterinary Journal* 58:35–36.

Balbo, T., P. Lanfranchi, L. Rossi, and P.G. Meneguz. 1987. Health management of a red deer population infected by *Fascioloides magna* (Bassi, 1875) Ward, 1917. *Anales Facultad de Medicina Veterinaria de Torino* 32:23–33.

Banfield, A.W.F. 1974. The mammals of Canada. Toronto: University of Toronto Press, 438 pp.

Barth, D., and K. Schaich. 1973. Zum vorkommen von *Fasciola hepatica* bei Reh- (*Capreolus capreolus*) und Rotwild (*Cervus elaphus*) und deren Bekämpfung mit Rafoxanid. *Deutsche Tierärztliche Wochenschrift* 80:448–450.

Bassi, R. 1875. Jaundiced verminous cachexy or pus of the stags caused by *Distoma magnum*. *Medico Veterinario* 4:497–515. [as reprinted in *Southeastern Veterinarian* 14:103–112.]

Behrend, D.F., G.F. Mattfeld, and J.E. Wiley. 1973. Incidence of liver flukes in a sample of white-tailed deer from the Adirondacks. *New York Fish and Game Journal* 20:158–161.

Berg, W.E. 1975. Management implications of natural mortality of moose in northwestern Minnesota. *North American Moose Conference and Workshop* 11:332–342.

Bergstrom, R.C. 1967. Sheep liver fluke, *Fasciola hepatica* (L., 1758) from buffalo, *Bison bison* (L., 1758) in western Wyoming. *The Journal of Parasitology* 53:724.

Bindernagel, J.A. 1972. Liver fluke *Fasciola gigantica*, in African buffalo and antelopes in Uganda, East Africa. *Journal of Wildlife Diseases* 8:315–317.

Bitakaramire, P.K. 1968. *Lymnaea natalensis* laboratory culture and production of *Fasciola gigantica* metacercariae. *Parasitology* 58:653–656.

Blažek, K., and F. Gilka. 1970. Contribution of the knowledge of the pigment found in infection with *Fascioloides magna*. *Folia Parasitoligica (Praha)* 17:165–170.

Blythe, C.B., and R.J. Hudson. 1987. *A plan for the management of vegetation and ungulates in Elk Island National Park.* Environment Canada Parks, Registration No. 87-04, 343 pp.

Bojovic, D., and L.K. Halls. 1984. Central Europe. In *White-tailed deer: Ecology and management.* Ed. L.K. Halls. Harrisburg, PA: Stackpole Books, pp. 557–568.

Boomker, J., and J.C. Dale-Kuys. 1977. First report of *Fascioloides magna* (Bassi, 1875) in South Africa. *Onderstepoort Journal of Veterinary Research* 44:49–52.

Boray, J.C. 1982. Chemotherapy of fasciolosis. *New South Wales Veterinary Proceedings* 18:42–47.

Brooks, D.R. 1989a. A summary of the database pertaining to the phylogeny of the major groups of parasitic platyhelminths, with a revised classification. *Canadian Journal of Zoology* 67:714–720.

———. 1989b. Erratum: A summary of the database pertaining to the phylogeny of the major groups of parasitic platyhelminths, with a revised classification. *Canadian Journal of Zoology* 67:2607–2608.

Browning, B.M., and E.M. Lauppe. 1964. A deer study in a redwood-Douglas fir forest type. *California Fish and Game* 50:132–147.

Bruce, E.A. 1930. As cited in Hilton (1930).

Bryant, L.D., and C. Maser. 1982. Classification and distribution. In *Elk of North America.* Ed. J.W. Thomas and D.E. Toweill. Harrisburg, PA: Stackpole Books, pp. 1–59.

Butler, W.J. 1932. Liver flukes. *Montana Livestock Sanitary Board* 1:18–19.

———. 1938. Wild animal disease investigation. *Montana Livestock Sanitary Board 1936/38,* pp. 14–16.

Butterworth, E., and M.J. Pybus. 1993. *Impact of the giant liver fluke* (Fascioloides magna) *on elk and other ungulates in Banff and Kootenay National Parks.* Calgary, Alberta: Canadian Parks Service, Contract #WR-91162, 81 pp.

Cameron, A.E. 1923. Notes on buffalo: Anatomy, pathological conditions, and parasites. *The Veterinary Journal* 79:331–336.

Cameron, T.W.M. 1944. The morphology, taxonomy, and life history of *Metorchis conjunctus* (Cobbold, 1860). *Canadian Journal of Research* 22:6–16.

———. 1945. Fish-carried parasites in Canada. I. Parasites carried by fresh-water fish. *Canadian Journal of Comparative Medicine* 9:302–311.

Cameron, T.W.M., I.W. Parnell, and L.L. Lyster. 1940. The helminth parasites of sledge-dogs in northern Canada and Newfoundland. *Canadian Journal of Research* 18D:325–332.

Campbell, W.C. 1960. Nature and possible significance of the pigment in fascioloidiasis. *Journal of Parasitology* 46:769–775.

———. 1961. Notes on the egg and miracidium of *Fascioloides magna*, (Trematoda). *Transactions of the American Microscopical Society* 80:308–319.

Campbell, W.C., and A.C. Todd. 1954. Natural infections of *Fascioloides magna* in Wisconsin sheep. *The Journal of Parasitology* 40:100.

Cheatum, E.L. 1951. Disease in relation to winter mortality of deer in New York. *Journal of Wildlife Management* 15:216–220.

Cheruiyot, H.K. 1987. Fascioliasis in Kenya: A review of its epidemiology in the hosts. *Tropical Veterinarian* 5:61–66.

Choquette, L.P.E., J.F. Gallivan, J.L. Byrne, and J. Pilipavicius. 1961. Parasites and diseases of bison in Canada. *Canadian Veterinary Journal* 2:168–174.

Choquette, L.P.E., G.G. Gibson, and B. Simard. 1971. *Fascioloides magna* (Bassi, 1875) Ward, 1917 (Trematoda) in woodland caribou, *Rangifer tarandus caribou* (Gmelin), of northeastern Quebec, and its distribution in wild ungulates in Canada. *Canadian Journal of Zoology* 49:280–281.

Christian, F.A., and J.A. Thompson. 1990. Sublethal effects of 2,2-dichloropropionic acid (dalapon) on *Fossaria cubensis,* intermediate host of the liver fluke, *Fasciola hepatica. Bulletin of Environmental Contamination and Toxicology* 45:343–349.

Christian, F.A., T.M. Tate, B. Eribo, and T. Tesfamichael. 1984. *Fascioloides magna* (Bassi 1875): Occurrence in white-tailed deer (Rafinesque, 1832) in Louisiana. *Proceedings of the Louisiana Academy of Sciences* 47:48–51.

Chroustová, E. 1979. Experimental infection of *Lymnaea palustris* snails with *Fascioloides magna. Veterinary Parasitology* 5:57–64.

Churcher C.S., P.W. Parmalee, G.L. Bell, and J.P. Lamb. 1989. Caribou from the late Pleistocene of northwestern Alabama. *Canadian Journal of Zoology* 67:1210–1216.

Cobbold, T.S. 1855. Description of a new species of trematode worm (*Fasciola gigantica*). *Edinburgh New Philosophical Journal* 2:262–267.

———. 1860. Synopsis of the Distomidae. *Journal of the Proceedings of the Linnean Society of London, Zoology* 5:1–56.

Conboy, G.A., T.D. O'Brien, and D.L. Stevens. 1988. A natural infection of *Fascioloides magna* in a llama (*Lama glama*). *The Journal of Parasitology.* 74:345–346.

Conklin, R.L., and A.D. Baker. 1930. Presence of the lancet fluke, *Dicrocoelium dendriticum* (Rudolphi, 1819), in Canada. *The Journal of Parasitology* 17:18–19.

Cowan, I.McT. 1946. Parasites, diseases, injuries, and anomalies of the Columbian black-tailed deer, *Odocoileus hemionus columbianus* (Richardson), in British Columbia. *Canadian Journal of Research, Series D,* 24:71–103.

————. 1951. The diseases and parasites of big game mammals of western Canada. *Proceedings of the Annual Game Convention* 5:37–64.

Craig, T.M., and R.L. Huey. 1984. Efficacy of triclabendazole against *Fasciola hepatica* and *Fascioloides magna* in naturally infected calves. *American Journal of Veterinary Research* 45:1644–1645.

Dick, T.A., and R.D. Leonard. 1979. Helminth parasites of fisher (*Martes pennanti*) (Erxleben) from Manitoba, Canada. *Journal of Wildlife Diseases* 15:409–412.

Dikmans, G. 1945. Check list of the internal and external animal parasties of domestic animals in North America. *American Journal of Veterinary Research* 6:211–241.

Dinaburg, A.G. 1939. Helminth parasites collected from deer, *Odocoileus Virginianus,* in Florida. *Proceedings of the Helminthological Society of Washington* 6:102–104.

Drabbick, J.J., J.E. Egan, S.L. Brown, R.G. Vick, B.M. Sandman, and R.C. Neafie. 1988. Dicrocoeliasis (lancet fluke disease) in an HIV seropositive man. *Journal of the American Medical Association* 259:567–568.

Drózdz, J. 1963. Helmintofauna zaaklimatyzowanego w Polsce jelenia sika (*Cervus nippon* L.). *Wiadomosci Parazytologiczne* 9:133–138.

Dutson, V. J., J.N.Shaw, and S.E. Knapp. 1967. Epizootiologic factors of *Fascioloides magna* (Trematoda) in Oregon and southern Washington. *American Journal of Veterinary Research* 28:853–860.

Erhardová, B. 1961. *Fascioloides magna* in Europe. *Helminthologia* 3:91–106.

Erhardová-Kotrlá, B. 1971. *The occurrence of Fascioloides magna (Bassi, 1875) in Czechoslovakia.* Prague: Czechoslovak Academy of Sciences, 155 pp.

Erhardová-Kotrlá, B., and K. Blaẑek. 1970. Artificial infestation caused by the fluke *Fascioloides magna. Acta Veterinaria (Brno)* 39:287–295.

Erhardová-Kotrlá, B., and A. Kotrly. 1968. Einschleppen eines Parasiten der Gattung *Fascioloides* beim Import lebenden Wildes aus anderen Kontinenten. *Zeitschrift für Jagdwissenschaft* 14:170–176.

————. 1970. Die Dauer des Parasitismus bei manchen Säugetiernematoden. *Helminthologia* 9:177–180.

Fabiyi, J.P. 1987. Production losses and control of helminths in ruminants of tropical regions. *International Journal of Parasitology* 17:435–442.

Facey, R.V., and P.D. Marsden. 1960. Fascioliasis in man: An outbreak in Hampshire. *British Medical Journal* 27(August): 619–625.

Fenstermacher, R. 1934. Diseases affecting moose. *The Alumni Quarterly* 22:81–94.

Fenstermacher, R., and O.W. Olsen. 1942. Further studies of diseases affecting moose III. *Cornell Veterinarian* 32:241–254.

Fenstermacher, R., O.W. Olsen, and B.S. Pomeroy. 1943. Some diseases of white-tailed deer in Minnesota. *Cornell Veterinarian* 33:323–332.

Flook, D.R., and J.E. Stenton. 1969. Incidence and abundance of certain parasites in wapiti in the national parks of the Canadian Rockies. *Canadian Journal of Zoology* 47:795–803.

Foreyt, W.J. 1981. Trematodes and cestodes. In *Diseases and parasites of white-tailed deer.* Ed. W.R. Davidson, F.A. Hayes, V.F. Nettles, and F.E. Kellogg., Tallahassee, FL: Tall Timbers Research Station Miscellaneous Publication No. 7, pp. 237–265.

————. 1988. Evaluation of clorsulon against immature *Fascioloides magna* in cattle and sheep. *American Journal of Veterinary Research* 49:1004–1006.

————. 1989. Efficacy of triclabendazole against experimentally induced *Fascioloides magna* infections in sheep. *American Journal of Veterinary Research* 50:431–432.

————. 1992. Experimental *Fascioloides magna* infections of mule deer (*Odocoileus hemionus hemionus*). *Journal of Wildlife Diseases* 28:183–187.

————. 1996a. Mule deer (*Odocoileus hemionus*) and elk (*Cervus elaphus*) as experimental definitive hosts for *Fascioloides magna. Journal of Wildlife Diseases* 32:603–606.

————. 1996b. Susceptibility of bighorn sheep (*Ovis canadensis*) to experimentally induced *Fascioloides magna* infections. *Journal of Wildlife Diseases* 32:556–559.

Foreyt, W.J, and D.L. Drawe. 1978. Anthelmintic activity of albendazole in white-tailed deer. *American Journal of Veterinary Research* 39:1901–1903.

————. 1985. Efficacy of clorsulon and albendazole against *Fascioloides magna* in naturally infected white-tailed deer. *Journal of the American Veterinary Medical Association* 187:1187–1188.

Foreyt, W.J., and K.M. Foreyt. 1980. Albendazole treatment of experimentally induced *Fascioloides magna* infection in goats. *Veterinary Medicine/ Small Animal Clinician,* September, pp. 1441–1444.

Foreyt, W.J., and R.L. Hunter. 1980. Clinical *Fascioloides magna* infection in sheep in Oregon on pasture shared by Columbian white-tailed deer. *American Journal of Veterinary Research* 41:1531–1532.

Foreyt, W.J., and C.W. Leathers. 1980. Experimental infection of domestic goats with *Fascioloides magna. American Journal of Veterinary Research* 41:883–884.

Foreyt, W.J., and S. Parish. 1990. Experimental infection of liver flukes (*Fascioloides magna*) in a llama (*Lama glama*). *Journal of Zoo and Wildlife Medicine* 21:468–470.

Foreyt, W.J., and A.C. Todd. 1972. The occurrence of *Fascioloides magna* and *Fasciola hepatica* together in the livers of naturally infected cattle in south Texas, and the incidence of the flukes in cattle, white-tailed deer, and feral hogs. *Journal of Parasitology* 58:1010–1011.

————. 1973. Action of oxyclozanide against adult *Fascioloides magna* (Bassi, 1875) infections in white-tailed deer. *The Journal of Parasitology* 59:208–209.

————. 1974. Efficacy of rafoxanide and oxyclozanide against *Fascioloides magna* in naturally infected cattle. *American Journal of Veterinary Research* 35:375–377.

————. 1976a. Development of the large American liver fluke, *Fascioloides magna,* in white-tailed deer, cattle, and sheep. *The Journal of Parasitology* 62:26–32.

————. 1976b. Effects of six fasciolicides against *Fascioloides magna* in white-tailed deer. *Journal of Wildlife Diseases* 12:361–366.

————. 1976c. Liver flukes in cattle. *Veterinary Medicine/ Small Animal Clinician,* June, pp. 816–822.

————. 1976d. Parental infection of white-tailed deer (*Odocoileus virginianus*) with metacercariae of *Fasciola hepatica* and *Fascioloides magna. The Journal of Parasitology* 62:144–145.

————. 1979. Selected clinicopathologic changes associated with experimentally induced *Fascioloides magna* infection in white-tailed deer. *Journal of Wildlife Diseases* 15:83–89.

Foreyt, W.J., A.C. Todd, and K. Foreyt. 1975. *Fascioloides magna* (Bassi, 1875) in feral swine from southern Texas. *Journal of Wildlife Diseases* 11:554–559.

Foreyt, W.J., W.M. Samuel, and A.C. Todd. 1977. *Fascioloides magna* in white-tailed deer (*Odocoileus virginianus*): Observations on the pairing tendency. *Journal of Parasitology* 63:1050–1052.

Forrester, D.J. 1992. *Parasites and diseases of wild mammals in Florida.* Gainsville: University Press of Florida, 459 pp.

Francis, M. 1891. Liver flukes. *Texas Agricultural Experimental Station Bulletin* 18:123–136.

Gardner, L.A., S. Hietla, and W.M. Boyce. 1996. Validity of using serological tests for diagnosis in wild animals. *Revue Scientifique et Technique of the Office International des épizooties* 15:323–335.

Griffiths, H.J. 1962. Fascioloidiasis of cattle, sheep, and deer in northern Minnesota. *Journal of the American Veterinary Medical Association* 140:342–347.

Griffiths, H.J., and C.A. Christensen. 1972. Survival of metacercariae of *Fascioloides magna* in water at room temperature and under refrigeration. *Journal of Parasitology* 58:404–405.

———. 1974. Further observations on the survival of metacercariae of *Fascioloides magna* in water at room temperature and under refrigeration. *Journal of Parasitology* 60:335.

Hadwen, S. 1916. A new host for *Fasciola magna,* Bassi, together with observations on the distribution of *Fasciola hepatica,* L. in Canada. *Journal of the American Veterinary Medical Association* 49:511–515.

———. 1939. Report on Elk Island Park and Wainwright. Ottawa, Ontario: Canadian National Parks Bureau Internal Report, August 23. 5 pp.

Hall, M.C. 1912. Our present knowledge of the distribution and importance of some parasitic diseases of sheep and cattle in the United States. United States Department of Agriculture, Bureau of Animal Industry, Circular 193.

———. 1914. Society proceedings of the Helminthological Society of Washington. *Journal of Parasitology* 1:106.

———. 1934. Outline for a campaign against the common sheep liver fluke and the large American cattle fluke in the United States. *North American Veterinarian* 15:48–55.

Haroun, E.M., and G.V. Hillyer. 1986. Resistance to fascioliasis—A review. *Veterinary Parasitology* 20:63–93.

Haroun, E.M., A.I. Yagi, S.A. Younis, A.A. El Sanhouri, H.A. Gadir, A.A. Gameel, and M.G. Taylor. 1988. Use of ionizing radiation in the development of vaccines against *Fasciola gigantica* and *Schistosoma bovis* in Sudanese cattle, sheep, and goats. In *Nuclear techniques in the study and control of parasitic diseases of livestock.* Vienna, Austria: International Atomic Energy Agency, pp. 1–21.

Herman, C.M. 1945. Some worm parasites of deer in California. *California Fish and Game* 31:201–208.

Hilton, G. 1930. Report of the Veterinary Director General, Department of Agriculture, Ottawa, Canada, 59 pp.

Hohorst, W., and G. Graefe. 1961. Ameisen—obligatorische Zwischenwirte des Lanzettegels (*Dicrocoelium dendriticum*). *Naturwissenschaften* 48:229–230.

Holland, J.B. 1959. Liver flukes in the southeastern white-tailed deer. *Annual Conference of the Southeast Association of Game and Fish Commissioners* 12:224–227.

Holmes, J.C., and R. Podesta. 1968. The helminths of wolves and coyotes from the forested regions of Alberta. *Canadian Journal of Zoology* 46:1193–1204.

Hood, B.R., M.C. Rognlie, and S.E. Knapp. 1997. Fascioloidiasis in game-ranched elk from Montana. *Journal of Wildlife Diseases* 33:882–885.

Huot, J. 1989. Body composition of the George River caribou (*Rangifer tarandus caribou*) in fall and late winter. *Canadian Journal of Zoology* 67:103–107.

Huot, J., and M. Beaulieu. 1985. Relationship between parasite infection levels and body fat reserves in George River caribou in spring and fall. In *Proceedings of the 2nd North American caribou workshop.* Ed. T.C. Meredith and A.M. Martell. McGill Subarctic Research Papers 40:317–327.

Jansen, J. 1965. Some problems related to the parasite interrelationship of deer and domestic animals. *Transactions of the Congress of International Ungulate Game Biologists* 6:127–132.

Jordan, H.E., and W.T. Ashby. 1957. Liver fluke (*Metorchis conjunctus*) in a dog from South Carolina. *Journal of the American Veterinary Medical Association* 131:239–240.

Karns, P.D. 1972. Minnesota's 1971 moose hunt: A preliminary report on the biological collections. *North American Moose Conference and Workshop* 8:115–123.

———. 1973. Minnesota's 1971 moose hunt: A preliminary report on the biological collections II. *North American Moose Conference and Workshop* 9:96–100.

Kendall, S.B. 1949. Nutritional factors affecting the rate of development of *Fasciola hepatica* in *Limnaea truncatula. Journal of Helminthology* 23:179–190.

Kendall, S.B., and J.W. Parfitt. 1959. Studies on the susceptibility of some species of *Lymnaea* to infection with *Fasciola gigantica* and *F. hepatica. Annals of Tropical Medicine and Parasitology* 53:220–227.

Kermode, F. 1916. Investigation of reported disease in the black-tail or Columbian coast deer (*Odocoileus columbianus*). *Annual Report of the British Columbia Provincial Museum, 1915,* pp. 12–13.

Kingscote, A.A. 1950. Liver rot (Fascioloidiasis) in ruminants. *Canadian Journal of Comparative Medicine* 14:203–208.

Kingscote, B.F., W.D. Yates, and G.B. Tiffin. 1987. Diseases of wapiti utilizing cattle range in southwestern Alberta. *Journal of Wildlife Diseases* 23:86–91.

Kistner, T.P., and L.D. Koller. 1975. Experimentally induced *Fasciola hepatica* infections in black-tailed deer. *Journal of Wildlife Diseases* 11:214–220.

Knapp. S.E., A.M. Dunkel, K. Han, and L.A. Zimmerman. 1992. Epizootiology of fascioliasis in Montana. *Veterinary Parasitology* 42:241–246.

Krull, W.H. 1958. The migratory route of the metacercaria of *Dicrocoelium dendriticum* (Rudolphi, 1819) Looss, 1899 in the definitive host. *Cornell Veterinarian* 48:17–24.

Krull, W.H., and C.R. Mapes. 1952. Studies on the biology of *Dicrocoelium dendriticum* (Rudolphi, 1819) Looss, 1899 (Trematoda: Dicrocoeliidae), including its relation to the intermediate host, *Cionella lubrica* (Muller). III. Observations on the slimeballs of *Dicrocoelium dendriticum. Cornell Veterinarian* 42:253–276.

Kotrlá, B., and A. Kotrly. 1977. Helminths of wild ruminants introduced into Czechoslovakia. *Folia Parasitologica (Praha)* 24:35–40.

———. 1980. Zur Verbreitung von Helminthen durch eingeführtes Wild. *Angewandte Parasitologie* 21:79–82.

Kotrly, A., and B. Kotrlá. 1980. Der einfluss der Lebensbedingungen des Schalenwildes auf das Parasitenvorkommen. *Angewandte Parasitologie* 21:70–78.

Lang, B.Z. 1977. Snail and mammalian hosts for *Fasciola hepatica* in eastern Washington. *Journal of Parasitology* 63:938–939.

Lankester, M.W. 1974. *Parelaphostrongylus tenuis* (Nematoda) and *Fascioloides magna* (Trematoda) in moose of southeastern Manitoba. *Canadian Journal of Zoology* 52:235–239.

Lankester, M.W., and S. Luttich. 1988. *Fascioloides magna* (Trematoda) in woodland caribou (*Rangifer tarandus caribou*) of the George River herd, Labrador. *Canadian Journal of Zoology* 66:475–479.

Lewis, P.D. 1974. Presence of *Dicrocoelium dendriticum* (Rudolphi, 1819) (Trematoda: Dicrocoeliidae) in western Canada. *Canadian Journal of Zoology.* 1974. 52:662–663.

Lloyd, H. 1927. Transfers of elk for re-stocking. *The Canadian Field-Naturalist* 41:126–127.

Locker, B. 1953. Parasites of bison in Northwestern USA. *The Journal of Parasitology* 39:58–59.

Longhurst, W.M., and J.R. Douglas. 1953. Parasite interrelationships of domestic sheep and Columbian black-tailed deer. *North American Wildlife Conference* 18:168–187.

Lorenzo, M., P. Ramirez, M. Mendez, M. Alonso, and R. Ramos.1989. Reporte de *Fascioloides magna,* Bassi, 1875, parasitando un wápiti (*Cervus canadensis*) en Cuba. *Revista Cubana de Ciencias Veterinarias* 20:263–266.

Lothian, W.F. 1981. *A history of Canada's national parks,* vol. 4. Ottawa, Ontario: Ministry of Environment, Parks Canada, 155 pp.

Mahato, S.N., L.J. Harrison, and J.A. Hammond. 1994. Efficacy of triclabendazole against *Fasciola gigantica* in buffaloes in eastern Nepal. *Veterinary Record* 135:579–580.

Majoros, G., and V. Sztojkov. 1994. Appearance of the large American liver fluke *Fascioloides magna* (Bassi, 1875) (Trematoda: Fasciolata) in Hungary. *Parasitologia Hungarica* 27:27–38.

Mapes, C.R. 1951. Studies on the biology of *Dicrocoelium dendriticum* (Rudolphi, 1819) Looss, 1899 (Trematoda: Dicrocoeliidae), including its relation to the intermediate host, *Cionella lubrica* (Muller). I. A study of *Dicrocoelium dendriticum* and *Dicrocoelium* infection. *Cornell Veterinarian* 41:382–432.

Mapes, C.R., and D.W. Baker. 1950. The white-tailed deer, a new host of *Dicrocoelium dendriticum* (Rudolphi, 1819) Looss, 1899 (Trematoda: Dicrocoeliidae). *Cornell Veterinarian* 40:211–212.

Marek, J. 1927. Neure beiträge zur Kenntnis der Leberegelkrankheit, mit besonderer Berücksichtigung der Infektionsweise, der Entwicklung der Distomen und der Therapie. *Deutsche Tierärztliche Wochenschrift* 32:513–519.

Mattes, O. 1936. Der Entwicklungsgang des Lanzettegels *Dicrocoelium lanceatum. Zeitschrift für Parasitenkunde* 8:371–430.

McCabe, R.E., And T.R. McCabe. 1984. Of slings and arrows: An historical retrospection. In *White-tailed deer ecology and management.* Ed. L.K. Halls. Harrisburg, PA: Stackpole Books, pp. 19–72.

Meunier, D.M., M.C. Georges, and A.J. Georges. 1984. Bilan des parasitoses intestinales de l'adulte dans un milieu urbain de la Republique Centrafricaine. *Bulletin de la Société de Pathologie Exotique.* 77:333–343.

Meyer, M.C. 1949. The presence of *Metorchis conjunctus* in Maine. *Journal of Parasitology* 35:39.

Migaki, G., D.E. Zinter, and F.M. Garner. 1971. *Fascioloides magna* in the pig—Three cases. *Journal of Veterinary Research* 32:1417–1421.

Mills, J.H.L., and R.S. Hirth. 1968. Lesions caused by the hepatic trematode, *Metorchis conjunctus,* Cobbold, 1860. *Journal of Small Animal Practice.* 9:1–6.

Mongeau, N. 1961. Hepatic distomatosis and infectious canine hepatitis in northern Manitoba. *Canadian Veterinary Journal* 2:33–38.

Morel, A.M. 1987. Detection of *Fasciola gigantica* eggs in faeces: A comparision of methods. *Veterinary Record* 120:90–91.

Mulvey, M., and J.M. Aho. 1993. Parasitism and mate competition: Liver flukes in white-tailed deer. *Oikos* 66:187–192.

Mulvey, M., J.M. Aho, C. Lydeard, P.L. Leberg, and M.H. Smith. 1991. Comparative population genetic structure of a parasite (*Fascioloides magna*) and its definitive host. *Evolution* 45:1628–1640.

Mustafovìc, A. 1983. Problemi dikrocelioze, bibliografski prikaz antiparazitika i njihovog u_inka [14] protiv *Dicrocoelium dendriticum. Veterinarski Glasnik* 37:955–964.

Nakamura, T., J. Nakahari, N. Machida, K. Kiryu, and M. Machida. 1984. Dicroceliasis in the wild Japanese serow, *Capricornis crispus. Japanese Journal of Veterinary Science* 46:405–408.

Nansen, P. 1975. Resistance in cattle to *Fasciola hepatica* induced by X-ray attentuated larvae: Results from a controlled field trial. *Research in Veterinary Science* 10:278–283.

Neuhaus, W. 1936. Untersuchungen über Bau und Entwicklung der Lanzettegel-Cercarien (*Cercaria vitrina*) und Klarstellung des Infektionsvorganges beim Endwirt. *Zeitschrift für Parasitenkunde* 8:431–473.

———. 1938. Die Invasionswege der Lanzettegelcercarie bei der Infektion des Endwirtes und ihre Entwicklung zum *Dicrocoelium lanceatum. Zeitschrift für Parasitenkunde* 10:476–512.

Nilsson, O. 1971. The inter-relationship of endo-parasites in wild cervids (*Capreolus capreolus* L. and *Alces alces* L.) and domestic ruminants in Sweden. *Acta Veterinaria Scandinavica* 12:36–68.

Olsen, O.W. 1948. Wild rabbits as reservoir hosts of the common liver fluke, *Fasciola hepatica,* in southern Texas. *The Journal of Parasitology* 34:119–123.

———. 1949. White-tailed deer as a reservoir host of the large American liver fluke. *Veterinary Medicine* 44:26–30.

Pfeiffer, H. 1983. *Fascioloides magna:* erster fund in Österreich. *Wiener Tierarztliche Monatsschrift* 70:168–170.

Presidente, P.J.A., B.M. McCraw, and J.H. Lumsden. 1974. Early pathological changes associated with *Fasciola hepatica* infection in white-tailed deer. *Canadian Journal of Comparative Medicine* 38:271–279.

———. 1975. Experimentally induced *Fasciola hepatica* infection in white-tailed deer I. Clinicopathological and parasitological features. *Canadian Journal of Comparative Medicine* 39:155–165.

———. 1980. Pathogenicity of immature *Fascioloides magna* in white-tailed deer. *Canadian Journal of Comparative Medicine* 44:423–432.

Prestwood, A.K., F.E. Kellogg, S.R. Pursglove, and F.A. Hayes. 1975. Helminth parasitisms among intermingling insular populations of white-tailed deer, feral cattle, and feral swine. *Journal of the American Veterinary Medical Association* 166:787–789.

Price, E.W. 1953. The fluke situation in American ruminants. *The Journal of Parasitology* 39:119–134.

Price, E.W., and W.D. Kinchelow. 1941. The occurrence of *Dicrocoelium dendriticum* in the United States. *Journal of Parasitology* 27(supplement): 14.

Pursglove, S.R., A.K. Prestwood, T.R. Ridgeway, and F.A. Hayes. 1977. *Fascioloides magna* infection in white-tailed deer of southeastern United States. *Journal of the American Veterinary Medical Association* 171:936–938.

Pybus, M.J. 1990. Survey of hepatic and pulmonary helminths of wild cervids in Alberta, Canada. *Journal of Wildlife Diseases* 26:453–459.

Pybus, M.J., D.K. Onderka, and N. Cool. 1991. Efficacy of triclabendazole against natural infections of *Fascioloides magna* in wapiti. *Journal of Wildlife Diseases* 27:599–605.

Pybus, M.J., E.W. Butterworth, and J. Woods. Forthcoming. *Giant liver fluke* (Fascioloides magna) *in elk and other ungulates in Banff and Kootenay National Parks.* Edmonton: Alberta Fish and Wildlife.

Qureshi, T., T.M. Craig, D.L. Drawe, and D.S. Davis. 1989. Efficacy of triclabendazole against fascioloidiasis (*Fascioloides magna*) in naturally infected white-tailed deer (*Odocoileus virginianus*). *Journal of Wildlife Diseases* 25:378–383.

Qureshi, T., D.S. Davis, and D.L. Drawe. 1990. Use of albendazole in feed to control *Fascioloides magna* infections in captive white-tailed deer (*Odocoileus virginianus*). *Journal of Wildlife Diseases* 26:231–236.

Qureshi, T., D.L. Drawe, D.S. Davis, and T.M. Craig. 1994. Use of bait containing triclabendazole to treat *Fascioloides magna* infections in free ranging white-tailed deer. *Journal of Wildlife Diseases* 30:346–350.

Qureshi, T., G.G. Wagner, D.L. Drawe, D.S. Davis, and T.M. Craig. 1995. Enzyme-linked immunoelectrotransfer blot analysis of excretory-secretory proteins of *Fascioloides magna* and *Fasciola hepatica*. *Veterinary Parasitology* 58:357–363.

Radostits, O.M., D.C. Blood, and C.C. Gay. 1994. *Veterinary medicine,* 8th ed. London: Ballière Tindall, 1763 pp.

Rajcevic, M. 1929. Wie lange bleiben die Cerkarien der Leberegel (*Distoma hepaticum*) am getrockneten alten Heu lebend und infektionsfähig? *Deutsche Tierärztliche Wochenschrift* 34:535–537.

Rajský, D., A. Patus, and K. Bukovjan. 1994. Prvý, nález *Fascioloides magna* Bassi, 1875 na Slovensku. *Slovak Veterinarsky Casopis* 19:29–30.

Reimers, E., T. Ringberg, and R. Sørumgård. 1982. Body composition of Svalbard reindeer. *Canadian Journal of Zoology* 60:1812–1821.

Rhode, K. 1990. Phylogeny of Platyhelminthes, with special reference to parasitic groups. *International Journal for Parasitology* 20:979–1007.

Roberts, J.A., and Suhardono. 1996. Approaches to the control of fasciolosis in ruminants. *International Journal for Parasitology* 26:971–981.

Rognlie, M.C., K.L. Dimke, and S.E. Knapp. 1994). Detection of *Fasciola hepatica* in infected intermediate hosts using RT-PCR. *The Journal of Parasitology* 80:748–755.

Ronald, N.C., T.M. Craig, and R.R. Bell. 1979. A controlled evaluation of albendazole against natural infections with *Fasciola hepatica* and *Fascioloides magna* in cattle. *American Journal of Veterinary Medicine* 40:1299–1300.

Round, M.C. 1968. Check list of the helminth parasites of African mammals. St. Albans, England: Commonwealth Agricultural Bureau, Technical Communication No. 38, 252 pp.

Sakamoto, T., S. Abe, M. Suga, I. Kuno, and N. Yasuda. 1982. *Dicrocoelium dendriticum* (Rudolphi, 1819) Looss, 1899 from pika *Ochotona hyperborea yesoensis* Kishida in Hokkaido, Japan [In Japanese]. *Bulletin of the Faculty of Agriculture, Kaposhiena University* 32:119–123.

Salomon, S. 1932. *Fascioloides magna* bei deutschem Rotwild. *Berliner Tierärztliche Wochenschrift* 48:627–628.

Samuel, W.M., and W.A. Low. 1970. Parasites of the collared peccary from Texas. *Journal of Wildlife Diseases* 6:16–23.

Schillhorn van Veen, T.W. 1980. Fascioliasis (*Fasciola gigantica*) in West Africa: A review. *The Veterinary Bulletin* 50:529–533.

Schillhorn van Veen, T.W. 1987. Prevalence of *Fascioloides magna* in cattle and deer in Michigan. *Journal of the American Veterinary Medical Association* 191:547–548.

Schulte, J.W., W.D. Klimstra, and W.G. Dyer. 1976. Protozoan and helminth parasites of Key deer. *The Journal of Wildlife Management* 40:579–581.

Schuster, V.R., and B. Neumann. 1988. Zum jahreszeitlichen Auftreten von *Dicrocoelium dendriticum* in Zwischenwirten. *Angewandte Parasitologie* 29:31–36.

Schwartz, J.E., and G.E. Mitchell. 1945. The Roosevelt elk on the Olympic Peninsula, Washington. *The Journal of Wildlife Management* 9:295–319.

Senger, C.M. 1963. Some parasites of Montana deer. *Montana Wildlife.* Autumn: 5–13.

Sewell, M.M., and J.A. Hammond. 1972. The detection of *Fasciola* eggs in faeces. *The Veterinary Record* 90:510–511.

Shah, B.H., M. Nawaz, and N.I. Chaudhry. 1984. Chemotherapy of fascioliasis. *Pakistan Veterinary Journal* 4:56–59.

Sinclair, K.B. 1967. Pathogenesis of *Fasciola* and other liver flukes. *Helminthological Abstracts* 36(2): 115–134.

Sinclair, L.J., and D.A. Wassall. 1988. Sero-diagnosis of *Fasciola hepatica* infections in cattle. *Veterinary Parasitology* 27:283–290.

Singh, A., and D.K. Singh. 1994. Pestoban, a potent herbal molluscicide. *Biological Agriculture and Horticulture.* 10:175–178.

Slusarski, W. 1955. Studia nad europejskimi przedstawicielami przywry *Fasciola magna* (Bassi, 1875) Stiles, 1894. I. Ponowne wykrycie ogniska inwazji u jeleni na `Sląc̨sku. *Acta Parasitologica Polonica* 3:1–59.

Slusarski, W. 1956. Dalsze studia nad Europejskimi przedstawicielami *Fasciola magna* (Bassi, 1875) Stiles, 1894. II. Rozmieszczenie I Biologia pasożyta w Polsce. *Wiadomo`sci Parazytologiczne* 5:165–166.

Smith, H.J. 1978. Parasites of red foxes in New Brunswick and Nova Scotia. *Journal of Wildlife Diseases* 14:366–370.

Špakulová, M., J. Čorba, M. Várady, and D. Rajskỳ. 1997. Biončmia, vỳskyt a vỳznam cicavice obrovskej (*Fascioloides magna*), závažného parazita vol'ne žij£cich prež£vacov. *Veterinárnej Medicíne—Czechoslovakia* 42:139–148.

Stiles, C.W., and A. Hassall. 1894. The anatomy of the large American fluke (*Fasciola magna*), and a comparison with other species of the genus *Fasciola*. *Journal of Comparative Medicine and Veterinary Archives* 15:161–178, 225–243, 299–313, 407–417, 457–462.

———. 1895. The anatomy of the large American liver fluke (*Fasciola magna*) and a comparison with other species of the genus *Fasciola*. *Journal of Comparative Medicine and Veterinary Archives* 16:139–147, 213–222, 277–282.

Stromberg, B.E., J.C. Schlotthauer, and P.D. Karns. 1983. Current status of *Fascioloides magna* in Minnesota. *Minnesota Veterinarian* 23:8–13.

Stromberg, B.E., G.A. Conboy, D.W. Hayden, and J.C. Schlotthauer. 1985. Pathophysiologic effects of experimentally induced *Fascioloides magna* infection in sheep. *American Journal of Veterinary Research.* 46:1637–1641.

Sugár, L. 1978. *Dicrocoelium dendriticum* (Stiles and Hassall, 1896) el¢fordulása és jelentösége vadállományunkban. *Parasitologia Hungarica* 11:145–146.

Swales, W.E. 1933. The present status of the knowledge of the helminth parasites of domestic and semidomesticated mammals and economically important birds in Canada, as determined from work published prior to 1933. *Canadian Journal of Research* 8:468–482.

———. 1935. The life cycle of *Fascioloides magna* (Bassi, 1875), the large liver fluke of ruminants in Canada. *Canadian Journal of Research,* Series D, *Zoological Sciences* 12:177–215.

———. 1936. Further studies on *Fascioloides magna* (Bassi, 1875) Ward, 1917, as a parasite of ruminants. *Canadian Journal of Research* 14:83–95.

Sweatman, G.K. 1952. Endoparasites of muskrats in the vicinity of Hamilton, Ontario. *Journal of Mammalogy* 33:248–250.

Sztojkov, V., Majoros, G., and K. Kámán. 1995. Szarvasokban ébö nagy amerikai májmétely (*Fascioloides magna*) megjelenése Magyarországon. *Magyar állatorvosok Lapja* 50:157–159.

Torbit, S.C., L.H. Carpenter, D.M. Swift, and A.W. Alldredge. 1985. Differential loss of fat and protein by mule deer during winter. *The Journal of Wildlife Management* 49:80–85.

Trainer, C.E. 1969. *Ecological study of Roosevelt elk.* Oregon State Game Commission, Job Completion Report, Project Number W-59-R-6, 25pp.

Trudgett, A., A. Anderson, and R.E. Hanna. 1988. Use of immunosorbent-purified antigens of *Fasciola hepatica* in enzyme immunoassays. *Research in Veterinary Science* 44:262–263.

Ullrich, K. 1930. Über das Vorkommen von seltenen oder wenig bekannten Parasiten der Sägetiere und Vögel in Böhmen und Mähren. *Prager Archiz für Tiermedizin und Vergleichende Pathologie* 10:19–43.

Unruh, D.H., J.E. King, R.D. Eaton, and J.R. Allen. 1973. Parasites of dogs from Indian settlements in northwestern Canada: A survey with public health implications. *Canadian Journal of Compariative Medicine* 37:25–32.

Waruiru, R.M., E.H. Weda, and W.K. Munyua. 1994. The efficacy of triclabendazole and oxyclozanide against *Fasciola gigantica* in naturally infected dairy cattle in Kenya. *Bulletin of Animal Health and Production in Africa* 42:205–209.

Watson, T.G. 1981a. Growth of *Metorchis conjunctus* (Cobbold, 1860) Looss, 1899 (Trematoda: Opisthorchiidae) in the bile ducts of various definitive hosts. *Canadian Journal of Zoology* 59:2014–2019.

———. 1981b. *Metorchis conjunctus* (Cobbold, 1860) Looss, 1899 (Trematoda: Opisthorchiidae): Isolation of metacercariae from fish hosts. *Canadian Journal of Zoology* 59:2010–2013.

Wetzel, V.R., and K. Enigk. 1936. Zur Würmfauna des Elches. *Deutsche Tierärztliche Wochenschrift* 44:576–577.

Whiting, T.L., and S.V. Tessaro. 1994. An abbatoir study of tuberculosis in a herd of farmed elk. *Canadian Veterinary Journal* 35:497–501.

Wikerhauser, T., and J. Brglez. 1961. Vitalnosti metacerkarija *Fasciola hepatica* iz silaze. *Veterinarski Archiv Zagreb* 31:315–318.

Wilson, R.A., G. Smith, and M.R. Thomas. 1982. In *The population dynamics of infectious diseases: Theory and application.* Ed. R.M. Anderson. London: Chapman and Hall, pp. 262–319.

Wobeser, G., W. Runge, and R.R. Stewart. 1983. *Metorchis conjunctus* (Cobbold, 1860) infection in wolves (*Canis lupus*), with pancreatic involvement in two animals. *Journal of Wildlife Diseases* 19:353–356.

Wobeser, G., A.A. Gajadhar, and H.M. Hunt. 1985. *Fascioloides magna:* Occurrence in Saskatchewan and distribution in Canada. *Canadian Veterinary Journal* 26:241–244.

Yoakum, J., W.P. Dasmann, H.R. Sanderson, C.M. Nixon, and H.S. Crawford. 1980. In *Wildlife management techniques manual.* Ed. S.D. Schemnitz. Washington DC: The Wildlife Society, pp. 329–409.

Záhoř, Z. 1965. Výskyt velké motolice (*Fascioloides magna* Bassi, 1875) u srncí zvěře. *Veterinárskví* 15:322–324.

Záhoř, Z., C. Prokš, and J. Vítovec. 1966. Nález vajíček motolice *Fascioloides magna* (Bassi, 1875) a fascioloidézních změn v játrech skotu. *Veterinárni Medicína Praha* 11(39) 6:397–404.

7

TAENIASIS AND ECHINOCOCCOSIS

ARLENE JONES AND MARGO J. PYBUS[1]

INTRODUCTION. Members of the cyclophyllidean family Taeniidae are the most important cestodes in terms of their significance for human and animal health, and as a cause of economic loss in livestock. Currently, two genera, *Taenia* L., 1758, and *Echinococcus* Rudolphi, 1801, are recognized in the family (Rausch 1994). The genus *Taenia* includes almost 80 nominal species, fewer than half of which are considered valid. The life cycles of approximately 25 species are wholly sylvatic (involve only wildlife), and the remainder are largely or entirely pastoral (involve domesticated animals) or have both pastoral and sylvatic components. In the latter species, wildlife act as a reservoir of infection wherever they are sympatric with infected livestock. The genus *Echinococcus* contains 4 valid species, 3 of which have predominantly sylvatic cycles. Taeniids are unusual cestodes in that both the definitive and intermediate hosts are mammals.

Adult worms occupy the small intestine of carnivorous and omnivorous mammals and the larval stages, called cysticercus or coenurus (*Taenia*) and hydatid (*Echinococcus*), occupy a variety of sites, generally skeletal muscle or other soft tissues, in large and small herbivores. The cycle is completed when eggs voided with the feces of infected final hosts contaminate vegetation that subsequently is eaten by the intermediate hosts. Larvae move to preferred sites within the herbivores, where they stay until ingested by a suitable final host. As with most cestodes, the adult stage causes little or no problem to its host, but the larval stages of some species are markedly pathogenic.

Much remains to be discovered about species with sylvatic cycles, so the absence of information on various aspects of their biology (e.g., pathology in wild intermediaries) does not imply the absence of detrimental effects. Details are provided where available for each species.

Terms for the disease condition caused by these cestodes have varied over time and to some extent reflect an early misinterpretation of larval stages as distinct species. Currently disease conditions in the definitive host are known as taeniasis and in the intermediate host as cysticerciasis for species with a cysticercus, coenuriasis for those that have a coenurus (*Taenia multiceps, T. serialis*), and hydatidiasis for those with a hydatid larval stage.

Diagnosis of species is by characteristic morphology of gravid segments from feces and/or examination of adults recovered after purging the host or at necropsy. Differentiation of species often involves the size, shape, and number of rostellar hooks. Occasionally, features of the larval stages are diagnostic.

In this chapter we provide a general review of valid species of Taeniidae, with emphasis on those known to have disease potential in wild mammals or that pose concerns for human or livestock health. Identity of the family and genus follow Rausch (1994). The species composition broadly follows that of Verster (1969), with the addition of several recently described species. In the last approximately 25 years, much information concerning new species, life cycles, application of biochemical and molecular techniques, pathology, and treatment has emerged. Leiby and Dyer (1971) provide a comprehensive source for information up to that time, and duplication has been avoided here. Thus, tables presented in this chapter are compiled from literature records published since about 1970 and are not intended as fully comprehensive host or geographical lists. Additional sources of information have been indicated where appropriate.

ETIOLOGIC AGENTS

Family Taeniidae Ludwig, 1886. Strobila are long with numerous segments, or tiny with very few segments. The scolex has four acetabulate suckers; the rostellum is normally present, rarely absent, and is armed with two alternating rows of hooks of characteristic taenioid shape; rarely, one or three rows are present. There are two pairs of longitudinal osmoregulatory canals, dorsal and ventral, with transverse anastomoses at the posterior margin of each segment. There is one set of reproductive organs per segment, and genital pores are marginal, alternating irregularly. Testes are numerous, in one or more horizontal layers. The ovary is posterior, bialate. The vitelline gland is compact, postovarian. The uterus has a median longitudinal stem and lateral branches. Eggs have a thick-walled embryophore composed of truncated blocks. Larval stage is a cysticercus or modified cysticercus (coenurus, strobilocercus) or a multilocular or unilocular hydatid that reproduces by asexual proliferation. Adults found in fissiped carnivores and man, larvae in various mammals. Type genus is *Taenia* L., 1758.

[1]Corresponding author.

Genus _Taenia_ L., 1758. Strobila are ribbon-like with numerous segments; segments usually are wider than long when mature, longer than wide when gravid. Rostellum usually has two alternating rows of taenioid hooks; rarely, there are one or three rows, or rostellum and hooks absent and the first row is longer than the second row, rarely equal. Genital ducts are between or ventral to dorsal and ventral longitudinal osmoregulatory canals. Testes are confluent in midline or not. Uterine lateral branches usually redivide. Eggs have striated embryophores. Larva is a cysticercus, strobilocercus, or coenurus. Type species _Taenia solium_ L., 1758.

1. _TAENIA ACINONYXI_ ORTLEPP, 1938. _Taenia acinonyxi_ has 34–42 rostellar hooks; the first-row hooks measure 205–232 μm, the second 119–148 μm. Testes are in one horizontal layer, not quite reaching the anterior margin of the segment and extending posteriorly to the level of the vitelline gland. They are confluent anteriorly by a narrow bridge, but not confluent posteriorly. Genital ducts are between the longitudinal osmoregulatory canals. The cirrus sac is club-shaped and reaches the longitudinal osmoregulatory canals. The genital pore is posterior to the midpoint of the lateral margin. The aporal lobe of the ovary is usually larger than the poral lobe; lobes may be subequal. A vaginal sphincter is absent. The uterus has 6–10 primary lateral branches on each side. The species can be distinguished from _T. ingwei_ (see below) by the absence of a vaginal sphincter and by testes that are not confluent behind the vitellarium.

Adult _T. acinonyxi_ occur in leopard (_Panthera pardus_) and cheetah (_Acinonyx jubatus_). Intermediate hosts are not definitely known, but cysticerci with rostellar hooks resembling those of the adults were found in the muscles of African herbivores and suids (Verster 1969). Possible intermediaries are impala (_Aepyceros melampus_), sable antelope (_Hippotragus niger_), gerenuk (_Litocranius walleri_), gemsbok (_Oryx gazella_), grey duiker (_Sylvicapra grimmia_), African buffalo (_Syncerus caffer_), and warthog (_Phacochoerus aethiopicus_). The species is limited to the range of leopard and cheetah in sub-Saharan and sub-Sahelian zones (Graber et al. 1973). Little more is known of this species, perhaps reflecting its occurrence only in endangered hosts.

2. _TAENIA BRACHYACANTHA_ BAER AND FAIN, 1951. _Taenia brachyacantha_ has 54 rostellar hooks: the first-row hooks are 23.5–28 μm, the second 26 μm. Testes are in 1–2 horizontal layers, extending from the anterior margin of the segment to the level of the vitellarium. The cirrus sac extends beyond the longitudinal osmoregulatory canals into the medulla. Genital ducts are ventral to the longitudinal osmoregulatory vessels. Ovary lobes are subequal. A vaginal sphincter is absent. Genital atrium is large and deep; its position in the lateral margin is not clear. The uterus has 14–17 primary lateral branches. Little is known of this species. It occurs in Africa in the white-naped weasel (_Poecilogale albinucha_).

3. _TAENIA CRASSICEPS_ (ZEDER, 1800) RUDOLPHI, 1810.
Synonyms: _Taenia hyperborea_ von Linstow, 1905; _Hydatigera hyperborea_ (von Linstow, 1905) Abuladze, 1964; _Cysticercus longicollis_ Rudolphi, 1819.

Taenia crassiceps has 28–34 rostellar hooks; first-row hooks are 172–200 μm, the second 121–155 μm. Testes are usually in two horizontal layers, not quite reaching the anterior margin of the segment; they are confluent anterior to the ovary and posterior to the vitelline gland. Genital ducts are between the dorsal and ventral longitudinal osmoregulatory canals. The cirrus sac is oval and extends beyond the osmoregulatory canals to enter the medulla. The genital pore is slightly anterior to the middle of the lateral margin; the pore region is prominent. Ovary lobes are approximately equal in size. A vaginal sphincter is absent. The uterus in fully gravid segments has 10–20 primary lateral branches on each side. Cysticercus is a thin-walled bladder up to 5 mm.

LIFE HISTORY. A comprehensive account of adult development in experimentally infected foxes and dogs and of larval development in experimentally infected white mice was presented by Freeman (1962) and reviewed by Leiby and Dyer (1971). Kroeze and Freeman (1983) described the development of cysticerci in experimentally infected mice. Within 24 hours, the majority of cysticerci evaginated the scolex and collapsed or detached the bladder. However, the hooks rarely everted while the worms remained in the gut lumen. At 12 and 24 hours postinfection, 34% and 68%, respectively, of the larvae reached the peritoneal cavity, but some were still in the gut lumen at 16 days. Only 2 of 1566 from the gut lumen had everted hooks, and more than 96% of those from the peritoneal cavity still had inverted rostellar hooks. Although segmentation and development of genital primordia occasionally commenced in the small intestine and peritoneal cavity, sexual maturity was not achieved. Conversely, some worms in the peritoneal cavity began to produce buds either from portions of bladder that had been pulled into the peritoneal cavity or from solid non-bladder tissue.

EPIZOOTIOLOGY. _Taenia crassiceps_ occurs commonly throughout North America, Europe, and the former USSR. Adults are found in canids, including Arctic fox (_Alopex lagopus, A. lagopus innuitus_), wolf (_Canis lupus_), coyote (_C. latrans_), red foxes (_Vulpes vulpes, V. vulpes caucasica, V. corsac_), and domestic dogs, but there are isolated records from felids: for example, wild cat (_Felis silvestris_) and lynx (_Felis lynx_) in the former USSR (Abuladze 1964). Cysticerci occur in the subcutaneous and muscle tissue of the body cavities of a wide spectrum of naturally infected mammals including rats and mice (_Rattus rattus, Mus musculus, Pitymys_ spp.), lagomorphs (_Lepus europaeus_), voles (_Arvicola terrestris, Microtus arvalis, M. oeconomus,_

TABLE 7.1—Some recent[a] records of *Taenia crassiceps*

Hosts	Number Examined	Prevalence (%)	Location	Reference
Definitive Hosts				
Alopex lagopus	50	78	Northwest Territory, Canada	Eaton and Secord 1979
Felis silvestris	25	8	Germany	Schuster et al. 1993
Martes foina	47	6	Germany	Loos-Frank and Zeyhle 1982
Vulpes vulpes	101	21.8	Germany	Lucius et al. 1988
	1300	17.7	Germany	Pfeifer 1996
	801	19.9	Germany	Wessbecher et al. 1994
	397	28.5	Germany	Ballek et al. 1992
	3575	24	Germany	Loos-Frank and Zeyhle 1982
	154	25	France	Deblock et al. 1988
	150	29	France	Petavy et al. 1990a
Intermediate Hosts				
Dicrostonyx torquatus	6	1 of 6	Northwest Territory, Canada	Webster 1974
Marmota marmota	1	1 of 1	Germany	Fatzer et al. 1976
Marmota monax	150	7.3	Maryland, USA	Albert et al. 1981
	55	9	Maryland, USA	Albert et al. 1972
	501	2.6	New York and Maryland, USA	Anderson et al. 1990
Microtus arvalis	3184	1.0	Germany	Loos-Frank 1981
	37	8	France	Petavy et al. 1996
Ondatra zibethica	670	0.5	Germany	Friedland et al. 1985
Rodents	?[b]	?[b]	Czech Republic	Tenora and Stanek 1994

[a]Since 1970.
[b]Original paper not accessible to the authors.

M. socialis, M. pennsylvanicus), marmots (*Marmota marmota*), woodchucks (*M. monax*), chipmunks (*Tamias striatus*), squirrels (*Sciurus vulgaris,*) sousliks (*Citellus suslicus, C. citellus*), moles (*Talpa europaea*), muskrats (*Ondatra zibethicus*), lemmings (*Lemmus trimucrocoronatum, Dicrostonyx groenlandi, D. torquatus, D. exsul*), and hamsters (*Cricetus cricetus, C. auratus*).

PREVALENCE AND INTENSITY. There are few reports since 1970 (Table 7.1). A coyote in Montana had 256 worms, but coyotes are rare hosts (Seesee et al. 1983). Prevalence of larvae in intermediaries generally is low (< 10%).

CLINICAL SIGNS. Cysticerci in the brain of *Microtus arvalis,* the most susceptible intermediary in Germany, interfered with host coordination and movements (Reitschel 1981). Nervous disorders also were found in a marmot that had cysticerci in the central nervous system, lungs, omentum, subcutaneous tissue, and psoas muscles (Fatzer et al. 1976). Infected intermediaries may have externally visible swellings at the sites where the larvae are located.

PATHOLOGY AND PATHOGENESIS. Fibrosarcomatous mesotheliomas were found in experimentally infected gerbils (Rausch et al. 1987). Woodchucks trapped in New York and Maryland had numerous larvae, which caused large subcutaneous masses in the axillary region and adjacent thoracic wall (Albert et al. 1981; Anderson et al. 1990). In addition, a focal parasitic granuloma was found in the lungs of one woodchuck; another had larvae in the liver parenchyma. The parasites were surrounded by fibrotic tissue, and mild scattered-to-coalescing lymphocytic aggregates occurred in adjacent subcutaneous tissue. There was minimal infiltration into the musculature. The authors did not find a connection between *T. crassiceps* infection and woodchuck hepatitis virus infection.

DIAGNOSIS. This species differs from others found in canids (except *T. pisiformis*) in having testes confluent posteriorly as well as anteriorly and from *T. pisiformis* in having shorter hooks in the first row. In the intermediary, diagnosis is by recovery of cysticerci from subcutaneous sites or in the thoracic or abdominal cavities; they characteristically have exogenous buds, and the rostellar hooks, if developed, conform in shape and size to those of *T. crassiceps.*

PUBLIC HEALTH CONCERNS. Intraocular infections of humans with larvae of *T. crassiceps* were first reported in North America (Canada) in the early 1970s (Fallis et al. 1973; Freeman et al. 1973; Shea et al. 1973). Natural infection in a pet dog probably was the source of infection in one case (Freeman et al. 1973). Larvae were surgically removed from the retinas of two patients. The cysticerci had an evaginated scolex and exogenous buds (Freeman et al. 1973). More recently, larvae were found in the subcutaneous tissue and muscles of an AIDS patient (Chermette et al. 1995).

This species is widespread in domestic canids, which pose the major zoonotic potential. Regular anthelmintic treatment of dogs and good hygiene practices would reduce risks of human cases.

4. TAENIA CROCUTAE METTRICK AND BEVERLEY-BURTON, 1961. *Taenia crocutae* has 36–40 rostellar hooks: first row 159–201 µm, second row 107–132 µm. The strobila is not markedly muscular, and reproductive organs usually are visible through the tegument. Testes are in 1–2 horizontal layers, not reaching the anterior margin, and extending posteriorly to the level of the ovary; they are confluent anteriorly by a relatively narrow band. Genital ducts are between the dorsal and ventral longitudinal osmoregulatory canals. The cirrus sac does not reach the longitudinal osmoregulatory canals. The genital pore is just behind the midpoint of the lateral margin of a mature segment, more posterior in a gravid segment. The aporal lobe of the ovary is larger than the poral lobe; lobes may be subequal. A vaginal sphincter is present. Gravid segments are rectangular, much longer than wide. The uterus has 19–50 primary lateral branches.

EPIZOOTIOLOGY. Adult *T. crocutae* occur in spotted (*Crocuta crocuta*) and brown hyenas *(Hyaena brunnea)* in Africa. Intermediaries include *Adenota kob, Aepyceros melampus, Alcelaphus lelwel, Alcelaphus buselaphus, Connochaetes taurinus, Damaliscus lunatus, D. korrigum, Hippotragus equinus, H. niger, Kobus leche, Oryx gazelli, Redunca arundinum, Taurotragus derbianus, Tragelaphus scriptus, T. strepsiceros, Sylvicapra grimmia,* and *Syncerus caffer.* Cysticerci are recorded from baboons (*Papio* sp.) in Kruger National Park, South Africa (Department of Agricultural Technical Services, South Africa, 1973). One example of the life cycle of *T. crocutae* involves cysticerci in Grant's gazelles and adults in spotted hyenas (Sachs 1977). Cysticerci are located in the skeletal muscles of the intermediaries that are killed by hyenas or stolen or scavenged after predation by large cats or hunting dogs.

T. crocutae only matures in hyenas despite the fact that lions and other predators are exposed to cysticerci in the same species and often in the same carcass. Similarly, domestic cats and dogs given muscle cysticerci from antelopes and goats, and sheep and cattle given gravid segments of tapeworms from hyena and lion did not become infected (Sachs 1970). Also, attempts to infect Ayrshire calves with eggs as well as hatched, unactivated or activated oncospheres did not succeed (Harrison et al. 1985), indicating that *T. crocutae* would be unlikely to establish in cattle sharing grazing with wild herbivores. Bongo et al. (1982) failed to infect guinea pigs, mice, rabbits, pigs, and a calf with embryonated eggs.

PREVALENCE AND INTENSITY. *Taenia crocutae* was found in 1 of 9 spotted hyena in Ethiopia (Graber et al. 1980) and 1 of 2 in the Central African Republic (Graber 1981). In the latter area, cysticerci of *T. hyaenae* were more common than those of *T. crocutae* (10% of muscle cysticerci were *T. crocutae*), but *T. crocutae* was more common in ruminants in Tanzania, South Africa, and Zambia (Graber et al. 1973). They were found in 1 of 97 African buffalo, 1 of 23 hartebeest, and

1 of 10 roan antelope. *Taenia crocutae* was common in spotted hyenas and wild herbivores collected in Kenya and Tanzania during the 1980s (A. Jones, unpublished), but *T. hyaenae* was not found in either host group.

DIAGNOSIS. Segments of *T. crocutae* are rectangular and much longer than wide. Gravid segments have a high number of primary uterine branches, distinguishing them from other taeniids in hyenas. It differs from *T. hyaenae* in having testes confluent only anteriorly, and from *T. hyaenae, T. olngojinei* and *T. dinniki* in having smaller rostellar hooks. Kamanga-Sollo et al. (1992) identified antigens that could be used for immunodiagnosis of *T. crocutae.*

IMMUNITY. An antibody response was detected in each of three previously unexposed calves given eggs or oncospheres of *T. crocutae* (Harrison et al. 1985). The response was most marked in a calf given 5000 hatched, unactivated oncospheres per os.

Sachs (1970) postulated that Thomson's gazelles may have a general immunity to muscle cysticercosis or may be unsuitable hosts for the *Taenia* spp. in Serengeti predators. None of 50 Thomson's gazelles from the Serengeti National Park had muscle cysticerci, but 60%–80% of Grant's gazelles, wildebeest, topi, kongoni, and dik-dik were infected (Sachs 1966).

PUBLIC HEALTH AND ANIMAL HEALTH CONCERNS. Cysticerci in wild ruminant flesh have implications for the marketability of game venison (Graber et al. 1973). Concern arises partly for aesthetic reasons and partly because cysticerci in flesh often are assumed to be those of *T. saginata,* a significant public health concern. Macroscopically, the species cannot be distinguished; however, microscopically, rostellar hooks are present on the scolex of *T. crocutae.* Estimated losses in game cropping schemes may be 15%–20% of total carcass yield if infected meat is condemned as unfit for human consumption (Schindler et al. 1969). These observations apply to the cysticerci of *T. crocutae, T. gonyamai, T. hyaenae* and *T. acinonyxi* in game venison.

5. TAENIA DINNIKI JONES AND KHALIL, 1984. *Taenia dinniki* has 38–42 rostellar hooks: the first row 240–277 µm, the second 134–171 µm. Testes are mainly in one horizontal layer, two irregular layers in lateral regions. They do not quite reach the anterior margin of the segment and extend posteriorly to the level of the vitelline gland; they are confluent anteriorly, but not posteriorly. The cirrus sac is pyriform to club-shaped, approaching or reaching the ventral osmoregulatory canal. The genital ducts are between the longitudinal osmoregulatory canals. The genital pore is at or just behind the midpoint of the lateral margin. The aporal ovarian lobe is larger than the poral lobe. A vaginal sphincter is present. The uterus has 6–13 primary uterine branches on each side.

EPIZOOTIOLOGY. This species has only been found twice. Its life cycle is unknown. It occurs in Africa in the Rift Valley, Tanzania, and Muguga, Kenya (Jones and Khalil, 1984). Known definitive hosts are striped hyena (*Hyaena hyaena*) and spotted hyena. Intermediate host(s) are unknown.

DIAGNOSIS. The adult differs from *T. olngojinei* in having generally fewer hooks and smaller hooks; from *T. hyaenae* in having longer first-row hooks, and testes not confluent posteriorly; and from *T. crocutae* in having longer first-row hooks, greater posterior extent of the testes, fewer primary uterine branches, and in the shape of the gravid segments.

6. *TAENIA ENDOTHORACICUS* (KIRSCHENBLATT, 1948).
Synonyms: *Multiceps endothoracicus* (Kirschenblatt, 1948) Dubnitsky, 1952; *Coenurus endothoracicus* Kirschenblatt, 1948.

Taenia endothoracicus has 52–64 rostellar hooks; first-row hooks are 300–378 μm, second 201–241 μm. Testes are mainly anterior to the ovary, extending close to the anterior margin of the segment and to the level of the vitellarium posteriorly. They are confluent anteriorly but not posteriorly; the number of layers is not documented. The cirrus sac extends to the longitudinal osmoregulatory canals. Genital ducts are between the longitudinal osmoregulatory canals. The genital pore is anterior to the midpoint of the lateral margin. Ovary lobes are subequal, almost spherical. A vaginal sphincter is apparently absent. The uterus has 10–12 primary lateral branches. Larva is polycephalic, described as a large branching coenurus with 3–19 invaginated scolices (Abuladze 1964).

EPIZOOTIOLOGY. Adult occurs in foxes (*Vulpes vulpes*) in North Africa, the former USSR, and Asia. The larva is located free or encapsulated in the thoracic and abdominal cavity of various rodents, including *Gerbillus pyramidus hirtipes*, *Meriones erythrourus*, *M. shawi*, *M. tamariscinus*, *M. tristrami* and *Rhombomys opimus*.

PATHOLOGY AND PATHOGENICITY. In the small intestine of experimentally infected *Vulpes corsac*, scolices of *T. endothoracicus* penetrated the crypts of Lieberkuhn, sometimes to the stratum compactum (Blazek et al. 1982). Villi and crypts were atrophied, and scattered hemorrhages and diffuse inflammatory infiltration of eosinophils occurred around the scolex.

DIAGNOSIS. In rodents, diagnosis is by recovery of the coenurus; the number and length of the rostellar hooks distinguishes this species from others with a coenurus larva. The adult resembles *T. laticollis*, but the latter is a parasite of *Lynx* spp. whereas *T. endothoracicus* is a parasite of foxes (Verster 1969).

7. *TAENIA GONYAMAI* ORTLEPP, 1938.
Synonym: *Taenia hlosei* Ortlepp, 1938.

Taenia gonyamai has 32–40 rostellar hooks: first row 183–222 μm, second row 120–144 μm. Testes are in one horizontal layer, extending from the anterior margin of the segment to the posterior margin; they are confluent anteriorly, not posteriorly. Genital ducts are between osmoregulatory canals. The cirrus sac is club-shaped or pyriform and usually reaches the osmoregulatory canals. Genital pore is posterior to the midpoint of the lateral margin; the pore region is not prominent. The aporal lobe of the ovary is larger than the poral lobe. A vaginal sphincter is present. The uterus has 14–22 primary lateral branches. Larva is a cysticercus.

EPIZOOTIOLOGY. Adult worms occur in lions (*Panthera leo*) and cheetah (*Acinonyx jubatus*) in central and eastern Africa. The cysticercus occurs in the muscles of *Alcelaphus buselaphus* and *Connochaetes taurinus*. It may also occur in the lymph nodes and lung tissue (Sachs 1970). Sachs (1969, 1977) postulated a host-parasite relationship between lion, impala, and wildebeest in the life cycle of *T. gonyamai* in East Africa. A lioness in Nairobi National Park, Kenya, had *T. gonyamai* as well as rabies and microbesnoitosis (Bwangamoi et al. 1990).

There appears to be a separating mechanism between *Taenia* spp. in lions and hyenas. Only *T. gonyamai*, *T. regis,* and *T. simbae* become gravid in lions, although immature specimens, some with hooks characteristic of the hyena parasites *T. crocutae* or *T. hyaenae* (cited as *T. lycaontis*) occur (Dinnik and Sachs 1972). The authors suggest that lions ingest cysticerci of other species, but for unknown reasons these cannot mature. Lions and hyenas frequently eat from the same carcass, and both must be exposed to a variety of *Taenia* species [except *T. olngojinei* (see below), the cysticerci of which are inaccessible to lions]. There are no reliable literature reports of lion-associated *Taenia* spp. in hyenas, jackals, or hunting dogs, or vice versa, and no such infections have been found in extensive collections from lions, canids, and hyaenids in East Africa (A. Jones, unpublished).

PREVALENCE AND INTENSITY. Information regarding prevalence and intensity is limited. Intensity of *T. gonyamai* was 38, 42, 62, and 81 in four lions from the Serengeti area of northern Tanzania (Dinnik and Sachs 1972). These authors also found immature *Taenia* sp., *T. regis,* and *T. simbae*. Graber (1981) found *T. gonyamai* in one of three lions in the Central African Republic.

DIAGNOSIS. Gravid segments of *T. gonyamai* have a greater number of primary uterine branches (14–30 on each side) than those of other species from lions: *T. regis* has 2–10, *T. simbae* has 7–12. The rostellar hooks are smaller than those of the other two species, and the species lacks the posteriorly confluent testes of *T. simbae*. The cysticercus locates in skeletal musculature, whereas those of *T. regis* and *T. simbae* occur in serosa. Hook number and length overlap those of the hyena parasites *T. hyaenae* and *T. crocutae,* which also have cysticerci in skeletal muscle, but the large hooks of *T. gonyamai* often, but not invariably, have a dorsal indentation near the junction of the blade and handle.

8. *TAENIA HYAENAE* BAER, 1926.
Synonyms: *Taenia lycaontis* Baer and Fain, 1995; *Cysticercus dromedarii* Pellegrini, 1945.

Taenia hyaenae has 28–38 rostellar hooks: the first row 202–223 µm, the second 127–165 µm. Testes are in one horizontal layer, extending between the anterior and posterior margins of the segment; they are confluent anteriorly and posteriorly to the female organs. Genital ducts are between the longitudinal osmoregulatory vessels. The cirrus sac is pyriform and reaches the longitudinal osmoregulatory vessels. The genital pore is posterior to the midpoint of the lateral margin; there are no conspicuous genital papillae. The aporal lobe of the ovary is larger than the poral lobe. A vaginal sphincter is present. The uterus has 10–14 primary lateral branches. The cysticercus locates in skeletal and cardiac muscles.

EPIZOOTIOLOGY. Adults occur in hyenas (*Crocuta crocuta, Hyaena brunnea*) or hunting dogs (*Lycaon pictus*) in Africa. Cysticerci occur in *Adenota kob, Alcelaphus lelwel, Camelus dromedarius, Gazella granti, G. thomsoni, G. soemmeringi, Hippotragus equinus, Sylvicapra grimmia, Syncerus caffer, Taurotragus derbianus, Tragelaphus scriptus,* and zebu cattle.

PREVALENCE AND INTENSITY. Adult worms have been found in 2 of 3 spotted hyaenas in the Central African Republic and in mixed infections with *T. crocutae* in 5 of 7 spotted hyaenas in Ethiopia (Graber 1978; Graber et al. 1973, 1980). Cysticerci of *T. crocutae* and *T. hyaenae* are difficult to distinguish. Muscle cysticerci with hooks corresponding in number and size to *T. hyaenae* were found in Grant's gazelle (Sachs 1969), but later revised to *T. crocutae* (see Sachs 1970). Despite mixed infections of the two species, Graber et al. (1973) estimated 90% of muscle cysticerci in ruminants in the Central African Republic were *T. hyaenae.* Prevalence was 19.5% in buffalo and 11% in antelopes in the Central African Republic (Graber 1981). Cysticerci have been found in 0.6% of 1000 camels in Egypt and in the following in the Central African Republic: 18% of 97 buffalo, 1 of 8 kob, 1 of 10 roan antelope, 13% of 23 hartebeest, 1 of 5 giant eland, and 1 of 3 bushbuck (Graber et al. 1973; Darwish and El Bahy 1991).

DIAGNOSIS. Adult *T. hyaenae* can be distinguished from *T. olngojinei* by the smaller rostellar hooks and by testes confluent anteriorly and posteriorly. It can be distinguished from *T. crocutae* by the generally smaller rostellar hooks and the smaller number of uterine branches in the gravid segment, and from *T. dinniki* by the generally smaller number and size of the hooks.

Cysticerci have hooks of the same number, length, and shape as those of the adults.

DOMESTIC ANIMAL HEALTH CONCERNS. Although there are reports of larvae in zebu cattle, there appears to be no risk to human health. Similarly, the adults appear to be restricted to hyenas and hunting dogs.

9. *TAENIA HYDATIGENA* PALLAS, 1766.
Synonyms: *T. ursina* von Linstow, 1893; *T. jakhalsi* Ortlepp, 1938; *Cysticercus tenuicollis* Rudolphi, 1810. For additional synonyms, see Abuladze (1964). Synonym of *T. jakhalsi* (proposed by Verster 1969) was confirmed by Jones et al. (1988).

Taenia hydatigena has 26–44 rostellar hooks: the first row 170–226 µm, the second 110–160 µm. Strobila have rectangular to square mature segments. Testes are in a single horizontal layer, extending to the anterior and posterior margins of segment; they are confluent anteriorly to the female organs but not posteriorly to the vitellarium, although rarely, some testes may be scattered behind the vitelline gland. The cirrus sac is elongated and club-shaped and reaches or just fails to reach the longitudinal osmoregulatory canals but does not cross them. Genital ducts are between the longitudinal osmoregulatory canals. The genital pore opens about midway along the lateral margin; the pore area is not prominent. The aporal lobe of the ovary is larger than the poral lobe. There is no vaginal sphincter. Fully gravid segments are wider than long, 10–14 x 4–7 mm, with 6–10 primary lateral uterine branches on each side. Cysticercus occurs in serosal tissue and is the largest *Taenia* cysticercus in this site; the thin-walled bladder is usually 25–40 mm in diameter but can attain the size of a hen's egg or larger. The invaginated scolex has a long 'neck' region.

LIFE HISTORY. *Taenia hydatigena* is a fecund species. There are no data for wild hosts, but gravid segments appeared in the feces of experimentally infected dogs after 48–65 days, each worm shed ~2 gravid segments/day and potentially about 100,000 eggs/day (Gregory 1976a). The point of attachment within the gut can affect egg production and environmental contamination (Coman and Rickard 1975). Shed segments in the gut lumen of dogs contained about 500 eggs; those still attached to the strobila contained about 31,000, indicating that most eggs were shed into the intestinal lumen. Eggs hatched and became activated, particularly if they were shed in the anterior part of the intestine. Although the infectivity of *T. hydatigena* was not studied, that of *T. pisiformis* eggs was reduced in these circumstances (Coman and Rickard 1975).

EPIZOOTIOLOGY. This species has a cosmopolitan distribution in a variety of domestic and wild carnivores, usually canids, and less frequently, felids: *Canis familiaris, C. lupus, C. latrans, C. mesomelas, C. aureus, Vulpes vulpes, Felis concolor, Lynx rufus* (Table 7.2).

TABLE 7.2—Some recent[a] records of *Taenia hydatigena*

Hosts	Number Examined	Prevalence (%)	Location	Reference
Definitive Hosts				
Canis lupus	25	16	Quebec, Canada	McNeill et al. 1984
	89	?[b]	Italy	Guberti et al. 1993
Felis concolor	39	10	Oregon, USA	Rausch et al. 1983
	1	1 of 1	California, USA	Jessup et al. 1993
Panthera leo	1	1 of 1	Nigeria [zoo]	Ogunbade and Ogunrinade 1984
Vulpes vulpes	397	0.8	Germany	Ballek et al. 1992
	140	8.6	Czechoslovakia	Letkova et al. 1989a
Intermediate Hosts				
Alces alces	51	75	Ontario, Canada	Addison et al. 1979
	191	61	Alberta, Canada	Pybus 1990
	177	70–100	European USSR	Mikhailova et al. 1983
Aplodontia rufa	26	23	Washington and Oregon, USA	Canaris and Bowers 1992
Capreolus capreolus	345	18	Hungary	Murai and Sugar 1979
	50	12	Czechoslovakia	Letkova et al. 1989b
	12	17	Spain	Navarrete et al. 1990
Castor fiber	1	1 of 1	Voronezh	Romashov 1973
Cephalophus monticola	3	2 of 3	South Africa	Boomker et al. 1991
Cercopithecus aethiops	52	19	Sudan	Sulaiman et al. 1986
Erythrocebus patas	26	39	Sudan	Sulaiman et al. 1986
Cervus dama	23	22	Czechoslovakia	Letkova et al. 1989b
Cervus elaphus	32	9	Czechoslovakia	Letkova et al. 1989b
Cervus elaphus hippelaphus	70	36	Hungary	Murai and Sugar 1979
Cervus elaphus nelsoni	97	2	Alberta, Canada	Pybus 1990
Dama dama	35	20	Hungary	Murai and Sugar 1979
Gazella subgutturosa	4	1 of 4	Turkmenia	Dobrynin 1987
Martes foina	67	4.5	Germany	Pfeiffer et al. 1989
Odocoileus h. hemionus	247	14	Alberta, Canada	Pybus 1990
Odocoileus virginianus	159	35	Ontario, Canada	Addison et al. 1988
	140	5	Alberta, Canada	Pybus 1990
	124	1	Florida, USA	Forrester and Rausch 1990
	30	20	Ohio, USA	Schurr et al. 1988
Ovibos moschatus	5	2 of 5	Northwest Territories, Canada	Webster and Rowell 1980
Ovis musimon	17	41	Hungary	Murai and Sugar 1979
	7	2 of 7	Czechoslovakia	Letkova et al. 1989b
Rangifer tarandus	510	24.5	Siberia	Mozgovoi et al. 1979
Rupicapra rupicapra	2	2 of 2	Czechoslovakia	Letkova et al. 1989b
Sus scrofa	44	43	Hungary	Murai and Sugar 1979
	96	"few"	Germany	Mennerich-Bunge et al. 1993
	60	10	Czechoslovakia	Letkova et al. 1989b
	91	3	Alberta, Canada	Dies 1979
Ursus americanus	141	4	Quebec, Canada	Frechette and Rau 1977

[a]Since 1970.
[b]Original paper not accessible to the authors.

There is one record of infection in a grizzly bear (*Ursus arctos*) (Dies 1979). Infection is reported from *Panthera leo* in a Nigerian zoo (Ogunbade and Ogunrinade 1984), but this probably reflects zoo conditions and feeding regimes; lions in the wild do not harbor this parasite as an adult although they are exposed to larvae in prey animals. The species also has a wide range of intermediate hosts, including domestic livestock (cattle and other bovids, sheep, goats, suids) and wild animals, principally cervids, *Alces alces*, *Odocoileus hemionus hemionus*, *O. virginianus*, *Cervus elaphus nelsoni* (Table 7.2). Cysticerci have been reported from primates (Sulaiman et al. 1986).

PREVALENCE AND INTENSITY. Despite the relatively large number of hosts identified, there is a degree of host specificity in the adult stage. *Taenia hydatigena* was not found in 7 lions from Tanzania, 1 from Kenya, 3 from Uganda, or 2 from Zambia, and reports from lions may be erroneous (Dinnik and Sachs 1972). Similarly, although recorded from foxes (Table 7.2), these hosts are not significant, at least in some countries. *Taenia hydatigena* was not found in foxes in Australia (Coman and Ryan 1974) or Wales, despite the fact that it occurred in 9.6% of 882 Welsh farm dogs and 6.5% of the 875 foxhounds examined during the same period (Jones and Walters 1992a,b). Foxes tend to prey on rabbits, but they will opportunistically scavenge sheep carcasses. Thus, their role in transmitting taeniids tends to be insignificant.

The dominant definitive and intermediate hosts differ in different geographical areas and localities (Table 7.2). In North American boreal forests, the cycle is mainly wolf-moose (Samuel et al. 1976; Addison et al. 1979; McNeill et al. 1984; Pybus 1990), a reflection of one of the primary predator-prey relationships in the boreal region. In other Canadian habitats, the cycle may involve coyotes (Samuel et al. 1976) or deer (Addison et al. 1988, Pybus 1990). In wolves, prevalence differed in different regions (Holmes and Podesta 1968; McNeill et al. 1984) and was higher than in coyotes (Holmes and Podesta 1968). In the intermediate hosts, prevalence and intensity differed among host species (Pybus 1990) and in different habitats (Samuel et al. 1976; Pybus 1990) and increased with age (Samuel et al. 1976; Addison et al. 1979, 1988), but did not differ between sexes. Although prevalence may be quite high (reaching 60%–70%), intensity usually remains low (< 10 cysticerci). Similarly, Mikhailova et al. (1983) found *T. hydatigena* in most moose from the former European USSR; however, mean intensities up to 26 cysticerci were recorded.

Taenia hydatigena (= *Cysticercus tenuicollis*) was not found during extensive studies of cysticerciasis in game animals in East Africa during the 1960s (Sachs and Sachs 1968; Sachs 1969, 1970). However, more recently it was identified frequently in large and small antelopes from East Africa and has extended its range, perhaps in conjunction with human migration and movements of domestic livestock (A. Jones, unpublished). There are occasional records from South Africa (Verster et al.1975; Boomker et al. 1991) and Turkmenistan (Dobrynin 1987), but information is limited.

Vervets (*Cercopithecus aethiops*) and African red monkeys (*Erythrocebus patas*) captured in central Sudan had cysticerci in the serosa and on the liver and other organs (Sulaiman et al. 1986) (Table 7.2). Mean intensity was 6.7 (range 1–30) and 5.1 (range 1–26) in vervet and red monkeys, respectively, but most animals had 1–3 cysticerci.

PATHOLOGY. There are no significant effects in definitive hosts, and intermediates also appear to tolerate infections without ill effect. There are few accounts of the pathology of the cysticerci in wild hosts. Migrating larvae may cause liver lesions similar to those seen in infected lambs (Trees et al. 1985), pigs (Blazek et al. 1985), and sheep (Sogoyan et al. 1982). Fibrous adhesions and localized hepatic peritonitis, retarded antler growth, and loss of body weight were seen in heavily infected moose in the European former USSR (Mikhailova et al. 1983); however, physical condition of moose in Ontario was not related to intensity of infection (Addison et al. 1979). A 3-week-old wapiti calf died with a grossly enlarged liver containing hundreds of *T. hydatigena* larvae (McKenna et al. 1980).

Migration tracks and subcapsular hemorrhages were found in the liver of four mature female wombats (*Vombatus ursinus*) experimentally infected with *T. hydatigena* eggs (see Presidente 1979). One animal also had an hepatic granuloma probably provoked by a degenerating larva. Similar lesions occurred in three of seven naturally infected wombats in Victoria, Australia; however, wombat probably is an aberrant host with no significance in perpetuating *T. hydatigena*.

DIAGNOSIS. Adults can be distinguished from those of *T. ovis, T. serialis, T. multiceps,* and *T. taeniaeformis* by the absence of a vaginal sphincter or pad, and from *T. pisiformis* and *T. crassiceps* in having testes confluent only anteriorly. It differs from *T. polyacantha* in the shape of the rostellar hooks and cirrus sac. In areas of Africa where more than one species may occur in the serosa of ungulates, *T. hydatigena* cysticerci are larger, and the number and length of the rostellar hooks differ from *T. regis* (see page 168).

Recently, molecular techniques were applied to this species. Characteristic patterns of ribosomal DNA of *T. hydatigena* (see Gasser and Chilton 1995) and isoelectric profiles indicated distinct differences among various African *Taenia* spp. (Allsopp et al. 1987).

CONTROL AND TREATMENT. Niclosamide [Phenasal] at 250 mg/kg body weight in two doses at a 35-day interval was effective against *T. hydatigena, T. multiceps,* and *Echinococcus* spp. in naturally or experimentally infected wolves, foxes, jackals, hyenas, and dogs (Bekirov and Dzhumaev 1976). However, control of cestodes in wild hosts generally is not feasible. Regular anthelmintic treatment of domestic dogs would reduce contamination of the environment with eggs. Safe disposal of carcasses and offal would render cysticerci inaccessible to scavenging wild or domestic carnivores. Because this is a common cosmopolitan species, the success of these measures would be limited.

MANAGEMENT IMPLICATIONS. Transmission of *Taenia* spp. among domestic and wild carnivores and herbivores will occur wherever ranges overlap, particularly in situations where human-related pressure on land and resources intensifies the competition with wild animals by encroaching on wildlife reserves. The recent appearance of *T. hydatigena* in East Africa, as mentioned above, is one example. Although there are no significant public health concerns associated with this species, cysticerci in the liver of game animals are relatively conspicuous and thus often a source of concern for the hunting public. These concerns can be alleviated easily by appropriate education programs.

10. *TAENIA INGWEI* ORTLEPP, 1938. *Taenia ingwei* has 30–40 rostellar hooks, first row 183–220 μm, second row 123–151 μm. Testes are in one horizontal layer, are confluent only anteriorly, and extend to the level of the vitelline gland posteriorly. Genital ducts are between the longitudinal osmoregulatory canals. The cirrus sac is club-shaped and reaches the longitudinal osmoregulatory canals or not. The genital pore is near the midpoint of the segment. The aporal lobe of the ovary is larger than the poral lobe. A vaginal sphincter is present. The uterus has 5–11 primary lateral branches.

EPIZOOTIOLOGY. Little is known about this species. Adults occur in leopards; larvae are unknown. The species differs from *T. acinonyxi,* the other taeniid in leopards, in having a vaginal sphincter.

11. *TAENIA KREPKOGORSKI* (SCHULZ AND LANDA, 1934).
Synonym: *Hydatigera krepkogorski* Schulz and Landa, 1934. Considered a *species inquirendum* by Verster (1969) but validated by Bray (1972).

Taenia krepkogorski has a rostellum armed with 60–76 hooks; the first-row hooks measure 265–354 µm, the second 182–222 µm. Unusually, first-row hooks alternate, giving the impression of a double row of long hooks (see also *T. macrocystis*). Testes are in 2–3 horizontal layers, confluent anteriorly not posteriorly. The cirrus sac is club-shaped and reaches the ventral osmoregulatory canal. Genital ducts are ventral to the osmoregulatory canals. The genital pore is near the midpoint of the lateral margin. The poral ovarian lobe is smaller than the aporal lobe. A vaginal sphincter is absent. The uterus has 4–5 primary lateral branches on each side.

EPIZOOTIOLOGY. The adult is parasitic in the gut of felids (*Felis lybica caudata, F. lybica ocreata, F. margarita, F. chaus, F. silvestris*) and, less commonly, canids (*Vulpes vulpes, V. vulpes karagan*). The larval stage is a strobilocercus in the abdominal mesentery of rodents (*Rhombomys opimus, Gerbillus meridianus, Meriones erythrourus*). Gerbils may be the primary intermediate (Bray 1972). This species occurs in Azerbaijan, Turkmenistan, and Bahrain and may be limited to the desert areas of southwest central Asia.

12. *TAENIA LATICOLLIS* RUDOLPHI, 1819. *Taenia laticollis* has 58–62 rostellar hooks, first row 370–407 µm, second row 183–247 µm. Testes are in 2–3 horizontal layers, extending from the anterior to the posterior margins of the segment; they are confluent anteriorly but not posteriorly. Genital ducts are between the osmoregulatory canals. The cirrus sac reaches and may cross the osmoregulatory canals. The genital pore is just behind the midpoint of the lateral margin. The aporal ovarian lobe is larger than the poral lobe. A vaginal sphincter is absent. The uterus has 15–20 primary lateral branches.

EPIZOOTIOLOGY. This species is known only from lynx in North America.

13. *TAENIA MACROCYSTIS* (DIESING, 1850).
Synonym: *Cysticercus macrocystis* Diesing, 1850.

The scolex of *T. macrocystis* is armed with 54–74 hooks: first-row hooks 297–430 µm, second 180–247 µm. There is an unusual arrangement of hooks in the first circle: alternate hooks are set more posteriorly, giving the appearance of a double row of long hooks. Handles of the anterior hooks are more robust than the posterior hooks, although they are similar in length. The strobila is small, up to 12 cm, with 90–100 segments. Testes are in two horizontal layers, extending to the anterior and posterior margins of the segment; they are confluent anteriorly to the female organs but not

posteriorly. Genital ducts are between the osmoregulatory canals. The cirrus sac is long, extending across the dorsal and ventral osmoregulatory canals into the medulla. The genital pore is prominent. The ovary lobes are subequal, or the aporal lobe is slightly larger. A vaginal sphincter is absent. Gravid segments have 8–16 primary uterine branches on each side.

EPIZOOTIOLOGY. This species is adapted to the close predator-prey relationship between felids and lagomorphs. Adults occur in *Felis tigrina, F. yagouarundi, F. macroura, F. baileyi, F. weidii weidii, F. geoffroyi paraguae, Lynx canadensis,* and *L. rufus* in South and North America. Reports from *Canis lupus* and *Vulpes vulpes* in the former USSR (Abuladze 1964) are doubtful (Verster 1969). The monocephalic strobilocercus larva occurs in or on the back muscles; on the abdominal mesenteries, diaphragm, and pericardium; and encapsulated on the liver of *Sylvilagus brasiliensis, Lepus americanus, L. californicus deserticola,* and *L. timidus.* Larvae also were found in *Sciurus vulgaris* in the former USSR. The life cycle was confirmed experimentally (Bursey and Burt 1970).

PREVALENCE AND INTENSITY. Bursey and Burt (1970) remarked on the high prevalence of *T. macrocystis* in the definitive and intermediate hosts. Adult worms were found in 86% of 129 bobcat, *Lynx rufus,* and 100% of 14 lynx, *L. canadensis,* and in some areas cysticerci occurred in nearly 100% of snowshoe hares.

DIAGNOSIS. Polyacrylamide gel electrophoresis was used to determine species-specific band patterns for total proteins (Bursey et al. 1980). Single segments were identified, and the technique can be used in field situations.

14. *TAENIA MADOQUAE* (PELLEGRINI, 1950) JONES, ALLSOPP, MACPHERSON AND ALLSOPP, 1988.
Synonym: *Cysticercus madoquae* Pellegrini, 1950.

Taenia madoquae rostellum is armed with 26–36 hooks: first row 165–194 µm, second row 106–132 µm. Testes extend from the anterior margin of the segment to the posterior margin or the level of the vitelline gland, mainly in one horizontal layer, and are confluent anteriorly but not posteriorly. Genital ducts are between the longitudinal osmoregulatory canals. The cirrus sac is flask-shaped and usually reaches the osmoregulatory canals. The genital pore is at or just behind the midpoint of the lateral margin of the segment; papilla is usually prominent. The aporal ovarian lobe is larger than the poral lobe. A vaginal sphincter is present. The uterus has 9–17 primary uterine branches on each side.

LIFE HISTORY. Although little is known of this species in the wild, it is one of the few taeniids from wild animals to have the life cycle completed experimentally (Jones et al. 1988). Cysticerci collected from the skeletal muscle of dik-dik (*Madoqua guentheri*) in Kenya were fed to a 5-week-old pup previously dosed with anthelmintics. A single adult worm was found at necropsy 42 days later. Scolex character and strobilar morphology were the same as those of previously undescribed adults from naturally infected silver-backed jackals (*Canis mesomelas*). Furthermore, isoenzyme profiles (glucose phosphate isomerase, hexokinase, and lactate dehydrogenase) of the cysticerci, adults from jackal, and the experimentally obtained adult were the same.

The location in the host, and the number and length of the hooks resemble those of *T. ovis*, but there are no reliable records of *T. ovis* in East Africa, and the adult morphology is quite different. *Taenia ovis* cysticerci from dik-dik in Somalia (Cornaglia 1984) probably are *T. madoquae*.

15. *TAENIA MARTIS* (ZEDER, 1803).

Synonyms: *T. intermedia* Rudolphi, 1810; *T. skrjabini* Romanov, 1952; *T. sibirica* Dubnitzky, 1952. Wahl (1967) erected two subspecies, subsequently accepted by Verster (1969): *T. martis martis* in Europe and *T. martis americana* in North America and the former USSR. Anterior row of rostellar hooks of the former are longer than those of the latter. However, Pence and Willis (1978) suggest the subspecies question should be reexamined. There is one report of *T. m. americana* in Germany (Schoo 1993). *T. sibirica* is a synonym of *T. m. americana* (see Verster 1969).

Taenia m. martis has 28–40 rostellar hooks: first row 175–220 μm, second row 130–169 μm. *Taenia m. americana* has 24–30 hooks, which are 134–157 μm and 125–141 μm. Testes are in two horizontal layers, confluent anteriorly but not posteriorly to female organs. The genital ducts are ventral to the longitudinal osmoregulatory canals. The cirrus sac reaches the ventral osmoregulatory canal but does not extend beyond. The genital pore is near the midpoint of the lateral segment margin; there are no prominent genital papillae. The aporal ovarian lobe is larger than the poral lobe. There is no vaginal sphincter. A fully gravid uterus has 6–15 primary uterine branches on each side. The larval stage is a monocephalic cysticercus.

LIFE HISTORY. Larvae in the thoracic cavity of naturally infected *Clethrionomys glareolus* and experimentally infected *Microtus agrestis* and white mice were infective to marten (*Martes martes*) (see Shakhmatova 1963). Adults began to shed segments 43 days after infection. Larvae also developed in small rodents (common voles, bank voles, white mice) experimentally infected with eggs from polecats (*Putorius putorius*) (see Prokopic 1970). Schuster and Benitz (1992) successfully infected mice with eggs.

EPIZOOTIOLOGY. Mustelids are the major definitive hosts, with reports from *Martes martes, M. foina,*

Mustela vison, M. erminea, M. nivalis, and *P. putorius* in Europe and the former USSR and from *Martes americana, M. pennanti,* and *Bassariscus astutus* in North America. Records from canids are doubtful (Verster 1969). A record from *Felis silvestris* (see Schuster et al. 1993) is considered spurious. Larvae occur in small rodents including *Apodemus agrarius, Clethrionomys glareolus, Lemmus sibiricus, Microtus agrestis, M. arvalis, M. xanthognathus, Mus musculus, Ondatra zibethicus,* and *Pitymys subterraneus.*

Prevalence differs markedly in different locations (Table 7.3). In fisher, prevalence was higher in males than females (Dick and Leonard 1979). Intensity of adult worms generally is low (< 5 worms) (Pence and Willis 1978; Dick and Leonard 1979; Hoberg et al. 1990).

16. *TAENIA MULTICEPS* LESKE, 1780.

Synonyms: *Multiceps multiceps* (Leske, 1780) Hall, 1919; *M. gaigeri* Hall, 1916; *M. skrjabini* Popov, 1937; *Coenurus cerebralis* (Batsch, 1786) Rudolphi, 1808.

The *T. multiceps* rostellum has 22–34 hooks; large hooks are 120–180 μm, small hooks 73–160 μm. The strobila is fairly delicate. Testes are in two horizontal layers, not extending to the anterior margin of the segment, but reaching the level of the vitelline gland posteriorly; they are confluent anteriorly, leaving a clear area in front of ovary, but not confluent behind vitelline gland. The cirrus sac is small, not reaching the longitudinal osmoregulatory canals. Genital ducts are between the canals. The genital pore is just behind the midpoint of the lateral margin, and the pore area is slightly elevated. The aporal lobe of the ovary is larger than the poral lobe. Vaginal pad present on the anterior wall of the vagina. The uterus has 9–26 primary lateral branches on each side; branches are bluntly rounded, giving gravid segments a characteristic appearance. The larva is a polycephalic coenurus, up to 10 cm in diameter. The bladder wall is delicate with scattered clusters of scolices.

EPIZOOTIOLOGY. *Taenia multiceps* has a well-established pastoral life cycle in dogs and domestic livestock and a sylvatic cycle in wild canids and wild herbivores. Canids acquire infection by preying on or scavenging infected herbivores or being fed their carcasses. The intermediaries, including large mammals, rodents, and lagomorphs, ingest eggs on contaminated pasture. In domestic livestock and large wild mammals, coenuri normally locate in the central nervous system, most often the cerebral hemispheres but also the spinal cord. In rodents and lagomorphs, coenuri invade the central nervous system or the subcutaneous or intermuscular connective tissue. Adult worms in carnivores can be numerous. A fertile cyst from *Oryx gazella* gave rise to over 100 adult worms when fed to a dog (Verster and Bezuidenhout 1972).

This species has a cosmopolitan distribution in domestic and wild canids (*Canis familiaris, C. lupus,*

TABLE 7.3—Some recent[a] records of *Taenia martis*

Hosts	Number Examined	Prevalence (%)	Location	Reference
Definitive Hosts				
Bassariscus astutus	15	20	Texas, USA	Pence and Willis 1978
Felis silvestris	25	4	Germany	Schuster et al. 1993
Martes americana	?	3	North America [arctic/subarctic]	Rausch 1977
	78	38	Washington, USA	Hoberg et al. 1990
Martes foina	152	14	Czechoslovakia	Prokopic 1970
	67	15	Germany	Pfeiffer et al. 1989
	259	2.3	Germany	Schoo 1993
	162	15	Manitoba, Canada	Dick and Leonard 1979
	47	36	Germany	Loos-Frank and Zeyhle 1982
	259	24.7	Germany	Schoo 1993
Martes martes	12	17	Czechoslovakia	Prokopic 1970
	5	3 of 5	Georgia	Rodonaya et al. 1985
Meles meles	84	2	Germany	Loos-Frank and Zeyhle 1982
Mustela erminea	24	4	Czechoslovakia	Prokopic 1970
Mustela vison	9	1 of 9	Spain	Miquel et al. 1992
Putorius putorius	305	18	Czechoslovakia	Prokopic 1970
Vulpes vulpes	397	0.3	Germany	Ballek et al. 1992
	3573	< 0.1	Germany	Ballek et al. 1992
	1	1 of 1	France	Deblock and Petavy 1993
Intermediate host				
Apodemus flavicollis	380	5.3	Germany	Loos-Frank 1981
Apodemus sylvaticus	124	1.6	Germany	Loos-Frank 1981
Clethrionomys glareolus	345	2	Czechoslovakia	Prokopic 1970
	436	4.8	Germany	Loos-Frank 1981
Microtus agrestis	215	0.5	Germany	Loos-Frank 1981
Microtus arvalis	802	0.3	Czechoslovakia	Prokopic 1970
	3184	0.1	Germany	Loos-Frank 1981
Microtus xanthognathus	1	1 of 1	Yukon Territory, Canada	Rausch 1977
Pitymys subterraneus	58	2	Czechoslovakia	Prokopic 1970

[a]Since 1970.

C. latrans, C. mesomelas, Alopex lagopus, Vulpes vulpes, Nyctereutes procyonoides), and rarely, felids (*Felis concolor*) (Table 7.4). Experimental infections have been established in *Vulpes corsak,* but this species is not as suitable as dogs (Zhuravets 1973). Coenuri are found in domestic cattle, sheep, goats, pigs, and many wild hosts (*Bos bonasus, B. grunniens, Camelus dromedarius, C. bactrianus, Capra sibirica, C. severtzowi, Capreolus capreolus, Gazella subgutturosa, Hippotragus equinus, Ovis orientalis, O. musimon, O. ammon, Oryx gazella, Rangifer tarandus, Rupicapra rupicapra, R. pyrenaica, Saiga tatarica, Sus scrofa, Lepus americanus*). There are occasional reports of the larva in primates in zoos; for example, gelada baboon, *Theropithecus gelada* (see Leith and Satterfield 1974; Tscherner et al. 1988).

CLINICAL SIGNS. Larvae in the central nervous system may cause a disease variously called gid, sturdy, or staggers. Clinical signs are associated with growing cysts in the brain (Kelly and Payne-Johnson 1993) and may take 6–8 months to appear. They vary slightly according to the number and location of the cysts. Lack of motor coordination is common. Sheep infected with one coenurus in the cerebral hemisphere may walk in circles in a direction opposite to the side of the brain in which the larva is located. Vision, posture, and gait also may be affected. Paralysis of the hindquarters may

occur if the coenurus is in the spinal cord. Depression, anorexia, emaciation, and death may occur in sheep (Soulsby 1982; Doherty et al. 1989). A lamb experimentally infected with eggs from *Vulpes corsak* died of acute coenuriasis (Zhuravets 1973). A naturally infected chamois caught in France lacked the normal escape reactions, inclined its head to one side, and had visual disturbances (Graber and Gevrey 1976).

PATHOLOGY AND PATHOGENESIS. Oncospheres are carried in the blood, and those that reach the central nervous system move through the nervous tissue, leaving migratory tracts. Acute meningoencephalitis results from heavy infections, with migratory tracts and encephalitis visible at necropsy. Necrotic lesions form around the coenuri, with leucocytic infiltration on the periphery. As the coenurus grows the skull may become soft or develop holes. After surgical removal of a cyst, a collapsed subcortical cavity lined by siderotic fibrovascular tissue and surrounded by gliomesodermal tissue remained (Kelly and Payne-Johnson 1993).

DIAGNOSIS. *Taenia multiceps* is the only species in canids to possess a vaginal pad rather than a sphincter. In large mammals, clinical signs may be suggestive of infection, but this is not specific; diagnosis must be confirmed at necropsy. PCR-based restriction fragment

TABLE 7.4—Some recent[a] records of *Taenia multiceps*

Hosts	Number Examined	Prevalence (%)	Location	Reference
Definitive Hosts				
Canis latrans	329	—[b]	Texas, USA	Radomski and Pence 1993
Canis lupus	89	?[c]	Italy	Guberti et al. 1993
	18	61	Tadzhikistan	Polishchuk and Dolgov 1979
Felis concolor	53	4	Texas, USA	Waid and Pence 1988
Vulpes vulpes	397	3.3	Germany	Ballek et al. 1992
Foxes	52	23	Tadzhikistan	Polishchuk and Dolgov 1979
Intermediate Hosts				
Ctenodactylus gundi	1	1 of 1	Tunisia	Bernard and Ben Rachid 1970
Oryx gazella	1	1 of 1	South Africa	Verster and Bezuidenhuit 1972
Ovis musimon	17	5.9	Hungary	Murai and Sugar 1979
Rupicapra pyrenaica	2	2 of 2	Spain	Lavin et al. 1995
	1	1 of 1	France	Graber and Gevrey 1976
Theropithecus gelada	1	1 of 1	Massachussetts, USA	Leith and Satterfield 1974
	1	1 of 1	Ethiopia (imported to Germany)	Tscherner et al. 1988

[a]Since 1970.
[b]Data not provided.
[c]Original paper not accessible to the authors.

techniques can be used to obtain characteristic patterns for *T. multiceps* (see Gasser and Chilton 1995).

CONTROL AND TREATMENT. Anthelmintic treatment of carnivores (Bekirov and Dzhumaev 1976) and safe disposal of carcasses to avoid scavenging would help reduce the problem. Surgical removal of the cyst from the brain of an infected sheep has been described (Kelly and Payne-Johnson 1993).

PUBLIC AND DOMESTIC ANIMAL HEALTH CONCERNS. Human infection with the coenurus occurs rarely (Graber 1976). As indicated above, infection in livestock can be debilitating or fatal.

17. *Taenia mustelae* Gmelin, 1790.

Synonyms: *Taenia tenuicollis* Rudolphi, 1819; *T. brevicollis* Rudolphi, 1819; *Halysis mustelae* Zeder, 1803.

The *T. mustelae* rostellum is armed with 38–66 hooks in a double row; all hooks are very small and more or less equal in length (12–21 μm). The strobila is small, up to 150 mm. Testes are confluent anteriorly but not posteriorly and extend from the anterior margin of the segment to the level of the ovary. The genital ducts are ventral to the longitudinal osmoregulatory canals. The cirrus sac extends beyond osmoregulatory canals into the medulla. The genital pore is just behind the midpoint of the lateral margin; genital papilla is prominent. Ovarian lobes are almost equal. A vaginal sphincter is absent. The uterus has 10–23 lateral branches on each side.

EPIZOOTIOLOGY. Adults occur in mustelids (*Mustela erminea, M. vison, M. nivalis, M. sibirica, M. altaica, M. eversmanni, Martes americana, M. martes, M. foina, M. zibellina, Putorius putorius*) throughout the northern hemisphere (Table 7.5). Cysticerci occur in various tissues in a wide range of sciurid and cricetid rodents (*Apodemus sylvaticus, Aplodontia rufa, Mus musculus, Rattus norvegicus, Microtus arvalis, M. socialis, M. oeconomus, M. majori, M. nivalis, M. agrestis, M. pennsylvanicus, M. miurus paneaki, M. schilovski, M. mirhanreini, Arvicola terrestris, Clethrionomys rufocanus, C. glareolus, C. gapperi, C. rutilus, Cricetus cricetus, Cynomys leucurus, Peromyscus maniculatus, P. leucopus, Synaptomys borealis, S. cooperi, Lemmus trimucronatus, Ondatra zibethicus, Pitymys subterraneus, Citellus fulvus, C. franklinii, Sciurus vulgaris, S. carolinensis, S. niger rufiventer, Marmota monax, Tamias striatus, Eutamias minimus, Aplodontia rufa,* and *Zapus hudsonius*).

Limited experimental study suggests some host specificity of adult *T. mustelae*, with mink apparently more suitable than ferret and with the production of singular or multiple scolices in rodents, despite the species of host (Freeman 1956). However, monocephalic larvae were seen in naturally infected muskrats (Todd et al. 1978) and fox squirrel (Langham et al. 1990).

PATHOLOGY AND PATHOGENESIS. Cysticerci can be associated with hepatic damage, including intraperitoneal hemorrhage prior to encapsulation of larvae (Freeman 1956) and parasitic granulomas in chronic infections (Roth et al. 1991). Excessive liver damage and hemorrhage killed some rodents (Freeman 1956). A fox squirrel, *Sciurus niger,* had many clear spherical cysts ~1 mm in diameter throughout the liver parenchyma (Langham et al. 1990). The larvae had provoked an intense inflammatory reaction, mainly lymphocytes with some eosinophils, and deposition of fibrous connective tissue. Migration routes were indicated by foci of necrosis and hemorrhage.

TABLE 7.5—Some recent[a] records of *Taenia mustelae*

Hosts	Number Examined	Prevalence (%)	Location	Reference
Definitive Hosts				
Marmota broweri	22	1	Alaska, USA	Rausch 1977
M. caligata	80	4	Alaska, USA	Rausch 1977
Martes americana	43	5	North America [arctic/subarctic]	Rausch 1977
Mustela erminea	50	?[b]	Spain	Feliu et al. 1991
	—[c]	—[c]	North America [arctic/subarctic]	Rausch 1977
	78	38	Washington, USA	Hoberg et al. 1990
Mustela nivalis	—[c]	—[c]	North America [arctic/subarctic]	Rausch 1977
Mustela vison	—[c]	—[c]	North America [arctic/subarctic]	Rausch 1977
	100	13	Montana, USA	Barber and Lockard 1973
Intermediate Hosts				
Aplodontia rufa	26	23	Washington and Oregon, USA	Canaris and Bowers 1992
Apodemus sp.	230	1	France	Le Pesteur et al. 1992
Clethrionomys glareolus	349	24	France	Le Pesteur et al. 1992
	436	1.2	Germany	Loos-Frank 1981
Cynomys leucurus	17	6	Wyoming, USA	Seville and Williams 1989
Marmota monax	1	1 of 1	Alaska, USA	Rausch 1977
Microtus agrestis	—[c]	—[c]	Finland	Haukisalmi et al. 1994
	47	9	France	Le Pesteur et al. 1992
	215	0.5	Germany	Loos-Frank 1981
Microtus arvalis	37	5	France	Petavy et al. 1996
	195	0.5	Hungary	Gubanyi et al. 1992
	2520	1	France	Le Pesteur et al. 1992
	3184	0.2	Germany	Loos-Frank 1981
Ondatra zibethica	1	1 of 1	Illinois, USA	Todd et al. 1978
Pitymys subterraneus	75	5	France	Le Pesteur et al. 1992
Sciurus niger rufiventer	1	1 of 1	Michigan, USA	Langham et al. 1990

[a]Since 1970.
[b]Original paper not accessible to the authors.
[c]Data not provided.

DIAGNOSIS. Adults and larvae of this species can be distinguished from other taeniids by the small size of the rostellar hooks and the similarity in length of hooks of the first and second rows.

18. *TAENIA OLNOJINEI* DINNIK AND SACHS, 1969. *Taenia olnojinei* has 42–48 rostellar hooks: the first row 274–314 μm, the second 167–222 μm. Testes are in one horizontal layer extending from the anterior margin of the segment to the level of the ovary, mainly in two lateral groups. Contrary to original description, they may be confluent anteriorly. Genital ducts are between the longitudinal osmoregulatory canals. The cirrus sac reaches the osmoregulatory canals. The aporal lobe of the ovary is larger than the poral lobe. A vaginal sphincter is absent. The uterus has 10–15 primary lateral branches.

EPIZOOTIOLOGY. Adults are known from spotted hyena (*Crocuta crocuta*) in Tanzania (Dinnik and Sachs 1969a) and the Central African Republic (Graber 1981) and in striped hyena (*Hyaena hyaena*) in the Central African Republic (Graber et al. 1972). It also occurs in Kenya (A. Jones, unpublished). Larvae occur in large antelope of the Alcelaphinae (hartebeeste group) (Sachs 1970, 1977), including *Alcelaphus buselaphus, Connochaetes taurinus, Damaliscus korrigum,* and *Gazella granti*. Its life cycle exhibits an extremely strong host-parasite relationship. Cysticerci occur only in the sacral epidural space. Prior to finding adult worms, it was reasoned that the definitive host was likely to be a hyena, the only animals with jaws powerful enough to crack the sacrum and gain access to the cysticerci (Sachs and Sachs 1968). Prevalence in hartebeests in Tanzania was 60%–90% (Sachs 1970, 1977).

DIAGNOSIS. *Taenia olnojinei* can be distinguished from other species in hyenas by the greater length of the anterior row of rostellar hooks; the testes typically, although not invariably, are in two lateral groups. The location of the cysticercus is unique to this species.

19. *TAENIA OMISSA* LUHE, 1910. *Taenia omissa* has 38–44 rostellar hooks: the first row is 232–297 μm, the second is 180–223 μm. The strobila is unusually wide, 9–11.5 mm. Testes are in a single horizontal layer, not reaching the anterior or posterior margins of the segment and extending posteriorly as far as the ovary. They are rarely confluent in front of the female organs and if so, only by a narrow bridge; they are not confluent posteriorly. Genital ducts are between the longitudinal osmoregulatory canals. The cirrus sac does not quite reach the longitudinal osmoregulatory vessels. The genital pore is just posterior to the midpoint of the lateral margin. The poral lobe of the ovary is smaller than the aporal lobe. A vaginal sphincter is present. The

uterus has up to eight primary lateral branches on each side. The cysticercus locates in lungs and pericardium.

EPIZOOTIOLOGY. *Taenia omissa* occurs in felids (*Felis concolor, F. tigrina, F. yaguarundi, F. azteca, F. oregonensis, F. hipploestes*) in North and South America. Larvae occur in deer (*Odocoileus virginianus, O. hemionus, Mazama* sp.).

PREVALENCE AND INTENSITY. Prevalence of adult *T. omissa* often approaches 100% in cougar throughout their range (Schmidt and Martin 1978; Rausch et al. 1983; Forrester et al. 1985; Waid and Pence 1988). In Texas, Oregon, and Alberta, mean intensity was 47, 54, and 33, respectively (Waid and Pence 1988; Rausch et al. 1983; and W.M. Samuel et al., unpublished; respectively).

Stubblefield et al. (1987) compared the prevalence and intensity of *T. omissa* cysticerci from the thoracic cavity in symmpatric Texas populations of white-tailed deer (29%, 3.8 ± 2.1) and mule deer (40%, 3.5 ± 0.6). Differences were attributed to the habitat preferences of the hosts and selective predation by cougar. In Florida, prevalence was 7% of 124 white-tailed deer, and intensity ranged from 1 to 15 (Forrester and Rausch 1990). Stock (1978) and Pybus (1990) found it in 1 of 60 and 2 of 263 mule deer, respectively, and 0 of 60 and 147 white-tailed deer, respectively, in Alberta.

DIAGNOSIS. The hook size and number overlap with those of *T. rileyi*, but *T. omissa* has fewer primary uterine branches and a wider strobila. A vaginal sphincter is consistently present in *T. omissa*, but in *T. rileyi* a sphincter and/or pad on the anterior wall of the vagina may be present in segments of the same strobila. *Taenia rileyi* is the only taeniid to show such variability in this character.

20. *TAENIA OVIS KRABBEI* (COBBOLD, 1869) VERSTER, 1969.

Synonyms: *Taenia krabbei* Moniez, 1879; *T. cervi* Christiansen, 1931; *T. djeirani* Boev, Sokolova and Tazieva, 1964; *Cysticercus tarandi* Villot, 1883. Verster (1969) split the species into two subspecies, *T. ovis ovis* and *T. ovis krabbei,* differentiated by their biological characteristics. They cannot be distinguished on morphological criteria. Most reports from wildlife are of *T. ovis krabbei,* but records of *T. ovis ovis* are included here when relevant.

Taenia ovis krabbei has 22–36 rostellar hooks: first row 137–195 µm , second row 85–141 µm. The strobila is broad and flat. Testes are in a single dorsal layer, extending from the anterior margin of the segment to the level of the ovary; they are confluent anteriorly but not posteriorly. Genital ducts are between the longitudinal osmoregulatory canals. The cirrus sac is oval and small, usually extending only halfway to the longitudi-

nal osmoregulatory canals; it may reach them if the strobila is contracted. The genital pore is just behind the midpoint of the lateral margin; the genital papilla is very prominent. The poral lobe of the ovary is smaller than the aporal lobe. A vaginal sphincter is present. The uterus has 8–24 primary lateral branches on each side. The cysticercus is usually found in skeletal and cardiac muscle.

EPIZOOTIOLOGY. *Taenia o. ovis* has a cosmopolitan distribution and a predominantly pastoral life cycle in dogs and sheep, whereas *T. o. krabbei* has a predominantly sylvatic life cycle and has a circumpolar distribution in wild canids and cervids. Specific hosts for adult *T. o. krabbei* include *Alopex lagopus, Canis familiaris, C. lupus, C. latrans, Felis concolor, Ursus americanus,* and *U. arctos* (Table 7.6). Recent records of interest include brown bear in Siberia (Odnokurtsev 1990) and black bear in New Brunswick, Canada (Duffy et al. 1994). Intermediate hosts include *Alces alces, Antilocapra americana, Capreolus capreolus, Cervus e. hippelaphus, Dama dama, Gazella subgutturosa, Odocoileus h. hemionus, Ovis musimon, Rangifer tarandus,* and *R. caribou silvestris. Cysticercus ovis* from a dik-dik (*Madoqua* sp.) in Somalia (Cornaglia 1984) may be misidentified (see *T. madoquae*), and *T. ovis* from wolves in Italy (Guberti et al. 1993) are likely *T. o. krabbei.* Reports of *T. o. krabbei* cysticerci in elk (*Cervus elaphus*) and Rocky Mountain bighorn sheep (*Ovis canadensis*) (Kingston and Honess 1982) are few and need to be confirmed.

Cattle, sheep, goats, and pigs are refractory to *T. o. krabbei,* and deer (*Dama dama, Cervus elaphus*) are refractory to *T. o. ovis* (Sweatman and Henshall 1962). Similarly, these taeniids show some specificity among wild canids. In Australia, where *T. o. ovis* is a major cause of economic loss in sheep, natural infections were not found in Tasmanian devil (*Sarcophilus harrisii*) and attempts to infect this host did not succeed (Coman and Ryan 1974). Foxes also are not significant in the life cycle of this species (Coman and Ryan 1974; Williams 1976; Jones and Walters 1992b). The primary host in North America is the wolf, although there are records from coyote (Seesee et al. 1983) and cougar (Rausch et al. 1983; Rickard and Foreyt 1992). Bears are considered insignificant in the epizootiology of the species (Choquette et al. 1968; Addison et al. 1979; Duffy et al. 1994). Although prevalence in wolves may reach 50%–70% (Rausch and Williamson 1959; Holmes and Podesta 1968; Volodina 1982), it rarely exceeds 5% in other definitive hosts.

There are many reports of *T. o. krabbei* cysticerci from reindeer; however, reindeer also are intermediate hosts *of T. parenchymatosa* and *T. hydatigena.* Although 26% of reindeer in the Yakut ASSR had cysticercosis, the prevalence of *T. o. krabbei* was < 1% (Isakov and Olesova 1979). Similarly, the species was found in only 2.6% of 6884 reindeer in the Magadan area of the former USSR (Zhidkov and Yurev 1984). Prevalence was higher in reindeer > 10 years old

TABLE 7.6—Some recent[a] records of *Taenia ovis krabbei*

Hosts	Number Examined	Prevalence (%)	Location	Reference
Definitive Hosts				
Canis lupus	89	?[b]	Italy	Guberti et al. 1993
	7	5 of 7	European	Volodina 1982
Canis latrans	219	1.4	Montana, USA	Seesee et al. 1983
Felis concolor	39	62	Oregon, USA	Rausch et al. 1983
	2	1 of 2	Washington, USA	Rickard and Foreyt 1992
Ursus americanus	91	1	Alberta, Canada	Dies 1979
	12	25	New Brunswick, Canada	Duffy et al. 1994
	55	4	Quebec, Canada	Frechette and Rau 1977
	83	2.4	Ontario, Canada	Addison et al. 1978
Ursus arctos	—[c]	—[c]	Montana, USA	Seesee and Worley 1986
	1	1 of 1	Siberia	Odnokurtsev 1990
	21	10	Yukon Territory, Canada	Choquette et al. 1968
Vulpes vulpes	100	?[b]	Austria	Hinaidy 1971
	101	1	Germany	Lucius et al. 1988
Intermediate Hosts				
Alces alces	54	74	Ontario, Canada	Addison et al. 1979
	—[c]	—[c]	Alberta, Canada	Samuel 1972
	80	4	Maine, USA	Gibbs and Eaton 1983
	—[c]	—[c]	Montana, USA	Seesee and Worley 1986
	470	4	European	Volodina 1982
Antilocapra americana	2	2 of 2	Wyoming, USA	Shults and Stanton 1986
Capreolus capreolus	345	33	Hungary	Murai and Sugar 1979
Cervus elaphus hippelaphus	70	19	Hungary	Murai and Sugar 1979
Dama dama	35	6	Hungary	Murai and Sugar 1979
Odocoileus h. hemionus	—[c]	—[c]	Montana, USA	Seesee and Worley 1986
Ovis musimon	17	12	Hungary	Murai and Sugar 1979
Rangifer tarandus	108	—	Norway	Bye 1985
	?[b]	?[b]	Siberia	Dorzhiev 1982a
	6884	2.6	Magadan area	Zhidkov and Yurev 1984

[a]Since 1970.
[b]Original paper not accessible to the authors.
[c]Data not provided.

(18–26%). Prevalence declined after anthelmintic treatment of dogs and safe disposal of dog feces and reindeer carcasses. In reindeer on Svalbard Island, Norway, *T. o. krabbei* was found only in animals > 1 year old; prevalence in females was highest in summer (Bye 1985).

Prevalence and intensity of cysticerci often is high in moose populations that are sympatric with infected wolves (e.g., Samuel 1972; Samuel et al. 1976). Prevalences in the range of 50%–70% have been reported, and prevalence and intensity increased with age (Samuel et al. 1976; Addison et al. 1979). In the latter study, degenerate cysts were found in all age classes. Pybus (unpublished) estimated an infection of 50,000 cysticerci in a yearling bull moose in Alberta. The cysticerci were essentially present in all skeletal muscles as well as the connective tissue fascia in and between the muscles.

Larvae of *T. o. krabbei* rarely are associated with significant tissue damage or loss of body condition, even in heavy infections (M.J. Pybus, unpublished). Infiltrating mononucleocytes, leucocytes, and plasma cells with a few polymorphonucleocytes, as well as perivascular cuffing, increased local gliosis, and tissue compression was seen adjacent to encapsulated cysticerci in the brain of three moose in Maine (Gibbs and Eaton

1983). Reinfection with *T. o. ovis* can occur (Coman and Rickard 1975), and field data suggest that intermediate hosts continue to accumulate cysts (Samuel et al. 1976; Addison et al. 1979).

DIAGNOSIS. There are no morphological differences between the two subspecies of *T. ovis;* they are distinguished on the basis of biological characteristics. In addition, *T. o. ovis* has been characterized by DNA analysis (Gasser and Chilton 1995). See *T. parenchymatosa* for further information.

CONTROL AND TREATMENT. Niclosamide at 250 mg/kg body weight or arecoline in gelatine capsules was effective against *T. o. krabbei* and *T. parenchymatosa* in working dogs (Shumilov and Dorzhiev 1982; Dorzhiev 1982b). Six annual treatments and provision of cooked or frozen meat also is recommended (Dorzhiev 1982a); however, some cysticerci embedded 2–2.5 cm in cooked meat may remain infective.

MANAGEMENT IMPLICATIONS. Cysticerci in the muscles of hunter-killed moose may be an aesthetic concern for the hunter and result in wastage of meat if infected animals are abandoned. Similarly, reindeer culled for human consumption may be unattractive if the flesh contains cysticerci. Removal of taeniid cysticerci reduced carcass weight by about 55 kg, resulting in annual loss of 50 tons of reindeer meat (Isakov and Olesova 1979). However, *T. o. krabbei* does not infect humans, and the cysticerci are killed by freezing and normal cooking temperatures. Unfrozen cysts should not be fed to domestic dogs.

21. *TAENIA PARENCHYMATOSA* PUSHMENKOV, 1945.

Taenia parenchymatosa has 30–34 rostellar hooks: first row 210–240 μm, second row 124–160 μm. Testes are confluent anteriorly, not posteriorly. Genital ducts are between the longitudinal osmoregulatory canals. The cirrus sac is oval and extends to the ventral osmoregulatory canal. The genital pore is just anterior to the midpoint of the lateral margin and is not very prominent. The aporal lobe of the ovary is bigger than the poral lobe. A vaginal sphincter may be absent. The uterus has 9–10 primary lateral branches on each side.

EPIZOOTIOLOGY. *Taenia parenchymatosa* occurs in arctic fox *(Alopex lagopus)* and domestic dogs in the northern regions of the former USSR. Cysticerci occur in the liver, heart, and lungs of *Rangifer tarandus* and *Cervus elaphus*. In reindeer, prevalence was 7.4%, 25.7%, and 59.2% in Magadan, Tyumen, and Siberia, respectively (Zhidkov and Yurev 1984; Kirichek and Belousov 1984; Mozgovoi et al. 1979; respectively). In Yakut ASSR, percent prevalence was 7.3 to 8.6 (Isakov and Olesova 1979). It also has been reported in the Koryak region (Zelinskii 1973).

DIAGNOSIS. Cysticerci of *T. parenchymatosa* are similar to those of *T. o. krabbei;* however, first-row hooks of *T. parenchymatosa* are distinctly longer. The predilection site for *T. o. krabbei* cysticerci is skeletal muscles; that for *T. parenchymatosa* is liver; but both can occupy other sites. In the adult stage, *T. o. krabbei* has a more prominent genital papilla, the cirrus sac does not reach the osmoregulatory canals, and the uterus has a greater number of primary uterine branches.

CONTROL AND TREATMENT. Anthelmintic treatment of dogs and safe disposal of dog feces and reindeer carcasses are the most effective means of control (Zhidkov and Yurev 1984). (See comments regarding *T. o. krabbei*).

MANAGEMENT IMPLICATIONS. Although there are no public health concerns, reindeer meat infected with cysticerci is unacceptable for human consumption.

22. *TAENIA PARVA* BAER, 1926.
Synonym: *Multiceps macracantha* Clapham, 1942.

Taenia parva has 36–48 rostellar hooks: first row 302–424 μm, second row 205–266 μm. The strobila is very small, up to 55 mm, and strongly muscular. Testes are in 1–3 horizontal layers, extending from the anterior to the posterior margins of the segment. They are confluent before and behind the female organs. Genital ducts are ventral to the longitudinal osmoregulatory canals. The cirrus sac extends across the osmoregulatory canals into the medulla. The genital pore is just anterior to the midpoint of the lateral margin. The aporal lobe of the ovary is larger than the poral lobe. A vaginal sphincter is absent. The uterus has 7–13 primary uterine branches on each side.

EPIZOOTIOLOGY. *Taenia parva* occurs in Europe and Africa in small wild felids and viverrids (*Genetta genetta, G. ludia, G. tigrina, Felis silvestris, Ictonyx striatus, Herpestes ichneumon*). The polycephalic larvae occur in the liver of rodents (*Apodemus sylvaticus, Arvicanthis niloticus, Mus musculus, M. minutoides, Rattus chrysophilus, R. namaquensis, R. paedulus, Rhabdomys pumilio, Praomys natalensis*). Recent reports include Alvarez et al. (1987), Elowni and Abu Samra (1988), and George et al. (1990), although information remains limited. The adult was found in 19 of 21 (Miquel et al. 1992) and 12 of 15 (Alvarez et al. 1990) *G. genetta* in Spain. The larva occurred in 2.47% of 242 *Apodemus sylvaticus* in Spain (Alvarez et al. 1987).

DIAGNOSIS. Adults can be distinguished from other taeniids in the same hosts (*T. endothoracicus, T. selousi*) by the small strobila and large rostellar hooks. *Taenia selousi* also has a polycephalic larva but has more and shorter hooks than *T. parva*.

23. *TAENIA PISIFORMIS* (BLOCH, 1780) GMELIN, 1790.
Synonyms: *Taenia serrata* Goeze, 1782; *Cysticercus pisiformis* (Bloch, 1780) Zeder, 1808. See Abuladze (1964) for a full list.

Taenia pisiformis has 32–48 rostellar hooks: first row 220–294 μm, second row 114–177 μm. The strobila is characteristically serrated. Testes are in 2–4 horizontal layers, extend to the anterior and posterior margins of the segment, and are confluent anteriorly and posteriorly. Genital ducts are between the longitudinal osmoregulatory canals. The cirrus sac reaches the longitudinal osmoregulatory canals and may intrude into medulla. The genital pore is behind the midpoint of the lateral margin and is not markedly prominent. The aporal lobe of the ovary is larger than the poral lobe. A vaginal sphincter is absent. The uterus has 8–16 primary lateral branches on each side.

LIFE HISTORY. *Taenia pisiformis* has a predominantly pastoral cycle, but also is well established in the wild. Adults occur in various canids and, rarely, felids. The cysticercus is found encapsulated in the serosa of the body cavity and viscera of rodents and lagomorphs (Pfaffenburger and Valencia 1988). Hatched, activated oncospheres inoculated into the duodenum of rabbits penetrated the intestine and reached the liver in 40 minutes and the body cavity in 13–26 days; larvae were infective at 28–32 days (Movsesyan et al. 1981; Keith et al. 1985). Adults recovered 56 days after experimental infection of dogs had a mean of 41,000 eggs per gravid segment, but detached segments from the intestinal lumen had only 1370 eggs. Eggs hatched and were activated in the intestinal lumen, especially if attachment was in the anterior half (Coman and Rickard 1975). Pups experimentally infected with cysticerci began to pass gravid segments in 35–45 days and continued up to 212 days (Yang et al. 1986). Prepatent period and subsequent infectivity of eggs in rabbits depended on the breed of dog (Movsesyan et al. 1981). Also, infectivity of eggs declined with the age of the worm.

Foxes (*Vulpes vulpes*) are refractory to experimental infection, and wild foxes rarely are infected (Beveridge and Coman 1978). Foxes appear to have an age resistance that is independent of previous exposure. Similarly, *T. pisiformis* did not establish in kittens or ferrets (Beveridge and Rickard 1975).

EPIZOOTIOLOGY. *Taenia pisiformis* has a cosmopolitan distribution in a wide range of hosts, including *Canis familiaris, C. lupus, C. aureus, C. latrans, C. mesomelas, C. nebraskensis, Lycaon pictus, Vulpes vulpes, Alopex lagopus, Lynx rufus, L. canadensis, Felis ocreata, F. tigrina, F. silvestris, Panthera leo, P. pardus, Putorius putorius,* and *Urocyon cinereoargenteus.* Intermediate hosts include *Oryctolagus cuniculus, Lepus americanus, L. californicus, L. capensis, L. europaeus, L. habessinicus, L. timidus, L. tolai, L. townsendi, Sylvilagus auduboni, S. brasiliensis, S. floridanus, S. nuttalli, S. palustris, S. transitionalis, Sciurus niger rufiventer, Mus musculus, Apodemus flavicollis, Rattus norvegicus, R. rattus, Clethrionomys glareolus, Microtus arvalis, Cavia porcella,* and *Ondatra zibethicus.*

PREVALENCE AND INTENSITY. Prevalence differs markedly among definitive hosts and geographic areas but generally is higher in North America than in other locations (Table 7.7). *Taenia pisiformis* was the dominant species in populations of coyotes from the U.S. Gulf Coast (Custer and Pence 1981). In Montana, mean intensity in coyotes was 9.8 (range 1–86) (Seesee et al. 1983). Prevalence may be dependent upon the proportion of lagomorphs in the diet.

Prevalence of cysticerci in over 8000 snowshoe hare (*Lepus americanus*) from Rochester, Alberta, was not related to age, sex, or month of collection (Keith et al. 1985, 1986). Seasonal prevalence rose to 53% in juveniles in April-May and fluctuated around 57% in adults. Prevalence in adults peaked later than in juveniles. It was stable in hares 1 to 3 years old, suggesting a balance between loss of old infections and acquisition of new ones (Keith et al. 1985). Alternately, visible infections may reach maximum prevalence in yearling hares and then persist. In this scenario, subclinical

infections may immunize adults that are not obviously infected with cysticerci (Keith et al. 1986; Bussche et al. 1987). Prevalence fluctuated markedly among years or groups of years and was linked to hare densities 1 to 2 years earlier. However, cyclic decline in hare populations could not be linked to *T. pisiformis* or any other parasites. Intensity was highest in juveniles. Similar patterns of infection were seen in cottontail rabbits (*Sylvilagus floridanus*) in the eastern United States (Strohlein and Christensen 1983; Lepitzki et al. 1992). Prevalence and intensity were higher in *S. audubonii* than in *Lepus californicus* sympatric in eastern New Mexico (Pfaffenburger and Valencia 1988).

PATHOLOGY AND PATHOGENICITY. Generally, cysticerci of *T. pisiformis* are not associated with tissue damage (Strohlein and Christensen 1983; Ryan et al. 1986). However, connective tissue surround the cysticerci, and there are yellow-white foci on the surface of the liver in some *S. floridanus* (see Lepitzki et al. 1992). Microscopically, coalescing and solitary granulomas with caseous cores of monocytes, giant cells, and eosinophils enclosed by a layer of mixed inflammatory cells and fibroblasts are seen. Migration and pathology in experimentally infected laboratory rabbits is described (Worley 1974).

DIAGNOSIS. There is a slight overlap in the number and length of the hooks of adult *T. pisiformis* and *T. hydatigena*, but in *T. pisiformis* the hooks are more robust and the first-row hooks generally are longer. The strobilae of *T. pisiformis* are narrower, with a serrated appearance, and the testes are always in several layers and confluent posteriorly as well as anteriorly. Cysticerci of both occur in the serosa of the intermediaries, but those of *T. hydatigena* are larger and rarely occur in rodents and lagomorphs (see Abuladze 1964). Characteristic patterns of ribosomal DNA (Gasser and Chilton 1995) and total proteins (Bursey et al. 1980) have been described.

24. *TAENIA POLYACANTHA* LEUCKART, 1856.
Synonyms: *Tetratirotaenia polyacantha* (Leuckart, 1856) Abuladze, 1964. Rausch and Fay (1988a,b) recognized two subspecies, *T. p. arctica* in the Holarctic tundra and *T. p. polyacantha* in Eurasia south of the tundra zone. *Taenia p. arctica* has a mean number of rostellar hooks < 50, and they are 200–234 µm and 140–182 µm. *Taenia p. polyacantha* has a mean number of hooks > 55 that measure 178–221 µm and 120–148 µm. *Monordotaenia alopexi* Obushenkov, 1983, is synonymous with *T. p. arctica* (see Rausch and Fay 1988b).

Taenia polyacantha has 44–68 rostellar hooks: first row 178–234 µm, second row 120–182 µm. Testes are in two horizontal layers, extend from the anterior margin of the segment to the level of the vitelline gland, and are confluent anteriorly but not posteriorly. The cirrus sac is characteristically rounded or subspherical

TABLE 7.7—Some recent[a] records of *Taenia pisiformis*

Hosts	Number Examined	Prevalence (%)	Location	Reference
Definitive Hosts				
Canis latrans	24	—[b]	Texas and Louisiana, USA	Custer and Pence 1981
C. latrans hybrids	46	—[b]	Texas and Louisiana, USA	Custer and Pence 1981
Canis rufus	8	—[b]	Texas and Louisiana, USA	Custer and Pence 1981
Canis latrans	267	51.3–81	Tennessee, USA	Bussche et al. 1987
	219	18	Montana, USA	Seesee et al. 1983
	329	—[b]	Texas, USA	Radomski and Pence 1993
Canis lupus	89	?[c]	Italy	Guberti et al. 1993
Felis silvestris	68	1.5	Spain	Torres et al. 1989
Vulpes vulpes	100	?[c]	Austria	Hinaidy 1971
	101	3	Germany	Lucius et al. 1988
	1300	0.2	Germany	Pfeifer 1996
	397	2	Germany	Ballek et al. 1992
	197	1.0	Britain	Jones and Walters 1992b
	131	12	Australia	Beveridge and Coman 1978
	154	1.3	France	Deblock et al. 1988
Intermediate Hosts				
Lepus americanus	346	55	Alberta, Canada	Keith et al. 1986
	7827	—[b]	Alberta, Canada	Keith et al. 1985
Lepus capensis	42	14	Spain	Moreno Montanez et al. 1979
Lepus timidus	103	12.3	European Karelia	Belkin et al. 1982
Oryctolagus cuniculus	245	60	Chile	Courtin et al. 1979
	116	51.7	Chile	Rubilar and Merello 1987
	42	7	Britain	Boag 1987
	324	14	Italy	Arru et al. 1967
Rodents	?[c]	?[c]	Czech Republic	Tenora and Stanek 1994
Sylvilagus auduboni	14	21	New Mexico, USA	De Bruin and Pfaffenberger 1984
	35	57	New Mexico, USA	Pfaffenberger and Valencia 1988
Sylvilagus californicus	35	9	New Mexico, USA	Pfaffenberger and Valencia 1988
Sylvilagus floridanus	1	1 of 1	Illinois, USA	Ryan et al. 1986
	45	53	Kentucky, USA	Strohlein and Christensen 1983
	96	32	Illinois, USA [penned]	Lepitski et al. 1992

[a]Since 1970.
[b]Data not provided.
[c]Original paper not accessible to the authors.

and reaches the ventral osmoregulatory canal. Genital ducts are between the longitudinal osmoregulatory canals. The genital pore is at or just anterior to the midpoint of the lateral margin and is not prominent. The aporal lobe of the ovary is larger than the poral lobe. A vaginal sphincter is absent. The vagina curves around the posterior wall of the cirrus sac. The uterus has 8–16 primary lateral branches on each side.

EPIZOOTIOLOGY. *Taenia polyacantha* occurs in canids of the Northern Hemisphere, primarily arctic fox, *Alopex lagopus,* in the tundra zone and red foxes and occasionally wolves and dogs in more southern regions. In arctic fox, adult worms may live at least 2 years (Rausch and Fay 1988a). Worms become patent in 2 months; the uterus did not contain eggs at 45 days, but they were present at 66 days. Intermediate hosts include *Lemmus sibiricus, Microtus oeconomus, M. arvalis, M. miurus, M. gregalis major, Clethrionomys glareolus, C. rufocanus, Lagurus lagurus, Ochotona pricei,* and *Oryctolagus cuniculi. Taenia p. arctica* occurs only in the peritoneal cavity of the intermediate host, but *T. p. polyacantha* often is found in the pleura and may grow larger than the northern subspecies (Rausch and Fay 1988b).

In laboratory-raised rodents, infections were established in *M. oeconomus, M. miurus, L. sibiricus,* and *O. zibethicus,* but not in *M. miurus/M. abbreviatus* intergrades or *Clethrionomys rutili* (see Rausch and Fay 1988a,b). Unique to this species, the larvae undergo asexual multiplication in arvicolid rodents. In experimentally infected voles and lemmings, the oncospheres reach the liver via the bloodstream and transform into tiny primary vesicles. In 6 to 10 days postinfection, they migrate to the peritoneal cavity and divide into several secondary vesicles. The vesicles dissociate, and each develops into a cysticercus ~30–40 days postinfection. After 60 days, further modifications transform the larva from a basic cysticercus to a larva with a posterior bladder, a flattened pseudosegmented body, and an evaginated scolex (similar to development of *Taenia martis*). Larvae are infective to voles at 41 days. Larvae from *C. rufocanus* in Czechoslovakia are described as an armatetrathyridium (Prokopic and Hulinska 1978).

Prevalence data are scarce and differ among different populations, but generally prevalences are low (< 15% in definitive hosts; < 3% in intermediates) (Table 7.8). Intensity of infection ranged from 2 to 65 in 25 voles and from 2 to 63 in 10 lemmings (Rausch and Fay 1988b).

TABLE 7.8—Some recent[a] records of *Taenia polyacantha*

Hosts	Number Examined	Prevalence (%)	Location	Reference
Definitive Hosts				
Alopex lagopus	1	1 of 1	Northwest Territory, Canada	Webster 1974
	—[b]	—[b]	Alaska, USA	Rausch and Fay 1988b
Vulpes vulpes	—[b]	—[b]	Alaska, USA	Rausch and Fay 1988b
	100	?[c]	Austria	Hinaidy 1971
	101	2	Germany	Lucius et al. 1988
	1300	11.9	Germany	Pfeifer 1996
	801	7	Germany	Wessbecher et al. 1994
	397	14.4	Germany	Ballek et al. 1992
	197	4.1	Britain	Jones and Walters 1992b
	3575	8	Germany	Loos-Frank and Zeyhle 1982
	154	11.4	France	Deblock et al. 1988
	150	14	France	Petavy et al. 1990a
Intermediate Hosts				
Apodemus flavicollis	380	0.3	Germany	Loos-Frank 1981
Clethrionomys glareolus	398	?	Norway	Tenora et al. 1979
Clethrionomys rufocanus	—[b]	in 3	Czechoslovakia	Prokopic and Hulinska 1978
Lagurus lagurus	?[c]	?[c]	Kazakhstan	Pleschev 1978
Lemmus sibiricus	421	2.4	Alaska, USA	Rausch and Fay 1988b
Microtus arvalis	37	2.7	France	Petavy et al. 1996
	3184	0.6	Germany	Loos-Frank 1981
Microtus oeconomus	6505	<1	Alaska, USA	Rausch and Fay 1988b
Ochotona pricei	?[c]	?[c]	Siberia	Fedorov and Potapkina 1975
Oryctolagus cuniculus	1	1 of 1	Czechoslovakia	Tenora et al. 1988
Rodents	?[c]	?[c]	Czech Republic	Tenora and Stanek 1994

[a]Since 1970.
[b]Data not provided.
[c]Original paper not accessible to the authors.

PATHOLOGY AND PATHOGENESIS. Chronic infections of *T. polyacantha* in naturally infected *M. oeconomus* are associated with fibrosarcomatous mesotheliomas (Rausch et al. 1987). In experimentally infected voles and lemmings, there was focal hepatitis around larvae 5 days postinfection, followed by acute to diffuse peritonitis when the larvae migrated into the peritoneal cavity on day 6 (Rausch and Fay 1988b). Smears of ascitic fluid included many eosinophils, segmented granulocytes, and mesothelial cells, some of which contained phagocytosed eosinophilic or basophilic material. Differential counts of leucocytes indicated neutrophilia from day 5 on and marked eosinophilia from day 9, to maxima of 59% and 69% on days 14 and 16, respectively. Sera and ascitic fluid from infected voles lacked alpha- and gamma-globulins on days 7 and 14.

Larvae in a rabbit were associated with enlarged liver and poor body condition (Tenora et al. 1988). The larvae were 6–13 mm but only one had hook rudiments, suggesting that full development would not be achieved in the liver. Naturally infected *C. glareolus* in southern Norway had ascites, peritoneal adhesions, and increased adrenal and spleen weights (Tenora et al. 1979). Larval development in experimentally infected *Meriones unguiculatus* and *C. rufocanus* was similar, but infections were relatively nonpathogenic in the former and fatal in the latter (Fujita et al. 1991). Larvae injected intraperitoneally into *M. unguiculatus* and mice developed at the inoculation sites, but development was delayed and was associated with much pathogenicity.

DIAGNOSIS. Adults cannot be differentiated from *T. hydatigena* by hook length; however, *T. polyacantha* has more hooks, and they have a distinctive shape. It also has a characteristically subspherical cirrus sac with the vagina applied to its posterior surface and testes in two horizontal layers. *Taenia crassiceps*, which occurs in the same host species in the same geographical areas, has fewer hooks (28–34), posteriorly confluent testes, and an elongated cirrus sac.

25. *TAENIA REGIS* BAER, 1923.
Synonym: *Taenia bubesei* Ortlepp, 1938.

Taenia regis has 32–46 rostellar hooks: first row 223–290 μm, second row 128–199 μm. Testes are in a horizontal layer and fail to reach the anterior margin of the segment, but extend to the vitellarium posteriorly. Genital ducts are between the longitudinal osmoregulatory canals. The cirrus sac extends to the longitudinal osmoregulatory canals. The prominent genital pore is located about midpoint of the lateral margin. The aporal lobe of the ovary is larger than the poral lobe. A vaginal sphincter is present. The uterus with 2–10 primary lateral branches on each side. Cysticerci are up to 20–25 mm in diameter.

EPIZOOTIOLOGY. Adults occur in *Panthera leo* and *P. pardus* in Africa; cysticerci in wildebeest, topi, and hartebeest, including *Alcelaphus buselaphus*, *Connochaetes taurinus*, *Damaliscus korrigum*, *Equus burchelli, Hippotragus niger, Kobus ellipsiprymnus, Oryx beisa, O. gazella, Redunca arundinum,* and *Phacochoerus aethiopicus* (see Sachs 1970). Larvae occur primarily in the abdominal cavity attached to the serosa of the digestive tract, omentum, and liver, but also occur in the thoracic cavity (Sachs and Sachs 1968; Young et al. 1969).

There is little information on prevalence and intensity of infections. One, 2, 7, and 28 *T. regis,* along with *T. gonyamai, T. simbae,* and immature *Taenia,* were collected from 4 lions in Serengeti (Dinnik and Sachs 1972). Each of 3 lions as well as 18% of warthogs and 9.9% of antelopes in the Central African Republic (Graber 1981), 4 *Redunca redunca* in the Sudan (El Din et al. 1986), and 77% of 33 adult blue wildebeest in Kruger National Park, South Africa (Young et al.1969) were infected with *T. regis.*

DIAGNOSIS. *Taenia regis* differs from the other taeniids in lions. It has larger rostellar hooks than *T. gonyamai* and fewer primary uterine branches (2–10 on each side, usually 2–7) than either *T. gonyamai* or *T. simbae.* It differs from *T. simbae* in having testes that are not confluent behind the vitellarium and in having a smaller cirrus sac and mature segments. Also, *T. regis* has characteristic isoenzymes (Allsopp et al. 1987) that differentiate it from *T. hydatigena* (see *T. hydatigena* above).

26. *TAENIA RILEYI* LOEWEN, 1929.
Synonym: *Hydatigera rileyi* (Loewen, 1929) Abuladze, 1964.

Taenia rileyi has 36–46 rostellar hooks: first row 207–258 μm, second row 159–198 μm. Testes are in a single layer, are confluent anteriorly, and extend to the posterior margin of the segment; some may occur behind vitelline gland. Genital ducts are between the longitudinal osmoregulatory canals. The cirrus sac does not reach the osmoregulatory canals. The genital pore is near the midpoint of lateral margin. Ovarian lobes are subequal or the aporal lobe is larger. A vaginal sphincter and/or vaginal pad is present. The uterus has 6–26 primary uterine branches on each side.

EPIZOOTIOLOGY. *Taenia rileyi* occurs in Nearctic felids (*Felis lynx, F. rufus, F. concolor*), although development in cougar may be unlikely (Rausch et al. 1983). Intermediate hosts include a variety of rodents (*Tamiasciurus hudsonicus, Aplodontia rufa, Neotoma cinerea, Oryzomys palustris, Sigmodon hispidus, Clethrionomys rutilus*). Red squirrels, common in the diet of lynx, were the only naturally infected intermediaries reported in Alaska (Rausch 1981). The life cycle was completed experimentally in various intermediates (*C. rutilus, M. oeconomus, T. hudsonicus*) and laboratory-reared *Felis silvestris* (see Rausch 1981). Larvae were distributed subcapsular and within the liver parenchyma. Bladders up to 1.4 mm and formation of the invaginal canal had begun by 23 days postinfection. Larvae were fully developed and infective at 68 days. The structure of the larva is unique in the genus, with an everted forebody and invaginated scolex. The scolex was evaginated and the rostellar hooks fully developed by 78 days. The posterior region of the forebody is pseudosegmented and anteriorly looks like a typical "neck" region. Rausch (1981) termed it a hemistrobilocercus. Larvae in *C. rutilus* were associated with hepatomegaly and fatty metamorphosis (Rausch 1981).

PREVALENCE AND INTENSITY. In west Texas, *T. rileyi* was found in 91% of 66 *Felis rufus* (see Stone and Pence 1978). In north central Alaska, 5% of 224 red squirrels were infected (mean intensity, 2.3). Only 1 of 800 *Clethrionomys rutilus* in Alaska was infected, with one larva, although the species is a good experimental host (Rausch 1981). In Texas, it occurred in 7% of 127 *S. hispidus,* but not in individuals infected with *T. taeniaeformis* (see Mollhagen 1979).

DIAGNOSIS. Larvae of *T. rileyi* are distinguished by the distinctive morphology (as above) (also see "diagnosis" of *T. omissa*).

27. *TAENIA SAGINATA* GOEZE, 1782.
Synonyms: *Cysticercus bovis* Cobbold, 1866; *Taenia confusa* Ward, 1896; *T. africana* von Linstow, 1900; *T. hominis* von Linstow, 1904; *T. tonkinensis* Railliet and Henry, 1905; *T. phillipina* Garrison, 1907; *T. cylindrica* Leon, 1922. See Abuladze (1964) for a comprehensive list.

In *T. saginata* the rostellum is absent, the scolex unarmed. Testes are in one horizontal layer, extend from the posterior margin of the segment, and are confluent anteriorly, not posteriorly. Genital ducts are between the longitudinal osmoregulatory canals. The cirrus sac does not reach the longitudinal osmoregulatory canals. The genital pore is posterior to the midpoint of the lateral margin of the segment. The aporal lobe of the ovary is larger than the poral lobe. A vaginal sphincter is present. The uterus has 14–33 pairs of primary lateral branches on each side.

EPIZOOTIOLOGY. *Taenia saginata* is one of two species of the genus to use humans as the definitive host. It has a cosmopolitan distribution. Eggs in human feces contaminate pasture and are ingested by cattle, the common intermediate host. The cysticerci occur in the skeletal muscles of bovines. The life cycle is well known, but recent recognition of strains of *T. saginata,* particularly one that involves semidomesticated intermediates, is of interest. The species also occurs in wild game (Graber 1974), although it is doubtful whether these are of great significance in transmission. The following account focuses on reports from wild hosts. Known intermediates include *Rangifer tarandus* for the northern strain. Cysticerci have been reported from *Damaliscus korrigum, Gazella rufifrons, G. dorcas, G.*

gutturosa, Kobus kob, Oryx gazella beisa, and *Tragelaphus scriptus,* but it is very unlikely that they have a significant role in transmission.

In northern regions of the former USSR, a strain of *T. saginata* occurs in the brain of reindeer (Kirichek and Belousov 1984), and the cycle from human to reindeer was completed (Kirichek et al. 1986). Cysticerci may occur in various tissues and organs in reindeer but only those in the meninges are infective (Kirichek 1985a; Blazek et al. 1986). The cysticerci provoked central nervous system disorders in reindeer (Kirichek et al. 1986). In domestic calves, larvae of the northern strain develop in the muscles, but in smaller numbers (Kirichek et al. 1986) and with a shorter lifespan (Kirichek 1985b) than the southern strain. Attempts to infect reindeer calves with the southern strain of *T. saginata* failed (Kirichek 1985b). Attempts to infect primates *(Pan schweinfurthii, Papio papio, Macaca irus, Cercopithecus aethiops)* and hamsters with the northern strain also proved unsuccessful (Kumar et al. 1977). Fall et al. (1995) failed to infect baboons *(Papio hamadryas)* with eggs of the Asian strain of *T. saginata.*

In East Africa, cysticerci in game animals are a deterrent to game ranching because of condemnation of carcasses. Larvae are aesthetically unacceptable for human consumption even though they pose no risk to health. Most cysticerci in wild herbivores are of species that mature in wild carnivores (see *Taenia crocutae, T. gonyamai, T. hyaenae*), but there are a few reports of *T. saginata,* and transmission might occur in pastoral landscapes. Cysticerci of *T. saginata* were found in 99% of 83 zebu cattle in west Chad (Graber 1959). However, no armed cysticerci were found in 524 cattle from areas in or near national parks and game reserves in Kenya, and wild species may have no role in transmission of *T. saginata* (see Gathuma and Mango 1976). Unarmed cysticerci have been reported in *Syncerus caffer* in Angola; *Gazella dorcas, G. rufifrons,* and *Adenota kob* in Chad; *Ourebia ourebi* in Zambia; *Tragelaphus scriptus* and *Connochaetes gnou* in Kenya; and *Giraffa camelopardalis* in various zoological gardens (Graber et al. 1973). Unarmed cysticerci also were found in topi *(Damaliscus korrigum)* living near human habitation in Kenya (Stevenson et al. 1982). Experimental infection of *T. saginata* was established in oryx *(Oryx gazella beisa)* but not in wildebeest *(Connochaetes taurinus)* (Stevenson et al. 1982).

PATHOLOGY AND PATHOGENESIS. In reindeer, nonpurulent leptomeningitis with formation of multinucleate symplasms occurred in the meninges along with lymphocytic encephalitis in the superficial layers of the cerebral cortex (Blazek et al. 1986). Survival of meningeal cysticerci was attributed to immunological tolerance in the brain. Cysticerci in other sites die and are encapsulated (Kirichek et al. 1986).

DIAGNOSIS. Gravid segments of *T. saginata* can be differentiated from *T. solium,* the other species in humans, by the number of uterine branches, the presence of a vaginal sphincter in *T. saginata,* and the distribution of the testes. Also, the scolex and larva of *T. saginata* are unarmed. Species-specific DNA probes for each species have been identified (Chapman et al. 1995).

CONTROL AND TREATMENT. Anthelmintic treatment of humans and hygienic disposal of feces to avoid pasture contamination are the most practical measures of control. Infection in reindeer and in African wild herbivores held in captivity is linked to infection in human handlers.

MANAGEMENT IMPLICATIONS. In Africa, segregation of grazing for domestic stock from that of wild herbivores might be desirable, but would be difficult to achieve as human settlements and agricultural practices encroach on the wild environment.

28. *TAENIA SELOUSI* METTRICK, 1962. *Taenia selousi* has 48–58 rostellar hooks: first row 256–290 μm, second row 160–187 μm. Testes are in 1–2 horizontal layers and extend from near the anterior margin of the segment to the level of the vitelline gland posteriorly. They are confluent anteriorly but not posteriorly. Genital ducts are ventral to the longitudinal osmoregulatory vessels. The cirrus sac crosses the osmoregulatory canals to enter the medulla. The aporal lobe of the ovary is larger than the poral lobe. A vaginal sphincter is absent. The uterus has 4–11 primary uterine branches on each side. Larvae are polycephalic.

EPIZOOTIOLOGY. The adults occur in wild cats, *Felis silvestris,* in southern Africa. Larvae occur in rodents, *Rhabdomys pumilio.* There is little information about this species.

DIAGNOSIS. *Taenia selousi* differs from *T. endothoracicus* in having smaller rostellar hooks; from *T. parva* in having more and shorter rostellar hooks as well as a smaller number of testes; and from *T. taeniaeformis* in lacking a vaginal sphincter.

29. *TAENIA SERIALIS* (GERVAIS, 1847) BAILLIET, 1863 *SENSU LATO.* Verster (1969) recognized two subspecies: *T. s. serialis* and *T. s. brauni* based largely on biological rather than morphological differences. Both are adult in canids, but *T. s. serialis* uses lagomorphs and, less frequently, rodents as intermediaries and has a cosmopolitan distribution, while *T. s. brauni* uses rodents and primates and occurs primarily in Africa.

Taenia serialis has 22–34 rostellar hooks: first row 110–177 μm, second row 85–160 μm. Testes are in 1–3 horizontal layers, are confluent anteriorly only, and extend to the level of the vitellarium posteriorly. Genital ducts are between the longitudinal osmoregulatory vessels. The cirrus sac extends to the longitudinal osmoregulatory vessels. The genital pore is posterior to the midpoint of the lateral margin; the genital papilla is prominent. The aporal lobe of the ovary is larger than the poral lobe. A vaginal sphincter is present. The uterus has 10–25 primary lateral branches. Larva is a coenurus in the body cavity, intermuscular connective tissue, and subcutaneous sites.

EPIZOOTIOLOGY. *Taenia s. brauni* has been found in *Canis mesomelas, C. familiaris,* and *Lycaon pictus.* A wide range of intermediate hosts includes *Gerbillus pyramidum hirtipus, Otomys irroratus vulcanius, Hystrix* sp., *Praomys natalensis, Mastomys coucha ugandae, Lemniscomys striatus, Grammomys* sp., *Tachyoryctes ruandae, Dendromus pumilio lineatus, Rattus rattus, Cercopithecus mitis doggetti* and, rarely, humans. *Taenia s. serialis* is found primarily in foxes, *Vulpes vulpes.* Larvae occur in *Lepus americanus, L. europeaus, Oryctolagus cuniculus, Sylvilagus californicus, Presbytis senex,* and *Mus musculus.* They also occur in domestic cats (Hayes and Creighton 1978; Kingston et al. 1984).

Adults mature in 1–3 months and live at least 1 year; coenuri are infective at 2–3 months and survive in the intermediate host up to 2 years (Abuladze 1964). There is little information regarding prevalence of the species (Table 7.9); however, Keith et al. (1985) suggested prevalence of larvae in snowshoe hare reflected the population density of red fox.

DIAGNOSIS. The species closely resembles *T. multiceps,* but is more robust and muscular. The testicular field extends into the preovarian space, and a vaginal sphincter, rather than a pad, is present. Recovery of a coenurus from the body cavity, intermuscular connective tissue, or subcutaneous tissue of lagomorphs is diagnostic. Characteristic patterns of ribosomal DNA have been identified (Gasser and Chilton 1995).

30. *TAENIA SIMBAE* DINNIK AND SACHS, 1972. *Taenia simbae* has 38–48 rostellar hooks: first row 242–290 μm, second row 147–186 μm. Testes are in a single horizontal layer, not quite reaching the anterior

margin of the segment and extending to the level of the vitelline gland posteriorly. They are confluent anteriorly by a broad arch and posteriorly by a single row. Genital ducts are between the longitudinal osmoregulatory canals. The cirrus sac is club-shaped and reaches the ventral osmoregulatory vessel. The genital pore is just anterior to the midpoint of the lateral margin. The aporal lobe of the ovary is larger than the poral lobe. A vaginal sphincter is present. The uterus has 7–12 primary lateral branches on each side.

EPIZOOTIOLOGY. The lion is the only known definitive host. Intermediate hosts are unknown. Dinnik and Sachs (1972) found 0, 20, 46, and 57 *T. simbae* in four lions in the Serengeti area of Tanzania. *Taenia regis, T. gonyamai,* and immature *Taenia* also were found.

DIAGNOSIS. *Taenia simbae* differs from *T. gonyamai* in having larger rostellar hooks and from *T. regis* and *T. gonyamai* in having testes confluent by a single row behind the vitellarium; it has more primary uterine branches than *T. regis* but fewer than *T. gonyamai.* Some *T. regis* specimens from lions in Kenya had some morphological characters intermediate between *T. regis* and *T. simbae,* but did not differ in isoenzyme profiles (Allsopp et al. 1987). This suggests some intraspecific variation or the species may not be distinct.

31. *TAENIA SOLIUM* L., 1758.
Synonyms: see Abuladze (1964) for a comprehensive list.

Taenia solium has 22–36 rostellar hooks: first row 139–200 μm, second row 93–139 μm. An accessory row of hooks, 86–118 μm, may be present in adults and larvae. Testes are in one horizontal layer, extend from the anterior to the posterior margins of the segment, and are confluent anteriorly and posteriorly behind the vitellarium. The genital ducts are between the longitudinal osmoregulatory vessels. The cirrus sac extends to

TABLE 7.9—Some recent[a] records of *Taenia serialis*

Hosts	Number Examined	Prevalence (%)	Location	Reference
Definitive Host				
Vulpes vulpes	1300	0.2	Germany	Pfeifer 1996
	397	2.3	Germany	Ballek et al. 1992
	3573	0.5	Germany	Loos-Frank and Zeyhle 1982
	197	0.5	Britain	Jones and Walters 1992b
	131	44	Australia	Beveridge and Coman 1978
Intermediate Hosts				
Lepus americanus	7827	< 1	Alberta, Canada	Keith et al. 1985
Lepus europaeus	121,531	< 0.1	Argentina	Gonzalez 1986
Mus musculus	75	1.37	Spain	Alvarez et al. 1987
Oryctolagus cuniculus	245	13	Chile	Courtin et al. 1979
	116	2.6	Chile	Rubilar and Merello 1987
Presbytis senex nestor	1	1 of 1	Louisiana, USA [zoo]	Lozano-Alarcon et al. 1985
Sylvilagus californicus	35	46	New Mexico, USA	Pfaffenberger and Valencia 1988

[a]Since 1970.

the longitudinal osmoregulatory vessels. The aporal lobe of the ovary is larger than the poral lobe, and a small third lobe is present porally. A vaginal sphincter is absent. The uterus has 7–16 primary lateral branches on each side.

EPIZOOTIOLOGY. Adults occur in humans and cysticerci in the muscles, heart, tongue, and brain of pigs, the usual intermediate host. Additional records include *Potamochoerus choeropotamus, Homo sapiens, Cercopithecus aethiops, C. cephus, C. patas, Hylobates lar, Papio ursinus, Macaca mulatta, M. inuus, Lepus timidus, Camelus bactrianus, Ursus arctos, Vulpes vulpes, Canis familiaris, Felis ocreata, Mustela putorius, Citellus citellus, Rattus rattus, Mesocricetus auratus, Oryctolagus cuniculus,* and *Mus* sp. Abuladze (1964) and Verster (1969) list a number of wild species as naturally infected with the cysticerci and record experimental infections in others. De Graaf et al. (1980) found cysticerci in a Cape fur seal, *Arctocephalus pusillus*. The species may mature only in humans and lar gibbons (Verster 1965).

Infections in humans are acquired by eating undercooked pork or by accidental ingestion of parasite eggs. In the human intermediary, cysticerci localize in the muscles, subcutaneous tissue, and occasionally in the eyes and brain. Cerebral cysticercosis with neurological symptoms similar to those of epilepsy may occur in the latter situation.

31. *TAENIA TAENIAEFORMIS* (BATSCH, 1786) WOLFFUGEL, 1911.
Synonyms: *Hydatigera taeniaeformis* (Batsch, 1786) Lamarck, 1816; *Cysticercus fasciolaris.*

The *T. taeniaeformis* rostellum has 26–52 hooks: first row 300–485 µm, second row 187–293 µm. Testes are in 1–2 horizontal layers, extending from close to the anterior margin of the segment to the level of the vitelline gland posteriorly. They are confluent anteriorly but not posteriorly. The genital ducts are ventral to the osmoregulatory canals. The cirrus sac crosses the osmoregulatory vessels to enter the medulla. The genital pore is at or just anterior to the midpoint of the segment and is not conspicuous. The ovary lobes are subequal, or the aporal lobe is larger than the poral lobe. The uterus has 5–11 primary lateral branches on each side.

EPIZOOTIOLOGY. Adults are widely distributed in felids (*Felis catus, F. rufus, F. silvestris*), with some spillover into foxes *(Vulpes vulpes)* and coyote/wolf hybrids (*Canis latrans* x *rufus*). Miscellaneous infections were found in two tigers in Indian game reserves (Gaur et al. 1980). Intermediate hosts include a variety of rodents (*Acomys cahirinus, Apodemus microps, Arvicanthis niloticus, Gerbillus gerbillus, Rattus norvegicus, R. rattus, Microtus agrestis, M. arvalis, M. pennsylvanicus, M. pinetorum, Mus musculus, M. spretus, Myocastor coypus, Ondatra zibethicus, Per-*

omyscus maniculatus, Pitymys savii, P. subterraneus, Sciurus carolinensis carolinensis, Sigmodon hispidus), and occasionally, birds (*Bubo bubo, Phasianus colchicus, Phyllotis xanthopygus*). The larva is a strobilocercus that develops in or on the liver. Strobilocerci from mice were infective to cats after 52 days and reached patency in 30–35 days (Movsesyan et al. 1981).

PREVALENCE AND INTENSITY. Prevalence of adult worms is considerably higher in felids than in canids (Table 7.10). Prevalence of the strobilocercus differs markedly in different rodent hosts, but generally is highest in rats, cotton rats, and muskrats. Prevalence in pine voles (*M. pinetorum*) was greater in adults (14.3%) than in juveniles (2.7%); however, intensities were higher in juveniles (4.5) than adults (1.8) (Lochmiller et al. 1982). Intensity in muskrats was < 20 (Abram 1972; Dvorakova and Prokopic 1984; Zabiega 1996).

Strong seasonal fluctuations in a population of *Peromyscus maniculatus* in northeast California were not accompanied by significant annual or seasonal fluctuations in *T. taeniaeformis* (Theis and Schwab 1992). Prevalence was significantly different in young (1.2%) and adult (4.2%) deer mice, but there were no significant differences in prevalence or intensity related to host sex. Theis and Schwab (1992) suggested differences may relate to different activity patterns in adults, passive immunity in juveniles, or capture of young deer mice before infections were established.

PATHOLOGY AND PATHOGENESIS. Infected deer mice have significantly increased liver weight (Lochmiller et al. 1982). Letonja and Hammerburg (1987a,b) describe the early inflammatory response in resistant and susceptible strains of mice, but there are no parallel accounts from wild rodents. Antibody titers were found in *Felis rufus* (see Heidt et al. 1988).

DIAGNOSIS. Strobilocerci have rostellar hooks corresponding in size and number to those of adult worms. Similarly, adults can be distinguished from other species in felids by the size and number of rostellar hooks. Species-specific protein patterns have been identified (Bursey et al. 1980).

PUBLIC HEALTH CONCERNS. A larva of *T. taeniaeformis* was found encapsulated in the liver of a 77-year-old man in Czechoslovakia (Sterba et al. 1977). However, the species is not considered a health risk.

32. *TAENIA TAXIDIENSIS* SKINKER, 1935.
Synonyms: *Fossor angertrudae* Honess, 1937; *Monordotaenia taxidiensis* (Skinker, 1935) Little, 1967.

Taenia taxidiensis has rostellar hooks in one row of 20–27 hooks measuring 79–104 µm. Testes are in one horizontal layer, extend from the anterior to the

TABLE 7.10—Some recent[a] records of *Taenia taeniaeformis*

Hosts	Number Examined	Prevalence (%)	Location	Reference
Definitive Hosts				
Canis latrans × *rufus*	46	2	Texas and Louisiana, USA	Custer and Pence 1981
	25	72	Germany	Schuster et al. 1993
Felis silvestris	68	60	Spain	Torres et al. 1989
	257	64	Czechoslovakia [Slovakia]	Mituch et al. 1988
	12	83	Yugoslavia	Brglez and Zeleznik 1976
Felis rufus	1	1 of 1	California, USA	Mueller 1973
	8	6 of 8	Arkansas, USA	Heidt et al. 1988
Vulpes vulpes	1300	0.2	Germany	Pfeifer 1996
	801	0.7	Germany	Wessbecher et al. 1994
	397	2.5	Germany	Ballek et al. 1992
	100	?[b]	Austria	Hinaidy 1971
	3573	0.6	Germany	Loos-Frank and Zeyhle 1982
Intermediate Hosts				
Acomys cahirinus	38	3	Egypt	Ramadan et al. 1988
Arvicanthus niloticus	498	0.4	Egypt	Ramadan et al. 1988
Rattus norvegicus	286	2.8	Egypt	Ramadan et al. 1988
Rattus rattus	54	2	Egypt	Ramadan et al. 1988
Apodemus flavicollis	380	1.3	Germany	Loos-Frank 1981
Apodemus sylvaticus	124	0.2	Germany	Loos-Frank 1981
Apodemus microps	201	—[c]	Hungary	Gubanyi et al. 1992
Bubo bubo	1	1 of 1	Switzerland	Gigon and Beuret 1991
Homo sapiens	1	1 of 1	Czechoslovakia	Sterba et al. 1977
Microtus agrestis	—[c]	—[c]	Finland	Haukisalmi et al. 1994
	47	4	France	Le Pesteur et al. 1992
	215	0.9	Germany	Loos-Frank 1981
Microtus arvalis	3184	0.3	Germany	Loos-Frank 1981
	3097	7.2	Hungary	Nechay 1973
	37	2.7	France	Petavy et al. 1996
	195	0.5	Hungary	Gubanyi et al. 1992
	2520	3.7	France	Le Pesteur et al. 1992
Microtus pennsylvanicus	89	17	Montana, USA	McBee 1977
Microtus pinetorum	298	11.4	Virginia, USA	Lochmiller et al. 1982
Mus musculus	36	2.8	Germany	Loos-Frank 1981
	73	13.4	Spain	Alvarez et al. 1987
Mus spretus	58	22.4	Portugal	Behnke et al. 1993
Myocastor coypus	?[b]	?[b]	Uzbekistan	Kashchanov 1972
Ondatra zibethica	670	44.3	Germany	Friedland et al. 1985
	72	29	Czechoslovakia	Rajsky 1985
	6	6 of 6	Czechoslovakia	Dvorakova and Prokopic 1984
	1	1 of 1	Germany	Schuster 1982
	1	1 of 1	Czechoslovakia	Sterba et al. 1977
	?[b]	?[b]	USSR	Vustina 1988
	50	22	Illinois, USA	Zabiega 1996
	?[b]	?[b]	Czech Republic	Stanek and Tenora 1992
	103	18	Maryland, USA	Abram 1972
Peromyscus maniculatus	4501	5.7	California, USA	Theis and Schwab 1992
Phasianus colchicus	1	1 of 1	Czechoslovakia	Sterba et al. 1977
	1	1 of 1	Czechoslovakia	Rysavy 1973
Pitymys savii	—[c]	—[c]	Spain	Tenora and Meszaros 1972
Pitymys subterraneus	75	16	France	Le Pesteur et al. 1992
Rattus norvegicus	37	8.1	Spain	Alvarez et al. 1987
	?[b]	40.9	Egypt	Wanas et al. 1993
Rattus rattus	?[b]	26.8	Egypt	Wanas et al. 1993
Gerbillus gerbillus	?[b]	33.3	Egypt	Wanas et al. 1993
Mus musculus	?[b]	25	Egypt	Wanas et al. 1993
Acomys cahirinus	?[b]	16.6	Egypt	Wanas et al. 1993
Arvicanthis niloticus	?[b]	7.2	Egypt	Wanas et al. 1993
Rattus norvegicus	510	11	Britain	Webster and Macdonald 1995
Sigmodon hispidus	129	23	Texas, USA	Mollhagen 1979

[a]Since 1970.
[b]Original paper not accessible to the authors.
[c]Data not provided.

posterior margin of the segment, and are confluent anteriorly and posteriorly. The genital ducts are ventral to the longitudinal osmoregulatory vessels. The cirrus sac fails to reach the osmoregulatory canals. The genital pore is near the midpoint of the lateral margin. The aporal ovary lobe is larger than the poral lobe. A vaginal sphincter is absent. The uterus has 10–23 primary lateral branches on each side.

EPIZOOTIOLOGY. This species has a North American distribution in badgers (*Taxidea taxus*) and coyotes (*Canis latrans*). Larvae occur in ground squirrels (*Spermophilus elegans, S. franklini, S. variegatus*). The species is uncommon. It was found in < 1% of 219 coyotes in Montana (Seesee et al. 1983), 2% of 154 *Spermophilus variegatus* in Utah (Jenkins and Grundmann 1973), and 2% of 46 *S. franklini* in Saskatchewan (McGee 1980). In Wyoming, it occurred in 1% of 335 *S. elegans* from xeric habitats, but in none of 419 from mesic habitats (Schults and Stanton 1987).

33. *TAENIA TWITCHELLI* SCHWARTZ, 1927.
Synonyms: *Multiceps twitchelli* Schwartz, 1927

Taenia twitchelli has 30–36 rostellar hooks: first row 184–218 μm, second row 143–178 μm. Testes are in two horizontal layers, extend from the anterior to the posterior margins of the segment, and are confluent anteriorly and posteriorly. The genital ducts are ventral to the longitudinal osmoregulatory canals. The cirrus sac extends to the osmoregulatory canals. The genital pore is at or anterior to the midpoint of the segment margin. The aporal lobe of the ovary is larger than the poral lobe. A vaginal sphincter is absent. The uterus has 7–12 primary lateral branches on each side. The larval stage has a branched coenurus (Rausch 1959).

EPIZOOTIOLOGY. Adults occur in wolverine (*Gulo gulo*). Larvae occur in porcupine (*Erethizon dorsatum, E. epixanthum*). Experimental infections have been achieved in various rodents (*Ondatra zibethicus, Lemmus sibiricus, Microtus pennsylvanicus, Citellus undulatus, Tamiasciurus hudsonicus*) (Rausch 1959). Eggs ingested by porcupines hatch in the gut and eventually reach the lungs via the liver. Intrapulmonary migration occurs at 11–12 days, and larvae penetrate the pleura and enter the thoracic cavity at 16–25 days (Rausch 1959). Heavily infected individuals may exhibit dyspnea. Larvae may undergo exogenous and endogenous budding. The buds form pedicels that develop scolices, usually 1 to 33 per bladder, averaging 10 pedicels. The shape and size of the larvae varies according to the host: the larger the host, the larger the larva. Prepatent period in wolverine is at least 75 days. Holmes and Podesta (1968) found an immature specimen in a coyote in Alberta but it is not clear whether the species can reach maturity in this host.

PREVALENCE AND INTENSITY. One of 55 porcupines and 75% of 80 wolverines in Alaska was infected

(Rausch 1959). Intensity was 9 in the porcupine and 1–61 in the wolverines.

DIAGNOSIS. The species appears to reach maturity only in wolverines and is the only species of *Taenia* reported from this host. Larval morphology is characteristic of the species.

Genus *Echinococcus* Rudolphi, 1801.
Synonyms: see Rausch (1994).

The strobila are tiny, up to 12 mm long, with 3–7 segments. Rostellum has two alternating rows of taenioid hooks, highly variable in number. Mature segments are usually longer than wide, and gravid segments are elongate. Genital pores alternate irregularly. Testes are relatively few, mostly lateral and anterior to female organs. The ovary is bialate, median, and posterior. The vitelline gland is compact and postovarian. The uterus is fully gravid only in the terminal segment. Lateral branches of the uterus are poorly developed or absent. Eggs have a striated embryophore. Larva is a unilocular, multivesicular, or polycystic hydatid; a laminated membrane is present; protoscolices are formed within brood capsules. The type species is *E. granulosus* (Batsch, 1786).

Recent reviews include Thompson and Lymbery (1988), Thompson (1992, 1995), Rausch (1993), and Thompson et al. (1994). Major advances in the last 25 to 30 years include the description of a new species, *E. vogeli;* the development of immunological, biochemical, and molecular techniques for identification and diagnosis; and the discovery of strains of *E. granulosus* distinguished by their biological, morphological, and molecular characteristics. Currently two Holarctic species (*E. granulosus* and *E. multilocularis*) and two Neotropical species (*E. oligarthrus* and *E. vogeli*) are recognized. Within *E. granulosus,* two biotypes and a number of host-adapted strains have been identified (see below); however, the topic is complicated and controversial. Species and strains can be differentiated molecularly, and there is evidence that *E. granulosus* is a complex of genetically distinct populations which may merit species status. Some studies suggest that *E. multilocularis* may not be distinct from *E. granulosus;* however, *E. vogeli* and *E. oligarthrus* are distant from them and quite distinct (Bowles and McManus 1993; Bowles et al. 1995). Strain differences have important implications for transmission, control, and treatment, but emphasis here is on sylvatic strains. Sources of further information are identified, in particular Thompson (1986) and Thompson and Lymbery (1990, 1995).

1. *ECHINOCOCCUS GRANULOSUS* (BATSCH, 1786).
Rostellar hooks are highly variable in number and are 25–49 μm (mean 32–42) and 17–31 μm (mean 22.6–27.8) long. The strobila is 2–11 mm long with 2–7 segments. The genital pore is posterior to the midpoint of the lateral margin of the segment. There are 25–80 testes, equally distributed anteriorly and posteri-

orly to the genital pore. The mature segment is penultimate or antepenultimate in the strobila. The uterus has small lateral sacculate diverticula. The ratio of the anterior part of the strobila to the gravid segment is 1:0.86–1.30. The larva is unilocular. Protoscolex hooks are 19.4–44 µm (mean 25.9–35) and 17–31 µm (mean 22.6–27.8) long.

Rausch (1995) identified two biological forms of *E. granulosus:* a northern biotype indigenous to Holarctic tundra and boreal forests (taiga), and a more southern European biotype. The latter form now has worldwide distribution, achieved as Europeans migrated throughout the world with their livestock. The northern biotype characteristically occurs as adults in wolves, *Canis lupus,* and larvae in cervids, particularly moose, *Alces alces.* This biotype also can infect domestic dogs. The European biotype occurs predominantly in domestic dogs and domestic ungulates, although variants of the cycle in different regions may involve wild canids and other carnivores, wild ungulates, macropodid marsupials and, rarely, lagomorphs. The cervid strain or northern biotype can be distinguished from other strains by its distinct genotype (Bowles et al. 1994).

There may be at least nine strains of *E. granulosus* adapted to different hosts and, in most cases, occupying a wide geographical area. Sylvatic strains include one in sheep, dingoes, and macropods in Australia and sheep, jackals, and hyenas in Africa; a cervid strain in wolf, coyote, dog, and cervids in North America and Eurasia; and a lion strain in Africa, with larvae in a wide range of prey species (Thompson 1995). Some strains infect humans, and of these the dog/sheep and dog/reindeer strains are the most significant. In northwest China, one homogeneous strain is believed to exist, indistinguishable from the sheep strain (McManus et al. 1994). European strains have been reviewed by Eckert and Thompson (1988) and African strains by Macpherson and Craig (1991). Isolates from different hosts and geographical areas have been characterized with DNA probes (McManus and Rishi 1989).

The complexity of strains in *Echinococcus* is illustrated in Australia. On the mainland, it appears that *E. granulosus* occurs in domestic (dogs and sheep) and sylvatic (feral dogs, dingoes, and foxes with larvae in kangaroos and wallabies) strains. However, there may be some overlap as most worms in feral dogs, dingoes, and foxes are of macropod origin, but many dogs and dingoes also have worms of sheep origin. This interaction between the sylvatic and synanthropic cycles has implications for control measures. Dingoes are highly susceptible to infection and provide a transmission route to Australian wildlife (Thompson and Kumaratilake 1985; Constantine et al. 1993). The discovery of hydatid cysts in 6 of 21 grey kangaroo, *Macropus fuliginosus,* and 11 of 24 feral pigs near Perth suggests recent introduction to western Australia with dogs used for pig hunting (Thompson et al. 1988).

However, restriction fragment length polymorphism failed to differentiate among *E. granulosus* from Aus

tralian macropods, Australian sheep, and U.K. sheep or between sheep material from mainland Australia and Tasmania. Also, DNA sequencing did not reveal differences between human cyst material and material from macropods, feral pigs, and dingoes, implying that the sheep/dog strain can infect Australian wildlife and suggesting that there is no distinct sylvatic dingo/macropod strain (Hope et al. 1991, 1992). Similarly, Bowles et al. (1992) found no evidence for a distinct Australian sylvatic strain, at least not in Queensland. These results have significant implications for public health and control.

A molecular phylogenetic reconstruction of the genus suggests that *E. granulosus* comprises at least three evolutionarily diverse groups (sheep, bovine, and horse strain groups) and may be a composite of more than one species. The cervid strain (the northern biotype) is not believed to be ancestral to the others, but its affinities have not yet been established (Bowles et al. 1995).

LIFE HISTORY. Life history and development in *Echinococcus granulosus* and other species of the genus were reviewed by Thompson (1995). The hydatid larva is unilocular with no exogenous budding. It occurs mainly in the liver and lungs of the intermediary, but can occur in a variety of sites including skeletal muscles and the eye. The fluid-filled cyst is surrounded by an elastic acellular laminated layer covered externally by a fibrous adventitial layer of host origin that forms a barrier between host and parasite tissue.

Worm burdens in the final host can exceed 300,000 in highly susceptible animals (Jenkins and Morris 1991). Patency occurs 34 to 48 days postinfection. Little is known about the number of eggs produced per gravid segment or per worm; there may be a cyclical pattern in egg shedding, but this is unclear. The genus compensates for comparatively low egg production by its massive asexual reproduction in the larval stage.

Development varies according to strain and host. The Australian sylvatic strain produces significantly greater worm burdens in dingoes than in domestic dogs; the worms grow to a significantly greater length in dingoes at 25 and 35 days postinfection, form segments at a faster rate in dingoes, and reach sexual maturity earlier (Thompson and Kumaratilake 1985). Patency in dogs in Kenya occurs in < 5 weeks, compared with 6–7 weeks in dogs in Nairobi, possibly a response to survival in an exceptionally arid area (Wachira et al. 1993).

EPIZOOTIOLOGY. The reader is directed to reviews of life cycle patterns, geographical distribution of species and strains, and epizootiology by Thompson and Lymbery (1990), Rausch (1995), and Schantz et al. (1995). Some recent prevalence data are provided in Table 7.11.

In southwestern Quebec, infection with *E. granulosus* is important in wolf-moose population dynamics. The prevalence, mean number, and mean total weight of cysts in moose lungs increased with increasing

TABLE 7.11—Some recent[a] records of *Echinococcus granulosus*

Hosts	Number Examined	Prevalence (%)	Location	Reference
Definitive Hosts				
Canis aureus	100	22	Iran	Dalimi and Mobedi 1992
Canis lupus	25	60	Quebec, Canada	McNeill et al. 1984
	52	55.8	Russia	Isakov and Safronov 1990
Canis mesomelas	7	1 of 7	Kenya	Nelson and Rausch 1963
Crocuta crocuta	19	16	Kenya	Nelson and Rausch 1963
Lycaon pictus	4	3 of 4	Kenya	Nelson and Rausch 1963
Vulpes vulpes	45	7	Australia	Jenkins and Craig 1992
	19	47.4	Australia	Obendorf et al. 1989
	197	1.0	Wales	Jones and Walters 1992b
Ursus arctos	32	3.1	Romania	Siko-Barabasi et al. 1995
Intermediate Hosts				
Alces alces	51	73	Alberta, Canada	Pybus 1990
	54	66.7	Ontario, Canada	Addison et al. 1979
	42	76.2	Russia	Isakov and Safronov 1990
Capreolus capreolus	88	6.8	Romania	Siko-Barabasi et al. 1995
Cervus elaphus	5114	1.9	Romania	Siko-Barabasi et al. 1995
	29	21	Alberta, Canada	Pybus 1990
Macropus fuliginosus	21	28.6	Australia	Thompson et al. 1988
Sus scrofa	44	36.4	Hungary	Murai and Sugar 1979
	635	22	Romania	Siko-Barabasi et al. 1995

[a]Since 1970.

moose density, and the infection in the moose population was overdispersed (Messier et al. 1989). Similarly, high intensity of infection in moose was correlated with high densities of wolves. The relationship may involve differential habitat use by wolves: in winter they congregate around kills and in summer they congregate at rendezvous sites, both patterns of activity leading to concentrated rather than random deposition of feces and therefore of parasite eggs in the environment. This in turn increased the chances of individual moose becoming infected or adding to established infections. Wolves may be able to recognize the vulnerability of infected animals (Rau and Caron 1979). Infection may regulate local moose (Messier et al. 1989) and/or wolf populations (Hadeler and Freedman 1989).

Where wolves are absent, other hosts maintain the life cycle. Hydatid cysts occur in moose in northwest Alberta (where wolves occur) and in central Alberta (where coyotes, but not wolves, occur) (Samuel et al. 1976; M.J. Pybus, unpublished). Red foxes are an important component of the life cycle in some countries (Australia) (Jenkins and Craig 1992), but not others (Britain) (Clarkson and Walters 1991; Jones and Walters 1992b).

Pybus (1990) found hydatid cysts in the lungs and liver of moose and wapiti in upland and northern mixed-wood habitats of northern Alberta (Table 7.11). Hydatid cysts were not found in mule deer or white-tailed deer in these habitats; Pybus (1990) concluded that moose and/or wapiti were required in order to maintain populations of *E. granulosus* in western Canada. Hydatid in reindeer in Finland is unusual (Oksanen and Laaksonen 1995) although it is common in northern regions of the former USSR.

In some places, human activity has transformed sylvatic foci into synanthropic foci or stimulated formation of new foci. For example, in Kamchatka the cycle is maintained mainly by dogs and reindeer, but introduced species such as elk [moose] and wolves may also be involved (Tranbenkova 1992). In Great Britain there is a wide distribution of hydatid in horses and fox hounds, with up to 60% prevalence in horses in some areas (Thompson and Smyth 1975). The cycle is reinforced by the feeding of raw horse meat and offal to the hounds. A few cases have been found in horses imported to United States (Rezabek et al. 1993), but recent evidence suggests the parasite may now be established in the northeast (Maryland) (Hoberg et al. 1994).

Infections can occur in unusual experimental hosts (vervets, *Cercopithecus aethiops,* and baboons, *Papio anubi)* (Rogan et al. 1993), in zoological settings (baboon: Goldberg et al. 1991; giant squirrel, *Ratufa indica:* Varma et al. 1995; ring-tailed lemur, *Lemur catta:* Shahar et al. 1995), and in free-ranging species (baboons, *P. hamadryas:* Ghandour et al. 1995). Vervets are suitable for immunological studies (Rogan et al. 1993).

Echinococcus granulosus is normally a parasite of canids rather than felids, but a lion-adapted strain is documented in Uganda, Kenya, Tanzania, South Africa, and the Central African Republic. Hydatid cysts occur in the liver, lungs, and heart of warthog, bushpig, zebras, buffalo, and wildebeest. Major intermediate host species differ in different geographical areas: zebra and buffalo are the most important in South Africa; warthog in the Central African Republic; and warthog, buffalo, and wildebeest in East African countries. The only other felid to harbour adults is the

African wild cat, *Felis lybica,* in South Africa. Although dogs are refractory to protoscolices from warthog cysts, infection can occur in spotted hyenas, Cape hunting dogs, and silver-backed jackals (Nelson and Rausch 1963; Rausch and Nelson 1963; Verster and Collins 1966; Sachs and Sachs 1968; Dinnik and Sachs 1969b, 1972; Woodford and Sachs 1973; Young 1975; Eugster 1978; Graber and Thal 1980; Macpherson et al.1983; Macpherson 1986).

PATHOLOGY AND PATHOGENESIS. The majority of hydatid cysts in moose develop in the lungs, where they often are superficial and may protrude into the pleural cavity. Infections generally occur without evidence of significant impact on lung capacity. However, heavily infected moose may have reduced stamina and be predisposed to predation when pursued by wolves (Messier et al. 1989). Lethargy, abdominal distension, and partial anorexia were observed in an infected ringtailed lemur. The infection was successfully treated with anthelmintics and surgical excision (Shahar et al. 1995).

DIAGNOSIS. Adult worms are identified to species and often to strain using morphological characters. *Echinococcus granulosus* can be distinguished from *E. multilocularis* by the more posterior position of the genital pore, the laterally lobed uterus, and the distribution of the testes in *E. granulosus.* Larvae of *E. granulosus* are unilocular and occur primarily in ungulates; those of *E. multilocularis* are multivesicular and occur in rodents.

Various molecular techniques for examining genotypes of adults, larvae, or eggs can be used to characterize and discriminate species and strains of *Echinococcus* (see McManus and Rishi 1989; Bowles et al. 1992; Bowles and McManus 1993; Scott and McManus 1994; Gasser and Chilton 1995), as reviewed by Lightowlers and Gottstein (1995). ELISA tests for detecting coproantigens in the feces of dogs, dingoes, and foxes can be used to test for both *E. granulosus* and *E. multilocularis* (see Deplazes et al. 1992; Walters and Craig 1992).

CONTROL AND TREATMENT. Control strategies must consider host-induced developmental variations in different hosts or the same host species in different environments (see Schantz et al. 1995). For example, early patency should be considered when treating dogs in arid areas (Wachira et al. 1993), and *E. granulosus* is uncommon in areas where hot dry seasons continue for longer than a few months (Gemmell 1990). Eggs are susceptible to desiccation and can die in 2 hours on dry ground in direct sunlight; however, survival time is increased in damp ground around water holes, where women, children, and dogs congregate (Wachira et al. 1991).

Education of dog owners is essential in any control program, but it can be difficult to persuade people to change their behavior. Continuous education programs in Kenya failed to change the attitude of local people towards their dogs, although it is clear that infection is positively correlated with the close proximity of dogs (Watson-Jones and Macpherson 1988). Twice as many women as men are infected, again reflecting a closer contact with dogs. In this region, prevalence of hydatid disease is the highest in the world despite the hostile arid environment.

Dogs should not be fed carcasses or allowed to scavenge (Wachira et al. 1990). Infected North American native children had contact with dogs fed moose entrails (Lamy et al. 1993). In some circumstances, infected humans can serve as intermediaries. Cysts in humans are large, with numerous protoscolices and are an important source of infection to dogs, particularly in societies that either do not bury their dead or inter them in shallow graves (Macpherson 1983).

2. ECHINOCOCCUS MULTILOCULARIS LEUCKART, 1863. Rostellar hooks in *E. multilocularis* are highly variable in number and are 25–34 µm and 20–31 µm long. The strobila is 1.2–4.5 mm long with up to six segments. The genital pore is anterior to the midpoint of the lateral margin of the segment. There are 16–35 testes, mainly posterior to the genital pore. The mature segment is antepenultimate in the strobila. The uterus is sac-like. The ratio of the anterior part of the strobila to the gravid segment is 1:0.31–0.80. The larva is a multivesicular (alveolar) hydatid. There are protoscolex hooks, 25–30 µm and 22–27 µm in length.

In contrast to *E. granulosus, E. multilocularis* exhibits little genetic variation (Thompson and Lymbery 1988, 1990; Bowles et al. 1992; Thompson et al. 1994), but there is biological variation in geographically separated populations (Eckert and Thompson 1988). Isolates from Alaska and Montana differ in rate of development in experimentally infected gerbils, length and number of protoscolex hooks, host response, and natural intermediate hosts (Bartel et al. 1992). Although the isolates may be biologically distinct, it is not clear if they are separate subspecies.

LIFE HISTORY. Although there are no data from wild hosts, patency of *E. multilocularis* in dogs occurs 32–33 days postinfection (Rausch et al. 1990) and can continue up to 111 days (Ishige et al. 1990). Multivesicular cysts occur in various locations in susceptible intermediates. They lack the adventitial layer that forms a host-tissue barrier in *E. granulosus* and thus invade the tissues and form a network of protrusions. Proliferation is both endogenous and exogenous, and detached germinal cells can be borne to new locations in blood or lymph fluid. Protoscolices develop in 2–3 months (Thompson 1995).

EPIZOOTIOLOGY. Typically, intermediate hosts of *E. multilocularis* are arvicoline rodents and definitive hosts are foxes (*Alopex, Vulpes*). Other canids, including Eastern grey fox (*Urocyon cinereoargenteus*), wolf (*Canis lupus*), coyote (*Canis latrans*), and domestic dogs and cats may be infected. Petavy et al. (1991) describe occurrence of sylvatic and synanthropic cycles in a focal area in the Massif Central, France. Zoonotic infections occur directly from foxes and domestic pets (Deblock and Petavy 1990).

Intermediate host species differ by geographic location. North American intermediates include *Ondatra zibethicus* in Montana; *Microtus oeconomus, Sorex* sp., *Clethrionomys rutilus,* and *Lemmus* spp. in Alaska; and *Peromyscus maniculatus* and *Microtus pennsylvanicus* in southern Canada and northcentral United States. In France, infections were identified in *M. arvalis, Arvicola terrestris* (mainly infertile cysts), *C. glareolus, O. zibethicus, Pitymys subterraneus,* and *Mus musculus.* A coypu (*Myocastor coypus*) on a private farm in Germany was infected; meat is used for human consumption (Worbes et al. 1989). In Japan, the main natural intermediate host is *C. rufocanus,* although recently infection in *C. rex* was reported (Takahashi and Nakata 1995). In a naturally infected *R. norvegicus* in Hokkaido, the protoscolices were incomplete; however, they did produce viable cysts when transplanted into the abdominal cavity in gerbils and a rat (Okamoto et al. 1992). Adult rats may be resistant to infection (Iwaki et al. 1995). In Russia (Kamchatka Peninsula), intermediates include *C. rutilus, C. rufocanus, M. oeconomus, O. zibethicus,* and *L. sibiricus;* foxes are the main definitive hosts, but wolves and dogs also are infected (Tranbenkova 1992). Brown rats (*Rattus norvegicus*), mink, and *Apodemus speciosus* are refractory to experimental infection (Ooi et al. 1992; Iwaki et al. 1995) and naturally infected wild boar are considered a dead-end host (Pfister et al. 1993).

Infections in rodents may also reflect differences in habitat, behavior, and food habits among rodent species. Deer mice are more exposed to infection because they are insectivorous and often live in or near abandoned fox dens, eat infected insects, and scavenge on feces (Leiby and Nickel 1968; Leiby et al. 1970). Small rodents are significantly more likely to become infected in habitats with poor ground cover (Leiby and Kritsky 1974), while species or individuals that live at the edges of fields, rural roads, and forest clearings are less likely to be infected (Delattre et al. 1988, 1990).

Although records are sporadic, *E. multilocularis* may cycle between house mice and domestic cats. Natural infections have been reported in cats in Canada, the United States, France, Germany, and Japan, and in mice in North America, France, and the former USSR (Leiby and Kritsky 1972; Deblock et al. 1989; Fesseler et al. 1989; Petavy et al. 1990b; Worbes 1992). Infected foxes may contaminate agricultural land and provide a source of eggs to infect mice and then cats. Cats could also acquire infection directly by predation on wild mice.

Humans are readily infected with *E. multilocularis,* and infections in captive primates occasionally are reported. These include a gorilla (*Gorilla gorilla*) and a ring-tailed lemur (*Lemur catta*) in a Japanese zoo (Kondo et al. 1996). Cysts in the lemur had calcareous corpuscles and protoscolices, but those in the gorilla had protoscolices only in one hepatic cyst. A crab-eating macaque (*Macaca fascicularis*) from a zoo in Stuttgart, an endemic area of Germany, had viable cysts in the liver (Reitschel and Kimmig 1994).

Echinococcus multilocularis continues to increase its geographical range in North America and Europe. Since the 1960s it has spread from the tundra zone of northern Canada to the central regions of continental United States. The current southern limits include parts of Wyoming, Nebraska, Iowa, Illinois, Indiana, and Ohio. In addition to natural dispersal, translocation of wild-caught foxes and coyotes from enzootic areas to fox-chasing enclosures in non-enzootic areas of the southeastern United States is considered a significant means of spread (Kazacos 1990; Davidson et al. 1992; Lee et al. 1993).

In Europe, the first report from Belgium was in 1991–1992 near the Luxembourg border (Brochier et al. 1992). Subsequent records near Gdansk, Poland, indicate that the affected area in central Europe is not isolated as previously believed, but is continuous with the large enzootic zone in Russia (Malczewski et al. 1995).

Using the ecological indicators of flora, climate, and lithology in a variety of habitats defined by altitude and minimum annual temperature, Gilot et al. (1988) found that two types of habitat were particularly good for completion of the life cycle in France: beech series on volcanic soil and locally acidophilous beech series on metamorphic soil.

PREVALENCE AND INTENSITY. Prevalence and intensity vary markedly among hosts and geographic locations in definitive and intermediate hosts (Table 7.12). In a serosurvey in Switzerland, 29% of 1252 red foxes had antibodies in serum or body fluid to the species-specific Em2-antigen (Ewald et al. 1992). In other studies, prevalence was lower in foxes from lowland areas than in those from forest and mountain locations and may reflect the distribution of intermediate hosts (Vos and Schneider 1994; Deutz et al. 1995). Sex-related differences were seen in prevalence in deer mice in North Dakota (Leiby and Kritsky 1974) but not in foxes in Germany (Vos and Schneider 1994; Deutz et al. 1995). Similarly, age-related differences in foxes may (Leiby and Kritsky 1974) or may not (Schott and Muller 1990) occur, perhaps affected by local or temporal variations. Prevalence of infection in deer mice was greater in spring (6.5% of 5638) than in summer (5.5%), autumn (2.2%), and winter (2%) (Leiby and Kritsky 1974).

Worm numbers tends to be higher in coyotes (mean 6579, range 1–52,000) than in foxes (mean 372, range 2–3640) and lower in southern portions of the species' range. In foxes in Illinois and Nebraska, the average intensity was 52 (range 1–320) (Ballard and Van de Vusse 1983; Ballard 1984).

PUBLIC HEALTH CONCERNS. Throughout the world, close contact between humans and dogs or cats is a

TABLE 7.12—Some recent[a] records of *Echinococcus multilocularis*

Hosts	Number Examined	Prevalence (%)	Location	Reference
Definitive Hosts				
Alopex lagopus	50	2	Northwest Territory, Canada	Eaton and Secord 1979
	129	40.3	Russia	Ageeva 1989
Canis latrans	219	4.1	Montana, USA	Seesee et al. 1983
	171	4.1	North central USA	Leiby et al. 1970
	70	18.6	Indiana, USA	Storandt and Kazacos 1993
	17	35.3	Illinois, USA	Storandt and Kazacos 1993
Canis lupus	2	1	China	Xu et al. 1992
Felis catus	498	1	Germany	Zeyhle et al. 1990
Vulpes corsac	6	2	China	Xu et al. 1992
Vulpes vulpes	313	34.8	Austria	Prosl and Schmid 1991
	500	3.6	Austria	Deutz et al. 1995
	139	4	Austria	Gottstein et al. 1991
	85	15.3	Belgium	Brochier et al. 1992
	79	33	China	Xu et al. 1992
	178	0.56	Czech Republic	Kolarova et al. 1996
	25	40	France	Petavy et al. 1991
	317	4.3	France	Pesson and Carbienier 1989
	150	23	France	Petavy et al. 1990a
	154	14.9	France	Deblock et al. 1988
	8425	14.2	Germany	Zeyhle et al. 1990
	244	55	Germany	Gottstein et al. 1991
	185	55.6	Germany	Schott and Muller 1989
	123	58.5	Germany	Schott and Muller 1990
	1300	0.3	Germany	Pfeifer 1996
	801	11.5	Germany	Wessbecher et al. 1994
	397	16.4	Germany	Ballek et al. 1992
	426	36.9	Germany	Welzel et al. 1995
	241	27.8	Germany	Vos and Schneider 1994
	679	44.8	Germany	Bilger et al. 1995
	805	12.7	Germany	Worbes 1992
	20	10	Poland	Malczewski et al. 1995
	1252	35	Switzerland	Ewald et al. 1992
	40	10	Illinois, USA	Ballard and Van de Vusse 1983
	71	22.5	Indiana, USA	Storandt and Kazacos 1993
	36	27.8	Nebraska, USA	Ballard and Van de Vusse 1983
	1540	8.5	North central USA	Leiby et al. 1970
	22	27.3	Ohio, USA	Storandt and Kazacos 1993
	72	8.3	Wisconsin, USA	Ballard 1984
Intermediate Hosts				
Arvicola terrestris	22	4.5	France	Petavy et al. 1996
	118	2.54	France	Petavy et al. 1991
	2010	0.2	France	Houin et al. 1982
Citellus dauricus	1500	0.2	China	Xu et al. 1992
Clethrionomys glareolus	436	0.2	Germany	Loos-Frank and Zeyhle 1982
Meriones unguiculatus	6	1	China	Xu et al. 1992
Microtus arvalis	37	2.7	France	Petavy et al. 1996
	3184	0.41	Germany	Loos-Frank and Zeyhle 1982
Microtus brandti	2635	2	China	Xu et al. 1992
Microtus pennsylvanicus	1033	2	North central USA	Leiby et al. 1970
Mus musculus	3	1	France	Petavy et al. 1991
	91	1.1	North central USA	Leiby et al. 1970
Myospalax fontanieri	320	0.3	China	Xu et al. 1992
Ochotona curzoni	214	4.2	China	Xu et al. 1992
Ondatra zibethicus	418	8.1	Germany	Seegers et al. 1995
	8403	2.9	Germany	Zeyhle et al. 1990
Papio hamadryas	67	13.4	Saudi Arabia	Ghandour et al. 1995
Peromyscus maniculatus	5638	4	North Dakota, USA	Leiby and Kritsky 1974
	4209	4.9	North central USA	Leiby et al. 1970
Rattus norvegicus	42	2.4	Japan	Okamoto et al. 1992

[a]Since 1970.

critical factor enhancing the risk of infection. Women in rural communities in China have a significantly greater chance than men of contracting infection, presumably reflecting greater exposure to dogs and dog feces (Craig et al. 1992). In Siberia, prevalence of infection is greatest in fur farmers, deer farmers, and dog owners (Ageeva 1989). In France, > 30% of foxes in foci may be infected, yet they are less important in domestic or peridomestic situations than dogs (Deblock and Petavy 1990).

As with *E. granulosus,* human activity has increased opportunities for transmission of *E. multilocularis.* Expansion of towns into a pastoral focus of alveolar hydatidosis in France resulted in infected microtine rodents in suburban and peri-urban sites (Laforge et al. 1992).

PATHOLOGY AND PATHOGENESIS. In humans, primary hepatic lesions associated with alveolar hydatid resemble hepatic carcinoma (D'Alessandro et al. 1979; Wilson and Rausch 1980). Little information is available about pathology in wild hosts, but the situation may be similar. In a bushy-tailed woodrat, *Neotoma cinerea rupicola,* tissue reactions in the liver were minimal, but the absence of calcareous corpuscles and protoscolices suggested that the woodrat is not a good host (Kritsky et al. 1977).

IMMUNITY. Very little is known about immunity in wild hosts. Brown rats naturally infected with *E. multilocularis* in Japan showed minimal immune response (Ito et al. 1996).

DIAGNOSIS. Morphological characters differentiating the adults and larvae of *Echinococcus multilocularis* and *E. granulosus* are provided above (see *E. granulosus*). In addition, *E. multilocularis* in foxes can be detected using the polymerase chain reaction to amplify DNA from eggs in fox feces. Sensitivity was estimated at 94% (Mathis et al. 1996) and at 1 egg/4 g feces (Bretagne et al. 1992), proving more sensitive than microscopic examination for detecting infection. Mucosal smear tests are used in Switzerland (Eckert et al. 1991; Ewald et al. 1992). ELISA using Em2-antigen was unreliable in detecting individuals but suitable for large-scale prescreenings of fox populations (Eckert et al. 1991). Assays with Em-2 antigen in Austria and Germany gave rather higher figures than parasitological examination of the same foxes (Gottstein et al. 1991). ELISA based on protein-A-purified polyclonal antibodies detects *E. multilocularis* coproantigens in fecal samples from dogs, dingoes, and foxes. In experimentally infected dogs, it gave positive results as early as 5 days after infection (Deplazes et al. 1992). Immunological diagnosis of *Echinococcus* spp. in domestic livestock is reviewed by Lightowlers and Gottstein (1995), but little information is available for sylvatic hosts. DNA probes are available to distinguish *E. multilocularis* and *E. granulosus* (see Vogel et al. 1990).

CONTROL. Control of infection in wild populations is unfeasible. However, regular anthelmintic treatment of domestic dogs and good hygiene practices are the best methods of control and prevention in humans. Translocation of infected canids from enzootic areas into captive enclosures in hydatid-free areas (e.g., southern United States) should be prohibited. Quarantine and treatment of wild-caught canids may mitigate the risks but should be verified prior to release of the animals. Monthly anthelmintic treatment of dogs was used as a control program in a hyperendemic area in Alaska (Rausch et al. 1990). The goal was to reduce the number of eggs in the environment, as expressed in lower prevalence of hydatid in northern voles. In the 10-year field trial, prevalence in voles was reduced from 53% to 5%, but success depended on a strict schedule of treatment for dogs and the elimination of unrestrained dogs.

3. *ECHINOCOCCUS OLIGARTHRUS* (DIESING, 1863).
Synonym: *E. cruzi* Brumpt and Joyeux, 1924.
Synonym confirmed by Sousa (1970) and Rausch et al. (1984).

Echinococcus oligarthrus has 26–40 rostellar hooks, 49–60 μm and 38.2–45 μm long. The strobila is 2.2–2.9 mm long, usually with three segments. The genital pore is at or anterior to the midpoint of the lateral margin of the segment. There are 15–46 (mean 29) testes, mainly posterior to the genital pore. The mature segment is antepenultimate. The uterus is sac-like and without diverticula. The ratio of the anterior part of the strobila to the gravid segment is 1:0.96–1.10. The larva is polycystic, in musculature and occasionally viscera. Protoscolex hooks are 29.1–37.9 μm (mean 30.5–33.40) and 22.6–29.2 μm (mean 25.4–27.2).

LIFE HISTORY. Gravid segments and adults from a naturally infected puma (*Felis concolor*) developed in the lungs, muscles, diaphragm, mesenteries, heart, and kidney of spiny rat (*Proechimys semispinosus*), Panama climbing rat (*Tylomys panamensis*), and brown agouti (*Dasyprocta punctata*) (Sousa and Thatcher 1969). Infective material from various intermediaries was fed to domestic cats, domestic dogs, margay (*F. tigrina*), raccoon (*Procyon lotor*), and coatimundi (*Nasua narica*). Adult worms in cats were normal, but those in dogs were not. No worms occurred in the other hosts. Over 1000 adult *E. oligarthrus* were recovered 121 days after a domestic cat was fed larvae from a naturally infected agouti (Sousa 1970).

EPIZOOTIOLOGY. Adult *E. oligarthrus* occur in wild felids [puma, jaguar (*F. onca*), jaguarundi (*F. yagouaroundi*), pampas cat (*F. colocolo*), and ocelot (*F. pardalis*)] in South and Central America: specifically Central America, Costa Rica, Panama, Columbia, and Brazil (D'Alessandro et al. 1981). Recently, the host and geographical range was extended by recovery of adults from a bobcat (*Lynx rufus texensis*) from Mexico

(Salinas-Lopez et al. 1996). Larvae are found in agouti [*Dasyprocta punctata, D. rubrata (=D. aguti cayana), D. leporina, D. fuliginosa*], pacas (*Cuniculus paca*), spiny rats (*Proechimys semispinosus, P. guyannensis*), and occasionally, in opossum (*Didelphis marsupialis*) and cottontail rabbit *(Sylvilagus floridanus)*. Prevalence in pacas increased with age but was not related to sex or geographical location (D'Alessandro et al. 1981). Larvae can also infect humans. Note that *E. vogeli* is sympatric with *E. oligarthrus* and uses similar intermediate hosts.

DIAGNOSIS. In heavily infected intermediate hosts, larvae can be detected by palpation; otherwise diagnosis is by removal and identification of the hydatid cyst. Brood capsules of *E. oligarthrus* are 267–517 μm x 224–445 μm (average 390 μm x 347 μm), with 6–30 protoscolices per brood capsule (average 18). Protoscolices are 125–168 μm x 95–142 μm (average 141 x 119 μm) (Rausch et al. 1981). The brood capsules are smaller and more delicate than those of *E. vogeli* with fewer and smaller protoscolices. Also, germinal tissue in *E. oligarthrus* tends to be columnar in appearance, and there is none of the proliferation of the laminated membrane in the vesicle which is characteristic of *E. vogeli*. Protoscolex rostellar hooks of *E. oligarthrus* are shorter and differ in shape from those of *E. vogeli* (see Rausch et al 1978). Hooks of *E. oligarthrus* have an almost straight dorsal surface, and the blade is about half the total hook length.

PUBLIC HEALTH CONCERNS. Only two cases of *E. oligarthrus* in humans are reported. One cyst was in the orbit (Lopera et al. 1989), the other in the heart (D'Alessandro et al. 1995). Each cyst was unilocular and may have been in an early developmental stage (D'Alessandro et al. 1995). The cyst in the eye was removed surgically.

4. *ECHINOCOCCUS VOGELI* RAUSCH AND BERNSTEIN, 1972. The rostellar hooks in *E. vogeli* are 38.2–57 μm and 30–47 μm long. The strobila is 3.9–5.5 mm long, with three segments. The genital pore is posterior to the midpoint of the segment margin. There are 50–67 testes, mainly posterior to the genital pore. The mature segment is antepenultimate. The uterus is long, tubular, and sac-like. The ratio of the anterior part of the strobila to the gravid segment is 1:1.9–3.0. The larva is a polycystic hydatid. The protoscolex hooks are 38.2–45.6 μm and 30.4–36.9 μm long.

LIFE HISTORY. When cysts of human origin were fed to dog and ocelot, one dog had about 250 immature and gravid worms 5 months later, and the ocelot had two partly developed worms 3 months later (D'Alessandro et al. 1979). Attempts to infect rice rats (*Oryzomys concolor*), spiny rats, gerbils (*Meriones unguiculatus*), and kittens with cyst material did not succeed. Similarly, oral inoculation of adult worms into paca, spiny rats, *Tylomys* sp., *Zygodontomys brevicauda, Thomomys fuscatus,* rabbit, and gerbils was unsuccessful.

EPIZOOTIOLOGY. *Echinococcus vogeli* is a Neotropical species distributed in Central and South America. Adults occur in bush dog (*Speothos venaticus),* but domestic dogs can also become infected; larvae occur in the liver of pacas (*Cuniculus paca).* Natural infections also occur in agoutis (*Dasyprocta* spp.), spiny rats (*Proechimys* spp.), and humans. The species is recorded from Panama, Ecuador, Colombia, Venezuela, Bolivia, and Brazil (D'Alessandro et al. 1981; Gardner et al. 1988; Rausch 1995) and probably occurs wherever bush dog and pacas are sympatric. Under zoo conditions, it will invade new intermediaries. Concurrent infections of *E. vogeli* and *E. oligarthrus* can occur.

PUBLIC HEALTH CONCERNS. *Echinococcus vogeli* is believed to be responsible for all cases of human polycystic hydatidosis reported from Colombia, Ecuador, Panama, Brazil, and perhaps Venezuela (D'Alessandro et al. 1979, 1996). Pacas are used as food by local human populations, and the viscera often are fed to domestic dogs (Rausch 1995). Similarly, patients with polycystic hydatid disease in Brazil had close contact with dogs fed on agouti viscera and were aware that the agoutis they hunted for food had a liver disease (Meneghelli et al. 1990). Rausch (1995) expressed concern that destruction of tropical forest habitat could precipitate development of a partly synanthropic life cycle, with increased prospects of human infection. Multilobed *E. vogeli* cysts from the liver, diaphragm, right iliac fossa, ileal mesentery, and peritoneum of a patient from Suriname who had lived in Guyana were surgically removed (Chigot et al. 1995).

PATHOLOGY AND PATHOGENESIS. Rausch et al. (1981) described larval development and pathology in the liver of naturally infected pacas and experimentally infected coypu (*Myocastor coypus).* The multilocular cyst is up to 30 mm in diameter, subspherical to asymmetrical, with a thick laminated membrane (3–50 μm). The interconnected chambers are produced by proliferation of the laminated membrane and germinal layer. The brood capsules arise in an irregular pattern from the germinal layer. In the natural host, there is no invasive growth into the liver by the exogenous proliferation which is characteristic of the infection in humans. Paca have a relatively long life span, and there is a marked tissue response to early, infective, and degenerating larvae.

DIAGNOSIS. Morphologic features of the hydatid larvae are distinctive (Rausch et al. 1981). Brood capsules are 424–1560 μm long by 389–1450 μm in diameter (average 817 μm x 781 μm). The average number of protoscolices per brood capsule is 81 (range 10–480), and the protoscolex dimensions are 158–203 μm x 108–145 μm (average 175 μm x 133 μm). The hydatid differs from that of *E. oligarthrus* in having a thicker laminated membrane, in the more extensive dispersal of brood capsules within the cyst (they tend to be peripheral in *E. oligarthrus*), and in the different shape and size of the protoscolex hooks. The protoscolex hooks of *E. vogeli* are 37–45.6 and 24.3–36.9 μm (Rausch et al. 1978; Gardner et al. 1988). They have a long, curved blade that occupies nearly two-thirds the total length of the hook (D'Alessandro et al. 1995).

LITERATURE CITED

Abram, J.B. 1972. A report of *Taenia taeniaeformis* from the muskrat, *Ondatra zibethicus zibethicus* in central Maryland. *Proceedings of the Helminthological Society of Washington* 39:264.

Abuladze, K.I. 1964. Taeniata of animals and man and diseases caused by them [In Russian]. In *Principles of cestodology*, vol. 4. Ed. K.I. Skryabin. Moscow: Izdatelstvo Nauka, 530 pp. [English Translation 1970. Israel Program for Scientific Translations, 549 pp.]

Addison, E.M.J., M.J. Pybus, and H.J. Rietveld. 1978. Helminth and arthropod parasites of black bear, *Ursus americanus*, in central Ontario. *Canadian Journal of Zoology* 56:2122–2126.

Addison, E.M.J., A. Fyvie, and F.J. Johnson. 1979. Metacestodes of moose, *Alces alces*, of the Chapleau Crown Game Preserve, Ontario. *Canadian Journal of Zoology* 57:1619–1623.

Addison, E.M.J., J. Hoeve, D.G. Joachim, and D.J. McLachlin. 1988. *Fascioloides magna* (Trematoda) and *Taenia hydatigena* (Cestoda) from white-tailed deer. *Canadian Journal of Zoology* 66:1359–1364.

Ageeva, N.G. 1989. Hydatidosis in the Nenets Autonomous Region [In Russian]. *Meditsinskaya Parazitologiya i Parazitarnye Bolezni* 5:65–68.

Albert, T.F., R.L. Schueler, J.A. Panuska, and A.L. Inging. 1972. Tapeworm larvae (*Taenia crassiceps*) in woodchucks. *Journal of the American Veterinary Medical Association* 161:648–651.

Albert, T.F., A. Chapman, and D. Pursley. 1981. Massive infection of tapeworm larvae (*Taenia crassiceps*) in woodchucks (*Marmota monax*). In *Worldwide Furbearer Conference Proceedings*, 3–11 August, 1980, Frostburg, MD, vol. II, pp. 670–677.

Allsopp, B.A., A. Jones, M.T.E.P. Allsopp, S.D. Newton, and C.N.L. Macpherson. 1987. Interspecific characterization of several taeniid cestodes by isoenzyme analysis using isoelectric focusing in agarose. *Parasitology* 95:593–601.

Alvarez, M.F., P. Quinteiro Alonso, M. Outeda Macias, and M.L. Sanmartin Duran. 1987. Larvas de cestodo de los muridos gallegos. In *Revista Iberica de Parasitologia, 1987*, Vol. Extraordinario: Enero, IV Congreso Nacional de la Asociacion de Parasitologos Espanoles (APE), pp. 91–96.

Alvarez, F., R. Iglesias, J. Bos, J. Tojo, and M.L. Sanmartin. 1990. New findings on the helminth fauna of the common European genet (*Genetta genetta* L.): First record of *Toxocara genettae* Warren, 1972 (Ascarididae) in Europe. *Annales de Parasitologie Humaine et Comparee* 65:244–248.

Anderson, W.I., D.W. Scott, W.E. Hornbuckle, J.M. King, and B.C. Tennant. 1990. *Taenia crassiceps* infection in the woodchuck: A retrospective study of 13 cases. *Veterinary Dermatology* 1:85–92.

Arru, E., S. Deiana, and A. Nuvole. 1967. Distomatosi epatica nei leporidi selvatici in Sardegna. *Atti della Societa Italiana delle Scienze Veterinaria* 21:762–766.

Ballard, N.B. 1984. *Echinococcus multilocularis* in Wisconsin. *The Journal of Parasitology* 70:844.

Ballard, N.B., and F.J. Van de Vusse. 1983. *Echinococcus multilocularis* in Illinois and Nebraska. *The Journal of Parasitology* 69:790–791.

Ballek, D., M. Takla, S. Volmer-Ising, and M. Stoye. 1992. Zur Helminthenfaune des Rotfuchses (*Vulpes vulpes* Linne 1758) in Nordhessen und Ostwestfalen. Teil I: Zestoden. *Deutsche Tierärztliche Wochenschrift* 99:362–365.

Barber, D.L., and L.L. Lockard. 1973. Some helminths from mink in southwestern Montana, with a checklist of their internal parasites. *Great Basin Naturalist* 33:53–60.

Bartel, M.H., F.M. Seesee, and D.E. Worley. 1992. Comparison of Montana and Alaska isolates of *Echinococcus multilocularis* in gerbils with observations of the cyst growth, hook characteristics, and host response. *The Journal of Parasitology* 78:529–532.

Behnke, J.M., C. Barnard, J.L. Hurst, P.K. McGregor, F. Gilbert, and J. Lewis. 1993. The prevalence and intensity of infection with helminth parasites in *Mus spretus* from the Setubal Peninsula of Portugal. *Journal of Helminthology* 67:115–122.

Bekirov, R.E., and Z. Dzhumaev. 1976. The role of wild animals in the epizootiology and epidemiology of larval taeniases [In Russian]. *Veterinariya, Moscow* 9:52–53.

Belkin, V.V., V.S. Anikhanova, T.A. Kolesova, and S.S. Shulman. 1982. The parasite fauna of the blue hare in Kareliya [In Russian]. *Ekologiya Paraziticheskikh Organizmov v Biogeotsenozakh Severa* 1982:151–156.

Bernard, J., and M.S. Ben Rachid. 1970. Presence d'un cenure de *Multiceps* sp. chez le goundi en Tunisie. *Archives de l'Institut Pasteur de Tunis* 47:337–341.

Beveridge, I., and B.J. Coman. 1978. Infection of foxes, *Vulpes vulpes*, with *Taenia pisiformis* (Cestoda). *Acta Parasitologica Polonica* 26:15–18.

Beveridge, I., and M.D. Rickard. 1975. The development of *Taenia pisiformis* in various definitive host species. *International Journal for Parasitology* 5:633–639.

Bilger, B., P. Veit, V. Muller, A. Merckelbach, D. Kersten, H. Stoppler, and R. Lucius. 1995. Weitere Untersuchungen zum Befall des Rotfuchses mit *Echinococcus multilocularis* im Regierungsbezirk Tübingen. *Tierärztliche Umschau* 50:465–470.

Blazek, K., D. Hulinska, and L.I. Lavrov. 1982. Pathological changes induced by *Multiceps endothoracicus* in the intestine of definitive host. *Folia Parasitologica* 29:333–336.

Blazek, K., J. Schramlova, and D. Hulinska. 1985. Pathology of the migration phase of *Taenia hydatigena* (Pallas, 1766) larvae. *Folia Parasitologica* 32:127–137.

Blazek, K., V.S. Kirichek, and J. Schramlova. 1986. Pathology of experimental *Cysticercus bovis* infection in the reindeer (*Rangifer tarandus* Linne, 1758). *Folia Parasitologica* 33:39–44.

Boag, B. 1987. The helminth parasites of the wild rabbit *Oryctolagus cuniculus* and the brown hare *Lepus capensis* from the Isle of Coll, Scotland. *Journal of Zoology* 212:352–355.

Bongo, G., G. Macchioni, A. Marconcini, M. Arispici, S. Rindi, F. Testi, D. Scaramella, M.A. Abulatif, M.H. Mohamed, and H.A. Abdulhamid. 1982. Prove di infestione sperimentale con uova do *Taenia crocutae* in animali domestici e di laboratorio. Nota preventiva. *Bolletino Scientifico della Facolta di Zootecnia e Veterinaria* 3:73–83.

Boomker, J., D.G. Booyse, and M.E. Keep. 1991. Parasites of South African wildlife. VI. Helminths of blue duikers, *Cephalophus monticola*, in Natal. *Onderstepoort Journal of Veterinary Research* 58:11–13.

Bowles, J., and D.P. McManus. 1993. Rapid discrimination of *Echinococcus* species and strains using a polymerase chain reaction-based RFLP method. *Molecular and Biochemical Parasitology* 57:231–239.

Bowles, J., D. Blair, and D.P. McManus. 1992. Genetic variants within the genus *Echinococcus* identified by mitochondrial DNA sequencing. *Molecular and Biochemical Parasitology* 54:165–173.

———. 1994. Molecular genetic characterization of the cervid strain ("northern form") of *Echinococcus granulosus. Parasitology* 109:215–221.

———. 1995. A molecular phylogeny of the genus *Echinococcus. Parasitology* 110:317–328.

Bray, R.A. 1972. The cestode *Taenia krepkogorski* (Schultz and Landa, 1934) in the Arabian sand-cat (*Felis margarita* Loche, 1858) in Bahrain. *Bulletin of the British Museum of Natural History (Zoology)* 24:183–194.

Bretagne, S., J.P. Guillou, M. Morand, and R. Houin. 1992. Detection of *Echinococcus multilocularis* DNA in fox faeces using DNA amplification. *Parasitology* 106:193–199.

Brglez, J., and Z. Zeleznik. 1976. Eine Übersicht über die Parasiten der Wildkatze (*Felis silvestris* Schreber) in Slowenien. *Zeitschrift für Jagdwissenschaft* 22:109–112.

Brochier, B., P. Coppens, B. Losson, M.F.A. Aubert, B. Bauduin, M.J. Barrat, F. Costy, D. Peharpre, L. Pouplard, and P.P. Pastoret. 1992. Prevalence of *Echinococcus multilocularis* infection in the red fox (*Vulpes vulpes*) in the province of Luxembourg (Belgium). *Annales de Medecine Veterinaire* 136:497–501.

Bursey, C.C., and M.D.B. Burt. 1970. *Taenia macrocystis* (Diesing, 1850), its occurrence in Eastern Canada and Maine, USA, and its life cycle in wild felines (*Lynx rufus* and *L. canadensis*) and hares (*Lepus americanus*). *Canadian Journal of Zoology* 48:1287–1293.

Bursey, C.C., J.A. McKenzie, and M.D.B. Burt. 1980. Polyacrylamide gel electrophoresis in the differentiation of *Taenia* (Cestoda) by total protein. *International Journal for Parasitology* 10:167–174.

Bussche, R.A. van den, M.L. Kennedy, and W.E. Willhelm. 1987. Helminth parasites of the coyote (*Canis latrans*) in Tennessee. *The Journal of Parasitology* 73:327–332.

Bwangamoi, O., D. Rottcher, and C. Wakesa. 1990. Rabies, microbesnoitosis and sarcocystis in a lion. *Veterinary Record* 127:411.

Bye, K. 1985. Cestodes of reindeer (*Rangifer tarandus platyrhynchus* Vrolik) on the Arctic islands of Svalbard. *Canadian Journal of Zoology* 63:2885–2887.

Canaris, A.G., and D. Bowers. 1992. Metazoan parasites of the mountain beaver, *Aplodontia rufa* (Rodentia: Aplodontidae), from Washington and Oregon, with a checklist of parasites. *The Journal of Parasitology* 78:904–906.

Chana, T.S. 1975. Muscle cysticercosis in wildebeeste in Kajiado District of Kenya. *Bulletin of Animal Health and Wildlife Diseases* 23:87–92.

Chapman, A., V. Vallejo, K.G. Mossie, D. Ortiz, N. Agabian, and A. Flisser. 1995. Isolation and characterization of species-specific DNA probes from *Taenia solium* and *Taenia saginata* and their use in an egg detection assay. *Journal of Clinical Microbiology* 33:1283–1288.

Chermette, R., J. Bussieras, J. Marionneau, E. Boyer, C. Roubin, B. Prophette, H. Maillard, and B. Fabiani. 1995. Cysticercose envahissante a *Taenia crassiceps* chez un patient atteint de SIDA. *Bulletin de l'Academie Nationale de Medecine* 179:777–783.

Chigot, J.P., F. Menegaux, R. Hammoud, J.P. Nozais, and C. Huang. 1995. A propos d'un cas d'hydatidose a *Echinococcus vogeli* ayant beneficie d'un traitement chirurgical complet. *Semaine des Hospitaux de Paris* 71:13–14, 429–431.

Choquette, L.P.E., G.G. Gibson, and A.M. Pearson. 1968. Helminths of the grizzly bear, *Ursus arctos* L., in northern Canada. *Canadian Journal of Zoology* 47:167–170.

Clarkson, M.J., and T.M.H. Walters. 1991. The growth and development of *Echinococcus granulosus* of sheep origin

in dogs and foxes in Britain. *Annals of Tropical Medicine and Parasitology* 85:53–61.

Coman, B.J., and M.D. Rickard. 1975. The location of *Taenia pisiformis, Taenia ovis* and *Taenia hydatigena* in the gut of the dog and its effect on net environmental contamination with ova. *Zeitschrift fur Parasitenkunde* 47:237–248.

Coman, B.J., and G. Ryan. 1974. The role of the fox as a host for *Taenia ovis* and *Taenia hydatigena* in Australia. *Australian Veterinary Journal* 50:12, 577–578.

Constantine, C.C., R.C.A. Thompson, D.J. Jenkins, R.P. Hobbs, and A.J. Lymbery. 1993. Morphological characterization of adult *Echinococcus granulosus* as a means of determining transmission patterns. *The Journal of Parasitology* 79:57–61.

Cornaglia, E. 1984. Parassitosi multipla nel dik-dik. (Nota preliminare). *Bolletino Scientifico della Facolta di Zootecnia e Veterinaria, Universita Nazionale Somalia* 5:107–114.

Courtin, S., H. Alcaino, J. Plaza, and G. Ferriere. 1979. Platelmintos del conejo silvestre (*Oryctolagus cuniculus*) en la Cordillera de Nahuelbuta, Chile. *Archivos de Medicina Veterinaria* 11:23–26.

Craig, P.S., D.S. Liu, C.N.L. Macpherson, D.Z. Shi, D. Reynolds, G. Barnish, B. Gottstein, and Z.R. Wang. 1992. A large focus of alveolar echinococcosis in central China. *Lancet* 340:826–831.

Custer, J.W., and D.B. Pence. 1981. Ecological analyses of helminth populations of wild canids from the Gulf Coastal Prairies of Texas and Louisiana. *The Journal of Parasitology* 67:289–307.

D'Alessandro, A., R.L. Rausch, C. Cuello, and N. Aristizabal. 1979. *Echinococcus vogeli* in man, with a review of polycystic hydatid disease in Colombia and neighboring countries. *American Journal of Tropical Medicine and Hygiene* 28:305–317.

D'Alessandro, A., R.L. Rausch, G.A. Morales, S. Collet, and D. Angel. 1981. *Echinococcus* infections in Colombian animals. *American Journal of Tropical Medicine and Hygiene* 30:1263–1276.

D'Alessandro, A., L.E. Ramirez, E. Chapadeiro, E.R. Lopes, and P.M. de Mesquita. 1995. Second recorded case of human infection by *Echinococcus oligarthrus. American Journal of Tropical Medicine and Hygiene* 52:29–33.

D'Alessandro, A., M.A.P. Moraes, and A.N. Raick. 1996. Polycystic hydatid disease in Brazil: Report of five new cases and a short review of other published observations. *Revista da Sociedade Brasileira de Medicina Tropical* 29:219–228.

Dalimi, A., and I. Mobedi. 1992. Helminth parasites of carnivores in northern Iran. *Annals of Tropical Medicine and Parasitology* 86:395–397.

Darwish, A.M., and M.M. El Bahy. 1991. Parasites in the muscles of slaughtered camels. *Veterinary Medical Journal, Giza* 39:221–229.

Davidson, W.R., M.J. Appel, F.L. Doster, O.E. Baker, and J.F. Brown. 1992. Diseases and parasites of red foxes, gray foxes, and coyotes from commercial sources selling to fox-chasing enclosures. *Journal of Wildlife Diseases* 28:581–589.

Deblock, S., and A.F. Petavy. 1990. Donnees recentes sur l'epidemiologie de l'echinococcose alveolaire en France. *Bulletin de la Société de Pathologie Exotique et de ses Filiales* 83:242–248.

Deblock, S., and A.F. Petavy. 1993. *Taenia intermedia* Rud., 1810 et ses crochets chez un renard de Bourgogne (France). *Bulletin de la Société Francaise de Parasitologie* 11:95–102.

Deblock, S., A.F. Petavy, and B. Gilot. 1988. Helminthes intestinaux du renard commun (*Vulpes vulpes* L.) dans le

Massif central (France). *Canadian Journal of Zoology* 66:1562–1569.

Deblock, S., C. Prost, S. Walbaum, and A.F. Petavy. 1989. *Echinococcus multilocularis,* a rare cestode of the domestic cat in France. *International Journal for Parasitology* 19:687–688.

De Bruin, D., and G.S. Pfaffenberg. 1984. Helminths of desert cottontail rabbits, *Sylvilagus auduboni* (Baird) inhabiting prairie dog towns in eastern New Mexico. *Proceedings of the Helminthological Society of Washington* 51:369–370.

De Graaf, A.S., P.D. Shaughnessy, R.M. McCully, and A. Verster. 1980. Occurrence of *Taenia solium* in a Cape fur seal (*Arctocephalus pusillus*). *Onderstepoort Journal of Veterinary Research* 47:119–120.

Delattre, P., P. Giraudoux, and J.P. Quere. 1990. Conséquences épidémiologique de la réceptivite d'un nouvel hôte intermediaire du taenia multiloculaire (*Echinococcus multilocularis*) et de la localisation spatiotemporelle des rongeurs infestes. *Comptes Rendus de l'Academie des Sciences,* Series 3, *Science de la Vie,* 310:339–344.

Delattre, P., M. Pascal, M.H. Le Pesteur, and J.P. Damange. 1988. Caracteristiques ecologiques et epidemiologiques de l'*Echinococcus multilocularis* au cours d'un cycle complet des populations d'un hote intermediaire (*Microtus arvalis*). *Canadian Journal of Zoology* 66:2740–2750.

Department of Agricultural Technical Services, South Africa. 1973. Annual Report of the Secretary for Agricultural Technical Services for the period 1 July 1971 to 30 June 1972, 270 pp.

Deplazes, P., B. Gottstein, J. Eckert, D.J. Jenkins, D. Ewald, and S. Jimenez-Palacios. 1992. Detection of *Echinococcus* coproantigens by enzyme-linked immunosorbent assay in dogs, dingoes and foxes. *Parasitology Research* 78:303–308.

Deutz, A., K. Fuchs, H. Lassnig, and F. Hinterdorfer. 1995. Eine Pravalenzstudie über *E. multilocularis* bei Fuchsen in der Steiermark unter Berücksichtigung biometrischer Methoden. *Berliner und Münchener Tierärztliche Wochenschrift* 108:408–411.

Dick, T.A., and R.D. Leonard. 1979. Helminth parasites of fisher *Martes pennanti* (Erxleben) from Manitoba, Canada. *Journal of Wildlife Diseases* 15:409–412.

Dies, K.H. 1979. Helminths recovered from black bears in the Peace River region of northwestern Alberta. *Journal of Wildlife Diseases* 15:49–50.

Dinnik, J.A., and R. Sachs. 1969a. Zystizerkose der Kreuzbeinwirbel bei Antilopen und *Taenia olngojinei* sp. nov. der Tupfelhyane. *Zeitschrift für Parasitenkunde* 31:326–339.

Dinnik, J.A., and R. Sachs. 1969b. Cysticercosis, echinococcosis and sparganosis in East Africa. *Veterinary Medicine Review* 2:104–114.

———. 1972. Taeniidae of lions in East Africa. *Zeitschrift für Tropenmedizin und Parasitologie* 23:197–210.

Dobrynin, M.I. 1987. The helminth fauna of *Gazella subgutturosa* in Turkmenistan [In Russian]. *Izvestiya Akademii Nauk Turkmenskoi SSR, Biologicheskikh Nauk* 3:64–67.

Doherty, M.L., H.F. Bassett, R. Breathnach, M.L. Monaghan, and B.A. McErlean. 1989. Outbreak of acute coenuriasis in adult sheep in Ireland. *Veterinary Record* 125:185.

Dokhnova, L.I., and A.S. Bessonov. 1987. Epizootiology of taeniases in the Chukotka region [In Russian]. *Byulleten Vsesoyuznogo Instituta Gelmintologii im K.I. Skryabina* 47:36–39.

Dorzhiev, D.D. 1982a. Transmission of taeniid infections to dogs and wild carnivores [In Russian]. *Nauchno Tekhnicheskii Byulleten, Sibirskoe Odtelenie VASKHNIL Voprosy veterinarii na krainem severo vostoke* 27:16–18.

———. 1982b. Treatment with phenasal of dogs with experimental *Taenia krabbei* and *T. parenchymatosa* infections [In Russian]. *Nauchno Tekhnicheskii Byulleten Sibirskogo Otdeleniya Vsesoyuznoi Selskokhozyaistvennoi Akademii* 27:21–25.

Duffy, M.S., T.A. Greaves, and M.D.B. Burt. 1994. Helminths of the black bear, *Ursus americanus,* in New Brunswick. *The Journal of Parasitology* 80:478–480.

Dvorakova, L., and J. Prokopic. 1984. *Hydatigera taeniaeformis* (Batsch, 1786) as the cause of mass deaths of muskrats. *Folia Parasitologica* 31:127–131.

Eaton, R.D.P., and D.C. Secord. 1979. Some intestinal parasites of Arctic fox, Banks Island, Northwest Territories. *Canadian Journal of Comparative Medicine* 43:229–230.

Eckert, J., and R.C.A. Thompson. 1988. *Echinococcus* strains in Europe: A review. *Tropical Medicine and Parasitology* 39:1–8.

Eckert, J., P. Deplazes, D. Ewald, and B. Gottstein. 1991. Parasitologische und immunologische Methoden von *Echinococcus multilocularis* bei Fuchsen. *Mitteilungen der Österreichischen Gesellschaft für Tropenmedizin und Parasitologie* 13:25–30.

El Din, M.H.T., M.B. Saad, and A.S. Mohamad. 1986. Cysticerci of *Taenia regis* Baer, 1923 in reedbucks, *Redunca redunca,* in Eldindir National Park, Sudan. *Journal of Wildlife Diseases* 22:118–119.

Elowni, E.E., and M.T. Abu Samra. 1988. Observations on a polycephalic cestode larva from a Nile rat (*Arvicanthis niloticus*). *Folia Parasitologica* 35:75–76.

Eugster, R.O. 1978. A contribution to the epidemiology of echinococcosis/hydatidosis in Kenya (East Africa) with special reference to Kajiado District. D.V.M. Thesis, University of Zurich.

Ewald, D., J. Eckert, B. Gottstein, M. Straub, and H. Nigg. 1992. Parasitological and serological studies on the prevalence of *Echinococcus multilocularis* Leuckart, 1863 in red foxes (*Vulpes vulpes* Linnaeus, 1758) in Switzerland. *Revue Scientifique et Technique Office International des Epizooties* 11:1057–1061.

Fall, E.H., S. Geerts, V. Kumar, T. Vervoort, R. De Deke, and K.S. Eom. 1995. Failure of experimental infection of baboons (*Papio hamadryas*) with the eggs of Asian *Taenia. Journal of Helminthology* 69:367–368.

Fallis, A.M., Freeman, R.S., and J. Walters. 1973. What eyes reveal. The light of the body is in the eye. *Canadian Journal of Public Health* 64:238–245.

Fatzer, R., B. Horning, and R. Fankhauser. 1976. Cysticercus von *Taenia crassiceps* (*Cysticercus longicollis*) im Zentralnervensystem eines Alpenmurmeltieres (*Marmota marmota*). In *Verhandlungsberichte des XVIII Internationalen Symposiums uber die Erkrankungen der Zootiere,* Innsbruck, 1976. Berlin: Akademie Verlag, pp. 111–113.

Fedorov, K.P., and A.F. Potapkina. 1975. The helminths of pikas (Ochotonidae) in the south of West Siberia [In Russian]. *Trudy Biologicheskogo Instituta Sibirskogo Otdeleniya Akademii Nauk SSSR* 23:203–211.

Feliu, C., J. Torres, J. Miquel, and J.C. Casanova. 1991. Helminthofauna of *Mustela erminea* Linnaeus, 1758 (Carnivora: Mustelidae) in the Iberian Peninsula. *Research and Reviews in Parasitology* 51:57–60.

Fesseler, M., E. Schott, and B. Muller. 1989. Zum Vorkommen von *Echinococcus multilocularis* bei der Katze, Untersuchungen im Regierungsbezirk Tübingen. *Tierärztliche Umschau* 44:766–75.

Forrester, D.J., and R.L. Rausch. 1990. Cysticerci (Cestoda: Taeniidae) from white-tailed deer, *Odocoileus virginianus,* in Southern Florida. *The Journal of Parasitology* 76:583–585.

Forrester, D.J., J.A. Conti, and R.C. Belden. 1985. Parasites of the Florida panther (*Felis concolor coryi*). *Proceedings of the Helminthological Society of Washington* 52:95–97.

Frechette, J.L., and M.E. Rau. 1977. Helminths of the black bear in Quebec. *Journal of Wildlife Diseases* 13:432–434.

Freeman, R.S. 1956. Life history studies on *Taenia mustelae* Gmelin, 1790 and the taxonomy of certain taenioid cestodes from Mustelidae. *Canadian Journal of Zoology* 34:219–242.

———. 1962. Studies on the biology of *Taenia crassiceps* (Zeder, 1800) Rudolphi, 1810 (Cestoda). *Canadian Journal of Zoology* 40:969–990.

Freeman, R.S., A.M. Fallis, M. Shea, A.L. Maberley, and J. Walters. 1973. Intraocular *Taenia crassiceps* (Cestoda). Part II. The parasite. *American Journal of Tropical Medicine and Hygiene* 22:493–495.

Friedland, T., B. Steiner, and W. Bockeler. 1985. Prävalenz der Cysticercose bei Bisams (*Ondatra zibethica* L.) in Schleswig-Holstein. *Zeitschrift für Jagdwissenschaft* 31:134–139.

Fujita, O., F. Oku, M. Okamoto, H. Sato, H.K. Ooi, M. Kamiya, and R.L. Rausch. 1991. Early development of larval *Taenia polyacantha* in experimental intermediate hosts. *Journal of the Helminthological Society of Washington* 58:100–109.

Gardner, S.L., R.L. Rausch, and O.C.J. Camacho. 1988. *Echinococcus vogeli* Rausch & Bernstein, 1972, from the paca, *Cuniculus paca* L. (Rodentia: Dasyproctidae), in the Departamento de Santa Cruz, Bolivia. *The Journal of Parasitology* 74:399–402.

Gasser, R.B., and N.B. Chilton. 1995. Characterisation of taeniid cestode species by PCR-RFLP of ITS2 ribosomal DNA. *Acta Tropica* 59:31–40.

Gathuma, J.M., and A.M. Mango. 1976. The role played by carnivores in the epidemiology of bovine cysticerciasis in Kenya. *Bulletin of Animal Health and Production in Africa* 24:149–155.

Gaur, S.N.S., H.C. Tewari, M.S. Seth, and O. Prakash. 1980. Helminths from tiger (*Panthera tigris*) in India. *Indian Journal of Parasitology* 4:71–72.

Gemmell, M.A. 1990. Australasian contributions to an understanding of the epidemiology and control of hydatid disease caused by *Echinococcus granulosus*—Past, present and future. *International Journal for Parasitology* 20:431–456.

George, T., B.A. Obiamiwe, and P.A. Anadu. 1990. Cestodes of small rodents of the rainforest zone of mid-western Nigeria. *Helminthologia* 27:47–53.

Ghandour, A.M., N.Z. Zahid, A.A. Banaja, K.B. Kamal, and A.I. Boug. 1995. First record of cystic echinococcus in free-ranging baboons, *Papio hamadryas*, in Saudi Arabia. *Annals of Tropical Medicine and Parasitology* 89:313–316.

Gibbs, H.C., and A. Eaton. 1983. Cysticerci of *Taenia ovis krabbei* Moniez, 1879, in the brain of moose, *Alces alces* (L.) in Maine. *Journal of Wildlife Diseases* 19:151–152.

Gigon, P., and J. Beuret. 1991. Contribution à la connaissance des helminthes d'oiseaux dans le nord-ouest de la Suisse. *Revue Suisse de Zoologie* 98:279–302.

Gilot, B., B. Doche, S. Deblock, and A.F. Petavy. 1988. Eléments pour la cartographie écologique de l'echinococcose alveolaire dans le Massif centrale (France): Essai de limitation d'un foyer. *Canadian Journal of Zoology* 66:696–702.

Goldberg, G.P., J.D. Fortman, F.Z. Beluhan, and B.T. Bennet. 1991. Pulmonary *Echinococcus granulosus* in a baboon (*Papio anubis*). *Laboratory Animal Science* 41:177–180.

Gonzalez, N.A. 1986. Finding *Coenurus serialis* in European hares in Patagonia. *Veterinaria Argentina* 3:788.

Gottstein, B., P. Deplazes, J. Eckert, B. Muller, E. Schott, O. Helle, P. Boujon, K. Wolff, A. Wandeler, U. Schwiete, and H. Moegle. 1991. Serological (Em2ELISA) and parasitological examinations of fox populations for *Echinococcus multilocularis* infections. *Journal of Veterinary Medicine*, Series B, 38:161–168.

Graber, M. 1959. Les parasites des animaux doméstiques et sauvages de la Republique du Tchad. 1. Regions du Kanem et du Bahr el Gazal. *Revue d'Elevage et Médecine Vétérinaire des Pays Tropicaux* 12:145–152.

———. 1974. *Cysticercus bovis* parasitizing wild ruminants in the Republic of Chad. *Bulletin of Epizootic Diseases of Africa* 22:345–348.

———. 1976. La cenurose des petits ruminants d'Afrique centrale. Les cenuroses africaines, humaines et animales. *Revue d' Elevage et de Médecine Vétérinaire des Pays Tropicaux* 29:323–335.

———. 1978. A propos de la cysticercose musculaire des ruminants sauvages et domestiques d'Ethiopie. *Revue d'Elevages et de Médecine des Pays Tropicaux* 31:33–37.

———. 1981. Endoparasites in domestic and wild animals of the Central African Republic (CAR). *Bulletin of Animal Health Production in Africa* 29:25–47.

Graber, M., and J. Gevrey. 1976. A propos de la cenurose cerebrale du chamois, *Rupicapra rupicapra* Linne. Confusion possible avec la rage. *Bulletin de la Societe des Sciences Veterinaires et de Medecine Comparee de Lyon* 78:209–214.

Graber, M., and J. Thal. 1980. L'echinococcose des artiodactyles sauvages de la Republique Centrafricaine: Existence probable d'un cycle lion-phacochoere. *Revue d'Elevage de Medecine Veterinaire Tropicale* 33:51–59.

Graber, M., P.M. Troncy and J. Thal. 1972. La cysticercose des sereuses de divers artiodactyles sauvages d'Afrique Centrale. *Bulletin of Epizootic Diseases of Africa* 20:126–142.

———. 1973. La cysticercose musculaire des ruminants sauvages d'Afrique Centrale. *Revue d'Elevage et de Medecine Veterinaire des Pays Tropicaux* 26:203–220.

Graber, M., P. Blanc, and R. Delaveney. 1980. Helminthes des animaux sauvages d'Ethiopie. I. Mammiferes. *Revue d'Elevage et Medecine Veterinaire des Pays Tropicaux* 33:143–158.

Gregory, G.G. 1976a. Fecundity and proglottid release of *Taenia ovis* and *T. hydatigena*. *Australian Veterinary Journal* 52:177–179.

Gubanyi, A., F. Meszaros, E. Murai, and A. Soltez. 1992. Studies on helminth parasites of the small field mouse (*Apodemus microps*) and the common vole (*Microtus arvalis*) from a pine forest in Hungary. *Parasitologica Hungarica* 25:37–51.

Guberti, V., L. Stancampiano, and F. Francisci. 1993. Intestinal helminth parasite community in wolves (*Canis lupus*) in Italy. *Parassitologia* 35:59–65.

Hadeler, K.P., and H.I. Freedman. 1989. Predator-prey populations with parasitic infection. *Journal of Mathematical Biology* 27:609–631.

Harrison, L.J.S., G.K.M. Muchemi, and M.M.H. Sewell. 1985. Attempted infection of calves with *Taenia crocutae* cysticerci and their subsequent response. *Research in Veterinary Medicine* 38:383–385.

Haukisalmi, V., H. Henttonen, and H. Pietiainen. 1994. Helminth parasitism does not increase the vulnerability of the field vole *Microtus agrestis* to predation by the Ural owl *Strix uralensis*. *Annales Zoologici Fennici* 31:263–269.

Hayes, M.A., and S.R. Creighton. 1978. A coenurus in the brain of a cat. *Canadian Veterinary Journal* 19:341–343.

Heidt, G.A., R.A. Rucker, M.L. Kennedy, and M.E. Baeyens. 1988. Haematology, intestinal parasites, and selected disease antibodies from a population of bobcats (*Felis rufus*) in Central Arkansas. *Journal of Wildlife Diseases* 24:180–183.

Hinaidy, H.K. 1971. Die Parasitenfauna des Rotfuchses, *Vulpes vulpes* (L.), in Österreich. *Zentralblatt fur Veterinärmedizin* 18B:21–32.

Hoberg, E.P., K.B. Aubry, and J.D. Brittell. 1990. Helminth parasitism in martens (*Martes americana*) and ermines (*Mustela erminea*) from Washington, with comments on the distribution of *Trichinella spiralis*. *Journal of Wildlife Diseases* 26:447–452.

Hoberg, E.P., S. Miller, and M.A. Brown. 1994. *Echinococcus granulosus* (Taeniidae) and autochthonous echinococcosis in a North American horse. *The Journal of Parasitology* 80:141–144.

Holmes, J.C., and R. Podesta. 1968. The helminths of wolves and coyotes from forested regions of Alberta. *Canadian Journal of Zoology* 46:1193–1204.

Hope, M., J. Bowles, and D.P. McManus. 1991. A reconsideration of the *Echinococcus granulosus* strain situation in Australia following RFLP analysis of cystic material. *International Journal for Parasitology* 21:471–475.

Hope, M., J. Bowles, P. Prociv, and D.P. McManus. 1992. A genetic comparison of human and wildlife isolates of *Echinococcus granulosus* in Queensland: Public health implications. *Medical Journal of Australia* 156:27–30.

Houin, R., M. Deniau, M. Liance, and F. Puel. 1982. *Arvicola terrestris*, an intermediate host of *Echinococcus multilocularis* in France: Epidemiological consequences. *International Journal for Parasitology* 12:593–600.

Isakov, S.I., and K.S. Olesova. 1979. Epizootiology of cysticerciasis of reindeer in Yakut ASSR [In Russian]. *Materialy Nauchnoi Konferentsii Vsesoyuznogo Obshchestva Gel'mintologov Tsestody i Tsestodozy* 31:46–49.

Isakov, S.I., and M.G. Safronov. 1990. The elk, an intermediate host of *Echinococcus granulosus* in Yakutiya [In Russian]. *Meditsinskaya Parazitologiya i Parazitarnye Bolezni* 2:58.

Ishige, M., K. Yagi, and M. Itoh. 1990. Egg production and life span of *Echinococcus multilocularis* in dogs, Hokkaido, Japan. In *Proceedings of an International Workshop on Alveolar Hydatid Disease*, Anchorage, Alaska, 1990, pp. 14–15.

Ito, A., M. Okamoto, H. Kariwa, A. Hashimoto, and M. Nakao. 1996. Antibody responses against *Echinococcus multilocularis* antigens in naturally infected *Rattus norvegicus*. *Journal of Helminthology* 70:355–357.

Iwaki, T., J. Inohara, Y. Oku, T. Shibahara, and M. Kamiya. 1995. Infectivity to rats of eggs of the *Echinococcus multilocularis* isolate from a Norway rat in Hokkaido, Japan. *Japanese Journal of Parasitology* 44:32–33.

Jenkins, D.J., and N.A. Craig. 1992. The role of foxes *Vulpes vulpes* in the epidemiology of *Echinococcus granulosus* in urban environments. *Medical Journal of Australia* 157:11–12, 754–756.

Jenkins, E., and A.W. Grundmann. 1973. The parasitology of ground squirrels of western Utah. *Proceedings of the Helminthological Society of Washington* 40:76–86.

Jenkins, D.J., and B. Morris. 1991. Unusually heavy infections of *Echinococcus granulosus* in wild dogs in south-eastern Australia. *Australian Veterinary Journal* 68:36–37.

Jessup, D.A., K.C. Pettan, L.J. Lowenstine, and N.C. Pedersen. 1993. Feline leukemia virus infection and renal spirochetosis in a free-ranging cougar (*Felis concolor*). *Journal of Zoo and Wildlife Medicine* 24:73–79.

Jones, A., and L.F. Khalil. 1984. *Taenia dinniki* sp. nov. (Cestoda: Taeniidae) from the striped and the spotted hyaena in East Africa. *Journal of Natural History* 18:803–809.

Jones, A., and T.M.H. Walters. 1992a. A survey of taeniid cestodes in farm dogs in mid-Wales. *Annals of Tropical Medicine and Parasitology* 86:137–142.

———. 1992b. The cestodes of foxhounds and foxes in Powys, mid-Wales. *Annals of Tropical Medicine and Parasitology* 86:143–150.

Jones, A., B.A. Allsopp, C.N.L. Macpherson, and M.T.E.P. Allsopp. 1988. The identity, life cycle and isoenzyme characteristics of *Taenia madoquae* (Pellegrini, 1950) n. comb. from silver-backed jackal (*Canis mesomelas* Schreber, 1775) in East Africa. *Systematic Parasitology* 11:31–38.

Kamanga-Sollo, E.I.P., K.J. Lindqvist, J.M. Gathuma, and A.J. Musoke. 1992. Antigens shared between metacestodes of *Taenia saginata* and *Taenia crocutae*. *Bulletin of Animal Health and Production in Africa* 41:25–32.

Kashchanov, E.K. 1972. The intermediate host of the cestode *Hydatigera taeniaeformis* (Batsch, 1786) Lamarck. 1816 [In Russian.] *Doklady Akademii Nauk Uzbekskoi SSR* 3:53–54.

Kazacos, K.R. 1990. *Echinococcus multilocularis* is identified in Indiana. *Large Animal Veterinary Report* 1: 6, 45.

Keith, I.M., L.B. Keith, and L.B. Cary. 1986. Parasitism in a declining population of snowshoe hares. *Journal of Wildlife Diseases* 22:349–363.

Keith, L.B., J.R. Cary, T.M. Yuill, and I.M. Keith. 1985. Prevalence of helminths in a cyclic snowshoe hare population. *Journal of Wildlife Diseases* 21:233–253.

Kelly, D.F., and C.E. Payne-Johnson. 1993. Cerebral healing after craniotomy to evacuate a *Coenurus cerebralis* cyst. *Journal of Comparative Pathology* 108:399–403.

Kingston, N., and R.F. Honess. 1982. Platyhelminthes. In *Diseases of wildlife in Wyoming,* second ed. Ed. E.T. Thorne, N. Kingston, W.R. Jolley, and R.C. Bergstrom. Cheyenne: Wyoming Game and Fish Department, pp. 155–187.

Kingston, N., E.S. Williams, R.C. Bergstrom, W.C. Wilson, and R. Miller. 1984. Cerebral coenuriasis in domestic cats in Wyoming and Alaska. *Proceedings of the Helminthological Society of Washington* 51:309–314.

Kirichek, V.S. 1985a. Localisation of *Cysticercus bovis* in the tissues and organs of experimentally infected reindeer [In Russian]. *Byulleten Vsesoyuznogo Instituta Gelmintologii im K.I. Skryabina* 40:37–43.

———. 1985b. Peculiarities of the biology of *Taenia saginata* and the disease that it causes [In Russian]. *Veterinariya, Moscow* 2:50–52.

Kirichek, V.S., and M.N. Belousov. 1984. Reindeer, a new host of *Cysticercus bovis* [In Russian]. *Byulleten Vsesoyuznogo Instituta Gelmintologii im K.I. Skryabina* 39:64–65.

Kirichek, V.S., A.S. Nikitin, A.A. Frolova, and L.S. Yarotskii. 1986. Some aspects of the biology of the northern strain of *Taenia saginata* [In Russian]. *Meditsinskaya Parazitologiya i Parazitarnye Bolezni* 6:37–39.

Kolarova, L., I. Pavlasek, and J. Chalupsky. 1996. *Echinococcus multilocularis* Leuckart, 1863 in the Czech Republic. *Helminthologia* 33:59–65.

Kondo, H., Y. Wada, G. Bando, M. Kosuge, K. Yagi, and Y. Oku. 1996. Alveolar hydatid in a gorilla and a ring-tailed lemur in Japan. *Journal of Veterinary Medical Science* 58:447–449.

Kritsky, D.C., P.D. Leiby, and G.E. Miller. 1977. The natural occurrence of *Echinococcus multilocularis* in the bushy-tailed woodrat, *Neotoma cinerea rupicola,* in Wyoming. *American Journal of Tropical Medicine and Hygiene* 26:1046–1047.

Kroeze, W.K, and R.S. Freeman. 1983. Growth and development of *Taenia crassiceps* (Cestoda) in the small intestine and peritoneal cavity of mice following oral infection. *Canadian Journal of Zoology* 61:1598–1604.

Kumar, V., S. Geerts, and J. Mortelmans. 1977. Failure of 74 days old *Cysticercus bovis* to develop in anthropoid apes, monkeys and hamsters. *Annales de la Societe Belge de Medecine Tropicale* 57:181–184.

Laforge, M.L., B. Gilot, B. Doche, S. Deblock, and A.F. Petavy. 1992. Urbanisation et populations de microtides dans le foyer Haut-Savoyard d'echinococcose alveolaire (Alpes francaises du Nord): L'exemple de La Roche sur Foron. *Revue Suisse de Zoologie* 99:373–394.

Lamy, A.L., B.H. Cameron, J.G. LeBlanc, J.A. Gordon-Culham, G.K. Blair, and G.P. Taylor. 1993. Giant hydatid lung cysts in the Canadian northwest: Outcome of conservative treatment in three children. *Journal of Pediatric Surgery* 28:1140–1143.

Langham, R.F., R.L. Rausch, and J.F. Williams. 1990. Cysticerci of *Taenia mustelae* in the fox squirrel. *Journal of Wildlife Diseases* 26:295–296.

Lavin, S., I. Marco, and J. Pastor. 1995. Cerebral coenurosis in chamois (*Rupicapra pyrenaica*). *Journal of Veterinary Medicine*, Series B, 42:205–208.

Lee, G.W., K.A. Lee, and W.R. Davidson. 1993. Evaluation of fox-chasing enclosures as sites of potential introduction and establishment of *Echinococcus multilocularis*. *Journal of Wildlife Diseases* 29:498–501.

Leiby, P.D., and W.G. Dyer. 1971. Cyclophyllidean tapeworms of wild Carnivora. In *Parasitic diseases of wild mammals*. Ed. Davis, J.W. and R.C. Anderson. Ames: The Iowa State University Press, pp. 174–234.

Leiby, P.D., and D.C. Kritsky. 1972. *Echinococcus multilocularis:* A possible domestic life cycle in central North America and its public health implications. *The Journal of Parasitology* 58:1213–1215.

———. 1974. Studies on sylvatic echinococcosis. IV. Ecology of *Echinococcus multilocularis* in the intermediate host, *Peromyscus maniculatus,* in North Dakota, 1965–1972. *American Journal of Tropical Medicine and Hygiene* 23:667–675.

Leiby, P.D., and M.P. Nickel. 1968. Studies on sylvatic echinococcosis. I. Ground beetle transmission of *Echinococcus multilocularis* Leuckart, 1863 to deer mice, *Peromyscus maniculatus* (Wagner). *The Journal of Parasitology* 54:536–537.

Leiby, P.D., W.P. Carney, and C.E. Woods. 1970. Studies on sylvatic echinococcosis. III. Host occurrence and geographic distribution of *Echinococcus multilocularis* in the north central United States. *The Journal of Parasitology* 56:1141–1150.

Leith, J.D., and W.C. Satterfield. 1974. Coenurus cysts of *Taenia multiceps* in a baboon, *Theropithecus gelada. Journal of Zoo Animal Medicine* 5:32–34.

Le Pesteur, M.H., P. Giraudoux, P. Delattre, J.P. Damange, and J.P. Quere. 1992. Spatiotemporal distribution of four species of cestodes in a landscape of mid-altitude mountains (Jura, France). *Annales de Parasitologie Humaine et Comparee* 67:155–160.

Lepitzki, D.A.W., A. Woolf, and B.M. Bunn. 1992. Parasites of cottontail rabbits of southern Illinois. *The Journal of Parasitology* 78:1080–1083.

Letkova, V., J. Mituch, J. Kocis, and G. Csizsmarova. 1989a. Occurrence of *Cysticercus tenuicollis* in cloven-footed game animals in Slovakia (Czechoslovakia) [In Slovakian]. *Folia Venatoria* 34:165–171.

———. 1989b. Importance of carnivores in the distribution of cysticercosis (*Taenia hydatigena* larvae) in cloven-footed game animals [In Slovakian]. *Folia Venatoria* 34:327–332.

Letonja, T., and C. Hammerberg. 1987a. *Taenia taeniaeformis:* Early inflammatory response around developing metacestodes in the liver of resistant and susceptible mice. I. Identification of leukocyte response with monoclonal antibodies. *The Journal of Parasitology* 73:962–970.

———. 1987b. *Taenia taeniaeformis:* Early inflammatory response around developing metacestodes in the liver of resistant and susceptible mice. II. Histochemistry and cytochemistry. *The Journal of Parasitology* 73:971–979.

Lightowlers, M.W., and B. Gottstein. 1995. Echinococcosis / hydatidosis: Antigens, immunological and molecular diagnosis. In Echinococcus *and hydatid disease.* Ed. R.C.A. Thompson and A.J. Lymbery. Wallingford, UK: CAB International, pp. 355–410.

Lochmiller, R.L., E.J. Jones, J.B. Whelan, and R.L. Kirkpatrick. 1982. The occurrence of *Taenia taeniaeformis* strobilocerci in *Microtus pinetorum. Journal of Parasitology* 68:975–976.

Loos-Frank, B. 1981. Larval cestodes in southwest German rodents. *Zeitschrift für Angewandte Zoologie* 74:97–105.

Loos-Frank, B., and E. Zeyhle. 1982. The helminths of the red fox and some other carnivores in southwest Germany. *Zeitschrift fur Parasitenkunde* 67:99–113.

Lopera, D.R., R.D. Melendez, I. Fernandez, I. Sirit, and P. Perera. 1989. Orbital hydatid cyst of *Echinococcus oligarthrus* in a human in Venezuela. *The Journal of Parasitology* 75:467–470.

Lozano-Alarcon, F., T.B. Stewart, and G.J. Pirie. 1985. Taeniasis in a purple-faced langur. *Journal of the American Veterinary Medical Association* 187:1271.

Lucius, R., W. Bockeler, and A.S. Pfeiffer. 1988. Parasiten der Haus-, Nutz- und Wildtiere Schleswig-Holsteins: Parasiten des inneren Organe des Rotfuchses (*Vulpes vulpes*). *Zeitschrift für Jagdwissenschaft* 34:242–255.

Macpherson, C.N.L. 1983. An active intermediate host role for man in the life cycle of *Echinococcus granulosus* in Turkana, Kenya. *American Journal of Tropical Medicine and Hygiene* 32:397–404.

———. 1986. *Echinococcus* infections in wild animals in Africa. In *Wildlife/livestock interfaces on rangelands.* Ed. S. MacMillan. Nairobi: Inter-African Bureau for Animal Resources, pp 73–78

Macpherson, C.N.L., and P.S. Craig. 1991. Echinococcosis—A plague on pastoralists. In *Parasitic helminths and zoonoses in Africa.* Ed. C.N.L. Macpherson and P.S. Craig. London: Unwin Hyman Ltd., pp. 25–53.

Macpherson, C.N.L., L. Karstad, P. Stevenson and J.H. Arundel. 1983. Hydatid disease in the Turkana District of Kenya (iii). The significance of wild animals in the transmission of *Echinococcus granulosus* with particular reference to Turkana and Masailand. *Annals of Tropical Medicine and Parasitology* 78:61–73.

Malczewski, A., B. Rocki, A. Ramisz, and J. Eckert. 1995. *Echinococcus multilocularis* (Cestoda), the causative agent of alveolar echinococcosis in humans: First record in Poland. *The Journal of Parasitology* 81:318–321.

Mathis, A., P. Deplazes, and J. Eckert. 1996. An improved test system for PCR-based detection of *Echinococcus multilocularis* eggs. *Journal of Helminthology* 70:219–222.

McBee, R.H., Jr. 1977. Varying prevalence of *Taenia taeniaeformis* strobilocerci in *Microtus pennsylvanicus* of Montana. *Great Basin Naturalist* 37:252.

McGee, S.G. 1980. Helminth parasites of ground squirrels (Sciuridae) in Saskatchewan. *Canadian Journal of Zoology* 58:2040–2050.

McKenna, P.B., I. Mackenzie, and D.D. Heath. 1980. Fatal hepatitis cysticercosa in a red deer fawn. *New Zealand Veterinary Journal* 28:124.

McManus, D.P., and A.K. Rishi. 1989. Genetic heterogeneity within *Echinococcus granulosus:* Isolates from different hosts and geographical areas characterized with DNA probes. *Parasitology* 99:17–29.

McManus, D.P., Z. Ding, and J. Bowles. 1994. A molecular genetic survey indicates the presence of a single, homogeneous strain of *Echinococcus granulosus* in northwestern China. *Acta Tropica* 56:7–14.

McNeill, M.A., M.E. Rau, and F. Messier. 1984. Helminths of wolves (*Canis lupus* L.) from southwestern Quebec. *Canadian Journal of Zoology* 62:1659–1660.

Meneghelli, U.G., A.L.C. Martinelli, and M.A.S.L. Velludo. 1990. Cistos de *Echinococcus vogeli* em figado de paca (*Cuniculus paca*). Originario do Estado do Acre, Brasil. *Revista da Sociedade Brasileira de Medicina Tropical* 3:153–155.

Mennerich-Bunge, B., K. Pohlmeyer, and M. Stoye. 1993. Zur Helminthenfauna der Wildschweine Westberliner Forsten. *Berliner und Münchener Tierärztliche Wochenschrift* 106:203–207.

Messier, F., M.E. Rau, and M.A. McNeill. 1989. *Echinococcus granulosus* (Cestoda: Taeniidae) infections and moose-wolf population dynamics in southwestern Quebec. *Canadian Journal of Zoology* 67:216–219.

Mikhailova, E.P., E.S. Kanakov, and N.I. Ovsyukova. 1983. Cysticerciasis of mammals in some areas of the RSFSR [In Russian]. *Parazitologicheskie issledovaniya v zapovednikakh-Sbornik Nauchnykh Trudov Tsentral'noi N.I. Laboratorii Okhotnich'ego Khozyaistva i Zapovednikov* 1983: 67–76.

Miquel, J., J. Torres, C. Feliu, J.C. Casanova, and J. Ruiz Olmo. 1992. On the helminth faunas of carnivores in Montseny massif (Catalonia, Spain). 1. Parasites of Viverridae and Mustelidae. *Vie et Milieu* 42:321–325.

Mituch, J., J. Sladek, and J. Hovorka. 1988. Helminth fauna of the wild cat in Slovakia [In Slovakian]. *Folia Venatoria* 18:353–358.

Mollhagen, T. 1979. The cysticercus of *Taenia rileyi* Loewen, 1929. *Proceedings of the Helminthological Society of Washington* 46:98–101.

Moreno Montanez, T., C. Becerra Martell, I.N. Lopez Cozar, T.M. Montanez, C.B. Martell, and I.N.L. Cozar. 1979. Contribucion al conocimiento de los parasitos de la liebre *Lepus capensis*. *Revista Iberica de Parasitologia* 39:1–4.

Movsesyan, S.O., F.A. Chubaryan, and A.V. Kurbet. 1981. Biological and morphological characteristics of the cestodes *Taenia pisiformis* (Bloch, 1780) and *Hydatigera taeniaeformis* (Batsch, 1786) [In Russian]. In *Raboty po gelmintologii. Materialy zasedaniya, posvyashchennogo 100 letiyu sodnya Akademika K.I. Skryabina.* Moscow: Nauka, pp. 128–137.

Mozgovoi, A.A., E.S. Kovalchuk, A.K. Gosteev, and V.I. Shakhmatova. 1979. Study of some population characteristics of *Taenia saginata* in West Siberia [In Russian]. *Trudy Biologicheskogo Instituta Sibirskogo Otdeleniya Akademii Nauk Ekologiya i morfologiya gelmintov zapadnoi Sibiri* 38:190–205.

Mueller, J.F. 1973. Accessory suckers (?) in *Taenia taeniaeformis* from the Californian bobcat. *The Journal of Parasitology* 59:562.

Murai, E., and L. Sugar. 1979. Taeniid species in Hungary (Cestoda: Taeniidae). 1. Cysticercosis, coenurosis and hydatidosis of wild ungulates. *Parasitologica Hungarica* 12:41–52.

Navarrete, I., D. Reina, M. Habela, G. Nito, F. Serrano, and E. Perez. 1990. Parasites of roe deer (*Capreolus capreolus*) in Caceres province, Spain. In *Erkrankungen der Zootiere. Verhandlungsbericht des 32. Internationalen Symposiums über die Erkrankungen der Zoo- und Wildtiere vom 23 Mai bis 27 Mai 1990 in Ekilstuna.* Berlin: Akademie Verlag, pp. 225–227.

Nechay, G. 1973. Seasonal incidence of larval *Hydatigera taeniaeformis* infection of *Microtus arvalis* in Hungary. *Parasitologica Hungarica* 6:117–129.

Nelson, G.S., and R.L. Rausch. 1963. *Echinococcus* infections in man and animals in Kenya. *Annals of Tropical Medicine and Parasitology* 57:136–149.

Obendorf, D.L., M.J. Matheson, and R.C.A. Thompson. 1989. *Echinococcus granulosus* infection of foxes in southeastern New South Wales. *Australian Veterinary Journal* 66:123–124.

Odnokurtsev, V.A. 1990. A first record of *Taenia krabbei* Moniez, 1879 in brown bears [In Russian]. *Redkie gelminty, kleshchi i nasemkomye. Series Novye i maloizvestnye Vidy Fauny Sibiri,* pp. 35–36.

Ogunbade, S.G., and A.F. Ogunrinade. 1984. Tapeworm infection (*Taenia hydatigena*) in lion (*Panthera leo*) in captivity. A case report. *Revue d'Elevage et de Médécine Vétérinaire des Pays Tropicaux* 37:30–31.

Okamoto, M., O. Fujita, J. Arikawa, T. Kurosawa, Y. Oku, and M. Kamiya. 1992. Natural *Echinococcus multilocularis* infection in a Norway rat, *Rattus norvegicus,* in southern Hokkaido, Japan. *International Journal for Parasitology* 22:681–684.

Oksanen, A., and S. Laaksonen. 1995. Ekinokokin jalkilypsy: Kuusamon koirien suuri ulostetutkimus talvella 1993. *Suomen Elainlaakarilehti* 101:168, 171–172.

Ooi, H.K., C. Inaba, and M. Kamiya. 1992. Experimental evaluation of mink and *Apodemus speciosus* in the *Echinococcus* life-cycle in Hokkaido, Japan. *Journal of Wildlife Diseases* 28:472–473.

Pence, D.B., and K.D. Willis. 1978. Helminths of the ringtail, *Bassariscus astutus,* from West Texas. *The Journal of Parasitology* 64:568–569.

Pesson, B., and R. Carbiener. 1989. Ecologie de l'echinococcose alveolaire en Alsace: Le parasitisme du renard roux (*Vulpes vulpes* L.). *Bulletin d'Ecologie* 20:295–301.

Petavy, A.F., S. Deblock, and C. Prost. 1990a. Epidemiologie de l'echinococcose alveolaire en France. I. Helminthes intestinaux du renard commun (*Vulpes vulpes* L.) en Haute-Savoie. *Annales de Parasitologie Humaine et Comparée* 65:22–27.

Petavy, A.F., S. Deblock, and S. Walbaum. 1990b. The house mouse: A potential intermediate host for *Echinococcus multilocularis* in France. *Transactions of the Royal Society of Tropical Medicine and Hygiene* 84:571–572.

———. 1991. Life cycles of *Echinococcus multilocularis* in relation to human infection. *The Journal of Parasitology* 77:133–137.

Petavy, A.F., F. Tenora, and S. Deblock. 1996. Contributions to knowledge on the helminths parasitizing several Arvicolidae (Rodentia) in Auvergne (France). *Helminthologia* 33:51–58.

Pfaffenberger, G.S., and V.B. Valencia. 1988. Helminths of sympatric black-tailed jack rabbits (*Lepus californicus*) and desert cottontails (*Sylvilagus audubonii*) from the high plains of eastern new Mexico. *Journal of Wildlife Diseases* 24:375–377.

Pfeifer, F. 1996. Zum Vorkommen von *Echinococcus multilocularis* und anderen Magen- Darm-Helminthen beim Rotfuchs (*Vulpes vulpes* L.) im Süden Sachsen-Anhalts. Thesis. Tierärztliche Hochschule, Hannover, Germany, 151 pp.

Pfeiffer, A.S., W. Bockeler, and R. Lucius. 1989. Parasiten der Haus-, Nutz- und Wildtiere Schleswig-Holsteins: Parasiten der inneren Organe des Steinmarders (*Martes foina*). *Zeitschrift für Jagdwissenschaft* 35:100–112.

Pfister, T., V. Schad, U. Schelling, R. Lucius, and W. Frank. 1993. Incomplete development of larval *Echinococcus multilocularis* (Cestoda: Taeniidae) in spontaneously infected wild boars. *Parasitology Research* 79:617–618.

Pleshchev, V.S. 1978. Morphological features of cestode larvae from rodents of northern Kazakhstan [In Russian]. *Zhiznennye tsikly, ekologiya morfologiya gelmintov zhivotnykh Kazakhstana* 1978:120–125.

Polishchuk, V.I., and V.V. Dolgov. 1979. *Multiceps* infection in carnivores and coenuriasis in sheep in southern and central Tadzhikistan, USSR [In Russian]. *Trudy Nauchno Issledovatelskogo Veterinarnogo Instituta Tadzhikiskoi SSR* 9:78–80.

Presidente, P.J.A. 1979. Liver lesions in the common wombat associated with migrating *Taenia hydatigena* larvae. *International Journal of Parasitology* 9:351–355.

Prokopic, J. 1970. Some notes on the distribution and life history of the cestode *Taenia martis* (Zeder, 1803). *Helminthologia* 11:187–193.

Prokopic, J., and D. Hulinska. 1978. Morphological structure of the larval cestode *Taenia polyacantha* Leuckart, 1856. *Folia Parasitologica* 25:241–246.

Prosl, H., and E. Schmid. 1991. Zum Vorkommen von *Echinococcus multilocularis* bei Fuchsen in Vorarlberg. *Mitteilung der Österreichischen Gesellschaft fur Tropenmedizin und Parasitologie* 13:41–46.

Pybus, M.J. 1990. Survey of hepatic and pulmonary helminths of wild cervids in Alberta, Canada. *Journal of Wildlife Diseases* 26:453–459.

Radomski, A.A., and D.B. Pence. 1993. Persistence of a recurrent group of intestinal helminth species in a coyote population from southern Texas. *The Journal of Parasitology* 79:371–378.

Rajský, D. 1985. *Ondatra zibethica,* an intermediate host in the life cycle of *Taenia taeniaeformis* [In Czech]. *Veterinarstvi* 35:136–138.

Ramadan, M.M., M.F.A. Saoud, and A.A.E. Shahawy. 1988. On the helminth parasites of rodents in the Eastern Delta. 2. A review of the cestode genus *Hydatigera* Lamarck, 1816. *Journal of the Egyptian Society of Parasitology* 18:141–147.

Rau, M.E., and F.R. Caron. 1979. Parasite-induced susceptibility of moose to hunting. *Canadian Journal of Zoology* 57:2466–2468.

Rausch, R.L. 1959. Studies on the helminth fauna of Alaska. XXXVI. Parasites of the wolverine, *Gulo gulo* L., with observations on the biology of *Taenia twitchelli* Schwartz, 1924. *The Journal of Parasitology* 45:465–484.

———. 1977. The specific distinction of *Taenia twitchelli* Schwartz, 1924 from *T. martis* (Zeder, 1803) (Cestoda: Taeniidae). *Excerta parasitologica en memoria del Doctor Eduardo Caballero y Caballero* 1977:357–366.

———. 1981. Morphological and biological characteristics of *Taenia rileyi* Loewen, 1929 (Cestoda: Taeniidae). *Canadian Journal of Zoology* 59:653–666.

———. 1993. The biology of *Echinococcus granulosus.* In *Compendium on cystic echinococcosis with special reference to the Xinjiang Uygur Autonomous Region, The People's Republic of China.* Ed. F.L. Andersen, J.J. Chai, and F.J Liu. Provo, UT: Brigham Young University, pp. 27–56.

———. 1994. Family Taeniidae. In *Keys to the cestode parasites of vertebrates.* Ed. L.F. Khalil, A. Jones, and R.A. Bray. Wallingford, UK: CAB International, pp. 665–672.

———. 1995. Life cycle patterns and geographic distribution of *Echinococcus* species. In Echinococcus *and hydatid disease.* Ed. R.C.A. Thompson and A.J. Lymbery. Wallingford, UK: CAB International, pp. 89–134.

Rausch, R.L., and F.H. Fay. 1988a. Postoncospheral development and cycle of *Taenia polyacantha* Leuckart, 1856 (Cestoda: Taeniidae). First part. *Annales de Parasitologie Humaine et Comparee* 63:263–277.

———. 1988b. Postoncospheral development and cycle of *Taenia polyacantha* Leuckart, 1856 (Cestoda: Taeniidae). Second part. *Annales de Parasitologie Humaine et Comparee* 63:334–348.

Rausch, R.L., and G.S. Nelson. 1963. A review of the genus *Echinococcus* Rudolphi, 1801. *Annals of Tropical Medicine and parasitology* 57:127–135.

Rausch, R.L., and F.S.L. Williamson. 1959. Studies on the helminth fauna of Alaska. XXXIV. The parasites of wolves, *Canis lupus* L. *The Journal of Parasitology* 45:395–403.

Rausch, R.L., V.R. Rausch, and A. D'Alessandro. 1978. Discrimination of the larval stages of *Echinococcus oligarthrus* (Diesing, 1863) and *E. vogeli* Rausch & Bernstein, 1972 (Cestoda: Taeniidae). *American Journal of Tropical Medicine and Hygiene* 27:1195–1202.

Rausch, R.L., A. D'Alessandro, and V.R. Rausch. 1981. Characteristics of the larval *Echinococcus vogeli* Rausch & Bernstein, 1972 in the natural intermediate host, the paca, *Cuniculus paca* L. (Rodentia: Dasyproctidae). *American Journal of Tropical Medicine and Hygiene* 30:1043–1052.

Rausch, R.L., C. Maser, and E.P. Hoberg. 1983. Gastrointestinal helminths of the cougar, *Felis concolor* L., in northeastern Oregon. *Journal of Wildlife Diseases* 19:14–19.

Rausch, R.L., A. D'Alessandro, and M. Ohbayashi. 1984. The taxonomic status of *Echinococcus cruzi* Brumpt & Joyeux, 1924 (Cestoda: Taeniidae) in an agouti (Rodentia: Dasyproctidae) in Brazil. *The Journal of Parasitology* 70:295–302.

Rausch, R.L., W.E. Giddens, and J.G. Bridgens. 1987. Mesothelial tumors associated with larval taeniid cestodes maintained by intraperitoneal inoculation in rodents. *Canadian Journal of Zoology* 65:1755–1758.

Rausch, R.L., J.F. Wilson, and P.M. Schantz. 1990. A programme to reduce the risk of infection by *Echinococcus multilocularis:* The use of praziquantel to control the cestode in a village in the hyperendemic region of Alaska. *Annals of Tropical Medicine and Parasitology* 84:239–250.

Reitschel, G. 1981. Beitrag zur Kenntnis von *Taenia crassiceps* (Zeder, 1800) Rudolphi, 1810 (Cestoda, Taeniidae). *Zeitschrift für Parasitenkunde* 65:309–315.

Rietschel, W., and P. Kimmig. 1994. Alveolare Echinokokkose bei einem Javaneraffen. *Tierärztliche Präxis* 22:85–88.

Rezabek, G.B., R.C. Giles, and E.T. Lyons. 1993. *Echinococcus granulosus* hydatid cysts in the liver of two horses. *Journal of Veterinary Diagnostic Investigations* 5:122–125.

Rickard, L.G., and W.J. Foreyt. 1992. Gastrointestinal parasites of cougars (*Felis concolor*) in Washington and the first report of *Ollulanus tricuspis* in a sylvatic felid from North America. *Journal of Wildlife Diseases* 28:130–133.

Rodonaya, T.E., G.V. Matsaberidze, and J. Prokopic. 1985. A new find of an adult *Taenia martis* (Zeder, 1803) in pine martens in Georgia [In Russian]. *Soobshcheniya Akademii Nauk Gruzinskoi SSR* 117:141–144.

Rogan, M.T., I. Marshall, G.D.F. Reid, C.N.L. Macpherson, and P.S. Craig. 1993. The potential of vervet monkeys (*Cercopithecus aethiops*) and baboons (*Papio anubis*) as models for the study of the immunology of *Echinococcus granulosus* infections. *Parasitology* 106:511–517.

Romashov, V.A. 1973. Occurrence of *Cysticercus tenuicollis* in the European beaver [In Russian]. *Parazitologiya* 7:294–295.

Roth, L., J.M. King, and B.C. Tennant. 1991. Hepatic lesions in woodchucks (*Marmota monax*) seronegative for woodchuck hepatitis virus. *Journal of Wildlife Diseases* 27:281–287.

Rubilar, C.L., and E. Merello. 1987. Endoparasitism in wild rabbits (*Oryctolagus cuniculus*) in the Florida zone, VIII region, Chile. *Agro-Ciencia* 3:31–34.

Ryan, M.J., J.P. Sundberg, R.J. Schauerschell, and K.S. Todd. 1986. Cryptosporidium in a wild cottontail rabbit (*Sylvilagus floridanus*). *Journal of Wildlife Diseases* 22:267.

Rysavy, B. 1973. Unusual finding of larval stages of the cestode *Hydatigera taeniaeformis* (Batsch, 1786) in the pheasant. *Folia Parasitologica* 20:15.

Sachs, R. 1966. Note on cysticercosis in game animals of the Serengeti. *East African Wildlife Journal* 4:152–153.

———. 1969. Serosal cysticercosis in East African game animals. *Bulletin of Epizootic Diseases of Africa* 17:337–339.

———. 1970. Cysticercosis of East African game animals. *Journal of the South African Veterinary Medical Association* 41:79–85.

———. 1977. Present and future parasite problems in African game. In *Origins of pest, parasite, disease and weed problems.* Ed. J.M. Cherrett, and G.R. Sagar. 18th Symposium British Ecological Society, Bangor, 12–14 April, 1976. Oxford, UK: Blackwell Scientific Publications, pp. 303–312.

Sachs, R., and C. Sachs. 1968. A survey of parasitic infestation of wild herbivores in the Serengeti region in northern Tanzania and the Lake Rukwa region in southern Tanzania. *Bulletin of Epizootic Diseases of Africa* 16:455–472.

Salinas-Lopez, N., F. Jimenez-Guzman, and A. Cruz-Reyes. 1996. Presence of *Echinococcus oligarthrus* (Diesing, 1863) Luhe, 1910 in *Lynx rufus texensis* Allen, 1895 from San Fernando, Tamaulipas State, in north-east Mexico. *International Journal for Parasitology* 26:793–796.

Samuel, W.M. 1972. *Taenia krabbei* in the musculature of moose: A review. *North American Moose Conference Workshop* 8:18–41.

Samuel, W.M., M.W. Barrett, and G.M. Lynch. 1976. Helminths in moose of Alberta. *Canadian Journal of Zoology* 54:307–312.

Schantz, P.M., J. Chai, P.S. Craig, J. Eckert, D.J. Jenkins, C.N.L. Macpherson, and A. Thakur. 1995. Epidemiology and control of hydatid disease. In Echinococcus *and hydatid disease.* Ed. R.C.A. Thompson, and A.J. Lymbery. Wallingford, UK: CAB International, pp. 232–331.

Schindler, R.R., Sachs, P.J. Hilton, and R.M. Watson. 1969. Some veterinary aspects of the utilisation of African game animals. *Bulletin of Epizootic Diseases of Africa* 17:215–221.

Schmidt, G.D., and R.L. Martin. 1978. Tapeworms of the Chaco Boreal, Paraguay, with two new species. *Journal of Helminthology* 52:205–209.

Schoo, G. 1993. Ein beitrag zur Helminthenfauna des Steinmarders (*Martes foina* Erxleben, 1777). Thesis. Tierärztliche Hochschule, Hannover, Germany, 92 pp.

Schott, E., and B. Muller. 1989. Zum Vorkommen von *Echinococcus multilocularis* beim Rotfuchs im Regierungsbezirk Tübingen. *Tierärztliche Umschau* 44:367–370.

———. 1990. *Echinococcus multilocularis*-Befall und Lebensalter beim Rotfuchs (*Vulpes vulpes*). *Tierärztliche Umschau* 45:620–623.

Schurr, K., F. Rabalais, and W. Terwilliger. 1988. *Cysticercus tenuicollis:* A new state record for Ohio. *Ohio Journal of Science* 88 104–105.

Schuster, R. 1982. *Cysticercus fasciolaris* in der Leber einer Bisamratte (*Ondatra zibethica*). *Angewandte Parasitologie* 23:223–227.

Schuster, R., and R. Benitz. 1992. On the development of *Taenia martis* (Zeder, 1802) in the intermediate host. *Helminthologia* 29:13–18.

Schuster, R., D. Heidecke, and K. Schierhorn. 1993. Beitrage zur parasitenfaune autochtoner Wirte. 10. Mitteilung: Zur Endoparasitenfauna von *Felis silvestris. Applied Parasitology* 34:113–120.

Scott, J.C., and D.P. McManus. 1994. The random amplification of polymorphic DNA can discriminate species and strains of *Echinococcus. Tropical Medicine and Parasitology* 45:1–4.

Seegers, G., S. Baumeister, K. Pohlmeyer, and M. Stoye. 1995. *Echinococcus multilocularis*-Metazestoden bei Bisamratten in Neidersachsen. *Deutsche Tierärztliche Wochenschrift* 102:256.

Seesee, F.M., and D.E. Worley. 1986. *Taenia ovis krabbei* from grizzly bears, *Ursus arctos,* in Montana and adjacent areas. *Proceedings of the Helminthological Society of Washington* 53:298–300.

Seesee, F.M., M.C. Sterner, and D.E. Worley. 1983. Helminths of the coyote (*Canis latrans* Say) in Montana. *Journal of Wildlife Diseases* 19:54–55.

Seville, R.S., and E.S. Williams. 1989. Endoparasites of the white-tailed prairie dog, *Cynomys leucurus,* at Meeteetse, Park County, Wyoming. *Proceedings of the Helminthological Society of Washington* 56:204–206.

Shahar, R., I.G. Horowitz, and I. Aizenburg. 1995. Disseminated hydatidosis in a ring-tailed lemur (*Lemur catta*): A case report. *Journal of Zoo and Wildlife Medicine* 26:119–122.

Shakhmatova, V.I. 1963. Helminths of martens of Karelia and the life cycle of *Taenia intermedia* Rudolphi, 1809 [In Russian]. Candidate Thesis. Biblioteka VIGIS, Moskva.

Shea, M., A.L. Maberley, J. Walters, R.S. Freeman, and A.M. Fallis. 1973. Intraocular *Taenia crassiceps* (Cestoda). *Transactions of the American Academy of Ophthalmology and Otolaryngology* 77:OP778–OP783.

Shults, L.M., and N.L. Stanton. 1986. *Taenia ovis krabbei* cysticerci in the pronghorn antelope, *Antilocapra americana. Proceedings of the Helminthological Society of Washington* 53:132.

Shumilov, M.F., and D.D. Dorzhiev. 1982. Prophylaxis of cysticerciasis in *Rangifer tarandus* [In Russian]. *Nauchno Tekhnicheskii Byulleten Sibirskoe Otdelenie VASKHNIL Voprosy veterinarii na krainem severo vostoke* 27:18–21.

Siko-Barabasi, S., E. Bokor, E. Fekeas, I. Nemes, E. Murai, and A. Gubanyi. 1995. Occurrence and epidemiology of *Echinococcus granulosus* and *E. multilocularis* in the Covasna County, East Carpathian Mountains, Romania. *Parasitologica Hungarica* 28:43–45.

Sogoyan, I.S., A.G. Chobanyan, A.V. Perkelyan, and G.M. Artunyan. 1982. The development of pathomorphological changes in sheep with *Cysticercus tenuicollis* infection [In Russian]. *Zoologicheskii Sbornik, Akademiya Nauk Armyanskoi SSR, Institut Zoologii Fauna parazitov zhivotnykh i vyzyvaemye imi zabolevaniya,* 18:102–109.

Soulsby, E.J.L. 1982. *Helminths, arthropods and protozoa of domesticated animals,* 7th ed. London: Balliere Tindall, 809 pp.

Sousa, O.E. (1970). Development of adult *Echinococcus oligarthrus* from hydatids of naturally infected agoutis. *The Journal of Parasitology* 56:197–199.

Sousa, O.E., and V.E. Thacher. 1969. Observations on the life cycle of *Echinococcus oligarthrus* (Diesing, 1863) in the Republic of Panama. *Annals of Tropical Medicine and Parasitology* 63:165–175.

Stanek, M., and F. Tenora. 1992. Larvae of cestode parasites of *Ondatra zibethicus* in the Czech Republic [In Czech]. *Acta Universitatis Agriculturae, Facultas Agronomica* 40:235–243.

Sterba, J., K. Blazek, and V. Barus. 1977. Contribution to the pathology of strobilocercosis (*Strobilocercus fasciolaris*) in the liver of man and some animals. *Folia Parasitologica* 24:41–46.

Stevenson P., G. Muchemi, and L. Karstadt. 1982. *Taenia saginata* infection in East African antelopes. *Veterinary Record* 111:322.

Stock, T.M. 1978. Gastro-intestinal helminths in white-tailed deer (*Odocoileus virginianus*) and mule deer (*Odocoileus hemionus*) of Alberta: A community approach. M.Sc. Thesis. Department of Zoology, University of Alberta, Edmonton, 111 pp.

Stone, J.E., and D.B. Pence. 1978. Ecology of helminth parasitism in the bobcat from West Texas. *The Journal of Parasitology* 64:295–302.

Storandt, S.T., and K.R. Kazacos. 1993. *Echinococcus multi-locularis* identified in Indiana, Ohio, and East-central Illinois. *The Journal of Parasitology* 79:301–305.

Strohlein, D.A. and B.M. Christensen. 1983. Metazoan parasites of the eastern cottontail rabbit in western Kentucky. *Journal of Wildlife Diseases* 19:20–23.

Stubblefield, S.S., D.B. Pence, and R.J. Warren. 1987. Visceral helminth communities of sympatric mule and white-tailed deer from the Davis Mountains of Texas. *Journal of Wildlife Diseases* 23:113–120.

Sulaiman, S., J.F. Williams, and D. Wu. 1986. Natural infections of vervet monkeys (*Cercopithecus aethiops*) and African red monkeys (*Erythrocebus patas*) in Sudan with taeniid cysticerci. *Journal of Wildlife Diseases* 22:586–587.

Sweatman, G.K., and T.C. Henshall. 1962. The comparative biology and morphology of *Taenia ovis* and *Taenia krabbei*, with observations on the development of *T. ovis* in domestic sheep. *Canadian Journal of Zoology* 40:1287–1311.

Takahashi, K., and K. Nakata. 1995. Note on the first occurrence of larval *Echinococcus multilocularis* in *Clethrionomys rex* in Hokkaido, Japan. *Journal of Helminthology* 69:265–266.

Tenora, F., and F. Meszaros. 1972. Data to the knowledge of the helminthofauna in *Pitymys* species occurring in Spain. *Parasitologica Hungarica* 5:159–161.

———. 1992. Second report of *Taenia martis* (Zeder, 1803) larvae (Cestoda), parasite of *Ondatra zibethicus* in Czechoslovakia [In Czech]. *Acta Universitatis Agriculturae, Facultas Agronomica* 40:229–234.

———. 1994. Changes in the helminth fauna in several Muridae and Arvicolidae at Lednice in Moravia. I. Systematics and taxonomy. *Acta Universitatis Agriculturae, Facultas Agronomica* 42:237–247.

Tenora, F., R. Wiger, and V. Barus. 1979. Seasonal and annual variations in the prevalence of helminths in a cyclic population of *Clethrionomys glareolus*. *Holarctic Ecology* 2:176–181.

Tenora, F., L. Beranek, and M. Stanek. 1988. Larvocysts of the cestode *T. polyacantha* (Leuckart, 1856) parasitizing *Oryctolagus cuniculus*. *Folia Parasitologica* 35:21–22.

Theis, J.H., and R.G. Schwab. 1992. Seasonal prevalence of *Taenia taeniaeformis:* Relationship to age, sex, reproduction and abundance of an intermediate host (*Peromyscus maniculatus*). *Journal of Wildlife Diseases* 28:42–50.

Thompson, R.C.A. 1986. Biology and systematics of *Echinococcus.* In *The biology of* Echinococcus *and hydatid disease.* Ed. R.C.A. Thompson. London: George, Allen and Unwin, pp. 5–43.

———. 1992. Parasitic zoonoses—Problems created by people, not animals. *International Journal for Parasitology* 22:556–561.

———. 1995. Biology and systematics of *Echinococcus.* In Echinococcus *and hydatid disease.* R.C.A. Thompson and A.J. Lymbery, (eds.). Wallingford, UK: CAB International, pp. 1–50.

Thompson, R.C.A., and L.M. Kumaratilake. 1985. Comparative development of Australian strains of *Echinococcus granulosus* in dingos (*Canis familiaris dingo*) and domestic dogs (*C. f. familiaris*), with further evidence for the origin of the Australian sylvatic strain. *International Journal for Parasitology* 15:535–542.

Thompson, R.C.A., and A.J. Lymbery. 1988. The nature, extent and significance of variation within the genus *Echinococcus. Advances in Parasitology* 27:210–258.

———. 1990. *Echinococcus:* Biology and strain variation. *International Journal for Parasitology* 20:457–470.

———. (eds). 1995. *Echinococcosis* and hydatid disease. Wallingford, UK: CAB International, 477 pp.

Thompson, R.C.A., and J.D. Smyth. 1975. Equine hydatidosis: A review of the current status in Great Britain and the results of an epidemiological survey. *Veterinary Parasitology* 1:107–127.

Thompson, R.C.A., A.J. Lymbery, R.P. Hobbs, and A.D. Elliott. 1988. Hydatid disease in urban areas of Western Australia: An unusual cycle involving western grey kangaroos (*Macropus fuliginosus*), feral pigs and domestic dogs. *Australian Veterinary Journal* 65:188–190.

Thompson, R.C.A., A.J. Lymbery, and C.C. Constantine. 1994. Variation in *Echinococcus:* Towards a taxonomic revision of the genus. *Advances in Parasitology* 35:145–176.

Todd, K.S., Jr., J.H. Adams, and J.H. Hoogeweg. 1978. The muskrat, *Ondatra zibethica,* as a host of *Taenia mustelae* in Illinois. *The Journal of Parasitology* 64:523.

Torres, J., J.C. Casanova, C. Feliu, J. Gisbert, and M.T. Manfredi. 1989. Contribucion al conocimiento de la cestodofauna de *Felis silvestris* Schreber, 1776 (Carnivora: Felidae) en la Peninsula Iberica. *Revista Iberica de Parasitologia* 49:307–312.

Tranbenkova, N.A. 1992. On the ecology of *Echinococcus multilocularis* (Leuckart, 1863) and *E. granulosus* (Batsch 1786) in the Kamchatka peninsula [In Russian]. *Meditsinskaya Parazitologiya i Parazitarnye Bolezni* 1:45–47.

Trees, A.J., R.R. Owen, P.S. Craig, and G.M. Purvis. 1985. *Taenia hydatigena:* A cause of persistent liver condemnations in lambs. *Veterinary Record* 116:512–516.

Tscherner, W., A.T. Movcan, J.S. Belkanija, I.S. Gvazava, and D. Schroder. 1988. Zwei neue Coenurus-Falle beim Blutbrustpavian (*Theropithecus gelada*). In *Erkankungen der Zootiere, Verhandlungs berichte des 30.* Internationalen Symposiums über die Erkrankungen der Zoo- und Wildtiere vom 11 Mai bis 15 Mai 1988 in Sofia. Berlin: Akademie Verlag, pp. 309–312.

Varma, T.K., B.M. Arora, and H.C. Malviya. 1995. On the occurrence of hydatid cyst in giant squirrel (*Ratufa indica). Indian Veterinary Journal* 72:1305–1306.

Verster, A. 1965. *Taenia solium* Lin., 1758 in the chacma baboon, *Papio ursinus* (Kerr, 1792). *Journal of the South African Veterinary Medical Association* 36:580.

———. 1969. A taxonomic revision of the genus *Taenia* Linnaeus, 1758 *s. str. Onderstepoort Journal of Veterinary Research* 36:3–58.

Verster, A., and J.D. Bezuidenhout. 1972. *Taenia multiceps* larva from a gemsbok. *Onderstepoort Journal of Veterinary Research* 39:123.

Verster, A., and M. Collins. 1966. The incidence of hydatidosis in the Republic of South Africa. *Onderstepoort Journal of Veterinary Research* 33:49–72.

Verster, A., G.D. Imes, and J.P.J. Smit. 1975. Helminths recovered from the bontbok, *Damaliscus dorcas dorcas* (Pallas, 1766). *Onderstepoort Journal of Veterinary Research* 42:29–32.

Vogel, M., N. Muller, B. Gottstein, K. Flury, J. Eckert, and T. Seebeck. 1990. *Echinococcus multilocularis:* Characterization of a DNA probe. *Acta Tropica* 48:109–116.

Volodina, L.L. 1982. Cysticerciasis in elks [In Russian]. *Veterinariya, Moscow* 7:45–46.

Vos, A., and L. Schneider. 1994. *Echinococcus multilocularis*—Befall beim Rotfuchs (*Vulpes vulpes*) im Landkreis Garmisch-Partenkirchen. *Tierärztliche Umschau* 49:225–228, 231–232.

Vustina, U.D. 1988. Infectious diseases of muskrats) *Ondatra zibethica*) [In Russian]. *Krolikovodstvo i Zverovodstvo* 1:23–24.

Wachira, T.M., C.N.L. Macpherson, and J.M. Gathuma. 1990. Hydatid disease in the Turkana District of Kenya, VII: Analysis of the infection pressure. *Annals of Tropical Medicine and Parasitology* 84:361–368.

———. 1991. Release and survival of *Echinococcus* eggs in different environments in Turkana and their possible impact on the incidence of hydatidosis in man and livestock. *Journal of Helminthology* 65:55–61.

Wachira, T.M., J. Bowles, E. Zeyhle, and D.P. McManus. 1993. Molecular examination of the sympatry and distribution of sheep and camel strains of *Echinococcus granulosus* in Kenya. *American Journal of Tropical Medicine and Parasitology* 48:473–479.

Wahl, E. 1967. Etude parasito-écologique des petits mammiferes (insectivores et ronguers) du val de l'Allandon (Geneve). *Revue Suisse de Zoologie* 74:129–188.

Waid, D.D., and D.B. Pence. 1988. Helminths of mountain lions (*Felis concolor*) from southwestern Texas, with a redescription of *Cylicospirura subaequalis* (Molin, 1860) Vevers, 1922. *Canadian Journal of Zoology* 66:2110–2117.

Walters, T.M.H., and P.S. Craig. 1992. Diagnosis of *Echinococcus granulosus* infection in dogs. *Veterinary Record* 131:39–40.

Wanas, M.Q.A., K.K. Shehata, and A.A. Rashed. 1993. Larval occurrence of *Hydatigera taeniaeformis* Batsch (1786) (Cestoda: Taeniidae) in the liver of wild rodents in Egypt. *Journal of the Egyptian Society of Parasitology* 23:381–388.

Watson-Jones, D.L., and C.N.L. Macpherson. 1988. Hydatid disease in the Turkana District of Kenya VI. Man: Dog contact and its role in the transmission and control of hydatidosis amongst the Turkana. *Annals of Tropical Medicine and Parasitology* 82:343–356.

Webster, J.P., and D.W. Macdonald. 1995. Parasites of wild brown rats (*Rattus norvegicus*) on UK farms. *Parasitology* 111:247–255.

Webster, W.A. 1974. Records of cestodes in varying lemmings and an arctic fox from Bathurst Island, Northwest Territories. *Canadian Journal of Zoology* 52:1425–1426.

Webster, W.A., and Rowell, J. 1980. Some helminth parasites from the small intestine of free-ranging muskoxen *Ovibos moschatus* (Zimmermann) of Devon and Ellesmere Islands, Northwest Territories. *Canadian Journal of Zoology* 58:304–305.

Welzel, A., G. Steinbach, M. von Keyserlingk, and M. Stoye. 1995. Zur Helminthenfauna des Rotfuchses (*Vulpes vulpes* L.) in Südniedersachsen. Teil 2: Zestoden. *Zeitschrift für Jagdwissenschaft* 41:100–109.

Wessbecher, H., W. Dalchow, and M. Stoye. 1994. Zur Helminthenfaune des Rotfuchses (*Vulpes vulpes* Linne 1758) im Regierungsbezirk Karlsruhe. Teil 1: Cestoden. *Deutsche Tierärztliche Wochenschrift* 101:322–326.

Williams, B.M. 1976. The intestinal parasites of the red fox in south west Wales. *British Veterinary Journal* 132:309–312.

Wilson, J.F., and R.L. Rausch. 1980. Alveolar hydatid disease. A review of clinical features of 35 indigenous cases of *Echinococcus multilocularis* infection in Alaskan Eski-mos. *American Journal of Tropical Medicine and Hygiene* 29:134–155.

Woodford, M.H., and R. Sachs. 1973. The incidence of cysticercosis, hydatidosis and sparganosis in wild herbivores of the Queen Elizabeth National Park, Uganda. *Bulletin of Epizootic Diseases of Africa* 21:265–271.

Worbes, H. 1992. Zum Vorkommen von *Echinococcus granulosus* und *E. multilocularis* in Thüringen. *Angewandte Parasitologie* 33:193–204.

Worbes, H., K.H. Schacht, and J. Eckert. 1989. *Echinococcus multilocularis* in a coypu (*Myocastor coypus*). *Angewandte Parasitologie* 30:161–165.

Worley, D.E. 1974. Quantitative studies on the migration and development of *Taenia pisiformis* larvae in laboratory rabbits. *Laboratory Animal Science* 24:517–522.

Xu, X.Y., M. Liance, Y.G. Lin, W.X. Li, and R. Houin. 1992. L'echinococcose alveolaire en Chine. Données actuelles. *Bulletin de la Societe de Pathologie Exotique* 85:241–246.

Yang, S.G., Z.K. Wang, and B.K. Shi. 1986. A study of the experimental infection and life-cycle of *Taenia pisiformis* [In Chinese]. *Chinese Journal of Veterinary Science and Technology* 6:16–19.

Young, E. 1975. *Echinococcus* (hydatidosis) in wild animals of the Kruger National Park. *Journal of the South African Medical Association* 46:285–286.

Young, E., J.J. Wagener, and P.J.L. Bronkhorst. 1969. The blue wildebeest as a source of food and by-products: The production potential, parasites and pathology of free living wildebeest of the Kruger National Park. *Journal of the South African Veterinary Medical Association* 40:315–318.

Zabiega, M.H. 1996. Helminths of mink, *Mustela vison,* and muskrats, *Ondatra zibethic,* in southern Illinois. *Journal of the Helminthological Society of Washington* 63:246–250.

Zelinskii, L.M. 1973. Larval cestode infections in reindeer in the Koryak region (USSR) [In Russian]. *Materialy Nauchnykh Konferentsii Vsesoyuznogo Obshchestva Gelmintologov* 25:113–119

Zeyhle, E., M. Abel, and W. Frank. 1990. Epidemiologische Untersuchungen zon Vorkommen von *Echinococcus multilocularis* bei End- und Zwischenwirten in der Bundesrepublik Deutschland. *Mitteilungen der Österreichischen Gesellschaft für Tropenmedizin und Parasitologie* 12:221–232.

Zhidkov, A.E., and N.A. Yurev. 1984. Prevalence and prophylaxis of larval cestode infections in reindeer in the Pevek State Farm, Magadan region [In Russian]. *Diagnostika, patogenez i lechenie infektsionnykh i invazionnykh zabolevanii selskokhozyaistvennykh zhivotnykh, Sbornik nauchnykh trudov.* 1984:3–8.

Zhuravets, A.K. 1973. The role of dog foxes in the epidemiology of coenurosis and echinococcosis [In Russian]. *Byulleten Vsesoyuznogo Instituta Gelmintologii* 10:49–52.

8 GASTROINTESTINAL STRONGYLES IN WILD RUMINANTS

ERIC P. HOBERG, A. ALAN KOCAN, AND LORA G. RICKARD

INTRODUCTION. Parasitologists have long studied helminth infections in wildlife species and have documented the existence of many organisms from a diversity of mammalian hosts. With this accumulation of information has come improved understanding of the significance of these organisms and the diseases they produce in their mammalian hosts. Some of the most notable examples include the metastrongyloid lungworms, *Trichinella spiralis,* and *Elaeophora schneideri,* which are covered separately in this volume. It is, however, for the group of parasites referred to as gastrointestinal nematodes that we have accumulated the most data. Only recently has progress been made in determining the significance of these strongylate nematodes with respect to their potential impact on the morbidity and mortality of the ruminants that they infect.

The accumulation of information on diseases of wild animals into a single combined volume has been slow, but progress has coincided with the proliferation of data for host and parasite interactions. Numerous references including *Alaskan Wildlife Diseases* (Dieterich 1981), *Manual of Common Wildlife Diseases in Colorado* (Adrian 1981), *Field Manual of Wildlife Diseases in the Southeastern United States* (Davidson and Nettles 1988*), Zoo and Wildlife Medicine* (Fowler 1993), and the previous editions of *Parasitic Diseases of Wild Mammals* (Davis and Anderson 1971) have all made significant contributions to our knowledge. Beyond North America, Dunn (1969) and Govorka et al. (1988) provided excellent compilations on the helminths in wild ruminants. In the 1971 printing of *Parasitic Diseases of Mammals,* however, there was no general coverage of gastrointestinal nematodes, and only *T. spiralis* was addressed. Herein, we present the first synoptic review of the strongylate nematodes that occur in the gastrointestinal system of wild ruminants from North America.

Context for Assessing the Nematode Fauna.
Strongylate nematodes are among the most characteristic parasites of the gastrointestinal system of ruminants throughout the world. A substantial literature encompassing systematics, ecology, and pathology has developed over the past century, particularly with reference to those species of direct veterinary importance that infect domestic bovids (e.g., Levine 1980; Lichtenfels and Hoberg 1993; Hoberg and Lichtenfels 1994; Lichtenfels et al. 1997). Although there is recognition of the potential influence of gastrointestinal nematodes on morbidity and mortality in sylvatic bovids and cervids, typically there have been only superficial assessments of these parasites within the context of wildlife management (e.g., Chapman and Feldhamer 1982).

Substantial research has been conducted on the systematics, diagnosis, and impact of gastrointestinal nematodes, but significant problems remain to be resolved. These include (1) standardization of methods for survey including sampling and necropsy of hosts; (2) uniformity in collection and preservation of nematode specimens; (3) consistency in parasite taxonomy; (4) adoption of a populational approach to studies of wildlife disease; and (5) application of a modern context for systematics, biodiversity assessment, and biogeography (Brooks and Hoberg 2000).

Although the procedures necessary for collection, identification, and enumeration of gastrointestinal nematodes in wild ruminants are often tedious and time consuming, they provide critical data for understanding epizootiology and the patterns of disease (see Eve and Kellogg 1977; Jordan and Stair 1983). It is necessary to document the significance of the parasite present and to carefully record the clinical signs that are observed. In keeping with a broader or population-based approach, it is also critical to derive information not associated with epizootics or mortality events. A standardized nomenclature for quantitative descriptors of parasite populations is encouraged (e.g., Bush et al. 1997).

Issues dealing with identification of eggs, free-living infective larvae, and early-stage parasitic larvae to the level of genus and species are of continuing importance (Lichtenfels et al. 1997). Lack of such reliable information represents a primary gap in our abilities to develop sound and predictive epizootiological models for the circulation of parasites in sylvatic host populations.

Consequently, the development of "epizootiological probes" derived from molecular biology and systematics will substantially influence our abilities to monitor the contemporary geographic range, patterns of transmission, and host distribution. The sensitivity and specificity of molecular markers applied to the identification of larvae and eggs could reduce reliance on current methods of parasite diagnosis that are dependent upon collection and necropsy of hosts and identification of adult helminths. Elimination of collecting has particular significance when linked to requisite studies of the influences of parasitism on morbidity, mortality, and population dynamics of endangered species. Such would represent a novel approach to simultaneously assess parasitism in wild ruminants across large geographic regions. Species-specific markers, for instance those that can be derived from the ITS region of genomic DNA [e.g., Christiansen et al. (1994a,b) for some trichostrongylids and Campbell et al. (1995) for some strongyles], are the primary requirement for development and realization of this methodology. This will provide an unprecedented application of molecular systematics and diagnostics, and for the first time make it feasible to develop a synoptic understanding of the scope of parasitism in populations of free-ranging sylvatic bovids and cervids.

Only recently have the theoretical and empirical implications of parasitism in wildlife and sylvatic ruminants, exclusive of direct mortality, been examined in greater detail (e.g., Grenfell 1988, 1992; Gulland 1992; Arneberg et al. 1996; Folstad et al. 1996). Through this body of research we have begun to recognize the often subtle influence of parasites and the feedback linkages between hosts, parasites, and habitat stability. They have also emphasized the importance of assessing the impacts of parasitic diseases at the level of host population within a rigorous theoretical framework (Gulland 1995; Grenfell and Gulland 1995; Hudson and Dobson 1995; Shaw and Dobson 1995). These areas of research are beyond the typical realm of investigating disease at the level of individual hosts. They are, however, an integral component in the development of an understanding of epizootiology, and the potential for density-dependent impacts on host demographics (Grenfell and Gulland 1995).

Biodiversity assessment and biogeographic analysis are important basic components to studies in parasitology and wildlife disease (Hoberg 1997; Brooks and Hoberg 2000). The nematode faunas in ruminants from North America and their relationships to those in Eurasia (see Govorka et al. 1988) are only now becoming adequately defined. Concepts developed from historical studies in the arctic and boreal zones can be applied directly to elucidating the evolution of nematode faunas among ruminants. We are only now beginning to unravel the anthropogenic and natural influences on diversification and distribution of this fauna (e.g., Hoberg et al. 1999). The origins and history of the North American fauna are complex, but must be elucidated in order to understand the distributional patterns for parasites and the potential for disease.

The contemporary strongylate fauna is a mosaic of archaic and introduced elements. Endemic (archaic) strongyles were influenced by historical movements of bovids and cervids across the Beringian nexus linking Eurasia and North America beginning 10–20 million years ago and extending into the Pliocene and Pleistocene. Secondarily, with the introduction of domestic stock starting in the fifteenth century and continuing today, numerous additional species associated with

bovids were introduced and became established in North America. The interaction between archaic and introduced faunas and the subsequent potential for exchange of strongyles between domestic and sylvatic hosts have in large part been determined by these historical and contemporary events. Thus, to understand the current strongylate fauna and its distribution in North American ruminants, it is necessary to recognize the context of biogeography and the historical constraints on the distribution of these host-parasite assemblages across the Holarctic (Hoberg and Lichtenfels 1994; Hoberg 1997). It is becoming apparent that a number of cryptic species representing this archaic fauna and currently unrecognized by science may be parasites in sylvatic hosts (Lichtenfels and Pilitt 1989; Lichtenfels et al. 1997; Hoberg et al. 1999). Both components of this fauna, however, have implications for management practices in North America and serve to reemphasize the importance of translocation of hosts on the distribution of parasites (see Hoberg 1997).

Recent studies among the ostertagiines, or medium stomach worms, and other nematodes have continued to identify the role of translocation of hosts and the introduction of parasites as factors determining the continental and international distribution of some pathogens (e.g., Thornton et al. 1973a,b; Rickard et al. 1993; Van Baren et al. 1996; Hoberg 1997). Studies of this type further emphasize the importance of systematics and taxonomy in providing a predictive framework for identification, documentation, and subsequently, surveillance (Brooks and Hoberg 2000). Incomplete documentation of the biodiversity of this fauna, including geographic range, host distribution, and the number of species involved (cryptic species), hampers the development of control measures to limit the impact of potentially pathogenic species of strongyles and other parasites. Accurate survey and inventory of the North American fauna is critical with respect to recognizing the potential emergence of pathogens and the interactions between parasite faunas circulating in domestic and sylvatic hosts.

Many of the changes that wildlife managers and parasitologists are now experiencing are related to overabundance of some bovids or cervids. Increased contact between domestic and sylvatic animals as well as the proliferation of game ranching and the farming of wild animals emphasize the importance of assessing wildlife diseases. Anthropogenically driven global change, particularly habitat alteration and the concomitant impact on the distribution of hosts, also highlights the significance of wildlife disease research, including parasitology, related to endangered species and conservation biology.

Strongylate Nematodes and Their Hosts. Strongylate nematodes representing three superfamilies, Ancylostomatoidea, Strongyloidea, and Trichostrongyloidea have been reported as parasites of the gastrointestinal system in wild bovids and cervids in North America.

The trichostrongyloid nematodes are dominant in terms of taxonomic, genealogical, and numerical diversity (e.g., Durette-Desset 1985; Hoberg and Lichtenfels 1994) and, consequently, are among the most significant as recognized or potential pathogens. Higher-level systematics for the Ancylostomatoidea and Strongyloidea is consistent with Lichtenfels (1980a,b) and disregards a recent proposal to elevate these and other related strongyles to the rank of suborder (Durette-Desset and Chabaud 1993). Systematics for the Trichostrongyloidea is consistent, in part, with that proposed by Durette-Desset (1983), with modifications related to the Trichostrongylidae based on Hoberg and Lichtenfels (1992, 1994). Phylogenetic relationships among the trichostrongylids and taxonomy within the family remain to be resolved, although current hypotheses share a high degree of similarity (Hoberg and Lictenfels 1994; Durette-Desset et al. 1999).

The following treatment presents a comprehensive view of the North American fauna including current knowledge for gastrointestinal strongyles in (1) six species of sylvatic bovids (pronghorn, *Antilocapra americana;* bison or buffalo, *Bison bison;* mountain goat, *Oreamnos americanus;* Rocky Mountain bighorn sheep, *Ovis canadensis;* Dall's sheep, *Ovis dalli;* and muskox, *Ovibos moschatus*), (2) five species of cervids (moose, *Alces alces;* elk or wapiti, *Cervus elaphus;* mule or black-tailed deer, *Odocoileus hemionus;* white-tailed deer, *O. virginianus;* and caribou, *Rangifer tarandus*), and (3) three species of primary domestic hosts (cattle, *Bos taurus;* sheep, *Ovis aries;* and llama, *Llama glama*) (Tables 8.1–8.12). Ancillary information is outlined on the occurrence of helminths in (1) introduced cervids (axis deer, *Axis axis;* red deer, *Cervus elaphus elaphus;* sambar, *C. unicolor;* fallow deer, *C. dama;* Pere David's deer, *Elaphurus davidianus;* and sika deer, *C. nippon*), (2) exotic bovids (addax, *Addax nasomaculatus;* blackbuck, *Antilope cervicapra;* sable antelope, *Hippotragus niger;* and gemsbok, *Oryx beisa*), and (3) camelids (*Llama glama*), pertinent to game ranching and maintenance of free-ranging herds (Tables 8.13 and 8.14). This provides the context for elucidating the occurrence of strongylate nematodes in wild and domestic bovids and the linkages within this assemblage of parasites and hosts.

Among wild ruminants in North America, 54 species of strongyles in 16 genera have been reported (Table 8.1); 21 in the abomasum, 28 in the small intestine, and 6 in the large intestine; some species occur in both the abomasum and the small intestine. This total does not include nematodes identified only at the level of family or genus reported in some studies. Additionally, not included among these, but discussed below, are a number of species and genera so far only associated with domestic or exotic hosts and several which could potentially be introduced from the Palearctic, Eurasia, and Africa (Tables 8.13 and 8.14). The relatively few species limited in occurrence solely to sheep or cattle are not addressed.

GASTROINTESTINAL STRONGYLES IN NORTH AMERICAN RUMINANTS

Genus *Monodontus* Molin, 1861
Classification: Ancylostomatoidea: Ancylostomatidae: Bunostominae.
Common Name: Hookworm of deer.
Monodontus louisianensis Chitwood and Jordan, 1965.

Monodontus louisianensis is a typical, but relatively uncommon parasite of the small intestine in *O. virginianus* across the southern United States (Prestwood and Pursglove 1981; Forrester 1992). It is the only hookworm known from sylvatic cervids or bovids in North America. The life cycle is currently unknown, but likely involves direct cutaneous penetration of the definitive host by third-stage larvae (L$_3$'s), similar to those documented for other hookworms (Prestwood and Pursglove 1981). Prevalence and intensity in white-tailed deer from Florida are 20%–100% and 1–13 worms per host (Forrester 1992). Disease associated with this nematode has seldom been documented in white-tailed deer and may be associated with weather conditions that concentrate deer in damp, fecal-contaminated areas that are conducive to transmission. Clinical signs would be expected to parallel those described for hookworm disease and anemia typical of other ruminants but are unlikely to be observed due to the low numbers of parasites usually present in parasitized hosts (Prestwood and Pursglove 1981).

Genus *Eucyathostomum* Molin, 1861
Classification: Strongyloidea: Strongylidae: Cyathostominae: Eucyathostominae.
Common Name: Colon worms.
Eucyathostomum webbi Pursglove, 1976. [Synonym: There are records of *E. longisubulatum* Molin, 1861 from white-tailed deer in Florida and South Carolina according to Pursglove (1976).]

Species of this genus are known as parasites in the colon of artiodactyls, particularly cervids, with one species being typical of white-tailed deer across the southern United States (Pursglove 1976; Prestwood and Pursglove 1981). Prevalence and intensity for white-tailed deer from Florida are 11%–80% and 1–26 worms per host (Forrester 1992). Diagnosis is based on the specific structure of the cephalic extremity (cervical inflation and leaf crowns) and the male copulatory organs, which are distinctive (Pursglove 1976; Lichtenfels 1980b). The life cycle is unknown, but consistent with other cyathostomes it is likely to be direct. Disease attributable to this nematode is apparently negligible, as infections generally are of low intensity.

Genus *Chabertia* Railliet and Henry, 1909
Classification: Strongyloidea: Chabertiidae: Chabertiinae.
Common Name: Large-mouthed bowel worms.

TABLE 8.1—Strongylate nematodes in North American ruminants: A comparison of faunas in wild bovids, cervids, and domesticated sheep, cattle, and camelids

	Bovidae						Cervidae					Domestic[a]		
	Prong-horn	Bison	Mountain Goat	Bighorn Sheep	Dall's Sheep	Musk-ox	Moose	Elk	Mule deer	White-tail	Cari-bou	Cattle	Sheep	Lama
Abomasum														
Haemonchus spp.	+	−	−	+	−	−	−	−	−	−	−	+	+	+
H. contortus	+	+	−	+	−	−	+	−	+	+	−	+	+	−
H. placei	+	−	−	+	−	−	−	−	−	+	−	+	+	−
H. similis	+	−	−	−	−	−	−	−	−	+	−	+	+	−
Marshallagia spp.	−	−	+	+	+	+	−	+	+	+	+	−	+	−
M. marshalli	+	−	+	+	+	+	+	+	+	+	+	−	−	−
Mazamastrongylus pursglovei	−	−	−	−	−	−	−	+	−	−	−	−	−	−
M. odocoilei	+	−	+	+	−	+	+	+	+	+	+	+	+	−
Obeliscoides cuniculi	+	+	−	+	−	+	+	−	+	−	+	+	+	+
Ostertagia spp.[b]	−	−	−	−	−	+	−	+	+	+	+	+	+	−
O. bisonis	+	+	−	−	−	−	−	−	−	−	−	+	−	−
O. gruehneri	−	−	−	−	+	−	−	+	+	+	+	+	+	+
O. leptospicularis	+	+	−	+	−	−	−	+	+	+	−	+	+	−
O. mossi	−	−	+	+	+	−	−	−	+	+	−	−	−	−
O. ostertagi	−	−	−	−	−	−	−	−	−	−	−	+	+	−
Pseudostertagia bullosa	+	−	−	+	−	+	+	+	+	+	+	+	+	−
Spiculopteragia spiculoptera	−	−	−	−	−	+	−	−	−	−	−	−	−	−
Teladorsagia spp.	+	−	+	+	−	+	+	+	+	+	+	+	+	+
T. boreoarcticus	+	−	−	−	+	+	+	+	+	+	+	−	−	−
T. circumcincta	−	−	+	+	+	+	−	−	−	−	+	+	+	+
Trichostrongylus spp.	+	−	+	+	+	+	+	+	+	+	+	+	+	−
T. askivali	−	+	−	+	−	−	−	+	+	+	+	+	+	+
T. axei	−	−	+	+	+	−	−	−	+	+	+	+	+	−
T. calcaratus	−	−	−	−	−	−	−	+	+	+	−	−	−	+
T. colubriformis	−	+	+	+	+	−	−	+	−	−	−	+	+	−
T. dosteri	−	−	−	−	−	−	−	−	−	+	−	−	−	−
T. longispicularis	−	−	−	+	+	−	−	−	−	+	−	+	+	+
Small Intestine														
Cooperia spp.	+	−	−	+	−	−	−	+	−	+	−	+	+	+
C. curticei	−	−	−	−	−	−	−	−	−	+	−	+	+	−
C. oncophora	+	+	−	+	−	−	−	+	+	+	−	+	+	+
C. pectinata	+	−	−	−	−	−	−	−	−	+	−	+	+	−

	C1	C2	C3	C4	C5	C6	C7	C8	C9	C10	C11	C12	C13	C14	C15
C. punctata	—	+	+	—	+	—	—	—	—	—	—	—	—	—	+
C. spatulata	—	+	+	—	+	—	—	—	—	—	—	—	—	—	—
C. surnabada	+	—	—	—	—	+	—	+	+	—	—	+	+	+	+
Cyathostominae gen. sp.	—	—	—	—	—	—	—	—	—	—	—	—	—	—	—
Monodontus louisianensis	—	+	+	+	+	—	+	+	+	+	—	—	—	—	—
Nematodirus spp.	—	+	—	+	+	+	+	+	+	+	+	+	+	+	+
N. abnormalis	—	—	—	+	+	—	+	—	+	+	—	+	+	+	+
N. andersoni	—	—	—	—	—	—	+	—	—	—	—	—	—	—	—
N. archari	—	—	—	—	—	—	+	—	—	—	—	—	—	—	—
N. becklundi	—	+	—	+	+	+	+	+	+	+	—	+	+	+	+
N. davtiani	+	+	—	+	+	+	+	+	+	+	—	+	+	+	+
N. filicollis	+	—	+	+	+	+	+	+	+	+	—	+	+	+	+
N. helvetianus	+	—	—	—	+	—	+	—	+	+	—	+	+	+	—
N. maculosus	—	—	—	—	—	—	+	—	—	—	—	—	—	—	—
N. odocoilei	—	+	—	—	+	—	+	—	+	—	—	—	+	—	—
N. oiratianus	—	+	—	+	—	+	+	+	+	+	+	+	+	+	—
N. oiratianus interruptus	+	+	—	—	+	—	+	—	+	—	—	—	+	+	+
N. spathiger	—	—	—	—	—	—	+	—	+	—	—	—	—	—	+
N. skrjabini	—	—	—	—	—	—	—	—	—	—	—	—	—	—	—
N. tarandi	—	—	—	—	—	—	—	—	—	—	—	—	—	—	—
Nematodirella spp.	—	—	—	—	—	—	—	—	—	—	—	—	—	—	—
N. alcidis	—	—	—	—	—	—	—	—	—	—	—	—	—	—	—
N. antilocaprae	—	+	—	—	+	+	—	+	+	+	+	+	+	—	+
N. gazelli	—	+	—	—	—	—	—	—	—	—	—	—	—	—	+
N. longissimespiculata	+	+	—	—	+	+	—	—	+	+	—	+	—	—	+
Trichostrongylus spp.	—	+	+	—	+	+	+	+	+	+	+	+	+	+	+
T. colubriformis	+	+	+	—	+	+	+	+	+	+	—	+	+	+	+
T. longispicularis	+	+	+	—	—	—	—	—	+	+	—	+	—	—	—
T. vitrinus	—	+	—	—	—	—	—	—	+	—	—	—	—	—	—
Large Intestine/Cecum															
Chabertia ovina	—	+	+	—	—	—	—	—	+	+	—	+	+	+	—
Eucyathostoma webbi	—	—	—	—	—	—	—	—	—	—	—	—	—	—	—
Oesophagostomum spp.	—	+	+	—	—	—	—	—	+	+	—	+	+	+	—
O. cervi	—	—	—	—	—	—	—	—	—	—	—	—	—	—	—
O. columbianum	—	+	—	—	—	—	—	—	—	—	—	+	—	—	—
O. radiatum	—	—	+	—	—	—	—	—	—	—	—	+	+	—	—
O. venulosum	+	+	+	—	+	+	+	+	+	+	+	+	+	+	+

[a] Data for domestic hosts primarily from Becklund (1964) and Rickard and Bishop (1991).

[b] Minor morphotypes for polymorphic species of ostertagiines are not listed.

197

TABLE 8.2—Strongylate nematodes in pronghorn, *Antilocapra americana*

Location/Species	Locality (State/Province)	Source[a]
Abomasum		
Haemonchus contortus	ND, SD, TX	2, 6, 9, 11, 16
H. placei	NM	14
Haemonchus sp.	WUS[b]	10
Marshallagia marshalli	MT, SD, WY, WUS[b]	1, 6, 9, 10, 13
Ostertagia bisonis	ND, SD, WY, WUS[b]	2, 7, 8, 9, 10, 16
O. ostertagi	MT, ND, NM, SD, WY, WUS[b]	2, 9, 10, 14, 16
Ostertagia sp.	SD, WY	9
Pseudostertagia bullosa	MT, NM, SD, WY, WUS[b]	2, 6, 9, 10, 14
Teladorsagia circumcincta/[c]	MT, ND, SD, WY, WUS[b]	2, 9, 10, 16
T. trifurcata		
Trichostrongylus axei	NM, WUS[b]	10, 14
Small Intestine		
Cooperia oncophora	ND, NM, SD, WUS[b]	2, 6, 10, 12, 14, 16
C. pectinata	NM, WUS[b]	10, 14
C. punctata	NM, WUS[b]	10, 14
C. surnabada	SD	2
Cooperia sp.	NM	14
Nematodirella antilocaprae[d]	AB, ID, MT, ND, NM, OR, SD, TX, WY	3, 4, 9, 11, 13, 14, 15, 16
N. longissimespiculata	SD	2
Nematodirus abnormalis	SD, WUS[b]	6, 9, 10
N. filicollis	ND, WUS[b]	10, 16
N. oratianus interruptus	NM	5, 14
N. spathiger	MT, ND, SD, WUS[b]	2, 6, 9, 10, 16
Nematodirus sp.	SD	2
Trichostrongylus colubriformis	MT, ND, NM, SD, WUS[b]	6, 9, 10, 14, 16
Trichostrongylus spp.	NM	14
Cyathostominae[e] gen. sp.	WY	9
Large Intestine		
None reported		

[a]1. Bergstrom (1975a). 2. Boddicker and Hugghins (1969). 3. Durette-Desset and Samuel (1989). 4. Lichtenfels and Pilitt (1983b). 5. Lichtenfels and Pilitt (1983a). 6. Lucker and Dikmans (1945). 7. Worley and Sharman (1966). 8. Lichtenfels and Pilitt (1991). 9. Unpublished records, U.S. National Parasite Collection. 10. Allen (1962). 11. Hailey et al. (1966). 12. Burtner and Becklund (1971). 13. Bergstrom (1975b). 14. Gilmore and Allen (1960). 15. Shaw (1947). 16. Goldsby and Eveleth (1954).
[b]Western United States.
[c]The distribution of *T. circumcincta* and associated minor morphotypes requires confirmation based on molecular analyses (Hoberg et al. 1999).
[d]Specimens identified as *Nematodirella longissimespiculata* by Boddicker and Hugghins (1969), were redetermined as *N. antilocaprae* by Lichtenfels and Pilitt (1983b).
[e]Unidentified "cylicostomes" collected by R. Bergstrom from Sweetwater County, WY.

Chabertia ovina (Fabricius, 1794). [Synonyms: *Strongylus ovinus* Fabricius, 1794; *S. hypostomus* Rudolphi, 1819; *S. cernuus* Creplin, 1819; *C. rishati* Akhtar, 1937]

Large bowel worms are considered rare or incidental parasites of wild bovids and cervids and have only been reported from *Odocoileus* spp., *Ovis canadensis,* and *B. bison.* It is probable that these parasites are acquired on common range with domesticated hosts including cattle and sheep. The life cycle is direct. Disease is unknown in wild hosts, possibly due to the low intensity and sporadic nature of infections. At high intensity, these blood-feeding parasites would be expected to cause severe diarrhea, loss of weight and condition, and the development of anemia (Levine 1980).

Genus *Oesophagostomum* Molin, 1861
Classification: Strongyloidea: Chabertiidae: Oesophagostominae.

Common Name: Nodular worms.
Oesophagostomum cervi Mertts, 1948. [Synonym: Considered by Baker and Pursglove (1976), and Levine (1980) to be a synonym of *O. venulosum,* this species has been reported from the southeastern United States, with an argument that it is distinguishable from the former (Payne et al. 1967). Govorka et al. (1988) list it as one of a number of species of *Oesophagostomum* in Eurasian cervids.]
Oesophagostomum columbianum Curtice, 1890.]
Oesophagostomum radiatum (Rudolphi, 1803). [Synonyms: *Bosicola radiatum* Sandground, 1929; *B. tricollaris* Sandground, 1929; *O. inflatum* (Schneider, 1866); *O. dilatum* (Railliet, 1884); *O. bovis* Schnyder, 1906; *O. biramosum* Cuillé, Marotel and Panisett, 1911; *O. vesiculosum* Rátz, 1898].
Oesophagostomum venulosum (Rudolphi, 1809). [Synonyms: *S. follicularis* Ostertag in Olt, 1898; *O.*

TABLE 8.3—Strongylate nematodes in buffalo or bison, *Bison bison*

Location/Species	Locality (State/Province)	Source[a]
Abomasum		
Haemonchus contortus	AB, KS, OK, SD	4, 5, 7
Ostertagia bisonis/	AB, AK, KS, SD, WY	2, 4, 6, 7, 9, 11, 12
O. cf. kazakhstanica[b]		
O. ostertagi/	AB, KS, WY	1, 4, 12
O. lyrata		
Trichostrongylus axei	AB, KS	4
Small Intestine		
Cooperia oncophora	AB, AK, SD, WY	3, 4, 7, 11, 12, 13
C. surnabada	AK, SD	7, 11
Nematodirus helvetianus	AB, WY	8, 12, 14
Strongylida??	UT, WY	10, 15
Large Intestine		
Chabertia ovina	SD	7
Oesophagostomum radiatum	AB, KS, MT, OK, WY	4, 5, 12
Oesophagostomum sp.	AB, MT	1, 12

[a]1. Cameron (1923, 1924). 2. Chapin (1925). 3. Cram (1925). 4. Dikmans (1939). 5. Locker (1953). 6. Becklund and Walker (1967b). 7. Boddicker and Hugghins (1969). 8. Bergstrom and Kass (1982). 9. Lichtenfels and Pillitt (1991). 10. Van Vuren and Scott (1995). 11. C. A. Nielsen, unpublished data. 12. Unpublished records, U.S. National Parasite Collection. 13. Burtner and Becklund (1971). 14. Card (1993). 15. Zaugg et al. (1993).

[b]Boddicker and Hugghins (1969) reported *O. trifurcata* in bison. The minor morphotype associated with *O. bisonis* is considered to be *O. kazakhstanica* according to Lichtenfels and Pilitt (1991). Reexamination of USNPC 59388 showed the specimen reported by Boddicker and Hugghins to be incorrectly identified, and it is tentatively referred to O. kazakhstanica, a new North American record for this ostertagiine. Drózdz (1995), however, has indicated that the minor morphotype associated with *O. bisonis* in North America may be undescribed.

TABLE 8.4—Strongylate nematodes in mountain goat, *Oreamnos americanus*

Location/Species	Locality (State/Province)	Source[a]
Abomasum		
Marshallagia marshalli/[b]	AB, AK, ID, WA, WY	3, 4, 5, 6, 10, 11, 13
M. occidentalis		
Ostertagia ostertagi	AB, SD	2, 4, 6
Ostertagia sp.	AB, WA, WY	11
Teladorsagia circumcincta/[c]	AB, SD	2, 4, 6, 11, 12, 13
T. davtiani		
T. trifurcata		
Trichostrongylus axei	SD	2
T. colubriformis	SD	2
Small Intestine		
Nematodirella antilocaprae	SD	7
Nematodirus becklundi	AB	9
N. davtiani	AB	13
N. filicollis	AB	4
N. helvetianus	AB, SD, WA	2, 11, 13
N. maculosus	AB, MT, SD	1, 2, 6, 13
N. odocoilei	AB, MT	11
N. oiratianus interruptus	AB	8
Nematodirus sp.	SD	12
Trichostrongylus sp.	ID	3
Large Intestine/Cecum		
Oesophagostomum venulosum	SD	2

[a]1. Becklund (1965). 2. Boddicker et al. (1971). 3. Brandborg (1955). 4. Cowan (1951). 5. Dikmans (1942). 6. Kerr and Holmes (1966). 7. Lichtenfels and Pilitt (1983b). 8. Lichtenfels and Pilitt (1983a). 9. Durette-Desset and Samuel (1992). 10. Lichtenfels and Pilitt (1989). 11. Unpublished records, U.S. National Parasite Collection. 12. Boddicker and Hugghins (1969). 13. Samuel et al. (1977).

[b]Specimens from *O. americanus* in Alberta, Alaska, Washington, and Wyoming may represent a distinct species of *Marshallagia* (see Lichtenfels and Pilitt 1989).

[c]Specimens of *T. circumcincta* and associated minor morphotypes should be confirmed based on analysis of morphometric and molecular date (see Hoberg et al. 1999).

TABLE 8.5—Strongylate nematodes in bighorn sheep, *Ovis canadensis*

Location/Species	Locality (State/Province)	Source[a]
Abomasum		
Haemonchus contortus	NM, WY	3, 10, 11
H. placei	NM	1
Haemonchus sp.	CO	19
Marshallagia marshalli/[b] *M. occidentalis*	AB, BC, CO, ID, MT, OR, SD, WY	3–8, 10, 11, 14, 15, 17, 18, 20, 22, 27, 29, 32, 33
Marshallagia sp.	AB, BC	20
Obeliscoides cuniculi	CO	29
Ostertagia ostertagi/ *O. lyrata*	BC, ID, MT, SD	3, 4, 14, 29, 32
Ostertagia sp.	BC, CO, OR, MT	6, 14, 19, 33
Pseudostertagia bullosa	CO, NM	1, 16
Teladorsagia circumcincta/[c] *T. trifurcata* *T. davtiani*	AB, BC, MT, SD, WY	3, 4, 6, 11, 20, 29, 32
Teladorsagia sp.	AB, BC	20
Trichostrongylus axei	OR, SD	14, 29
T. colubriformis	SD	29
Trichostrongylus sp.	MT	29
Small Intestine		
Cooperia oncophora	MT, OR, WY	3, 11, 14, 31
C. surnabada	MT	3
Cooperia sp.	MT	33
Nematodirella antilocaprae	AB	9
Nematodirus abnormalis	MT, WY	11, 32
N. andersoni	AB	9
N. archari[d]	BC, MT, WY	3, 20, 21, 26
N. davtiani	AB, BC, MT, WY	3, 20, 23, 26, 30, 32
N. filicollis	AB, MT	6, 23
N. helvetianus	MT, SD, WY	3, 24, 26, 29
N. maculosus	AB, BC, SD, WY	20, 26, 29
N. odocoilei	MT	28
N. oiratianus	BC, OR	14, 20
N. oiratianus interruptus[e]	AB, CO, MT	3, 16, 23
N. spathiger	BC, CO, MT, NM, WY	2, 3, 11,16, 20, 23
Nematodirus sp.	AB, BC, CA, MT, OR, SD, WA	4, 5, 12, 13, 14, 20, 22, 24, 25, 29
Large Intestine		
Chabertia ovina	MT	32
Oesophagostomum sp.	NM, OR, WA	1, 12, 13, 14

[a]1. Allen (1955). 2. Allen and Kennedy (1952). 3. Becklund and Senger (1967). 4. Blood (1963). 5. Couey (1950). 6. Cowan (1951). 7. Dikmans (1932). 8. Dikmans (1942). 9. Durette-Desset and Samuel (1989). 10. Honess and Scott (1942). 11. Honess and Winter (1956). 12. Johnson (1974). 13. Johnson (1975). 14. Kistner et al. (1977). 15. Marsh (1938). 16. Pilmore (1961). 17. Quortrup and Sudheimer (1944). 18. Rush (1932). 19. Spencer (1943). 20. Uhazy and Holmes (1971). 21. Rickard and Lichtenfels (1989). 22. Boddicker and Hugghins (1969). 23. Lichtenfels and Pilitt (1983a). 24. McCullough and Schneegas (1966). 25. Capelle (1966). 26. Bergstrom and Kass (1982). 27. Bergstrom (1975a). 28. Becklund and Walker (1967a). 29. Unpublished records, U.S. National Parasite Collection. 30. Becklund (1966). 31. Burtner and Becklund (1971). 32. Hoar et al. (1996). 33. Worley and Seesee (1992).

[b]Dróżdż (1995) considers that some *Marshallagia* in *O. canadensis* represent an undescribed species.

[c]Some specimens identified as *T. circumcincta* may represent an undescribed cryptic species; specimens of *T. circumcincta* require confirmation based on morphometric and molecular data (see Hoberg et al. 1999).

[d]Specimens identified as *N. archari* may be referrable to *N. andersoni* [see Durette-Desset and Samuel (1989), Rickard and Lichtenfels (1989)].

[e]Specimens of *N. lanceolatus* from North America are considered synonyms of *N. oiratianus interruptus* by Lichtenfels and Pilitt (1983a).

TABLE 8.6—Strongylate nematodes in Dall's sheep, *Ovis dalli*[b]

Location/Species	Locality (State/Province)	Source[a]
Abomasum		
Marshallagia marshalli/ M. occidentalis	AK, NWT	1, 4
Ostertagia ostertagi	AK	1
Teladorsagia circumcincta/[c]	AK	1
T. trifurcata		
T. davtiani		
Small Intestine		
Nematodirella sp.(c.f. *N. alcidis*)[d]	AK	1
Nematodirus andersoni	AK	3
N. archari[e]	AK	1, 5
N. davtiani	AK	1
N. oiratianus	AK	1
N. oiratianus interruptus	AK	2
N. spathiger	AK	1
Nematodirus sp.	NWT	1
Large Intestine		
None reported		

[a]1. Nielsen and Neiland (1974). 2. Lichtenfels and Pilitt (1983a). 3. Durette-Desset and Samuel (1989). 4. Unpublished records, U.S. National Parasite Collection. 5. Rickard and Lichtenfels (1989).

[b]Nematodes apparently only reported from *Ovis dalli dalli* and not from *O. d. stonei.*

[c]Specimens identified as *T. circumcincta* require confirmation based on molecular analyses and may represent an undescribed species (Hoberg et al. 1999).

[d]Specimens referred to as *N. longispiculata* by Nielsen and Neiland (1974).

[e]Specimens referred to *N. archari* may actually represent *N. andersoni* (see Durette-Desset and Samuel 1989; Rickard and Lichtenfels 1989).

TABLE 8.7—Strongylate nematodes in muskox, *Ovibos moschatus*[b,c]

Location/Species	Locality (State/Province)	Source[a]
Abomasum		
Marshallagia marshalli/M. occidentalis	AK, NU[h]	1, 4, 6, 7, 9
Marshallagia sp.	NU	4, 7,
Ostertagia gruehneri/ O. arctica	AK, NU	7, 8
Ostertagia sp.	AK, NU	4
Teladorsagia boreoarcticus[d]	NU, NWT	11
T. circumcincta/[d]	AK, NU	2, 6, 8
T. trifurcata		
T. davtiani		
Trichostrongylus spp.	AK	3
Small Intestine		
Nematodirella alcidis	NU	7
N. gazelli[e]	NU	2, 4, 5
N. longissimespiculata[f]	AK	5, 8
Nematodirella sp.	AK, NU	4
Nematodirus helvetianus	NU	4, 6
N. skrjabini[g]	AK	8
N. tarandi	AK, NU	7, 10
Nematodirus sp.	AK, NU	4, 7
Large Intestine		
None reported		

[a]1. Dikmans (1939). 2. Gibbs and Tener (1958). 3. Bos (1967). 4. Samuel and Gray (1974). 5. Lichtenfels and Pilitt (1983b). 6. Webster and Rowell (1980). 7. E. Hoberg, S. Kutz, and J. Nishi, unpublished data from Victoria Island and Cox Lake and Rae River, near Kugluktuk, NU. 8. C. A. Nielsen, unpublished data from Barter Island; specimens in introduced population of white-faced musk ox, *Ovibos moschatus wardi* translocated from East Greenland in 1935 to Nunivak Island and subsequently to the Arctic coastal plain in 1969 (see Hoberg et al. 1999). 9. Lichtenfels and Pilitt (1989). 10. Unpublished records, U.S. National Parasite Collection. 11. Hoberg et al. 1999.

[b]Including barrenground musk ox, *Ovibos moschatus moschatus,* and white-faced musk ox, *O. m. wardi.*

[c]See Alendal and Helle (1983) for a review of records from captive herds; also see MacDonald et al. (1976).

[d]Specimens collected from Victoria Island and the mainland on the Rae and Richardson Rivers, near Kugluktuk, NU, represent a recently described cryptic species (Hoberg et al. 1999). *Teladorsagia boreoarcticus* is represented by two male morphotypes, designated respectively as *T. boreoarcticus* forma major and *T. boreoarcticus* f. minor. Previous records of *T. circumcincta* from Arctic Canada, and those from other wild bovids across the Holarctic require confirmation (Hoberg et al. 1999).

[e]Specimens reported as *Nematodirella longispiculata* by Samuel and Gray (1974) were redetermined as *N. gazelli* by Lichtenfels and Pilitt (1983b); records by Gibbs and Tener (1958) may represent this species.

[f]Specimens from Nunivak Island, Alaska, examined by C.A. Neilsen (unpublished) and identified as *N. longispiculata,* may represent this species (see Lichtenfels and Pilitt 1983b).

[g]There is continuing disagreement over the validity of *N. skrjabini,* with some authorities reducing it as a synonym of *N. tarandi.*

[h]NU = Nunavut, Canada, a former region of the eastern Northwest Territories.

TABLE 8.8—Strongylate nematodes in moose, *Alces alces*

Location/Species	Locality (State/ Province)	Source[a]
Abomasum		
Haemonchus contortus	NWT	8
Ostertagia sp.	AB	3
Trichostrongylus sp.	MN	12
Small Intestine		
Nematodirella alcidis[b]	AB, AK, BC, MN, MT NF, ON	1–7, 9, 10
N. longissimespiculata	WY	11
Nematodirus tarandi	MN	11
Nematodirus sp.	AK	5
Trichostrongylus longispicularis	AB	3
Large Intestine		
Oesophagostomum venulosum	MN	6

[a]1. Lichtenfels and Pilitt (1983b). 2. Samuel et al. (1976). 3. Stock and Barrett (1983). 4. Cowan (1951). 5. C.A. Nielsen, unpublished data. 6. Anderson and Lankester (1974). 7. Threlfall (1969). 8. Unpublished records, U.S. National Parasite Collection. 9. Fruetel and Lankester (1988). 10. Hoeve et al. (1988). 11. Unpublished records, U.S. National Parasite Collection. 12. Loken et al. (1965).
[b]It is apparent that *N. alcidis* represents the correct name for the species that occurs most commonly in moose across North America; *N. alcidis* is a species established for *N. longispiculata alcidis* Dikmans, 1935. Specimens reported as *N. longispiculata* by Cowan (1951) and Samuel et al. (1976) were redetermined as *N. alcidis* by Lichtenfels and Pilitt (1983b). Andersen and Lankester (1974) summarized reports of *N. longispiculata* from moose across North America.

TABLE 8.9—Strongylate nematodes in elk or wapiti, *Cervus elaphus*

Location/Species	Locality (State/ Province)	Source[a]
Abomasum		
Marshallagia marshalli	WY	6, 7, 9
Mazamastrongylus odocoilei	MI	5, 7
M. pursglovei	CA	3
Ostertagia leptospicularis/ O. kolchida	CA	3
Ostertagia ostertagi	NM	8
Ostertagia sp. (reported as *Skrjabinagia*)	AB, WY	2, 9, 10
Trichostrongylus axei	AB, CA, NM	2, 3, 8, 10
T. colubriformis	NM	8
Small Intestine		
Cooperia oncophora	AB	2, 10
Cooperia sp.	MI, WY	7, 9
Nematodirella alcidis	AB	2, 10
N. antilocaprae	SD[b]	1, 4
Nematodirus helvetianus	AB, SD	1, 2, 10
N. odocoilei	MI	7
Nematodirus sp.	WY	9
Trichostrongylus sp.	WY	9
Large Intestine		
Oesophagostomum venulosum	MI, SD	1, 7

[a]1. Boddicker and Hugghins (1969). 2. Stock and Barrett (1983). 3. Van Baren et al. (1996). 4. Lichtenfels and Pilitt (1983b). 5. Lichtenfels et al. (1993). 6. Bergstrom (1975a). 7. Unpublished records, U.S. National Parasite Collection. 8. Wilson (1969). 9. Worley (1979). 10. Thorne et al. (2001).
[b]Specimens reported as *N. longissimespiculata* by Boddicker and Hugghins (1969) were redetermined as *N. antilocaprae* by Lichtenfels and Pilitt (1983b).

TABLE 8.10—Strongylate nematodes in black-tailed or mule deer, *Odocoileus hemionus*

Location/Species	Locality (State/Province)	Source[a]
Abomasum		
Haemonchus contortus	BC, CA, MT, SD, TX	1, 4, 6, 7, 9, 14
Marshallagia marshalli/M. occidentalis	WY	1, 5
Ostertagia bisonis	MT, SD, WY	1, 4, 8, 12, 14
O. leptospicularis/O. kolchida	OR	3
O. ostertagi	MT, SD, WY	1, 4, 14
Ostertagia sp.	OR	14
Pseudostertagia bullosa	MT	4, 14
Teladorsagia circumcincta/[b]	AK, BC, CA, OR, WY, UT	1, 2, 7, 13, 14
T. trifurcata		
T. davtiani		
Trichostrongylus axei	CA, MT, OR	1, 7, 14
Small Intestine		
Cooperia oncophora	AZ, MT	1, 4, 10
C. surnabada	CA	1
Nematodirella antilocaprae	WY	14, 15
N. longissimespiculata	BC	1
Nematodirus abnormalis	CA, WY	1
N. filicollis	BC, CA	1
N. helvetianus	WY	14
N. odocoilei	BC, CA, MT, OR, WY	1, 4, 11, 14
N. spathiger	CA, WY	1, 7
Trichostrongylus colubriformis	CA, WY, MT	1, 4, 7
T. longispicularis	MT	4
T. vitrinus	CA	1, 7
Trichostrongylus sp.	BC, CA	1
Large Intestine		
Chabertia ovina	CA, OR	1, 7
Oesophagostomum venulosum	AK, BC, CA, OR	1, 7, 14
Oesophagostomum sp.	AK	2

[a]1. Walker and Becklund (1970). 2. C. A. Nielsen, unpublished records, Kodiak Island and Sitka. 3. Hoberg et al. (1993b). 4. Worley and Eustace (1972). 5. Bergstrom (1975a). 6. Stubblefield et al. (1987). 7. Longhurst and Douglas (1953). 8. Worley and Sharman (1966). 9. Gray et al. (1978). 10. Allen and Erling (1964). 11. Becklund and Walker (1967a). 12. Becklund and Walker (1967b). 13. Jensen et al. (1982). 14. Unpublished records, U.S. National Parasite Collection. 15. Lichtenfels and Pilitt (1983b).
[b]Records of *T. circumcincta* require confirmation (Hoberg et al. 1999).

acutum Molin, 1861; *O. inflatum* var. *ovis* Carità, 1887; *O. vigentimembrum* Canavan, 1931.]

Four species of nodular worms are known from the large intestine in wild bovids or cervids from North America. *Oesophagostomum venulosum* and *O. cervi* are the most commonly occurring species reported in cervids; *O. columbianum* and *O. radiatum* have rarely been reported from wild ruminants. Wild cervids, particularly elk and deer, are the probable source of *O. venulosum* reported in cattle from the western United States (e.g., Baker and Fisk 1986; Hoberg et al. 1988). Wild cervids and bovids, however, are unlikely to be important in the epizootiology of other species, which circulate primarily among domestic hosts.

Diagnosis is based on the examination of adult nematodes. Important characters include the structure of the leaf crowns, relative degree of development of the cephalic vesicle, placement of the cervical papillae, and specific attributes of the copulatory bursa and spicules (e.g., Levine 1980).

Adult nodular worms reside in the lumen of the large intestine, and larvae are found in walls of the small and large intestine, where development of typical nodules may occur. The life cycle for species of *Oesophagosto-*

mum is direct and with respect to free-living larval stages is largely identical to those documented for other strongyloid nematodes (e.g., Levine 1980); L_3's are infective. In contrast to other strongyles, fourth-stage larvae develop within nodules in the small and large intestine, and near 17–22 days postinfection, they migrate back to the large intestine for the final molt; the prepatent period is 32–42 days.

Disease attributable to *O. venulosum* or other species has not been documented for infections in wild ruminants (e.g., Prestwood and Pursglove 1981). This may reflect generally moderate levels of prevalence and low intensity as documented in deer from Florida (27%–60%; 1–9 per host) (Forrester 1992). Oesophagostomiosis in domestic hosts, however, is associated with inflammation and the development of characteristic nodules in the intestinal wall. Severe infections in cattle are typified by edema of the intestinal wall, anorexia, weight loss, and diarrhea. Pathogenesis is linked to the level of exposure, with 20,000–250,000 larvae being required to elicit clinical signs (Levine 1980). Consequently, in the relatively sporadic and low intensity infections in deer and other wild ruminants (e.g., Prestwood and Pursglove 1981; Forrester 1992), the probability of significant disease is rare.

TABLE 8.11—Strongylate nematodes in white-tailed deer, *Odocoileus virginianus*

Location/Species	Locality (State/ Province)	Source[a]
Abomasum		
Haemonchus contortus	AL, AR, FL, GA, IL, LA, MI, MS, OK, PA, SC, SD, TN TX, WI, WV	1, 4, 5, 8, 11, 12, 13, 21
H. placei	FL, TX	4, 18
H. similis	FL	1, 4
Mazamastrongylus odocoilei	AL, AR, FL, GA, IL, KY, LA, MA, MD, ME, MS, NC, NJ, NY, SD, TX, VA, WI	1, 3–5, 7, 9,12, 13, 15, 16, 19, 21
M. pursglovei	AL, AR, FL, GA, KY, LA, MS, NC, SC, VA	3–5, 7, 16,19
Obeliscoides cuniculi	AR, GA	1
Ostertagia mossi/ O. dikmansi	AL, AR, GA, IL, KY, LA, MA, ME, MD, MS, NC, NJ, NY, OK, ON, PA, SC, TN, TX, VA, WI, WV	1–3, 5, 7–9, 13, 15, 16, 21
Ostertagia ostertagi	AR, FL, GA, KY, MA, MS, NY, TX, WV	1, 4, 5, 12, 14, 15, 20
Ostertagia sp.	FL, MT, NY, SD, TX	1
Spiculopteragia spiculoptera	QE	6
Teladorsagia circumcincta/ T. trifurcata	NY	1
Trichostrongylus askivali	AL, AR, FL, GA, KY, LA, ME, MS, NC, OK, SC, TN, TX	4, 5, 7, 15, 21
T. axei	AL, AR, FL, GA, KY, LA, MD, ME, MS, OK, SC, TN, TX, WI	1, 4, 5, 7, 15, 21
T. calcaratus	GA	5
T. dosteri	FL, GA	4, 5
T. longispicularis	AL, FL, GA, LA, SC, VA, WV	5
Small Intestine		
Cooperia curticei	KY	5, 20
C. oncophora	SC	5
C. pectinata	TX	5
C. punctata	AL, FL, GA, LA, MS, SC, TX, VA, WV	4, 5
C. spatulata	SC	5
Cooperia sp.	NY, TX	1, 12
Monodontus louisianensis	FL, GA, LA, MS, SC, WV	1, 4, 5
Nematodirus filicollis[b]	MI, PA, WI	1
N. odocoilei	AL, AR, FL, GA, KY, LA, MA, MD, MI, MS, NC, NY, PA, QE, SC, TX, VA, WA, WI	1, 4, 5, 7, 10, 21
Nematodirus sp.	NY, WI	1
Trichostrongylus sp.	TX	1
Large Intestine		
Chabertia ovina	NY	1
Eucyathostomum webbi[c]	AR, FL, GA, OK, SC	1, 4, 5, 17
Oesophagostomum cervi[d]	AL, LA, MD, MS, NC, VA, WV	1
O. columbianum	TX	1
O. venulosum[d]	AL, FL, GA, KY, LA, MD, MI, MS, NC, NY, OK, ON, PA, TX, VA, WV	1, 4, 5, 7, 8, 9, 12, 20, 21

[a]1. Walker and Becklund (1970). 2. Hoberg et al. (1993b). 3. Lichtenfels et al. (1993). 4. Forrester (1992). 5. Pursglove et al. (1976); Prestwood and Pursglove (1981). 6. Doster and Friend (1971). 7. Davidson et al. (1985). 8. Richardson and Demarais (1992). 9. Davidson and Crow (1983). 10. Foreyt and Trainer (1970). 11. Stubblefied et al. (1987). 12. Waid et al. (1985). 13. Cook et al. (1979). 14. Conti and Howerth (1987). 15. Xiao and Gibbs (1991). 16. Belem et al. (1993). 17. Pursglove (1976). 18. Lichtenfels et al. (1994). 19. Strohlein et al. (1988). 20. Heuer et al. (1975). 21. Foreyt and Samuel (1979).

[b]Records of *N. filicollis* from deer may represent *N. odocoilei* (see Becklund and Walker 1967a).

[c]Records of *Eucyathostomum longisubulatum* are included under *E. webbi,* consistent with observation by Pursglove (1976).

[d]*Oesophagostumum cervi* may represent a synonym of *O. venulosum* (see Baker and Pursglove, 1976), possibly refuting Payne et al. (1967) who provided justification for the validity of the former species.

TABLE 8.12—Strongylate nematodes in caribou, *Rangifer tarandus*[b,c]

Location/Species	Locality (State/ Province)	Source[a]
Abomasum		
Marshallagia marshalli	AK, NU[g]	7, 8
Ostertagia gruehneri/ O. arctica	AK, NF, NU, NWT, ON	1, 2, 7, 8, 12
O. mossi[d]	NF	2
Ostertagia sp.	AK, BC, QE	3, 4, 5, 9, 16
Teladorsagia boreoarcticus[e]	NU	14
Teladorsagia circumcincta/[f]		
T. trifurcata	AK, BC, NU, NWT, QE	1, 3, 4, 6, 8, 9, 13, 15
Trichostrongylus axei	NF	1
Small Intestine		
Nematodirella alcidis	NWT	9
N. longissimespiculata	AK, BC, NF, NWT, ON, QE	1, 2, 4, 5, 9, 11
Nematodirus filicollis	NF	2
N. odocoilei	NF	1
N. skrjabini	AK	8
N. tarandi	AK, NWT, QE	1, 5, 9, 10
Nematodirus sp.	AK, BC	4, 16

[a]1. Fruetel and Lankester (1989) 2. Bergerud (1971). 3. Cowan (1951). 4. Low (1976). 5. Hout and Beaulieu (1984). 6. Jean et al. (1982). 7. E. P. Hoberg, J. Nishi, and S. Kutz unpublished records, near Kugluktuk, NU. 8. C.A. Nielsen, unpublished records. 9. Unpublished records, U.S. National Parasite Collection. 10. Hadwen (1922) in introduced reindeer. 11. Lichtenfels and Pilitt (1983b). 12. Lichtenfels et al. (1990). 13. Becklund (1962). 14. Hoberg et al. (1999). 15. Choquette et al. (1957), in introduced reindeer. 16. Hadwen and Palmer (1922), in introduced reindeer.

[b]Includes barrenground caribou, *Rangifer tarandus groenlandicus;* woodland caribou, *R. t. caribou;* Alaskan barrenground caribou, *R. t. granti;* and introduced reindeer from the Palearctic, *R. t. tarandus;* records from Peary caribou, *R. t. pearyi,* are apparently lacking.

[c]Additional records from Fruetel and Lankester (1989) include parasites from a captive herd at Kakabeka Falls, Ontario: *Ostertagia gruehneri/O. arctica, O. ostertagi, O. leptospicularis/ O. kolchida, Spiculopteragia asymmetrica, S. spiculoptera, Nematodirella longissimespiculata, Nematodirus odocoilei, N. helvetianus, Trichostrongylus axei, T. vitrinus,* and *Oesophagostomum venulosum.*

[d]The report of *O. mossi* from Newfoundland could represent either *O. gruehneri* or *O. leptospicularis* (see Hoberg et al. 1993b; Lichtenfels et al. 1990).

[e]Specimens of *Teladorsagia* in barrenground caribou from the central Canadian arctic appear referable to *T. boreoarcticus.*

[f]The identity of specimens in caribou and reindeer from North America and across the Holarctic requires reevaluation (Hoberg et al. 1999).

[g]NU = Nunavut, Canada, a former region of the eastern Northwest Territories.

TABLE 8.13—Strongylate nematodes in introduced and exotic Cervidae

Host Species	Parasite	Locality (State/Province)	Source[a]
Cervus elaphus	*Spiculopteragia spiculoptera*	TX	1
	S. asymmetrica	TX	1
Cervus nippon	None reported	MD, VA	7
	Oesophagostomum venulosum	TX	8
Cervus dama	*Cooperia punctata*	AL	5
	Haemonchus contortus	AL, TX	5, 8
	Mazamastrongylus odocoilei	AL, KY	2, 5
	M. pursglovei	KY	2
	Nematodirus odocoilei	KY	2
	Oesophagostomum venulosum	KY, TX	2, 8
	Ostertagia mossi	KY	4
	Spiculopteragia asymmetrica	GA, KY	2, 3
Cervus unicolor	*Trichostrongylus askivali*	FL	6
Axis axis	*Haemonchus contortus*	TX, HI	8, 9
	Cooperia punctata	HI	9
	Oesophagostomum venulosum	TX	8
	Trichostrongylus axei	HI	9
Elaphurus davidianus	*Spiculopteragia suppereri*	TX	10

Nematodes with potential for introduction in cervids:
Ashworthius sidemi Schul'ts, 1933—Palearctic
Schulzinema spp. Krastin, 1937—Asia
Spiculopteragia spp.—Palearctic

[a]1. Rickard et al. (1993). 2. Davidson et al. (1985). 3. Doster and Friend (1971). 4. Phillips et al. (1974). 5. Brugh (1971). 6. Davidson et al. (1987). 7. Davidson and Crow (1983). 8. Richardson and Demarais (1992). 9. McKenzie and Davidson (1989). 10. T. M. Craig and J. H. Johnson, unpublished record (Abstract No. 61, Southern Conference on Animal Parasites, Louisiana State University, Baton Rouge, 1994).

TABLE 8.14—Strongylate nematodes in introduced and exotic Bovidae and Camelidae

Host Species	Parasite	Locality (State/Province)	Source[a]
Bovidae:			
Addax nasomaculatus	*Haemonchus contortus*	TX	1
	Longistrongylus curvispiculum	TX	1
Antilope cervicaprae	*Camelostrongylus mentulatus*	TX	2
	H. contortus	TX	2
	Nematodirus spathiger	TX	2
	Oesophagostomum sp.	TX	2
	Trichostrongylus axei	TX	2
	T. colubriformis	TX	2
	T. probolurus	TX	2
Hippotragus niger	*H. contortus*	TX	1
	L. curvispiculum	TX	1
Oryx beisa	*H. contortus*	TX	1
	L. curvispiculum	TX	1
Camelidae:			
Llama glama	*Camelostrongylus mentulatus*	OR	3
	Cooperia oncophora	OR	3
	C. surnabada	OR	3
	Haemonchus sp.	OR	3
	Nematodirus filicollis	OR	3
	N. helvetianus	OR	3
	N. spathiger	OR	3
	Ostertagia ostertagi	OR	3
	Oesophagostomum venulosum	OR	3
	T. axei	OR	3
	T. longispicularis	OR	3
	T. vitrinus	OR	3

Nematodes with potential for introduction in bovids and camelids:
Agriostomum spp. Railliet, 1902—Asia, Africa; bovids
Cooperiinae, genera and species— Africa; bovids
Haemonchus spp.—Africa; bovids
Lamanema chavezi Becklund, 1963—S. America; camelids
Longistrongylus spp.—Africa; bovids
Mecistocirrus digitatus (Linstow, 1906)—S. America, Central America, Asia; bovids
Sarwaria bubalis (Sarwar, 1956)—India, S. America; bovids

[a]1. Craig (1993). 2. Thornton et al. (1973a, 1973b). 3. Rickard and Bishop (1991).

Genus *Cooperia* Ransom, 1907
Classification: Trichostrongyloidea:
Trichostrongylidae: Cooperiinae.
Common Name: Cooperias.
Cooperia oncophora (Railliet, 1898). [Synonyms: *Strongylus radiatus* Rudolphi, 1803 in part; *S. ventricosus* Rudolphi, 1809 in part; *S. oncophorus* Railliet, 1898; *C. bisonis* Cram, 1925.]
Cooperia curticei (Railliet, 1893). [Synonyms: *Strongylus ventricosus* Rudolphi, 1809; *S. curticei* Giles, 1892; *S. curticei* Railliet, 1893.]
Cooperia punctata (Linstow, 1897). [Synonyms: *Strongylus* sp. Schneider, 1906; *S. punctatus* Linstow, 1896 in Schneider, 1907; *S. bovis* Vrijburg, 1907; *C. brasiliensis* Travassos, 1914.]
Cooperia pectinata (Ransom, 1907). [Synonym: *C. nicoli* Baylis, 1929.]
Cooperia spatulata (Baylis, 1938).
Cooperia surnabada (Antipin, 1931). [Synonym: *C. mcmasteri* Gordon, 1932.]

Species of *Cooperia* are well defined morphologically and can be identified based on the structure of the spicules and copulatory bursa in males and by the synlophe (the system of cuticular ridges characteristic of most trichostrongylids) in males and females (Lichtenfels 1977; Gibbons and Khalil 1982; Durette-Desset 1983). There are six species known from North America, although there is compelling evidence based on biochemical and nucleotide data that *C. surnabada* is a morphological form of *C. oncophora* (see Isenstein 1971; Humbert and Cabaret 1995).

Consistent with other trichostrongylids, the life cycle is direct; adults reside in the small intestine. The prepatent period may be 17–22 days (Levine 1980). Species are primarily parasites of sheep and cattle, but are relatively minor parasites in sylvatic bovids and cervids. All species known from domesticated hosts have been found in wild ruminants, the most commonly reported being *C. oncophora*. Particularly in sylvatic bovids, species of *Cooperia* are usually found in association with other trichostrongyles acquired on common range with cattle or sheep. Most records show that intensity and prevalence are minimal in wild hosts, and these nematodes are unlikely to occur at levels considered pathogenic. In contrast, heavy infections in calves may lead to serious disease

TABLE 8.15—Number of adult nematodes needed to produce clinical signs in calves less than one year in age: monospecific infections[a]

Parasite	Morbidity	Mortality
Cooperia spp.	140,000	?
Haemonchus spp.	5,000–9,000	>10,000
Ostertagia ostertagi	5,000–15,000 (Type II)	12,000–15,000 (Type II)
Nematodirus spp.	600–13,000	?
Trichostrongylus spp.	100,000	> 140,000

[a]Modified from Jordan and Stair (1983).

(Levine 1980) (Tables 8.15 and 8.16). Geographically, climatological factors may limit the distribution of *Cooperia* spp. to the southern temperate and boreal zones as they have only rarely been recognized among sylvatic hosts at higher latitudes of the subarctic and arctic regions.

Genus *Haemonchus* Cobb, 1898
Classification: Trichostrongyloidea: Trichostrongylidae: Haemonchinae.
Common Name: Large stomach worms; barber pole worms.
Haemonchus contortus (Rudolphi, 1803). [Synonyms: *H. bispinosus* Molin, 1860; *H. lunatus* Travassos, 1914; *H. cervinus* Baylis and Daubney, 1922; *H. atectus* Lebedev, 1929; *H. pseudocontortus* Lebedev, 1929; *H. fuhrmanni* Kamensky, 1929; *H. okapiae* van den Berghe, 1937 in part; *H. tartaricus* Evranova, 1940; *H. contortus contortus* Das and Whitlock, 1960; *H. contortus cayugensis* Das and Whitlock, 1960; *H. contortus bangelorensis* Rao and Rahman, 1967; *H. contortus hispanicus* Martínez and Gómez, 1968; *H. contortus kentuckiensis* Sukhapesna, 1974; and *H. contortus* var. *uktalensis* Das and Whitlock, 1960.]
Haemonchus placei (Place, 1893).
Haemonchus similis Travassos, 1914. [Synonym: *H. bubalis* Chauhan and Pande, 1968.]

Haemonchines that could be introduced: *Ashworthius sidemi* Schulz, 1933 is a species that could be introduced with Palearctic cervids such as red deer.

Species of *Haemonchus* are parasites of the abomasum and are broadly distributed nematodes in ruminants throughout the world. Among the ten currently valid species, three have been documented in wild bovids or cervids from North America; all are typical parasites of either domestic sheep or cattle (see Lichtenfels et al. 1994). Considering these, *H. contortus* has been widely reported from both bovid and cervid hosts across the boreal and southern regions of North America (Levine 1980; Prestwood and Pursglove 1981; Forrester 1992); records of *H. placei* and *H. similis* apparently are rare.

Nematodes of this genus are characterized by a prominent buccal tooth, well-developed synlophe, and copulatory bursa in the male. Identification to species, until recently somewhat equivocal, is now based on structural characteristics of adult worms, particularly the configuration of the synlophe in the cervical region of males and females, the length of the spicules in males [see Lichtenfels et al. (1994) for review], and differences in the ITS region of rDNA (Zarlenga et al. 1994). This has eliminated the controversy over the validity of *H. placei*, which has often been listed as a synonym of *H. contortus* (e.g., Gibbons 1979). A potential problem is now evident, however, with respect to records of *H. contortus* and *H. placei* from wild hosts in the United States and Canada. Prior to the studies by Lichtenfels et al. (1994) it was not possible to unambiguously distinguish between *H. placei* and *H. contortus* based on morphological characters. Thus, although the latter is the most commonly reported species in deer, bison, pronghorn, bighorn sheep, and exotic cervids, the records must be considered suspect and may not reflect accurate identifications. Additionally, the contention that *Haemonchus* represents an "actively evolving" group in the sense presented by Das and Whitlock (1960) and Prestwood and Pursglove (1981) is no longer supportable. This concept for *H. contortus* had been based on the premise of a number of diagnosable subspecies (Das and Whitlock 1960) defined by morphological characters that have since been found to be influenced by broad intraspecific variation (Gibbons 1979).

The life cycle for species of *Haemonchus* is direct, with blood-feeding adults producing eggs that are shed in the feces. Infective L_3's develop in ~3 days under optimum conditions. Following ingestion by the ruminant host, development to the fourth stage is completed in ~48 hours. Larvae, situated at the surface of the

TABLE 8.16 Number of adult nematodes needed to produce clinical signs in calves less than one year in age: multispecies infections[a]

Parasite	Intensity	Other Parasites and Intensity		Outcome
Cooperia	6000—25,000	*Ostertagia*	2000—10,000	Morbidity
		Nematodirus	300—1000	
		Trichostrongylus	200	
Trichostrongylus	10,000—65,000	*Ostertagia*	12,000—20,000	Morbidity
Trichostrongylus	20,000—50,000	*Ostertagia*	12,000—20,000	Morbidity
		Cooperia	20,000—40,000	

[a]Modified from Jordan and Stair (1983).

mucosa, feed on blood and complete development to the adult stage; the prepatent period is ~18–21 days (Levine 1980).

Species of *Haemonchus,* but particularly those identified as *H. contortus,* are widely distributed in North America and have been reported from bovids (*Bison bison, Ovis canadensis*), cervids (*Odocoileus* spp.; and exotic species), and *Antilocapra americana* in a range extending north to British Columbia and Alberta. When found in white-tailed deer it is most common in the southeastern United States (Prestwood and Pursglove 1981). Species of *Haemonchus* are not known from the subarctic and arctic regions, a pattern similar to that known for *Cooperia* spp.

Data for prevalence and intensity of *Haemonchus* suggest that among wild ruminants these are relatively uncommon parasites except in deer and pronghorn. *Haemonchus contortus* was the most commonly occurring nematode reported by Boddicker and Hugghins (1969) in *A. americana* examined in South Dakota (68% of 60 animals). With respect to other recorded hosts, prevalence and intensity have been relatively minimal except in *Odocoileus* spp., and in deer appear to vary geographically. The highest levels of infection by *H. contortus* in white-tailed deer have been observed in the sandy, coastal plain localities of the southeastern United States (Prestwood and Pursglove 1981). In this region prevalence approached 100%, and the maximum intensity documented exceeded 4300 worms (Pursglove et al. 1976; Prestwood and Pursglove 1981). Forrester (1992) summarized records from Florida, where overall prevalence in fawns was near 100% (with up to 10,545 worms) and in adults near 80% (maximum 2083 worms). Morbidity and direct mortality in deer, particularly fawns, has been attributed to infections ranging from over 1000 nematodes to a maximum of 16,540, the former possibly synergistic with malnutrition and the presence of other parasites (Prestwood and Kellogg 1971; Davidson et al. 1980; Forrester 1992).

Based on reports from white-tailed deer, species of *Haemonchus* must be considered as recognized and potential primary pathogens in wild ruminants (Davidson et al. 1980; Prestwood and Pursglove 1981; Forrester 1992). Boddicker and Hugghins (1969) reported hemorrhagic lesions when *H. contortus,* along with other trichostrongyles, were present in large numbers in pronghorn. In deer, and presumably other wild ruminants, haemonchosis is associated with severe blood loss (Foreyt and Trainer 1970). Typical clinical signs include stunting and emaciation, pale mucous membranes, and "bottle jaw" with the accumulation of fluid in the submandibular region. Internally, tissues and organs are pale, and ascitic fluid is commonly found in the body cavity. The mucosa of the abomasum is reddened, ulcerated, and eroded, and large numbers of nematodes may be visible (Prestwood and Pursglove 1981).

Although clearly pathogenic, diagnosis is problematic as the clinical signs of infection may develop prior to patency, and the eggs of *Haemonchus* cannot be reliably distinguished from those of related trichostrongylids using traditional methods (Georgi and McCulloch 1989; Sommer 1996). Clinical signs, particularly anemia, in conjunction with animals originating in areas where *Haemonchus* may be enzootic, continue to be among the most useful criteria for diagnosis (Prestwood and Pursglove 1981). With the advent of molecular markers for *Haemonchus* and other genera of trichostrongylids, it should now be possible to unequivocally identify eggs in feces (Zarlenga et al. 1994; Lichtenfels et al. 1997), thus replacing the laborious task of distinguishing among L_3's recovered from fecal cultures. As outlined above, adult males and females of the three species known from North America can now be reliably identified based on morphological and molecular criteria (Lichtenfels et al. 1994).

Currently, control and treatment remain problematic. An array of efficacious anthelmintics, including benzimidazoles and avermectins, with significant activity against adults and larvae of *Haemonchus* and other trichostrongyles are available; however, few have "label approval" for applications in wild bovids or cervids (e.g., "Safe-Guard" a formulation of fenbendazole released by Hoechst-Roussel is listed for use in zoo and wild animals as a broad spectrum nematocide). Accordingly, effective dosages, routes of administration, potential toxicity, side effects, and predictable efficacies generally have not been determined for most wild ruminants. The difficulties are compounded by the problems of attempting anthelmintic therapy in free-ranging ruminants (Prestwood and Pursglove 1981), which indeed may only be practical when dealing with confined or endangered species. The use of anthelmintics in game animals is further complicated by the "withdrawal" periods that would be required for some compounds. Management practices that limit competition with other ruminants and overpopulation on areas used for foraging appear to be most appropriate to control and limit the impact of haemonchosis (Prestwood and Pursglove 1981).

Genus *Pseudostertagia* Orloff, 1933
Classification: Trichostrongyloidea: Trichostrongylidae: Libyostrongylinae.
Pseudostertagia bullosa (Ransom and Hall, 1912).
[Synonyms: *Ostertagia bullosa* Ransom and Hall, 1912; *Ostertagia* (*Pseudostertagia*) *bullosa* Orloff, 1933.]

Originally described in the genus *Ostertagia,* this nematode was later transferred to the Libyostrongylinae and is currently the only member of the subfamily known as a typical parasite in ruminants from North America (Durette-Desset and Chabaud 1977). Unlike most members of the Libyostrongylinae, the synlophe is well developed (Durette-Desset 1983). *Pseudostertagia bullosa* was originally described from domestic sheep in Colorado (Ransom and Hall 1912). This is primarily a parasite of the abomasum in *A. americana*

from western North America and is seldom observed in
O. hemionus and *O. canadensis.* There have been subsequent records from domestic sheep in this region, but
none from cattle (Becklund 1964). It has been suggested that the occurrence of this nematode in domestic stock is dependent on the presence of pronghorn
(Lucker and Dikmans 1945). Morbidity and mortality
in wild or domestic ruminants has not been observed.

Genus *Obeliscoides* Graybill, 1924
Classification: Trichostrongyloidea:
 Trichostrongylidae: Libyostrongylinae.
Obeliscoides cuniculi (Graybill, 1923). [Synonym:
 Obeliscus cuniculi Graybill 1923.]

Lagomorphs, particularly *Lepus* spp. and *Sylvilagus*
spp., are the characteristic hosts for *O. cuniculi* in
North America. There are only two reports of this
species in the abomasum of white-tailed deer, and as a
consequence this is considered an atypical parasite in
white-tailed deer (Maples and Jordan 1966; Prestwood
and Pursglove 1981). It was also found in *O. canadensis* transported from Colorado to North Dakota (unpublished records, U.S. National Parasite Collection).

Subfamily Ostertagiinae
Classification: Trichostrongyloidea:
 Trichostrongylidae.
Common Name: Medium stomach worms.

The ostertagiines, or medium stomach worms, are
among the most pathogenic of the strongyles known
from ruminants (Levine 1980). In North America and
across the Holarctic region, nematodes of this subfamily parasitize both cervids and bovids and represent a
dominant component of the abomasal nematode fauna
(Drózdz 1965, 1966; Govorka et al. 1988; Lichtenfels
and Hoberg 1993). Taxonomy and systematics among
the ostertagiine nematodes have been particularly confused and are still open to resolution with respect to
nomenclature and relationships at the generic and
species level (e.g., Drózdz 1965, 1995; Gibbons and
Khalil 1982; Durette-Desset 1982, 1983; Lichtenfels
and Hoberg 1993; Hoberg et al. 1993a,b; Hoberg
1996). A considerable divergence in opinion exists over
the number of genera in the Ostertagiinae. Gibbons and
Khalil (1982) recognized 17 genera, Durette-Desset
(1982, 1983) included 5 or 6 genera, Jansen (1989)
proposed 7 genera, and most recently Drózdz (1995)
presented arguments for inclusion of 9 genera in the
subfamily. The diversity of opinions for generic level
taxonomy relates in part to rejection or acceptance of
the hypothesis for polymorphism among male nematodes in this group (Lichtenfels and Hoberg 1993;
Lichtenfels et al. 1997). Lack of resolution over the
generic-level taxonomy and systematics is not a trivial
issue as it directly impacts our abilities to formulate
any comprehensive understanding of parasite-host
biology.
A key in addressing the generic limits within the
ostertagiine subfamily is recognition of polymorphism,

arguably the most important concept related to taxonomy in this group over the past 20 years (Drózdz 1974;
Daskalov 1974; Lancaster and Hong 1981; Lancaster et
al. 1983). The polymorphism hypothesis was based on
the following observations: (1) pairs of male morphotypes consistently occur together, with one constituting
a "major" proportion and the other a "minor" proportion of the combined population; and (2) consistent
structural differences allow recognition of each of the
morphological types. In the past this led to the recognition of separate genera and species for major and minor
morphotypes (e.g., Drózdz 1965; Gibbons and Khalil
1982). These are now regarded as a series of polymorphic species distributed among a reduced number of
genera (Drózdz 1995). The proposal for polymorphism
has been corroborated based on morphological, biochemical, and molecular grounds (for review see Lichtenfels and Hoberg 1993; Lichtenfels et al. 1997). Consistent with the hypothesis for polymorphism in males,
the number of valid genera probably will not exceed
nine (see Drózdz 1995), but definitive resolution is
dependent on phylogenetic studies of this group now in
progress (Hoberg et al. 1993a; Hoberg and Lichtenfels
1994).
 In North American ruminants, species of seven genera have been recognized. The endemic fauna in wild
bovids and cervids includes species of *Ostertagia* (containing *Orloffia* in this review), *Teladorsagia, Marshallagia,* and *Mazamastrongylus.* Species of *Spiculopteragia, Camelostrongylus,* and *Longistrongylus* have
been introduced coincidental with importation of
exotic bovids and cervids from the Palearctic, Sub-
Saharan Africa, and possibly South America (Tables
8.13 and 8.14) (Lichtenfels and Hoberg 1993; Lichtenfels et al. 1997). Among these, polymorphism has been
recognized in *Ostertagia, Marshallagia, Teladorsagia,*
and *Spiculopteragia,* whereas it is considered to be
absent in *Mazamastrongylus, Camelostrongylus,* and
Longistrongylus (Drózdz 1995). Keys for the identification of genera and species in North American ruminants are presented in Lichtenfels et al. (1988a,b) and
Lichtenfels and Hoberg (1993). It should be noted that
nomenclature for the genera and species of ostertagiines as proposed by Durette-Desset (1989) is inconsistent with the hypothesis for polymorphism (see Lichtenfels and Hoberg 1993; Drózdz 1995).
 Medium stomach worms are characterized by a
reduced buccal capsule and well-developed copulatory
bursa in the male. The cervical papillae are prominent
and thorn-like. The synlophe is composed of a large
number of cuticular ridges that are perpendicular to the
body surface; in the cervical region one of three patterns, consistent with either generic- or species-level
groups can be recognized (Lichtenfels and Hoberg
1993). The genital cone always has paired "0" papillae
ventrally, and an accessory bursal membrane containing the paired "7" papillae dorsally. The lateral rays of
the copulatory bursa are in a pattern of 2-1-2 or 2-2-1,
considered characteristic for specific generic groups
(Durette-Desset 1982, 1983).

Identification of medium stomach worms is based on the structure of the bursa, genital cone, and spicules in males and on the dimensions of the esophageal valve and the configuration of the synlophe in males and females. Application of the synlophe has allowed accurate identification of females of most species for the first time (Lichtenfels et al. 1988a,b; Lancaster and Hong 1990). The identification of infective and parasitic larval stages continues to remain problematic (e.g., Belem et al. 1993) but is vital for developing an understanding of epizootiological patterns such as arrested development. It continues to be difficult to reliably identify eggs of any ostertagiines other than *Marshallagia,* and diagnosis of infection is still linked to necropsy, recovery, and identification. Quantification is best achieved by the application of an aliquot method such as that outlined in Prestwood and Pursglove (1981).

The life cycles for medium stomach worms found in sylvatic ruminants in North America are direct, but specific details of larval development and adult longevity are undetermined (for data from the Palearctic see Semenova and Korosteleva 1980; Semenova 1987; Govorka et al. 1988). Patterns of development of free-living and parasitic stages should parallel those elucidated for congeners in domestic bovids (Levine 1963; Herd 1986). Adults reside in the abomasum, embryonated eggs are passed in feces, and the first through third larval stages are free-living. The infective third stage is ensheathed, and parasitic development and the prepatent period require between 2 and 3 weeks, depending on the species involved. The potential for arrested development in response to seasonal and perhaps other factors (e.g., parasite density or immune status of host) may substantially prolong development time in the definitive host (but see Halvorsen 1986). In these instances, early fourth-stage larvae are retained in the abomasal mucosa for extended periods of time prior to resuming maturation to the adult stage. Evidence for seasonally defined inhibition (e.g., a summer or winter pattern) in wild hosts has been limited primarily to data from deer, some being equivocal or problematic to interpret (Baker and Andersen 1975; Conti and Howerth 1987; Borgsteede 1988; Xiao and Gibbs 1991; Belem et al. 1993). Also, life history patterns for species of *Marshallagia, Ostertagia,* and *Teladorsagia* in the Arctic may be adapted to high-latitude environments and, thus, differ from those observed in the mid-latitude boreal zones (Halvorsen and Bye 1999; Halvorsen et al. 1999; Irvine et al. 2000).

In general, specific morbidity and mortality has not been linked to the ostertagiines that parasitize wild ruminants. Data for prevalence and intensity of infection, however, have been difficult to document. It is probable that "subclinical" effects (e.g., alteration of foraging behavior, host physiology, and body weight) may be recognized that are similar to those documented for the influence of ostertagiines in domestic hosts. In particular, modification of food intake and body weight can be linked directly to prasitism by abo-

masal nematodes (e.g., Arneberg et al. 1996; Arneberg and Folstad 1999). Clinical signs of ostertagiosis in cattle are characterized by anemia, emaciation, submandibular edema, and diarrhea. In such cases, in excess of 40,000 nematodes may be present in the abomasum, and a minimum of 10,000 is considered necessary for development of severe gastric disease (Tables 8.15 and 8.16) (Levine 1980). In contrast, intensities of infection in *Odocoileus* spp. rarely exceed several hundred, with a maximum near 4000 for *Ostertagia* spp. (e.g., Prestwood and Pursglove 1981; Waid et al. 1985; Conti and Howerth 1987; Belem et al. 1993). Similar low intensities occur in *R. tarandus* (hundreds to several thousand for *Ostertagia* and *Teladorsagia*) (e.g., Bye 1987; Arneberg et al. 1996) and other cervids and bovids. In sylvatic hosts, environmental factors may result in fewer parasites being required to produce disease than in domestic stock (Pursglove et al. 1976). A confounding factor in understanding the distribution and potential for disease is the paucity of epizootiological information on patterns of transmission and the occurrence of Type I and Type II ostertagiasis in wild hosts (e.g., Gibbs and Herd 1986; Conti and Howerth 1987; Connan 1991, 1996).

Manifestations of ostertagiasis in deer have been associated with infections in excess of 1000 nematodes. In these instances, edema and pin-point ulcerations of the abomasal mucosa may be observed, which in heavier infections may coincide with nodular thickening of the abomasal mucosa (e.g., Conti and Howerth 1987). Generally, lesions are not evident in hosts with lower numbers of ostertagiines (Prestwood and Pursglove 1981).

Control of these and other nematodes in cervids has received some attention, particularly due to the commercial aspects of game ranching in New Zealand, North America, and the United Kingdom. Benzimidazoles and avermectins have been shown to be efficacious against ostertagiines and other gastrointestinal strongyles in red deer, and some recommendations for dosages have been outlined (e.g., MacKintosh et al. 1985; Kutzer 1987; Andrews and Lancaster 1988; Connan 1996). Pharmicokinetics, however, remains poorly understood (e.g., Lancaster and Andrews 1991). As indicated above, for *Haemonchus* spp., application of anthelmintics continues to be problematic, and label approval is generally lacking for helminths in wild ruminants.

Specific aspects of the biology and host and geographic distribution of ostertagiines in North America are addressed below. It should be noted that most genera and species have somewhat specific distributions linked to either cervids or bovids; the occurrence of some ostertagiines is associated with importation of exotic ruminants.

Genus *Marshallagia* Orloff, 1933
Classification: Trichostrongyloidea:
    Trichostrongylidae: Ostertagiinae.
Marshallagia marshalli (Ransom, 1907) Orloff,
    1933/*M. occidentalis* (Ransom, 1907) Durette-

Desset, 1982. [Synonyms of *M. marshalli:*
Ostertagia marshalli (Ransom, 1907) Orloff, 1933;
O. brignatiaca Blanchard, 1909; *O. tricuspis*
Marotel, 1912; *Haemonchus* sp. Marshall, 1904; *O.
orientalis* Bhalero, 1932.] [Synonyms of *M.
occidentalis: Grosspiculagia occidentalis* of Jansen,
1958; *Ostertagiella occidentalis* (Ransom, 1907)
Andreeva, 1957; *Grosspiculagia trifida* (Cuillé,
Marotel, and Panisset, 1912) Sarwar, 1956;
Grosspiculagia skrjabini (Kamenskii, 1929)
Sarwar, 1956.]

Marshallagia marshalli/M. occidentalis represent a
single polymorphic species, the only member of this
genus currently recognized in North America (Lichtenfels and Pilitt 1989). Specimens designated as *Marshallagia* sp./*Ostertagia* sp. in mountain goat from
western North America may represent a distinct
species, but confirmation will require comparison to
congeners known from Eurasia (Lichtenfels and Pilitt
1989). Additionally, Drózdz (1995) considers *Marshallagia* sp. in bighorn sheep to represent a species distinct
from *M. marshalli.*
Pending resolution of the taxonomy for *Marshallagia* spp. in the Nearctic, *M. marshalli* has a broad host
distribution in bovids and cervids extending from the
northwestern regions into the Arctic. In Wyoming it
was found to be a common parasite in bighorn sheep
(67%–80% prevalence based on fecal examination and
necropsy, respectively) and pronghorn (36%–47%), but
rare or absent in moose, elk, and mule deer (Bergstrom
1975a). In the Northwest Territories and Nunavut,
Canada, it was found in muskoxen and caribou (Webster and Rowell 1980; E.P. Hoberg et al., unpublished).
It is considered a parasite more typical of wild sheep
and bovids than of cervids. For example, it was suggested that the presence of *M. marshalli* in reindeer
from Spitzbergen was the result of introduction of the
parasite with muskoxen (Bye et al. 1987).
Adults of this species can be identified based on the
structure of the copulatory bursa and spicules in males
and by the synlophe in males and females (Lichtenfels
and Pilitt 1989; Lichtenfels and Hoberg 1993). Eggs
are recognizable in fecal examination by their large
size (> 150 µm in length) and would potentially be confused only with those of *Nematodirus* spp. or *Nematodirella* spp.
This is a nearly ubiquitous parasite of bighorn sheep,
often with 100% prevalence at some localities (Becklund and Senger 1967; Uhazy and Holmes 1971; Kistner et al. 1977) (Table 8.5); maximum reported intensity was near 1300 nematodes. Despite relatively high
prevalence and intensity in some hosts, there are no
specific reports of pathogenicity related to infections of
Marshallagia in wild ruminants. In domestic sheep in
Eurasia, however, marshallagiasis may result in significant disease (see Bye and Halvorsen 1983). *Marshallagia marshalli* has been reported from sheep but not
cattle in North America. Substantial prevalence (100%)
and intensity (near 11,000) have been documented in

reindeer from Svalbard, Norway, exceeding that
reported from North American caribou (C.A. Nielsen,
unpublished). The intensity of infection may be sufficient to adversely influence host productivity and life
expectancy (Bye and Halvorsen 1983).

Genus *Mazamastrongylus* Jansen, 1986
Classification: Trichostrongyloidea:
   Trichostrongylidae: Ostertagiinae.
Mazamastrongylus odocoilei (Dikmans, 1931) Jansen,
   1986. [Synonyms: *Ostertagia odocoilei* Dikmans,
   1931; *Skrjabinagia odocoilei* (Dikmans, 1931)
   Kassimov, 1942; *Ostertagiella odocoilei* (Dikmans,
   1931) Andreeva, 1956; *Spiculopteroides odocoilei*
   (Dikmans, 1931) Jansen, 1958; *Apteragia odocoilei*
   (Dikmans, 1931) Drózdz, 1965; *Camelostrongylus
   odocoilei* (Dikmans, 1931) Durette-Desset, 1989.]
Mazamstrongylus pursglovei (Davidson and
   Prestwood, 1979) Jansen, 1986. [Synonyms:
   Apteragia pursglovei Davidson and Prestwood,
   1979; *Spiculopteroides pursglovei* (Davidson and
   Prestwood, 1979) Hinaidy and Prosl, 1981;
   Teladorsagia pursglovei (Davidson and Prestwood,
   1979) Durette-Desset, 1989.]

Species of *Mazamastrongylus* are largely host-
specific parasites in cervids from the Holarctic
(Drózdz 1995; Hoberg 1996; Hoberg and Khrustalev
1996). Two species of *Mazamastrongylus* occur in
Odocoileus virginianus from eastern North America
(Lichtenfels et al. 1993). The distribution of *M.
odocoilei* coincides with that of white-tailed deer,
whereas that of *M. pursglovei* is restricted to the
southeastern United States, such that the two species
have overlapping but distinct geographic ranges
(Strohlein et al. 1988; Lichtenfels et al. 1993).
Records from other cervid hosts are rare (fallow deer
and wapiti) (Tables 8.9 and 8.13), and there are no
reports of either species in domestic stock.
Morphologically, species of *Mazamastrongylus* have
a characteristic tapering synlophe and club-shaped
esophagus. They can only be confused with species of
Spiculopteragia from which they are separated by the
structure of the spicules (Lichtenfels et al. 1993; Hoberg
1996). Only two characters, spicule length and structure,
are useful in distinguishing between males of *M. pursglovei* and *M. odocoilei;* females cannot be identified.
Mazamastrongylus spp. are the most commonly
occurring parasites in white-tailed deer, with
20%–100% prevalence and a maximum of 10–9060
worms reported at specific localities (Davidson and
Prestwood 1979; Prestwood and Pursglove 1981; Forrester 1992); mixed infections are not uncommon.
There are no specific reports of pathogenicity associated with infections of either species.

**Genus *Ostertagia* Ransom, 1907 (including *Orloffia*
Drózdz, 1965)**
Classification: Trichostrongyloidea:
   Trichostrongylidae: Ostertagiinae.

Ostertagia bisonis Chapin, 1925/*O. kazakhstanica*
(Dikov and Nekipelova, 1963). [Synonyms of *O.
bisonis: Ostertagia orloffi* Sankin, 1930; *Ostertagia
bellae* Landrum, 1951 nomen nudum;
Camelostrongylus bisonis (Chapin, 1925) Durette-
Desset, 1989; *Orloffia orloffi* (Sankin, 1930)
Drózdz, 1995; *Orloffia bisonis* (Chapin, 1925)
Drózdz, 1995.] [Synonym of *O. kazakhstanica:
Orloffia* sp. of Drózdz, 1995.]
Ostertagia gruehneri Skrjabin, 1929/*O. arctica*
Mitzkewitsch, 1929. [Synonym of *O. gruehneri:
Grühneria grühneri* Sarwar, 1956.] [Synonyms of
O. arctica: Sjobergia arctica (Mitzkewitsch, 1929)
Sarwar, 1956; *Ostertagiella arctica* (Mitzkewitsch,
1929) Andreeva, 1957; *Skrjabinagia arctica*
(Mitzkewitsch, 1929) Drózdz, 1965.]
Ostertagia leptospicularis Asadov, 1953/*O.kolchida*
Popova, 1937. [Synonyms of *O. leptospicularis:
Capreolagia skrjabini* Shul'ts, Andreeva and
Kadenazii, 1954; *Ostertagia capreoli* Andreeva,
1957; *Ostertagia taurica* Kadenazii and Andreeva,
1956 nomen nudum; *Ostertagia crimensis*
Kadenazii and Andreeva, 1956 nomen nudum;
Capreolagia antipini Kadenazii, 1957; *Capreolagia
paraskrjabini* Kadenazii, 1957; *Ostertagia
paracapreoli* Kadenazii and Andreeva, 1957;
Ostertagia capreolagi Jansen, 1958.] [Synonyms of
O. kolchida: Ostertagia (Ostertagia) kolchida
Popova, 1937; *Sjobergia kolchida* (Popova, 1937)
Sarwar, 1956; *Ostertagia (Skrjabinagia) popovi*
Kassimov, 1942; *Skrjabinagia popovi* Kassimov,
1942; *Grosspiculagia popovi* (Kassimov, 1942)
Jansen, 1958; *Grosspiculagia kolchida* (Popova,
1937) Jansen, 1958; *Ostertagia (Grosspiculagia)
lasensis* Assadov, 1953; *Grosspiculagia lasensis*
Asadov, 1953; *Skrjabinagia lasensis* (Asadov,
1953) Andreeva, 1957; *Muflonagia podjapolskyi*
Shul'ts, Andreeva and Kadenazii, 1954;
Skrjabinagia podjapolskyi (Shul'ts, Andreeva, and
Kadenazii, 1954) Andreeva, 1957; *Grosspiculagia
podjapolskyi* (Shul'ts, Andreeva, and Kadenazii,
1954); Jansen, 1958; *Skrjabinagia kolchida*
(Popova, 1937) Andreeva, 1957.]
Ostertagia mossi Dikmans, 1931/*O.dikmansi*
Becklund and Walker, 1968. [Synonym of *O.
dikmansi: Skrjabinagia dikmansi* (Becklund and
Walker, 1968) Drózdz, 1971.]
Ostertagia ostertagi (Stiles, 1892) Ransom,
1907/*O.lyrata* Sjöberg, 1926. [Synonyms of *O.
ostertagia: Strongylus ostertagi* Stiles, 1892; *O.
caprae* Andreeva and Nikolsky, 1957.] [Synonyms
of *O. lyrata: O. (Grosspiculagia) lyrata* Sjöberg,
1926; *Sjöbergia lyrata* (Sjöberg, 1926) Sarwar,
1956; *Grosspiculagia lyrata* (Sjöberg, 1926)
Jansen, 1958; *Skrjabinagia lyrata* (Sjöberg, 1926;
Andreeva, 1957; *Ostertagia occidentalis* Gebauer,
1932 nec. Ransom, 1907; *Camelostrongylus lyratus*
(Sjöberg, 1926) Durette-Desset, 1989.]

Species of *Ostertagia* are characteristic abomasal
nematodes in ruminants throughout the world. The current cosmopolitan distribution for some species, particularly those in domestic stock, has been strongly influenced by translocation and introduction of hosts and
parasites from Europe (Hoberg 1997). In contrast,
species endemic to either the Palearctic or the Nearctic
generally have characteristic distributions associated
either with bovids or cervids (Drózdz 1965; Govorka et
al. 1988). As noted earlier, there are five polymorphic
species of *Ostertagia* recognized in wild ruminants
from North America (Lichtenfels and Hoberg 1993).

Ostertagia bisonis circulates in pronghorn, bison, and
mule deer across the northcentral plains into Canada.
Morphologically, it is most similar to *Teladorsagia circumcincta* and *O. ostertagi,* but can be distinguished by
the structure of the spicules, the copulatory bursa, and
the dimensions of the esophageal valve (Becklund and
Walker 1967b; Lichtenfels and Pilitt 1991); the minor
male morphotype is *O. kazakhstanica* (see Lichtenfels
and Pilitt 1991; Drózdz 1995). This ostertagiine is
referred to the genus *Orloffia* by Drózdz (1995). It is not
known to be pathogenic in wild ruminants but has been
associated with significant clinical gastritis in cattle
sharing common range with deer, pronghorn, and bison
(Worley and Sharman 1966). Contrary to Worley and
Sharman (1966), nematodes depicted in photomicrographs of tissue sections were mature adults rather than
parasitic stages of larvae. This ostertagiine is known
from cattle in Wyoming, Montana, and Colorado (Becklund 1964; Lichtenfels and Pilitt 1991).

Ostertagia gruehneri is restricted in distribution to
the high latitudes of the Northern Hemisphere, and is a
typical abomasal nematode in caribou and muskox
across the Holarctic (Bye and Halvorsen 1983; Bye et
al. 1987; Fruetel and Lankester 1989). Morphologically, *O. gruehneri* is most similar to *O. leptospicularis*
and *O. mossi,* from which it can be distinguished based
on the structure of the genital cone and spicules (Lichtenfels et al. 1990; Hoberg et al. 1993b; Lichtenfels and
Hoberg 1993). Disease associated with infections of
this species has not been observed. Irvine et al. (2000),
however, suggested that *O. gruehneri* may have a role
as a determinant of population fluctuations or cycles
for reindeer. There are no records of this ostertagiine
from cattle, sheep, or other domesticated hosts.

Ostertagia leptospicularis and its minor morphotype, *O. kolchida,* are distributed across the western
Palearctic and occur in cervids and bovids (e.g.,
Drózdz 1965). Only recently has this species been
reported in North America, with records being from
cattle or caribou maintained in a captive herd (Rickard
and Zimmerman 1986; Fruetel and Lankester 1989;
Mulrooney et al. 1991). Records from wild cervids in
North America are limited to mule deer and elk, but the
parasite is considered to have an historically broader
geographic distribution, particularly in the western
United States (Hoberg et al. 1993b; Van Baren et al.
1996). The significance of *O. leptospicularis* is in its
reported pathogenicity in cervids. It was implicated in
winter mortality in red deer (Dunn 1983), where there
was an apparent shift in the abundance (dominance) of
O. leptospicularis relative to species of *Spiculoptera-*

gia. Additionally a concern is its potential for cross-transmission from cervids and its association with ostertagiosis in cattle in the United Kingdom and New Zealand (Borgsteede 1982; Hoberg et al. 1993b).

Ostertagia mossi and the associated minor morphotype, *O. dikmansi,* have a distribution restricted to eastern North America and have only been reported from white-tailed deer (Dikmans 1931; Becklund and Walker 1967b, 1968; Prestwood and Pursglove 1981, Forrester 1992; Hoberg et al. 1993b); it appears to be absent in the southeastern United States. Morphologically, this species is difficult to distinguish from *O. leptospicularis,* but can be identified based on the structure of the genital cone and terminal processes of the spicules in males (Hoberg et al. 1993b). Nematodes of this species are not considered to be pathogenic in the numbers typically encountered in white-tailed deer (prevalence to 70% and maximum of over 1000 nematodes at some localities) (Prestwood and Pursglove 1981; Forrester 1992).

Ostertagia ostertagi and the associated minor morphotype, *O. lyrata,* are ubiquitous parasites of domestic stock, principally cattle, throughout the world (Levine 1980). There are numerous records in wild ruminants in North America, and some reports have been linked to significant ostertagiosis (e.g., Conti and Howerth 1987). Generally, however, this ostertagiine occurs at low levels of intensity in wild bovids and cervids and would be unlikely to cause disease (see Prestwood and Pursglove 1981). It appears that *O. ostertagi* is found in wild ruminants only when range is shared with cattle.

Genus *Spiculopteragia* Orloff, 1933
Classification: Trichostrongyloidea:
   Trichostrongylidae: Ostertagiinae.
Spiculopteragia asymmetrica (Ware, 1925) Orloff, 1933/*S. quadrispiculata* (Jansen, 1958) Durette-Desset, 1982. [Synonym: *S. asymmetrica: Ostertagia asymmetrica* Ware, 1924; *S. cervi* (Cameron, 1931).][Synonyms: *S. quadrispiculata: Apteragia quadrispiculata* (Jansen, 1958) Durette-Desset, 1982; *Skrjabinagia monodigitata* Andrews, 1964.]
Spiculopteragia spiculoptera (Guschanskaia, 1931) Orloff, 1933/*S. mathevossiani,* Ruchliadeu, 1948.
[Synonyms: *Ostertagia spiculoptera* Guschanskaia, 1931; *O. boehmi* Gebauer, 1932; *S. kotkascheni* Asadov, 1952; *S. (Petrowiagia) pigulski* Ruchliadev, 1961; many authors list *S. spiculoptera* and *S. boehmi* as synonyms, Hinaidy et al. (1972) presented the argument that the later species name had priority.] [Synonyms: *S. mathevossiani: Rinadia mathevossiani* (Ruchliadev, 1948) Andreeva, 1957; *Rinadia schulzi* Grigorian, 1951; *Rinadia caucasica* Asadov, 1955; *Rinadia pavlovskyi* Kadenazii and Andreeva, 1957; *Rinadia quadrifurcata* Andrews, 1964.]
Spiculopteragia suppereri Hinaidy and Prosl, 1978.

Among parasites that could be introduced with wild cervids from the Palearctic and New Zealand (e.g., *C. elaphus elaphus, C. dama, C. nippon;* roe deer, *Capre-*

olus capreolus) are additional species of *Spiculopteragia* and other ostertagiines (e.g., Drózdz 1965, 1967; Kutzer and Hinaidy 1969; Govorka et al. 1988; Mason 1994).

Species of *Spiculopteragia* are typical parasites in the abomasum of cervids in the Palearctic (Drózdz 1965, 1966, 1967; Govorka et al. 1988). The occurrence of three species in North America can be attributed to introduction of cervids of exotic origin (Rickard et al. 1993). There are no records of *S. asymmetrica* from white-tailed deer on common range with fallow deer; *S. spiculoptera* has been reported once from white-tailed deer and from captive caribou (Tables 8.11, 8.13). *Spiculopteragia suppereri* was found in Pere David's deer imported to Texas (T.M.Craig, unpublished) and is recognized as a host-specific parasite in this cervid (Drózdz 1998). Disease conditions attributable to these species have not been observed in North America. Species of *Spiculopteragia* are generally restricted to cervid hosts, although records from *Bos* and *Bison* in Europe have been documented (Drózdz 1965, 1966, 1967, 1995; Suarez and Cabaret 1991).

Genus *Teladorsagia* Andreeva
and Satubaldin, 1954
Classification: Trichostrongyloidea:
   Trichostrongylidae: Ostertagiinae.
Teladorsagia boreoarcticus Hoberg, Monsen, Kutz, and Blouin, 1999, with *T. boreoarcticus* forma major and *T. boreoarcticus* f. minor, respectively, for major and minor morphotype males.

Teladorsagia circumcincta (Stadleman, 1894) Drózdz, 1965/ *T. trifurcata* (Ransom, 1907) Drózdz, 1965/ *T. davtiani* Andreeva and Satubaldin, 1954.
[Synonyms of *T. circumcincta: Strongylus circumcincta* Stadleman, 1894; *Ostertagia circumcincta* (Stadleman, 1894) Ransom, 1907; *Stadelmania circumcincta* (Stadleman, 1894) Sarwar, 1956; *Ostertagiella circumcincta* (Stadleman, 1894) Andreeva, 1957; *Strongylus vicarius* Stadleman, 1893; *Strongylus cervicornis* McFadyean, 1897 in part; *Strongylus instabilis* Julien, 1897; *Ostertagia turkestanica* Petrov and Shakhovtsova, 1926; *Stadelmania turkestanica* (Petrov and Shakhovtsova, 1926) Sarwar, 1956.]
[Synonyms of *Teladorsagia trifurcata: Ostertagia trifurcata* Ransom, 1907; *Stadelmania trifurcata* (Ransom, 1907) Sarwar, 1956.] Lancaster and Hong (1981) and Drózdz (1965) consider *T. davtiani* to be a synonym of *T. trifurcata;* Daskalov (1974) and Becklund and Walker (1971) consider them separate. Based on ITS-2 sequences from rDNA, *T. circumcincta* is trimorphic (Stevenson et al. 1996).

Teladorsagia circumcincta and associated minor morphotypes now have a cosmopolitan distribution. This ostertagiine is a characteristic abomasal parasite in wild and domesticated bovids, and only occasionally is reported from cervid hosts in North America (Lichtenfels et al. 1988a,b; Hoberg et al. 1999). In a recent hypothesis, E.P. Hoberg (in Lictenfels et al. 1997) suggested that forms designated as *T. circumcincta* from historically isolated populations of wild bovids may represent a complex of cryptic but distinct species. Such may be indicated by the exceptionally broad morphological variation documented for *T. circumcincta* and respective morphotypes in wild and domestic bovids across the Holarctic (e.g., Becklund and Walker 1971). Supportive of this hypothesis, collections in muskox and caribou from the central Arctic of Canada revealed a cryptic polymorphic species which was described as *Teladorsagia boreoarcticus* by Hoberg et al. (1999).

Discovery of *T. boreoarcticus* raises questions about the identity of nematodes reported as *T. circumcincta* (or associated morphotypes) in wild ruminants across the Holarctic and suggests a broader complex of sibling species in wild ruminants of the Nearctic (e.g., in Dall's sheep, bighorn sheep, mountain goats, pronghorn, and cervids) (Hoberg et al. 1999). Detailed studies of nematodes reported as *T. circumcincta* in wild bovids and cervids from North America and the Palearctic are requisite and should include molecular level analyses.

In sheep, *T. circumcincta* is considered one of the most significant pathogens throughout the world (Levine 1980). Generally, levels of intensity observed in domestic sheep are not attained in wild hosts (Nielsen and Neiland 1974). There have been no records of disease attributable to this species in wild ruminants in North America.

Other species of ostertagiines also have been introduced with exotic bovids from Sub-Saharan Africa, India, and possibly South America and the Palearctic. In some cases the original source can no longer be determined; they are mentioned here because of the potential for cross-transmission to endemic North American bovids or to cattle and sheep.

Genus *Camelostrongylus* Orloff, 1933
Classification: Trichostrongyloidea:
Trichostrongylidae: Ostertagiinae:
Camelostrongylus mentulatus (Railliet and Henry, 1909) Orloff, 1933. [Synonyms: *Ostertagia mentulata* Railliet and Henry, 1909; *Marshallagia mentulata* (Railliet and Henry, 1909) Durette-Desset, 1982.]

Camelostrongylus mentulatus is a pathogenic ostertagiine with a broad host range (camelids, bovids, and some cervids) and geographic distribution outside of North America. The exceptionally long and vermiculated spicules of the male are diagnostic for this ostertagiine (Gibbons and Khalil 1982). In the United States it has been reported in blackbuck antelope and llamas, but currently is not considered a common or widespread parasite (Rickard and Bishop 1991). This parasite, introduced into the United States (currently no records from Canada), is circulating in free-ranging herds of African bovids and llamas; there is considerable potential for dissemination to wild or domestic ruminants coinciding with transport of animals within North America. Thornton et al. (1973a,b) successfully

infected sheep and goats with larvae of *C. mentulatus* from antelope; cattle were apparently refractory to infection. Parasitic gastritis, chronic emaciation, and death of the host may be the consequences of infection (see Rickard and Bishop 1991).

Genus *Longistrongylus* LeRoux, 1931
Classification: Trichostrongyloidea:
Trichostrongylidae: Ostertagiinae.
Longistrongylus curvispiculum (Gibbons, 1973) Gibbons, 1977. [Synonym: *Bigalkenema curvispiculum* Gibbons, 1973.]

Species of *Longistrongylus* are parasites of bovids in the region of Sub-Saharan Africa (Gibbons 1977). Currently, *L. curvispiculum* is established in free-ranging herds of exotic bovids in Texas (Craig 1993) (Table 8.14). Although species of *Longistrongylus* appear to be relatively host specific, there is the potential for cross-transmission to wild and domestic ruminants in North America. Disease associated with infections by species of *Longistrongylus* has not been reported.

Genus *Trichostrongylus* Looss, 1905
Classification: Trichostrongyloidea:
Trichostrongylidae: Trichostrongylinae.
Common Name: Intestinal hair–worms.
Trichostrongylus askivali Dunn, 1964.
Trichostrongylus axei (Cobbold, 1879) Railliet and Henry, 1909. [Synonyms: *Strongylus gracilis* MacFadyean, 1896; *S. tenuissimus* Mazzanti, 1891; *T. extenuatus* (Railliet, 1898).]
Trichostrongylus calcaratus Ransom, 1911.
Trichostrongylus colubriformis (Giles, 1892). [Synonyms: *T. instabilis* (Railliet, 1893); *T. delicatus* Hall, 1916; *S. subtilis* Looss, 1895.]
Trichostrongylus dosteri Maples and England, 1971.
Trichostrongylus longispicularis Gordon, 1933.
Trichostrongylus vitrinus Looss, 1905.
Trichostrongylus probolurus (Railliet, 1896). [Synonym: *Strongylus probolurus* Railliet, 1896.]

Species of *Trichostrongylus* are parasites of either the abomasum or the small intestine and generally are uncommon. These are the smallest of the trichostrongylid nematodes that will be encountered as adult worms in bovid and cervid hosts. At the generic level, adults are readily identified by the prominent notch in the cuticle at the level of the excretory pore. In North America, these are the only trichostrongylids in which the synlophe is absent (Gibbons and Khalil 1982). Levine (1980), Maples and England (1971), and Pursglove et al. (1974) provide important diagnostic information at the species level.

The life cycle for trichostrongylines is direct, but there is no information for species such as *T. askivali* or *T. dosteri,* which are typical parasites of deer (Prestwood and Pursglove 1981). In *T. axei* and *T. colubriformis,* the third-stage infective larvae develop within 7–9 days under optimum conditions of temperature and moisture. Following ingestion of infective larvae, the prepatent period is ~15–23 days; patency extends up to 15 months for *T. axei* (see Levine 1980). Current evidence suggests that arrested development of the third- or early fourth-stage larva is of limited significance among *Trichostrongylus* spp.

Prevalence and intensity of infection are generally low and usually appear to be under the threshold where disease might be expected. In cattle, usually in excess of 100,000 worms (single species infections) or 10,000 worms (multispecies infections) are required to produce clinical disease (Table 8.15 and 8.16). In these instances, infections can be associated with weight loss, general weakness, inappetence, and watery diarrhea and occasionally can lead to mortality of the host. Lesions have not been described in wild bovids or cervids but may be expected to resemble those typical of trichostrongylosis in cattle. In heavy infections, there may be hyperemia of the abomasum and the development of whitish, necrotic plaques (Levine 1980).

Species of *Trichostrongylus* other than *T. askivali* and *T. dosteri* are likely acquired on range shared with domestic sheep or cattle. There are few records of *Trichostrongylus* occurring in ruminants at subarctic to arctic latitudes.

Genus *Nematodirus* Ransom, 1907
Classification: Trichostrongyloidea: Molineidae: Nematodirinae.
Common Name: Thread-necked strongyles.
Nematodirus abnormalis May, 1920.
Nematodirus andersoni Durette-Desset and Samuel, 1989. [Synonyms: c.f. *N. archari,* North American records, see Durette-Desset and Samuel (1989).]
Nematodirus archari Sokolova, 1948.
Nematodirus becklundi Durette-Desset and Samuel, 1992.
Nematodirus davtiani Grigorian, 1949. [Synonym: *N. rufaevastitatis* Durbin and Honess, 1951.]
Nematodirus filicollis (Rudolphi, 1802) Ransom, 1907. [Synonyms: *Ascaris filicollis* Rudolphi, 1802; *Strongylus filicollis* (Rudolphi, 1802) Rudolphi, 1803; *Fusaria filicollis* (Rudolphi, 1802) Zeder, 1803; *Oesophagostomum filicollis* (Rudolphi, 1802) Stossich, 1899; *N. furcatus* May, 1920.]
Nematodirus helvetianus May, 1920.
Nematodirus maculosus Becklund, 1965.
Nematodirus odocoilei Becklund and Walker, 1967. [Synonym: records of *N. filicollis* in *Odocoileus* spp. may represent this species according to Becklund and Walker (1967a).]
Nematodirus oiratianus Raevskaia, 1929. [Synonyms: *N. lanceolatus* Ault, 1944. Lichtenfels and Pilitt (1983a) consider all North American records referable to the subspecies *N. oiratianus interruptus;* however, not all specimens were examined so some records of this species are equivocal.]
Nematodirus oiratianus interruptus Lichtenfels and Pilitt, 1983. [Synonyms: North American records of *N. oiratianus* Raevskaia, 1929; *N. lanceolatus* Ault, 1944.]

Nematodirus spathiger (Railliet, 1896). [Synonym: *Strongylus spathiger* Railliet, 1896.]
Nematodirus skrjabini Mizkewitsch, 1929.
Nematodirus tarandi Hadwen, 1922. [Synonyms: *N. skrjabini* Mizkewitsch, 1929? Dikmans (1936) listed this species as a synonym of *N. tarandi;* however, Skrjabin et al. (1954) considered it distinct, but with *N. tarandi* referable to the genus *Nematodirella.*]

The genus *Nematodirus* is a speciose group that includes nematodes characteristic of either bovid or cervid hosts across the Holarctic (Kulmamatov 1974). There are in excess of 40 valid species, with 13 or 14 being found in wild ruminants from North America. These are among the largest of the trichostrongyloids in the small intestine (rarely abomasum) of bovids and cervids. They usually are recognized by the prominent cephalic vesicle, long, filiform spicules, a large copulatory bursa in the male, and large eggs, generally near 200 µm in length. The synlophe and the spicule tips and bursa are diagnostic characters for distinguishing among the species. Lichtenfels and Pilitt (1983a) provided keys for species occurring primarily in domesticated hosts; additional pertinent information on sylvatic species can be found in Hoberg and Rickard (1988), Hoberg et al. (1989), Rickard and Lichtenfels (1989), and Durette-Desset and Samuel (1989, 1992). Infective third-stage and parasitic larvae can be recognized based on characters of the tail (Fruetel and Lankester 1989).

Consistent with other trichostrongyloids, the life cycle is direct; however, development to the infective third larval stage occurs entirely within the egg. Development time is from 3–4 weeks at optimum temperatures for *N. filicollis, N. spathiger,* and *N. battus;* following ingestion, the minimum prepatent period is 2–3 weeks (Kates and Turner 1955; Thomas 1959). Epizootiological patterns for these species in the Pacific Northwest have been investigated by Rickard et al. (1989); data for other species are lacking.

Eggs and larvae are resistant to desiccation and low temperature, and overwinter survival has been documented. A limiting factor may be maximum temperatures attained in the summer, as larvae are intolerant to high temperatures. Transmission to the definitive host may have a marked seasonality and, in part, is mediated by precipitation and temperature (Marquardt et al. 1959; Gibson and Everett 1976, 1981; Rickard et al. 1989). Seasonally defined peaks of larval abundance are typical for *Nematodirus* spp. (e.g., Rickard et al. 1989). Thus, for some species in particularly harsh environments there may be only a single parasitic generation per year. This epizootiological picture would strongly influence the patterns of geographic and host distribution and the potential for disease associated with infections of *Nematodirus* spp.

Each species of *Nematodirus* has a well-defined host spectrum, such that species are usually limited in distribution to either cervids or bovids (Tables 8.1–8.12). Levels of prevalence and intensity vary according to the host, parasite, and geographic locality. For example in *Odocoileus* spp., the characteristic *N. odocoilei* has a widespread geographic range coinciding with its hosts. Prevalence generally ranges from 10%–20% with a maximum of 60% reported; intensity usually does not exceed several hundred worms (Pursglove et al. 1976; Forrester 1992). The maximum reported from one white-tailed deer was near 18,000, but was considered to be exceptional (Pursglove et al. 1976). Species of *Nematodirus* are abundant in wild sheep, with 100% prevalence and a maximum of 70–6000 adult worms and 3000 larvae reported (Kistner et al. 1977). These levels of infection would not be atypical across the range of bighorn sheep (Becklund and Senger 1967; Uhazy and Holmes 1971); comparable levels have been documented for Dall's sheep in Alaska (Nielsen and Neiland 1974). These levels are considered to be below that where substantial disease might be observed, but in a synergistic manner could become significant in the presence of other strongyles and malnutrition (Becklund and Senger 1967).

Among nematodirines, overlap in the faunas of domestic and sylvatic hosts are related to the sharing of parasites characteristic of cattle and sheep (*N. filicollis, N. spathiger, N. abnormalis* and *N. helvetianus)* (Table 8.1). Generally, a degree of host specificity is observed for those species found either in wild bovids (e.g., *N. becklundi* and *N. maculosus* in mountain goat and *N. andersoni* in Dall's and bighorn sheep) or cervids (e.g., *N. odocoilei* in deer) (Tables 8.1, 8.5, 8.6, 8.10, and 8.11). None of these species has been reported in domestic ruminants. Although the recently introduced and highly pathogenic *N. battus* has so far only been reported from sheep, cattle, and llamas in North America, there is some expectation that it could successfully parasitize such endemic cervids as deer or elk (Hoberg et al. 1986; Hoberg 1997).

Genus *Nematodirella* Yorke and Maplestone, 1926
Classification: Trichostrongyloidea: Molineidae:
    Nematodirinae.
Nematodirella alcidis (Dikmans, 1935). [Synonym: *N.*
    longispiculata alcidis Dikmans, 1935.]
Nematodirella antilocaprae (Price, 1927). [Synonyms:
    N. antilocaprae Price, 1927; *N. longispiculata*
    antilocaprae Dikmans, 1935; *Nematodirella*
    longissimespiculata antilocaprae of Skrjabin and
    Shikhobalova, 1952.]
Nematodirella gazelli (Sokolova, 1948). [Synonym:
    N. longispiculata gazelli Sokolova, 1948.]
Nematodirella longissimespiculata (Romanovich,
    1915). [Synonyms: *Microcephalus longissime*
    spiculatus Romanovich, 1915; *N. longispiculata*
    Yorke and Maplestone, 1926; *N. longispiculata*
    longispiculata Dikmans, 1935; *N.*
    longissimespiculata longissimespiculata Skrjabin
    and Skhikobalova, 1952.]

Systematics and taxonomy for this genus have been reviewed by Lichtenfels and Pilitt (1983b). Similar to *Nematodirus*, specimens of *Nematodirella* spp. are large strongyles generally from 10–40 mm in length.

Males are characterized by exceptionally long spicules, in excess of 4 mm (maximum over 12 mm in *N. gazelli*). The structure of the synlophe is diagnostic for males and females of the five Holarctic species; four species are known in wild ruminants from North America. Eggs are generally > 240 μm in length; among infective, ensheathed larvae the caudal structure is diagnostic for some species (Fruetel and Lankester 1989).

These are typically parasites of the small intestine in cervids and bovids at high boreal to arctic latitudes across the Northern Hemisphere. Some species such as *N. alcidis* in moose appear to be largely host specific; in contrast, *N. antilocaprae* is known from mule deer, elk, and pronghorn. Additionally, *N. alcidis* is one of the few trichostrongyloids that is commonly found in moose throughout North America. Records of *Nematodirella* spp. from domestic hosts are exceptional.

Life cycles for species of *Nematodirella* currently are unknown, but likely are similar to those documented for *Nematodirus*. Detailed information for prevalence and intensity of infection generally are not available or are based on small, host sample sizes. For *N. alcidis,* Stock and Barrett (1983) reported 52% prevalence and intensity ranging from 1 to 250 among 140 moose in Alberta; 1% of 186 elk were infected. There is no direct evidence of pathogenesis associated with infections of *Nematodirella* spp., and intensity and prevalence appear to be typically low.

STRONGYLATE FAUNA: A GENERAL OVERVIEW. Strongylate nematodes are common parasites in wild ruminants from North America. Numerical diversity ranges from a maximum of 28 species in *Odocoileus virginianus* to a minimum of 8 reported from *Alces alces;* the mean is 15 species per host (Tables 8.2–8.12). The range in species richness may in part reflect the degree of sampling effort and geographic distribution, particularly with the historical emphasis on parasitological studies of *Odocoileus* spp. This situation is likely to be more complex, however, as very few parasites are known from moose even though relatively large samples have been examined in some areas (Anderson and Lankester 1974). For example, Bergstrom (1975a) did not find *Marshallagia* in 60 moose from Montana; Spencer and Chatelain (1953) mention no parasites from moose in the Kenai Peninsula of Alaska; Stock and Barrett (1983) examined 140 moose from southeastern Alberta and found 3 species of strongyles; and C. A. Nielsen (unpublished) found 2 species in 25 moose from Alaska (Table 8.8).

This numerical diversity emphasizes the influence of host specificity (e.g., *Spiculopteragia* and *Mazamastrongylus* in *Cervus* spp. and *Odocoileus* spp., respectively) and apparent geographic limitations on the distribution of the relatively characteristic faunas associated with each host (e.g., Prestwood et al. 1975) (Tables 8.2–8.12). The importance of specificity, however, is variable, and in some instances the absence of this phenomenon accounts for the extensive host range documented for some strongyles (e.g., Suarez and

Cabaret 1991) (Table 8.1). Consequently, the faunas in wild ruminants are only partially segregated from those in domesticated sheep and cattle (Baker et al. 1957), but a relatively low percentage of the entire fauna is shared among these host groups. For example, cattle and sheep are the general source of infections by *Haemonchus* spp., *O. ostertagi, Trichostrongylus* spp., *N. filicollis, N. spathiger, N. helvetianus,* and *Cooperia* spp. in wild hosts; there is some suggestion based on high prevalence and intensity that circulation of *H. contortus* in white-tailed deer may not require cattle (see Forrester 1992). In contrast, *M. marshalli, O. bisonis, O. leptospicularis, P. bullosa, N. oiratianus interruptus,* and *O. venulosum* may be maintained primarily in wild bovids or cervids. These, along with *T. circumcincta,* would be expected on common range shared by wild and domesticated ruminants; however, *"T. circumcincta"* in wild bovids may represent an extensive complex of cryptic species which will further complicate our understanding of host distribution. A notable example of broad susceptibility to parasitism is seen in the infections of strongyles recorded in translocated muskoxen in contact with either domestic, semidomestic, or other sylvatic hosts (Alendal and Helle 1983).

On a worldwide basis, a comparison of the helminth faunas in a number of wild ruminants indicates that cross-transmission to domestic hosts may, in fact, be common (Dunn 1969). In most instances, however, helminth parasites of wild animals to which domestic stock are exposed appear to be of low pathogenicity. As a result, wild ruminants appear to be more likely to suffer from the effects of endoparasitism than do domestic cattle, sheep, and goats in areas of common grazing. For example, morbidity and mortality in captive and wild herds of muskoxen in contact with helminths derived from domestic hosts is documented (MacDonald et al. 1976; Alendal and Helle 1983). In general, it appears that in most free-ranging conditions, wild ruminants do not generally play a significant role in the spread or maintenance of helminth infections in domestic stock (Semenova 1984); one exception may be *O. leptospicularis* circulating among cervids, cattle, and sheep (Borgsteede 1982).

In some cases, significant disease may be associated with parasitism in an atypical host, such as that reported for *O. bisonis* in cattle, *O. ostertagi* in deer, or *M. marshalli* in domestic sheep (Worley and Sharman 1966; Oripov 1970; Conti and Howerth 1987). Additionally, it is possible that species currently recognized only as parasites of exotic and introduced bovids and cervids (Tables 8.13 and 8.14) may be capable of infecting both wild and domestic ruminants in North America.

Although cross-transmission of strongyles between host species does not appear to be a common occurrence in North America (Table 8.1), the basic biology associated with development and transmission of the various species of parasitic nematodes is similar (Govorka et al. 1988). For example, arrested development, as a mechanism for survival during periods of unfavorable environmental conditions, is a common phenomenon for many abomasal nematodes infecting domestic

ruminants (Gibbs and Herd 1986; Williams 1986). Nematodes such as *Mazamastrongylus* and other ostertagiines that infect white-tailed deer also appear to undergo similar developmental changes as an integral part of their transmission. The seasonal timing of inhibition generally coincides with that of related genera and species in bovine hosts (Belem et al. 1993). In contrast, Halvorsen (1986) suggested that larval inhibition may not be critical in the transmission and survival of gastrointestinal strongyles in reindeer that exist in harsh winter environments of the Arctic.

Management strategies for most game species are constantly being modified or are subject to local custom or national and international jurisdiction (e.g., Gunn 1982; Klein 1996). Such strategies as translocation and reintroduction can be expected to directly influence the distribution of parasites and the potential for disease (Hoberg 1997; Hoberg et al. 1999). Likewise, changes in associations between wild species and humans, domestic species, and introduced or farmed exotic ruminants may also alter the significance for a diversity of parasitic organisms (Haigh 1996). Consequently, we are now making significant observations related to the importance of gastrointestinal parasites of wild mammals and are beginning to determine that many species may be important contributors to the health of their mammalian hosts. Some specific examples of the significance of parasitism can be derived from the studies conducted on white-tailed deer.

MANAGEMENT IMPLICATIONS: MORBIDITY AND MORTALITY. The best documented parasite fauna among North American ruminants is that found in white-tailed deer (Table 8.11). In North America, *Odocoileus virginianus* is perhaps the most abundant species of ruminant, and one that has shown a remarkable ability to adapt to changing or modified habitats within its potential range. Although information documenting the occurrence of gastrointestinal strongyles is notable, it is important to recall that parasites are not equal in their pathogenic potential. Consequently, it is of fundamental importance not only to identify the specific organism(s) present, but also to determine the approximate intensity of infection. Clinical signs such as weight loss, diarrhea, anorexia, anemia, and poor pelage can be indicative of, or associated with, endoparasitism in both domestic and wild ruminants. Other health problems, however, including malnutrition, toxicities, concurrent hemoparasitic infections, and numerous infectious diseases can lead to similar clinical signs. Thus, in investigations of endoparasitic infections in wild species, we are not always able to unequivocally determine the role of a variety of factors or disease agents that have influenced the range of observed clinical signs. As a result, we are often limited in our ability to make precise statements related to the parasite fauna and its direct association with morbidity and mortality.

Veterinary medicine has made some contributions in this area, particularly for the range of nematode species that may be found in the abomasum (Tables 8.15 and

8.16: modified from Jordan and Stair 1983). For example, infection with 5000 to 9000 *H. contortus* is reported to result in notable morbidity in calves < 1 year of age; infections > 10,000 result in mortality. Among other genera the numbers of adult nematodes needed to produce mortality in calves of a similar age range from >140,000 for *Trichostrongylus* and 12,000–15,000 for *O. ostertagi* (in Type II ostertagiasis). Synergistic effects between species of strongyles may result in morbidity at lower levels of intensity (Table 8.16).

Experimental and/or field data for clinical effects of strongyles in wild ruminants has been limited (e.g., Johnston et al. 1984) but is available for parasites such as *H. contortus*. For example, a naturally infected and malnourished deer was found to have 16,540 adult *H. contortus* (Prestwood and Kellogg 1971); additional mortality was seen in deer with average worm burdens of > 1000 *H. contortus* (Prestwood et al. 1973). A general guideline has been proposed where 75 adults of *H. contortus* per kg body weight is the level of infection where clinical signs become apparent (Foreyt and Trainer 1970; McGhee et al. 1981). These studies are consistent with those in domestic animals where 500–>1000 adults of *H. contortus* are considered pathogenic (Herlich 1962; Anderson et al. 1966; Jordan and Stair 1983). Thus, it appears that in some cases extrapolation of values from domestic hosts to wild ruminants may be valid.

We emphasize that the values for intensity of infection and their linkage to pathogenicity must not be overinterpreted, and it is vital not to focus on a particular numerical range as being of significance in the etiology of disease. We suggest this due to the array of factors that may influence the interaction between hosts and parasites, including different species of nematodes, host species, weight, age, immune status, nutritional plain, and environmental setting (e.g., ambient temperatures, availability of water and forage). Consequently, although these values may serve as rough baselines, each situation and species of bovid or cervid must be evaluated independently. In the absence of controlled studies with specific species of parasites in wild ruminants, cautious extrapolation from domestic stock may represent the only source of information on pathogenicity; these data must be interpreted in a conservative manner. Additionally, as addressed in the subsequent section, the subclinical effects of parasitism, specifically at the level of host population, must also be recognized.

An extension of studies of gastrointestinal nematodes, particularly in white-tailed deer, was the development of the "abomasal parasite count" or APC (Eve and Kellogg 1977). In the southeastern United States wildlife biologists have employed this method to correlate the intensity of infection by abomasal parasites with the local population density of deer. This was accomplished by comparing the APC with an independent rating of deer density relative to the carrying capacity of the habitat (Eve and Kellogg 1977). Using a graded scale correlating these factors, APCs were used to assist

in management decisions related to manipulation of population density for deer. Specifically, management was tied to enhancing nutrition and natural immunity while reducing environmental contamination and minimizing the potential for transmission of parasites and related density-dependent disease conditions (Eve 1981). This procedure has been employed with mixed success in the southeastern United States, and its application to other regions has been problematic due to seasonal fluctuations in the abundance of parasites (Demarias et al. 1983; Waid et al. 1985). In Norway, Bye (1987) postulated an association linking poor physical condition, high population density, and high-intensity infections by ostertagiine nematodes in reindeer. Thus, it appears that variation in seasonal prevalence and abundance and other factors should be considered in the application and validity of the APC.

PARASITES AND HOST POPULATIONS: THEORETICAL ISSUES. The potential for interaction of the sylvatic and domestic fauna is important in evaluating the potential for disease attributable to gastrointestinal strongyles. Of additional and critical importance is consideration of the synergistic interactions of parasites and habitat. Rather than pathogenesis and mortality, associated with exceptional or monospecific infections (e.g., haemonchiasis and ostertagiasis in deer: Conti and Howerth 1987; Forrester 1992), it may be the cumulative effects of mixed species that induce disease or reduce performance (e.g., Bye and Halvorsen 1983). The subclinical effects of strongyle infections and impairment of gastrointestinal function have been documented in domestic sheep (Sykes 1978; Coop and Angus 1981), and it would be expected that these observations represent a generality among wild and domestic ruminants. Additionally, in circumstances of a high prevalence of infection such as those reported for reindeer, strongyles may be important as a determinant of population dynamics of the host (Bye and Halvorsen 1983; Halvorsen 1986).

A dynamic linkage between hosts, parasites, and habitat stability related to density-dependent effects of parasitism by gastrointestinal nematodes was postulated by Grenfell (1988, 1992). In these instances, parasites may influence plant-host interactions by regulation of host population density. Feedback mechanisms would exist where increasing intensity of parasitism would be expected with increasing host density (e.g., Eve and Kellogg 1977; Bye 1987; Arneberg et al. 1996); high levels of parasitism lead to reduced food intake and reduced impact on habitat (Grenfell 1992). Empirical support for this contention derives from observations of depression of food intake in *R. tarandus* related to the intensity of infection by gastrointestinal nematodes (Arneberg et al. 1996). This can be linked in a density-dependent manner to mortality and future fecundity within the host population. For example, reindeer calves reared in high-density areas are lighter than those from comparatively underpopulated regions, an observation previously emphasized solely for food availability (Skogland 1990). Thus, infections of high intensity by ostertagiines in the abomasum can lead to reduced food intake and efficiency and can eventually influence growth in calves; such effects could be pronounced during lactation (Bye 1987). Eventual impacts on host demography and the potential for limitation in the growth of the host population would be predicted (Anderson 1980; Bye 1987). Reduced foraging activity also may result in altered patterns of exposure that influence transmission of parasites to hosts. Ultimately a reduction in food intake may constitute a constraint on parasite abundance in individuals and in host populations.

Parasites can exacerbate the effects of malnutrition and food availability, which is indicative of the complex association linking herbivores, nematodes, foraging dynamics, and habitat stability (Grenfell 1992; Arneberg et al. 1996). This association has been demonstrated in studies of parasitism in caribou and in feral populations of the Soay sheep (Bye 1987; Gulland 1992; Arneberg et al. 1996). The synergism of food shortage and immunosuppression may result in pathogenic infections resulting in host mortality (Gulland 1992). Obvious implications are evident with respect to the effects of subclinical and clinical parasitism among a diversity of sylvatic ruminants. Thus, it is necessary to also consider the importance of aggregation of parasite populations and the distribution of parasites in natural host populations (e.g., Shaw and Dobson 1995; Hudson and Dobson 1995) rather than focusing on disease in individual animals.

CONSERVATION BIOLOGY, GLOBAL CHANGE, AND PARASITISM.

Human activities constitute a major control on the distribution and dissemination of helminth parasites and other pathogens (Vitousek et al. 1996; Hoberg 1997; Hoberg et al. 1999). The cosmopolitan ranges for many strongyles have largely resulted from the breakdown of isolating mechanisms or ecological barriers. Thus, alteration of historical associations through ecological disruption and long-range translocation will figure prominently in the continued emergence of pathogenic nematode parasites (Dobson and May 1986a,b; Scott 1988; Woodford and Rossiter 1994; Hoberg 1997; Daszek et al. 2000).

Translocation and introduction exposes indigenous wildlife to new disease organisms and concomitantly can expose introduced animals to novel pathogens. Rapid and long distance transport, introduction and maintenance of domesticated stock, or establishment of free-ranging or captive herds on small reserves can be important factors in the dissemination and amplification of pathogenic nematodes and other parasites (Dobson and May 1986b; Haigh 1996; Daszek et al. 2000). Woodford and Rossiter (1994) outlined protocols for minimization of risk by screening and intervention related to management practices for wild hosts. Careful planning, site selection (e.g., physical, ecological, presence of alternative hosts), quarantine, screening, and monitoring are requisite to controlling the introduction of potential pathogens (Haigh 1996). Development of comprehensive databases on host and geographic distribution of strongyles and other infectious agents can lead to a predictive framework that can be used as the basis for prevention (e.g., current development of a database for nematode parasites of Holarctic bovids and cervids) (E.P. Hoberg, unpublished). In conjunction with modern systematics to elucidate aspects of host-parasite evolutionary history, these become powerful tools in limiting the potential impacts of pathogenic nematodes (Hoberg 1997).

Baseline information on host behavior and ecology also aid in the control process. For example, Syroechkovskii (1995) identified the role of long-range migrations by reindeer and caribou as important determinants on the distribution of pathogens. Grazing and foraging behavior are also important factors to consider with respect to how different species of ruminants may be exposed to infection by parasites with direct life cycles. Habitat use influences prevalence and intensity, particularly in situations where animals are confined. There is an expectation of pathogenicity due to nematodes in hosts in relatively restricted conservation areas where the effects of crowding, concentration at waterholes, malnutrition, and heavy range exploitation (often in conjunction with domestic hosts) may be observed. A shift from the use of optimal to suboptimal forage or habitats may expose animals to parasitism; for example, a shift from a browsing to a grazing behavior. There is also a particular concern about the impact of host density in natural conservation reserves where transmission of parasites may be enhanced (Dobson and May 1986a,b; Scott 1988; Aguirre and Starkey 1994).

Only recently has the synergistic influence of anthropogenic and climatologically driven global change been discussed with reference to helminths and other parasites (e.g., Dobson and Carper 1992). Peters (1992) addressed a range of biotic responses to climate change (increase in global temperature), including alteration of habitat, and latitudinal shifts in distribution and abundance of plants and animals. For host-parasite systems in temperate regions, Dobson and Carper (1992) postulated that increasing temperatures and desiccation could limit the distribution of some parasites. Epizootiological patterns would be altered, possibly leading to reduced levels of parasitism or to the wider dissemination of species tolerant of higher ambient temperatures. Alternatively, the response of hosts to pathogens would also be modified (Dobson and Carper 1992) where (1) increased stress can change the degree of susceptibility to parasitism and parasite-induced mortality (Esch et al. 1975); (2) changes in host and parasite distribution can lead to overlapping ranges and increased host-switching; and (3) broader dissemination of some pathogens would be expected. In the Arctic and subarctic, however, changes may be particularly pronounced and radically different from those in boreal regions. At high latitudes, climatological changes and impacts may lead to (1) latitudinal shifts in geographic ranges; (2) extension of the growth season, with earlier springs, and a broadened window for transmission; (3) reduction in developmental times linked to higher temperatures; (4) decrease in generation times; (5) increase in rates of transmission, larval survival, and availability; and (6) increases in prevalence and intensity for some parasites.

The potential for amplification of parasite populations and emergence of subclinical or clinical effects is dependent on the degree to which ambient environmental and ecological conditions are limiting factors of parasite abundance in Arctic host-parasite systems. Genetics of *Teladorsagia boreoarcticus* are compatible with a small effective population in muskox and caribou from the central Canadian Arctic. Constraints on parasite abundance may result from small and dispersed host populations (particularly for muskox), ephemeral reservoirs of infective larvae, and a combination of limiting physical and environmental factors acting synergistically to define seasonal windows for transmission (Hoberg et al. 1999). Further, mechanisms controlling the population dynamics for such species as *Marshallagia marshalli* and *Ostertagia gruehneri* are complex; the intrinsic environment within the host may be most significant for the former, whereas extrinsic abiotic factors may limit the latter (Halvorsen et al. 1999; Irvine et al. 2000). Abundance and transmission also are affected by where and how populations of nematodes are sequestered during the winter, whether as adults and arrested larvae in ruminant hosts or as infective larvae in the external environment (Irvine et al. 2000). Such shifts in parasite abundance and patterns of transmission could have an impact on populations of large ruminants that serve as the primary food resources of native and subsistence cultures in the Arctic (Hoberg 1997) and other regions. The linkage of anthropogenic and climatological global change must be recognized in future management plans for wild ruminants in North America and throughout the world.

STRONGYLES, SYSTEMATICS, AND RUMINANT HOSTS: A SYNTHESIS.

Strongylate nematodes are significant components of global biodiversity and can represent potential and real threats to economically important wild and domestic ruminants. The North American strongylate fauna is a relatively diverse assemblage distributed among both wild and domestic hosts. These parasites are ubiquitous and have characteristic relationships, host and geographic distributions, and predictable life cycles and patterns of transmission. Documentation of parasite biodiversity through survey and inventory is the first step in defining the relationships of endemic and introduced faunas in ruminants. Systematics provides the foundation for elucidating the phylogenetic, coevolutionary, and biogeographic history of host-parasite assemblages (Brooks and Hoberg 2000). This historical database constitutes the predictive framework for recognizing contemporary interactions with naive-host groups, and the behavior of parasites introduced into new geographic and ecological settings. This information, in conjunction with ongoing research, which examines pathogenesis of strongyles in individual hosts and host populations, will become increasingly important with the escalation of environmental change across a diversity of ecosystems. An understanding of pathogenic parasites such as the strongylate nematodes characteristic of ruminants will remain critical within the context of wildlife biology, conservation, and the management of recovering, threatened, or endangered species.

ACKNOWLEDGMENTS. We thank Dr. Carol Nielsen for allowing access to records of parasitological studies in Alaskan ruminants. Dr. Anne Gunn, Mr. Alasdair Veitch, Mr. John Nishi, and Dr. Brett Elkin of the Department of Resources, Wildlife and Economic Development, Government of the Northwest Territories, Canada, and Dr. Susan Kutz of the University of Saskatchewan contributed to studies of helminth parasites of ruminants in the Arctic. Improvements of this manuscript resulted from critical reviews kindly prepared by Dr. Lydden Polley and Dr. S. Kutz of the University of Saskatchewan and Dr. Dante Zarlenga of the Agricultural Research Service, Beltsville, Maryland.

LITERATURE CITED

Adrian, W.J. (Ed). 1981. *Manual of common wildlife diseases in Colorado*. Denver: Colorado Division of Wildlife.

Aguirre, A.A., and E.E. Starkey. 1994. Wildlife disease in U.S. national parks: Historical and coevolutionary perspectives. *Conservation Biology* 8:654–661.

Allen, R.W. 1955. Parasites of mountain sheep in New Mexico, with new host records. *The Journal of Parasitology* 41:583–587.

———. 1962. Extent and sources of parasitism in pronghorn antelope. *Transactions of the Interstate Antelope Conference 1962*, pp. 48–51.

Allen, R.W., and H.G. Erling. 1964. Parasites of bighorn sheep and mule deer in Arizona with new host records. *The Journal of Parasitology* 50:38.

Allen, R.W., and C.B. Kennedy. 1952. Parasites of bighorn sheep in New Mexico. *Proceedings of the Helminthological Society of Washington* 19:39.

Alendal, E., and O. Helle. 1983. Helminth parasites of muskoxen *Ovibos moschatus* in Norway incl. Spitsbergen and in Sweden, with a synopsis of parasites reported from this host. *Fauna Norveigica* 4:41–52.

Anderson, N., J. Armour, R.M. Eadie, W.F.H. Jarrett, F.W. Jennings, J.S.D. Ritchie, and G.M. Urquhart. 1966. Experimental *Ostertagia ostertagi* infections in calves: Results of single infections with five graded dose levels of larvae. *American Journal of Veterinary Research* 27:1259–1265.

Anderson, R.C., and M.W. Lankester. 1974. Infectious and parasitic diseases and arthropod pests of moose in North America. *Naturaliste Canada* 101:23–50.

Anderson, R.M. 1980. Depression of host population abundance by direct life cycle macroparasites. *Journal of Theoretical Biology* 82:283–311.

Andrews, S.J., and M.B. Lancaster. 1988. Use of ivermectin in deer. *Veterinary Record* 123:354.

Arneberg, P., and I. Folstad. 1999. Predicting effects of naturally acquired abomasal nematode infections on growth rate and food intake in reindeer using serum pepsinogen levels. *Journal of Parasitology* 85:367–369.

Arneberg, P., I. Folstad, and A.J. Karter. 1996. Gastrointestinal nematodes depress food intake in naturally infected reindeer. *Parasitology* 112:213–219.

Baker, M.R., and R.C. Anderson. 1975. Seasonal changes in abomasal worms (*Ostertagia* sp.) in white-tailed deer (*Odocoileus virginianus*) at Long Point, Ontario. *Canadian Journal of Zoology* 53:87–96.

Baker, M.R., and S.R. Pursglove, Jr. 1976. *Oesophagostomum* Molin 1861 in white-tailed deer (*Odocoileus virginianus*) of North America. *The Journal of Parasitology* 62:166–168.

Baker, N.F., and R.A. Fisk. 1986. Seasonal occurrence of infective nematode larvae in California Sierra foothill pastures grazed by cattle. *American Journal of Veterinary Research* 47:1680–1685.

Baker, N.F., W.M. Longhurst, and J.R. Douglas. 1957. Experimental transmission of gastrointestinal nematodes between domestic sheep and Columbian black-tailed deer. *22nd North American Wildlife Conference*, pp. 160–168.

Becklund, W.W. 1962. Distribution and hosts of the ruminant parasite *Teladorsagia davtiani* Andreeva and Satubaldin, 1954 (Nematoda: Trichostrongylidae) in the United States. *The Journal of Parasitology* 48:469.

———. 1964. Revised checklist of internal and external parasites of domestic animals in the United States and possessions and in Canada. *American Journal of Veterinary Research* 25:1380–1416.

———. 1965. *Nematodirus maculosus* sp. n. (Nematoda: Trichostrongyloidea) from the mountain goat, *Oreamnos americanus*, in North America. *The Journal of Parasitology* 51:945–947.

———. 1966. Suppression of *Nematodirus rufaevastitatis* Durbin and Honess, 1951, a nematode described from *Ovis aries*, as a synonym of *Nematodirus davtiani* Grigorian, 1949. *Proceedings of the Helminthological Society of Washington* 33:199–201.

Becklund, W.W., and C. Senger. 1967. Parasites of *Ovis canadensis* in Montana, with a checklist of the internal and external parasites of Rocky Mountain bighorn sheep in North America. *The Journal of Parasitology* 53:157–165.

Becklund, W.W., and M.L. Walker. 1967a. *Nematodirus odocoilei* sp. n. (Nematoda: Trichostrongylidae) from the black-tailed deer, *Odocoileus hemionus*, in North America. *The Journal of Parasitology* 53:392–394.

———. 1967b. Redescriptions of the nematodes *Ostertagia bisonis* Chapin, 1925, of cattle and wild ruminants, and *Ostertagia mossi* of deer. *The Journal of Parasitology* 53:1273–1280.

———. 1968. *Ostertagia dikmansi* sp. n. (Nematoda: Trichostrongylidae) from deer, *Odocoileus virginianus*, with a key to species of medium stomach worms of *Odocoileus* in North America. *The Journal of Parasitology* 54:441–444.

———. 1971. Nomenclature and morphology of *Ostertagia trifurcata* Ransom, 1907, with data on spicule lengths of five stomach worms of ruminants. *The Journal of Parasitology* 57:508–516.

Belem, A.M.G., C.E. Couvillion, C. Siefker, and R.N. Griffin. 1993. Evidence for arrested development of abomasal nematodes in white-tailed deer. *Journal of Wildlife Diseases* 29:261–265.

Bergstrom, R.C. 1975a. Prevalence of *Marshallagia marshalli* (Orlov, 1933) in wild ruminants in Wyoming. *Proceedings of the Oklahoma Academy of Sciences* 55:101–102.

———. 1975b. Incidence of *Marshallagia marshalli* Orloff, 1933 in Wyoming sheep, *Ovis aries*, and pronghorn antelope, *Antilocapra americana*. *Proceedings of the Helminthological Society of Washington* 42:61–63.

Bergstrom, R.C., and T. Kass. 1982. Nematodes and nematodirosis. In *Diseases of wildlife in Wyoming,* 2nd ed. Ed. E.T. Thorne, N. Kingston, W.R. Jolley, and R.C. Bergstrom. Cheyenne: Wyoming Game and Fish Department Special Publication, pp. 199–201.

Bergerud, A.T. 1971. The population dynamics of Newfoundland caribou. *Wildlife Monographs* 25:1–55.

Blood, D.A. 1963. Parasites from California bighorn sheep in southern British Columbia. *Canadian Journal of Zoology* 41:9133–918.

Boddicker, M.L., and E.J. Hugghins. 1969. Helminths of big game mammals in South Dakota. *The Journal of Parasitology* 55:1067–1074.

Boddicker, M.L., E.J. Hugghins, and A.H. Richardson. 1971. Parasites and pesticide residues of mountain goats in South Dakota. *The Journal of Wildlife Management* 35:94–103.

Borgsteede, F.H.M. 1982. The infectivity of some nematode parasites of reindeer (*Rangifer tarandus* L) and elk (*Alces alces* L) for cattle and sheep. *Zeitschrift für Parasitenkunde* 67:211–215.

———. 1988. Studies on the epidemiological pattern and control of nematode infection in Cervidae. In *The management and health of farmed deer.* Ed. H.W. Reid. Dordrecht, Netherlands: Kluwer Academic Publishers, pp. 13–22.

Bos, G.N. 1967. Range types and their utilization by muskox on Nunivak Island, Alaska: A reconnaissance study. M.Sc. Thesis, University of Alaska, Fairbanks, 113 pp.

Brandborg, S.M. 1955. *Life history and management of the mountain goat in Idaho.* Idaho Department of Fish and Game, Wildlife Bulletin 2, 142 pp.

Brooks, D.R., and E.P. Hoberg. 2000. Triage for the biosphere: The need and rationale for taxonomic inventories and phylogenetic studies of parasites. *Comparative Parasitology* 67:1–25.

Brugh, T.H., Jr. 1971. A survey of internal parasites of a feral herd of fallow deer (*Dama dama*) in Alabama. *Journal of the Alabama Academy of Sciences* 42:133.

Burtner, R.H., and W.W. Becklund. 1971. Prevalence, geographic distribution, and hosts of *Cooperia surnabada* Antipin, 1931, and *C. oncophora* (Railliet, 18988) Ransom, 1907 in the United States. *The Journal of Parasitology* 57:191–192.

Bush, A.O., K.D. Lafferty, J.M. Lotz, and A.W. Shostak. 1997. Parasitology meets ecology on its own terms: Margolis et al. revisited. *The Journal of Parasitology* 83:575–583.

Bye, K. 1987. Abomasal nematodes from three Norwegian wild reindeer populations. *Canadian Journal of Zoology* 65:677–680

Bye, K., and O. Halvorsen. 1983. Abomasal nematodes in the Svalbard reindeer (*Rangifer tarandus platyrhynchus* Vrolik). *Journal of Wildlife Diseases* 19:101–105.

Bye, K., O. Halvorsen, and K. Nilssen. 1987. Immigration and regional distribution of abomasal nematodes of Svalbard reindeer. *Journal of Biogeography* 14:451–458.

Cameron, A.E. 1923. Notes on buffalo: Anatomy, pathological conditions and parasites. *British Veterinary Journal* 79:331–336.

———. 1924. Some further notes on buffalo. *Veterinary Journal* 80:413–417.

Campbell, A.J.D., R.B. Gasser, and N.B. Chilton. 1995. Differences in ribosomal DNA sequence of *Strongylus* species allows identification of single eggs. *International Journal of Parasitology* 25:359–365.

Capelle, K.J. 1966. The occurrence of *Oestris ovis* L. (Diptera: Oestridae) in the bighorn sheep from Wyoming and Montana. *The Journal of Parasitology* 52:618–621.

Card, C.S. 1993. Report of the committee on infectious disease of cattle, bison, and llama. *Proceedings of the U.S. Animal Health Association* 97:171–185.

Chapin, E.A. 1925. New nematodes from North American mammals. *Journal of Agricultural Research* 30:677–681.

Chapman J.A., and G.A. Feldhamer (Eds). 1982. *Wild mammals of North America, biology, management, and economics.* Baltimore: Johns Hopkins University Press, 1147 pp.

Choquette, L.P.E., L.K. Whitten, G. Rankin, and C.M. Seal. 1957. Note on parasites found in reindeer (*Rangifer tarandus*) in Canada. *Canadian Journal of Comparative Medicine* 21:199–203.

Christiansen, C.M., D.S. Zarlenga, and L.C. Gasbarre. 1994a. *Ostertagia, Haemonchus, Cooperia,* and *Oesophagostomum:* Construction and characterization of genus-specific DNA probes to differentiate important parasites of cattle. *Veterinary Parasitology* 78:93–100.

———. 1994b. Identification of a *Haemonchus placei*-specific DNA probe. *Journal of the Helminthological Society of Washington* 61:249–252.

Connan, R.M. 1991. Type II ostertagiosis in farmed red deer. *Veterinary Record* 128:233–235.

———. 1996. Hypobiosis in the ostertagids of red deer and the efficacy of ivermectin and fenbendazole against them. *Veterinary Record* 140:203–205.

Conti, J.A., and E.W. Howerth. 1987. Ostertagiosis in a white-tailed deer due to *Ostertagia ostertagi. Journal of Wildlife Diseases* 23:159–162.

Cook, T.W., B.T. Ridgeway, R. Andrews, and J. Hodge. 1979. Gastro-intestinal helminths of white-tailed deer (*Odocoileus virginianus*) of Illinois. *Journal of Wildlife Diseases* 15:405–408.

Coop, R.L., and K.W. Angus. 1981. How helminths affect sheep. *Veterinary Record* 108:4–11.

Couey, F.M. 1950. *Rocky Mountain bighorn sheep of Montana.* Montana Fish and Game Commission, Big Game Biologist Bulletin 2, 90 pp.

Cowan, I.McT. 1951. The diseases and parasites of big game animals of western Canada. *Report of the 5th Annual Game Conference, Victoria, British Columbia,* pp. 37–64.

Craig, T.M. 1993. *Longistrongylus curvispiculum* (Nematoda: Trichostrongyloidea) in free-ranging exotic antelope in Texas. *Journal of Wildlife Diseases* 29:516–517.

Cram, E.B. 1925. *Cooperia bisonis* a new nematode from buffalo. *Journal of Agricultural Research* 30:571–573.

Das, K.M., and J.H. Whitlock. 1960. Subspeciation in *Haemonchus contortus* (Rudolphi, 1803) Nemata, Trichostrongyloidea. *Cornell Veterinarian* 50:182–197.

Daskalov, P. 1974. On the reproductive relationships between *Ostertagia circumcincta, Teladorsagia davtiani,* and *O. trifurcata* (Nematoda: Trichostrongylidae) [In Bulgarian]. *Izvestiya na Tsentralnata Kheminthologichna Laboratoriya, Sofia* 17:59–72.

Daszak, P. A.A. Cunningham, and A.D. Hyatt. 2000. Emerging infectious diseases of wildlife—Threats to biodiversity and human health. *Science* 287:443–449.

Davidson, W.R., and C.B. Crow. 1983. Parasites, diseases and health status of sympatric populations of sika deer and white-tailed deer in Maryland and Virginia. *Journal of Wildlife Diseases* 19:345–348.

Davidson, W.R., and V.F. Nettles. 1988. *Field manual of wildlife diseases in the southeastern United States.* Athens, GA: Southeastern Cooperative Wildlife Disease Study.

Davidson, W.R., and A.K. Prestwood. 1979. *Apteragia pursglovei* sp. n. (Trichostrongyloidea: Trichostrongylidae) from the white-tailed deer, *Odocoileus virginianus. The Journal of Parasitology* 65:280–284.

Davidson, W.R., M.B. McGhee, V.F. Nettles, and L.C. Chappell. 1980. Haemonchosis in white-tailed deer in the southeastern United States. Journal of Wildlife Diseases 16:499–508.

Davidson, W.R., J.M. Crum, J.L. Blue, D.W. Sharp, and J.H. Philips. 1985. Parasites, diseases and health status of sympatric populations of fallow deer and white-tailed deer in Kentucky. *Journal of Wildlife Diseases* 21:1533–159.

Davidson, W.R., J.L. Blue, L.B. Flynn, S.M. Shea, R.L. Marchinton, and J.A. Lewis. 1987. Parasites, diseases and health status of sympatric populations of sambar deer and white-tailed deer in Florida. *Journal of Wildlife Diseases* 23:267–272.

Davis, J.W., and R.C. Anderson (Eds). 1971. *Parasitic diseases of wild mammals.* Ames: Iowa State University Press.

Demarais, S., H.A. Jacobson, and D.C. Guynn. 1983. Abomasal parasites as a health index for white-tailed deer in Mississippi. *The Journal of Wildlife Management* 47:247–252.

Dieterich, R.A. (Ed). 1981. *Alaskan wildlife diseases.* Fairbanks: University of Alaska.

Dikmans, G. 1931. Two new species of nematode worms of the genus *Ostertagia* from Virginia deer, with a note on *Ostertagia lyrata. Proceedings of the United States National Museum* 79:1–6.

———. 1932. Abstract of report before the Helminthological Society of Washington. *The Journal of Parasitology* 19:83–84.

———. 1936. A note on the identity of *Nematodirus tarandi* Hadwen, 1922, and *Nematodirus skrjabini* Mitzkevitsch, 1929 (Nematoda: Trichostrongyloidea). *Proceedings of the Helminthological Society of Washington* 2:56.

———. 1939. Helminth parasites of North American semidomesticated and wild ruminants. *Proceedings of the Helminthological Society of Washington* 6:97–101.

———. 1942. New host-parasite records. *Proceedings of the Helminthological Society of Washington* 9:65.

Dobson, A., and R. Carper. 1992. Global warming and potential changes in host-parasite and disease vector relationships. In *Global warming and biological diversity.* Ed. R.L. Peters and T.E. Lovejoy. New Haven: Yale University Press, pp. 201–220.

Dobson, A.P., and R.M. May. 1986a. Patterns of invasions by pathogens and parasites. In *Ecological Studies.* Vol. 58, *Ecology of biological invasions of North America and Hawaii.* Ed. H.A. Moore and J.A. Drake. New York: Springer-Verlag, pp. 58–76.

Dobson, A.P., and R.M. May. 1986b. Disease and conservation. In *Conservation biology and the science of scarcity and diversity.* Ed. M.E. Soulé. Sunderland, MA: Sinaeur Associates, pp. 345–365.

Doster, G.L., and M. Friend. 1971. *Spiculopteragia* (Nematoda) from deer of North America. *The Journal of Parasitology* 57:468.

Drózdz, J. 1965. Studies on helminths and helminthiases in Cervidae I. Revision of the subfamily Ostertagiinae Sarwar, 1956, and an attempt to explain phylogenesis of its representatives. *Acta Parasitological Polonica* 13:445–481.

———. 1966. Studies on the helminths and helminthiases in Cervidae II. The helminth fauna in Cervidae in Poland. *Acta Parasitological Polonica* 14:1–13.

———. 1967. Studies on helminths and helminthiases in Cervidae III. Historical formation of helminthofauna in Cervidae. *Acta Parasitological Polonica* 14:27–300.

———. 1974. The question of genetic isolation and of permanent coincidence of some species of the subfamily Ostertagiinae. In *Proceedings of the Third International Congress of Parasitology,* Munich, Germany, vol. 1, pp. 477–478.

———. 1995. Polymorphism in the Ostertagiinae Lopez-Neyra, 1947, and comments on the systematics of these nematodes. *Systematic Parasitology* 32:91–99.

———. 1998. A record of *Spiculopteragia suppereri* (Nematoda: Trichostrongylidae) in farmed *Elaphurus davidianus* Cervidae in Poland. *Acta Parasitologica Polonica* 43:109–110.

Dunn, A.M. 1969. The wild ruminant as reservoir host of helminth infection. In *Diseases in free-living wild animals.* Ed. A. McDiarmid. New York: Academic Press, pp.221–246.

————. 1983. Winter deaths in red deer: A preliminary report on abomasal parasite burdens. *Publication of the Veterinary Deer Society* 1:17–25.

Durette-Desset, M.-Cl. 1982. Sur les divisions génériques des nématodes Ostertagiinae. *Annales de Parasitologie Humaine et Comparee* 57:375–381.

————. 1983. Keys to the genera of the superfamily Trichostrongyloidea. In *CIH keys to the nematode parasites of vertebrates,* No. 10. Ed. R.C. Anderson and A.G. Chabaud. Farnham Royal, UK: Commonwealth Agricultural Bureaux, pp. 1–86.

————. 1985. Trichostrongyloid nematodes and their vertebrate hosts: Reconstruction of the phylogeny of a parasitic group. *Advances in Parasitology* 24:239–306.

————. 1989. Nomenclature proposée pour les espèces décrites dans la sous-famille des Ostertagiinae Lopez-Neyra, 1947. *Annales de Parasitologie Humaine et Comparee* 64:356–373.

Durette-Desset, M.-Cl., and A.G. Chabaud. 1977. Essaie de classification des nématodes Trichostrongyloidea. *Annales de Parasitologie Humaine et Comparee* 52:539–558.

————. 1993. Nomenclature des Strongylida au-dessus du groupe-famille. *Annales de Parasitologie Humaine et Comparee* 68:111–112.

Durette-Desset, M.-Cl., and W.M. Samuel. 1989. Nematodirinae (Nematoda: Trichostrongyloidea) d'*Antilocapra* et d'*Ovis* en Alberta, Canada. *Annales Parasitologie Humaine et Comparee* 64:469–477.

————. 1992. Nematodirinae (Nematoda: Trichostrongyloidea) chez l'*Oreamnos americanus* en Alberta, Canada, description du *Nematodirus becklundi* sp. nov. *Canadian Journal of Zoology* 70:212–219.

Durette-Desset, M.-Cl., J.P. Hugot, P. Darlu, and A.G. Chabaud. 1999. A cladistic analysis of the Trichostrongyloidea (Nematoda). *International Journal for Parasitology* 29:1065–1086.

Esch, G.W., J.W. Gibbons, and J.E. Bourque. 1975. An analysis of the relationship between stress and parasitism. *The American Midland Naturalist* 93:339–353.

Eve, J.H. 1981. Management implications of disease. In *Diseases and parasites of white-tailed deer.* Ed. W.R. Davidson, F.A. Hayes, V.F. Nettles, and F.E. Kellogg. Tallahassee, FL: Tall Timbers Research Station Miscellaneous Publication No. 7, pp. 413–423.

Eve, J.H., and F. Kellogg. 1977. Management implications of abomasal parasites of southeastern white-tailed deer. *The Journal of Wildlife Management* 41:169–177.

Folstad, I., P. Arneberg, and A.J. Karter. 1996. Antlers and parasites. *Oecologia* 105:556–558.

Foreyt, W., and W.M. Samuel. 1979. Parasite of white-tailed deer of the Welder Wildlife Refuge in southern Texas: A review. In *Proceedings of the First Welder Wildlife Foundation Symposium.* Ed. D.L. Drawe. Sinton, TX: Welder Wildlife Foundation, pp. 105–132.

Foreyt, W., and D.O. Trainer. 1970. Seasonal parasitism changes in two populations of white-tailed deer in Wisconsin. *The Journal of Wildlife Management* 44:758–764.

Forrester, D.J. 1992. *Parasites and diseases of wild mammals in Florida.* Gainesville: University Press of Florida, 459 pp.

Fowler, M. (Ed). 1993. *Zoo and wildlife animal medicine. Current therapy 3.* Philadelphia, PA: W.B. Saunders Co.

Fruetel, M., and M.W. Lankester. 1988. *Nematodirella alcidis* (Nematoda: Trichostrongyloidea) in moose of northwestern Ontario. *Alces* 24:159–163.

————. 1989. Gastrointestinal helminths of woodland and barren ground caribou (*Rangifer tarandus*) in Canada, with key to species. *Canadian Journal of Zoology* 67:2253–2269.

Georgi, J.R., and C.E. McCulloch. 1989. Diagnostic morphometry: Identification of helminth eggs by discriminant analysis of morphometric data. *Journal of the Helminthological Society of Washington* 56:44–57.

Gibbons, L.M. 1977. Revision of the genera *Longistrongylus* LeRoux, 1931, *Kobusinema* Ortlepp, 1963, and *Bigalkenema* Ortlepp, 1963 (Nematoda: Trichostrongylidae). *Journal of Helminthology* 51:41–62.

————. 1979. Revision of the genus *Haemonchus* Cobb, 1898 (Nematoda: Trichostrongylidae). *Systematic Parasitology* 1:3–24.

Gibbons, L.M., and L.F. Khalil. 1982. A key for the identification of genera of the nematode family Trichostrongylidae Leiper, 1912. *Journal of Helminthology* 56:185–233.

Gibbs, H.C., and R.P. Herd. 1986. Nematodiasis in cattle, importance, species involved, immunity and resistance. *Veterinary Clinics of North America: Food Animal Practice* 2:211–224.

Gibbs, H.C., and J.S. Tener. 1958. On some helminth parasites collected from the musk ox (*Ovibos moschatus*) in the Thelon Game Sanctuary, Northwest Territories. *Canadian Journal of Zoology* 36:529–532.

Gibson, T.E., and G. Everett. 1976. The ecology of freeliving stages of *Nematodirus filicollis*. Research in Veterinary Science 20:158–161.

————. 1981. Ecology of freeliving stages of *Nematodirus battus. Research in Veterinary Science* 31:233–327.

Gilmore, R.E., and Allen, R.W. 1960. Helminth parasites of pronghorn antelope (*Antilocapra americana*) in New Mexico with new host records. *Proceedings of the Helminthological Society of Washington* 27:69–73.

Goldsby, A.I., and Eveleth, D.H. 1954. Internal parasites in North Dakota antelope. *The Journal of Parasitology* 40:637–648.

Govorka, Ia., L.P. Maklakova, Ia. Mitukh, A.N. Pel'gunov, A.S Rykovskii, M.K. Semenova, M.K. Sonin, B. Erkhardova-Kotrla, and V. Iurashek. 1988. *Gel'minty dikikh kopytnykh Vostochnoi Evropy.* Moskva: Akademiia Nauk SSSR, Laboratoria Gel'mintologii, Izdatel'stvo Nauka, 207 pp.

Gray, G.G., D.B. Pence, and C.D. Simpson. 1978. Helminths of sympatric Barbary sheep and mule deer in the Texas panhandle. *Proceedings of the Helminthological Society of Washington* 45:139–141.

Grenfell, B.T. 1988. Gastrointestinal nematode parasites and the stability and productivity of intensive ruminant grazing systems. *Philosophical Transactions of the Royal Society of London,* Series B 321:541–563.

————. 1992. Parasitism and the dynamics of ungulate grazing systems. *American Naturalist* 139:907–929.

Grenfell, B.T., and F.M.D. Gulland. 1995. Introduction: Ecological impact of parasitism on wildlife host populations. *Parasitology* 111(supplement): S3–S14.

Gulland, F.M.D. 1992. The role of parasites in soay sheep (*Ovis aries* L) mortality during a host population crash. *Parasitology* 105:493–503.

————. 1995. The impact of infectious diseases on wildlife populations—A review. In *Ecology of infectious diseases in natural populations.* Ed. B.T. Grenfell and A.P. Dobson. Cambridge: Cambridge University Press, pp. 20–51.

Gunn, A. 1982. Muskox, *Ovibos moschatus*. In *Wild mammals of North America: Biology management and economics.* Ed. J.A. Chapman and G.A. Feldhammer. Baltimore: Johns Hopkins University Press, pp. 1021–1035.

Hadwen, I.A.S. 1922. *Nematodirus tarandi* a new species of nematode from the reindeer. *The Journal of Parasitology* 9:35.

Hadwen, S., and L.J. Palmer. 1922. *Reindeer in Alaska.* United States Department of Agriculture Bulletin No. 1089. Washington, D.C.: U.S. Government Printing Office, 74 pp.

Haigh, J.C. 1996. Management practices to minimise infectious and parasitic diseases of farmed and ranched cervids and bison. *Revue Scientifique et Technique Office International des épizooties* 15:209–226.

Hailey, T.L., J.W. Thomas, and R.M.Robinson. 1966. Pronghorn die-off in the Trans-Pecos, Texas. *The Journal of Wildlife Management* 30:488–496.

Halvorsen, O. 1986. Epidemiology of reindeer parasites. *Parasitology Today* 12:334–339.

Halvorsen, O., and K. Bye. 1999. Parasites, biodiversity, and population dynamics in an ecosystem in the high Arctic. *Veterinary Parasitology* 84:205–227.

Halvorsen, O., A. Stein, J. Irvine, R. Langvatn, and S. Albon. 1999. Evidence for continued transmission of parasitic nematodes in reindeer during the Arctic winter. *International Journal for Parasitology* 29:567–579.

Herd, R.P. 1986. Epidemiology and control of nematodes and cestodes in small ruminants, northern United States. *Veterinary Clinics of North America: Food Animal Practice.* 2:355–362.

Herlich, H. 1962. Studies on calves experimentally infected with four nematode species. *American Journal of Veterinary Research* 23:521–528.

Heuer, D.E., J.H. Phillips, W.J. Rudersdorf, and J.P. Harley. 1975. Range extension records for *Cooperia curticei, Ostertagia ostertagi, Setaria yehi,* and *Trichuris ovis* in white-tailed deer from Kentucky. *Proceedings of the Helminthological Scoiety of Washington* 42:141–143.

Hinaidy, H.K., V.C. Guttieres, and R. Supperer. 1972. Die Gastrointestinal-Helminthen des Rindes in Österreich. *Zentralblatt für Veterinámedizin* 19:679–695.

Hoar, K.L., D.E. Worley, and K.E. Aune. 1996. Parasite loads and their relationship to herd health in the highlands bighorn sheep herd in southwestern Montana. *Biennial Symposium North American Wild Sheep and Goat Council* 10:57–65.

Hoberg, E.P. 1996. Emended description of *Mazamastrongylus peruvianus* (Nematoda: Trichostrongylidae), with comments on the relationships of the genera *Mazamastrongylus* and *Spiculopteragia. The Journal of Parasitology* 82:470–477.

———. 1997. Parasite biodiversity and emerging pathogens: A role for systematics in limiting impacts on genetic resources. In *Global genetic resources: Access ownership and intellectual property rights.* Ed. K.E. Hoagland and A.Y. Rossman. Washington, DC: Association of Systematics Collections, pp. 77–89.

Hoberg, E.P., and A.V. Khrustalev. 1996. Re-evaluation of *Mazamastrongylus dagestanica* (Trichostrongylidae) with descriptions of the synlophe, genital cone and other structural characters. *The Journal of Parasitology* 82:778–787.

Hoberg, E.P., and J.R. Lichtenfels. 1992. Morphology of the synlophe and genital cone of *Parostertagia heterospiculum* (Trichostrongylidae) with comments on the subfamilial placement of the genus. *Systematic Parasitology* 22:1–16.

———. 1994. Phylogenetic systematic analysis of the Trichostrongylidae (Nematoda), with an initial assessment of coevolution and biogeography. *The Journal of Parasitology* 80:976–996.

Hoberg, E.P. and L.G. Rickard. 1988. Morphology of the synlophe of *Nematodirus maculosus* (Trichostrongyloidea) with comments on the evolution of *Nematodirus* spp. among the Caprinae (Artiodactyla). *Proceedings of the Helminthological Society of Washington* 55:160–164.

Hoberg, E.P., G.L. Zimmerman, and J.R. Lichtenfels. 1986. First report of *Nematodirus battus* (Nematoda: Trichostrongyloidea) in North America: Redescription and comparison to other species. *Proceedings of the Helminthological Society of Washington* 53:80–88.

Hoberg, E.P., G.L. Zimmerman, L.G. Rickard, and D.J. Schons. 1988. Efficacy of febantel against naturally acquired gastrointestinal nematodes in calves, and recognition of *Oesophagostomum venulosum* in Oregon cattle. *American Journal of Veterinary Research* 49:1540–1542.

Hoberg, E.P., M. Fruetel, and L.G. Rickard. 1989. Synlophe of *Nematodirus odocoilei* (Trichostrongyloidea) from deer and caribou in North America with comments on the evolution of *Nematodirus* spp. among the Cervidae (Artiodactyla). *Canadian Journal of Zoology* 67:1489–1494.

Hoberg, E.P., J.R. Lichtenfels, and P.A. Pilitt. 1993a. Synlophe of *Hyostrongylus rubidus* (Trichostrongylidae), with evaluation of structural characters supporting affiliation with the Ostertagiinae. *Journal of the Helminthological Society of Washington* 60:219–233.

———. 1993b. Comparative morphology of *Ostertagia mossi* and *Ostertagia dikmansi* (Trichostrongylidae) from *Odocoileus virginianus* and comments on other *Ostertagia* spp. from the Cervidae. *Systematic Parasitology* 24:111–127.

Hoberg, E.P., K. Monsen, S. Kutz, and M.S. Blouin. 1999. Structure, biodiversity and historical biogeography of nematode faunas in Holarctic ruminants: Morphological and molecular diagnoses for *Teladorsagia boreoarcticus* sp. n. (Nematoda: Ostertagiinae), a dimorphic cryptic species in muskoxen (*Ovibos moschatus*). *Journal of Parasitology* 85:910–934.

Hoeve, J., D.G. Joachim, and E.M. Addison. 1988. Parasites of moose (*Alces alces*) from an agricultural area of eastern Ontario. *Journal of Wildlife Diseases* 24:371–374.

Honess, R.F., and J.W. Scott. 1942. Annual Report, Wyoming Agricultural Experiment Station (1941–1942), pp. 27–28.

Honess, R.F., and K.B. Winter. 1956. *Diseases of Wildlife in Wyoming.* Wyoming Game and Fish Commission, Bulletin 9, 279 pp.

Hout, J., and M. Beaulieau. 1984. Relationship between parasitic infection levels and body fat reserves in George River caribou. In *Proceedings of the 2nd North American Caribou Workshop.* Ed. T.C. Meredith and A.M. Martell. pp. 317–327.

Hudson, P.J., and A.P. Dobson. 1995. Macroparasites: Observed patterns in naturally fluctuating animal populations. In *Ecology of infectious diseases in natural populations.* Ed. B.T. Grenfell and A.P. Dobson. Cambridge: Cambridge University Press, pp. 144–176.

Humbert, J.F., and J. Cabaret. 1995. Use of random amplified polymorphic DNA for identification of ruminant trichostrongylid nematodes. *Parasitology Research* 81:1–5.

Irvine, R.J., A. Stein, O. Halvorsen, R. Langvatn, and S. Albon. 2000. Life-history strategies and population dynamics of abomasal nematodes in Svalbard reindeer (*Rangifer tarandus platyrhynchus*). *Parasitology* 120:297–311.

Isenstein, R.S. 1971. The polymorphic relationship of *Cooperia oncophora* (Railliet, 1898) Ransom, 1907, to *Cooperia surnabada* Antipin, 1931 (Nematoda: Trichostrongylidae). *The Journal of Parasitology* 57:316–319.

Jansen, J. 1989. A concise history of the Ostertagiinae Lopez-Neyra, 1947 (Nematoda: Trichostrongyloidea) and a discussion on its composition. *Acta Leidensia* 58:151–159.

Jean, M., R. Petanaude, J. Frechette, Y. Elazhary, Y.R. Higgins, A. Tremblay, and I. Juniper. 1982. *Exploratory study of the health status of caribou of the George River herd.* Quebec City: Quebec Department of Recreation, Fish and Game, Wildlife Research Branch.

Jensen, L.A., J.A. Short, and F.L. Andersen. 1982. Internal parasites of *Odocoileus hemionus* of central Utah. *Proceedings of the Helminthological Society of Washington* 49:317–319.

Johnson, R.L. 1974. *Bighorn sheep 1973. A biological evaluation of the Tucannon Bighorn with notes on other Washington sheep.* Olympia: Washington Department of Game, 69 pp.

———. 1975. *Bighorn sheep 1974. An evaluation of bighorn sheep in the Sinlahekin area of northcentral Washington with notes on other Washington sheep.* Olympia: Washington Department of Game, 39 pp.

Johnston, J.T., A.S. Familton, R. McAnulty, and A.R. Sykes. 1984. Pathogenicity of *O. circumcincta, O. ostertagi,* and *H. contortus* in weanling stag fawns (*Cervus elaphus*). *New Zealand Veterinary Journal* 32:177–179.

Jordan, H., and E.L. Stair. 1983. Documenting clinical gastrointestinal parasitism: Worm burdens—A valuable tool. *American Association of Laboratory Diagnosticians* 26:241–248.

Kates, K.C., and J.H. Turner. 1955. Observations on the life cycle of *Nematodirus spathiger,* a nematode parasitic in the intestine of sheep and other ruminants. *American Journal of Veterinary Research* 16:105–115.

Kerr, G.R., and J.C. Holmes. 1966. Parasites of mountain goats in west-central Alberta. *The Journal of Wildlife Management* 30:786–790.

Kistner, T.P., S.M. Matlock, D. Wyse, and G.E. Mason. 1977. Helminth parasites of bighorn sheep in Oregon. *Journal of Wildlife Diseases* 13:125–130.

Klein, D.R. 1996. Structures for caribou management and their status in the circumpolar north. *Rangifer* (special issue) 9:245–251.

Kulmamatov, A. 1974. O vidovom sostave roda *Nematodirus* Ransom, 1907. *Materialy Nauchnykh Konferentsii Vsesoiuznogo Obshchestva Gel'mintologii.*26:1337–140.

Kutzer, E. 1987. The application of the anthelmintic Ivomec (ivermectin) in game animals [In German]. In *Verhandlungsbericht des XXI Internationalen Symposiums des Österreichischen Wildgehegeverbandes,* Vienna, Austria, pp. 7–17.

Kutzer, E., and H. K. Hinaidy. 1969. Die Parasiten der wildlebenden Widerkäuer Österreichs. *Zeitschrift für Parasitenkunde* 32:354–368.

Lancaster, M.B., and S.J. Andrews. 1991. Red deer, nematodes, and anthelmintics. *Veterinary Record* 128:411.

Lancaster, M.B., and C. Hong. 1981. Polymorphism in nematodes. *Systematic Parasitology* 3:28–31.

———. 1990. The identification of females within the subfamily Ostertagiinae Lopez-Neyra 1947. *Veterinary Parasitology* 35:21–27.

Lancaster, M.B., C. Hong, and J.F. Michel. 1983. Polymorphism in the Trichostrongylidae. In *Concepts in nematode systematics.* Ed. A.R. Stone, H.M. Platt, and L.F. Khalil. London, UK: Academic Press, pp. 293–302.

Levine, N. 1963. Weather, climate and bionomics of ruminant nematode larvae. *Advances in Veterinary Science* 8:215–261.

———. 1980. *Nematode parasites of domestic animals and man,* 2nd ed. Minneapolis, MN: Burgess Publishing Co., 477 pp.

Lichtenfels, J.R. 1977. Differences in cuticular ridges among *Cooperia* spp. of North American ruminants with an illustrated key to species. *Proceedings of the Helminthological Society of Washington* 44:111–119.

———. 1980a. Keys to the genera of the superfamilies Ancylostomatoidea and Diaphanocephaloidea. In *CIH keys to the nematode parasites of vertebrates,* No. 8. Ed. R.C. Anderson, A.G. Chabaud, and S. Wilmott. Farnham Royal, UK: Commonwealth Agricultural Bureaux, pp. 1–26.

———. 1980b. Keys to the genera of the superfamily Strongyloidea. In *CIH keys to the nematode parasites of vertebrates,* No. 7. Ed. R.C. Anderson, A.G. Chabaud, and S. Wilmott. Farnham Royal, UK: Commonwealth Agricultural Bureaux, pp. 1–41.

Lichtenfels, J.R., and E.P. Hoberg. 1993. The systematics of nematodes that cause ostertagiasis in domestic and wild ruminants in North America: An update and a key to species. *Veterinary Parasitology* 46:33–53.

Lichtenfels, J.R., and P.A. Pilitt. 1983a. Cuticular ridge patterns of *Nematodirus* (Nematoda: Trichostrongyloidea) parasitic in domestic ruminants of North America, with a key to species. *Proceedings of the Helminthological Society of Washington* 50:261–274.

———. 1983b. Cuticular ridge patterns of *Nematodirella* (Nematoda: Trichostrongyloidea) of North American ruminants, with a key to species. *Systematic Parasitology* 5:271–285.

———. 1989. Cuticular ridge patterns of *Marshallagia marshalli* and *Ostertagia occidentalis* (Nematoda: Trichostrongyloidea) parasitic in ruminants of North America. *Proceedings of the Helminthological Society of Washington* 56:173–182.

———. 1991. A redescription of *Ostertagia bisonis* (Nematoda: Trichostrongyloidea) and a key to species of Ostertagiinae with a tapering lateral synlophe from domestic ruminants in North America. *Journal of the Helminthological Society of Washington* 58:231–244.

Lichtenfels, J.R., P.A. Pilitt, and M.B. Lancaster. 1988a. Cuticular ridge patterns of seven species of Ostertagiinae (Nematoda) parasitic in domestic ruminants. *Proceedings of the Helminthological Society of Washington* 55:77–86.

———. 1988b. Systematics of the nematodes that cause ostertagiasis in cattle, sheep, and goats in North America. *Veterinary Parasitology* 27:33–12.

Lichtenfels, J.R., P.A. Pilitt, and M.Fruetel. 1990. Cuticular ridge pattern in *Ostertagia gruehneri* and *Ostertagia arctica* (Nematoda: Trichostrongyloidea) from caribou, *Rangifer tarandus. Journal of the Helminthological Society of Washington* 57:61–68.

Lichtenfels, J.R., E.P. Hoberg, P.A. Pilitt, and A.M.G. Belem. 1993. A comparison of the cuticular ridge patterns and other morphological characters of *Mazamastrongylus odocoilei* and *Mazamastrongylus pursglovei* (Nematoda: Trichostrongyloidea) from white-tailed deer, *Odocoileus virginianus. Systematic Parasitology* 24:1–15.

Lichtenfels, J.R., P.A. Pilitt, and E.P. Hoberg. 1994. New morphological characters for identifying individual specimens of *Haemonchus* spp. (Nematoda: Trichostrongyloidea) with a key to species in ruminants of North America. *The Journal of Parasitology* 80:107–119.

Lichtenfels, J.R., E.P. Hoberg, and D.S. Zarlenga. 1997. Systematics of gastrointestinal nematodes of domestic ruminants: Advances 1992–1995, and proposals for future research. *Veterinary Parasitology* 72:225–245.

Locker, B. 1953. Parasites of bison in northwestern USA. *The Journal of Parasitology* 3:58–59.

Loken, N.I., J.C. Schlotthauer, H.J. Kurtz, and P.D Karns. 1965. *Pneumostrongylus tenuis* in Minnesota moose (*Alces alces*). *Bulletin Wildlife Disease Association* 1:7.

Longhurst, W.M., and J.R. Douglas. 1953. Parasite interrelationships of domestic sheep and columbian black-tailed deer. *18th North American Wildlife Conference,* pp.168–188.

Low, W.A. 1976. Parasites of woodland caribou in Tweedsmuir Provincial Park, British Columbia. *Canadian Field Naturalist* 90:189–191.

Lucker, J.T., and G. Dikmans. 1945. The distribution of *Pseudostertagia bullosa* and some new records of nematodes from pronghorn antelope (*Antilocapra americana*). *Proceedings of the Helminthological Society of Washington* 12:2–4.

MacDonald, D.W., W.M. Samuel, and J.O.C. Hunter. 1976. Haemonchosis in a captive muskox calf. *Canadian Veterinary Journal* 17:138–139.

MacKintosh, C.G., P.C. Mason, T. Manley, K. Baker, and R. Littlejohn. 1985. Efficacy and pharmacokinetics of febantel and ivermectin in red deer (*Cervus elaphus*). *New Zealand Veterinary Journal* 33:127–131.

Maples, W.P., and R.B. England. 1971. *Trichostrongylus dosteri* sp. n. (Nematoda: Trichostrongylidae): A parasite of the white-tailed deer, *Odocoileus virginianus* (Zimmermann). *American Midland Naturalist* 86:506–508.

Maples, W.P., and H.E. Jordan. 1966. A new host record for *Obeliscoides cuniculi* (Graybill, 1923) Graybill, 1924. *The Journal of Parasitology* 52:49.

Marquardt, W.C., D.H. Fritts, C.M. Senger, and L. Seghetti. 1959. The effect of weather on the development and survival of the free-living stages of *Nematodirus spathiger* (Nematoda: Trichostrongyloidea). *The Journal of Parasitology* 45:431–439.

Marsh, H. 1938. Pneumonia in Rocky Mountain bighorn sheep. *Journal of Mammalogy* 19:214–219.

Mason, P. 1994. Parasites of deer in New Zealand. *New Zealand Journal of Zoology* 21:39–47.

McCullough, D.R., and E.R. Schneegas. 1966. Winter observations on the Sierra Nevada bighorn sheep. *California Fish and Game* 52:68–84.

McGhee, M.B., V.F. Nettles, E.A. Rollor, A.K. Prestwood, and W.R. Davidson. 1981. Studies on cross-transmission and pathogenicity of *Haemonchus contortus* in white-tailed deer, domestic cattle and sheep. *Journal of Wildlife Diseases* 17:353–364.

McKenzie, M.E., and W.R. Davidson. 1989. Helminth parasites of intermingling axis deer, wild swine and domestic cattle from the island of Molokai, Hawaii. *Journal of Wildlife Diseases* 25:252–257.

Mulrooney, D.M., J.K. Bishop, and G.L. Zimmerman. 1991. First report of *Ostertagia leptospicularis* (Nematoda: Trichostrongyloidea) in calves (*Bos taurus*) from North America. *Journal of the Helminthological Society of Washington* 58:260–262.

Nielsen, C.A., and K.A. Neiland. 1974. *Sheep disease report,* vol. 14. Juneau: Alaska Department of Fish and Game, 104 pp.

Oripov, A.O. 1970. Marshallagiosis of sheep [In Russian]. In *Materialy Pyatoi Ob'edinennoi Konferentsii,* pp. 12–137.

Payne, R.L., W.P. Maples, and J.F. Smith. 1967. The occurrence of *Oesophagostomum cervi* Mertts, 1948, in white-tailed deer (*Odocoileus virginianus*) of the southeastern United States. *The Journal of Parasitology* 53:691.

Peters, R.L. 1992. Conservation of biological diversity in the face of climate change. In *Global warming and biological diversity.* Ed. R.L. Peters and T.E. Lovejoy. New Haven: Yale University Press, pp. 15–30.

Pilmore, R.E. 1961. General investigations of diseases and parasites. Colorado Department of Fish and Game Report No. 10, pp. 101–102.

Phillips, J.H., J.P. Harley, and W.J. Rudersdorf. 1974. New host records for *Setaria yehi* Disset, 1966, and range extension records for *Dictyocaulus viviparus* (Bloch, 1782) and *Ostertagia mossi* Dikmans, 1931, in fallow deer (*Dama dama* L). *Proceedings of the Helminthological Society of Washington* 41:250.

Prestwood, A.K., and F.E. Kellogg. 1971. Naturally occurring haemonchosis in a white-tailed deer. *Journal of Wildlife Diseases* 7:133–134.

Prestwood, A.K., and S.R. Pursglove. 1981. Gastrointestinal nematodes. In *Diseases and parasites of white-tailed deer.* Ed. W.R. Davidson, F.A. Hayes, V.F. Nettles, and F.E. Kellogg. Tallahassee, FL: Tall Timbers Research Station Miscellaneous Publication No. 7., pp. 318–349.

Prestwood, A.K., H.A. Hayes, J.H. Eve, and J.F. Smith. 1973. Abomasal helminths of white-tailed deer in southeastern United States, Texas, and the Virgin Islands. *Journal of the American Veterinary Medical Association* 163:556–561.

Prestwood, A.K., F.E. Kellogg, S.R. Pursglove, and F.A. Hayes. 1975. Helminth parasitisms among intermingling insular populations of white-tailed deer, feral cattle and feral swine. *Journal of the American Veterinary Medical Association* 166:787–789.

Pursglove, S.R., Jr. 1976. *Eucyathostomum webbi* sp. n. (Strongyloidea: Cloacinidae) from white-tailed deer (*Odocoileus virginianus*). *The Journal of Parasitology* 62:574–578.

Pursglove, S.R., Jr., G.L. Doster, and A.K. Prestwood. 1974. *Trichostrongylus askivali* Dunn, 1964, and *Ostertagia ostertagi* (Stiles, 1892) in white-tailed deer (*Odocoileus virginianus*) of the southeastern United States. *The Journal of Parasitology* 60:1059–1060.

Pursglove, S.R., A.K. Prestwood, V.F. Nettles, and F.A. Hayes. 1976. Intestinal nematodes of white-tailed deer in southeastern United States. *Journal of the American Veterinary Medical Association* 169:896–900.

Quortrup, E.R., and R.L. Sudheimer. 1944. Some wildlife cases of particular interest. *Journal of the American Veterinary Medical Association* 104:29.

Ransom, B.H., and M.C. Hall. 1912. A new nematode, *Ostertagia bullosa,* parasitic in the alimentary tract of sheep. *Proceedings of the United States National Museum* 42:175–179.

Richardson, M.L., and S. Demarais. 1992. Parasites and condition of coexisting populations of white-tailed and exotic deer in south-central Texas. *Journal of Wildlife Diseases* 28:485–489.

Rickard, L.G., and J.K. Bishop. 1991. Helminth parasites of llamas (*Lama glama*) in the Pacific Northwest. *Journal of the Helminthological Society of Washington* 58:110–115.

Rickard, L.G., and J.R. Lichtenfels. 1989. *Nematodirus archari* (Nematoda: Trichostrongyloidea) from ruminants in North America with a description of the synlophe and the female. *Canadian Journal of Zoology* 67:1708–1714.

Rickard, L.G., and G.L. Zimmerman. 1986. First report of *Ostertagia kolchida* (Nematoda: Trichostrongyloidea) from North America. *Proceedings of the Helminthological Society of Washington* 53:136–138.

Rickard, L.G., E.P. Hoberg, J.K. Bishop, and G.L. Zimmerman. 1989. Epizootiology of *Nematodirus battus, N. filicollis,* and *N. spathiger* (Nematoda: Trichostrongyloidea) in western Oregon. *Proceedings of the Helminthological Society of Washington* 56:104–115.

Rickard, L.G., E.P. Hoberg, N.M. Allen, G.L. Zimmerman, and T.M. Craig. 1993. *Spiculopteragia spiculoptera* and *S. asymmetrica* (Nematoda: Trichostrongyloidea) from red deer (*Cervus elaphus*) in Texas. *Journal of Wildlife Diseases* 29:512–515.

Rush, W.M. 1932. *Northern Yellowstone elk study.* Montana Fish and Game Commission, 131 pp.

Samuel, W.M., and D.R. Gray. 1974. Parasitic infection in muskoxen. *The Journal of Wildlife Management* 38:775–782.

Samuel, W.M., M.W. Barrett, and G.M. Lynch. 1976. Helminths in moose of Alberta. *Canadian Journal of Zoology* 54:307–312.

Samuel, W.M., W.K. Hall, J.G. Stelfox, and W.D. Wishart. 1977. Parasites of mountain goat, *Oreamnos americanus* (Blainville), of west central Alberta with a comparison of the helminths of mountain goat and Rocky Mountain bighorn sheep, *Ovis c. canadensis* Shaw. In *Proceedings of the First International Mountain Goat Symposium, Kalispell, MT.* Ed. W. Samuel and W.G. MacGregor. Victoria, BC: British Columbia Ministry of Recreation and Conservation, pp. 212–225.

Scott, M.E. 1988. The impact of infection and diseases on animal population: Implications for conservation biology. *Conservation Biology* 2:40–56.

Semenova, M.K. 1984. Studies on the circulation of Strongylata of domestic animals [In Russian]. In *Gel'minty sel'skokhozyaistvennykh i okhotnich'e-promyslovykh zhivotnykh.* Ed. M.D. Sonin. Moscow: Akademiia Nauk, SSSR, pp. 128–134.

———. 1987. Survival of larval trichostrongylids of wild ruminants [In Russian]. *Trudy Gel'mintologicheskoi Laboratorii* 35:127–134.

Semenova, M.K., and Iu.E. Korosteleva. 1980. Study of the life cycle of *Spiculopteragia alcis* (Stongylata: Trichostrongylidae) a parasite of wild ungulates [In Russian]. In *Fauna nechernozem'ia ii okhrana vosproizvedenie I ispol'zovanie.* Moscow: Kalinin, SSSR, Gel'mintologicheskii Laboratorii, pp. 126–131.

Shaw, D.J., and A.P. Dobson. 1995. Patterns of macroparasite abundance and aggregation in wildlife populations: A quantitative review. *Parasitology* 111 (supplement): S111–S133.

Shaw, J.N. 1947. *Some parasites of Oregon wild life.* Oregon Agricultural Experiment Station, Technical bulletin No. 11, 16 pp.

Skogland, T. 1990. Density dependence in a fluctuating wild reindeer herd; maternal versus offspring effects. *Oecologia* 84:442–450.

Skrjabin, K.I., N.P. Shikhobalova, and R.S. Schul'ts. 1954. Trichostrongyloidea of animals and man [In Russian]. *Osnovy nematology III.* Moscow: Akad Nauk SSSR, 683 pp. [English Translation (1960). Springfield, VA: National Technical Information Service No. OTS60-21124.]

Sommer C. 1996. Digital image analysis and identification of eggs from bovine parasitic nematodes. *Journal of Helminthology* 70:143–151.

Spencer, C.C. 1943. Notes on the life history of Rocky Mountain sheep in the Tarryall Mountains of Colorado. *Journal of Mammalogy* 24:1–11.

Spencer, D.L., and E.F. Chatelain. 1953. Progress in management of the moose of southcentral Alaska. In *Transactions of the 18th North American Wildlife Conference,* pp. 541–552.

Stevenson, L.A., R.B. Gasser, and N.B. Chilton. 1996. The ITS-2 rDNA of *Teladorsagia circumcincta, T. trifurcata* and *T. davtiani* (Nematoda: Trichostrongylidae) indicates that these taxa are one species. *International Journal for Parasitology* 26:1123–1126.

Stock, T.M., and M.W. Barrett. 1983. Helminth parasites of the gastrointestinal tracts and lungs of moose (*Alces alces*) and wapiti (*Cervus elaphus*) from Cypress Hills, Alberta, Canada. *Proceedings of the Helminthological Society of Washington* 50:246–251.

Strohlein, D.A., C.B. Crow, and W.R. Davidson. 1988. Distribution of *Spiculopteragia pursglovei* and *S. odocoilei* (Nematoda: Trichostrongyloidea) from white-tailed deer (*Odocoileus virginianus*) in the southeastern United States. *The Journal of Parasitology* 74:347–349.

Stubblefield, S.S., D.B. Pence, and R.J. Warren. 1987. Visceral helminth communities of sympatric mule and white-tailed deer from the Davis Mountains of Texas. *Journal of Wildlife Diseases* 23:113–120.

Suarez, V.H., and J. Cabaret. 1991. Similarities between species of the Ostertagiinae (Nematoda: Trichostrongyloidea) in relation to host-specificity and climatic environment. *Systematic Parasitology* 20:179–185.

Sykes, A.R. 1978. The effect of subclinical parasitism in sheep. *Veterinary Record* 102:32–34.

Syroechkovskii, E.E. 1995. *Wild reindeer.* Washington, DC: Smithsonian Institution Libraries, 290 pp.

Thomas, R.J. 1959. A comparative study of the life histories of *Nematodirus battus* and *N. filicollis,* nematode parasites of sheep. *Parasitology* 49:374–386.

Thorne, E.T., E.S. Williams, W.M. Samuel, and T.P. Kistner. 2001. Diseases and parasites. In *Ecology and management of the North American elk,* 2nd ed. Ed. J.W. Thomas and D.E. Toweill. Washington, D.C.: Smithsonian Institution Press. Forthcoming.

Thornton, J.E., T.J. Galvin, and R.R. Bell. 1973a. Parasites of the blackbuck antelope (*Antilope cervicapra*) in Texas. *Journal of Wildlife Diseases* 9:160–162.

Thornton, J.E., T.J. Galvin, R.R. Bell, and C.S. Ramsey. 1973b. Transmissibility of gastrointestinal nematodes from blackbuck antelope to cattle, sheep and goats. *Journal of the American Veterinary Medical Association* 163:554–555.

Threlfall, W. 1969. Further records of helminths from Newfoundland mammals. *Canadian Journal of Zoology* 47:197–201.

Uhazy, L.S., and J.C. Holmes. 1971. Helminths of the Rocky Mountain bighorn sheep in western Canada. *Canadian Journal of Zoology* 49:507–512.

Van Baren, D.C., E.P. Hoberg, and R.G. Botzler. 1996. Abomasal parasites in tule elk (*Cervus elaphus nannodes*) from Grizzly Island, California. *Journal of the Helminthological Society of Washington* 63:222–225.

Van Vuren, D., and C.A. Scott. 1995. Internal parasites of sympatric bison, *Bison bison,* and cattle, *Bos taurus.* *Canadian Field Naturalist* 109:467–469.

Vitousek, P.M., C.M. D'Antonio, L.L. Loope, and R. Westbrooks. 1996. Biological invasions as global environmental change. *American Scientist* 84:468–478.

Waid, D.D., D.B. Pence, and R.J. Warren. 1985. Effects of season and physical condition on the gastrointestinal helminth community of white-tailed deer from the Texas Edwards plateau. *Journal of Wildlife Diseases* 21:264–273.

Walker, M.L., and W.W. Becklund. 1970. *Checklist of the internal and external parasites of deer, Odocoileus hemionus and O. virginianus, in the United States and Canada.* Special Publication 1. *Index Catalogue of Medical and Veterinary Zoology.* Washington, DC: U.S. Department of Agriculture, Agricultural Research Service, U.S. Government Printing Office, 45 pp.

Webster, W.A., and J. Rowell. 1980. Some helminth parasites from the small intestine of free-ranging muskoxen *Ovibos moschatus* (Zimmermann) of Devon and Ellsemere Islands, Northwest Territories. *Canadian Journal of Zoology* 58:304–305.

Williams, J.E. 1986. Epidemiological patterns of nematodiasis in cattle. *Veterinary Clinics of North America: Food Animal Practice* 2:235–246.

Wilson, G.I. 1969. Some parasites of elk in New Mexico. *Journal of Wildlife Diseases* 5:23–24.

Woodford, M.H., and P.B. Rossiter. 1994. Disease risks associated with wildlife translocation projects. In Creative conservation: Interactive management of wild and captive animals. Ed. P.J.S. Olney, G.M. Mace, and A.T.C. Feistner. London, UK: Chapman and Hall, pp. 179–200.

Worley, D.E. 1979. Parasites and parasitic diseases of elk in the Northern Rocky Mountain region: A review. *In North American elk: Ecology, behavior and management.* Ed. M.S. Boyce and L.D. Hayden-Wing. Laramie: University of Wyoming Press, pp. 206–211.

Worley, D.E., and C.D. Eustace. 1972. Prevalence of helminth parasites in mule deer from eastern Montana. *Proceedings of the Helminthological Society of Washington* 39:135–138.

Worley, D.E., and F.M. Seesee. 1992. Gastrointestinal parasites of bighorn sheep in western Montana and their relationships to herd health. *Biennial Symposium North American Wild Sheep and Goat Council* 8:202–212.

Worley, D.E., and G.A.M. Sharman. 1966. Gastritis associated with *Ostertagia bisonis* in Montana range cattle. *Journal of the American Veterinary Medical Association* 149:1291–1294.

Xiao, L. and H.C. Gibbs. 1991. Abomasal nematodes from white-tailed deer (*Odocoileus virginianus*) in Maine. *Journal of the Helminthological Society of Washington* 58:198–201.

Zarlenga, D.S., F. Stringfellow, M. Nobary, and J.R. Lichtenfels. 1994. Cloning and characterization of ribosomal RNA genes from three species of *Haemonchus* (Nematoda: Trichostrongyloidea) and identification of PCR primers for rapid differentiation. *Experimental Parasitology* 78:28–36.

Zaugg, J.L., S.K. Taylor, B.C. Anderson, D.L. Hunter, J. Ryder, and M. Divine. 1993. Hematologic, serologic values, histopathologic and fecal evaluations of bison from Yellowstone Park. *Journal of Wildlife Diseases* 29:453–457.

9

EXTRAPULMONARY LUNGWORMS OF CERVIDS

MURRAY W. LANKESTER

INTRODUCTION. Of mammalian lungworms, none has attracted as much attention as members of the genera *Parelaphostrongylus* and *Elaphostrongylus*. These genera comprise a small but important group of parasites found in ruminants, notably members of the Cervidae. This chapter reviews the six known species in these genera, with emphasis on recent literature.

PARELAPHOSTRONGYLUS TENUIS (DOUGHERTY 1945)

Classification: Nematoda: Metastrongyloidea: Protostrongylidae.

Synonyms: *Odocoileostrongylus tenuis* (Dougherty) Schulz, 1951; *Elaphostrongylus odocoilei* Anderson, 1956 (not Hobmaier and Hobmaier, 1934); *Neurofilaria cornellensis* Whitlock, 1952; *Elaphostrongylus tenuis* (Dougherty) Whitlock, 1959, Smith and Archibald, 1967.

Common Names: Cerebrospinal nematodiasis, parelaphostrongylosis, meningeal worm, brain worm, moose sickness, moose disease.

Parelaphostrongylus tenuis is common almost everywhere white-tailed deer (WTD) (*Odocoileus virginianus*) occur in eastern North America (Fig. 9.1). Little or no disease is apparent in white-tails, but when other native cervids, and some bovids and camelids, encounter the parasite, debilitating neurological signs may result. Since the discovery that *P. tenuis* was the causative agent of "moose sickness" (Anderson 1964a,b), considerable knowledge about this parasite has accumulated in the literature. Yet our understanding of its past and present impact on populations of wild moose (*Alces alces*) and other native cervids remains incomplete. In certain areas, parelaphostrongylosis causes financial loss to owners of llamas, sheep, and goats that share range with white-tailed deer, and it is an important concern in zoos and game farm settings. Fear of spreading this parasite to western North America has led to legislation restricting the translocation of white-tails and other hosts in which the parasite occasionally matures.

Previous reviews of *P. tenuis* include Anderson (1968, 1971a), Anderson and Prestwood (1981), Lankester (1987), Anderson (1992), Lankester and Samuel (1998) (also, see annotated bibliography on members of *Parelaphostrongylus* and *Elaphostrongy-*

lus by Samuel 1991). The present account defers to Anderson (1971a) and Anderson and Prestwood (1981) for some earlier references, but attempts to cite most recent literature, particularly that on the biology and epizootiology of *P. tenuis* in white-tailed deer, the impact of this parasite on other species, and advancements in diagnostic methods. For information on the parasite's morphology and phylogeny, readers are referred to Anderson (1963a,b), Platt (1984), Carreno and Lankester (1993, 1994), and Carreno and Hoberg (1999).

Life History. Adult *P. tenuis* are long and thread-like. Males are up to 6.2 cm long x 0.2 mm wide and greenish-yellow to brown in color (Table 9.1, Fig. 9.2). Females are up to 9 cm x 0.25 mm and coloured darker brown to black by the contents of their intestine (Carreno and Lankester 1993). In white-tailed deer, adult worms are found most frequently in the veins and venous sinuses of the cranial meninges. These include the cavernous and intercavernous blood sinuses in the floor of the cranium, as well as the connecting sagittal and transverse venous sinuses in the overlying dura membrane (Anderson 1963a; Slomke et al. 1995). Worms also occur free in the cranial subdural space, where they are easily detected on the surface of the brain or on the inner surface of the dura (Gilbert 1973). Few worms are found adhering to or beneath the pia in white-tailed deer (Slomke et al. 1995). In abnormal hosts such as moose, worms may be associated with the cranial nerves, and their eggs and larvae have been found in the eyes (Anderson 1965a; Kurtz et al. 1966). Rarely, worms are swept from the blood sinuses to other locations in the body. This probably explains the recovery of the holotype specimen of *P. tenuis* from the lung of a white-tailed deer and its original assignment to *Pneumostrongylus* by Dougherty (1945).

Unembryonated eggs released by females into the venous blood are carried to the heart and then to the lungs, where they lodge in alveolar capillaries and complete their development to the first larval stage (L_1) (Table 9.2). Eggs laid by females extravascularly within the cranium develop and hatch, but whether these larvae can enter the circulation and reach the lungs is unknown. L_1's move into the alveolar air space and are propelled out of the lungs in the layer of mucous that moves upwards on the so-called ciliary escalator lining most of the respiratory tree. Upon

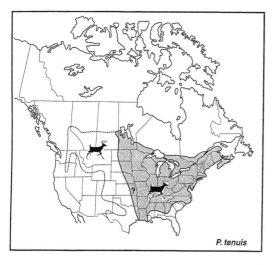

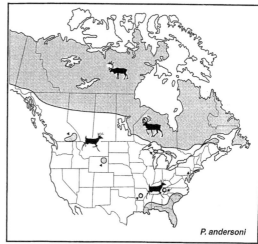

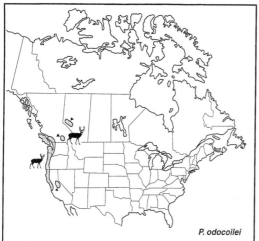

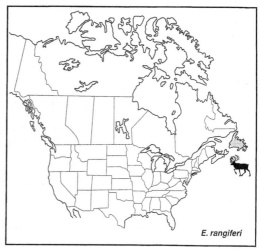

FIG. 9.1—Distribution of the four species of elaphostrongyline nematodes of cervids in North America. Shaded areas indicate the known distribution of the parasite in the cervid hosts illustrated (*P. tenuis* in white-tailed deer, *P. andersoni* with a disjunct distribution in white-tailed deer and more continuous distribution in woodland and barrenground caribou, *P. odocoilei* in mule deer [larger silhouette] and black-tailed deer [smaller silhouette], and *E. rangiferi* in woodland caribou). There are no published reports of *P. tenuis* in Kansas (?). The dotted line approximates the western limits of the distribution of white-tailed deer. Arrowheads accentuate the location of isolated reports.

reaching the pharynx, larvae are swallowed and pass unharmed through the digestive tract and out with the feces (Anderson 1963a).

Most L_1's are located on the surface of fecal pellets in a thin layer of mucous (Lankester and Anderson 1968; Forrester and Lankester 1997a). This contrasts, for example, with the location of larval *Protostrongylus* spp. of bighorn sheep (*Ovis canadensis*) that are most numerous toward the center of pellets (Forrester and Lankester 1997b). L_1's of *P. tenuis* readily leave pellets immersed in water and presumably are also removed by rain and melting snow. To develop further, they must penetrate, or be eaten by, a terrestrial snail or slug. A large variety of species are capable of serving as intermediate hosts (Anderson and Prestwood 1981) (Table 9.3). Terrestrial gastropods may become infected most frequently when they encounter larvae dispersed in the soil. This method of infection has been demonstrated to occur under laboratory conditions (Lankester and Anderson 1968) and might explain why most naturally infected gastropods contain few larvae. Natural infections have not been found in aquatic snails but *Lymnea* sp. has been infected experimentally (Anderson 1963a).

TABLE 9.1—Adult dimensions of elaphostrongyline nematodes in North American cervids (μm), unless otherwise indicated

	P. tenuis[a]		*P. andersoni*[b]		*P. odocoilei*[c]		*E. rangiferi*[d]	
	Mean	Range	Mean	Range	Mean	Range	Mean	Range
Males								
Length (mm)	55	(31–62)	20	(19–23)	23	(18–26)	35	(31–38)
Width	162	(92–200)	111	(87–140)	147	(138–156)	199	(175–220)
Espohagus length	640	(562–770)	726	(670–770)	653	(565–717)	681	(650–740)
Nerve ring[f]	—	(110–150)[e]	85	(80–100)	88	(68–94)	132	(100–170)
Excretory pore[f]	—	(100–140)[e]	103	(87–120)	75	(56–94)	153	(115–175)
Spicule length	223	(202–249)	104	(87–115)	149	(132–170)	220	(205–232)
Gubernaculum length	109	(89–137)	47	(42–52)	93	(73–112)	75	(63–85)
Females								
Length (mm)	79	(66–90)	31	(30–35)	44	(39–48)	47	(47)
Width	209	(120–250)	113	(95–130)	163	(141–179)	223	(220–240)
Espohagus length	694	(623–796)	747	(670–900)	627	(588–658)	698	(635–770)
Nerve ring[f]	104	(90–126)	90	(70–100)	92	(79–106)	131	(120–150)
Excretory pore[f]	139	(109–164)	—	(67–130)	78	(71–82)	145	(118–170)
Vulva[g]	181	(138–233)	122	(97–170)	178	(161–194)	300	(300)
Tail	53	(35–62)	53	(40–75)	48	(44–65)	68	(68)

[a]Measurements according to Carreno and Lankester (1993). Others available from Anderson (1956).
[b]Measurements according to Prestwood (1972). Others available from Pybus and Samuel (1981), Lankester and Hauta (1989), Carreno and Lankester (1993), Lankester and Fong (1998).
[c]Measurements according to Platt and Samuel (1978b). Others available from Hobmaier and Hobmaier (1934), Brunetti (1969).
[d]Measurements according to Lankester and Fong (1998). Others available from Lankester and Northcott (1979), Carreno and Lankester (1993).
[e]From Anderson (1956).
[f]Position measured from anterior end.
[g]Position measured from posterior end.

In the foot tissue of gastropods, L_1's molt to the L_2 and then to the L_3, or infective stage. The rate of development is temperature dependent. Almost 4 weeks were required to reach the infective stage at temperatures fluctuating between 18° C and 30° C (Anderson 1963a). It probably takes 2–3 times as long at lower field temperatures likely experienced by terrestrial gastropods, although this has never been investigated. Development is slowed or stopped in snails that estivate to avoid dessication, but resumes with the return of favorable conditions. L_3's can survive freezing temperatures over winter in gastropods and probably remain viable for the life of the intermediate host (Lankester and Anderson 1968).

White-tailed deer become infected when they accidentally ingest terrestrial gastropods along with vegetation. L_3's released by digestion from gastropod tissues penetrate through the gastrointestinal wall (particularly of the abomasum) and reach the peritoneal cavity (Anderson 1963a, 1965b,c). Their migration to the central nervous system is thought to be direct. Migrating dorsally in the abdominal cavity and following lateral spinal nerves, mostly in the lumbar region, larvae reach the vertebral canal in about 10 days (Anderson and Strelive 1967, 1969). Still in the third larval stage, they enter tissue of the spinal cord (dorsal horns of grey matter) and molt twice to the fourth and then to the fifth, or subadult stage. By 40 days after infection, most worms have left the spinal cord, apparently via dorsal nerve roots. They move anteriorly in the spinal subdural space to reach the cranium and enter the venous sinuses. The presence of developing worms in the neural parenchyma of the brain of white-tailed deer apparently is rare (Anderson 1968).

The prepatent period of *P. tenuis* in white-tailed deer varies from 82 to 137 days (Anderson and Prestwood 1981; Rickard et al. 1994). It apparently varies inversely with the infecting dose (Rickard et al. 1994), but white-tailed deer age at the time of infection may also be important (M.W. Lankester and A.A. Gajadhar, unpublished). Fawns born in early June become naturally infected and pass larvae as early as mid-October (Peterson and Lankester 1991), but most do not become patent until mid-December or January, a prepatent period estimated to be ~4.5 months (Slomke et al. 1995). The ensuing production of larvae by newly infected white-tailed deer has not been studied thoroughly. In one experimentally infected fawn, larval output increased rapidly following patency, peaked 1 month later, and then declined (Samuel et al. 1992).

Most white-tailed deer acquire a small number of worms within the first or second summer of their life, and intensity does not increase appreciably thereafter (Slomke et al. 1995). Up to 71% of fawns were infected within 5–6 months of birth, and 91% by the time they were 17–18 months old. Average intensities by host age were 2.7 (fawns), 3.0 (yearlings), 3.5 (2 to 6 years) and 4.1 (7 to 15 years). Similar observations were made by Anderson and Prestwood (1981), who first suggested that white-tailed deer acquire a protective immune response against repeated infection. The high proportion of unisexual *P. tenuis* infections in white-tailed

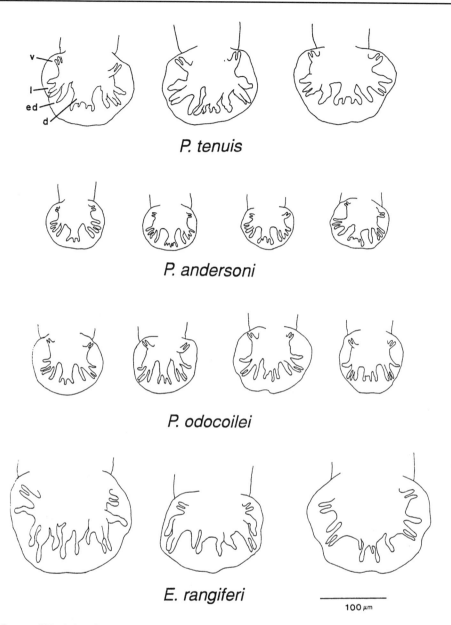

P. tenuis

P. andersoni

P. odocoilei

E. rangiferi

100 μm

FIG. 9.2—Bursae of North American elaphostrongyline nematodes, ventral view: *v,* ventral ray; *l,* lateral ray; *ed,* externaldorsal ray; *d,* dorsal ray. *Parelaphostrongylus tenuis* from white-tailed deer; *P. andersoni* from white-tailed deer and barren ground caribou; *P. odocoilei* from black-tailed deer and mule deer; *Elaphostrongylus rangiferi* from caribou (bottom right specimen) and moose (After Carreno and Lankester 1993; used with permission of NRC Research Press.).

deer provides additional evidence of an acquired immunity. As many as one-third of infected white-tailed deer pass no larvae in their feces because adult worms of only one sex are present (Slomke et al. 1995). If repeated infections were possible, the proportion of these unisexual infections would decrease in older animals, but this was not observed. As well, since the mean number of worms acquired by fawns during their first summer and fall was unchanged during their second summer as yearlings, this protection must develop during winter. Variations in the length of the frost-free period when transmission to fawns is possible will, therefore, influence both the mean intensity and the proportion of patent infections. White-tailed deer in

TABLE 9.2—Larval dimensions of elaphostrongyline nematodes in North American cervids (µm)

Larva	*P. tenuis*[a]	*P.andersoni*[b]	*P. odocoilei*	*E. rangiferi*[c]
First Stage				
Length	348(310–380)	351(308–382)	378[d]	426(381–490)
Width	18(16–19)	17(17–18)	17	20(17–24)
Nerve ring	94(80–112)	94(66–109)	—	110(95–130)
Excretory pore	94(80–112)	94(66–109)	98	109(97–125)
Esophagus	165(132–181)	175(163–183)	166	191(163–230)
Genital prim.	224(210–246)	234(216–249)	—	267(245–325)
Tail	32(29–41)	32(27–36)	40	44(32–53)
Third Stage				
Length	971(900–1080)	1019(966–1200)	890(738–977)[e]	1004(937–1041)
Width	42(36–45)	36(33–50)	44(36–52)	46(42–49)
Nerve ring	114(100–125)	117(100–133)	141(135–154)	139(120–150)
Excretory pore	133(122–149)	117(100–133)	—	153(138–163)
Esophagus	352(300–400)	358(300–420)	323(282–399)	381(338–421)
Genital prim.	629(569–707)	681(600–800)	561(521–586)	615(574–648)
Tail	35(31–45)	35(33–45)	47(45–50)	52(40–70)

[a]Anderson (1963).
[b]Prestwood (1972).
[c]Lankester and Northcott (1979).
[d]Hobmaier and Hobmaier (1934).
[e]Ballantyne and Samuel (1984).

some southern areas reportedly have slightly greater numbers of worms than deer near the northern limit of their range (Anderson and Prestwood 1981).

Field evidence provided by Slomke et al. (1995) supports the hypothesis that *P. tenuis* is long-lived in white-tailed deer and that worms acquired by fawns may persist for life. This is consistent with observation by others on the related nematodes, *E. cervi* and *P. odocoilei* that are known to live at least 6 and 8.5 years, respectively (Watson 1984; W.M. Samuel, personal communication).

Epizootiology

DISTRIBUTION. Meningeal worm is common in white-tailed deer of the deciduous forest biome and deciduous-coniferous ecotone of eastern and central North America (Fig. 9.1). It is rare or absent in the coastal plains region of the southeastern United States and is not documented in western North America. New distribution records not listed by Anderson and Prestwood (1981) include Foreyt and Trainer (1980) (Wisconsin), Beaulieu-Goudreault (1981) and Claveau and Fillion (1984) (Quebec), Garrison et al. (1987) (Missouri), Platt (1989) (Indiana), Comer et al. (1991) (South Carolina), Jarvinen and Hedberg (1993) (Iowa), Wasel (1995) (North Dakota, Saskatchewan), Davidson et al. (1996) (Wassaw Island, Geogia), and Oates et al. (1999) (South Dakota and Nebraska).

In 1968, *P. tenuis* was recovered from one white-tailed deer in Collier Co., Florida, where it was probably introduced with white-tailed deer from Wisconsin (Prestwood and Smith 1969). However, it has not been found there since, despite large numbers of white-tailed deer having been examined (Comer et al. 1991). Its occurrence on Wassaw Island off the coast of Georgia

was also attributed to an introduction of white-tailed deer from Pennsylvania, further adding credence to concerns that *P. tenuis* can be spread through the translocation of infected hosts (Davidson et al. 1996).

It is not known what limits the natural spread of the parasite westward. The drier central grasslands of North America are presumed to be a barrier by being less hospitable for gastropods, but it is more difficult to imagine why the more northerly aspen parklands did not provide a corridor (Anderson 1972). It is equally unclear why *P. tenuis* is rare or absent in white-tailed deer of the coastal plains portion of the Atlantic and Gulf coast states of Alabama, Georgia, Mississippi, South Carolina, and Florida. Prestwood and Smith (1969) suggested that this might be due to a scarcity of suitable species of gastropod intermediate hosts or to other factors associated with the predominantly sandy soil, pine forest habitat. However, Davidson et al. (1996) rejected this hypothesis on finding a high prevalence of *P. tenuis* in white-tailed deer occupying similar habitat on Wassaw Island, Georgia, where the worm appears to have persisted for almost 90 years. Since the related nematode, *P. andersoni,* is successfully transmitted among white-tailed deer in the coastal plains region (Forrester 1992), yet concurrent infections of *P. andersoni* and *P. tenuis* are rare (Prestwood et al. 1974), some form of host cross-immune response might prevent the geographical overlap of the two parasites (Lankester and Hauta 1989).

HOST RANGE. White-tailed deer is the normal definitive host in which *P. tenuis* becomes patent without causing disease. However, the parasite develops to varying degrees in a variety of abnormal hosts that have contracted infection on natural white-tailed deer range, in proximity to white-tailed deer in zoos or game

TABLE 9.3—Terrestrial gastropods found naturally infected with *Parelaphostrongylus tenuis*

Reference	Location	Deer Density/km² (% Infected)	Overall Prevalence of *P. tenuis* % (Number of Gastropods Examined)	Mean Number Larvae/Gastropod (Range)	Species of Gastropods Infected[a]
Beach (1992)	New Brunswick, Canada	1.2–3.6 (50%–60%)	0.2%–2.0% (1960)	NR[b] (1–28)	*Zonitoides arboreus* (0.5% of 635), *Deroceras laeve* (1.5% of 589), *Discus cronkhitei* (1.6% of 249), *Pallifera dorsalis* (0.8% of 118), *Triodopsis albolabris* (9.5% of 21), *Strobilops labyrinthica* (5.3% of 38)
Gleich et al. (1977)	Central Maine (USA)	1.6–3.1[c] (63%–80%)	0.1% (1700)	2.0 (2)	*P. dorsalis* (0.8% of 225)
Kearney and Gilbert (1978)	Near North Bay, Ontario, Canada	2.0–6.4[d]	0.05%–0.12% (16,450)	2.4	NR
Lankester (1967)	Algonquin Park, Ontario, Canada	<4[e] (41%)	1.0% (1540)	NR	*T. albolabris* (18% of 39), *D. cronkhitei* (2% of 256), *Z. arboreus* (0.4% of 562), *Succinea ovalis* (1.5% of 66), *D. laeve* (0.3% of 385)
Lankester and Anderson (1968)	Navy Island near Niagara Falls, Ontario, Canada	94 (61%)	4.2% (9940)	2.9 (1–97[f])	*D. laeve* (8.2% of 2434), *Zonitoides nitidus* (4.3% of 4719), *Anguispera alternata* (2.5% of 121), *S. ovalis* (4% of 195), *Cochlicopa lubrica* (0.4% of 249), *Deroceras reticulatum* (0.3% of 1,097), *Arion circumscriptus* (0.1% of 1064)
Lankester and Peterson (1996)	Near Grand Marais, Minnesota (USA)	19 (for 5 months) 4 (for 7 months) (80%)	0.1% (12,095)	3.2 ± 2.5 (1–7)	*A. alternata* (1.2% of 81), *D.cronkhitei* (0.4% of 968), *S. ovalis* (0.3% of 393), *D. laeve* (0.2% of 1212), *D. reticulatum* (0.03% of 6949)
Maze and Johnstone (1986)	Northcentral Pennsylvania (Elk State Forest) (USA)	12–15 (54%)	9.0% (808)	3.0 (1–44)	*T. albolabris* (20% of 70), *Triodopsis tridentata* (12% of 17), *Ventridens intertextus* (20% of 118), *D. laeve* (1.6% of 61), *Z. arboreus* (12% of 41), *D. cronkhitei* (15% of 143), *Stenotrema fraturnum* (12% of 50)

(continued)

TABLE 9.3 (*continued*)

Reference	Location	Deer Density/km² (% Infected)	Overall Prevalence of *P. tenuis* % (Number of Gastropods Examined)	Mean Number Larvae/Gastropod (Range)	Species of Gastropods Infected[a]
Parker (1966)	Nova Scotia, Canada	2.6[g] (63%)	2.6% (509)	NR	*D. cronkhitei, Z.arboreus, D. reticulatum, Striatura exigua, Phylomycus carolinianus*
Pitt and Jordan (1994)	Northeastern Minnesota (USA)	4–5 (57%)	0.8% (744)	NR	NR
Platt (1989)	Northwestern Indiana (USA)	40 (over winter) (38%)	1.9% (736)	2.5–3.8 (1–26[f])	*Cochlicopa* spp (5.5% of 163), *D. cronkhitei* (1.2% of 252), *D. laeve* (2.8% of 71)
Raskevtiz et al. (1991)	Eastern Oklahoma (USA)	17 (39%)	8.0% (959)	65 larvae in 8/15 species	*Discus patulus* (0.8% of 129), *Helicina orbicula* (3.1% of 293), *Mesopmphix cupreus* (10% of 10), *Mesodon inflectus* (24% of 33), *Triodopsis divesta* (30% of 83), *Strenotrema strenotrema* (4.3% of 70), *Polygyra dorenilliana* (10% of 113), *Polygyra jacksoni* (8.8% of 194)
Rowley et al. (1987)	National Zoological Park near Front Royal, Virginia (USA)	NR	2.2% (670)	2.5 ± 2.9 (1–10)	*D. laeve* (1.5% of 338), *T. tridentata* (33% of 9), *Z. arboreus* (4.3% of 69), *P. carolinianus* (9% of 31), *Vallonia collisella* (20% of 5)
Upshall et al. (1987)	Near Fredericton, New Brunswick, Canada	2.3[g] (78%)	2.5% (569)	6.0	*D. laeve* (5.3% of 225), *Z. arboreus* (0.4% of 229), *D. cronkhitei* (2.2% of 45)
Whitlaw et al. (1996)	Northcentral New Brunswick, Canada	12 (in winter) 2–3 (in summer) (67%)	0.4% (10,343)	1.5 (1–3)	*Arion* spp. (0.04% of 2377), *D. laeve* (0.5% of 438), *D. cronkhetei* (0.02% of 4671)

[a]Number gastropods infected/number examined (%).
[b]NR, not reported.
[c]Gilbert (1973).
[d]Kearney and Gilbert (1976).
[e]Wilton (1987).
[f]In three different studies individual *D. laeve* had high numbers of larvae (97, 26).
[g]Whitlaw and Lankester (1994b).

farms, and by experimental infection. These include moose, wapiti (*Cervus elaphus canadensis*), red deer (*C. e. elaphus*), woodland caribou (*Rangifer tarandus caribou*), reindeer (*R. t. tarandus*), mule-deer (*Odocoileus hemionus hemionus*), black-tailed deer (*O. h. columbianus*) and black-tails × white-tailed deer hybrids, fallow deer (*Dama dama*), and the non-cervids, bighorn sheep (*Ovis canadensis*), domestic sheep and goats, llamas, guanocos, alpacas, camels, pronghorns (*Antilocapra americana*), eland (*Taurotragus oryx*), sable antelope (*Hippotragus niger*), and possibly bongo antelope (*Tragelaphus eurycercus*), scimitar-horned oryx (*Oryx dammah*), blackbuck antelope (*Antilope cervicapra*), and domestic cattle (see Anderson 1992; Rickard et al. 1994; Oliver et al. 1996; Yamini et al. 1997). The parasite causes neurologic disease in most of these, and occasionally becomes patent, passing small numbers of larvae, as in moose and wapiti.

Guinea pigs have proven to be useful laboratory hosts for investigating the hematological response to infection and the parasite's tissue migration route; a few L_3's may reach the central nervous system, develop to the subadult stage, and produce paresis (Anderson and Strelive 1966b; Spratt and Anderson 1968; Bresele 1990). A single worm was found in the brainstem of a domestic rabbit (*Oryctolagus cuniculus*) given 100 L_3's, but none was recovered from cotton-tails (*Sylvilagus floridanus*) or a swamp rabbit (*S. aquaticus*), each given 25 L3's (Nettles and Prestwood 1979).

PREVALENCE AND INTENSITY IN WHITE-TAILED DEER AND GASTROPODS. The reported prevalence of meningeal worm in white-tails varies widely (1%–94%) (see review by Anderson and Prestwood 1981 and additional reports by Foreyt and Trainer 1980; Beaulieu-Goudreault 1981; Kocan et al. 1982; Rau 1984; Upshall et al. 1987; Thomas and Dodds 1988; Dew 1988; Comer et al. 1991; Foreyt and Crompton 1991; Garner and Porter 1991; Bogaczyk et al. 1993; Jarvinen and Hedberg 1993; Pitt and Jordan 1994; Slomke et al. 1995; Davidson et al. 1996; Peterson et al. 1996; Gogan et al. 1997). This wide variation in prevalence may, however, be due mostly to sampling error. Instead, most or all white-tailed deer in a population may eventually become infected as was suggested several years ago by Karns (1967) and Behrend and Witter (1968). This was recently confirmed by Slomke et al. (1995) for a low density white-tailed deer population in northern Minnesota. Ninety-one percent of yearlings and 96% of animals 7–15 years old were infected. Lower percent infection has been observed in habitats near the extreme limits of the parasite's distribution (Kocan et al. 1982; Comer et al. 1991; Whitlaw and Lankester 1994b; Wasel 1995).

Underestimates of prevalence may be due to a lack of care and skill required to find adult worms in venous sinuses, the inclusion of traumatized heads that cannot be reliably examined, or sampling at the wrong time of the year. Young, infected animals available from hunters in autumn may not yet have either adults in the head or first-stage larvae in feces. Their inclusion in calculations may grossly underestimate the overall population prevalence. Considerable discrepancy also occurs between prevalence determined by examining heads and that from feces (Anderson and Prestwood 1981; Thomas and Dodds 1988; Bogaczyk 1990; Garner and Porter 1991). Much of this is due to unisexual, occult infections that are not identified by fecal examination (Slomke et al. 1995). In addition, prevalence may be underestimated by examining feces in fall and early winter when larval output by older animals is at its lowest and may have fallen below levels detectable using the Baermann technique (Peterson et al. 1996). White-tailed deer heads and feces are best collected for examination from February to April, and only data standardized for age and season should be compared.

The prevalence of infection does not appear to vary with host sex (Garner and Porter 1991; Slomke et al. 1995; Peterson et al. 1996), although some earlier authors suspected this to be the case (Gilbert 1973; Thurston and Strout 1978). There is some evidence that overall sample prevalence in white-tailed deer does vary annually in relation to summer precipitation (Gilbert 1973; Bogaczyk 1990; Peterson and Lankester 1991; Bogaczyk et al. 1993), but workers have failed to find a consistent relationship between prevalence and white-tailed deer population density (Karns 1967; Behrend and Witter 1968; Gilbert 1973; Brown 1983; Thomas and Dodds 1988; Bogaczyk 1990; Garner and Porter 1991; Peterson and Lankester 1991; Bogaczyk et al. 1993).

Only the white-tailed deer fawn cohort is useful for investigating environmental factors that may alter rates of transmission of the parasite. Significant annual variation in the prevalence of first-stage larvae measured in fawns in late winter correlated best with the number of days prior to snow accumulation the previous fall (Peterson et al. 1996). Extended periods for transmission in the fall were thought to increase the number of animals becoming infected and to reduce the number of unisexual infections.

The intensity of adult *P. tenuis* in white-tailed deer usually is quite low. Anderson and Prestwood (1981) reviewed the accumulated literature and reported intensities of 1–20 worms with mean intensity ranging from 1.5 to 8.7 worms. Mean intensity changes little with deer density or with age after 1 year (Behrend 1970; Gilbert 1973; Slomke et al. 1995). In fact, a threshold number of adult worms may be reached that is not exceeded appreciably as white-tail densities and the probability of infection increase. Slomke et al. (1995) found the same mean intensity of adult worms in white-tailed deer confined year-round in a fenced area at a density of $30/km^2$ (3.5 ± 1.8 worms) as in those at a summer density of about $2/km^2$ (3.0 ± 2 worms). Occasionally, individual white-tailed deer acquire large numbers of worms (Prestwood 1970).

Although the number of adult worms changes little with white-tail age and time of year, the number of L_1's detectable in feces varies considerably. Young, recently infected white-tailed deer pass more larvae than older animals, and animals of all ages pass the greatest numbers of larvae in spring (Anderson 1963a; Anderson and Prestwood 1981; Slomke et al. 1995; Peterson et al. 1996; Forrester and Lankester 1998). The number of larvae passed in feces cannot be correlated, however, with the total number of adult worms in the cranium (Bogaczyk 1990) or with the total number of female worms present (Slomke et al. 1995). Although expected intuitively, such a relationship may be masked by the combined effects of infection age, season, location of female worms, and possibly, individual host immune response. For example, naturally infected fawns approaching 1 year old passed 132 ± 133 larvae/g of fresh feces and had 2.0 ± 1.2 adult worms in the cranium (Slomke et al. 1995), while an experimentally infected fawn with 3 females and 1 male worm passed 4800 larvae/g at 200 days postinfection (M.W. Lankester, unpublished).

Mean intensity of larvae in white-tailed deer feces provides a useful measure of the productivity of the parasite suprapopulation in an area and may be the best estimator of disease risk to cohabiting susceptible animals (Whitlaw and Lankester 1994b). However, of the many factors known to affect larval numbers, the most important is probably the method used to extract them from feces (Welch et al. 1991). Forrester and Lankester (1997a) demonstrated that the traditional Baermann technique may recover as few as 13% of the P. tenuis larvae actually present and does not provide a repeatable result (see Diagnosis section of this chapter).

The prevalence of P. tenuis in gastropods is probably determined primarily by white-tailed deer density, as well as by microclimatic conditions that favor snails and slugs. A large number of studies conducted throughout the range of P. tenuis, report an overall prevalence of infection in gastropods ranging from 0.01% to 9.0% and reaching 33% in certain species (Table 9.1). Generally, prevalences of < 1% are reported near the northern limits of white-tail distribution, while values of 1.9%–2.6% found in the Canadian maritime provinces and eastern United States may reflect greater white-tailed deer densities as well as a slightly warmer climate with longer seasons for gastropod activity. Higher values of 4.2%–9.0% are unusual and are reported only where white-tailed deer may be at exceptionally high densities or restricted in their seasonal movements (Lankester and Peterson 1996).

High prevalence in Triodopsis spp. suggests that this snail is attracted to fresh fecal material, although no such attraction was found for the closely related Mesodon sp. (McCoy 1997). Whether white-tailed deer actually ingest snails as large as mature adult Triodopsis spp., Anguispira alternata, and Mesodon spp., either for extra protein or mistakenly as mast, remains to be investigated. Infective larvae are thought to survive as long as their gastropod host. Consequently, more seasonal and annual fluctuation in prevalence can be expected in shorter-lived species like D. laeve than

in Zonitoides and Discus spp. that live 2–3 years (Lankester and Anderson 1968).

Most snails and slugs contain only a few infective larvae (means of 2–6) (Table 9.1). Since the mean number of adult worms in white-tailed deer (2.8 ± 1.8) (Slomke et al. 1995) can be similar to the mean number of larvae per infected gastropod in the same area (3.2 ± 2.5) (Lankester and Peterson 1996), many infections in white-tailed deer may be the result of ingesting a single infected snail or slug. Prestwood and Nettles (1977) hypothesized that white-tailed deer may similarly acquire P. andersoni as a result of a single exposure. In three separate reports (Table 9.1), individual D. laeve were found to contain unusually large numbers of larvae (26, 75, and 97). These individuals probably lingered on fresh feces. Possibly the ingestion of such a heavily infected slug accounts for the rare reports of massive infection in white-tailed deer and some of the more severe cases of parelaphostrongylosis in susceptible hosts.

Although a large variety of wild gastropods is found naturally infected with P. tenuis, important species in field transmission will be those most frequently infected and most abundant in areas used by susceptible age classes of white-tailed deer. In the northern parts of the white-tail range, these species include the snails Zonitoides spp. and Discus cronkhitei and the slugs Deroceras spp. (Lankester and Anderson 1968; Lankester and Peterson 1996; Whitlaw et al. 1996). In addition, marked seasonal changes in the abundance of terrestrial gastropods will affect the relative importance of different species (Lankester and Peterson 1996). Reasonable estimates of the numbers and kinds of terrestrial gastropods encountered by deer can be obtained by sampling during damp weather conditions using corrugated cardboard sheets (Hawkins et al. 1998).

It is important to recognize in future studies that wild gastropods frequently contain a variety of larval and adult nematodes, some of which are easily mistaken for those of P. tenuis. For example, Gleich et al. (1977) found nematodes in 19% of Pallifera spp. and in 7% of gastropods overall, but only 0.1% had larvae of P. tenuis. Similarly, Lankester and Peterson (1996) found larvae of other nematodes species in 4% of a sample of over 12,000 gastropods, while only 0.1% had developing P. tenuis larvae.

TRANSMISSION AND ENVIRONMENTAL LIMITATIONS. The ability of L$_1$'s to survive adverse natural conditions and remain infective to gastropods has not been thoroughly studied. In the laboratory L$_1$'s survive constant, subzero temperatures several months (Lankester and Anderson 1968), but repeated freezing and thawing greatly reduces survival (Shostak and Samuel 1984), as does repeated drying and wetting at room temperature. The latter authors cautioned that some survivors that regain motility may have lost their ability to infect gastropods.

Survival of larvae beneath snow in northeastern Minnesota was relatively low (16%), despite moderated and stable subnivean temperatures (-0.2° C to -2.5° C compared to ambient air temperatures of 6.5° C to –24.0° C) (Forrester and Lankester 1998). Even those larvae produced during the "spring rise" in mid-March experienced high mortality (70%), since winter conditions at this northern location continued until late April. Nothing is known of the ability of L_1's to survive summer or winter conditions in the soil. This information, along with more knowledge of the life span of various gastropods, is needed to determine when an area, previously occupied by white-tails, would be free of risk to other susceptible host species.

Transmission may be more likely in particular areas within white-tailed deer range, but whether distinct foci of infection exist is uncertain. Such areas might have a higher than usual density of infected gastropods and be used by young, susceptible white-tailed deer. Small foci were reported by Lankester and Anderson (1968) and Maze and Johnstone (1986), but none could be clearly identified in a study by Platt (1989). Based solely on the availability of intermediate hosts, Kearney and Gilbert (1978) concluded that all forested habitats in central Ontario had approximately equal potential to serve as transmission sites, while open areas have a lower potential except during late summer and fall. The use of open fields and meadows where gastropods were less numerous was thought to explain the persistence of wapiti in an area with infected white-tailed (Raskevitz et al. 1991). Rather than the existence of particular foci of infection, Anderson and Prestwood (1981) suggested that the large volume of vegetation eaten daily by ungulates probably explains the high prevalence of infection in white-tailed deer, even in areas with few infected gastropods. Lankester and Peterson (1996) examined this hypothesis in an area where most fawns became infected within 6 months of birth, yet fewer than 0.1% of gastropods were infected. Fawns were estimated to consume at least one infected gastropod within 51 days, even when infected gastropods were assumed to be distributed randomly and ingested accidentally. White-tailed deer wintering yards were not thought to be especially important in transmission, despite higher densities of infected gastropods (Lankester and Peterson 1996). Deer arrive in yards after snowfall, and by early spring, when gastropods become available, many are immune to reinfection.

Clinical Signs and Pathology in White-tailed Deer. Signs of parelaphostrongylosis are rare in white-tailed deer. Circling and progressive loss of motor function were described in a wild doe with 30–40 adult worms in the cranium (Prestwood 1970), and in an animal raised on a game farm that had 10 worms in the subdural space and others deep in the cerebral cortex (Eckroade et al. 1970). Even large experimental doses of *P. tenuis* in white-tailed deer resulting in as many as 65 adult worms in the cranium produce only transitory lameness or limb weakness (Anderson 1968; Pybus et al. 1989; M.W. Lankester and A.A. Gajadhar, unpub-

lished data). These experimental results are remarkable in indicating that white-tails generally show no ill effects of the spinal cord tissue damage associated with the presence of many more developing worms than are ever likely to be encountered in nature. They also raise the possibility that susceptible species such as moose and wapiti may be less affected by the physical trauma caused by a few worms in the spinal cord than by the meningoencephalitis and perineuritis resulting from infection.

In the spinal cord of experimentally infected white-tailed deer fawns, worms develop in the dorsal horns of grey matter (Anderson 1965b,c). They usually are found in cell-free tunnels surrounded by compressed neural tissue. Malacia is absent except for tiny areas occasionally seen in white matter. The central canal remains undamaged. In white matter, scattered, single myelin sheath degeneration as well as degeneration and disappearance of axis cylinders are common. Infiltrations of eosinophils, lymphocytes, and plasma cells are observed in and on the dura mater, the epineurium, ganglion capsules, and other tissues of the epidural space. Mature worms accumulate in the subdural space over the brain where they are found free or partially embedded in the dura (Anderson 1963a). Areas on the surface of the dura are covered by yellowish exudate unevenly colored by blood. The dura may be thickened and inflamed with patches of eggs and larvae surrounded by giant cells and fibrous tissue visible in sections. Eggs are disseminated to all regions of the lung and found in all stages of development, usually singly or in groups of two or three (Anderson 1963a). Larvae are numerous in alveoli. Heavily infected areas of the lung are considerably altered with congested vessels, collapsed alveoli, fibrosed alveolar walls, petechiae, and collateral vessel formation. Numerous agranulocytes and giant cells are invariably applied to the remains of hatched eggs and clumps of eosinophils and macrophages with hemosiderin-like material are common.

Epizootiology in Abnormal Cervid Hosts. The severity of infection in hosts other than white-tailed deer generally is thought to be due to the higher proportion of invading worms that reach the central nervous system, their longer developmental period in the spinal cord, their resulting larger size and coiling behaviour, and frequent invasion of the ependymal canal (Anderson 1968). Occasionally, naturally infected moose and wapiti pass larvae, but in most abnormal hosts either the worms die or the host dies before infections become patent. Pathogenesis and clinical signs are known from infections produced experimentally as well as those acquired naturally.

MOOSE. Nearly 500 cases of moose sickness have been reported in the literature since the syndrome was first described by Thomas and Cahn (1932). The disease has been reported only in the Canadian provinces of New Brunswick (*n* = 27), Nova Scotia

(137), Quebec (84), Ontario (50), and Manitoba (12) and the northern states of Maine (69), Minnesota (97), and Michigan (13) where moose share range with infected white-tails (Anderson 1965a,b; Aho and Hendrickson 1989; Whitlaw and Lankester 1994a,b, Dumont and Créte 1996; M.W. Lankester and W.J. Peterson, unpublished). The frequency of the disease seems reasonably well correlated with the density of cohabiting white-tailed deer (Karns 1967; Gilbert 1974; Dumont and Créte 1996).

Despite a relatively large number of opportunistic reports of sick moose, only a few studies provide estimates of *P. tenuis* prevalence in wild moose populations. Smith and Archibald (1967) found adult worms in the crania of 5% of 115 clinically normal moose examined over a 4-year period in Nova Scotia and New Brunswick, while 80% of 45 moose showing clinical signs had worms. Similarly, of 153 moose examined in Maine over a 4-year period by Gilbert (1974), *P. tenuis* could be recovered from the cranium of 25% of those killed by poachers, 10%–15% of those killed by vehicles and other miscellaneous causes, and in 80% of those showing signs of parelaphostrongylosis. Thomas and Dodds (1988) found worms in the head of 6.5% of moose shot by hunters and dying of other causes.

In Minnesota, larvae presumed to be those of *P. tenuis* were found in 0.6% of 361 moose fecal samples (Karns 1977), in 0.3% of feces from 617 hunter-killed moose (M.S. Lenarz, personal communication: cited in Gogan et al. 1997), and in 5% of 22 field-collected, moose fecal samples from Voyageurs National Park (Gogan et al. 1997). Higher prevalences reported by Clark and Bowyer (1986) in moose feces in Maine (up to 31%) and by Thomas and Dodds (1988) in Nova Scotia (13%) could not be confirmed in subsequent studies (Upshall et al. 1987; McCollough and Pollard 1993). Estimating the prevalence of *P. tenuis* by examining fecal samples for larvae has serious limitations. Dorsal-spined larvae cannot be identified with certainty, and those of both *P. tenuis* and *P. andersoni* may be passed by moose (Lankester and Fong 1998). As well, the proportion of infected moose that pass larvae can vary. Karns (1977) found larvae in feces of 29% of moose diagnosed as being sick. In a sample of 27 sick moose examined by M.K. Lankester and W.J. Peterson (unpublished) in Minnesota, 15% were passing larvae. How many clinically normal moose, if any, pass larvae is unknown. Lastly, the habit of sick moose remaining for extended periods in the same area makes it difficult to avoid overrepresenting them in fecal collections.

The intensity of adult *P. tenuis* in naturally infected moose usually is very low (mean of ~2; range 1–10) (Anderson 1965a; Smith and Archibald 1967; Gilbert 1974; Thomas and Dodds 1988; M.W. Lankester and W.J. Peterson, unpublished). Animals showing severe signs may have as few as one grossly visible worm. Others may have none. Adult worms were found in the heads of only one-third of sick moose examined by Lankester (1974) and a presumptive diagnosis of parelaphostrongylosis was made based on scattered inflammatory and degenerative lesions in the meninges and parenchyma of the brain and spinal cord.

Moose of all ages can be affected, but reports of younger animals have tended to predominate (Anderson and Prestwood 1981; M.W. Lankester and W.J. Peterson, unpublished data). In this regard, the overhanging muzzle that becomes accentuated in older moose may reduce their feeding low to the ground where there is a greater likelihood of ingesting gastropods. On the other hand, Dumont and Créte (1996) noted that cases in calves were lower, proportionately (3%), than would be expected from their percentage in the population (28%).

Wild moose may show any or all of the following signs: swaying and weakness in the hindquarters, wide base stance of the legs, standing with weight forward on the front legs, tilting or turning of the head and neck to one side (torticollis), knuckling, overextension of the rear fetlock joints and spreading of the toes, circling, fearlessness, depression, rapid eye movements (nystagmus), apparent blindness, ataxia, paresis, difficulty in rising, inability to stand, and weight loss. Peterson (1989) noted the presence of abnormal antlers and kidney stones in moose displaying signs of moose sickness. Worms in moose are frequently found within or beneath the pia-arachnoid (Smith et al. 1964; Lankester 1974). In this location, they may more easily reenter nerve tissue of the brain causing clinical signs. This may explain the slight preponderance of clinical cases in mid- to late winter, several months after gastropods were available (Anderson 1965a,b).

Histopathological lesions in experimentally infected moose killed within 60 days of infection included focal traumatic malacia caused by developing nematodes in dorsal horns of the spinal cord, gliosis and giant cell response, disruption of the ependyma, neuronal loss and single-fiber myelin degeneration, and perivascular infiltrations primarily of lyphocyctes, plasma cells, and eosinophils (Anderson 1964a,b). In wild moose with parelaphostrongylosis, the brain is more extensively involved than the spinal cord (Smith and Archibald 1967; Anderson 1965a; Kurtz et al. 1966). Lesions in the brain parenchyma include cuffing with round cells; disrupted areas or tracts with swollen axis cylinders; gitter cells; congestion; infiltrations of eosinophils, lymphocytes, and plasma cells; and calcified remains of worms. Eggs and larvae may be found associated with the eyes or the roots of cranial nerves, on the leptomeninges, and in brain tissue. Only small glial scars and scattered areas of malacia, degenerating axis cylinders, and microcavitation occur in the spinal cord.

Historically, many authors have associated marked declines in moose populations and reports of sick moose with incursions by white-tailed deer (see Anderson 1972; Lankester and Samuel 1998). However, the implicit hypothesis that *P. tenuis* was the major cause of the declines was never tested (Nudds 1990) until Whitlaw and Lankester (1994a) attempted a retrospective study using published historical data from six jurisdictions where moose sickness has been repeatedly seen. An inverse relationship between moose and white-tailed deer numbers was evident, with moose declining when white-tailed deer exceeded 5/km². However, despite a coincidence of relatively high white-tailed deer densities, moose declines, and reports of sick moose in at least 5 of 13 population cycles examined, these factors were not consistently related. Although the test was probably weakened by the poor reliability of opportunistic reporting of sick animals, the hypothesis could not be supported by available historical data. They concluded that the precise role of *P. tenuis* in past declines of moose may never be known.

In present times, white-tailed deer densities are relatively low in most areas shared with moose because of hunting and winter snow depths (Whitlaw and Lankester 1994b). Throughout much of Ontario where moose and white-tailed deer coexist, white-tailed deer numbers seldom exceeded 6/km² throughout the 1980s, and populations of both cervids were either stable or increasing moderately with only sporadic reports of neurologic disease in moose (Whitlaw and Lankester 1994b). However, moose densities were greatest when white-tailed deer were < 4/km² and varied inversely with the mean numbers of first-stage larvae being passed by white-tailed deer. In Voyageurs National Park, Minnesota, where no hunting occurs, white-tailed deer reached densities of 8/km² during the 1980s, yet no cases of parelaphostrongylosis in sympatric moose were reported (Gogan et al. 1997). At white-tailed deer densities approaching 13/km² in southern Quebec, the annual mortality rate of sympatric moose due to meningeal worm was estimated to be < 1% (Dumont and Créte 1996). Although moose still persisted, the disease was considered a limiting factor, diminishing their demographic vigour. Similar low estimates of moose mortality were made by Lenarz and Kerr (1987) in Minnesota. In 1985, moose were reintroduced into Michigan. Despite *P. tenuis* initially causing 38% of the observed mortality, the moose population continued to grow in the presence of infected white-tailed deer at 5/km² (Aho and Hendrickson 1989). Introduced moose experienced high twinning rates, and no wolf or bear predation was suspected. No hunting or poaching occurred. This experiment has demonstrated that a moose population coexisting at moderate white-tailed deer densities can increase, despite some mortality due to meningeal worm, at least while other factors are exceptionally favourable.

A belief that *P. tenuis* was invariably lethal to moose, probably led earlier authors to reason that moose appearing to cohabit successfully with white-tailed deer must be isolated spatially or temporally from infection. Rather compelling evidence thought to support this view included areas where both cervids existed but were separated at different altitudes during winter in response to snow depths (Telfer 1967; Kelsall and Prescott 1971), the existence of refugia where moose were thought to experience lower rates of infection (Telfer 1967; Gilbert 1974), and areas with considerable habitat heterogeniety thought to reduce overlap between moose and white-tailed deer (Kearney and Gilbert 1976). Nudds (1990) and Gilbert (1992) debated the relative strengths of these data, while more recent moose workers have failed to find strong evidence for the existence of such isolating mechanisms (Whitlaw and Lankester 1994b; Dumont and Créte 1996; Gogan et al. 1997).

If moose are not separated spatially from white-tailed deer and if their feeding habits do not differ substantially, particularly when young, they likely ingest similar numbers of infected gastropods when cohabiting. The number of larvae consumed would be low (Lankester and Peterson 1996), but the effects of such low doses on moose have only recently been investigated (M.W. Lankester, unpublished data). Each of two 5-month-old calves infected with 3 L_3's developed some lameness and hindquarter weakness after 6 weeks, but signs were hardly noticeable at 3 months when a single adult worm was found subdurally in each animal. Two moose infected at 9.5 months with 5 and 10 L_3's, respectively, showed no lasting locomotory signs, and only a single worm was found in one moose after 8 months, despite each having been challenged with 15 L_3's, 199 days after the initial infection. Two other moose given 5 and 15 larvae, respectively, showed persistent lameness and hindquarter weakness and had zero and three worms in the cranium when killed after 3 months. Apparently the severity of parelaphostrongylosis in moose is dose and age dependant. In addition, infection with low numbers of larvae, approximating those found in naturally infected gastropods, is not immediately lethal. Results also suggest that some moose can overcome such infections and that an acquired immunity may protect surviving individuals. Unfortunately, this experiment had to be terminated before the ultimate fate of animals with live worms still in the cranium could be determined with more certainty (M.W. Lankester, unpublished).

In light of this study, it is not altogether clear why some wild moose develop terminal neurologic disease with only one or two worms apparent in the cranium. An additional worm in a vital area within the brain or cord could be responsible, but experiments indicate that the immediate effects of small numbers of worms developing in the spinal cord can sometimes be overcome. Of greater consequence may be the trauma and inflammation caused by persistent adult worms in the subdural space or by those that reenter and oviposit in tissues of the brain as reported by Anderson (1965a). The outcome of infection may also be determined by an individual's innate and acquired immune response to larvae ingested throughout its life.

Overall, the impact of meningeal worm on moose in an area may in large part be a function of dose and age at first exposure for individuals as well as prior experience of older animals with the parasite. The density and age composition of the cohabiting white-tailed deer population will, in turn, determine the numbers of *P. tenuis* larvae being produced, provided that conditions are suitable for terrestrial gastropods. Since the frequency of the disease is independent of moose numbers, the parasite cannot regulate moose populations in the strict sense of this word, but it may be an important limiting factor (Whitlaw and Lankester 1994a; Dumont and Crete 1996). Whether the parasite plays a significant role in the observed inverse relationship between moose and white-tailed deer numbers is still unclear. Moose numbers are also affected by changes in habitat and weather, hunting, predation, and other parasites such as winter tick (*Dermacentor albipictus*) (Lankester and Samuel 1998). The extent to which moose are limited by *P. tenuis* can only be determined by measuring survival and reproductive rates of individuals in relation to their experience with the parasite under various conditions. Although relatively low rates of overt disease are observed in moose at moderate white-tailed deer densities, the possible importance of subclinical effects cannot be discounted. For example, an interesting modeling exercise by Ives and Murray (1997) demonstrated that sublethal effects of a parasite on snowshoe hare can have a destabilizing effect through increased vulnerability to predation, making population cycles more likely.

WAPITI/RED DEER. Meningeal worm can cause debilitating neurologic disease and death in free-ranging wapiti, and it has probably limited the success of past wapiti reintroductions into eastern North America (Anderson and Prestwood 1981; Raskevitz et al. 1991). Nonetheless, despite sporadic cases of parelaphostrongylosis, a few native populations and some introduced herds do persist on range with infected white-tails (Samuel et al. 1992). Infected wapiti or red deer have been reported in eastern Oklahoma (Carpenter et al. 1973; Raskevitz et al. 1991), Pennsylvania (Woolf et al. 1977; Olsen and Woolf 1978, 1979), northcentral Pennsylvania (Devlin and Drake 1989), Michigan and Virginia (Anderson and Prestwood 1981), and Manitoba (Pybus et al. 1989).

Prevalence and intensity of infection in wapiti in areas with sympatric infected white-tailed deer are not well documented. However, contact rates with the parasite can be fairly high while cases of overt disease are less frequent. Histological lesions suggestive of infection were seen in 34% of clinically normal wapiti sampled over a 5-year period in Pennsylvania, but only 11 cases of neurologic disease were recorded (Olsen and Woolf 1979). Infection was most frequent in 1.5 to 2.5-yr-old animals. Four sick wapiti with a history of circling, ataxia, adipsia, or vision impairment were seen within a year or two of being released in eastern Oklahoma (Carpenter et al. 1973). Most were yearlings, and each had 1–3 adult *P. tenuis* in tissues of the brain. The parasite is presumed to behave similarly in red deer.

Experimentally, the development of worms in wapiti is similar to that in white-tailed deer (Anderson et al. 1966). Worms and microcavitations were seen mostly in dorsal horns of grey matter along the entire length of the spinal cord; some worms entered the central canal.

Although a few lesions were found in the medulla, choroid plexus, and cerebellum, their relative scarcity in the brain, compared to that in the spinal cord, is in accordance with results seen in experimentally infected moose (Anderson 1964b). As in moose, developing worms stayed an abnormally long time in the spinal cord, but tissue invasion and heavy infiltrations of lymphocytes, eosinophils, and plasma cells in the epineurium and connective tissue surrounding spinal nerve roots were more marked than in moose (Anderson et al. 1966).

Lesions seen in naturally infected wapiti with adult worms in the cranium consisted mostly of meningitis with focal, disseminated areas of lymphocytes, macrophages, eosinophils, and some giant cells (Carpenter et al. 1973). Adult nematodes were found only in the meninges and elicited little inflammatory response. Lesions in the brain and spinal cord included mild cuffing and gliosis with little reaction visible around clumps of nematode eggs and larvae in brain parenchyma. There was no evidence of nematode-induced trauma as seen in the cord of experimental animals by Anderson et al. (1966).

The severity and outcome of infection in wapiti is dose dependent (Samuel et al. 1992). All animals (2 or 7 months old) given 125 or more L_3's died, while only six of eight given 25 or 75 L_3's showed neurologic signs (two died). Several elk shed L_1's in their feces 78–165 days postinfection. Five given 15 larvae showed no clinical signs nor shed larvae, even though two animals had 2 and 3 adult worms in the cranium when killed up to 158 days postinfection. Clearly, some wapiti can resist or recover from doses of infective larvae (Anderson et al. 1966; Samuel et al. 1992) that are much greater than those likely to be encountered in nature. Nonetheless, mortality of wapiti is probably related to the number of infective larvae ingested, the age at infection, and possibly the specific damage caused by worms within the central nervous system. It has yet to be demonstrated whether a degree of acquired immunity will, in time, reduce observed herd mortality following an introduction.

Potentially, wapiti could introduce *P. tenuis* to areas where white-tailed deer are presently free of infection (Samuel et al. 1992). Although only a few larvae appear intermittently in the feces of experimentally infected elk (Anderson et al. 1966; Welch et al. 1991), both the worm and the host are long-lived, thereby increasing the potential for the parasite to become established. In nature, the presence of dorsal-spined larvae of *P. tenuis* have been presumed in wapiti feces in Minnesota (Karns 1966) and proven in samples from central and southwestern Manitoba (Pybus et al. 1989). There is, however, no evidence that *P. tenuis* can persist in wapiti populations without the continued presence of white-tailed deer.

CARIBOU/REINDEER. There are no reports of *P. tenuis* in free-ranging caribou but there is considerable evidence that caribou and reindeer are particularly susceptible to meningeal worm. The parasite has been suspected of being a factor in the failure of several caribou introductions in areas with white-tailed deer, including the Cape Breton Highlands, Nova Scotia (Dauphiné 1975); Red Lake Refuge, Minnesota (Karns 1979); Liscombe Game Sanctuary, Nova Scotia (Benson and Dodds 1977); and Baxter State Park, Maine (McCollough and Connery 1990). After reviewing 33 reintroduction attempts in eastern North America, Bergerud and Mercer (1989) concluded that caribou cannot be reintroduced to ranges where white-tailed deer have a high frequency of meningeal worm infection. Presently, there are few places in eastern North America, with the exception of eastern Quebec, where infected white-tails even threaten to encroach on caribou habitat.

Even holding caribou or reindeer in enclosures in areas occupied by white-tailed deer has had dire consequences in Ontario (Anderson 1971b), central Wisconsin (Trainer 1973), Virginia (Nichols et al. 1986), and Maine (McCollough and Connery 1990). Anderson (1971b) provided a detailed account of the fate of a shipment of reindeer from Norway placed in an enclosure that had been recently constructed on white-tailed deer range. Neurologic disease was first seen 3 months after their release, and within 5 months, 8 of the 12 were showing signs. In Wisconsin, all of 14 woodland caribou (including 10 adults) released into a 2640 ha enclosure with 600 white-tails, died within 6 months. Trainer (1973). Typically, caribou that were otherwise in good condition showed lumbar weakness, posterior ataxia, circling, severe torticollis, and bulging eyes.

Anderson and Strelive (1968) experimentally infected each of two woodland caribou calves with 200 L3's of *P. tenuis*. Slight neurological signs began 5–7 days postinfection. One died shortly thereafter of a mycotic infection while the second showed progressively severe signs including severe ataxia with knuckling and posterior weakness and was euthanised 29 days postinfection. Developing worms were in dorsal horns of grey matter of the spinal cord and in the medulla oblongata and brain stem. Traumatic lesions and worms were unusually numerous in lateral and dorsal funiculi of white matter, compared to other experimentally infected cervids.

The feasibility of reintroducing caribou into parts of their former habitat now occupied by white-tails has been examined more recently by Gogan et al. (1990) and Pitt and Jordan (1994), but no such introductions have been attempted. This is probably contraindicated unless white-tailed deer can be kept at extremely low densities and caribou can be protected from most other causes of mortality.

MULE DEER/BLACK-TAILED DEER. There are no reports of parelaphostrongylosis in wild mule deer, despite their proximity to infected white-tailed deer in areas such as southwestern Manitoba. Nonetheless, their susceptibility, as well as that of black-tail χ whitetail hybrids, has been demonstrated experimentally

(Anderson et al. 1966; Nettles et al. 1977a; Tyler et al. 1980). Mule deer given 75–200 larvae showed neurologic signs after 35 days that progressed rapidly to paralysis within 80 days postinfecton (Tyler et al. 1980). All died or had to be euthanised, except one adult that showed only slight signs before recovering. Tyler et al. (1980) suggested that mule deer show a weaker cellular response to *P. tenuis* than black-tailed deer as described by Nettles et al. (1977a). Anderson et al. (1966) noted that worms from an experimentally infected mule deer were fertilized, suggesting that *P. tenuis* might become patent in this host if individuals survived long enough. Nematode eggs were found in the cranial dura of a mule deer killed at 87 days postinfection by Tyler et al. (1980), but no larvae were found in lungs or feces.

Histological findings in an experimentally infected mule deer fawn were considered noteworthy since some worms were still in nerve tissue 62 days postinfection (Anderson et al. 1966). Traumatic lesions were intermediate in size and number between moose and wapiti, and white-tailed deer. Cellular infiltration of the neural parenchyma was slight or absent, but worms and tracks left by worms were relatively numerous in the brain. Lesions found in fawns were also most severe in the brain, while those in adult mule deer were more marked in the spinal cord (Tyler et al. 1980). These authors concluded that adult mule deer are more likely to succumb within 40 days to the initial effects of the parasite developing in the spinal cord, whereas fawns may survive this phase, only to have signs reappear later, possibly when large adult worms reenter brain tissues.

Black-tailed deer and their hybrids will not prosper on range with appreciable numbers of infected white-tailed deer (Nettles et al. 1977a). A herd brought to Tennessee grew in number and rarely had sick animals as long as they were held in an enclosure with relatively few white-tailed deer. When some were released into an area where white-tails were increasing, neurologic disease was more frequent, and numbers steadily declined. Black-tails found dead or unable to stand had up to three adult *P. tenuis* in the cranial and spinal subdural space, in the lateral ventricle, or associated with the optic nerve. Multiple foci of malacia, gliosis, and microhemorrhage were seen mostly in white matter of the brain and spinal cord. No eggs or larvae were detected in lungs or feces.

FALLOW DEER. Parelaphostrongylosis has been reported in fallow deer on a game ranch in Georgia (Kistner et al. 1977) and in the Land between the Lakes area bordering Kentucky and Tennessee (Nettles et al. 1977b). In one instance the rapid onset of hindquarter weakness and paresis was seen in adult deer following strenuous capture efforts. Up to four adult worms were found in the cranial and spinal subdural space of other animals found with advanced neurologic impairment, but no eggs or larvae were observed in lungs or feces. The persistence of fallow deer in the Land between the

Lakes area with white-tailed deer at 13/km^2 later led Davidson et al. (1985) to hypothesize that fallow deer may have a degree of innate resistance to *P. tenuis* and that lightly infected individuals may acquire protective immunity against reinfection. Evidence supporting this idea included mild degenerative and inflammatory central nervous system lesions (considered indicative of prior *P. tenuis* infection) in several adult animals that were otherwise normal and in good physical condition.

Histological lesions in fallow deer showing neurologic signs include thickening and chronic lymphocytic inflammation with mineralization of the dura and microcavitations, and lymphocytic and eosinophillic cuffing, within the cervical and lumber cord (Kistner et al. 1977). Scattered foci of malacia, gliosis, microhemorrhage, and mononuclear cuffing are evident in brains (Nettles et al. 1977b). Small round nodules (2–3 mm diameter) visible on the surface of the cord represent granulomatous accumulations of mononuclear cells and often surround cross sections of dead nematodes.

Pybus et al. (1992) infected six fallow deer fawns with 25 or 150 L$_3$'s, and all died. The three fawns given the higher dose died of peritonitis 6–23 days postinfection. Those given lower doses showed progressive paralysis and had to be euthanized 54–67 days postinfection; a mean of ~20 adult worms was recovered from the nerve tissue and subdural space of the central nervous system. A strong lymphoid response and the presence of dead worms were considered evidence of some innate immunity. Small, fleshy lymphoid nodules were seen along the thoracic cord and epidurally around nerve roots, as were widespread, multifocal meningitis and myelitis of the central nervous system. Adult worms remained in the spinal grey matter and cerebral white matter well after 40 days when they leave the cord of white-tailed deer.

Sporadic mortality can be expected in fallow deer held on farms with infected white-tails. Survival of individuals will probably depend on the number of infective larvae ingested, possibly the age at first exposure, and the time elapsing between reinfection. Although fallow deer have never been known to pass *P. tenuis* larvae, the feces of few survivors of infection have been examined. Caution is urged in translocating fallow deer from enzootic areas (Pybus et al. 1992).

Diagnosis. Recovering adult worms from the central nervous system is presently the only way to confirm infection with *P. tenuis*. Dimensions, particularly of the male spicules and gubernaculum, will distinguish *P. tenuis* from close relatives (Carreno and Lankester 1993). Clinical neurological signs in susceptible species held near white-tails are suggestive of infection, as is the presence of nematode eggs (50 (m diameter) and larvae in washings of the cranium or in histological sections of central nervous system tissues.

Dorsal-spined larvae in cervid lungs or feces are not diagnostic of *P. tenuis* infection. The dimensions of the first-stage larvae of several closely related species are similar (Prestwood 1972; Pybus and Shave 1984;

Lankester and Hauta 1989). The Baermann funnel technique is unreliable for detecting and quantifying larvae in feces, and a more sensitive method using fecal pellets held in screen envelopes and submerged in water-filled, straight-sided beakers has been described (Forrester and Lankester 1997a). Forrester and Lankester (1997a) also emphasized the importance of expressing numbers of larvae on a dry weight basis since the weight of "fresh" feces changes rapidly in air. Even this improved methods has limitations. A fecal test cannot be relied upon to identify those animals that pass larvae in very low numbers, or only intermittently (Welch et al. 1991). In addition, a fecal test is of no diagnostic value in a case of clinical illness due to unisexual infection. Apparatus used in fecal examinations is easily contaminated. Larvae from previous samples can remain viable on glassware, but a hot soapy wash and a vigorous alcohol rinse will effectively remove them (Whitlaw and Lankester 1995). In the absence of fecal samples, washes of the oral cavity can be used to detect white-tailed deer passing larvae (Slomke et al. 1995).

Larvae from feces can be used to infect gastropods and to produce L$_3$'s. The distinctive C- or J-shape assumed by lungworm larvae when they are heat-relaxed helps to distinguish L$_1$'s and L$_3$'s from other nematode larvae that occur commonly in fecal material and in gastropods, respectively (Anderson 1963a). The dimensions of L$_3$'s, however, also overlap with those of closely related species, and the size and position of a dorsal bump near the tip of the tail, considered to be diagnostic (Ballantyne and Samuel 1984), may be too variable in this and other species to be useful (Lankester and Hauta 1989). Many of the problems associated with the identification of larvae may be superseded by the application of molecular techniques.

Progress has been made using polymerase chain reaction (PCR) to identify elaphostrongyline larvae in feces (Gajadhar et al. 2000). Amplification of ITS-2 DNA of both L$_1$'s and L$_3$'s, as well as adult worms, allowed the separation of *Parelaphostrongylus* spp. from closely related genera. Available primers also distinguished all three species of the genus: *P. tenuis, P. odocoilei,* and *P. andersoni*.

Hematology and blood chemistry are of limited value in detecting infection. Eosinophilic pleocytosis of the cerebrospinal fluid was used in conjunction with clinical signs to make a presumptive antemortem diagnosis of meningeal worm infection in llamas in an endemic area (Lunn and Hinchcliff 1989). However, Rickard et al. (1994) concluded that cerebrospinal fluid and serum chemistry values were too variable to be of diagnostic value in llamas, as was concluded for goats and white-tailed deer (Dew et al. 1992).

The lack of a reliable conventional test for *P. tenuis* infection in cervids has stimulated considerable interest in the development of a blood test using immunological and molecular techniques. Dew et al. (1992), using antigen extracts from adult *P. tenuis* in an enzyme-linked immunosorbent assay (ELISA), demonstrated antibodies in both serum and cerebrospinal fluid of two goats, but only in cerebrospinal fluid of two white-tail fawns, 4–8 weeks after infection. Using similar methods, Duffy et al. (1993) detected a serum antibody response in two experimentally infected white-tail fawns 75 days after they received 20 *P. tenuis* L_3's, and in nine naturally infected white-tailed deer.

Using sera obtained from rabbits immunized with *P. tenuis* soluble extracts, Neumann et al. (1994) identified two larval (L_3) and seven adult somatic antigens of *P. tenuis* that differed from those in *Dictyocaulus viviparus* and *Trichinella spiralis*. A continuation of this work led to detection of serum antibodies to *P. tenuis* antigens in wapiti (Bienek et al. 1998). When reactivity of sera was tested using an ELISA, larval and adult antigens were consistently recognized by serum from wapiti given 300 L_3's, but only larval antigens were recognized by those given 15. When these sera were further tested by immunoblot analysis, samples (collected from elk with adult worms in the central nervous system) consistently recognized the 25–27, 28–30, and 34–35 kDa antigens of infective larvae after 83 days. However, several *D. viviparus* molecules also were recognized by antibodies directed at *P. tenuis*.

Recent studies show continued progress toward a more sensitive and specific blood test for *P. tenuis* in white-tailed deer using excretory-secretory and somatic antigen preparations from L_3's and somatic antigens from adult worms (Ogunremi et al. 1999a,b). Larval preparations, particularly excretory-secretory antigens, were superior in that they detected infections earlier and more consistently, while somatic antigens prepared from adult worms failed to detect all *P. tenuis* infected animals. This work also revealed considerable cross-reactivity between unfractionated antigen preparations of *P. tenuis* and sera from other cervids infected with the related nematodes *P. andersoni* and *E. rangiferi*. Anti-*P. tenuis* L_3 antibodies were detected as early as 21 days after infection of white-tailed deer given as few as six infective larvae (and later found to have only three adult worms in the cranium). Immunoblotting demonstrated that a total of six *P. tenuis* antigens were recognized, but only one, a 37 kDa protein present in both larval and adult antigen preparations, reacted specifically with serum from infected white-tailed deer. This antigen may be indistinguishable from the 36 kDa protein identified by Neumann et al. (1994) and may be unique to *P. tenuis*. Its reliability in a routine serological test is being examined more closely (O. Ogunremi et al., unpublished).

A satisfactory blood test for *P. tenuis* in white-tailed deer and wapiti requires a high level of sensitivity, allowing early detection of lightly infected and prepatent animals, and a degree of specificity that will not produce false positives in animals infected with other parasites. With helminth infections these standards are difficult to meet and will require rigorous field validation. Yet, such a test will be of great value in veterinary practice and wildlife management.

Immunity. An acquired or concomitant immunity following low-dose infections in white-tailed deer

(Slomke et al. 1995) and fallow deer (Davidson et al. 1985) is suggested by field studies but has not been confirmed experimentally. Protection against a challenge infection with *P. tenuis* may also occur in moose (M.W. Lankester, unpublished). The nature of this apparent protection is just beginning to be understood. Antibody titers against larval *P. tenuis* antigens continued to increase in some infected white-tailed deer throughout 147 days of experimentation but declined in others after 2 months (Ogunremi et al. 1999a). This decline might be expected as worms mature to the adult stage. However, if the 37 kDa antigen found in both L3's and adult *P. tenuis* are similar, either adult worms or repeated exposure to L_3's in nature may maintain or continually boost the antibody response in many animals (Ogunremi et al. 1999b).

Innate differences in the susceptibility of various cervids to *P. tenuis* apparently exist. In part this is reflected by the relative success of larvae in reaching the central nervous system. For example, at least when relatively high doses are given (> 150 L_3) about 1 of every 5 larvae given to moose reaches the spinal cord to begin development while only 1 in 20 do so in white-tailed deer (Anderson 1963a, 1964a, 1965c; M.W. Lankester, unpublished). Host species with the least innate defense against migrating larvae can be expected to succumb most frequently to low-level, natural infection when sharing range with infected white-tailed deer. Rickard et al. (1994) recognized that resistance to the parasite, whether innate or acquired, appears to be more effective when animals are exposed to few infective larvae. Although the minimum dose required to produce sustained neurologic disease is unknown for most susceptible hosts, available field and experimental data suggest that caribou, mule deer, and black-tailed deer are the most likely to exhibit signs of parelaphostrongylosis following exposure to low-level infection under field conditions. The next most susceptible hosts are moose, followed by fallow deer and wapiti and red deer. Similarly for domestic species, llamas are more susceptible than goats and goats more than sheep. A dearth of cases in domestic cattle suggests that they may be the least susceptible, yet exotic bovids housed near white-tails clearly are vulnerable.

Evidence of age immunity is equivocal. Although parelaphostrongylosis tends to be seen more frequently in young moose, older animals also become infected (Whitlaw and Lankester 1994a; Dumont and Crête 1996). When adult moose were introduced into Michigan, 38% of mortality seen over the first few years was due to *P. tenuis* (Aho and Hendrickson 1989). Thereafter, fewer sick animals were reported, and the herd continued to grow. Dispersal of animals and decreased surveillance could have accounted for fewer reports of disease, but some of the surviving animals may have acquired a degree of protection. Disease is reportedly seen most frequently in younger wapiti (Olsen and Woolf 1979).

A strong immune response by white-tailed deer might also explain in part why *P. tenuis* has not spread westward. As prevalence and intensity drop in drier grassland habitat that is marginal for transmission, an increasing number of white-tailed deer may acquire only a single worm and become immune. A high proportion of single-sex infections producing no larvae would depress parasite productivity and contribute to the low prevalence often seen near the parasite's distributional limits (Kocan et al. 1982; Whitlaw and Lankester 1994b; Wasel 1995).

Control and Treatment. Rates of disease may be controlled in cohabiting wild cervids by reducing white-tailed deer numbers, through liberal hunting, for example. Risk of infection by captive stock can be reduced by the use of white-tailed deer–proof fencing and gravel or paved barriers treated with molluscicides. Zoos should choose neonatal white-tails when acquiring new stock. Otherwise, susceptible species should be separated from white-tailed deer by mollusc barriers. It is not known how much time must elapse before ground that has previously held infected white-tailed deer is safe. However, some *P. tenuis* larvae probably live in the soil at least 1 year, and some snail hosts live 2 or 3 years. Small enclosures with little or no ground vegetation can probably be freed of risk sooner by the replacement of soil or by tilling to promote drying.

Considerable effort has been made by owners and clinicians to save valuable exotic and domestic species, particularly llamas. Treatments have included various anthelminthics (levamisole, albendazole, diethylcarbamazine, subcutaneous ivermectin, oral fenbendazole, and intramuscular flunixine meglumine) as well as steroids and anti-inflammatory agents. None of these has been tested in controlled studies, but when used with good supportive care, they may contribute toward recovery, at least of lightly infected animals (Krogdahl et al. 1987; Lunn and Hinchcliff 1989; Rickard et al. 1994). Kocan (1985) demonstrated that ivermectin (at 0.1–0.4 mg/kg) will protect white-tailed deer and fallow deer if given 24 hours after experimental infection with *P. tenuis*. If not given until 10 days after infection, worms develop normally. By 10 days, migrating larvae have entered the spinal cord and appear to be protected by the so-called blood-brain barrier. Treatment has no effect on adult worms already in the central nervous system but depresses the number of larvae developing in the lungs and being passed in feces. Larvae reappear in feces, however, within a month of treatment (Kocan 1985). Ivermectin combined with banamine shows some promise in stopping the progression of signs in sick llama, although controlled studies have yet to be conducted (A. Kocan, personal communication).

Domestic Animal Health Concerns. Sheep have some innate resistance to infection. Reports of parelaphostrongylosis are infrequent, although some may go unrecognized or be misdiagnosed (Anderson 1965b). Sporadic cases of neurologic disease in sheep attributed to *P. tenuis* have been reported in New Hampshire, Connecticut, West Virginia, and Minnesota (Anderson and Prestwood 1981; Jortner et al. 1985; O'Brien et al. 1986). Morbidity in infected flocks has ranged from 2% (Alden et al. 1975) to 59% (Jortner et al. 1985). The worm does not mature in sheep, and spontaneous recovery from clinical signs has been observed (Alden et al. 1975). Progressive hind limb weakness leading to total paresis has been produced experimentally in lambs given ≥ 150 larvae (Anderson and Strelive 1966a). Cross sections of worms or their remains were seen in dorsal and ventral horns of grey matter with microcavitations, swollen axis cylinders, demyelination, giant cells, and gliosis in lateral and ventral funiculi of white matter. The amount of trauma to the central nervous system was surprisingly slight in view of the severity of signs, even in animals receiving 1000 L_3's. The authors suggested that worm secretions, excretions, or breakdown products of moribund and dead worms might account for some of the signs observed. In a study by Pybus et al. (1996), each of 12 domestic sheep lambs received 15–300 larvae; only 1 lamb (given 125 L_3's) showed mild transitory signs.

The response of bighorn sheep to *P. tenuis* is similar to that of domestic sheep (Pybus et al. 1996). Bighorns resist light infections but show neurologic signs or die if exposed to high numbers of larvae. In both domestic and bighorn sheep, most migrating larvae seem to be killed before reaching the central nervous system, thereby avoiding fatal damage to the host (Pybus et al. 1996).

Goats are somewhat more susceptible to meningeal worm infection than sheep. Neurologic disturbance caused by *P. tenuis* in naturally infected goats has been reported in New York, Texas, and Michigan (Anderson and Prestwood 1981; Kopcha et al. 1989). Infected animals usually were in good condition but frequently became separated from the flock (Guthery and Beasom 1979). They often stood in a "humped up" position and exhibited posterior weakness or ataxia that predisposed them to accidental death and coyote predation. Central nervous system lesions consisted of scattered malacic areas with adjacent clusters of gitter cells and blood vessels cuffed with lymphocytes and occasional eosinophils and plasma cells. One kid given only 50 larvae developed progressive hind limb weakness after about 40 days and died (Anderson and Strelive 1969, 1972). Goats given doses of 200 larvae or more, developed fatal necrotizing colitis and bacterial peritonitis within about a week. Worms can reach the adult stage in the central nervous system of this host. Similar results were reported by Dew et al. (1992).

Parelaphostrongylosis is either rare or largely overlooked in domestic cattle. A 3-month-old calf off pasture in Michigan was recumbent with a suspected thoracolumbar spinal cord lesion (Yamini et al. 1997). A coiled worm seen in histological sections of the lumbar region was associated with extensive vacuolation, necrosis, disintegration and swelling of axons in the funiculi, gitter cells in grey matter, and multifocal lymphoplasmacytic and eosinophilic, perivascular cuffing. In Virginia, a 7-month-old heifer presented with acute-onset, rear-limb ataxia that progressed over 10 days to sternal recumbency (Duncan and Patton 1998). Sections of coiled nematodes resembling *P. tenuis* were present in nerve parenchyma of cervical and lumbar regions of the spinal cord. Perivascular, eosinophilic, and lymphoplasmacytic infiltrates were seen in the meninges and in white and gray matter, as were tracts and varying degrees of axonal degeneration at all levels of the cord. Grayish-white nodules (up to 7 mm diameter) visible grossly at the surface and within cervical, thoracic, and lumbar regions were characterised microscopically as nodular lymphoid hyperplasia.

Exotic Bovids and Camelids. Meningeal worm infection was confirmed in one, and suspected in a second, adult sable antelope in Virginia where white-tailed deer frequented the fence line of a zoological park (Nichols et al. 1986). Both animals showed a rapidly progressing hind limb ataxia. Hemorrhage and perivasculitis were seen in the dura over the brain and spinal cord as well as tracts, cuffing with lymphocytes, plasma cells, and eosinophils in nerve tissue; remains of a nematode were seen in the medulla of one animal. Oliver et al. (1996) reported a cluster of cases of neurologic disease in blackbuck antelope on two game farms in southwestern Louisiana that also held white-tailed deer. Clinical signs included a protracted course of weakness, staggering, trembling, torticollis, and eventual recumbency. Adult nematodes identified as *P. tenuis* and nematode larvae were found in the meninges and neural parenchyma of some animals; others were diagnosed on the basis of clinical signs and histological examination. Lesions in the meninges were remarkably slight, with perivascular cuffing and a few foci of granulocytic and lymphocytic infiltrates surrounding larvae. Foci of necrotic cells, glial cells, and areas of swollen axons were seen in the cerebral hemispheres. Sections of a worm were seen in the dorsal horn of gray matter of the spinal cord. Blackbuck antelope are a commonly raised exotic species in southwestern Louisiana and are often allowed to range freely with white-tailed deer on game farms (Oliver et al. 1996). Either infection is not widespread in white-tailed deer, or neurologic disease caused by *P. tenuis* may until recently have gone unnoticed.

Llamas and their relatives are susceptible to *P. tenuis* at doses that can be acquired on pastures frequented by white-tailed deer. Reports in New York (Brown et al. 1978), Ohio (Baumgartner et al. 1985), Minnesota (O'Brien et al. 1986), Virginia (Krogdahl et al. 1987), and Wisconsin (Lunn and Hinchcliff 1989) may underrepresent the frequency of cases in routine veterinary practice. The variety of camelids frequently held in zoological parks should be considered at risk unless isolated from infected white-tails.

The disease progresses rapidly and is often fatal. Signs include head tilting, arching of the neck, incoordination, difficulty rising, posterior paresis, and gradual loss of weight (Brown et al. 1978; O'Brien et al. 1986). Adult nematodes may be found associated with

hemorrhage in the cranial meninges. Microscopic lesions in the brain and along much of the spinal cord include swollen and demyelinated axons, necrotic tracts with debris, perivascular cuffing, and small cavitations in white matter surrounded by macrophages and glial cells (O'Brien et al. 1986). Experimentally, adult llamas given 5–7 infective larvae develop signs of neurologic deficit with incoordination and hypermetria about 50 days after infection (Foreyt et al. 1992; Rickard et al. 1994). Younger animals were affected first. Two of six animals survived after showing only slight neurologic signs; a dead nematode was found in the central nervous system of one when the experiment was terminated at 146 days postinfection (Rickard et al. 1994). The presence of adult nematodes was associated with severe meningoencephalomyelitis and eosinophilia of cerebralspinal fluids. Histological lesions were found primarily in the cervical spinal cord and consisted of nonsymmetrical microcavitations of grey matter, and spongiosis of white matter accompanied by gliosis, infiltrates of lymphocyctes, and some plasma cells, histiocytes, and eosinophils. Llamas are considered to pose little risk of spreading meningeal worm to nonendemic areas, since either they or the worms usually die before infections are patent (Foreyt et al. 1992; Rickard et al. 1994).

Management Implications. Every effort should be made by government regulation and game ranching industry practice to prevent the introduction of *P. tenuis* into western North America. The highly adaptable white-tailed deer presently flourishes in a variety of habitats throughout the western United States and Canada and shares range with mule deer, black-tailed deer, moose, wapiti, woodland caribou, and pronghorns, all of which are susceptible to parelaphostrongylosis. Currently, meningeal worm is absent from western North America, but there is no reason to believe that conditions there are unsuitable for transmission if it were to arrive there with infected cervids. White-tails from enzootic areas represent the greatest threat of accidental introduction, but wapiti, and possibly other cervids, could be responsible (Samuel et al. 1992). To prevent such an occurrence, strict interstate/interprovincial and international monitoring of all ungulate translocations in conjunction with a reliable test are needed to exclude *P. tenuis*–infected animals (de With et al. 1998).

Ecosystyem restoration projects that involve the reintroduction of extirpated species are highly publicized events and normally are not undertaken lightly. Their failure can have high economic as well as political costs. The complete failure of past attempts to introduce caribou, reindeer, and black-tailed deer into enzootic areas should clearly discourage any future efforts, unless white-tails are virtually absent and are guaranteed to remain so. A definitive assessment has yet to be made on the advisability of reintroducing moose into areas where *P. tenuis* occurs. The current experiment in upper Michigan will provide valuable information if the interest and financial support needed to monitor white-tailed deer density and the growth of the moose herd can be sustained. The persistence of a few localized wapiti herds within white-tailed deer range has recently encouraged new introductions of several hundred wapiti from Alberta into Ontario and Kentucky. Introduced moose and wapiti will experience some initial mortality that may later diminish and involve mostly immunologically naive recruits to the population. Long-term monitoring of white-tail densities, intensity of *P. tenuis,* growth of the introduced population, and serological evidence of contact with the parasite will help determine the likelihood of success for future reintroductions.

The sizes of indigenous moose populations historically have varied inversely with white-tailed deer over the medium to long term, but the role of *P. tenuis* in these fluctuations still is not fully understood. The impact of the parasite may be relatively low in areas of eastern North America where range of moose and white-tailed deer overlap. Here, white-tailed deer numbers are periodically reduced by severe winters, and most populations are hunted. However, white-tail numbers are less restricted in parks and areas with extensive secondary forest succession following commercial harvesting or fire. Local conditions allowing increased white-tailed deer densities predictably will increase the number of sick moose. Possible subclinical effects of *P. tenuis* ultimately may prove to be important in understanding the long-term interaction between moose and infected white-tailed deer.

PARELAPHOSTRONGYLUS ANDERSONI PRESTWOOD, 1972

Classification: Nematoda: Metastrongyloidea: Protostrongylidae.
Common Name: muscleworm, parelaphostrongylosis.

Parelaphostrongylus andersoni is a widely distributed muscleworm of caribou (*Rangifer tarandus* var.) in North America and may also occur in reindeer in Eurasia (Fig. 9.1). Its occurrence in white-tailed deer, the host in which it was originally found (Prestwood 1972), probably is incompletely known. Infection runs a rapid course in young animals; first-stage larval production is high for several weeks and then subsides to low levels in older animals. Clinical disease has not been reported in naturally infected caribou or deer but a resulting interstitial pneumonia may compromise normal respiratory function. This parasite is also of interest because it shares cervid hosts with more pathogenic protostrongylids, namely *P. tenuis* and *E. rangiferi,* from which it must be distinguished.

Life History. Adult *P. andersoni* are delicate, thread-like nematodes (Table 9.1, Fig. 9.2) associated with blood vessels and connective tissue deep within loin (longissimus dorsi and psoas) and thigh muscles (Prest-

wood 1972; Pybus 1983; Pybus and Samuel 1984a; Lankester and Hauta 1989). A few may be seen on the surface of the lateral abdominal and intercostal muscles, but those located within larger muscles are only visible upon teasing muscle samples apart under a stereomicroscope. Adult worms are relatively short (females 23–36 mm long, males 17–23 mm) and only about 100 µm wide. Males and females are often paired. They may be loosely coiled or outstretched, with much of the body length oriented parallel to adjacent muscle fibers. Female worms are commonly seen lying partially within small veins where they deposit eggs. Eggs are carried as emboli to the lungs, where they lodge in alveolar capillaries and later hatch. First-stage larvae (L_1's) emerge into the alveolar spaces, move up the bronchial escalator, and are swallowed and passed in feces.

Larvae must penetrate the foot of a terrestrial gastropod in order to molt twice and develop to the L_3 or infective stage (Table 9.2). Natural infections have been found in the snail, *Mesodon* sp. (Anderson and Prestwood 1981), and the slug, *D. laeve* (Lankester and Fong 1998), but other species likely become infected as well. Experimentally, larvae developed to the infective stage within 3–4 weeks in *Mesodon* spp. and *Triodopsis* spp. held at 20° C–26° C (Prestwood 1972; Prestwood and Nettles 1977; Pybus and Samuel 1981). Snails probably remain infected for life, but intensity decreases with time (Anderson and Prestwood 1981). Cervids are infected upon accidentally ingesting gastropods with vegetation.

The migration and development of adult *P. andersoni* within cervid hosts is incompletely known. The best information comes from Pybus (1983) and Pybus and Samuel (1984a), who studied both *P. andersoni* and the related nematode *P. odocoilei* and concluded that both species behave similarly. An impressive 54% of infective larvae given to deer were recovered during necropsies. At 46 days postinfection, when animals were first examined, most worms were found in the backstrap muscles. They had already reached the fifth stage, but none was gravid. In animals examined at later intervals, some worms appeared to move away from this location and were found in a variety of skeletal muscles (hind legs, abdominal wall, thorax, and neck), in epidural fat within the lumbar and sacral regions of the spinal canal, and in an enlarged spinal lymph node in the cauda equina. Curiously, some adults were found in abdominal fat deposits immediately ventral to the sacral vertebrae and overlying the ventral curvature of the abomasum (Pybus and Samuel 1984a). Prestwood (1972) also mentioned finding a fragment of an adult worm in washings of the abomasum. These results suggest that migrating L_3's of *P. andersoni* and *P. odocoilei* do not have to reach a particular site or tissue in which to molt, as has been demonstrated for related neurotropic forms (namely *P. tenuis* and *Elaphostrongylus* spp.). Studies in guinea pigs and rabbits likewise suggest that L_3's migrate in the body cavity and penetrate tissues directly, but some also go via the circulatory system. All became encapsulated and died before reaching skeletal muscles (Pybus and Samuel 1984a,b).

The prepatent period for *P. andersoni* is short relative to that of related nematode species and appears similar in all known cervid hosts. In experimentally infected white-tailed deer, larvae are first passed in feces after 51–69 days (Prestwood 1972; Nettles and Prestwood 1976; Pybus and Samuel 1981, 1984a). In mule deer they are passed after 49–54 days (Pybus and Samuel 1984a), in fallow deer in 69–75 days (Lankester et al. 1990), and in caribou within 66 days of infection (Lankester and Hauta 1989). Larvae passed after 64 days by a moose calf given a mixture of larvae originating off range in Newfoundland were probably *P. andersoni* (Lankester 1977). The prepatent period and the duration of larval production in any host species appears, however, to be inversely related to dose (Prestwood and Nettles 1977; Pybus and Samuel 1984a). Therefore, in naturally infected animals that probably ingest only a few larvae, a slightly longer prepatent period might be expected. Interestingly, each of two white-tailed deer given five L_3's each weekday for 13 weeks did not become patent for 99 and 113 days, possibly because of an unusually strong immune response (Prestwood and Nettles 1977).

The numbers of *P. andersoni* larvae passed in feces rises quickly following patency, peaks at relatively high numbers in 2–8 weeks, and then declines (Nettles and Prestwood 1976; Pybus and Samuel 1981). Details depend on dose and host species. In white-tailed deer given > 1000 L_3's, mean larval output peaked at about 2500/g of fresh feces, but all adult worms eventually were killed, and larval production fell to zero after about 12 weeks. In those given moderate doses (200–350), mean numbers of larvae peaked at about 1000/g before subsiding. Small numbers of adult worms persisted, and larval production continued at low levels for at least a year (Nettles and Prestwood 1976). Similar peaks of *P. andersoni* larval output were reported by Pybus and Samuel (1984a). By comparison, an experimentally infected caribou given 385 L_3's, was passing only 124 larvae/g of fresh feces 14 days after patency and by 32 days, output had declined to 7/g (Lankester and Hauta 1989).

Epizootiology

DISTRIBUTION. *Parelaphostrongylus andersoni* appears to be widely distributed among woodland and barren-ground caribou across northern Canada (Newfoundland and Labrador, northern Quebec, northwestern Ontario, central Manitoba, central Northwest Territories) (Lankester and Hauta 1989; Lankester and Fong 1989; Lankester and Fong 1998) and is present in Alaska (M.W. Lankester and R.L. Zarnke, unpublished). Its widespread occurrence in *Rangifer* led Lankester and Hauta (1989) to speculate that *P. andersoni* may have come to North America with this host and may as yet be overlooked in reindeer of northern

Europe and Asia (discussed further in *E. rangiferi* section). Notwithstanding, host-parasite coevolutionary analyses suggest that *P. andersoni* originated in North America (Carreno and Lankester 1994).

In white-tailed deer, *P. andersoni* has been reported at disjunct locations spanning the entire distribution of this host in North America. It has been found in white-tailed deer of the southeastern United States (Alabama, Arkansas, Florida, Georgia, Louisiana, Mississippi, Tennessee, and North and South Carolina) (Prestwood et al. 1974; Anderson and Prestwood 1981; Forrester 1992), New Jersey (Pursglove 1977), Michigan (Pybus et al. 1990), southeastern and southcentral British Columbia (Pybus and Samuel 1981; M.W. Lankester, R. Lincoln, and W. Samuel, unpublished), and northeastern Wyoming (Edwards 1995). In spite of reasonable effort, it has not been found in Alabama, Arkansas, Maryland, Mississippi, Virginia, and West Virginia (Prestwood et al. 1974), Maine (Bogaczyk 1992), and northeastern Minnesota (Peterson and Lankester 1991). This disjunct distribution may simply reflect the underreporting of an inconspicuous parasite or, as suggested by Lankester and Hauta (1989), results from a degree of cross-immunity in deer that discourages the sympatry of *P. andersoni* and *P. tenuis* (discussed fully elsewhere).

HOST RANGE. Muscleworm has been found in naturally infected woodland and barren-ground caribou, white-tailed deer, a black-tail χ white-tail hybrid, and possibly, moose (Prestwood 1972; Lankester and Hauta 1989; Nettles et al. 1977a; Lankester and Fong 1998). Additional hosts known to be suitable experimentally include mule deer, fallow deer, and probably moose (Lankester 1977; Pybus and Samuel 1984a; Lankester et al. 1990). Infective larvae given to guinea pigs and rabbits did not develop, and no larvae were passed by experimentally infected domestic goats (Pybus and Samuel 1984b). Attempts to infect calves were unsuccessful (Anderson and Prestwood 1981).

PREVALENCE AND INTENSITY. Reliable prevalence and intensity data are scarce, because of the difficulty in finding these small, inconspicuous worms and in distinguishing larvae in feces. Prevalence is typically up to 50% in a population, but intensity usually is low. Adult worms were detected in 20%–40% of white-tailed deer in areas of the southeastern United States, but prevalence based on finding adult worms must be considered minimal (Prestwood et al. 1974). In coastal South Carolina, where only *P. andersoni* was thought to occur, adult worms were found in muscles of 37% of white-tailed deer examined, yet 77% had histological evidence of protostrongylid eggs and larvae in the lungs (Anderson and Prestwood 1981). The mean intensity of adult worms in naturally infected white-tailed deer in the southeastern United States was 3.1, but moribund deer collected in the Mississippi floodplain region had up to 20 hemorrhagic lesions in loin muscles, each containing at least one *P. andersoni*. Pybus and Samuel

(1984a) demonstrated that the number of adult female *P. andersoni* found at necropsy was correlated with the number of larvae being passed in feces. First-stage larvae believed to be those of *P. andersoni* were found in up to 58% of white-tailed deer feces in Florida (Forrester 1992) and in 74% of white-tailed deer feces in southeastern British Columbia at a mean intensity of 40 larvae/g (0.1–837 larvae/g) (Pybus and Samuel 1981). The prevalence of larvae in feces was lowest in late summer and fall (Forrester 1992). It reached about 40% in 2-year-olds and did not change in older animals.

Similar data were obtained for *P. andersoni* in several caribou herds (Lankester and Hauta 1989). Prevalence of larvae in feces ranged from 4%–56%, and mean numbers of larvae were low (up to 13 larvae/g). Animals < 3 years old were more frequently infected and passed more larvae than older animals. There was a tendency for more larvae to be passed in spring by animals of all ages. No differences were attributable to host sex. Of 12 caribou examined for *P. andersoni* in Newfoundland, adult worms could be found in only the 2 youngest; a 7-month-old had 29 worms (Lankester and Fong 1998). Thirty-three percent of feces contained a mean of 94 larvae/g in an area that at that time had only *P. andersoni*. A diminishing number of worms residing in inconspicuous locations is probably responsible for the low numbers of larvae that continue to be passed by older animals in the population.

TRANSMISSION AND ENVIRONMENTAL LIMITATIONS. Almost nothing is known about climatic and biological factors that may affect the transmission of *P. andersoni*. Nonetheless, the existence of this parasite across extreme environments ranging from the sandy, pine forests of the southeastern United States to the Arctic region of Canada and Alaska attests to its hardiness.

Clinical Signs and Pathology. Clinical signs have only been observed in animals given massive numbers of larvae (5000) (Nettles and Prestwood 1976). Symptoms included a reluctance to stand, weakness, panting, walking with short steps and arched back, and sinking to the ground when light pressure was applied to the loin muscles.

In white-tailed deer, areas of hemorrhage may be visible grossly on the surface or within back and thigh muscles (Prestwood 1972; Pybus and Samuel 1981). In these lesions, adult worms can be seen between muscle fibers or partially within the lumen of small venules. In heavily infected animals, pale green tracts and caseous green abscesses up to a centimeter in diameter with nematode eggs or dead worms may be seen (Nettles and Prestwood 1976). Microscopically, these areas are characterized by a granulomatous reaction around larvae or eggs. Inflammatory reaction is absent in muscle around live worms or includes only a few eosinophils and mononuclear cells. Nettles and Prestwood (1976) concluded that granulomatous foci in the lungs and interstitial thickening probably represent the most significant effect of *P. andersoni* on wild white-tailed

deer. Red or grey-white palpable nodules up to 1 mm in diameter were evenly distributed throughout the lung parenchyma (Nettles and Prestwood 1976; Pybus and Samuel 1981). Histologically these were foreign body granulomas containing nematode eggs. In recently occluded alveolar capillaries, eggs, singly or in groups, were surrounded by a thin band of large and small monocytes and a few eosinophils. The number of histiocyctes, fibroblasts, lymphocytes, and plasma cells increased over time. Alveolar septae adjacent to large granulomas became thickened by fibroblasts, histiocytes, eosinophils, and the proliferation of alveolar epithelium. Bronchial lymph nodes contained numerous eosinophils (Nettles and Prestwood 1976).

Mule deer potentially may be more severely affected than white-tailed deer; experimentally, more worms could be recovered and lung pathology was more severe (Pybus 1983). Muscle and lung lesions seen in naturally and experimentally infected caribou were similar to those reported for white-tailed deer (Lankester and Hauta 1989; Lankester and Fong 1998).

Diagnosis. Examination of adult male worms is necessary to confirm infections of *P. andersoni*, but specimens are very difficult to find in infected animals. Thin (0.75 cm), transverse sections of muscle must be teased apart while being viewed at 15X using a stereoscopic microscope. The use of a moderately sharp knife will cleanly sever the body of the adult worm, but not the more supple, black-coloured intestine. Instead, the intestine is stretched out onto the surface of the muscle section and becomes visible as a fine black thread (lighter color in males), but only with the aid of a microscope (Lankester and Hauta 1989). Small areas of hemorrhage (0.5–1 cm diameter) visible under a bright light in well-bled animals may signal the location of some worms (Prestwood 1972). Examining only the longissimus dorsi muscles (backstraps) is a reliable way of surveying for the presence of *P. andersoni* (Prestwood et al. 1974; Pybus and Samuel 1984a), but the muscle must be dissected close to the vertebrae since worms are often situated medially.

Although concurrent infections are thought to be rare, *P. andersoni* has been found with *P. tenuis* in white-tailed deer (Prestwood et al. 1974), with *Elaphostrongylus rangiferi* in caribou and moose (Lankester and Fong 1998), and might be expected with *P. odocoilei* in mule deer (Pybus and Samuel 1984a). Adult *P. andersoni* can readily be distinguished from those of *P. odocoilei* and *P. tenuis* by body dimensions and by the greatly reduced gubernacular crurae and shorter spicules of the males (Prestwood 1972; Lankester and Hauta 1989; Carreno and Lankester 1993). The morphology of spicules and the gubernaculum also distinguish *P. andersoni* from *E. rangiferi*. The predominant location of adult *P. andersoni* is within muscles, whereas that of *E. rangiferi* is on the surface of muscles; *P. odocoilei* also occurs within muscles.

The L_1's of *P. andersoni* are similar in size and appearance to those of all other *Parelaphostrongylus* spp. Their mean length is shorter then that of *E. rangiferi*, but overlapping measurements prevent their specific identification in mixed infections. Prestwood (1972) and Ballantyne and Samuel (1984) suggested that the shape of the tail might be used to distinguish the infective larvae of *Parelaphostrongylus* spp., but Lankester and Hauta (1989) found this character highly variable and cautioned against relying on the method. Progress has been made using PCR to identify elaphostrongyline larvae in feces (Gajadhar et al. 2000) (see Diagnosis section, *P. tenuis*, this chapter).

Immunity. An immune response is suggested by a decline in larval output with age and the difficulty of finding adult worms in animals older than 1 year. A stronger immune response was manifest in white-tailed deer given repeated low-level infections than in animals given large single doses. Repeated infection resulted in a sharp decline in larval numbers shortly after patency, a strong cellular response to adult worms in muscles, reduced viability of eggs and larvae, and sustained leukocytosis with an absolute eosinophilia (Prestwood and Nettles 1977). The evidence is mixed on whether previously infected animals can resist a challenge infection in the wild (Nettles and Prestwood 1976; Prestwood and Nettles 1977).

Control and Treatment. It is impractical and probably unnecessary to prevent infection of wild cervids with *P. andersoni*. On the other hand, treatment to rid captive animals of infection may be desirable, but apparently is difficult to accomplish. A single subcutaneous injection of ivermectin (200–400 µg/kg) reduced larval output in white-tailed deer to 0 within 18 days, but L_1's reappeared again from 1.5 to 6 weeks later (Samuel and Gray 1988). Repeated injections delayed the time for reappearance of larvae and reduced their numbers. The authors concluded that ivermectin has a limited efficacy against *P. andersoni* and may primarily suppress larval production by adult females or destroy L_1's in the lungs.

Management Implications. Natural infections of *P. andersoni* seem to be tolerated well by both white-tailed deer and caribou, but the intense granulomatous reaction seen particularly in young animals may compromise them during periods of stress and when avoiding predators. The translocation of infected animals is of no concern because of the parasite's wide distribution in North America, but its presence in certain stock may confound efforts to identify *P. tenuis*-free animals for shipment. A better understanding of the significance of this parasite to the health and management of wild cervids will not be forthcoming until an easier and more reliable method of detecting *P. andersoni* is developed.

PARELAPHOSTRONGYLUS ODOCOILEI (HOBMAIER AND HOBMAIER, 1934)
Classification: Nematoda: Metastrongyloidea: Protostrongylidae.

Synonym: *Elaphostrongylus odocoilei* Hobmaier and Hobmaier, 1934.
Common Names: mule deer muscleworm, parelaphostrongylosis.

Parelaphostrongylus odocoilei is a common parasite of black-tailed deer and mule deer in the western regions of Canada and the United States (Fig. 9.1). Mule deer in particular have heavy infections that persist throughout much of their lives. Although distinctive signs of disease have not been attributed to infection in free-ranging animals, a hemorrhagic myositis and interstitial pneumonia seen at necropsy suggest that *P. odocoilei* has the potential to impact populations of these and other native cervids as well as bovids.

Current knowledge of the biology and pathogenicity of *P. odocoilei* comes largely from Platt (1978), Platt and Samuel (1978a), Pybus (1983), Pybus and Samuel (1984a,b,c), and Samuel et al. (1985). Morphology, taxonomy, and systematics have been reviewed (Platt and Samuel 1978b; Platt 1984; Carreno and Lankester 1993, 1994).

Life History. Adult *P. odocoilei* are relatively small, hair-like worms found within muscles, primarily of the back (longissimus dorsi and psoas) and upper hind legs (Homaier and Hobmaier 1934; Pybus 1983; Pybus and Samuel 1984a). Males are up to 3.5 cm long and 0.12 mm wide and females 5.6 cm long and 0.22 mm wide (Platt and Samuel 1978b) (Table 9.1, Fig. 9.2). They are whitish in color except for the reddish-brown to black intestine. Adult worms are closely associated with veins in connective tissue between muscle bundles (Pybus and Samuel 1984a). Females may have their tails extending into a vessel in order to deposit eggs. Some adults apparently are swept away and have been found in the heart of black-tailed deer (Hobmaier and Hobmaier 1934; Brunetti 1969). A few females may associate with lymphatic vessels, accounting for eggs and larvae found in lymph nodes (Brunetti 1969; Pybus and Samuel 1980).

Nematode eggs are carried as emboli in venous blood to the lungs where they embryonate and hatch. First-stage larvae (L_1's) move into the alveolar spaces and up the bronchial tree and are swallowed and passed with the feces (Platt 1978; Pybus 1983). To develop to the infective stage, L_1's enter the tissues of a terrestrial gastropod, mostly by direct penetration of the foot epithelium, but some are ingested (Platt and Samuel 1984). L_3's can develop as early as 21 days at temperatures of 15°C–19° C, but most need up to 5.5 weeks (Hart 1983; Shostak and Samuel 1984). Seven of 14 species of terrestrial gastropods examined in Jasper National Park, Alberta, were naturally infected, including *Deroceras laeve, Euconulus fulvus, Zonitoides arboreus, Z. nitidus, Vitrina limpida, Discus cronkhitei,* and *D. shimeki* (Samuel et al. 1985). The slug *D. laeve* was considered the most important because of its abundance and relatively high percent infection (5.3%). Additional species that have been infected in the laboratory include *Agriolimax* spp., *Helix aspersa,* and *Epigramorpha arrosa* (Hobmaier and Hobmaier 1934) and *Triodopsis multilineata* and *Deroceras reticulatum* (poorly) (Platt and Samuel 1978a, 1984).

Deer become infected when they accidentally ingest infected gastropods with food. The route taken by developing worms to muscles is not fully understood but is believed to be similar to that of *P. andersoni* (Pybus and Samuel 1984a) (see earlier description). Worms move across the peritoneal cavity and reach muscles of the back within 46 days. From there some move to muscles of the hind legs while others appear in muscles of the abdominal wall, thorax, and neck. Most worms are coiled within connective tissue of the deep and superficial perimysium, where females can be found with their posterior body inserted into an adjacent vein. Some eggs are found in the lymphatics, but most are released into the blood circulation and filtered out in the capillary beds of the lungs. Some worms can complete their development to the adult stage among the mesentery of the peritoneal cavity. Although mature worms and eggs were found in epidural fat of the spinal canal (Pybus and Samuel 1984a,c), there is no reason to believe that this species must enter nerve tissue to molt to the adult stage (Platt and Samuel 1978a). Studies using guinea pigs also revealed a direct migration through the peritoneal cavity, but some larvae appeared to go via the blood (Pybus and Samuel 1984b).

The prepatent period for *P. odocoilei* is similar to that of *P. andersoni,* taking 45–62 days in mule deer, up to 72 days in black-tailed deer (Platt and Samuel 1978a; Pybus and Samuel 1984a; Gray and Samuel 1986), and 67–72 days in moose (Platt and Samuel 1978a; Pybus and Samuel 1980). Prepatent periods of 2.5–5 months estimated by earlier authors (Hobmaier and Hobmaier 1934; Brunetti 1969) are less precise. There is an inverse relationship between the dose of L3's given and the prepatent period (Platt and Samuel 1978a). In addition, the numbers of larvae passed in feces increase logarithmically during the first 2–4 weeks following patency. In mule deer larval output remains high for almost a year, while in black-tailed deer initial larval numbers decline somewhat but are equally persistent. Only small numbers of larvae are passed by experimentally infected moose. Larval output over 20,000 larvae/g of feces in mule deer is much higher than noted for any other related protostrongylid nematode, regardless of dose given (Pybus and Samuel 1984a). Interestingly, mule deer held without an opportunity for repeated infection have been known to pass larvae up to 8.5 years (W.M. Samuel, personal communication).

Transmission of *P. odocoilei* in mule deer populations depends on an interesting synchrony of seasonal fluctuations in host migration, parasite larval output, and gastropod reproduction and life span (Samuel et al. 1985). Mule deer in Jasper National Park aggregate over winter along river valleys and are still present during March-April when the larval output from adult deer peaks. The slug *D. laeve* is active in May, and mature

individuals infected the previous year are a potential source of L_3's to deer that graze at this time of year. By early June most deer disperse and have their fawns. From June-August adult slugs lay eggs and die as immature individuals are recruited into the population and accumulate infections. In the period August-October, mule deer return to the winter range at a time when prevalence is rising in young *D. laeve* and when fawns are being weaned. By November over 80% of fawns are passing larvae, and all have patent infections by January. Considering a prepatent period of about 53 days, most fawns are thought to become infected upon their return to the winter range (Samuel et al. 1985). It is not known if mule deer can be infected repeatedly.

Epizootiology

DISTRIBUTION. This parasite has a disjunct distribution in the extreme western regions of the United States and Canada in a variety of cervids and one bovid host. It has been reported from the coastal mountains of central California (Hobmaier and Hobmaier 1934) and on Vancouver Island (Pybus et al. 1984) in Columbian black-tailed deer and may occur extensively over the range of this coastal deer found from southern California to the Alaskan panhandle. The parasite also is known in the western Sierra Nevada mountains of California (in California mule deer, *O. hemionus californicus*) (Brunetti 1969), Jasper National Park, western Alberta (Samuel et al. 1985), and the Okanagan Valley of British Columbia (in mule deer) (M.W. Lankester et al., unpublished). It occurs in northern Alberta (in woodland caribou) (Gray and Samuel 1986), northern Washington, and Jasper National Park (in mountain goat, *Oreamnos americanus*) (Pybus et al. 1984). Adults and dorsal-spined larvae morphologically consistent with those of *P. odocoilei* have been found in Dall's sheep from the Mackenzie Mountains, Northwest Territories, Canada; further molecular and morphological analyses are in progress (S.J. Kutz et al., unpublished).

HOST RANGE. The principal hosts of *P. odocoilei* are mule deer and Columbian black-tailed deer (Hobmaier and Hobmaier 1934; Brunetti 1969; Platt and Samuel 1978a), although patent infections have also been found in woodland caribou, mountain goat, and a white-tail χ mule deer hybrid (Gray and Samuel 1985b; Pybus et al. 1984). Moose can be infected experimentally (Platt and Samuel 1978a; Pybus and Samuel 1980), but results for white-tailed deer were inconclusive (Platt and Samuel 1978a; Pybus and Samuel 1984a); neither has been found naturally infected. In guinea pigs, L_3's migrated only as far as the peritoneal and pleural cavities and did not develop further (Pybus and Samuel 1984b).

PREVALENCE AND INTENSITY. Adult *P. odocoilei* were found in the muscles of 25% of black-tailed deer in California (Hobmaier and Hobmaier 1934), and Pybus et al.(1984) found 56% of black-tailed deer on

Vancouver island passing small numbers of larvae in their feces in June (0.7 larvae/g). Mule deer appear to be a more suitable host (Platt and Samuel 1978a). They are more frequently infected and pass relatively large numbers of larvae. Samuel et al. (1985) found 93% of mule deer in Jasper National Park infected. In spring (March and April), fawns passed a mean of almost 2000 larvae/g, and adults passed over 800 larvae/g. During the summer months, larval output dropped close to zero. Eighty-two percent of mule deer near Penticton, British Columbia, were passing 1–41 larvae/ g of *P. odocoilei* larvae in August (M.W. Lankester et al., unpublished).

The parasite also appears well established in populations of other non-deer hosts. Larvae were found in 28% of woodland caribou feces in northwestern Alberta (Gray and Samuel 1986) and in 55% of mountain goat feces from Alberta, central British Columbia, and Washington state (Pybus et al. 1984). One goat found in a weakened condition had about 65 *P. odocoilei* in skeletal muscles.

In naturally infected gastropods, the prevalence ranged from 0.6% to 5.3% in seven species examined in Alberta (Samuel et al. 1985). Prevalence was highest in *Deroceras laeve*. This slug lives ~1 year, and the largest individuals were most frequently infected.

Transmission and Environmental Limitations. The survival of *P. odocoilei* L$_1$'s was greatest at low relative humidity and cooler temperatures (Shostak and Samuel 1984). Those frozen in water at –25° C experienced little mortality after 280 days, whereas mortality was higher in those dried prior to freezing. Survival of larvae decreased with repeated freeze-thaw and desiccation-rehydration cycles. Drying, increased temperature, and duration of treatment reduced the ability of active larvae to develop in snails. Laboratory results suggested that *P. odocoilei* L$_1$'s are well adapted to survive dry, cold habitats, but field studies are required to completely understand the effects of variable microclimatic factors (Shostak and Samuel 1984).

Clinical Signs and Pathology. No distinct disease signs have been associated with natural infections of *P. odocoilei*, but Brunetti (1969) attributed the moribund condition of a 12-mo-old California mule deer to an infection of *P. odocoilei*. Dyspnea following minimal exercise was observed 75 days after infection of mule deer fawns with 300 L$_3$'s (Pybus 1983). One fawn with labored breathing and gasping following minor exercise, died of respiratory stress at 104 days postinfection with hemorrhagic foam being discharged at the nares. This parasite is considered to have the potential to affect populations of free-ranging mule deer, and it may have caused the death of mountain goats in Washington and Alberta (Pybus 1983; Pybus et al. 1984).

Infections with *P. odocoilei* largely have been studied experimentally using relatively large single infecting doses. In black-tailed deer and mule deer, worms within muscles were often associated with hemorrhage

and localized tissue damage (Pybus and Samuel 1984c; Pybus et al. 1984). Focal necrosis of muscles was evident in older infections. Cellular response to adult worms in connective tissue was minimal. In contrast, adjacent eggs and larvae in muscles evoked an intense granulomatous inflammation with subsequent necrosis and calcification, which intensified with duration of infection. Muscle lesions were considered serious enough to interfere with movement in free-ranging deer. Histological lesions in lungs of mule deer included a granulomatous inflammation around eggs and larvae within alveolar walls throughout all lobes of the lungs (Hobmaier 1937; Pybus and Samuel 1984c). A mild bronchitis and bronchiolitis was associated with larvae in the lumen or mucosa of small airways. Lobules without parasites were mildly emphysematous. Granulomas consisting of large mononuclear cells and some eosinophils and neutrophils became progressively larger and confluent with some focal necrosis and calcification, totally obscuring the normal architecture of the lung parenchyma. Extensive vasculitis, particularly arteritis, was noted in all lung sections. Generalized lymphadenosis was seen with hemorrhage and inflammation only in deep inguinal nodes.

Lesions in moose included myositis in the back and hindquarters with general softening of tissues, lymph node hypertrophy, and petechiae throughout the lungs (Pybus and Samuel 1980). Chronic, progressive myositis and increased lymphoid activity was confirmed histologically. An intense lymphocytic response around clusters of eggs in the perimysium extended into adjacent muscle bundles. Atelectasis, interstitial pneumonia, and interlobular edema characterized lung sections. The overall severity of *P. odocoilei* infection was judged to be low in white-tailed deer, low to moderate in black-tailed deer, moderate in moose, and highest in mule deer (Pybus and Samuel 1984a). Differences between hosts were thought to reflect primarily their relative susceptibility to infection and the numbers of female worms maturing in muscles.

A naturally infected mountain goat in weakened condition had no visible body fat and extensive hemorrhaging throughout the skeletal musculature (Pybus et al. 1984). A total of 65 *P. odocoilei* was recovered adjacent to the hemorrhages. Lung lesions were indicative of a verminous pneumonia. Pathology in caribou has not been studied.

Diagnosis. Specific identification of *P. odocoilei* is possible only by examining adult male worms from muscles. It is distinguished from other members of the genus by the length of the male spicules and gubernaculum (Platt and Samuel 1978b; Carreno and Lankester 1993). Otherwise, the prepatent period, location in muscles of the host, and other body dimensions are similar to those of *P. andersoni*. The L$_1$'s and L$_3$'s cannot be distinguished from those of close species (see Diagnosis section, *P. tenuis*, above). Progress has been made using PCR to identify elaphostrongyline larvae in feces (Gajadhar et al. 1999) (see Diagnosis section, *P. tenuis,* above).

Management Implications. The presence of muscleworm has important implications for the management of large ungulates in western North America. Infection is widespread in mule deer and black-tailed deer and appears to be established in rather fragile populations of woodland caribou and mountain goats. Infections can be intense and long-lasting, and the potential to cause severe myositis and verminous pneumonia likely depends, among other things, on host movements and densities.

ELAPHOSTRONGYLUS RANGIFERI MITSKEVICH, 1958
Classification: Nematoda: Metastrongyloidea: Protostrongylidae.
Synonyms: *Elaphostrongylus cervi rangiferi* (Pryadko and Boev 1971, Kontimavichus et al. 1976); *Elaphostrongylus cervi* (Kutzer and Prosol 1975; Lankester 1977; Lankester and Northcott 1979; **not** Cameron 1931).
Common Name: Cerebrospinal elaphostrongylosis (CSE), elaphostrongylosis, staggers, ataxia, stiffneck, posterior paresis of reindeer, brainworm, muscleworm.

Elaphostrongylus rangiferi is a common parasite of semidomesticated and wild reindeer (*Rangifer tarandus tarandus*) in northern Fennoscandinavia and Russia where these gregarious hosts exceed 3 million animals (Nordkvist 1971). The parasite is responsible for periodic epizootics of a debilitating neurologic disease (Fig. 9.3). An intensive verminous pneumonia is also a consequence of infection. The severity of clinical disease is probably dose-dependant, and primarily affects the young and other immunologically naive animals in the population. During epizootics, considerable economic loss may occur in the reindeer industry due to winter deaths, unthriftiness, forced culling for slaughter, and carcass trimming. Domestic stock, including goats and sheep kept on reindeer pasture, may become infected. This parasite was spread from Norway to the island of Newfoundland, Canada, by translocated reindeer (Fig. 9.1).

Earlier reviews of the biology and pathogenesis of *E. rangiferi* are provided in Roneus and Nordkvist (1962), Bakken and Sparboe (1973), Kontrimavichus et al. (1976), Halvorsen (1986a), Anderson (2000), and Mason (1989, 1995). Recent contributions to our understanding of the parasite's morphology and systematics include Stéen et al. (1989), Stéen and Johansson (1990), Gibbons et al. (1991), and Carreno and Lankester (1993, 1994).

Life History. Adult *E. rangiferi* are slender, dark brown nematodes found on the surface of or just beneath the epimysium of skeletal muscles of the shoulders, chest, belly, and hind limbs (Roneus and Nordkvist 1962; Lankester and Northcott 1979; Hemmingsen et al. 1993). Males are up to 3.9 cm long and 0.19 mm wide; females 5.5 cm x 0.24 mm (Mitskevich 1958; Carreno and Lankester 1993) (Table 9.1). Some occur immediately beneath the skin, while others can only be found after separating major muscle groups. The parasite is also found in the central nervous system, usually in the arachnoid or the subdural space over the spinal cord and brain. Specimens in this location are lighter in colour than those occurring among muscles (Lankester and Fong 1998). In the course of their development, worms migrate first to the central nervous system and then into the musculature. Infection of calves in late summer and fall probably explains why most worms found during winter are in the central nervous system, while increasingly toward spring and summer, they are found exclusively among muscles. Previously infected adult animals have worms among muscles throughout the year.

Eggs are released by gravid females into blood vessels and are carried to the lungs. Those deposited

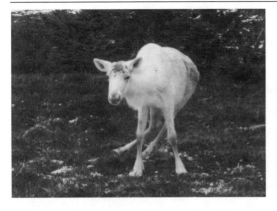
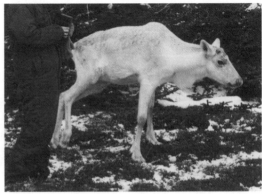

FIG. 9.3—Cerebrospinal elaphostrongylosis (CSE) in a caribou. (Photograph by Ms. Abra Whitney.)

carelessly by females beneath muscle fascia or on the meninges embryonate and hatch, but whether they enter the blood circulation and reach the lungs is unknown. Larvae hatching in the lungs are swept up the bronchial escalator, swallowed, and passed in the feces. Their position on or within fecal pellets has not been determined.

First-stage larvae (L_1's) develop to the L_2 and then to the L_3 or infective stage in both terrestrial and freshwater gastropods (Tables 9.2, 9.4, and 9.5). In the laboratory, development can occur in a variety of species (Mitskevich 1958; Lankester and Northcott 1979; Skorping and Halvorsen 1980; Skorping 1982, 1985a), but the number of larvae able to penetrate and their rate of development vary in each (Skorping and Halvorsen 1980). Of the freshwater snails, Mitskevich (1958) found species of *Galba* and *Lymnaea* most readily infected in the laboratory, but natural infections in aquatic snails are not known. Development in *L. stagnalis* is comparable to that in the most favorable terrestrial species, but juveniles are more readily infected than adults (Skorping 1985a). Gastropods important in Norway include slugs (*Arion subfuscus* and *Deroceras* spp.) and the snail, *Oxyloma pfeifferi* (Skorping and Andersen 1991). Only the small dark slug, *D. laeve*, has been found infected in Newfoundland (Lankester and Fong 1998).

Development of *E. rangiferi* in gastropods is temperature-dependent and varies among species (Skorping and Halvorsen 1980; Skorping 1982; Halvorsen and Skorping 1982). For example, development to the L_3 in *Arianta arbustorum* at 12° C takes 75 days, but at 28° C takes only 11 days; in *Euconulus fulvus*, development at 12° C takes 49 days. At temperatures below 10° C, larval development in *A. arbustorum* and *E. fulvus* stopped, and over time, L_1's survived better than L_2's and L_3's (Halvorsen and Skorping 1982). Schjetlein and Skorping (1995) suggested that this apparent developmental threshold around 10° C could be of adaptive significance by reducing larval mortality over winter. Such a threshold is not absolute, however, in all intermediate hosts. Bodnar (1998) found that L_1's molted to L_2's after 20 weeks in *D. laeve* at 7.5° C, and no differential mortality was evident. As well, L_1's in *D. laeve* at 4.5° C for 10 weeks developed normally when returned to higher temperatures. The presence of L_3's in gastropods in early spring indicates they can survive winter in gastropods (Skorping and Andersen 1991) and probably persist for the life of the intermediate host (Mitskevich 1964).

Reindeer become infected by accidentally eating gastropods. Third-stage larvae released in the abomasum migrate to the central nervous system in order to develop to adults, but there is disagreement on the route by which they get there. Handeland and Skorping (1992a,b) and Handeland et al. (1993) concluded that *E. rangiferi* follows an hematogenous route to the central nervous system of sheep and goats. However, numerous subpleural nodules and foci of necrosis seen on the surface of the diaphragm and the visceral organs

could be caused by larvae penetrating from the peritoneal and pleural cavities rather than arriving there via blood. In a later study using reindeer, Handeland (1994) concluded that *E. rangiferi* penetrate venules of the abomasal wall, travel via the hepatic-portal circulation to the heart and lungs, and then disperse via the general circulation to all tissues, including the brain. Some larvae lodging in arterioles close to the vertebral column may reach the vertebral canal directly along lateral nerves. An hematogenous route also was assumed by Kontrimavichus et al. (1976), Prosl and Kutzer (1980a), and Demiaszkiewicz (1989) studying *E. cervi*. Recently, Olsson et al. (1998) followed the migration of *E. cervi* and *E. alces* in guinea pigs by pressing and digesting all organs. The absence of larvae in blood and skeletal muscles and the length of time required to reach the central nervous system (11 days) were considered inconsistent with an hematogenous route. These authors concluded, instead, that infective larvae of *Elaphostrongylus* spp. undergo a direct tissue migration via the abdominal and thoracic cavities, entering the central nervous system along lateral nerves.

In the central nervous system, L_3's reach the adult stage and mate (Handeland and Skorping 1992a). Females may become gravid as early as 52 days postinfection (Hemmingsen et al. 1993; Handeland 1994). Precisely where maturation occurs needs clarification. Based on histological examination of the entire central nervous system of 12 reindeer given 200–1000 *E. rangiferi*, Handeland (1994) concluded that larvae develop primarily in the arachnoid along the spinal cord, as well as in the spinal canal and ventricles, but sections of worms also were found deeper in nerve parenchyma. In this regard it may be useful to recall the suggestion of Anderson (1968) that *Elaphostrongylus* spp., like *P. tenuis*, may have to enter nerve parenchyma in order to undergo the third and fourth molts. Thus, it might be prudent to examine a greater number of reindeer within the first 40 days of infection and use tissue pressing techniques, as well as histology, to determine precisely where molting occurs.

Initially, developing worms may migrate anteriorly into the cranium (Hemmingsen et al. 1993). Over one-half of those in the central nervous system of reindeer examined at 48 days postinfection were in the cranium, and these were significantly larger than specimens found along the spinal cord. Adult worms leave the central nervous system and appear among skeletal muscles between 90 and 196 days postinfection. Variation in their size in the central nervous system and in the time of their departure may reflect individual differences in the time taken by invading larvae to get there. Their presence in the perineuria of cranial nerves (Handeland 1994) and the inner ear (Roneus and Nordkvist 1962) probably indicates that some exit the central nervous system via cranial nerves. Others are thought to move posteriorly in the subdural space and leave via lateral nerves anywhere along the length of the spinal canal (Handeland 1994). Worms found near

TABLE 9.4 Dimensions of first-stage larvae of *Elaphostrongylus alces*, *E. cervi*, and *E. rangiferi*

Reference	Number of Larvae	Length	Width	Nerve[a] Ring	Excretory[a] Pore	Esophagus	Genital[a] Primordium	Tail
Elaphostrongylus alces								
Lankester et al. (1998)	30	417±16[b] (377–445)	19±1 (17–21)	90±7 (83–106)	112±7 (104–132)	188±12 (173–236)	262±16 (204–289)	42±5 (32–49)
Elaphostrongylus cervi								
Panin (1964a) (as *E. panticola*)	100	(352–425)	(19–22)	?	(101–117)	(165–190)	n.a.	(34–42)
Barus and Blazek (1973)	21	(342–408)	(18–20)	(82–89)	(95–112)	(160–178)	(214–271)	(26–35)
Kutzer and Prosl (1975)	n.a.[c]	407 (364–452)	(17–21)	109	n.a.	183	263	43 (35–50)
Hale (1980)	n.a.	412 (368–448)	n.a.	(98–120)	109 (98–120)	183 (164–197)	263 (235–285)	43 (35–50)
Demiaszkiewicz (1986)	500	434 (382–463)	19 (16–24)	n.a.	n.a.	188 (171–208)	286[d] (235–285)	43 (38–50)
Resác (1990)	12	422 (390–459)	19 (16–23)	103 (92–120)	109 (101–113)	186 (183–193)	n.a.	44 (41–49)
Present study	30	420±13 (392–445)	19±1 (17–22)	114±5 (106–125)	111±4 (104–121)	187±7 (175–206)	270±10 (253–288)	43±3 (37–47)
Elaphostrongylus rangiferi								
Mitskevich (1958)	n.a.	349	15.9	n.a.	n.a.	169	n.a.	31
Kontrimavichus et al. (1976)	n.a.	(288–403)	(15–17)[e]	n.a.	n.a.	(168–170)	n.a.	(29–32)
Lankester and Northcott (1979) as *E. cervi*	15	426 (381–490)	20 (17–24)	110 (95–130)	109 (97–125)	191 (163–230)	267 (245–325)	44 (32–53)
Lorentzen (1979)	39	421±13 (370–445)	20±0.7 (18–22)	n.a.	109±4 (100–114)	n.a.	n.a.	44±2 (37–49)

[a]Position measured from the anterior end.
[b]Mean ± S.D. subtended by range in brackets.
[c]n.a.= not available.
[d]Converted from original work which gave position from posterior end.
[e]Value given as 15–170 in translation; likely 15–17 in original.

Table 9.5 Dimensions of third-stage larvae of *Elaphostrongylus alces*, *E.cervi* and *E. rangiferi*

Reference	Number of Larvae	Length	Width	Nerve[a] Ring	Excretory[a] Pore	Esophagus	Genital[a] Primordium	Tail
Elaphostrongylus alces								
Lankester et al. (1998)	34	714±23[b] (675–756)	38±2 (34–43)	108±1 (107–110)[c]	126±5 (112–136)	238±10 (222–258)	440±16 (409–468)	40±4 (33–47)
Elaphostrongylus cervi								
Panin (1964a) (as *E. panticola*)	n.a.[d]	(910–1110)	(42–50)		(134–137)	(308–336)	(308–528)	(53–61)
Hale (1980)	n.a.	997 (687–1291)	49 (37–73)		152 (101–194)	64 (230–480)	607 (405–772)[e]	54 (33–80)
Demiaszkiewicz (1986)	500	1006 (902–1182)	46 (42–52)	133 (114–157)		384 (320–447)	567[e]	52 (44–63)
Present study	30	831±78 (726–954)	39±2 (33–42)	122±11 (103–147)	131±12 (112–158)	324±33 (256–392)	511±52 (409–600)	44±6 (34–54)
Elaphostrongylus rangiferi								
Kontrimavichus et al. (1976)	n.a.	933	39	139 (120–150)	147	342		51
Lankester and Northcott (1979) (as *E. cervi*)	15	1004 (937–1041)	46 (42–49)		153 (138–163)	381 (338–421)	615 (574–648)	52 (40–70)

[a]Position measured from anterior end.
[b]Mean ± S.D. subtended by range in brackets.
[c]Four measurements.
[d]n.a.= not available.
[e]Converted from original work which gave position from posterior end.

intercostal nerves and the brachial plexus of caribou 3–4 months after infection (Lankester 1977) probably left along thoracic nerves. Hemmingsen et al. (1993) noted that about one-half the worms in the musculature of reindeer were associated with the latissimus and external oblique muscles and one-third with the longissimus dorsi. The remainder were on the belly and among muscles of the thighs (this distribution also seen by Roneus and Nordkvist 1962; Mitskevich 1964; Lankester and Northcott 1979).

The prepatent period of *E. rangiferi* in reindeer has been estimated at 3–9 months (Mitskevich 1958, 1964; Kontimavichus et al. 1976), but a more precise determination is that of Handeland et al. (1994) at 4–4.5 months in experimentally infected reindeer calves. This was corroborated by Stéen et al. (1997), who found *E. rangiferi* larvae passed by moose calves after 133 days. A prepatent period of 74 days in caribou (Lankester 1977) is unreliable since infections were later found to include both *E. rangiferi* and *P. andersoni* (Lankester and Fong 1989).

Generally, many reindeer calves born in early May become infected by autumn. Some pass larvae in their feces as early as September or October (Wissler and Halvorsen 1976), but others do not pass large numbers until January or February (Polyanskaya 1963; Mitskevich 1964). Prevalence increases quickly with age, with most animals becoming infected within 2 years (Halvorsen et al. 1980). There is a marked seasonal cycle of larval output (Halvorsen et al. 1985). In fawns, patency in mid-winter is initially followed by a logarithmic increase, but larval numbers decline during the following summer. In older animals, a sex-specific, annual cycle occurs, with maximum numbers of larvae apparently passed by males in autumn (September and October) and females in winter and spring (January to July).

There is an inverse relationship between seasonal changes in larval numbers and the titer of a larval-specific, circulating antibody believed to fluctuate in relation to stress (Gaudernack et al. 1984). The highest numbers of larvae were shed by adult bucks during the rut and by females experiencing late winter weather conditions in conjunction with pregnancy (Gaudernack et al. 1984; Halvorsen 1986a). Otherwise, the number of shed larvae remains the same in individual animals, year after year. A tendency toward declining larval numbers with increasing host age is thought to reflect reduced fecundity of female worms or the gradual mortality of long-lived worms (Halvorsen et al. 1985).

Epizootiology

DISTRIBUTION. *Elaphostrongylus rangiferi* probably occurs throughout the range of reindeer in the coniferous forest and highlands of northern Fennoscandinavia (Lapland) and northern Russia, above about 62° north latitude (Roneus and Nordkvist 1962). This includes Finnmark County of northern Norway, Sweden northward from the northern part of Dalecarlia, the Karelia region of northern Finland, and in Russia, from the Murmansk region of the Kola or Kol'skii Peninsula east to at least the Buryat region near Lake Baikal (Mitskevich 1958; Roneus and Nordkvist 1962; Polyanskaya 1963; Nordkvist 1971; Kontrimavichus et al. 1976; Holmstrom et al. 1989). Bye and Halvorsen (1984) also found *E. rangiferi* in wild reindeer populations on the mountain plateau of Hardangervidda in southern Norway.

The parasite was introduced into Newfoundland, Canada, with reindeer brought from Altenfjord, Norway, in 1908 (Lankester and Fong 1989). Reindeer were landed at the northern tip of the island and herded southward into the middle part of the province, where some escaped to mix with native caribou. By 1990 the parasite had spread across the province and reached an isolated herd on the southern Avalon Peninsula (Lankester and Fong 1998). Despite later importations of reindeer from Norway and Newfoundland to mainland Canada and the United States, the parasite does not appear to have become established anywhere in mainland Canada (Lankester and Fong 1989).

HOST RANGE. Reindeer and caribou are the usual hosts, but moose (*Alces alces*) also are naturally infected. Care must be taken in identifying *Elaphostrongylus* from moose since the discovery of *E. alces* in Sweden and Norway (Stéen et al. 1989; Gibbons et al. 1991). However, specimens recovered from the musculature of moose in Newfoundland (Lankester and Fong 1998) are identical to *E. rangiferi* in caribou on the same range; and *E. alces* is not known to occur in North America. Moose have been experimentally infected with *E. rangiferi* (Lankester 1977; Stéen et al. 1997).

Fallow deer (*Dama dama*) were infected using *E. rangiferi* from caribou, but only a few subadult worms were later recovered from the central nervous system (Lankester et al. 1990). Muskoxen (*Ovibos moschatus*) in northern Norway showing ataxia and having immature *Elaphostrongylus*-like nematodes in the central nervous system may have been infected with *E. rangiferi* (Holt et al. 1990). Various domestic animals become infected on reindeer range or have been exposed experimentally. These include calves, sheep, and goats (Bakken et al. 1975; Handeland 1991; Handeland and Sparboe 1991). Guinea pigs died 5 days after getting 5000 larvae (Mitskevich 1964), and only a single immature larva was found in guinea pigs given about 100 larvae (Bresele 1990).

PREVALENCE AND INTENSITY. Little field data exists on the prevalence and intensity of *E. rangiferi* in reindeer and caribou, possibly because of problems associated with getting and interpreting representative samples. The detection of patent animals and the number of adult worms found varies with host age, season, and tissues available for examination. In addition, recently acquired worms in the central nervous system are difficult to see, and complete counts of worms in muscles are impossible if only commercially and hunter-harvested animals are available. Estimates based on larvae in feces require more field studies to understand age-related and seasonal fluctuations. The interpretation of such data also is confounded by the possible presence of other protostrongylid nematodes whose larvae are indistinguishable from those of *E. rangiferi.*

In an extensive survey of feces from various regions in northern Russia, 20%–61% of reindeer passed dorsal-spined nematode larvae (Mitskevich 1958). In Norway, the prevalence of *E. rangiferi* larvae in reindeer feces examined in April increased with host age; all animals in the 2+ age group were infected (Wissler and Halvorsen 1976; Halvorsen et al. 1980). Prevalence in the calf cohort varied among years, dropping steadily from 68% in April 1975 to 7% four years later. The prevalence of dorsal-spined larvae in caribou of Newfoundland, determined from feces collected from January to April, ranged from 30%–88% (Lankester and Northcott 1979; Lankester and Fong 1998), but larvae from some animals were probably a mixture of *E. rangiferi* and *P. andersoni.*

Roneus and Nordkvist (1962) reported up to 20 adult *E. rangiferi* in the central nervous system of reindeer showing neurologic signs. In a sample of sick caribou (mostly male calves) examined in Newfoundland from January to April, up to 46 adult worms were present in the central nervous system and musculature (Lankester and Fong 1998). The numbers of larvae in feces of these animals (2–277/g fresh feces) were not correlated with the number of adult worms found or with the severity of neurologic signs. Intensity in reindeer in Norway increased with age up to the oldest age group (2+ years) that passed a mean of 451 larvae/g of fresh feces (Wissler and Halvorsen 1976). The seasonal patterns and numbers of larvae produced by a few captive individuals changed little over 3–4 years (Halvorsen et al. 1985).

Studies of naturally infected gastropods suggest that the dynamics of *E. rangiferi* transmission in semidomesticated and wild herds may differ markedly. Surprisingly high levels of infection were found in nine gastropod species on reindeer pastures in Finnmark County, Norway (70°15′N, 25°30′E) (Skorping and Andersen 1991). The slugs *Arion subfuscus* and *Deroceras* spp. and the semiaquatic snail *Oxyloma pfeifferi* were the most frequently infected (up to 21%, 16%, and 10%, respectively), with protostrongylid larvae resembling *E. rangiferi;* a maximum of 49 larvae was found in one *O. pfeifferi.* On caribou range in Newfoundland, however, only 0.6% of *D. laeve* was found infected (maximum intensity = 15 larvae) (Lankester and Fong 1998).

Transmission and Environmental Limitations. The ability of L_1's to survive long periods under various conditions of temperature and moisture was first studied by Mitskevich (1964). Infected fecal pellets on pastures were sampled weekly over a period of about 3 years. Survival varied with the degree of drying, but even under the most severe conditions some larvae were still alive after 27 months. However, Lorentzen and Halvorsen (1986) found only 17% of larvae placed on reindeer pastures in June were still alive 1 year later.

At constant conditions in the laboratory, Lorentzen and Halvorsen (1986) demonstrated that L_1's in water at 6° C survive for up to ~200 days, while those frozen in water or on feces at –20° C or –80° C, survive for at least 1 year. However, when larvae were repeatedly frozen to –15° C and thawed to 6° C, all died within 77 days. When dried in air at 22° C and 20% relative humidity, all died within 11 days. A derived exponential function describing larval survivorship in water predicted that as many as 50% of larvae held near 0° C might still be alive after 615 days. In practical terms, at least some first-stage *E. rangiferi* larvae can probably persist on contaminated pastures for almost 2 years (Lorentzen and Halvorsen 1986). Skorping (1982) cautioned that tests to determine larval survivorship under different conditions should be interpreted carefully since many larvae stored in water at 12° C remained motile, but their ability to infect snails was reduced by about 50% over 2 months, and to zero after 3 months.

In other laboratory studies, larval growth rate and development in snails was slowed, and mortality and tissue response by snails was increased in more heavily infected snails (Skorping 1984). Several other density-dependent effects were seen. Penetration of L_1's into snails increased directly with density of larvae in exposure dishes (Skorping 1988), and snail fecundity and survivorship of younger individuals decreased with heavy infections (Skorping 1985b). Most snail deaths occurred in the first 8–12 days postinfection, the time at which larvae were molting from the first to the second stage. Although these effects were only seen at relatively high intensities of infection (up to a mean of 67 larvae in snails 6.0 mm long), they were considered to be of potential importance under field conditions (Skorping 1988).

The abundance and distribution of gastropods in northern Norway in relation to the seasonal movements of reindeer was examined by Halvorsen et al. (1980). Although the greatest densities of snails were found on the routes taken by reindeer going to and from summer range, the ground was usually frozen or snow-covered when they did so. Gastropods were scarce in areas dominated by ground lichens. Most reindeer were probably infected, they concluded, in late summer and early autumn in the calcium-rich bogs above the timberline where the amphibious snail *Lymnaea truncatula* was abundant, although gastropods also occurred in the wooded parts of range used by reindeer in spring and summer. Andersen and Halvorsen (1984) found the greatest abundance and diversity of gastropods in calcium-rich bogs and birch woods, while gastropods were scarce in areas with sandstone bedrock. Variety was greatest in coastal habitats of northern Norway and decreased inland, presumably because of lower continental temperatures and a lack of protective snow cover. Almendingen et al. (1993) suggested that the slug *Arion subfuscus* may be of special importance in the transmission of *E. rangiferi.* It is a suitable experimental host and was the most likely of several gastropods observed to be associated with mushrooms, which are readily eaten by reindeer.

Periodic outbreaks of cerebrospinal elaphostrongylosis (CSE) in reindeer of northern Norway appear to follow unusually warm summers (Halvorsen 1986a). Such epizootics have been explained in terms of laboratory studies of larval development and survivorship in gastropods (Halvorsen et al. 1980; Halvorsen 1986a). No development occurred below 10° C, and L_1's survived better than other stages. Therefore, in cool summers on reindeer pastures, the number of larvae reaching the infective stage by autumn would be limited, and L_2's and L_3's would decline over winter. After warmer than usual summers, more infective stage larvae would be available to reindeer by late summer, resulting in heavier infections and more young animals exhibiting CSE the following winter. For reindeer pastures in Norway that lie mostly above the Arctic Circle, the validity of this explanation was strengthened by historical records. An epizootic of CSE around 1970 was preceded by a series of unusually warm summers; the number of cases subsequently subsided as summer temperatures cooled (Halvorsen et al. 1980). A total of seven separate outbreaks of clinical CSE in reindeer over the period 1960–1993 were found to be strongly associated (but not correlated) with higher than average temperatures, and to some extent with higher rainfall, during the preceding summer (Handeland and Slettbakk 1994). Higher than usual mean temperatures were also seen in summers immediately preceding reports of CSE in goats and sheep on reindeer pastures (Handeland and Slettbakk 1995).

Two epizootics of CSE have been observed among caribou of Newfoundland, one in central Newfoundland in the winters of 1981–1985 and another on the Avalon Peninsula during 1995–1997 (McBurney et al. 1996; Lankester and Fong 1998). Here, *D. laeve* is the main source of infection. Larval development in this slug is slowed but not stopped at temperatures as low as 4.5° C, and no larval mortality is observed at low temperatures (Bodnar 1998). As well, *D. laeve* continues to be active on vegetation at temperatures approaching 0° C (Lankester and Peterson 1996). Therefore, epizootics in this more temperate, maritime location are probably less affected by summer temperatures than by weather conditions in autumn and early winter that determine how long slugs remain available on vegetation. The outbreak of CSE on the Avalon Peninsula coincided with unusually mild winters with little snow (Lankester and Fong 1998).

Epizootics also are probably linked to high host population densities and patterns of range utilization, but no field data are available to test this. A method of accurately estimating levels of infections in individual animals is first needed in order to make valid comparisons between herds living under different density and range conditions. Understanding epizootics of CSE will also require knowledge of the biology of the particular gastropods involved in transmission, in particular, their life span. For example, some snails involved in the transmission of protostrongylids live for 2–3 years and are capable of carrying infection over more than one summer. The slug *D. laeve,* on the other hand, lives for only 1 year in the temperate zone (Lankester and Anderson 1968), but may live longer in northern regions. Its life span in Newfoundland has not been determined.

Clinical Signs. Two related forms of the disease have been described, mostly in calves and yearlings. In reindeer, the more common is a subacute verminous pneumonia characterized by restlessness, unsteadiness, dyspnea, general weakness, poor condition, and sometimes coughing, with 8–12-month-old animals dying of inanition in winter and early spring (Roneus and Nordkvizt 1962; Polyanskaya 1965; Nordkvist 1971). Some showing these signs may recover (Handeland et al. 1994). Similarly affected caribou are underweight, stand alone, hold the head low and back arched, and stay in the same general area for long periods (Lankester and Fong 1998).

Other animals develop a more debilitating form of the disease characterized by lack of fear and more conspicuous neurologic signs including somnolence, mental confusion, suspected reduced vision, tilting of the head, lameness, poor coordination, weakness, ataxia, and partial or total paralysis of the hind quarters (Roneus and Nordkvist 1962; Polyanskaya 1963, 1965; Nordkvist 1971; Lankester and Northcott 1979; Handeland and Norberg 1992; Lankester and Fong 1998) (Fig. 9.3). Such clinical signs are also observed in experimentally infected animals given large numbers of infective larvae (Lankester 1977; Handeland et al. 1994). Mitskevich (1964) described emaciation, poor growth, and delayed molting of antlers in experimentally infected reindeer.

The severity of infection in naturally infected animals is probably dose dependant, but only indirect evidence is available. Halvorsen (1986b) demonstrated that the level of infection is correlated with weight, and weight is determined largely by the amount of food eaten. Thus, male reindeer were found infected more frequently than females, and bigger females were more frequently infected than smaller ones. Although other factors may be involved, it seems reasonable to conclude, therefore, that animals most likely to show neurologic signs have in fact ingested more infective larvae than those without signs. The number of worms in the cranium of caribou calves could not be correlated with the severity of neurologic signs (Lankester and Fong 1998), but all sick animals were males. A closer relationship between the severity of disease and intensity of infection might yet be shown when whole-body worm counts are made on animals with infections of similar duration.

Pathology. Infected animals showing neurologic signs have grossly visible lesions in the central nervous system ranging from slight edema and yellowish discoloration of the leptomeninges to firm adhesions between the dura and pia over much of the brain surface (Roneus and Nordkvist 1962; Bakken and Sparboe 1973; Lankester and Northcott 1979; Lankester and Fong 1998). A few small nodules (1–2 mm diam) are often visible ventrally on the spinal cord, particularly in the region of the cauda equina. Worms and parenchymal lesions are not always evident in the central nervous system of clinically ill animals. Worms may only recently have left, or as suggested by Roneus and Nordkvist (1962), neurologic signs may sometimes result from toxins or metabolites produced by worms. A macroscopically visible otitis media was believed related to *E. rangiferi* infection in one reindeer (Roneus and Nordkvist 1962).

Significant histological lesions are often visible in both the central and peripheral nervous systems. Infiltrations of lymphocytes, plasma cells, and a few eosinophils in the leptomeninges of the brain and spinal cord are usually most intense ventrally, around vessels, deep in the sulci, and around nematode eggs. Inflammation often is pronounced in the region of the cauda equina and may include granulomas and foreign-body giant cells around remains of nematodes. Scattered axon demyelinization and swelling may be seen in the nerve roots of the sciatic and other spinal nerves and in branches of the brachial plexus. Malacic foci and tracts containing macrophages, erythrocytes, swollen or disintegrated axons, and clumps of nematode eggs may be seen in the white matter of the brain and spinal cord (Roneus and Nordkvist 1962; Lankester and Northcott 1979; Handeland and Norberg 1992; Handeland 1994).

In the skeletal muscles of animals examined in winter and spring, small foci of hemorrhage and slight yellowish-green discoloration may be visible beneath the epimysium in the vicinity of worms (Lankester and Northcott 1979). In contrast, animals examined in late June have considerable wet, yellowish-red, subcutaneous edema and caseous exudate near worms over muscles of the chest, lateral abdomen, and lower limbs (Lankester and Fong 1998). To what extent the migrating larvae of the warble fly, *Hypoderma tarandi*, might contribute to such lesions is unclear. Histologically, little reaction is seen immediately around sections of worms beneath the epimysium and in intermuscular fascia, although edema and accumulations of eosinophils, lymphocytes, histiocytes, and blood cells occur around clumps of nematode eggs (Lankester and Northcott 1979; Handeland 1994).

All lobes of the lungs of infected animals may have numerous pinpoint-sized red spots or be more mottled, with firm, reddish-grey patches and conspicuous interlobular septae. Histological sections reveal diffuse interstitial pneumonia, with disrupted and thickened alveolar walls infiltrated by eosinophils and lymphocytes, and the presence of eosinophilic granulomas, with giant cells surrounding eggs and larvae. Such lesion may be particularly intense in the subpleural and interlobular spaces. Occasional, consolidated lobules show intense proliferation of interstitial cells and fibroblasts interspersed with histiocyctes, eosinophils, and red blood cells (Bakken and Sparboe 1973; Lankester and Northcott 1979; Handeland and Norberg 1992).

Biology in Moose. Moose in Newfoundland are naturally infected with *E. rangiferi*. Adult worms were recovered among muscles and fascia of the shoulders of four adult animals, but no larvae were present in feces (Lankester and Fong 1998). Unidentified protostrongylid eggs and larvae were reported in the lungs of yearling moose in Newfoundland (Daoust and McBurney 1994), and larvae long enough to be those of *E. rangiferi* occurred in 1 of 28 field-collected fecal samples (Lankester and Fong 1998). Halvorsen and Wissler (1983a) found larvae that may have been those of *E. rangifer* in moose that shared range with reindeer in northern Norway, and a calf moose experimentally infected with *E. rangifer* passed larvae after 133 days (Stéen et al. 1997). Patent infections of *E. rangiferi* in moose may be restricted to younger animals. Although no cases of neurologic disease attributable to *E. rangifer* have been reported in wild moose, neurologic disease has been produced experimentally in this host (Lankester 1977; Stéen et al. 1997).

Diagnosis. The recovery of bursate nematodes among muscles and in the central nervous system of *Rangifer* is suggestive of *E. rangiferi* infection, but in some localities the presence of other protostrongylids may have to be excluded. In Fennoscandia, *E. alces* and *E. cervi* both coexist with *E. rangiferi* (Stéen et al. 1989; Gibbons et al. 1991). The former species matures in reindeer (Stéen et al. 1997), while the latter apparently does not (Halvorsen et al. 1989). To distinguish adults of the three species of *Elaphostrongylus,* it is necessary to compare the form and dimensions of the male bursa and the shapes of the esophagus, anterior and posterior ends, and female genital cone (Stéen et al. 1989; Gibbons et al. 1991). In Newfoundland, adult *E. rangiferi* must be distinguished from *P. andersoni*. Although specimens of the latter usually occur deep within muscle bundles of the back and thighs, they may also occur more superficially, like *E. rangiferi*. Males of these two species are easily distinguished by a simple gubernaculum lacking crurae and longer spicules in *E. rangiferi* (Carreno and Lankester 1993).

First-stage larvae can be extracted from fecal pellets using a method described by Halvorsen and Wissler (1983a) that proved to be a significant improvement over the Baermann technique, at least for previously frozen pellets. The method of Forrester and Lankester (1997) is also applicable. The L_1's of all three species of *Elaphostrongylus* are indistinguishable, but the L_3's of *E. alces* are shorter than those of the other two species (Lankester et al. 1998). The L_1's of *E. rangiferi* tend to be longer (mean, > 400 μm) than those of *P. andersoni* (mean, ~360 μm), but this is of less diagnostic value in mixed infections because of considerable overlap in length measurements (Lankester and Fong 1998). It has been suggested that reindeer in Russia might also be infected with *P. andersoni* or another protostrongylid with relatively short larvae (Lankester and Hauta 1989; Lankester et al. 1998). This is based on reports by Mitskevich (1958) and Polyanskaya (1963) of unusually short dorsal-spined larvae in reindeer (up to 349 µm, and 288–360 µm, respectively) that were much shorter than measurements of *E. rangiferi* provided by Lorentzen (1979) from reindeer in Norway (421 ± 13; 370–445).

The prepatent period may be useful in distinguishing the species involved. For example, *E. rangiferi* takes ~4 months before larvae are passed in feces of reindeer (Handeland et al. 1994), while *P. andersoni,* which coexists with it in caribou of Newfoundland, takes only about 64–71 days (Lankester and Hauta 1989). This approach, however, has less application in Fennoscandia since the prepatent period of *E. cervi* (86–125 days) reportedly can be as long as that of *E. rangiferi* (Anderson 2000). The prepatent period of E. *alces* appears to be shorter in some animals (39–73 days in moose; 39–133 days in reindeer) (Stéen et al. 1997).

Immunity. Field experience suggests that animals respond immunologically to *E. rangiferi.* Naive calves and yearlings usually show the most severe signs of disease, while infection in older animals probably is mitigated by prior or current experience with the parasite. There is no evidence of age immunity. During an epizootic on the Avalon caribou herd in Newfoundland, where the parasite had only recently become established, cerebrospinal elaphostrongylosis (CSE) was seen in adults as well as younger animals (Lankester and Fong 1998). It is not known if animals can be repeatedly infected with *E. rangiferi.* Moose and caribou appear equally susceptible to experimental infection, but some innate resistance is seen in sheep and, to a lesser extent, in goats (Handeland 1994).

Gaudernack et al. (1984), using an indirect immunofluorescence technique, demonstrated that serum from reindeer infected with *E. rangiferi* contained antibodies against L_1 cuticular antigens and that antibody titers varied inversely with the number of larvae being passed in feces. Ogunremi et al. (1999a,b) demonstrated reactivity between unfractionated *P. tenuis* antigen preparations and the serum of caribou infected with *E. rangiferi.*

Control and Treatment. Considerable local knowledge undoubtedly is relied upon to manage *E. rangiferi* infections in the long-established reindeer industry of Fennoscandia and northern Russia, yet little is accessible in the literature. Mitskevich (1964) recommended stringent pasture management with 3-year rotation to reduce infection. Halvorsen (1990) suggested that the clumped distribution of infection in young male reindeer theoretically makes selective harvesting an effective means of reducing infection in herds.

Rehbinder et al. (1982) reported the effective use of mebendazole against larvae of *E. rangiferi* when presented to reindeer in feed. A few animals that continued to pass larvae were thought to have been undermedicated, possibly because of their low social status. Nordkvist et al. (1983) also found that mebendazole administered as medicated feed for 10 days was superior to three other anthelminthics used against *E. rangiferi* in reindeer calves. Feces and lungs were free of larvae by 50 days after treatment, and no adult worms were found at necropsy. Fenbendazole acted similarly, but not all adult worms were killed. Ivermectin injected subcutaneously did not eliminate larvae from feces or from lungs, and adults worms persisted in the cranium. Fenthion had no measurable effect. In another field trial using ivermectin, Nordkvist et al. (1984) reported 100% efficacy against *E. rangiferi.* Oksanen et al. (1993) found subcutaneous injections of ivermectin (200 µg/kg) to be superior to oral or topical applications for dipteran parasites, but none had a demonstrable effect on *E. rangiferi.* Results of using ivermectin vary considerably and may depend on time of treatment and whether some worms are still in the central nervous system and protected by the so-called blood-brain barrier.

Domestic Animal Health Concerns. Sheep and goats that share pastures with reindeer in northern Norway became infected with *E. rangiferi,* and those showing signs of neurologic disturbance had 1–4 adult worms and some eggs in the cranium (Handeland and Sparboe 1991; Handeland 1991). Goats of all ages are more seriously affected than sheep, and lambs are more susceptible than older animals. Most cases occur in November and December. In naturally infected sheep, clinical signs of paresis, paralysis, and vestibular system disease are observed (Handeland 1991). A common feature of infection in goats is pruritus caused by rubbing and scratching. This is followed by motor weakness, lameness, paresis, reduced vision, circling, abnormal head positions, bulging eyes, and scoliosis (Handeland and Sparboe 1991; Handeland and Skorping 1993).

Bakken et al. (1975) observed no clinical disease in two calves and two sheep given fewer than 100 *E. rangiferi* larvae, but inflammatory lesions in the central nervous system were similar to those seen in infected reindeer. Effects in sheep were limited, even at much higher doses. Although some worms matured, they failed to leave the central nervous system and eventually were overcome (Handeland et al. 1993). A sheep given 1000 L_3's first showed signs of ataxia 21 days postinfection and was killed on day 24, after rapidly becoming lethargic and unwilling to rise (Stéen et al. 1998b). In goats given up to 1000 larvae, eosinophils in the cerebral spinal fluid and the onset of neurologic signs were positively related to the infecting dose (Handeland and Skorping 1992a,b, 1993). Up to 16 worms were recovered from the central nervous system of kids killed within a few months of infection, but none was found after 5 months.

Microscopic lesions in the central nervous system of experimentally infected sheep included focal, traumatic encephalomyelomacia caused by migrating worms, with eosinophilic meningitis and choroiditis, lymphohistiocytic granulomas, and perineural infiltrations (Handeland 1991; Stéen et al. 1998b). In goats, accumulations of inflammatory cells and granulomas were seen in the peri- and epineurium of the spinal nerve roots, in nerve fascicles, in the dura and epidural tissue of the cord, choroid plexus of the brain, and leptomeninges over the entire central nervous system. Nerve parenchyma, mostly in the spinal cord, contained foci of traumatic encephalomyelomacia, microgliosis, secondary axon degeneration, perivascular cuffs, and granulomas (Handeland and Skorping 1992b).

Management Implications. Elaphostrongylosis is of major importance in the management of semidomesticated reindeer and wild caribou herds. It is responsible for high mortality in epizootics, losses due to poor growth and weight gain, and unsightly carcasses of harvested animals. Possible impacts of subclinical infection are more difficult to assess. Halvorsen and Skorping (1982) compared the age-dependent prevalence and intensity of *E. rangiferi* larvae in the feces of animals in two reindeer herds with different levels of infection. The mean life expectancy of mature nematodes was thus calculated to be ~1 year in a heavily infected herd, and ~3 years in a more lightly infected herd. This analysis suggested that parasite-induced mortality occurs in a dose-related manner, even at herd infection levels where few cases of overtly sick animals are seen. Subclinical infection may also affect population growth. Before the arrival of *E. rangiferi*, the isolated Avalon caribou herd in Newfoundland consistently showed a greater rate of growth than all other herds in which the parasite had been present for many years (Lankester and Fong 1998).

Several features of reindeer and caribou biology may intensify infection with *E. rangiferi* under present-day conditions. Whether herded or wild, these animals are gregarious for much of the year and repeatedly use the same seasonal grazing areas, often in high numbers. They also exist largely in the absence of predators that would otherwise cull heavily infected individuals shedding the most larvae. Throughout Fennoscandia, and much of Russia where reindeer are herded, wolves (*Canis lupus*) and other predators are controlled. In Newfoundland, lynx (*Lynx canadensis*) and black bears (*Ursus americanus*) occur, but there are no wolves.

Proper management of herds parasitized by *E. rangiferi* requires a better understanding of the roles of herd density and weather in determining infection levels and the onset of epizootics. Herd density can be adjusted by harvest rates, but it is difficult to monitor a species that has such a clumped distribution, is migratory, and segregates by sex and age for periods of the year. Weather conditions that promote the survivorship and development of larvae and the abundance and

mobility of gastropods also must be better understood. Reindeer and caribou may be unable to flourish in areas where conditions habitually are ideal for transmission. Finally, care must be taken to prevent the translocation of infected animals from endemic areas to mainland North America, where susceptible hosts include the widely distributed bands of woodland caribou (*R. t. caribou*) of the boreal forest, the large northern herds of barren ground caribou (*R. t. groenlandicus*), the descendants of introduced reindeer in Alaska, and moose.

ELAPHOSTRONGYLUS CERVI CAMERON, 1931

Classification: Nematoda: Metastrongyloidea: Protostrongylidae.

Synonyms: *Protostrongyloides cervi,* Baudet and Verwey, 1951; *Elaphostrongylus panticola* Lubimov, 1945; *Elaphostrongylus cervi cervi* (Pryadko and Boev 1971), *Elaphostrongylus cervi panticola* (Pryadko and Boev 1971).

Common Name: Tissue worm.

Elaphostrongylus cervi is found in the skeletal musculature and central nervous system of wild and semidomesticated varieties of red deer (*Cervus elaphus*) in Great Britain, Europe, and Asia. It was introduced into New Zealand from Great Britain around the turn of the century (Mason and McAllum 1976). More recently, its introduction into Australia and Canada with infected red deer from New Zealand is believed to have been prevented at points of quarantine (Presidente 1986a,b; Gajadhar et al. 1994; respectively). Interstitial pneumonia, neurologic disease and lowered carcass value are of greatest concern in farming situations. Experimentally this parasite is also pathogenic to certain North American deer (Gajadhar and Tessaro 1995). Without appropriate vigilance, further spread of *E. cervi* by the translocation of live animals in the game farming industry is likely (de With et al. 1998).

Earlier reviews of the biology and pathogenicity of *E. cervi* are provided by Anderson (1968), Kontrimavichus et al. (1976), Watson (1981), Mason (1989), Anderson (2000), Burt and McKelvey (1993), and Mason (1995).

Disagreement persists among specialists regarding the name of this parasite. The issue cannot be resolved here, but may be pertinent to understanding reported differences in pathogenicity across its range. Throughout Europe, Fenoscandinavia, and New Zealand, infected animals rarely show disease signs, while on deer farms in Asia, epizootics of elaphostrongylosis periodically cause considerable economic loss. The name *E. cervi* was first given to a form from red deer (*Cervus elaphus*) in Scotland (Cameron 1931) and the name *E. panticola* to a form from Siberian red deer or maral deer (*C. e. sibericus*) and sika deer (*C. nippon*) farmed in the Altai region of Kazakhstan. However, citing the lack of consistent morphological differences, several authors consider *E. panticola* to be a synonym of *E. cervi* (Barus and Blazek 1973; Kutzer and Prosl 1975; Pryadko 1976a; Demiaszkiewicz 1987a; Gibbons et al. 1991), while others advocate using the subspecies designations *E. c. cervi* and *E. c. panticola* (Pryadko and Boev 1971) in recognition of host and locality differences and possible differences in pathogenicity (Kontimavichus et al. 1976). For simplicity in this review, the name *E. cervi* is used, and either a European or Asian origin is specified when considered important.

Life History. Adult worms are thin and brown to yellowish and are found beneath the epimysium and in the intermuscular connective tissue of the shoulders, chest, back, and upper limbs. Males are up to 4.5 cm long and 0.13 mm wide, females 5.9 cm x 0.16 mm (Cameron 1931; Kutzer and Prosl 1975, 1976; Gibbons et al. 1991). Mature worms also occur in the central nervous system, in the subdural and subarachnoid spaces and occasionally in the ventricles. Adults or larvae may be associated with the eyes (Kontrimavichus et al. 1976). Female worms among muscles presumably are located close to vessels into which they release eggs that are transported via blood to the lungs. Panin (1964a,b) believed that larvae hatching from eggs on the meninges also traveled to the lungs in the blood, while Barus and Blazek (1973) suggested they move out of the cranium along olfactory nerves and directly into the nasal sinuses. In the lungs, first-stage larvae hatch, move into alveoli, travel up the mucociliary escalator, and are swallowed and passed in feces.

First-stage larvae survive on pastures up to 1.5 years and reportedly move away from feces, especially on wet days (Panin 1964a). They penetrate the foot of gastropods (Rezác et al. 1994) and undergo two molts to the L_3 (Panin 1964b; Svarc et al. 1985) (Tables 9.4 and 9.5). A variety of terrestrial gastropod species have been found naturally infected (Panin 1964a,b; Hale 1980), and the aquatic snails *Radix ovata* and *Arianta arbustorum* have been infected experimentally (Panin and Rusikova 1964; Rezác et al. 1994). Gastropods considered most important in transmission, because of their abundance and high infection rates, include *Zenobiella nordenskioldi, Bradybaena fruticum,* and *Succinea altaica* in the Altai region of Kazakhstan (Panin 1964a; Panin and Rusikova 1964) and *B. fruticum* and *Cepaea vindobonensis* in Austria (Hale 1980). In New Zealand, Watson and Kean (1983) found five common species of slug and two species of snails susceptible to infection in laboratory studies. The North American species *Triodopsis multilineata* and the Holarctic *Deroceras reticulatum* have been shown experimentally to be suitable hosts (Gajadhar and Tessaro 1995).

Development of larvae to the infective stage is temperature dependent and varies among intermediate host species (Liubimov 1959a,b). Thirty to 50 days were required in *Z. nordenskioldi* at unpublished temperatures (Panin and Rusikova 1964). In *C. hortensis,* Hale (1980) predicted that development to the L_3 in mollusks under natural conditions would require as much as 2–3 months since it took 3 months at a laboratory temperature of 15° C, but only 23–26 days at 20° C or 30° C; no development was observed at 10° C. Watson and Kean (1983) found L_3's as early as 28 days postinfection in *Deroceras panormitanum* held at 20° C, and by 40 days all had completed development to L_3. The survivorship of infective larvae in snails has not been studied carefully. Some were found alive in *B. fruticum* after 15 months (Liubimov 1959a,b), but none was present in snails collected where infected deer had been pastured 3 years earlier (Panin 1964b). Some L3's probably survive in snails over winter (Panin 1965; Hale 1980).

Cervids are infected by ingesting gastropods. The route taken by infective larvae to the central nervous system has been assumed to be hematogenous (Kontrimavichus et al. 1976; Prosl and Kutzer 1980a), but this has not been investigated in red deer. Using guinea pigs, Demiaszkiewicz (1989) concluded that L_3's reach the central nervous system via the blood. Olsson et al. (1998) argued instead that L_3's of *E. cervi* undergo a direct tissue migration via the abdominal cavity into the thoracic cavity and thereafter enter the central nervous system along lateral nerves. This conclusion was supported by the absence of disseminated larvae in muscles of guinea pigs and by 11 days being required for larvae to reach the central nervous system. A better understanding of the precise route and timing of migration may allow for the more efficacious use of anthelminthics during periods of high transmission.

The presence of numerous *E. cervi* in the cranium of maral deer during winter, but fewer in late summer and autumn (Liubimov 1959a,b), suggested to Anderson (1968) that the parasite may require development in nerve tissue of the central nervous system before moving out into skeletal muscles. In fact single specimens of *E. cervi* have been found within the cerebellum of three hinds (Demiaszkiewicz 1985). On the other hand, the observations of Prosl and Kutzer (1980b) suggest that worms may not need to enter nerve tissue. They noted the absence of lesions in the cerebral parenchyma and the rarity of neurologic signs in the normal host (*C. e. hippelaphus*), even in animals with numerous worms on the meninges. The same can be said, however, of standing infections of *P. tenuis* in white-tailed deer. Even heavy infections are asymptomatic, yet larval development occurs in spinal nerve parenchyma for almost a month before worms enter the subdural space and move anteriorly into the cranium (Anderson 1963). Careful examination of the central nervous system of red deer killed at intervals of 10–40 days postinfection is required to determine precisely where *E. cervi* undergoes the last two molts.

The prepatent period in maral deer is ~120 days (Panin 1964a; Pryadko 1976a,b), but apparently varies inversely with infecting dose. Eighteen-month-old red deer calves given 400–500 larvae were patent after 86–98 days, while those given 200 infective larvae were patent after 107–125 days (Watson 1983, 1986).

The prepatent period in a red deer given only 7 infective larvae, a dose that more closely approximates that likely in nature, was 206 days (Gajadhar et al. 1994). Like other nematodes in this group, *E. cervi* may be long-lived. Adults persist in maral deer for at least 2 years (Kontrimavichus et al. 1976) and produce eggs and larvae in red deer for up to 6 years (Watson 1986).

Larval output increases rapidly in newly infected animals, reaches high levels about 2 months postpatency (5–6 months after infection), and then plateaus (Panin 1964a; Watson 1983). Larval production typically peaks in January to March and is relatively low from May to October; young animals pass the greatest numbers (Liubimov 1959a,b; Pryadko et al. 1963; Prosl and Kutzer 1980a, 1982; Demiaszkiewicz 1987a). The extent of annual reinfection is unclear, although it seems clear that animals develop a degree of postinfection immunity (Pryadko 1976b, Kontrimavichus et al. 1976).

Epizootiology

DISTRIBUTION. *Elaphostrongylus cervi* occurs in Britain, Europe, and Fennoscandinavia, and in Asia from the Altai region to the Far East (where it has been known as *E. panticola*). It has been reported from Britain (Cameron 1931; Hollands 1985; English et al. 1985), Austria (Kutzer and Prosl 1975; Prosl and Kutzer 1980a,b), Switzerland (Pusterla et al. 1997, 1998), Poland (Demiaszkiewicz 1985, 1987a), Hungary (Sugar and Kavai 1977), Czechoslovakia (Dykova 1969; Barus and Blazek 1973; Kotrla and Kotrly 1977; Rezác 1990, 1991), Denmark (Jorgensen and Vigh-Larsen 1986; Eriksen et al. 1989), Norway (Helle 1980; Ottestad 1983; Gibbons et al. 1991), Sweden (Stéen et al. 1989), Kazakhstan (Liubimov 1948, 1959a,b; Panin 1964a; Pryadko et al. 1963; Pryadko 1976a; Kontrimavichus et al. 1976), and New Zealand (Sutherland 1976; Mason 1975, 1979; Mason and Gladden 1983; Watson 1984). Watson's (1980) suggestion that *E. cervi* is in Canada is incorrect. All other references to *E. cervi* (sensu Kutzer and Prosl 1975) in caribou of Canada refer instead to *E. rangiferi* in Newfoundland or to *P. andersoni*, now known to be widespread in North America (Lankester and Fong 1989; Carreno and Lankester 1993).

HOST RANGE. This parasite infects European red deer (including *Cervus elaphus elaphus, C. e. scoticus, C. e. hippelaphus*), Siberian red deer or marals (*C. e. sibiricus*), wapiti (*C. e. nelsoni*), sika deer or spotted deer (*C. nippon*), and possibly roe deer (*Capreolus capreolus*). A report of *E. cervi* in Scotland's only reindeer herd near Aviemore (Invernesshire) is based on larvae in feces and needs confirmation (English et al. 1985). Reindeer experimentally infected with larvae originating from red deer in Norway did not become patent (Halvorsen et al. 1989). Patent infections were produced experimentally in mule deer (*Odocoileus hemionus*) exposed to *E. cervi* originating from red

deer from New Zealand (Gajadhar and Tessaro 1995). A few worms developed in the central nervous system of guinea pigs (Watson and Gill 1985; Demiaszkiewicz 1989).

A report of a single *E. cervi* in a fallow deer in Hungary (Sugar 1978) is inconsistent with findings elsewhere in Europe and New Zealand where this deer remains free of infection when sharing pastures with infected hosts (Mason 1995). Reports that moose are infected (Kontrimavichus et al. 1976) should be confirmed. Experimental infection of moose in Norway (Stuve 1986, 1987; Stuve and Skorping 1987) apparently involved the newly described species *E. alces* (see Gibbons et al. 1991).

PREVALENCE AND INTENSITY. The prevalence of infection generally is high whether in wild or farmed populations. Intensity, however, has not been thoroughly documented but tends, as expected, to be highest in captive herds. On deer farms in the Altai region, Panin (1964a) reported 60%–82% of marals and 52% of sika deer passing larvae. Prevalence in young marals rose quickly with age from 6% in 4–6-month-olds, to 55% in 6–8-month-olds and 95–100% in 18-month-old animals; in sika it rose to 60% by 18 months. Data provided by Kontimavichus et al. (1976) suggest that infection levels eventually decline in older animals. The prevalence in sika deer up to 5 years was 44%, from 5 to 10 years was 15%, and older than 10 years was 21%. Similar figures for farmed sika deer in the Far East were 39% in 1-year-olds, 20% in 2–3-year-olds, 17% in 5–10-year-olds, and 13% in 12–17-year-olds. No differences were found between the sexes when grazed on the same pastures. In farmed facilities, intensities in maral deer exceeded 300 adult worms, and some individuals passed up to 300,000 larvae/day. (Kontimavichus et al. 1976).

High prevalences of infection are also seen in deer facilities in Europe. From 64% to 91% of red deer from various hunting grounds in Poland were passing larvae (Demiaszkiewicz 1987b), but adult worms (up to 20) were found in only 14% of deer carcasses available for examination from one area (Demiaszkiewicz 1985). In northern Scotland, 83% of wild red deer and 40% of treated deer on farms were passing larvae believed to be those of *E. cervi*, but adult worms could not be found (English et al. 1985). The parasite was originally described from Scotland (Cameron 1931) and is still believed to be widespread in wild and captive deer there (Munro and Hunter 1983). Only recently, however, have additional adult specimens been recovered and, apparently for the first time in Britain, reported from within the cranial meninges, primarily of calves (Hollands 1985).

In Hungary, Sugar (1978) found 45% of red deer (*C.e. hippelaphus*) infected with little difference evidenced among age groups. The numbers of worms recovered from the cranium and musculature ranged from 1 to 7 and 1 to 40, respectively. On farms in Denmark, infected red deer had from 1 to 10 adult worms in the skeletal muscles and one had 2 worms in the cranial meninges (Eriksen et al. 1989). Small numbers of *E. cervi* were frequently encountered by Dykova (1969) in red deer in Czechoslovakia; 3–6 was most common in musculature (max. = 12), and 2 were found in the brain of one of the most heavily infected animals. On a farm in Austria with 150 red deer on 220 ha, the prevalence in untreated animals approached 100%, and larval output in calves peaked in February–March at around 350 larvae/g and in adults at 100 lpg (Prosl and Kutzer 1982). Several authors noted that seasonally high larval production may occur despite low numbers of adult worms detectable in muscles.

In New Zealand, Mason and Gladden (1983) found *E. cervi* larvae in red deer and wapiti-red deer hybrids on 35% of farms. Frequency of infection was highest on farms that had received feral stock captured in the Southland/Fiordland region, where the parasite was first discovered (Mason et al. 1976). Prevalence was higher in adult deer than in calves. Most positive animals were passing < 5 larvae/g. One percent or less of carcasses inspected at slaughter and packing facilities were considered infected based on detection of a greenish discolouration or worms on muscle (Mason 1994). Up to 13 worms were seen on carcasses (Sutherland 1976).

The prevalence and intensity of *E. cervi* infection in gastropods has been studied mostly in situations where deer densities are high. In a sample of almost 9000 snails and slugs collected from deer farms (marals and sika) in the Altai, 5.7% were infected, including 15 of 20 species (Panin 1964b; Panin and Rusikova 1964). The most abundant were *Zenobiella nordenskiolda, Bradybaena fruticum,* and *Succinea* sp., with percent prevalences of 24%, 9%, and 8%, respectively. In one experimental deer park, 93% of the gastropods contained larvae. Percent prevalences in gastropods collected near feeding areas on a red deer facility in Austria were 22% (*B. fruticum*), 22% (*Cepaea vindobonensis*), and 54% (*Euomphalium strigella*); mean intensity was 1.9 larvae (Hale 1980). These rather high prevalences existed despite the fact that deer were treated with anthelminthics in February, which reduced numbers of larvae in feces (hence, exposure to gastropods) over summer. Infection was most common in *Succinea putris* (27%) and *Perforatella bidentata* (17%) in Poland (Demiaszkiewicz 1987b).

Transmission and Environmental Limitations. Periods of maximum transmission probably are determined by a number of factors, some of which will vary annually. These include, among others, the seasonal rhythm of larval output by deer of different ages, survivorship of larvae on pastures, temperature requirements for development in intermediate hosts, and annual cycles of gastropod activity and abundance, as well as their life span. Factors that cause major epizootics like those seen on farms in Asia apparently have not been studied in detail.

The release of L_1's by pastured red deer was followed over a 4-year period (Prosl and Kutzer 1980b, 1982; Hale 1980). Output from May to October was low but began to increase in November and peaked from February to March. Calves passed many more larvae than adult deer. Demiaszkiewicz (1987a,b) also found L_1's passed by two wild red deer to peak in February and May.

Although little studied, L_1's of *E. cervi* probably are as resistant to adverse environmental conditions as most other protostrongylids. First-stage larvae can withstand freezing and drying in feces on pastures in the Altai for more than a year and survive in water at ~20° C for 4 months (Liubimov 1959a,b). Larvae exposed on pastures for a year were still capable of developing to L_3's in snails but took longer than normal (Panin 1964b). Infective larvae are equally tenacious, surviving on pastures in gastropod hosts for 1.5–2 or more years (Panin 1964b, 1965), probably determined by the life span of the gastropod host.

In the Altai, gastropods are active only from May to October (Kontimavichus et al. 1976). Parasite prevalence in them is low in spring, with mostly preinfective larvae, but the number with L_3's increases over summer. Most transmission is thought to occur in July and August when gastropods are abundant on the open larch forests, on grassy slopes, and along stream banks. The prevalence of infective larvae continues to increase, but gastropod numbers decline markedly in autumn.

Infection of gastropods in Austria occurred mostly in spring following the peak of larval output by deer in February and March (Hale 1980). However, both preinfective and fully developed infective forms were found in early April. Since no larval development occurs at temperatures below 11° C, some infective larvae must have developed the previous autumn and survived winter. One particular snail, *B. fruticum,* became active in Austria on mild days in January, a behavior contributing to its importance as a source of infection. At normal spring and summer temperatures, L_3's were estimated to require 2–3 months to develop. Accordingly, they became increasingly prevalent in snails in June and July when calves were grazing, but declined abruptly in mid-August, probably because older snails in the population died. Demiaszkiewicz (1987b) also found that snails in Poland mostly became infected from June to August and declined in September. In these areas, therefore, the peak of transmission occurs in late summer, but probably continues at a lower rate at other times of the year when deer can access infected gastropods.

Clinical Signs. Workers in Britain, Europe, and New Zealand rarely see neurologic disease in native deer, and many emphasize that interstitial pneumonia and occasionally the discoloration of meat are the principal concerns of *E. cervi* infection (Burg et al. 1953; Sutherland 1976; Borg 1979; Munro and Hunter 1983; Hollands 1985; Watson and Gill 1985; Mason 1989, 1995).

On the other hand, elaphostrongylosis characterized by varying degrees of neurologic impairment has been considered one of the most serious helminth diseases of farmed cervids in central and eastern Asia, with periodic epizootics causing serious economic loss (Pryadko et al. 1963; Kontimavichus et al. 1976).

Infection of Siberian maral deer is common and often subclinical, but when large numbers of worms are present (sometimes more than 300) neurologic disturbance is evident, particularly in younger animals (Kontrimavichus et al. 1976). Sick deer often stand away from the herd. The head may be held low or turned to the side; animals may circle aimlessly, walk sideways, have an unsteady gait, and fall down, eventually being unable to rise (Kontimavichus et al. 1976). The pathogenicity of *E. cervi* is considered more severe in Siberian maral deer than in sika deer (Liubimov 1959b; Pryadko 1976a). This was attributed to differences in what were considered final sites favored by adult worms in the two hosts. On examination of marals, most worms were found in the central nervous system, while in sika deer, most were in the musculature. Notwithstanding, the pathogenicity of *E. cervi* probably is related primarily to the numbers of worms passing through the central nervous system. In this regard, however, differences in parasite strain, host susceptibility, exposure rates, and animal management techniques, are likely important contributing factors.

Experimental infections of red deer in New Zealand with 200 L_3's resulted in severe pulmonary hemorrhage, exercise intolerance, posterior paresis, nervous disorders, blindness, verminous pneumonia, and death (Watson 1983). Mule deer given ~100 and 400 L_3's originating from New Zealand red deer developed progressive neurologic disease including posterior ataxia, knuckling, loss of proprioception, and hyperextension of the fetlocks beginning 104 days postinfection. Both had to be killed 4 and 7 weeks later (Gajadhar and Tessaro 1995).

Pathology. Most adult worms in fascia or epimysium cause no gross tissue changes other than occasional associated focal hemorrhaging or slightly elevated green caseous plaques or nodules (Sutherland 1976; Mason 1994). Regional lymph nodes when cut may be moist with a greenish discoloration. The lungs of red red deer from Fiordland National Park, New Zealand, had a number of emphysematous blebs scattered over the costal surface, particularly of the diaphragmatic lobes (Sutherland 1976). Some lungs were firm with scattered areas of consolidation. Histologically, a diffuse, mild interstitial pneumonia was characterized by infiltrating eosinophils, leucocytes, lymphocytes, and mild fibrosis. In consolidated areas, alveoli with thickened walls were flooded with an intensely pink eosinophilic exudate. The author saw no lesions in the few brains and spinal cords examined.

The cellular response seen in the meninges of red deer calves with small numbers of *E. cervi* in the cerebral subdural space and sulci and on the spinal cord was considered insignificant (Hollands 1985). Rather, the diffuse interstitial pneumonia in most deer older than 6 months was considered the most important aspect of infection. Study of lung lesions was usually complicated by concurrent infections of *E. cervi* and *Dictyocaulus* spp. as well as by an exudative bronchopneumonia associated with fungal infections (Munro and Hunter 1983). The response attributable to *E. cervi* was stronger around eggs than larvae. Alveolar walls were thickened by invading mononuclear cells and eosinophils, and collapsed alveoli were diffuse and infiltrated by macrophages, eosinophils, neutrophils, and multinucleated giant cells.

More marked histopathology was seen in the central nervous system of red deer in Czechoslovakia with only 1 or 2 worms in the cranium (as many as 12 among muscles) (Dykova 1969). Findings included lymphocyctic and eosinophilic infiltrations, granules of hemosiderin, and perivascular cuffing in the meninges over the cerebrum and cerebellum and in the choroid plexus. In an animal with a worm along the sciatic nerve, the spinal cord showed loss of ganglial cells, nodular gliosis, focal demyelinization in the ventral and lateral funiculi at several levels, and focal proliferation of the arachnoid. Extensive demyelinization of the funiculi was seen in one animal in which worms could only be found among muscles. This was said to be typical of a condition referred to as spinal ataxia of cervids.

In maral deer that had died of elaphostrongylosis (possibly complicated by concurrent *Setaria* sp. infections), worms were present in the subdural space and foci of inflammatory exudate, hemorrhage and engorged vessels were visible in the cranial meninges, and excess clear fluid filled the ventricles (Pryadko et al. 1963). Microscopic lesions were described as hemorrhagic leptomeningitis, productive pachymeningitis, and aseptic encephalomyelitis spreading over the brain and spinal cord. Despite clear evidence of the potential to cause serious disease, the pathogenesis of *E. cervi*, surprisingly, has not been studied in detail.

Diagnosis. Infection of cervids is suggested by neurologic disturbance or verminous pneumonia and adult nematodes among skeletal muscle or in the cranium. The form and dimensions of the male gubernaculum and spicules defines the genus *Elaphostrongylus*, and host and locality will assist specific diagnosis. *Setaria* sp. and gadfly infection also cause neurologic disturbance in cervids of central Asia and must be differentiated from *E. cervi* infection (Kontrimavichus et al. 1976). First-stage larvae are shorter than those of *Varestrongylus* spp. (Demiaszkiewicz 1986; Rezác 1990) and the dorsal spine on the tail distinguishes them from *Dictyocaulus*. They may be depressed in number by drug treatment or only be passed intermittently (Presidente 1986b; Gajadhar et al. 1994). Cervid feces are best examined for elaphostrongyline larvae using the Baermann beaker extraction method (Forrester and Lankester 1997) and the examination method of

Gajadhar et al. (1994). Animal importation regulations presently require lengthy quarantine and repeated sampling of feces.

Considerable progress has been made using PCR to identify elaphostrongyline larvae in feces (Gajadhar et al. 2000). Amplification of ITS-2 rDNA of both L_1 and L_3, as well as adult worms, allowed the separation of *Elaphostrongylus* spp. and *Parelaphostrongylus* spp. Available primers distinguished *E. alces* but were not useful in separating *E. rangiferi* from *E. cervi*. A blood test using methods similar to those described for *P. tenuis* in white-tailed deer (Ogunremi et al. 1999a,b) is being tested for *E. cervi*. The Western blot technique using excretory-secretory and somatic antigens from L_3's, detected anti- *E. cervi* antibodies in red deer as early as 23 days after infection (Ogunremi et al. 1998).

Control and Treatment. Mason and Gladden (1983) and Mason (1995) concluded that no effective drug treatment is known to rid animals of *E. cervi,* although benzimidazole and ivermectin may suppress or decrease larval production. Nonetheless, a measure of parasite control has been achieved by a variety of anthelminthic treatments using ivermectin (Watson 1986; Presidente 1986b; Kutzer 1987; Sugar and Sarkozy 1988), fenbedazole (Prosl and Kutzer 1982; Mason and Gladden 1983), oxfendazole (Mason and Gladden 1983; Watson 1986), albendazole (Mason and Gladden 1983; Sugar and Sarkozy 1988), thiabendazole (Pryadko et al. 1968, 1971; Shol et al. 1969), and phenthiozine (Osipov 1964). Planned pasture rotation was recommended by Kontrimavichus et al. (1976) as the most effective control of *E. cervi* in farmed species. This involved leaving animals on the same ground during summer for no more than ~30 days (minimum time required for L_3 to develop in gastropods) and not reusing those pastures for at least 2 years.

Domestic Animal Health Concerns. Apart from farmed deer, *E. cervi* is not otherwise a problem in domestic stock. Panin (1964a) concluded from experimental infections that *E. cervi* does not develop in sheep. This was confirmed by the absence of infection in these hosts pastured with infected maral deer on Altai farms. Kontrimavichus et al. (1976) concurred. Recently, however, *E. cervi* has been reported in goats of Switzerland (Pusterla et al. 1997, 1998). Clinical disease was seen mostly in winter in different areas of Switzerland where goats were in close contact with red deer. Animals exhibited progressive pelvic limb ataxia, recumbency, vestibular disease, circling, proprioceptive deficits, reduced skin sensation, and cranial nerve reflex deficit. Infection with *E. cervi* was diagnosed from clinical signs, mononuclear cells and eosinophils in the cerbrospinal fluid, and finding sections of nematodes in the brains of two animals.

Management Implications. Intensity of infection apparently determines the severity and outcome of elaphostrongylosis. Disease is most evident on deer farms in Europe. Accordingly, appropriate stocking densities and animal mangement techniques should be established in concordance with knowledge of the parasite's seasonal transmission and local climatic conditions. On deer farms in central and eastern Asia, this parasite is an important cause of economic loss due to reduced quantity and quality of deer products, forced slaughter, and abortion (Pryadko 1976a; Kontrimavichus et al. 1976). In one particularly bad epizootic in the winter of 1961–1962, 64% of the animals on one farm were lost due to *E. cervi* infection (Pryadko et al. 1963). Its importance in wild red deer populations probably deserves careful vigilance, particularly in relation to possible climate change and improved conditions for transmission in particular areas.

The parasite is considered important in New Zealand, not because of health risks to red deer but because its presence prevents the export of live animals to Australia, Canada, and possibly elsewhere because of concerns for the health of native cervids in receiving countries (Presidente 1986a,b; Gadjadhar et al. 1994; Mason 1995).

ELAPHOSTRONGYLUS ALCES STÉEN, CHABAUD AND REHBINDER, 1989

Classification: Nematoda: Metastrongyloidea: Protostrongylidae.

Synonyms: *Elaphostrongylus cervi* (Stuve 1986, 1987; Stuve and Skorping 1987; Halvorsen and Wissler 1983a; **not** Cameron 1931).

Common Names: Brain worm, elaphostrongylosis, cerebrospinal nematodiasis.

Elaphostrongylus alces is known only from moose of Sweden, Norway, and Finland (Stéen et al. 1989; Gibbons et al. 1991; Stéen et al. 1998a). In this host it causes neurologic disease and has been associated with emaciation and death, particularly of calves and yearlings. Experimental infection of other native cervids is possible, but the extent to which this occurs in nature is unknown. Domestic animals may not be susceptible.

Earlier reviews of the biology and pathogenesis of *E. alces* are provided by Stéen (1991) and Stéen et al. (1998a) and of the morphology by Stéen and Mørner (1985), Stéen and Johansson (1990), Stéen (1991), and Gibbons et al. (1991).

Life History. Adult *E. alces* are found immediately beneath the epimysium or in fasciae between muscle bundles (Stéen and Rehbinder 1986, Stuve and Skorping 1987). Predilection sites include the superficial thoracic muscles and between the gracilis and sartorius muscles. Worms associated with the central nervous system are found outside of the dura in the fat and loose connective tissue within the vertebral canal. Males are up to 4.7 cm x 0.15 mm wide and females up to 7.0 cm x 0.22 mm (Gibbons et al. 1991; Stéen et al. 1998b).

Eggs released by females, both within the epidural space and on muscles, may hatch in situ or are transported to the lungs by the venous circulation. First-stage larvae developing in the lungs move up the respiratory tree and are swallowed and passed in feces. Nothing is known of their ability to survive external conditions. Larvae must penetrate a terrestrial gastropod to develop to the L_2 and then the L_3 or infective-stage larva (Tables 9.4 and 9.5). In the snail *Arianta arbustorum* held at 20° C, almost all L_1's developed to L_3 within 40 days (Lankester et al. 1998). Snails known to become naturally infected in Sweden include *Arion subfuscus, Deroceras agreste, D. reticulatum, Limax cinereoniger, Succinea* spp., *Vitrina pellucida,* and *Zonitoides nitidus* (Olsson et al. 1995).

Moose become infected by accidentally ingesting infected gastropods. The route taken by migrating L_3's is not known, but they may undergo a direct tissue route to the vertebral canal and then into the skeletal muscles, somewhat like that of *E. rangiferi* (Olsson et al. 1998). An important difference, however, is that most worms do not penetrate beneath the dura (Stéen and Rehbinder 1986; Stuve and Skorping 1987; Stéen 1991). Instead, they appear to develop to the adult stage epidurally near lateral nerves and surrounding fat and connective tissue within the vertebral canal. Whether some L_3's migrate directly to muscles (without being associated with peripheral nerve tissue) is yet to be determined. Adult worms were found in the epidural space and on muscle of moose as early as 6 weeks after experimental infection (Stéen 1991; Stéen et al. 1997). In an animal killed almost 7 months after infection, 32 worms were found in the musculature, compared to 12 still in the epidural space (Stuve and Skorping 1987). A wild moose calf killed at 8–10 months had 8 worms in the epidural space and only 2 among muscles (Stuve 1987).

The prepatent period of *E. alces* is relatively short compared to other *Elaphostrongylus* spp. One moose calf passed larvae 63 days postinfection (Stuve and Skorping 1987). Five other infected calves first passed larvae at 39–73 days postinfection (Stéen et al. 1997).

Several studies indicate that many calves become infected in their first summer of life (Stéen and Rehbinder 1986; Stuve 1987; Olsson et al. 1995). Apparently, the output of L_1's quickly peaks following patency and then declines. One calf given 360 L_3's passed peak numbers of L_1's (1920 larvae/g) 67 days after patency, but numbers quickly declined thereafter by almost two-thirds (Stuve and Skorping 1987).

Epizootiology

DISTRIBUTION AND HOST RANGE. The parasite is so far known throughout Norway and Sweden, and probably Finland (Stéen et al. 1989; Gibbons et al. 1991; Stéen et al. 1998a). Adult *Elaphostrongylus* sp. have been reported in moose of Sweden by Nilsson (1971), Roneus et al. (1984), and Stéen and M.rner (1985); in moose of southern Norway by Holt (1982) and Stuve (1980b, 1987); and in moose of northern Norway by Halvorsen and Wissler (1983a). Halvorsen et al. (1989)

failed to infect reindeer with larvae originating from wild moose, but Stéen et al. (1997, 1998b) succeeded. Six reindeer calves given 1000 L_3's of *E. alces* became patent 39–133 days postinfection, but only low numbers of larvae were shed intermittently. In guinea pigs, only 4% of administered L_3's pentrated the gut wall, and only 1 larva moved beyond the abdominal cavity into the mediastinal tissue of the thorax (Olsson et al. 1998). None reached the spinal canal or associated musculature.

PREVALENCE AND INTENSITY. As with other elaphostrongylines, estimates of prevalence and intensity can be influenced greatly by the age and sex composition of the sample, as well as by sampling time. The prevalence of larvae was as high as 35% in both southern and northern Norway (Stuve 1986; Halvorsen and Wissler 1983a; respectively) and 49% in central Sweden (Stéen and Rehbinder 1986) on examining feces and lungs of mostly adult moose shot by hunters in late September and October. However, when samples included mostly calves taken from January to April (8–11 months old), the prevalence of adult worms and larvae in feces was as high as 88% in southern Norway (Stuve 1987) and 71% in southeastern Sweden (Olsson et al. 1995). Yearlings were most frequently infected, and prevalence declined with increasing age; no moose older than 4.5 years passed larvae (Stuve 1986). Males may be more frequently infected than females (Stuve 1986; Halvorsen and Wissler 1983a). Prevalence was not correlated with moose density or with the presence of other cervids (Stuve 1986).

Calves in southern Norway had 1–9 adult *E. alces* associated with the spinal canal (mean = 4) (Stuve 1987), and the majority of infected calves examined from the Swedish island of Uto had 4–10 (Olsson et al. 1995); carcasses were not available for examination in either study. Up to 30 adult worms in total were recovered in the central nervous system and musculature of naturally infected calves (Stéen and Rehbinder 1986). Mean larval counts in southern Norway were 39 larvae/g (max. = 1215) in calves, 33 larvae/g in yearlings, and 53 larvae/g (max. = 1415) in adults (2.5–4.5 years) (Stuve 1986); and in calves from Uto the larval count was 20 larvae/g (max. = 174) (Olsson et al. 1995).

Levels of infection in gastropods were studied by Olsson et al. (1995) at Uto, where only moose had *E. alces.* One percent of 2025 snails and slugs had a mean of 4.3 ± 5.2 larvae; 8 had only 1 larva, while 1 had 20. The snails, *Succinea* spp., and the slugs, *Deroceras* spp., were the most numerous and frequently infected (1.2% and 2.4%, respectively). They were also the species most frequently found crawling high on vegetation in damp weather (Olsson et al. 1995).

Clinical Signs. Although the majority of infected animals show no signs of clinical disease, some may exhibit pronounced neurologic disturbance. Naturally infected moose calves were described as being weak, displaying uncoordinated movements and lameness, rising with difficulty, and having hindquarters that are lowered, unsteady, and swaying (Stéen and Rehbinder 1986; Stéen and Roepstorff 1990; Stéen 1991). The hind limbs had a broad-base stance, and much of the body weight was borne by the forelegs. Animals were notably alert. A calf given 360 L_3's first showed lameness of a hind leg 75 days postinfection (Stuve and Skorping 1987). Mild signs of ataxia and stiffness that followed gradually faded and were no longer apparent when the animal was killed at 202 days. The intermittent lameness and moderate neurologic disturbance observed were attributed to worms moving within the epidural space and to possible compression and inflammation of spinal nerves.

Infection with *E. alces* frequently has been associated with emaciation, slow growth, and underdevelopment of calves (Stéen et al. 1998a), yet mean carcass weights of infected calves shot in southern Norway (Stuve 1987) and Uto (Olsson et al. 1995) did not differ from those of uninfected calves. Stuve (1986), however, found carcass weights of infected adult moose ($\geq$ 2.5 years) to be significantly lower than those of noninfected adults. Those with clinical neurologic disease usually are emaciated, probably as a result of impaired feeding (Stéen and Rehbinder 1986).

Pathology. Principal gross lesions include edema, hemorrhage, and yellowish-brown discoloration with serous atrophy of fat associated with worms in the epidural space of the vertebral canal (Stéen and Rehbinder 1986; Stuve 1987; Stuve and Skorping 1987). Such lesions usually are not seen in the cervical spine or cranium. In fascia and on skeletal muscles, worms often are associated with focal hemorrhage. Scattered subpleural and interstitial petechiae are notable in lungs.

Generally, the inflammatory response toward adults and larvae in the central nervous system is slight or absent, but much more intense around eggs (Stéen and Rehbinder 1986). The epidural connective tissue may contain focal accumulations of granulocytes, mononuclear cells, neutrophils, and giant cells extending close to spinal nerves and the outer dura (Stuve and Skorping 1987). Small veins and lymph vessels are occasionally thrombotic and surrounded with accumulations of eosinophils and macrophages containing hemosiderin. Lesions were not found in the leptomeninges or in the neural parenchyma of naturally infected calves by Stuve and Skorping (1987). In contrast, Stéen and Rehbinder (1986) noted several cases with mild infiltrations of lymphocytes, plasma cells, and macrophages in the cranial and spinal leptomeninges, and one calf with an adult worm in the subdural space of the cerebrum had associated mild cerebral gliosis.

Histological examination of the skeletal muscles reveals moderate infiltrations of eosinophils, macrophages, neutrophils, and lymphocytes in the endomysium, epimysium, and loose connective tissue adjacent to adult worms. A mild bronchopneumonia is common in infected calves (Stuve 1987). Eggs disseminated throughout the lungs appear to be in capillaries, causing embolic occlusions with infiltrating macrophages, neurtrophils, and lymphocyctes (Stuve and Skorping 1987).

Pathology of *E. alces* in reindeer, sheep, and goats was described by Stéen et al. (1998b). Despite relatively heavy experimental infection of a reindeer, histopathological lesions were rare and included only a mild response with granulocytes and mononuclear cells on the outer surface of the spinal dura and epidurally around lateral nerves and lymph nodes. Inflammatory lesions attributable to *E. alces* in infected sheep and goats were mild and nonspecific (Stéen et al. 1998b) or absent (Stuve and Skorping 1990).

Diagnosis. Developing adult worms occur in the epidural rather than in the subdural spaces as is seen with other *Elaphostrongylus* spp. (Stéen and Rehbinder 1986). Characteristic of the genus, males have a simple gubernaculum lacking crura. The bursa is oval and longer and has more slender bursal rays than other *Elaphostrongylus* spp. Females are longer and wider, have a bottle-shaped esophagus not seen in congeners, a more pointed distal end, and a less well-developed genital cone (Stéen et al. 1989; Stéen and Johansson 1990; Gibbons et al. 1991). The morphometrics of L_1's are similar to those of related species, but the mean length of L_3's is significantly shorter than both *E. cervi* and *E. rangiferi*, although the range of some measurements overlap (Table 9.5) (Lankester et al. 1998). Isoelectric focusing of adult and larval proteins has been used to separate *E. alces* from *E. rangiferi* (Stéen et al. 1994). *Varestrongylus alcis* is a common parasite of moose in Fennoscandia and produces dorsal-spined L_1's that differ from those of *E. alces* only by being slightly shorter. Progress has been made using PCR to identify elaphostrongyline larvae in feces (Gajadhar et al. (2000) (see Diagnosis section for *E. cervi,* above).

Immunity. Some form of acquired immunity probably explains the observed decline in prevalence and intensity with age and the absence of larvae in feces of moose older than 4.5 years (Stuve 1986).

Domestic Animal Health Concerns. Attempts by Stuve and Skorping (1990) to infect domestic sheep and goats with *E. alces* from moose in Norway were unsuccessful. However, finding protostrongylid eggs in the lungs of an experimentally infected kid led Stéen et al. (1998b) to suggest that *E. alces* might be capable of maturing in this host.

Management Implications. The parasite apparently is of little concern to the health of cervids other than moose or to domestic livestock. It is, however, a widespread parasite of moose in Fennoscandia (and likely further east), and conditions that promote transmission periodically will increase the frequency of neurologic disease observed, particularly in young animals. The short- and long-term impact of such disease on moose populations is difficult to measure, as it is for almost all other helminth diseases of wildlife. Yet in the 1980's, several authors attributed increased moose mortality during winter, particularly of calves, to elaphostrongylosis (Holt 1982; Stéen and Mørner 1985; Stéen 1991). Others, however, consider it to be only of moderate (Stuve 1986; Stuve and Skorping 1987) or little importance (Nikander in Stéen et al. 1998a).

LITERATURE CITED

Parelaphostrongylus

Aho, R.W., and J. Hendrickson. 1989. Reproduction and mortality of moose translocated from Ontario to Michigan. *Alces* 25:75–80.

Alden, C., F. Woodson, R. Mohan, and S. Miller. 1975. Cerebrospinal nematodiasis in sheep. *Journal of the American Veterinary Medical Association* 166:784–786.

Anderson, R.C. 1956. *Elaphostrongylus odocoilei* Hobmaier and Hobmaier, 1934 in the cranial case of *Odocoileus virginianus borealis* Miller. *Canadian Journal of Zoology* 34:167–173.

———. 1963a. The incidence, development, and experimental transmission of *Pneumostrongylus tenuis* Dougherty (Metastrongyloidea: Protostrongylidae) of the meninges of the white-tailed deer (*Odocoileus virginianus borealis*) in Ontario. *Canadian Journal of Zoology* 41:775–802.

———. 1963b. Studies on *Pneumostrongylus tenuis* Dougherty, 1945 of *Odocoileus virginianus*. *The Journal of Parasitology* 49:40–47.

———. 1964a. Motor ataxia and paralysis in moose calves infected experimentally with *Pneumostrongylus tenuis* (Nematoda: Metastrongyloides). *Northeastern Wildlife Conference,* Hartford, Connecticut, January 21, pp. 1–7.

———. 1964b. Neurologic disease in moose infected experimentally with *Pneumostrongylus tenuis* from white-tailed deer. *Veterinary Pathology* 1:289–322.

———. 1965a. An examination of wild moose exhibiting neurologic signs, in Ontario. *Canadian Journal of Zoology* 43:635–639.

———. 1965b. Cerebrospinal nematodiasis (*Pneumostrongylus tenuis*) in North American cervids. *Transactions of the North American Wildlife and Natural Resources Conference* 13:156–167.

———. 1965c. The development of *Pneumostrongylus tenuis* in the central nervous system of white-tailed deer. *Pathologia Veterinaria* 2:360–379.

———. 1968. The pathogenesis and transmission of neurotropic and accidental nematode parasites of the central nervous system of mammals and birds. *Helminthological Abstracts* 37:191–210.

———. 1971a. Lungworms. In *Parasitic diseases of wild mammals.* Ed. J.W. Davis and R.C. Anderson. Ames: The Iowa State University Press, pp. 81–126.

———. 1971b. Neurologic disease in reindeer (*Rangifer tarandus tarandus*) introduced into Ontario. *Canadian Journal of Zoology* 49:159–166.

———. 1972. The ecological relationships of meningeal worm and native cervids in North America. *Journal of Wildlife Diseases* 8:304–310.

———. 2000. *Nematode parasites of vertebrates: Their development and transmission,* 2nd ed. Cambridge: C.A.B. International, University Press, Cambridge, 650 pp.

Anderson, R.C., and A.K. Prestwood. 1981. Lungworms. In *Diseases and parasites of white-tailed deer.* Ed. W.R. Davidson, F.A. Hayes, V.F. Nettles, and F.E. Kellogg.

Miscellaneous Publications Number 7. Tallahassee, FL: Tall Timbers Research Station, pp. 266–317.

Anderson, R.C., and U.R. Strelive. 1966a. Experimental cerebrospinal nematodiasis (*Pneumostrongylus tenuis*) in sheep. *Canadian Journal of Zoology* 44:889–894.

———. 1966b. The transmission of *Pneumostrongylus tenuis* to guinea pigs. *Canadian Journal of Zoology* 44:533–540.

———. 1967. The penetration of *Pneumostrongylus tenuis* into the tissues of white-tailed deer. *Canadian Journal of Zoology* 45:285–289.

———. 1968. The experimental transmission of *Pneumostrongylus tenuis* to caribou (*Rangifer tarandus terraenovae*). *Canadian Journal of Zoology* 46:503–510.

———. 1969. The effect of *Pneumostrongylus tenuis* (Nematoda: Metastrongyloidea) on kids. *Canadian Journal of Comparative Medicine* 33:280–286.

———. 1972. Experimental cerebrospinal nematodiasis in kids. *The Journal of Parasitology* 58:816.

Anderson, R.C., M.W. Lankester, and U.R. Strelive. 1966. Further experimental studies of *Pneumostrongylus tenuis* in cervids. *Canadian Journal of Zoology* 44:851–861.

Ballantyne, R.J., and W.M. Samuel. 1984. Diagnostic morphology of the third-stage larvae of three species of *Parelaphostrongylus* (Nematoda, Metastrongyloidea). *The Journal of Parasitology* 70:602–604.

Baumgartner, W., A. Zajac, B.L. Hull, F. Andrews, and F. Garry. 1985. Parelaphostrongylosis in llamas. *Journal of the American Veterinary and Medical Association* 187:1243–1245.

Beach, T.D. 1992. Transmission of meningeal worm: An analysis of sympatric use of habitat by white-tailed deer, moose and gastropods. M.Sc. Thesis, University of New Brunswick, Fredericton, New Brunswick, 214 pp.

Beaulieu-Goudreault, M. 1981. Etude des endoparasites et plus specialement du ver des meninges (*Parelaphostrongylus tenuis*) du cerf de virginie (*Odocoileus virginianus*) a l'ile d'Anticosti. M.S. Thesis, Universite McGill, Montreal, Quebec, 65 pp.

Behrend, D.F. 1970. The nematode, *Pneumostrongylus tenuis,* in white-tailed deer in the Adirondacks. *New York Fish and Game Journal* 17:45–49.

Behrend, D.F., and J.F. Witter. 1968. *Pneumostrongylus tenuis* in white-tailed deer in Maine. *The Journal of Wildlife Management* 32:963–966.

Benson, D.A., and G.D. Dodds. 1977. *The deer of Nova Scotia.* Department of Lands and Forests, Nova Scotia, 92 pp.

Bienek, D.R., N.F. Neumann, W.M. Samuel, and M. Belosevic. 1998. Meningeal worm evokes a heterogenous immune response in elk. *Journal of Wildlife Diseases* 34:334–341.

Bergerud, A.T. and W.E. Mercer. 1989. Caribou introductions in eastern North America. *Wildlife Society Bulletin* 17:111–120.

Bogaczyk, B. 1990. A survey of metastrongyloid parasites in Maine cervids. M.Sc. Thesis, University of Maine, Orono, Maine, 60 pp.

Bogaczyk, B.A. 1992. A search for *Parelaphostrongylus andersoni* in white-tailed deer from Maine. *Journal of Wildlife Diseases* 28:311–312.

Bogacyzk, B.A., W.B. Krohn, and H.C. Gibbs. 1993. Factors affecting *Parelaphostrongylus tenuis* in white-tailed deer (*Odocoileus virginianus*) from Maine. *Journal of Wildlife Diseases* 29:266–272.

Bresele, L.M. 1990. Attempts to differentiate elaphostrongyline larvae (Nematoda: Protostrongylidae) using guinea pigs (*Cavia porcellus*) as alternate hosts. M.Sc. Thesis, Lakehead University, Thunder Bay, Ontario, 87 pp.

Brown, J.E. 1983. *Parelaphostrongylus tenuis* (Pryadko and Boev) in the moose and white-tailed deer of Nova Scotia.

M.Sc. Thesis, Acadia University, Wolfville, Nova Scotia, 117 pp.

Brown, T.T., Jr., H.E. Jordan, and C.N. Demorest. 1978. Cerebrospinal parelaphostrongylosis in llamas. *Journal of Wildlife Diseases* 14:441–444.

Brunetti, O.A. 1969. Redescription of *Parelaphostrongylus* (Boev and Schulz, 1950) in California deer, with studies on its life history and pathology. *California Fish and Game* 55:307–316.

Carpenter, J.W., H.E. Jordan, and B.C. Ward. 1973. Neurologic disease in wapiti naturally infected with meningeal worms. *Journal of Wildlife Diseases* 9:148–153.

Carreno, R.A., and E.P. Hoberg. 1999. Evolutionary relationships among the protostrongylidae (Nematoda: Metastrongyloidea) as inferred from morphological characters, with consideration of parasite-host coevolution. *The Journal of Parasitology* 85:638–648.

Carreno, R.A., and M.W. Lankester. 1993. Additional information on the morphology of the Elaphostrongylinae (Nematoda: Protostrongylidae) of North American Cervidae. *Canadian Journal of Zoology* 71:592–600.

———. 1994. A re-evaluation of the phylogeny of *Parelaphostrongylus* Boev & Schulz, 1950 (Nematoda, Protostrongylidae). *Systematic Parasitology* 28:145–151.

Clark, R.A., and R.T. Bowyer. 1986. Occurrence of protostrongylid nematodes in sympatric populations of moose and white-tailed deer in Maine. *Alces* 22:313–322.

Claveau, R., and J.-P. Fillion. 1984. Fréquence et distribution du ver des méninges (*Parelaphostrongylus tenuis*) chez le cerf de virginie de l'est du Quebec. *Naturaliste Canadien* 111:203–206.

Comer, J.A., W.R. Davidson, A.K. Prestwood, and V.F. Nettles. 1991. An update on the distribution of *Parelaphostrongylus tenuis* in the southeastern United States. *Journal of Wildlife Diseases* 27:348–354.

Dauphiné, T.C. 1975. The disappearance of caribou reintroduced to Cape Breton Highlands National Park. *Canadian Field-Naturalist* 89:299–310.

Davidson, W.R., J.M. Crum, J.L. Blue, D.W. Sharp, and J.H. Phillips. 1985. Parasites, diseases, and health status of sympatric populations of fallow deer and white-tailed deer in Kentucky. *Journal of Wildlife Diseases* 21:153–159.

Davidson, W.R., G.L. Doster, and R.C. Freeman. 1996. *Parelaphostrongylus tenuis* on Wassaw Island, Georgia: A result of translocating white-tailed deer. *Journal of Willife Diseases* 32:701–703.

Devlin, D. and W. Drake. 1989. Pennsylvania Elk Census— 1989. Annual Unpublished Report, Pennsylvania Game Commission, Harrisburg, Pennsylvania, 8pp.

Dew, T.L. 1988. Prevalence of *Parelaphostrongylus tenuis* in a sample of hunter-harvested white-tailed deer from a tri-county area in northeastern Wisconsin. *Journal of Wildlife Diseses* 24:720–721.

Dew, T.L., D.D. Bowman, and R.B. Grieve. 1992. Parasite-specific immunoglobulin in the serum and cerebrospinal fluid of white-tailed deer (*Odocoileus virginianus*) and goats (*Capra hircus*) with experimentally induced parelaphostrongylosis. *Journal of Zoo and Wildlife Medicine* 23:281–287.

de With, N., C. Ribble, J.J. Aramini, F.A. Leighton, G. Wobeser. 1998. Risk assessment for the importation of farmed elk to Saskatchewan from Ontario with respect to *Elaphostrongylus cervi* and *Parelaphostrongylus tenuis*. A report of the Canadian Cooperative Wildlife Health Centre, 37 pp.

Dougherty, E.C. 1945. The nematode lungworms (suborder Strongylina) of North American deer of the genus *Odocoileus*. *Parasitology* 36:199–208.

Duffy, M.S., C.E. Tanner, and M.D.B. Burt. 1993. Serodiagnosis of *Parelaphostrongylus tenuis* in white-tailed deer

Odocoileus virginianus. Proceeding of the International Union of Game Biologists XXI Congress, Halifax, Nova Scotia, vol. 2, pp. 92–95.

Dumont, A. and M. Créte. 1996. The meningeal worm, *Parelaphostrongylus tenuis,* a marginal limiting factor for moose, *Alces alces,* in southern Quebec. *Canadian Field Naturalist* 110:413–418.

Duncan, R.B. and S. Patton. 1998. Naturally occurring cerebrospinal parelaphostrongylosis in a heifer. *Journal of Veterinary Diagnostic Investigation* 10:287–291.

Eckroade, R.J., G.M. ZuRhein, M. Gabriele, and W. Foreyt. 1970. Meningeal worm invasion of the brain of a naturally infected white-tailed deer. *Journal of Wildlife Diseases* 6:430–436.

Edwards, W.H. 1995. *Parelaphostrongylus andersoni* (Nematoda: Protostrongylidae) in white-tailed deer (*Odocoileus virginianus*) of northeastern Wyoming. M.Sc. Thesis, University of Wyoming, Laramie, Wyoming, 83 pp.

Foreyt, W.J., and B.B. Compton. 1991. Survey for meningeal worm (*Parelaphostrongylus tenuis*) and ear mites in white-tailed deer from northern Idaho. *Journal of Wildlife Diseases* 27:716–718.

Foreyt, W.J., and D.O. Trainer. 1980. Seasonal parasitism changes in two populations of white-tailed deer in Wisconsin. *Journal of Wildlife Management* 44:758–764.

Foreyt, W.J., L.G. Rickard, S. Dowling, S. Parish, and M. Pipas. 1992. Experimental infections of two llamas with the meningeal worm (*Parelaphostrongylus tenuis*). *Journal of Zoo Wildlife Medicine* 22:339–344.

Forrester, D.J. 1992. *Parasites and diseases of wild mammals in Florida.* Gainsville: University Press of Florida, Gainsville, 459 pp.

Forrester, S.G., and M.W. Lankester. 1997a. Extracting protostrongylid nematode larvae from ungulate feces. *Journal of Wildlife Diseases* 33:511–516.

———. 1997b. Extracting *Protostrongylus* spp. larvae from bighorn sheep feces. *Journal of Wildlife Diseases* 33:868–872.

———. 1998. Over-winter survival of first-stage larvae of *Parelaphostrongylus tenuis* (Nematoda: Protostrongylidae). *Canadian Journal of Zoology* 76:704–710.

Gajadhar, A., T. Steeves-Gurnsey, J. Kendall, M. Lankester, and M. Steen. 2000. Differentiation of dorsal-spined elaphostrongyline larvae by polymerase chain reaction amplification of ITS-2 rDNA. *Journal of Wildlife Diseases* 36:713–723.

Garner, D.L., and W.F. Porter. 1991. Prevalence of *Parelaphostrongylus tenuis* in white-tailed deer in northern New York. *Journal of Wildlife Diseases* 27:594–598.

Garrison, R.C., D.C. Ashley, and D.J. Robbins. 1987. The 1986 survey for meningeal worm in white-tailed deer in northwestern Missouri. *Transactions of the Missouri Academy of Science* 21:149.

Gilbert, F.F. 1973. *Parelaphostrongylus tenuis* (Dougherty) in Maine: I—The parasite in white-tailed deer (*Odocoileus virginianus,* Zimmermann). *Journal of Wildlife Diseases* 9:136–143.

———. 1974. *Parelaphostrongylus tenuis* in Maine: II—prevalence in moose. *The Journal of Wildlife Management* 38:42–46.

———. 1992. Retroductive logic and the effects of meningeal worm: A comment. *The Journal of Wildlife Management* 56:614–616.

Gleich, J.G., F.F. Gilbert, and N.P. Kutscha. 1977. Nematodes in terrestrial gastropods from central Maine. *Journal of Wildlife Diseases* 13:43–46.

Gogan, P.J.P., P.A. Jordan, and J.L. Nielson. 1990. Planning to reintroduce woodland caribou to Minnesota. *Transactions of the North American Wildlife and Natural Resources Conference* 55:599–608.

Gogan, P.J.P., K.D. Kozie, E.M. Olexia and N.S. Duncan. 1997. Ecological status of moose and white-tailed deer at Voyageurs National Park, Minnesota. *Alces* 33:187– 201.

Gray, J.B., and W.M. Samuel. 1986. *Parelaphostrongylus odocoilei* (Nematoda: Protostrongylidae) and a protostrongylid nematode in woodland caribou (*Rangifer tarandus caribou*) of Alberta, Canada. *Journal of Wildlife Diseases* 22:48–50.

Guthery, F.S., and S.L. Beasom. 1979. Cerebrospinal nematodiasis caused by *Parelaphostrongylus tenuis* in angora goats in Texas. *Journal of Wildlife Diseases* 15:37–42.

Hart, M. 1983. The effect of diurnal temperature variation on the larval development of *Parelaphostrongylus odocoilei*. Unpublished Report, Department of Zoology, University of Alberta, Edmonton.

Hawkins, J.W., M.W. Lankester, and R.A. Nelson. 1998. Sampling terrestrial gastropods using cardboard sheets. *Malacologia* 39:1–9.

Hobmaier, A., and M. Hobmaier. 1934. *Elaphostrongylus odocoilei* n.sp., a new lungworm in black-tailed deer (*Odocoileus columbianus*). Description and life history. *Proceedings of the Society for Experimental Biology and Medicine* 31:509–514.

Hobmaier, M. 1937. Studies on the pathology of *Elaphostrongylus odocoilei* in *Odocoileus columbianus columbianus*. *Raboty Gel'mint* 22:235–240.

Ives, A.R., D.L. Murray. 1997. Can sublethal parasitism destabilize predator-prey population dynamics? A model of snowshoe hares, predators and parasites. *Journal of Animal Ecology* 66:265–278.

Jarvinen, J.A., and W.A. Hedberg. 1993. *Parelaphostrongylus tenuis* (Nematoda) in white-tailed deer (*Odocoileus virginianus*) in central Iowa. *The Journal of Parasitology* 79:116–119.

Jortner, B.S., H.F. Troutt, T. Collins, and K. Scarratt. 1985. Lesions of spinal cord parelaphostrongylosis in sheep. Sequential changes following intramedullary larval migration. *Veterinary Pathology* 22:137–140.

Karns, P.D. 1966. *Pneumostrongylus tenuis* from elk (*Cervus canadensis*) in Minnesota. *Bulletin of the Wildlife Disease Association* 2:79–80.

———. 1967. *Pneumostrongylus tenuis* in deer in Minnesota and implications for moose. *Journal of Wildlife Management* 31:299–303.

———. 1977. Deer-moose relationships with emphasis on *Parelaphostrongylus tenuis*. *Minnesota Wildlife Research Quarterly* 37:40–61.

———. 1979. Survey of *Parelaphostrongylus tenuis* as a potential limiting factor to woodland caribou (*Rangifer tarandus*) in northern Minnesota. Unpublished Report, Minnesota Department of Natural Resources, Grand Rapids.

Kearney, S.R., and F.F. Gilbert. 1976. Habitat use by white-tailed deer and moose on sympatric range. *The Journal of Wildlife Management* 40:645–657.

———. 1978. Terrestrial gastropods from the Himsworth Game Preserve, Ontario, and their significance in *Parelaphostrongylus tenuis* transmission. *Canadian Journal of Zoology* 56:688–694.

Kelsall, J.P., and W. Prescott. 1971. *Moose and deer behaviour in snow in Fundy National Park, New Brunswick*. Report Series Canadian Wildlife Service, No. 15, 25 pp.

Kistner, T.P., G.R. Johnson, and G.A. Rilling. 1977. Naturally occurring neurologic disease in a fallow deer infected with meningeal worms. *Journal of Wildlife Diseases* 13:55–58.

Kocan, A.A. 1985. The use of ivermectin in the treatment and prevention of infection with *Parelaphostrongylus tenuis* (Dougherty) (Nematoda: Metastrongyloidea) in white-tailed deer (*Odocoileus virginianus* Zimmermann). *Journal of Wildlife Diseases* 21:454–455.

Kocan, A.A., M.G. Shaw, K.A. Waldrup, and G.J. Kubat. 1982. Distribution of *Parelaphostrongylus tenuis* (Nematoda: Metastrongyloidea) in white-tailed deer from Oklahoma. *Journal of Wildlife Diseases* 18:457–460.

Kopcha, M., J.V. Marteniuk, R. Sills, B. Steficek, and T.W. Schillhorn van Veen. 1989. Cerebrospinal nematodiasis in a goat herd. *Journal of the American Veterinary Medical Association* 194:1439–1442.

Krogdahl, D.W., J.P. Thilsted, and S.K. Olsen. 1987. Ataxia and hypermetria caused by *Parelaphostrongylus tenuis* infection in llamas. *Journal of the American Veterinary and Medical Association* 190:191–193.

Kurtz, H.J., K. Loken, and J.C. Schlotthauer. 1966. Histopathologic studies on cerebrospinal nematodiasis of moose in Minnesota naturally infected with *Pneumostrongylus tenuis*. *American Journal of Veterinary Research* 27:548–558.

Lankester, M.W. 1967. Gastropods as intermediate hosts of *Pneumostrongylus tenuis* Dougherty, of white-tailed deer. M.Sc. Thesis, University of Guelph, Guelph, Ontario, 68pp.

———. 1974. *Parelaphostrongylus tenuis* (Nematoda) and *Fascioloides magna* (Trematoda) in moose of southeastern Manitoba. *Canadian Journal of Zoology* 52:235–239.

———. 1977. Neurologic disease in moose caused by *Elaphostrongylus cervi* Cameron, 1931 from caribou. *Proceedings of the 13th North American Moose Conference and Workshop,* Jasper, Alberta, pp. 177–190.

———. 1987. Pests, parasites and diseases of moose (*Alces alces*) in North America. *Swedish Wildlife Research (Viltrevy). Supplement* 1:461–489.

Lankester, M.W., and R.C. Anderson. 1968. Gastropods as intermediate hosts of *Pneumostrongylus tenuis* Dougherty. *Canadian Journal of Zoology* 46:373–383.

Lankester, M.W., and D. Fong. 1989. Distribution of elaphostrongyline nematodes (Metastrongyloidea: Protostrongylidae) in cervidae and possible effects of moving *Rangifer* spp. into and within North America. *Alces* 25:133–145.

———. 1998. Protostrongylid nematodes from caribou (*Rangifer tarandus caribou*) and moose (*Alces alces*) in Newfoundland. *Rangifer,* Special Issue No. 10, pp. 73–83.

Lankester, M.W., and P.L. Hauta. 1989. *Parelaphostrongylus andersoni* (Nematoda: Elaphostrongylinae) in caribou (*Rangifer tarandus*) of northern and central Canada. *Canadian Journal of Zoology* 67:1966–1975.

Lankester, M.W., and W.J. Peterson. 1996. The possible importance of deer wintering yards in the transmission of *Parelaphostrongylus tenuis* to white-tailed deer and moose. *Journal of Wildlife Disease* 32:31–38.

Lankester, M.W., and W.M. Samuel. 1998. Pests, parasites, and diseases. In *Ecology and management of the moose.* Ed. A.W. Franzmann and C.C. Schwartz. Washington, DC: A Wildlife Management Institute Book, pp. 479–517.

Lankester, M.W., J.E. G. Smits, M.J. Pybus, D. Fong, and J.C. Haigh. 1990. Experimental infection of fallow deer (*Dama dama*) with elaphostrongyline nematodes (Nematoda: Protostrongylidae) from caribou (*Rangifer tarandus caribou*) in Newfoundland. *Alces* 26:154–162.

Lenarz, M.S., and K.D. Kerr. 1987. An evaluation of *Parelaphostrongylus tenuis* as a source of mortality of moose. Annual Report of the Minnesota Department of Natural Resources, Populations and Research Unit, Grand Rapids, pp. 34–36.

Lunn, D.K., and K.W. Hinchcliff. 1989. Cerebrospinal fluid eosinophilia and ataxia in five llamas. *Veterinary Record* 124:302–305.

Maze, R.J., and C. Johnstone. 1986. Gastropod intermediate hosts of the meningeal worm *Parelaphostrongylus tenuis* in Pennsylvania: Observations on their ecology. *Canadian Journal of Zoology* 64:185–188.

McCollough, M., and B. Connery. 1990. An evaluation of the Maine caribou reintroduction project. Maine Caribou Project Report, University of Maine, Orono, 54 pp.

McCollough, M.A., and K.A. Pollard. 1993. *Parelaphostrongylus tenuis* in Maine moose and the possible influence of faulty Baermann procedures. *Journal of Wildlife Diseases* 29:156–158.

McCoy, K.D. 1997. Prevalence of *Parelaphostrongylus tenuis* in gastropod populations: Ecological and behavioural factors affecting transmission. M.Sc. Thesis, University of Guelph, Guelph, Ontario, 104 pp.

Nettles, V.F., and A.K. Prestwood. 1976. Experimental *Parelaphostrongylus andersoni* infections in white-tailed deer. *Veterinary Pathology* 13:381–393.

———. 1979. Experimental infection of rabbits with meningeal worm. *The Journal of Parasitology* 65:327–328.

Nettles, V.F., A.K. Prestwood, R.G. Nichols, and C.J. Whitehead. 1977a. Meningeal worm-induced neurologic disease in black-tailed deer. *Journal of Wildlife Diseases* 13:137–143.

Nettles, V.F., A.K. Prestwood, and R.D. Smith. 1977b. Cerebrospinal parelaphostrongylosis in fallow deer. *Journal of Wildlife Diseases* 13:440–444.

Neumann, N.F., W.S. Pon, A. Nowicki, W.M. Samuel, and M. Belosevic. 1994. Antigens of adults and third-stage larvae of the meningeal worm, *Parelaphostrongylus tenuis* (Nematoda, Metastrongyloidea). *Journal of Veterinary Diagnostic Investigations* 6:222–229.

Nichols, D.K., R.J. Montali, L.G. Phillips, T.P. Alvarado, M. Bush, and L. Collins. 1986. *Parelaphostrongylus tenuis* in captive reindeer and sable antelope. *Journal of the American Veterinary and Medical Association* 188:619–621.

Nudds, T.D. 1990. Retroductive logic in retrospect: The ecological effects of meningeal worms. *The Journal of Wildlife Management* 54:396–402.

Oates, D.W., M.C. Sterner, and D.J. Steffen. 1999. Meningeal worm in free-ranging deer in Nebraska. *Journal of Wildlife Diseases* 35:101–104.

O'Brien, T.D., T.P. O'Leary, J.R. Sherman, D.L. Stevens, and C.B. Wolf. 1986. Cerebrospinal parelaphostrongylosis in Minnesota. *Minnesota Veterinarian* 26:18–22.

Ogunremi, O., M.W. Lankester, S. Loran, and A. Gajadhar. 1999a. Evaluation of excretory-secretory products and somatic worm antigens for the serodiagnosis of experimental *Parelaphostrongylus tenuis* infection in white-tailed deer. *Journal Veterinary Diagnostic Investigations.* 11:515–521.

Ogunremi, O., M.W. Lankester, and A. Gajadhar. 1999b. Serological diagnosis of *Parelaphostrongylus tenuis* infection in white-tailed deer and identification of a potentially unique parasite antigen. *The Journal of Parasitology* 85:122–127.

Oliver, J.L., S.R. Trosclair, J.M. Morris, D.B. Paulsen, D.E. Duncan, D.-Y. Kim, A.C. Camus, T.J. Vicek, and M.-C. Azara Nasarre. 1996. Neurologic disease attributable to infection with *Parelaphostrongylus tenuis* in blackbuck antelope. *Journal of the American Veterinary Medical Association* 209:140–142.

Olsen, A., and A. Woolf. 1978. The development of clinical signs and the population significance of neurological disease in a captive wapiti herd. *Journal of Wildlife Diseases* 14:263–268.

Olsen, A., and A. Woolf. 1979. A summary of the prevalence of *Parelaphostrongylus tenuis* in a captive wapiti population. *Journal of Wildlife Diseases* 15:33–35.

Parker, G.R. 1966. Moose disease in Nova Scotia. M.Sc. Thesis, Acadia University, Wolfville, Nova Scotia, 126 pp.

Peterson, W.J. 1989. Abnormal antlers and kidney stones in moose displaying symptoms of parelaphostrongylosis. *Alces* 25:11–14.

Peterson, W.J., and M.W. Lankester. 1991. Aspects of the epizootiology of *Parelaphostrongylus tenuis* in a white-tailed deer population. *Alces* 27:183–192.

Peterson, W.J., M.W. Lankester, and M. Riggs. 1996. Seasonal and annual changes in shedding of *Parelaphostrongylus tenuis* larvae by white-tailed deer in northeastern Minnesota. *Alces* 32:61–73.

Pitt, W.C., and P.A. Jordan. 1994. A survey of the nematode parasite *Parelaphostrongylus tenuis* in the white-tailed deer, *Odocoileus virginianus,* in a region proposed for caribou, *Rangifer tarandus caribou,* re-introduction in Minnesota. *Canadian Field Naturalist* 108:341–346.

Platt, T.R. 1978. The life cycle and systematics of *Parelaphostrongylus odocoilei* (Nematoda: Metastrongyloidea), a parasite of mule deer (*Odocoileus hemionus hemionus*), with special reference to the molluscan intermediate host. Ph.D. Thesis, Univesity of Alberta, Edmonton, 233 pp.

———. 1984. Evolution of the Elaphostrongylinae (Nematoda: Metastrongyloidea: Protostrongylidae) parasites of cervids (Mammalia). *Proceedings of the Helminthological Society Washington* 51:196–204.

———. 1989. Gastropod intermediate hosts of *Parelaphostrongylus tenuis* (Nematoda: Matastrongyloidea) from northwestern Indiana. *The Journal of Parasitology* 75:519–523.

Platt, T.R., and W.M. Samuel. 1978a. *Parelaphostrongylus odocoilei:* Life cycle in experimentally infected cervids including the mule deer, *Odocoileus h. hemionus. Experimental Parasitology* 46:330–338.

———. 1978b. A redescription and neotype designation for *Parelaphostrongylus odocoilei* (Nematoda: Metastrongyloidea). *The Journal of Parasitology* 64:226–232.

———. 1984. Mode of entry of first-stage larvae of *Parelaphostrongylus odocoilei* (Nematoda: Metastrongyloidea) into four species of terrestrial gastropods. *Proceedings of the Helminthological Society of Washington* 51:205–207.

Prestwood, A.K. 1970. Neurologic disease in a white-tailed deer massively infected with meningeal worm (*Pneumostrongylus tenuis*). *Journal of Wildlife Diseases* 6:84–86.

———. 1972. *Parelaphostrongylus andersoni* sp.n. (Metastrongyloidea: Protostrongylidae) from the musculature of the white-tailed deer (*Odocoileus virginianus*). *The Journal of Parasitology* 58:897–902.

Prestwood, A.K., and V.F. Nettles. 1977. Repeated low-level infection of white-tailed deer with *Parelaphostrongylus andersoni. The Journal of Parasitology* 63:974–978.

Prestwood, A.K., and J.F. Smith. 1969. Distribution of meningeal worm (*Pneumostrongylus tenuis*) in deer in the southeastern United States. *The Journal of Parasitology* 55:720–725.

Prestwood, A.K., V.F. Nettles, and F.E. Kellogg. 1974. Distribution of muscle worm, (*Parelaphostrongylus andersoni*), among white-tailed deer of the southeastern United States. *Journal of Wildlife Diseases* 10:404–409.

Pursglove, S.R. 1977. Helminth parasites of white-tailed deer (*Odocoileus virginianus*) from New Jersey and Oklahoma. *Proceedings of the Helminthological Society of Washington.* 44:107–108.

Pybus, M.J. 1983. *Parelaphostrongylus andersoni* Prestwood 1972 and *P. odocoilei* (Hobmaier and Hobmaier 1934) (Nematoda: Metastrongyloidea) in two cervid definitive hosts. Ph.D. Thesis, University of Alberta, Edmonton, 185 pp.

Pybus, M.J., and W.M. Samuel. 1980. Pathology of the muscleworm, *Parelaphostrongylus odocoilei* (Nematoda:

Metastrongyloidea), in moose. *Proceedings of the North American Moose Conference and Workshop* 16:152–170.

———. 1981. Nematode muscleworm from white-tailed deer of southeastern British Columbia. *The Journal of Wildlife Management* 45:537–542.

———. 1984a. *Parelaphostrongylus andersoni* (Nematoda: Protostrongylidae) and *P. odocoilei* in two cervid definitive hosts. *The Journal of Parasitology* 70:507–515.

———. 1984b. Attempts to find a laboratory host for *Parelaphostrongylus andersoni* and *Parelaphostrongylus odocoilei* (Nematoda: Protostrongylidae). *Canadian Journal of Zoology* 62:1181–1184.

———. 1984c. Lesions caused by *Parelaphostrongylus odocoilei* (Nematoda: Metastrongyloidea) in two cervid hosts. *Veterinary Pathology* 21:425–431.

Pybus, M.J., and H. Shave. 1984. *Muellerius capillaris* (Mueller, 1889)(Nematoda: Protostrongylidae): An unusual finding in Rocky Mountain bighorn sheep (*Ovis canadensis canadensis* Shaw) in South Dakota. *Journal of Wildlife Diseases* 20:284–288.

Pybus, M.J., W.J. Foreyt, and W.M. Samuel. 1984. Natural infections of *Parelaphostrongylus odocoilei* (Nematoda: Protostrongylidae) in several hosts and locations. *Proceedings of the Helminthological Society of Washington* 51:338–340.

Pybus, M.J., W.M. Samuel, and V. Crichton. 1989. Identification of dorsal spined larvae from free-ranging wapiti (*Cervus elaphus*) in southwestern Manitoba, Canada. *Journal of Wildlife Diseases* 25:291–293.

Pybus, M.J., W.M. Samuel, D.A. Welch, and C.J. Wilke. 1990. *Parelaphostrongylus andersoni* (Nematoda: Protostrongylidae) from white-tailed deer in Michigan. *Journal of Wildlife Diseases* 26:535–537.

Pybus, M.J., W.M. Samuel, D.A. Welch, J. Smits, and J.C. Haigh. 1992. Mortality of fallow deer (*Dama dama*) experimentally-infected with meningeal worm, *Parelaphostrongylus tenuis*. *Journal of Wildlife Diseases* 28:95–101.

Pybus, M.J., S. Groom, and W.M. Samuel. 1996. Meningeal worm in experimentally infected bighorn and domestic sheep. *Journal of Wildlife Diseases* 32:614–618.

Raskevitz, R.F., A.A. Kocan, and J.H. Shaw. 1991. Gastropod availability and habitat utilization by wapiti and white-tailed deer sympatric on range enzootic for meningeal worm. *Journal of Wildlife Diseases* 27:92–101.

Rau, M. 1984. Report on the prevalence of parasitic helminths in the lungs, brains, spinal cords and livers of moose shot during an experimental hunt on Anticosti Island in the autumn of 1983. Unpublished Report, Institute of Parasitology of McGill University, Montreal, Quebec, 3 pp.

Rickard, L.G., B.B. Smith, E.J. Gentz, A.A. Frank, E.G. Pearson, L.L. Walker, and M.J. Pybus. 1994. Experimentally induced meningeal worm (*Parelaphostrongylus tenuis*) infection in the llama (*Lama glama*): Clinical evaluation and implications for parasite translocation. *Journal of Zoo and Wildlife Medicine* 25:390–402.

Rowley, M.A., E.S. Loker, J.F. Pagels, and R.J. Montali. 1987. Terrestrial gastropod hosts of *Parelaphostrongylus tenuis* at the National Zoological Park's Conservation and Research Center. *The Journal of Parasitology* 73:1084–1089.

Samuel, W.M. 1991. A partially annotated bibliography of meningeal worm, *Parelaphostongylus tenuis* (Nematoda), and its close relatives. *Synopsis of the parasites of vertebrates.* Ed. M.J. Kennedy. Edmonton: Alberta Agriculture, Animal Health Division, 36 pp.

———. 1988. Efficacy of ivermectin against *Parelaphostrongylus andersoni* (Nematoda, Metastrongyloidea) in white-tailed deer (*Odocoileus virginianus*). *Journal of Wildlife Diseases* 24:491–495.

Samuel, W.M., T.R. Platt, and S.M. Knispel-Krause. 1985. Gastropod intermediate hosts and transmission of *Parelaphostrongylus odocoilei*, a muscle-inhabiting nematode of mule deer, *Odocoileus h. hemionus,* in Jasper National Park, Alberta. *Canadian Journal of Zoology* 63:928–932.

Samuel, W.M., M.J. Pybus, D.A. Welch, and C.J. Wilke. 1992. Elk as a potential host for meningeal worm: Implications for translocation. *The Journal of Wildlife Management* 56:629–639.

Shostak, A.W., and W.M. Samuel. 1984. Moisture and temperature effects of survival and infectivity of first-stage larvae of *Parelaphostrongylus odocoilei* and *P. tenuis* (Nematoda: Metastrongyloidea). *Journal of Parasitology* 70:261–269.

Slomke, A.M., M.W. Lankester, and W.J. Peterson. 1995. Infrapopulation dynamics of *Parelaphostrongylus tenuis* in white-tailed deer. *Journal of Wildlife Diseases* 31:125–135.

Smith, H.J., and R.M. Archibald. 1967. Moose sickness, a neurological disease of moose infected with the common cervine parasite, *Elaphostrongylus tenuis*. *Canadian Veterinary Journal* 8:173–177.

Smith, H.J., R.M. Archibald, and A.H. Corner. 1964. Elaphostrongylosis in maritime moose and deer. *Canadian Veterinary Journal* 5:287–296.

Spratt, D.M., and R.C. Anderson. 1968. The guinea pig as an experimental host of the meningeal worm, *Pneumostrongylus tenuis* Dougherty. *Journal of Helminthology* 42:139–156.

Telfer, E.S. 1967. Comparison of moose and deer winter range in Nova Scotia. *Journal of Wildlife Management* 31:418–425.

Thomas, J.E., and D.G. Dodds. 1988. Brainworm, *Parelaphostrongylus tenuis* in moose *Alces alces,* and white-tailed deer *Odocoileus virginianus* of Nova Scotia. *Canadian Field-Naturalist* 102:639–642.

Thomas, L.J., and A.R. Cahn. 1932. A new disease of moose. I. Preliminary report. *The Journal of Parasitology* 18:219–231.

Thurston, D.R., and R.G. Strout. 1978. Prevalence of meningeal worm (*Parelaphostrongylus tenuis*) in white-tailed deer from New Hampshire. *Journal of Wildlife Diseases* 14:89–96.

Trainer, D.O. 1973. Caribou mortality due to the meningeal worm (*Parelaphostrongylus tenuis*). *Journal of Wildlife Diseases* 9:376–378.

Tyler, G.V., C.P. Hibler, and A.K. Prestwood.1980. Experimental infection of mule deer with *Parelaphostrongylus tenuis*. *Journal of Wildlife Diseases* 16:533–540.

Upshall, S.M., M.D.B. Burt, and T.G. Dilworth. 1987. *Parelaphostrongylus tenuis* in New Brunswick: The parasite in white-tailed deer (*Odocoileus virginianus*) and moose (*Alces alces*). *Journal of Wildlife Diseases* 23:683–685.

Wasel, S.M. 1995. Meningeal worm, *Parelaphostrongylus tenuis* (Nematoda), in Manitoba, Saskatchewan, and North Dakota: Distribution and ecological correlates. M.Sc. Thesis, University of Alberta, Edmonton, 100 pp.

Watson, T.G. 1984. *Tissue worm in red deer: Symptoms and control.* AgLink FPP 249 (1st Revise). Wellington, New Zealand: Media Services, MAF.

Welch, D.A., M.J. Pybus, W.M. Samuel, and C.J. Wilke. 1991. Reliability of fecal examination for detecting infections of meningeal worm in elk. *Wildlife Society Bulletin* 19:326–331.

Whitlaw, H.A., and M.W. Lankester. 1994a. A retrospective evaluation of the effects of parelaphostrongylosis on moose populations. *Canadian Journal of Zoology* 72:1–7.

———. 1994b. The co-occurrence of moose, white-tailed deer and *Parelaphostrongylus tenuis* in Ontario. *Canadian Journal of Zoology* 72:819–825.

————. 1995. A practical method for cleaning Baermann glassware. *Journal of Wildlife Diseases* 31:93–95.

Whitlaw, H.A., M.W. Lankester, and W.B. Ballard. 1996. *Parelaphostrongylus tenuis* in terrestrial gastropods from white-tailed deer winter and summer range in northern New Brunswick. *Alces* 32:75–83.

Wilton, M. 1987. How the moose came to Algonquin. *Alces* 23:89–106.

Woolf, A., C.A. Mason, and D. Kradel. 1977. Prevalence and effects of *Parelaphostrongylus tenuis* in a captive wapiti population. *Journal of Wildlife Diseases* 13:149–154.

Yamini, B., J.C. Baker, P.C. Stromberg, and C.H. Gardiner. 1997. Cerebrospinal nematodiasis in vertebral chondrodysplasia in a calf. *Journal of Veterinary Diagnostic Investigation* 9:451–454.

Elaphostrongylus

Almendingen, Siv F., A. Skorping, and J. Andersen. 1993. Ecological interactions between gastropods, mushrooms and the nematode *Elaphostrongylus rangiferi*. *Bulletin Scandinavian Society of Parasitolology* 3:37.

Andersen, J., and O. Halvorsen. 1984. Species composition, abundance, habitat requirements and regional distribution of terrestrial gastropods in Arctic Norway. *Polar Biology* 3:45–53.

Anderson, R.C. 1963. Studies on *Pneumostrongylus tenuis* Dougherty, 1945 of *Odocoileus virginianus*. *The Journal of Parasitology* 49:40–47.

————. 1968. The pathogenesis and transmission of neurotropic and accidental nematode parasites of the central nervous system of mammals and birds. *Helminthological Abstracts* 37:191–210.

————. 2000. *Nematode parasites of vertebrates, their development and transmission,* 2nd ed. Cambridge: C.A.B. International, University Press, Cambridge. 650 pp.

Bakken, G., and O. Sparboe. 1973. Elaphostrongylosis in reindeer. *Nordisk Veterinaermedicin* 25:203–210.

Bakken, G., O. Selle, O. Sparboe, and T. Solhoy. 1975. Experimental *Elaphostrongylus rangiferi* infection in calves and lambs. *Nordisk Veterinaermedicin* 27:220–223.

Barus, V., and K. Blazek. 1973. Report on the finding of larval nematodes *Elaphostrongylus cervi* (Protostrongylidae) in the cranial cavity of a stag. *Folia Parasitologia* 20:279–280.

Bodnar, T. 1998. Development and survivorship of *Elaphostrongylus rangiferi* at different temperatures in the slug, *Deroceras laeve*. H.B.Sc. Thesis, Lakehead University, Thunder Bay, Ontario, 19 pp.

Borg, K. 1979. Symptome der Kreuzlahme (Schleuderkrankheit) bei Elaphostrongylusbefall des Kleinhirns bei einem Rotwildkalb. *Zeitschrift für Jagdwissenschaft* 25:237–238.

Bresele, L.M. 1990. Attempts to differentiate elaphostrongyline larvae (Nematoda: Protostrongylidae) using guinea pigs (*Cavia porcellus*) as alternate hosts. M.Sc. Thesis, Lakehead University, Thunder Bay, Canada, 87 pp.

Burg, W.B., E.A. Baudet, and J.H. Verwey. 1953. Lethal bleeding in the cranial cavity of deer (*Cervus elaphus*) caused by a nematode belonging to the family Metastrongylidae. *Proceedings of the 15th International Veterinary Congress, Stockholm,* vol. 1, pp. 414–416.

Burt, M.D.B., and P.F. McKelvey. 1993. An assessment of research needs to support the farming of alternative livestock species (deer and bison). A report to Agriculture Canada and New Brunswick Department of Agriculture, 164 pp.

Bye, K., and O. Halvorsen. 1984. Isolation of *Elaphostrongylus rangiferi* from wild reindeer in Scandinavia. *Veterinary Record* 115:87.

Cameron, T.W.M. 1931. On two new species of nematodes from the Scottish red deer. *Journal of Helminthology* 9:213–216.

Carreno, R.A., and M.W. Lankester. 1993. Additional information on the morphology of the Elaphostrongylinae (Nematoda: Protostrongylidae) of North American Cervidae. *Canadian Journal of Zoology* 71:592–600.

————. 1994. A re-evaluation of the phylogeny of *Parelaphostrongylus* Boev & Schulz, 1950 (Nematoda, Protostrongylidae). *Systematic Parasitology* 28:145–151.

Daoust, P.-Y., and S. McBurney. 1994. Protostrongylid infection in a Newfoundland moose. *Wildlife Health Centre Newsletter, Canadian Cooperative Wildlife Health Centre* 2:4.

Demiaszkiewicz, A.W. 1985. Elaphostrongylosis—a new parasitic disease of Cervidae in Poland [In Polish]. *Medycyna Weterynaryjna* 41:616–618.

————. 1986. Laboratory diagnosis of protostrongylid infections in Cervidae [In Polish]. *Medycyna Weterynaryjna* 42:660–663.

————. 1987a. *Elaphostrongylus cervi* Cameron, 1931 in European red deer (*Cervus elaphus*) in Poland. *Acta Parasitologica Polonica* 32:171–178.

————. 1987b. Epizootiology of *Elaphostrongylus* infection of red deer in the Bialowieza forest [In Polish]. *Medycyna Weterynaryjna* 43:208–211.

————. 1989. Migration of invasive larvae of *Elaphostrongylus cervi* Cameron, 1931 and their development to maturity in the guinea pig. *Acta Parasitologica Polonica* 34:39–43.

de With, N., C. Ribble, J.J. Aramini, F.A. Leighton, G. Wobeser. 1998. Risk assessment for the importation of farmed elk to Saskatchewan from Ontario with respect to *Elaphostrongylus cervi* and *Parelaphostrongylus tenuis*. A Report of the Canadian Cooperative Wildlife Health Centre, 37 pp.

Dykova, I. 1969. *Elaphostrongylus cervi* Cameron, 1931 in the central nervous system of red deer (*Cervus elaphus*) [In Czech]. *Folia Parasitologica (Prague)* 16:74

English, A.W., C.F. Watt, and W. Corrigall. 1985. Larvae of *Elaphostrongylus cervi* in the deer of Scotland. *Veterinary Record* 116:254–256.

Eriksen, L., J. Monrad, and M. Stéen. 1989. *Elaphostrongylus cervi* in Danish wild red deer (*Cervus elaphus*). *Veterinary Record* 124:124.

Forrester, S.G., and M.W. Lankester. 1997. Extracting protostrongylid nematode larvae from ungulate feces. *Journal of Wildlife Diseases* 33:511–516.

Gajadhar, A.A., and S.V. Tessaro. 1995. Susceptibility of mule deer (*Odocoileus hemionus*) and two species of North American molluscs to *Elaphostrongylus cervi* (Nematoda: Metastrongyloidea). *The Journal of Parasitology* 81:593–596.

Gajadhar, A.A., S.V. Tessaro, and W.D.G. Yates. 1994. Diagnosis of *Elaphostrongylus cervi* infection in New Zealand red deer (*Cervus elaphus*) quarantined in Canada, and experimental determination of a new extended prepatent period. *Canadian Veterinary Journal* 35:433–437.

Gajadhar, A., T. Steeves-Gurnsey, J. Kendall, M. Lankester, and M. Steen. 2000. Differentiation of dorsal-spined elaphostrongyline larvae by polymerase chain reaction amplification of ITS-2 rDNA. *Journal of Wildlife Diseases* 36:713–723.

Gaudernack, G., O. Halvorsen, A. Skorping and K.A. Stokkan. 1984. Humoral immunity and output of firststage larvae of *Elaphostrongylus rangiferi* (Nematoda, Metastrongyloidea) by infected reindeer, *Rangifer tarandus tarandus*. *Journal of Helminthology* 58:13–18.

Gibbons, L.M., O. Halvorsen, and G. Stuve. 1991. Revision of the genus *Elaphostrongylus* Cameron (Nematoda:

Metastrongyloidea) with particular reference to the species of the genus occurring in Norwegian cervids. *Zoologica Scripta* 20:15–26.

Hale, I. 1980. Development of *Elaphostrongylus cervi* Cameron, 1931 in intermediate host [In German]. (Abstract of Dissertation). *Wiener Tierärztliche Monatsschrift* 67:378.

Halvorsen, O. 1986a. Epidemiology of reindeer parasites. *Parasitology Today* 2:334–339.

———. 1986b. On the relationship between social status of host and risk of parasitic infection. *Oikos* 47:71–74.

———. 1990. The influence of parasites on game populations. A question of methods of investigation? *Transactions of the 19th International Union of Game Biologists Congress*, Trondheim, Norway, pp. 205–208.

Halvorsen, O., and A. Skorping. 1982. The influence of temperature on growth and development of the nematode *Elaphostrongylus rangiferi* in the gastropods *Arianta arbustorum* and *Euconulus fulvus. Oikos* 38:285–290.

Halvorsen, O., and K. Wissler. 1983a. *Elaphostrongylus* sp. (Nematoda, Protostrongylidae) and other helminths in faeces of moose (*Alces alces* (L.)) in north Norway. *Fauna Norvegica,* Series A 4:37–40.

———. 1983b. Methods for estimating the density of *Elaphostrongylus rangiferi* Mitskevich (nematoda, Metastrongyloidea) larvae in faeces from reindeer, *Rangifer tarandus* L. *Rangifer* 3:33–39.

Halvorsen, O., J. Andersen, A. Skorping, and G. Lorentzen. 1980. Infection in reindeer with the nematode *Elaphostrongylus rangiferi* Mitskevich in relation to climate and distribution of intermediate hosts. In *Proceeding of the 2nd International Reindeer/Caribou Symposium,* Röros, Norway. Ed. Reimers, E., E. Gaare, and S. Skjenneberg, pp. 449–455.

Halvorsen, O., A. Skorping, and K. Hansen. 1985. Seasonal cycles in the output of first-stage larvae of the nematode *Elaphostrongylus rangiferi* from reindeer, *Rangifer tarandus tarandus. Journal of Polar Biology* 5:49–54.

Halvorsen, O., A. Skorping, and K. Bye. 1989. Experimental infection of reindeer with *Elaphostrongylus* (Nematoda: Protostrongylida) originating from reindeer, red deer, and moose. *Canadian Journal of Zoology* 67:1200–1202.

Handeland, K. 1991. Cerebrospinal elaphostrongylosis in sheep in northern Norway. *Journal of Veterinary Medicine* 38:773–780.

———. 1994. Experimental studies of *Elaphostrongylus rangiferi* in reindeer (*Rangifer tarandus tarandus*): Life cycle, pathogenesis, and pathology. *Journal of Veterinary Medicine B* 41:351–365.

Handeland, K., and H.S. Norberg. 1992. Lethal cerebrospinal elaphostrongylosis in a reindeer calf. *Journal of Veterinary Medicine B* 39:668–671.

Handeland, K., and A. Skorping. 1992a. The early migration of *Elaphostrongylus rangiferi* in goats. *Journal of Veterinary Medicine B* 39:263–272.

———. 1992b. Experimental cerebrospinal elaphostrongyosis (*Elaphostrongylus rangiferi*) in goats: II. Pathological findings. *Journal of Veterinary Medicine B* 39:713–722.

———. 1993. Experimental cerebrospinal elaphostrongylosis (*Elaphostrongylus rangiferi*) in goats: I. Clinical observations. *Journal of Veterinary Medicine B* 40:141–147.

Handeland, K. and T. Slettbakk. 1994. Outbreaks of clinical cerebrospinal elaphostrongylosis in reindeer (*Rangifer tarandus tarandus*) in Finnmark, Norway, and their relations to climatic conditions. *Journal of Veterinary Medicine B* 41:407–410.

———. 1995. Epidemiological aspects of cerebrospinal elaphostrongylosis in small ruminants in northern Norway. *Journal of Veterinary Medicine B* 42:110–117.

Handeland, K., and O. Sparboe. 1991. Cerebrospinal elaphostrongylosis in dairy goats in northern Norway. *Journal of Veterinary Medicine B* 38:755–763.

Handeland, K., A. Skorping, and T. Slettbakk. 1993. Experimental cerebrospinal elaphostrongylosis (*Elaphostrongylus rangiferi*) in sheep. *Journal of Veterinary Medicine B* 40:181–189.

Handeland, K., A. Skorping, S. Stuen, and T. Slettbakk. 1994. Experimental studies of *Elaphostrongylus rangiferi* in reindeer (*Rangifer tarandus tarandus*): Clinical observations. *Rangifer* 14:83–87.

Helle, O. 1980. *Elaphostrongylus cervi* in red deer (*Cervus elaphus*) in Norway [In Norwegian]. *Norsk Veterinaertidsskrift* 92:677–678.

Hemmingsen, W., O. Halvorsen, and A. Skorping. 1993. Migration of adult *Elaphostrongylus rangiferi* (Nematoda: Protostrongylidae) from the spinal subdural space to the muscles of reindeer (*Rangifer tarandus*). *The Journal of Parasitology* 79:728–732.

Hollands, R.D. 1985. *Elaphostrongylus cervi cervi* in the central nervous system of red deer (*Cervus elaphus*) in Scotland. *Veterinary Record* 116:584–585.

Holmstrom, S., P. Korhonen, S. Nikander, and T. Rahko. 1989. On the occurrence of lungworm infection in reindeer in Finnish Eastern Lapland. *Suomen Elainlaakarilehti* 95:178–181.

Holt, G. 1982. Demonstration of elaphostrongylosis in moose in South Norway gives reason for some anxiety [In Norweigian]. *Jakt fiske og friluftsliv* 9:33–34.

Holt, G., C. Berg, and A. Haugen. 1990. Nematode related spinal myelomeningitis and posterior ataxia in muskoxen (*Ovibos moschatus*). *Journal of Wildlife Diseases* 26:528–531.

Jorgensen, R.J., and F. Vigh-Larsen. 1986 . Preliminary observations on lungworms in farmed and feral red deer (*Cervus elaphus*) in Denmark. *Nordisk Veterinaermedicin* 38:173–179.

Kontrimavichus, V.L., S.L. Delyamure, and S.N. Boev. 1976. Metastrongyloidea of domestic and wild animals. In *Principles of nematology.* Ed. K.M. Ryzhikov. Moscow, USSR: Osnovy Nematodologii, Izdatel'stvo "Nauka", 240 pp. [Translated from Russian by the U.S. Department of Agriculture and NSF, 1985].

Kotrla, R., and A. Kotrly. 1977. Helminths of wild ruminants introduced into Czechoslovakia. *Folia Parasitologica Praha* 24:35–40.

Kutzer, E. 1987. The application of the anthelmintic Ivomec (ivermectin) in game animals [In German]. *Verhandlungsbericht des XXI Internationalen Symposiums des Österreichischen Wildgehegeverbandes,* 19 und 20 Juni, 1987, Bad Mitterndorf (Steiermark), Austria. Vienna, Austria: Veterinarmedizinsche Universität, pp.7–17.

Kutzer, E., and H. Prosl. 1975. Zur Kenntnis von *Elaphostrongylus cervi* Cameron, 1931. I. Morphologie und Diagnose (Contribution to the knowledge of *Elaphostrongylus cervi* Cameron, 1931. 1: Morphology and diagnosis). *Wiener Tierärztliche Monatschrift* 62:258–266.

———. 1976. Knowledge of *Elaphostrongylus cervi* Cameron, 1931. II. Biology [In German]. In *Erkrankungen der Zootiere.* Ed. R. Ippen, and H.D. Schroder. Verhandlungsbericht des XVIII Internationalen Symposiums über die Erkrankungen der Zootiere, 16–20 June, 1976, Innsbruck, Germany. Berlin: Akademie-Verlag, pp. 239–243.

Lankester, M.W. 1977. Neurologic disease in moose caused by *Elaphostrongylus cervi* Cameron 1931 from caribou. *Proceedings of the 13th Annual North American Moose Conference and Workshop,* Jasper, Alberta, pp. 177–190.

Lankester, M.W., and R.C. Anderson. 1968. Gastropods as intermediate hosts of *Pneumostrongylus tenuis* Dougherty. *Canadian Journal of Zoology* 46:373–383.

Lankester, M.W., and D. Fong. 1989. Distribution of elaphostrongyline nematodes (Metastrongyloidea: Protostrongylidae) in cervidae and possible effects of moving *Rangifer* spp. into and within North America. *Alces* 25:133–145.

———. 1998. Protostrongylid nematodes in caribou (*Rangifer tarandus caribou*) and moose (*Alces alces*) of Newfoundland. *Rangifer,* Special Issue No. 10, pp. 73–83.

Lankester, M.W., and P.L. Hauta. 1989. *Parelaphostrongylus andersoni* (Nematoda: Elaphostrongylinae) in caribou (*Rangifer tarandus*) of northern and central Canada. *Canadian Journal of Zoology* 67:1966–1975.

Lankester, M.W., and T.H. Northcott. 1979. *Elaphostrongylus cervi* Cameron 1931 (Nematoda: Metastrongyloidea) in caribou (*Rangifer tarandus*) of Newfoundland. *Canadian Journal of Zoology* 57:1384–1392.

Lankester M.W., and W.J. Peterson. 1996. The possible importance of deer wintering yards in the transmission of *Parelaphostrongylus tenuis* to white-tailed deer and moose. *Journal of Wildlife Diseases* 32:31–38.

Lankester, M.W., I.-M. Olsson, M. Stéen, and A. Gajadhar. 1998. Extra-mammalian larval stages of *Elaphostrongylus alces* (Nematoda: Protostrongylidae), a parasite of moose (*Alces alces)* in Fennoscandia. *Canadian Journal of Zoology* 76:33–38.

Lankester, M.W., J.E.B. Smits, M.J. Pybus, D. Fong, and J.C. Haigh. 1990. Experimental infection of fallow deer (*Dama dama*) with elaphostrongyline nematodes (Nematoda: Protostrongylidae) from caribou(*Rangifer tarandus caribou*) in Newfoundland. *Alces* 26:154–162.

Lorentzen, G. 1979. The ecology of *Elaphostrongylus rangiferi* (Nematoda, Metastrongyloidea): The free-living larval stage. University of Tromsø Thesis, Tromsø, Norway.

Lorentzen, G., and O. Halvorsen. 1986. Survival of the first-stage larva of the metastrongyloid nematode *Elaphostrongylus rangiferi* under various conditions of temperature and humidity. *Holarctic Ecology* 9:301–304.

Liubimov, M.P. 1948. New helminths in the brain of maral deer [In Russian]. *Trudy Gel'mintologicheskoi Laboratorii Akademii Nauk SSSR* 1:198–201.

———. 1959a. Seasonal dynamics of elaphostrongylosis and setariasis in *Cervus elaphus maral* [In Russian]. *Trudy Gel'mintologicheskoi Laboratorii Akademii Nauk SSSR* 9:155–156.

———. 1959b. New observations on the epizootiology, prophylaxis, and therapy of elaphostrongylosis in maral deer [In Russian]. Sbornik Nauchnykh Rabot Nauchnye-Issledovatel'skoi Laboratorii Pantovogo Olenovodstvo, Gorno-Altai, pp. 164–214.

Mason, P.C. 1975. *Elaphostrongylus cervi* (Protostrongylidae: Elaphostrongylinae) in New Zealand cervids. *Proceedings of the 1975 Conference of the New Zealand Society for Parasitology,* Massey University, Palmerston North, 21–22 August, 1975, pp. 45–51.

———. 1979. Tissue worm in red deer: Biology and significance. AgLink FPP 249. Wellington, New Zealand: Media Services, MAF.

———. 1989. *Elaphostrongylus cervi*—A review. *Surveillance* 16:3–10.

———. 1994. Identification of *Elaphostrongylus cervi* lesions at routine meat inspection of deer carcasses. *Surveillance* 21:27–28.

———. 1995. *Elaphostrongylus cervi* and its close relatives; a review of protostrongylids (Nematoda, Metastrongyloidea) with spiny-tailed larvae. *Surveillance* 22:19–24.

Mason, P.C., and N.R. Gladden. 1983. Survey of internal parasitism and anthelmintics used in farmed deer. *New Zealand Veterinary Journal* 31:217–220.

Mason, P.C., and H.J.F. McAllum. 1976. *Dictyocaulus viviparus* and *Elaphostrongylus cervi* in wapiti. *New Zealand Veterinary Journal* 24:23.

Mason, P.C., N.R. Kiddey, R.J. Sutherland, D.M. Rutherford, and A.G. Green. 1976. *Elaphostrongylus cervi* in red deer. *New Zealand Veterinary Journal* 24:22–23.

McBurney, S, H. Whitney, and M. Lankester. 1996. Fatal infection with *Elaphostrongylus rangiferi* in Newfoundland caribou. *Canadian Cooperative Wildlife Health Centre Newsletter* 4:5–6.

Mitskevich, V.Y. 1958. On the interpretation of the developmental cycle of the nematode *Elaphostrongylus rangiferi* n. sp. from a reindeer [In Russian]. *Doklady Akademii Nauk SSSR* 119:621–624.

———. 1964. Life cycle of *Elaphostrongylus rangiferi* Mitskevich 1958. In *Parasites of farm animals in Kazakhstan* [In Russian]. Ed. S.N. Boev. *Izdatel'stvo Akademii Nauk SSR Alma-Ata* 3: 49–60.

Munro, R. and A. R. Hunter. 1983. Histopathological findings in the lungs of Scottish red deer and roe deer. *Veterinary Record* 112:194–197.

Nilsson, O. 1971. The inter-relationship of endo-parasites in wild cervids (*Capreolus capreolus* L. and *Alces alces* L.) and domestic ruminants in Sweden. *Acta Veterinaria Scandinavia* 12:36–68.

Nordkvist, M. 1971. The problems of veterinary medicine in reindeer breeding. *Veterinary Medical Review Numbers* 2/3:405–413.

Nordkvist, M., C. Rehbinder, D. Christensson, and C. RönnbÑck. 1983. A comparative study of the efficacy of four anthelmintics on some important reindeer parasites. *Rangifer* 3:19–38.

Nordkvist, M., D. Christensson, and C. Rehbinder. 1984. A de-worming field trial with ivermectin in reindeer. *Rangifer* 4:10–15.

Ogunremi, O., M.W. Lankester and A. Gajadhar. 1998. Serological diagnosis of *Elaphostrongylus cervi* and *Parelaphostrongylus tenuis* in North American cervids. (Abstract) Annual Meeting of the American Society of Parasitolology, Hawaii, August, 1998, p. 52.

Ogunremi, O., M.W. Lankester, S. Loran, and A. Gajadhar. 1999a. Evaluation of excretory-secretory products and somatic worm antigens for the sero-diagnosis of experimental *Parelaphostrongylus tenuis* infections in white-tailed deer. *Journal of Veterinary Diagnostic Investigations* 11:515–521.

Ogunremi, O., M.W. Lankester, and A. Gajadhar. 1999b. Serological diagnosis of *Parelaphostrongylus tenuis* infection in white-tailed deer and identification of a potentially unique parasite antigen. *The Journal of Parasitology* 85:122–127.

Oksanen, A., M. Nieminen, and T. Soveri. 1993. A comparison of topical, subcutaneous and oral administrations of ivermectin to reindeer. *The Veterinary Record* 133:312–314.

Olsson, I.-M., R. Bergström, M. Stéen, M., and F. Sandegren. 1995. A study of *Elaphostrongylus alces* in an island moose population with low calf body weights. *Alces* 31:61–75.

Olsson, I.-M. C., M.W. Lankester, A.A. Gajadhar, and M. Stéen. 1998. Tissue migration of *Elaphostrongylus* spp. in guinea pigs (*Cavia porcellus*). *The Journal of Parasitology* 84:968–975.

Osipov, P.P. 1964. Effect of feeding phenothiazine to *Cervus elaphus* on the fecal counts of *Elaphostrongylus, Dictyocaulus,* and *Bicaulus* larvae. In *Parasites of farm animals in Kazakhstan* [In Russian]. Ed. S.N. Boev. Alma-Ata: Izdatel'stvo Akademii Nauk Kazakhskoi SSR, 3:98–100.

Ottestad, A.K. 1983. The occurrence of *Elaphostrongylus cervi* in a population of red deer (*Cervus elaphus*) [In

Norweigian]. Candidatus Realium Thesis, University of Tromsø, Tromsø, Norway.

Panin, V.Y. 1964a. Developmental cycle of *Elaphostrongylus panticola* Lubimov, 1945. In *Parasites of farm animals in Kazakhstan* [In Russian]. Ed. S.N. Boev. Alma-Ata: Izdatel'stvo Akademii Nauk Kazakhskoi SSR, 3:34–48.

———. 1964b. Role of terrestrial molluscs in spreading *Elaphostrongylus* in deer. In *Parasites of farm animals in Kazakhstan* [In Russian]. S.N. Boev (Ed.). Alma-Ata: Izdatel'stvo Akademii Nauk Kazakhskoi SSR, 3:79–83.

Panin, V.Y. 1965. Epizootiology and prophylaxis of elaphostrongylosis of Siberian maral [In Russian]. *Izdatel'stvo Akademii Nauk SSR, Alma-Ata*, Series B, 2:56–63.

Panin, V.Y., and O.I. Rusikova. 1964. Susceptibility of molluscs to infection with larvae of *Elaphostrongylus panticola* Lubimov, 1945. In *Parasites of farm animals in Kazakhstan* [In Russian]. S.N. Boev (Ed.). Alma-Ata: Izdatel'stvo Akademii Nauk Kazakhskoi SSR, 3:84–89.

Polyanskaya, M.V. 1963. On elaphostrongylosis in reindeer. In (*Helminths of man, animals, and plants and their control*). Papers presented to Academician K.I. Skrjabin on his 85th birthday. Moscow: Izdatel'stvo Akademii Nauk SSSR, pp. 424–425.

———. 1965. On the forms of elaphostrongylosis of reindeer. *Materialy Nauchnye Konferentsii Vsesoyuznogo Obschch. Gel'mintologov. Moscow,* part 2, pp. 205–207.

Presidente, P.J.A. 1986a. First report of the tissue worm in Australia. *The Federal Deerbreeder* 5:13–17.

———. 1986b. Tissue worm: Implications for live deer exports. In *Deer farming into the nineties*. Ed. P. Owen. Based on the proceedings of the Australian Deer 86 conference. Brisbane: Owen Art and Publishing, pp. 192–202.

Prosl, H., and E. Kutzer. 1980a. Biology and control of *Elaphostrongylus cervi* [In German]. *Zeitschrift für Jagdwissenschaft* 26:198–207.

———. 1980b. Zur pathologie des *Elaphostrongylus befalles beim Rothirsch (Cervus elaphus hippelaphus)*. *Monatshefte für Veterinäermedizin* 35:151–153.

———. 1982. Annual rhythm in the excretion by red deer (*Cervus elaphus*) of *Dictyocaulus viviparus, Varestrongylus sagittatus* and *Elaphostrongylus cervi* larvae. *Angewandte Parasitologie* 23:9–14.

———. 1976a. Helminths of deer [In Russian]. *Izdatel'stvo Akademii Nauka Kazahkskoi SSR,* 229 pp.

———. 1976b. The susceptibility of marals to reinfection with *Elaphostrongylus cervi panticola* [In Russian]. *Third International Symposium of the Helminthological Institute,* Kosice, Czechoslovakia. 2 pp.

Pryadko, E.I., and S.N. Boev. 1971. Systematics, phylogeny and evolution of Elaphostrongylinae—Nematodes of deer [In Russian]. *Izdatel'stvo Akademii Nauk Kazakhskoi SSSR, Seriya Biologicheskaya,* No. 5, pp. 74–85.

Pryadko, E.I., S.N. Visokov, and V.S. Frolov. 1963. Helminths of ungulates of Kazakhstan. Epizootiology of *Elaphostrongylus* in maral deer. In *Parasites of farm animals in Kazakhstan* [In Russian]. Ed. S.N. Boev. Alma-Alta: Izdatel'stvo Akademii Nauk Kazakhskoi SSR, 3:74–85.

Pryadko, E.I., N.I. Drobishchenko, V.I. Teterin, and V.A. Shol. 1968. Efficacy of thiabendazole against *Elaphostrongylus* infection of marals [In Russian]. *Materialy Konferentsii Posvyashchennoi Pamyati N.V. Badanina,* Tashkent, pp. 248–249.

Pryadko, E.I., V.A. Shol, V.I. Teterin, and N.I. Drobishchenko. 1971. Screening for therapeutic compounds to control *Elaphostrongylus* infection of maral deer [In Russian]. *Sbornik Rabot po Gel'mintologicheskoi 90—letiyu so dnya rozhderiya Akademika K.I. Skryabin.* Moscow: Izdatel'stvo 'Kolos,' pp. 313–316.

Pusterla, N., P. Caplazi, and U. Braun. 1997. Cerebrospinal nematodiasis in seven goats. *Schweizer Archiv für Tierheilkunde* 139:282–287.

Pusterla, N., H. Hertzberg, M. Viglezio, T. Vanzetti, and U. Braun. 1998. The incidence of lumbar paralysis in goats and the occurrence of *Elaphostrongylus cervi* in red deer in the Canto Ticno. *Schweizer Archiv für Tierheilkunde* 140:76–82.

Rehbinder, C., I. Forssell, M. Nordkvist, and P. von Szokolay. 1982. Efficacy of mebendazole on *Elaphostrongylus rangiferi* in reindeer. In *Wildlife diseases of the Pacific Basin and other countries.* Ed. M.E. Fowler. Proceedings of the Fourth International Congress of the Wildlife Disease Association, Sydney, Australia, pp. 208–212.

Rezác, P. 1990. Differential diagnosis of 1st-stage larvae of the nematodes *Varestronylus sagittatus* and *Elaphostrongylus cervi* [In Czech]. *Veterinárstvu* 40:311–313.

———. 1991. Occurrence of lungworms in red deer under different types of management [In Czech]. *Folia Venatoria* 21:37–50.

Rezác, P., L. Palkovik, E. Holasova, and J. Busta. 1994. Modes of entry of the first-stage larvae of *Elaphostrongylus cervi* (Nematoda: Protostrongylidae) into pulmonate snails *Arianta arbustorum* and *Helix pomatia. Folia Parasitologica* 41:209–214.

Roneus, O., and M. Nordkvist. 1962. Cerebrospinal and muscular nematodiasis (*Elaphostrongylus rangiferi*) in Swedish reindeer. *Acta Veterinaria Scandinavica* 3:201–225.

Roneus, O., N.-G. Nilsson, and C. Rehbinder. 1984. *Onchocerca* lesions in moose (*Alces alces* L.) *Nordisk Veterinaermedicin* 36:367–370.

Schjetlein, J., and A. Skorping. 1995. The temperature threshold for development of *Elaphostrongylus rangiferi* in the intermediate host: An adaptation to winter survival? *Parasitolgy* 111:103–110.

Shol, V.A., E.I. Pryadko, V.I. Teterin, and N.I. Drobishchenko. 1969. Thiabendazole against some helminthiases of marals (*Cervus elaphus maral*). In *Work on helminthology in Kazakhstan* [In Russian]. Ed. Sh.E. Esenov. Alma-Ata: Izdatel'stvo Nauk Kazakhstoi SSR, pp. 103–112.

Skorping, A. 1982. *Elaphostrongylus rangiferi:* Influence of temperature, substrate, and larval age on the infection rate in the intermediate snail host, *Arianta arbustorum. Experimental Parasitology* 54:222–228.

———. 1984. Density-dependent effects in a parasitic nematode, *Elaphostrongylus rangiferi,* in the snail intermediate host. *Oecologia* 64:34–40.

———. 1985a. *Lymnea stagnalis* as experimental intermediate host for the protostrongylid nematode *Elaphostrongylus rangiferi. Zeitschrift für Parasitenkunde* 71:265–270.

———. 1985b. Parasite-induced reduction in host survival and fecundity: The effect of the nematode *Elaphostrongylus rangiferi* on the snail intermediate host. *Parasitology* 91:555–562.

———. 1988. The effect of density of first-stage larvae of *Elaphostrongylus rangiferi* on the infection rate in the snail intermediate host. *Parasitology* 96:487–492.

Skorping, A., and J. Andersen. 1991. Sluttrapport for Projektet "Fordelingsmoenster og Infeksjonsnivaa av Reinens Hjernemark, *Elaphostrongylus rangiferi,* i Naturlige Populasjoner av Snegl i et Reinbeiteomraade i Finnmark." Report—University of Tromsø, Norway, pp. 1–16.

Skorping, A., and O. Halvorsen. 1980. The susceptibility of terrestrial gastropods to experimental infection with *Elaphostrongylus rangiferi* Mitskevich (Nematoda: Metastrongyloidea). *Zeitschrift für Parasitenkunde* 62:7–14.

———. 1991. Elaphostrongylosis: A clinical, pathological, and taxonomical study with special emphasis on the infection in moose. Ph.D. Dissertation, Swedish University of Agricultural Sciences, Uppsala, Sweden, 128 pp.

Stéen, M., and C. Johansson. 1990. *Elaphostrongylus* spp. from Scandinavian Cervidae—A scanning electron microscope study (SEM). *Rangifer* 10:39–46.

Stéen, M., and T. M.rner. 1985. Brainworm—A new serious disease of wild game [In Swedish]. *Svensk Jakt* 7/8:601–603.

Stéen, M., and C. Rehbinder. 1986. Nervous tissue lesions caused by elaphostrongylosis in wild Swedish moose. *Acta Veterinaria Scandinavica* 27:326–342.

Stéen, M., and L. Roepstorff. 1990. Neurological disorder in two moose calves (*Alces alces* L.) naturally infected with *Elaphostrongylus alces*. *Rangifer,* Special Issue No. 3, pp. 399–406.

Stéen, M., A.G. Chabaud, and C. Rehbinder. 1989. Species of the genus *Elaphostrongylus* parasite of Swedish cervidae. A description of *E. alces* n. sp. *Annals de Parasitologie Humaine et Comparee* 64:134–142.

Stéen, M., S. Persson, and L. Hajdu. 1994. Protostrongylidae in Cervidae and *Ovibos muscatus:* A clustering based on isoelectric focussing on the nematode body proteins. *Applied Parasitology* 35:193–206.

Stéen, M., C.G.M. Blackmore, and A. Skorping. 1997. Cross-infection of moose (*Alces alces*) and reindeer(*Rangifer tarandus*) with *Elaphostrongylus alces* and *Elaphostrongylus rangiferi* (Nematoda, Protostrongylidae): Effects on the parasite morphology and prepatent period. *Veterinary Parasitology* 71: 27–38.

Stéen, M., W.E. Faber, and A. Oksanen. 1998a. Disease and genetical investigations of Fennoscandian cervids—A review. *Alces* 34:287–310.

Stéen, M., I. Warsame, and A. Skorping. 1998b. Experimental infection of reindeer, sheep and goats with *Elaphostrongylus* spp. (Nematoda, Protostrongylidae) from moose and reindeer. *Rangifer* 18:73–80.

Stuve, G. 1986. The prevalence of *Elaphostrongylus cervi* infection in moose (*Alces alces*) in southern Norway. *Acta Veterinaria Scandinavica* 27:397–409.

———. 1987. *Elaphostrongylus cervi* infection in moose (*Alces alces*). Prevalence and pathological changes in relation to age and season. *Acta Veterinaria Scandinavica* 28:157–164.

Stuve, G., and A. Skorping. 1987. Experimental *Elaphostrongylus cervi* infection in moose (*Alces alces*). *Acta Veterinaria Scandinavica* 28:165–171.

———. 1990. Attempts to transfer *Elaphostrongylus alces* from moose (*Alces alces*) to sheep and goats. *Acta Veterinaria Scandinavica* 31:409–412.

Sugar, L. 1978. Nematode infection of wild ruminants in Hungary [In Hungarian]. *Parasitologia Hungarica* 11:146–148.

Sugar, L., and A. Kavai. 1977. The occurrence of *Elaphostongylus cervi* Cameron, 1931 in a red deer population in Hungary [In Hungarian]. *Parasitologia Hungarica* 10:95–96.

Sugar, L., and P. Sarkozy. 1988. Lungworm control with albendazole (Vermitan[R]) in captive red deer herds. *Verhandlungsbericht des 30 Internationalen Symposiums über die Erkrankungen der Zoo- und Wildtiere Sofia 1988.* Berlin: Akademie-Verlag, pp. 149–152.

Sutherland, R.J. 1976. *Elaphostrongylus cervi* in cervids in New Zealand 1. The gross and histological lesions in red deer (*Cervus elaphus*). *New Zealand Veterinary Journal* 24:263–266.

Svarc, R., E.I. Pryadko, Z. Kh. Tazieva, and A. Pajersky. 1985. The larval stages of *Elaphostrongylus cervi panticola* Lubimov, 1945. *Helminthologia* 22:171–180.

Watson, T.G. 1980. *Elaphostrongylus cervi* Cameron in Canada and New Zealand; an historical overview. Proceedings of the 8th Annual Meeting of the New Zealand Society for Parasitology, Palmerston North, 20–22 August, 1980. Abstract, *New Zealand Journal of Zoology* 7:604.

———. 1981. *Elaphostrongyulus cervi* Cameron, 1931 and elaphostrongylosis: A review. *Proceedings of a Deer Seminar for Veterinarians, Deer Advisory Panel,* Queenstown: New Zealand Veterinary Association, pp. 94–103.

———. 1983. Some clinical and parasitological features of *Elaphostrongylus cervi* infections in *Cervus elaphus*. *New Zealand Journal of Zoology* 10:129 (Abstract only).

———. 1984. Tissue worm in red deer: Symptoms and control. AgLink FPP 249 (1st Revise). Wellington, New Zealand: Media Services, MAF.

———. 1986. Efficacy of drenching red deer and wapiti with particular reference to *Elaphostrongylus cervi* and *Dictyocaulus viviparus. Proceedings of Deer Course for Veterinarians, Rotorua, July 1986.* Rotorua, New Zealand: Deer Branch, New Zealand, Veterinary Association. Deer Branch Course No. 3, pp. 170–182.

Watson, T.G., and J.M. Gill. 1985. The experimental infection of guinea pigs with the tissue worm of deer—*Elaphostrongylus cervi. New Zealand Veterinary Journal* 33:81–83.

Watson, T.G., and A.C. Kean. 1983. Some potential intermediate hosts of *Elaphostrongylus*. *New Zealand Journal of Zoology* 10:127.

Wissler, K., and O. Halvorsen. 1976. Infection of reindeer with *Elaphostrongylus rangiferi* (Nematoda: Metastrongyloidea) in relation to age and season. *Norwegian Journal of Zoology* 24:462–463.

10

LUNGWORMS OF MARINE MAMMALS

LENA N. MEASURES

Most published works about lungworms of marine mammals describe new species or pathologic lesions found in captive pinnipeds and cetaceans. Currently there is renewed interest in these helminths as a reflection of increased research with marine mammals and their diseases as well as a worldwide proliferation of "rehabilitation programs" for stranded animals. This chapter is a compilation of current knowledge with respect to these important parasites in seals and cetaceans.

LUNGWORMS OF PINNIPEDS

Otostrongylus circumlitus
Synonyms: *Strongylus circumlitus* (Railliet 1899); *Kutastrongylus andreewoi* (Skrjabin 1933); *Kutassicaulus andreewoi* (Skrjabin 1933).

Otostrongylus circumlitus (Railliet 1899; de Bruyn 1933) is a large parasitic roundworm (Metastrongyloidea: Crenosomatidae) found in the principal airways of phocid pinnipeds. Occasionally worms are found in the pulmonary artery, right ventricle of the heart, and more rarely, blood vessels of the liver. Distribution is Holarctic, and infections are primarily confined to young seals less than 1 year old. This large bronchial worm is believed to influence the health and diving ability of seals, subsequently affecting feeding, growth, and survival (Onderka 1989; Bergeron et al. 1997a,b; Gosselin et al. 1998). Fatal infections have been documented in some hosts (Gulland et al. 1997).

LIFE HISTORY. The life cycle of *O. circumlitus* is incompletely understood. Adults occur in the lungs. Cephalic extremities are deeply embedded in peribronchial tissue (5–10 mm deep), and posterior extremities are free in bronchioles and primary and secondary bronchi, often extending as far anteriorly as the bifurcation of the trachea (Onderka 1989; Bergeron et al. 1997b) (Fig. 10.1). Adult females are ovoviviparous and release first-stage larvae (L_1's) into airways where they are observed in mucus. First-stage larvae are also observed in feces. Presumably they are moved passively up the bronchial escalator by mucociliary action, swallowed into the stomach, and passed with feces into the external environment.

In experimentally infected American plaice (*Hippoglossoides platessoides*) larvae enter the intestinal wall and encapsulate in the serosa (Bergeron et al. 1997a). The first molt occurs 3 days and the second molt 56 days after infection. Third-stage larvae (785–1007 µm long) retain cuticles of the first and second stages (L_2, 211–428 µm long). Experimental infection of invertebrates (gastropods and crustaceans) was unsuccessful (Bergeron et al. 1997a). Invertebrates such as gastropods and crustaceans apparently are not required as intermediate hosts, but fish are obligate intermediate hosts. Although invertebrates could be paratenic, or transport hosts, for L_1's, there is no evidence that this occurs (Bergeron et al. 1997a).

Development within the seal definitive host is unknown. Mature worms are usually found in the lungs, less frequently in the heart and pulmonary artery. Small or immature worms are sometimes seen in the heart and pulmonary artery (Menschel et al. 1966; Onderka 1989; Gulland et al. 1997; Bergeron et al. 1997b). Skrjabin (1933) reported *O. circumlitus* (= *Kutassicaulus andreewoi*) in blood vessels of the liver in ringed seals (*Phoca hispida*). These data suggest that *O. circumlitus* may migrate to the lungs via the hepatic-portal, heart, and pulmonary circulation, as with *Crenosoma vulpis* in dogs (Stockdale and Hulland 1970). The longevity of *O. circumlitus* in seals is not known but is likely a matter of months. Infection is confined primarily to young seals < 1 year old, but Onderka (1989) observed worms in two 1-year-old, one 5-year-old and one 8-year-old ringed seal (in thin body condition). Gosselin et al. (1998) found an infected 25-year-old grey seal (*Halichoerus grypus*).

EPIZOOTIOLOGY

DISTRIBUTION. *Otostrongylus circumlitus* appears restricted to the northern hemisphere, but there are few studies on lungworms of pinnipeds in the southern hemisphere (Dailey 1975). Distribution is Holarctic and circumpolar, including coastal waters of Canada (western Arctic, eastern Arctic, and the western Atlantic), the United States (Washington, Oregon, California, and New England), the former USSR (Sea of Okhotsk, White Sea, Bering Sea, Lake Baikal), Sea of Japan, Europe (France, Holland, Denmark, Germany, Scotland, Ireland), and Iceland. Lungworms also have been observed in crabeater (*Lobodon carcinophagus*) and Weddell seals (*Leptonychotes weddelli*) (see Schumacher et al. 1990) and in Antarctic

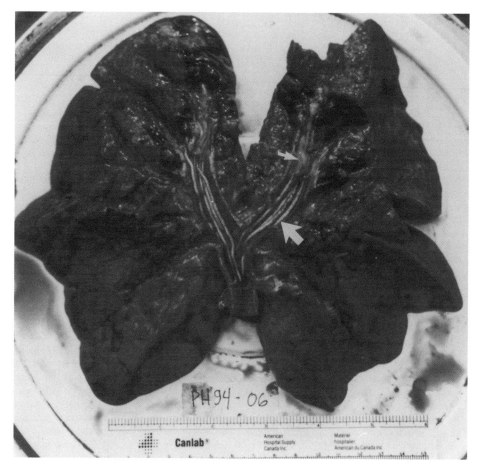

FIG. 10.1—Ventral view of lungs from a young ringed seal (*Phoca hispida*). Bronchi and bronchioles are opened and contain 14 adult *Otostrongylus circumlitus* (large arrow) and mucus (small arrow). (Reprinted by permission National Research Council.)

fur seals (*Arctocephalus gazella*) (see Baker and McCann 1989), but worms were not identified.

HOST RANGE. Final hosts are phocid pinnipeds including harbor seal (*Phoca vitulina*), ringed seal, spotted seal (*Phoca largha*), ribbon seal (*Phoca fasciata*), Baikal seal (*Phoca sibirica*), grey seal, bearded seal (*Erignathnus barbatus*), and northern elephant seal (*Mirounga angustirostris*) (see Railliet 1899; de Bruyn 1933; Delyamure 1955; Van den Broek and Wensvoort 1959; Belopol'skaia 1960; Menschel et al. 1966; Sweeney 1972; Schroeder et al. 1973; Vauk 1973; Zimmerman and Nebel 1975; Delyamure and Popov 1975; Popov 1975; Dunn and Wolke 1976; Stroud and Dailey 1978; Stroud and Roffe 1978; Clausen 1978; Geraci 1979; Dailey and Otto 1982; Van Haaften 1982; Delyamure et al. 1982; Delyamure et al. 1984; Baker 1987; Breuer et al. 1988; Onderka 1989; Dailey and Fallace 1989; Kennedy et al. 1989; Skirnisson and Olafsson 1990; Borgsteede et al. 1991;

Claussen et al. 1991; Heide-Jørgensen et al. 1992; Measures and Gosselin 1994; Gulland et al. 1997; Bergeron et al. 1997b; Gosselin et al. 1998). *Otostrongylus circumlitus* has been observed in three young hooded seals (*Cystophora cristata*) from Newfoundland, Nova Scotia, and Sable Island (P.-Y. Daoust and G. Conboy, personal communication). The apparent absence of this lungworm in other northern phocids such as harp seal (*Phoca groenlandica*) and Caspian seal (*Phoca caspica*) probably reflects the low number of seals examined at 3 months to 1 year old (see Gosselin et al. 1998).

PREVALENCE AND INTENSITY. Prevalence and intensity of *O. circumlitus* in phocid populations must be interpreted with caution. Samples excluding young animals will be biased. Seals up to 25 years old can be infected, but this is considered rare and may be related to immune incompetence. Conversely, stranded animals are often young and thus not representative of infections in free-ranging populations. Stranded old animals, on the other hand, often have chronic disease conditions resulting in poor resistance to pathogens and parasites. For example, prevalence of *O. circumlitus* in stranded seals includes up to 78% of harbor seals in the Wadden Sea (Van den Broek and Wensvoort 1959; Van den Broek 1963; Clausen 1978; Borgsteede et al. 1991; Claussen et al. 1991), 17% of 18 harbor seals from the North Sea (Menschel et al. 1966), 35% of 94 harbor seals off New England (Geraci and St. Aubin 1979), 4 of 8 elephant seals off Oregon (Stroud and Dailey 1978; Dailey and Otto 1982), as well as 89% of 73 northern elephant seals and 12% of 304 harbor seals off the California coast (Gulland et al. 1997). These stranded animals were mostly less than 1 year old or juveniles.

Baker (1987) reported that 57% of 35 grey seals drowned in fishing nets off the Outer Hebrides, Scotland, had lungworm infections (88% of infected seals were < 1 year old), but no distinction was made between *O. circumlitus* and *Parafilaroides* sp. (see Baker 1989). Van der Kamp (1987) reported no lungworm infections (*O. circumlitus* nor *Parafilaroides* spp.) in stranded harbor seals younger than 3 months old, but over 60% of older seals were infected. Prevalence of *O. circumlitus* in hunted seals include 1 each of 228 ribbon seals from the Sea of Okhotsk (Popov 1975), 33 bearded seals from off Sakhalin (Delyamure and Popov 1975) and 77 harbor seals from the Washington coast (Dailey and Fallace 1989); 58% of 19 ringed seals (all infected seals were less than 1 year old) from the eastern Arctic (Smith et al. 1979); 10% of 382 ringed seals (32% of infected seals were less than 1 year old) from western Arctic Canada (Onderka 1989); 3 of 5 ringed seals (infected seals were less than 1 year old) from Arctic Quebec (Measures and Gosselin 1994); and 10% of 190 ringed seals (36% of infected seals were less than 1 year old) and 1 of 3 bearded seals (the infected seal was less than 1 year old) from eastern Arctic Canada (Bergeron et al. 1997b). Gosselin et al. (1998) found *O. circumlitus* in young harbor and grey seals (82% of infected seals were less than 1 year old) hunted on the east coast of Canada. Clausen (1978) reported 7 of 37 hunted and 8 of 28 stranded, drowned, or abandoned harbor seals (most examined seals were less than 2 years old) infected with this large bronchial worm in Danish waters. Hunting also introduces sampling bias, particularly for young, naive seals that are more easily shot. In addition, infected young seals may require longer recovery time at the surface following a dive, further increasing their susceptibility to hunting or predation (Gosselin et al. 1998).

Reported intensities range from 1–280 worms in stranded northern elephant and harbor seals less than 1 year old (Gulland et al. 1997). In hunted ringed seals, mean intensity was 14 (Onderka 1989) and 9.4 (Bergeron et al. 1997b). Intensities in stranded harbor seals are generally 1–87 worms (see Van den Broek and Wensvoort 1959; Van den Broek 1963; Claussen et al.

1991). Infections with greater than 40 worms may be fatal (Clausen 1978). Mean intensity was 55 and 2 in the airways and 5 and 58 in the right heart and pulmonary arteries in stranded harbor seals and northern elephant seals, respectively (Gulland et al. 1997). The location and immature stage of worms and the severe pathologic lesions in northern elephant seals (Stroud and Dailey 1978; Gulland et al. 1996, 1997) suggest a poorly adapted host.

Almost no seasonal data on *O. circumlitus* in seals exist. However, some limited data from young seals collected in Europe and North America suggest that they acquire infections after weaning. This suggests transmission is horizontal via the food chain. The youngest reported infected ringed and grey seals were 3.5 and 6.5 months old, respectively (Onderka 1989; Gosselin et al. 1998). Northern elephant seals < 1 year old examined in California had infections as early as April (when 3–4 months old), but prevalence of larvae in feces was not high until October. Harbor seals off California had larvae in feces as early as May (Gulland et al. 1997). Prevalence of adult and larval *O. circumlitus* in California harbor seals increased from May to December, with 100% of 17 seals passing larvae in August. If the time of transmission is known, this may help determine which seasonal prey may serve as intermediate hosts.

ENVIRONMENTAL LIMITATIONS. The importance of environmental conditions during development and transmission of lungworms of marine mammals has not been investigated thoroughly. The wide distribution in arctic, subarctic, and boreal seals suggests wide environmental tolerances or local adaptation. Similarly, the presence of *O. circumlitus* in Lake Baikal indicates adaptation to a freshwater ecosystem (Delyamure et al. 1982). First-stage larvae remained alive in seawater at 5° C for 3–6 months and were infective to fish up to 23 days (Bergeron et al. 1997a). First-stage larvae sink in seawater, but whether larvae infect primarily benthic fish is unknown (Bergeron et al. 1997a).

CLINICAL SIGNS. Observations are made primarily on naturally infected, stranded seals. Also, these animals often have multiple infections including *O. circumlitus, Parafilaroides* spp., and the heartworm, *Acanthocheilonema spirocauda;* therefore, attributing clinical signs to one particular parasite is difficult. Clinical signs also may be inapparent if infections are light. In contrast, various signs are reported in stranded animals that eventually died with heavy infections (Van den Broek and Wensvoort 1959; Claussen et al. 1991; Gulland et al. 1996, 1997). These signs include anorexia, emaciation, dehydration, depression, dyspnea, bronchiospasm, cough with expectoration of blood-flecked bronchial mucus, and blood-tinged nasal discharge. Breathing through the mouth may occur if nasal passages are filled with mucus (Moesker 1987). Mucus and worms could be expelled by coughing (Van den Broek and Wensvoort (1959). Growth may be stunted in young infected seals (Smith 1987); however, this also may result from other factors (Measures and Gosselin 1994; Bergeron et al. 1997b). There was a weak negative relationship between infection with *O. circumlitus* and sternal blubber thickness in hunted ringed seals of < 1-year-old (Bergeron et al. 1997b).

PATHOLOGY AND PATHOGENESIS. Although, pathogenesis of *O. circumlitus* has not been studied, pathological lesions are described from hunted (Onderka 1989) and stranded animals (Stroud and Dailey 1978; Van der Kamp 1987; Breuer et al. 1988; Munro et al. 1992; Gulland et al. 1996, 1997). Severity of lesions caused by *O. circumlitus* depend on intensity of infections and host susceptibility. Obliterative bronchitis with extensive bronchial mucosal hyperplasia occurred in infected ringed seals (Onderka 1989). All infected seals had pulmonary arteritis of variable degree, and some infected seals had periarteritis. In one case a mineralized worm occluded a blood vessel. Onderka (1989) indicated that while there was locally extensive pulmonary consolidation, infected seals had only a slight reduction in respiratory parenchyma compared to uninfected seals; however, he thought the abundant mucus in bronchi may pose respiratory difficulties for a diving animal. However, Munro et al. (1992) found that *O. circumlitus* in the pulmonary arteries of young harbor seals elicited no inflammatory reaction.

According to Dungworth (1985) inflammation of the large bronchi is of less clinical significance than inflammation of the small bronchi and bronchioles. In these deeper regions of the lung, airways may easily be occluded by copious exudate and are too far distal for an effective cough reflex. Furthermore, inflammation of large airways such as bronchi often resolves without any granulation tissue forming. This may account for the apparent lack of evidence of infection in seals older than 1 year.

Bronchial and bronchiolar obstruction and inflammation due to *O. circumlitus* is observed in stranded harbor seals (Geraci 1979; Van der Kamp 1987; Claussen et al. 1991; Munro et al. 1992). Concurrent bacterial or viral infections such as phocine morbillivirus may confound observed pathologies (Menschel et al. 1966; Breuer et al. 1988; Kennedy et al. 1989; Munro et al. 1992; Heide-J.rgensen et al. 1992). Purulent tracheobronchitis in dead or moribund infected harbor seals is reported (Breuer et al. 1988). Abscess formation due to secondary bacterial infection also is reported (Van der Kamp 1987; Claussen et al. 1991; Gulland et al. 1997). In heavily infected stranded harbor seals, airways were blocked with mucus, blood, and worms. Lesions included severely congested lungs, multiple pulmonary abscesses, severe obstructive suppurative bronchitis, and severe bronchopneumonia (Gulland et al. 1997). Cephalic extremities of adult worms deeply embedded in pulmonary tissue elicit markedly visible lesions such as pulmonary hemorrhage and edema.

Severe pathologic lesions due to *O. circumlitus* and leading to death have been documented in northern ele-

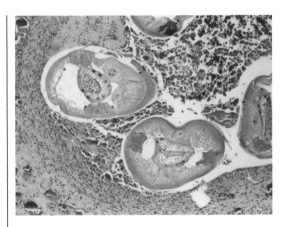

FIG. 10.2—Histologic section from a young elephant seal (*Mirounga angustirostris*) with pulmonary arteritis due to *Otostrongylus circumlitus* (prepatent infection). (Hematoxylin and eosin stain) (63X magnification) (Provided by Linda Lowenstine, University of California at Davis.)

phant seals, suggesting that this species is a poorly adapted host. Verminous or suppurative interstitial pneumonia associated with *O. circumlitus* occurs in northern elephant seals (Stroud and Dailey 1978; Gulland et al. 1996). Sepsis in conjunction with verminous arteritis likely led to disseminated intravascular coagulation and death in one stranded elephant seal. In a larger study, lesions in stranded northern elephant seals included severe suppurative arteritis of the pulmonary vasculature, occasional bronchiolar epithelial necrosis, multiple thromboses, and areas of pulmonary hemorrhage (Fig. 10.2) (Gulland et al. 1997). Various bacteria also were isolated from lung tissues. It was suggested that severe vasculitis or bacterial septicemia secondary to *O. circumlitus* infection led to disseminated intravascular coagulation.

DIAGNOSIS. Adult specimens are described by Railliet (1899), de Bruyn (1933), Delyamure (1955), Menschel et al. (1966), and Bergeron (1996). Adult worms are large: females 32–140 mm long and 0.64–2.4 mm wide, males 30–115 mm long and 0.53–1.3 mm wide. When alive, adult worms are yellowish white in colour. Eggs in utero are 72–129 μm long and 51–76 μm wide with a thin transparent shell. First-stage larvae are 393–469 μm by 19–27 μm (Bergeron et al. 1997a). Freshly collected feces or pulmonary/nasal mucus can be examined for L_1's using smears or suspension in seawater. Larvae can be washed and concentrated using centrifugation followed by examination with a dissecting microscope. Gulland et al. (1997) used a modified filtration/sedimentation method to find larve in a detergent-water mixture. Alternatively, a modified Baermann apparatus (Bergeron et al. 1997b) and staining of bronchial swabs (Claussen et al. 1991) have also been used.

First-stage *O. circumlitus* are described by Railliet (1899), Menschel et al. (1966) and Bergeron et al. (1997a) and should be differentiated from those of *Parafilaroides decorus* and *P. gymnurus* (see Dailey 1970; Gosselin and Measures 1997). All described species possess a dorsally curved or bent tail tip. First-stage larvae of *O. circumlitus* are longer (393–469 µm) and wider (19–27 µm) than those of *P. decorus* (240–279 µm long, 13–18 µm wide) or *P. gymnurus* (220–304 µm long, 11–19 µm wide).

IMMUNITY. Absence of *O. circumlitus* in older seals may be due to mortality of severely infected animals (Onderka 1989); however, there is no evidence that infections last only a few months. Previously infected young seals may develop an acquired immunity (see Claussen et al. 1991; Bergeron et al. 1997b). Older unexposed seals may be resistant, but experimental evidence is lacking. Contaminants or other infectious agents that compromise the immune system may account for infections seen occasionally in older seals.

CONTROL AND TREATMENT. Control of lungworms in free-ranging pinnipeds is not practical. In aquaria or in rehabilitation centers, infections can be treated with anthelminthics, but care must be taken with the choice of drug and dose used (see Dierauf 1990). Allergic reactions may occur when drugs kill large numbers of worms in situ (Munro et al. 1992). Low initial doses in conjunction with antihistamines and adrenocorticotropic agents are recommended (Hubbard 1969). Levamisole and diethylcarbamazine are primarily larvicidal (Sweeney 1972, 1974). Additional treatment to control secondary bacterial infections, dissolve mucus in airways, stimulate expectoration of worms, remove or reduce respiratory distress and shock, and effect rehydration is recommended in some cases (Moesker 1987; Van der Kamp 1987).

PUBLIC HEALTH CONCERNS. There are no reports of human infections with this lungworm. The eating of raw marine fish containing infective larval stages may be a concern for consumers; however, as larvae appear to be restricted to the visceral organs of fish (Bergeron et al. 1997a), it is unlikely that humans would ingest larvae by consuming raw fillets.

MANAGEMENT IMPLICATIONS. *Otostrongylus circumlitus* may have serious implications for recruitment in ringed seal populations in arctic regions (Onderka 1989; Measures and Gosselin 1994; Bergeron et al. 1997b). Impact in young ringed seals could be exacerbated as they dive under the ice to feed and escape predators during winter. However, effects on individual seals and free-ranging populations are difficult to demonstrate (Bergeron et al. 1997b; Gosselin et al. 1998). Northern elephant seals (Gulland et al. 1997) or stranded seals that may be immunocompromised (Geraci 1979; Geraci and St. Aubin 1986; Breuer et al. 1988; Claussen et al. 1991; Munro et al. 1992; Heide-

Jørgensen et al. 1992; Gulland et al. 1996) may be particularly susceptible, with some infections producing severe clinical disease (Menschel et al. 1966; Van Haaften 1982; Gulland et al. 1997).

In captive situations there are no reports of pinnipeds being infected with *O. circumlitus* as most fish given as food is frozen previously, which may kill larvae. However, wild young pinnipeds brought into captivity for display in aquaria or for rehabilitation purposes frequently are naturally infected.

Nematodes are known as vectors of some viral, bacterial, and protozoan pathogens (see Bird and Bird 1991). Lungworms such as *O. circumlitus* and *Parafilaroides decorus* may be vectors for viral or bacterial infections such as *Brucella* spp.(Garner et al. 1997) and calicivirus (Smith et al. 1980). However, evidence of germinal cell infection and subsequent transmission has not been demonstrated ultrastructurally or experimentally. Nematodes may simply serve as mechanical vectors between intermediate and final hosts.

Filaroides (Parafilaroides) spp.

Synonyms: *Pseudalius gymnurus* Railliet, 1899; *Halocercus gymnurus* (Railliet, 1899) Baylis and Daubney, 1925; *Filaroides gymnurus* (Railliet, 1899) Dougherty, 1943; *Filaroides (Parafilaroides) arcticus* (Delyamure and Alekseev, 1966) Kennedy, 1986; *Filaroides (Parafilaroides) krascheninnikovi* (Yurakhno and Skrjabin, 1971) Kennedy, 1986; *Parafilaroides nanus* Dougherty and Herman, 1947; *Parafilaroides prolificus* Dougherty and Herman, 1947.

Small parasitic nematodes belonging to *Filaroides (Parafilaroides)* (Metastrongyloidea: Filaroididae) are found coiled in the respiratory parenchyma of pinnipeds (otariids and phocids). Gosselin and Measures (1997) recognized four valid species of the subgenus *Parafilaroides* (Dougherty, 1946) Anderson 1978: *F. (P.) gymnurus* (Railliet, 1899) Anderson 1978; *F. (P.) decorus* (Dougherty and Herman, 1947) Anderson 1978; *F. (P.) hydrurgae* (Mawson, 1953) Kennedy, 1986; and *F. (P.) hispidus* Kennedy, 1986. *Filaroides (Parafilaroides) caspicus* (Kurochkin and Zablotsky, 1958) Kennedy, 1986 is considered a *species inquirendum* (see Gosselin and Measures 1997).

LIFE HISTORY. *Filaroides (Parafilaroides)* spp. are located throughout the lung (Fleischman and Squire 1970; Onderka 1989; Gosselin et al. 1998); however, adult *Parafilaroides* spp. generally are confined to alveoli and small bronchioles (Migaki et al. 1971; Stroud and Dailey 1978; Nicholson and Fanning 1981; Van der Kamp 1987). A few worms are in the bronchi (see Kontrimavichus and Delyamure 1979, 48) and interlobular septa (Fleischman and Squire 1970; Onderka 1989). Microscopic examination of lung tissue is needed to detect most infections of *Parafilaroides* due to their location and small size. Schumacher et al. (1990) observed *P. gymnurus* in the lungs and pulmonary arteries and apparently in the liver, thymus, and lymph nodes.

Adult females are ovoviviparous and release L_1's into the airways. As the larvae are seen in pulmonary mucus and in feces, it is presumed that larvae are moved passively up the bronchial escalator by mucociliary action, swallowed into the stomach, and passed with feces into the external environment.

Dougherty and Herman (1947) suspected that an intermediate host was required in metastrongyloids infecting marine mammals, and *Parafilaroides decorus* was the first for which a vertebrate intermediate was demonstrated experimentally. Dailey (1970) exposed 8 species of mollusk, 1 species of copepod, and 1 species of teleost fish to first-stage *P. decorus* from naturally infected California sea lions (*Zalophus californianus*). Invertebrates did not become infected; however, larvae molted to the third infective stage in the opaleye fish, *Girella nigricans*. The first molt apparently occurred 12–15 days postinfection, and an L_2 (341 µm long) was observed in the intestinal muscles at 18 days postinfection. The second molt occurred 24–36 days postinfection, after which L_3's (329–384 µm long) were found in the serosa or mesenteric adipose tissue. Third-stage larvae from *G. nigricans* could not be passaged to previously unexposed *G. nigricans* or California killifish (*Fundulus parvipinnis*). A California sea lion whose feces were negative for *Parafilaroides* larvae over 21 days was given *G. nigricans* experimentally infected with *P. decorus*. Prepatent period in the sea lion was 21 days. Apparently, infections remain patent up to 1 year (Sweeney and Gilmartin 1974) and may persist for years (Dailey 1986).

Hill (1971) exposed a Steller sea lion pup (*Eumetopias jubatus*) to 2000–3000 L_3 *P. decorus* from an experimentally infected *G. nigricans*. At 60 days postinfection the sea lion died of pneumonia. Thirty-five worms were recovered; 44% of the females were gravid. The life history of other species of *Parafilaroides* is unknown but is likely similar to that of *P. decorus*. Mollusks and crustaceans may be paratenic or transport hosts of L_1's, but further experimental work is required. Mozgovoi et al. (1963, in Kontrimavichus and Delyamure 1979) exposed a variety of marine invertebrates to ringed seal (*Phoca hispida*) feces containing larval *P. gymnurus*. After 47 days, larvae of similar morphology, but larger and more developed than those in the seal feces, were found in the body cavity of nereid polychaetes. No larvae were found in other invertebrates. This experiment conducted in the tidal zone requires confirmation in a controlled laboratory situation.

EPIZOOTIOLOGY

DISTRIBUTION. Species of *Filaroides* (*Parafilaroides*) are primarily reported from pinnipeds in the northern hemisphere, except *F. (P.) hydrurgae* reported from the Southern Ocean (Heard Island) and an undescribed, apparently new, species of *Parafilaroides* reported from South Australia (see Mawson 1953; Nicholson and Fanning 1981). *Filaroides (P.) gymnurus* is reported from phocids in coastal waters of Canada (western Arctic, eastern Arctic, western Atlantic), Europe (France, Holland, Gulf of Finland), and the former USSR. (White Sea, Chukchi Sea, Bering Sea, Sea of Okhotsk, Lake Baikal). *Filaroides (P.) decorus* is reported from otariids in Pacific waters of the United States. *Filaroides (P.) hispidus* is reported from phocids in coastal waters of Canada (western Arctic and western Atlantic). *Filaroides (P.) caspicus sp. inq.* is reported in the Caspian seal from the Caspian Sea (see Gosselin and Measures 1997). Pulmonary nematodes have been reported in Antarctic fur seals (Baker and McCann 1989) as well as crabeater and Weddell seals (Schumacher et al. 1990), but worms were not identified. Similarly, Hanni et al. (1997) reported verminous pneumonia in a stranded Guadalupe fur seal (*Arctocephalus townsendi*) in California, but worms were not identified. Due to the paucity of parasitological work with the 11 species of otariids and 5 species of phocids known in the southern hemisphere (see Dailey 1975), it is likely that new species of *Parafilaroides* remain to be discovered.

HOST RANGE. Final hosts of *F. (P.) gymnurus* are phocid seals including harbor seal, ringed seal, harp seal, spotted seal, grey seal, bearded seal, and Baikal seal (Railliet 1899; Van den Broek and Wensvoort 1959; Van den Broek 1963; Delyamure and Alekseev 1966; Yurakhno and Skrjabin 1971; Delyamure and Popov 1975; Delyamure et al. 1980, 1982, 1984; Van der Kamp 1987, Schumacher et al. 1990; Claussen et al. 1991; Borgsteede et al. 1991; Measures and Gosselin 1994; Gosselin and Measures 1997; Gosselin et al. 1998). Final hosts of *F. (P.) decorus* are otariid pinnipeds including California sea lion, Steller sea lion, and northern fur seal (*Callorhinus ursinus*) (Dougherty and Herman 1947; Dailey 1970; Migaki et al. 1971; Schroeder et al. 1973; Sweeney and Gilmartin 1974; Ridgway et al. 1975; Stroud and Dailey 1978; Stroud and Roffe 1979; Dailey and Otto 1982; Joseph and Cornell 1986; Gage et al. 1993; Roletto 1993). Final hosts of *F. (P.) hispidus* are phocid seals including ringed seal and grey seals (Kennedy 1986; Onderka 1989; Gosselin et al. 1998). The final host of *F. (P.) hydrurgae* is the leopard seal (*Hydrurga leptonyx*) (Mawson 1953). The final host of *F. (P.) caspicus sp. inq.* is the Caspian seal (Kurochkin and Zablotsky 1958; Kurochkin 1975), and the final host of an unidentified species of *Parafilaroides* is the Australian sea lion (*Neophoca cinerea*) (Nicholson and Fanning 1981). The report of *Parafilaroides* in the Pacific harbor seal (Garner et al. 1997) requires verification. Unidentified or tentatively identified *Parafilaroides* spp. are reported in Steller sea lion (Margolis 1956; Dailey and Hill 1970), California sea lion (Johnson and Ridgway 1969; Gerber et al. 1993), northern elephant seal (Johnson and Ridgway 1969; Stroud and Dailey 1978; Stroud and Roffe 1979; Dailey and Otto 1982;

Gerber et al. 1993; Gulland et al. 1996), northern fur seal (Gerber et al. 1993), Atlantic harbor seal (Munro et al. 1992), and grey seal (Baker 1987, 1989).

PREVALENCE AND INTENSITY. Prevalence and intensity data must be interpreted with caution as *Parafilaroides* spp. are very difficult to remove from tissues and as some reports are based on histologic evidence only. Also, prevalence data often is obtained from stranded animals which are not representative of infections in free-ranging populations. Small gravid worms seen in cross sections of alveoli are likely *Parafilaroides* spp. as the only other lungworm found in pinnipeds, *Otostrongylus circumlitus,* is large and is located in large bronchioles and bronchi. Morphology of larvae in histologic sections of lung tissue from pinnipeds has not been studied. Identification of species of *Parafilaroides* is often based on host (e.g., only *P. decorus* has been reported in the California sea lion), but morphological study is required to verify the species, delimit host and geographic range, and estimate prevalence (see Host Range section).

Prevalence of *P. gymnurus* in stranded seals ranged from 8% to 88% (Van den Broek and Wensvoort 1959; Van den Broek 1963; Schumacher et al. 1990; Borgsteede et al. 1991). Borgsteede et al. (1991) observed up to 143 worms in stranded harbor seals from the Wadden Sea but also indicated that intensities may be higher based on limitations of the techniques used. Prevalence of *P. decorus* in stranded pinnipeds from the Pacific coast of the United States was 8%–85% in California sea lions (Dailey 1970; Sweeney and Gilmartin 1974; Stroud and Dailey 1978; Dailey and Otto 1982; Dierauf et al. 1985; Gage et al. 1993), 14%–56% in Steller sea lions (Dailey and Hill 1970; Stroud and Dailey 1978; Dailey and Otto 1982), and 9% in the northern fur seal (Gage et al. 1993). There are no estimates of intensity of infection with *P. decorus.*

Prevalence of *P. gymnurus* in hunted seals was 5%–81% in ringed seals (Yurakhno 1972; Yurakhno and Popov 1976; Delyamure et al. 1980; Measures and Gosselin 1994; Gosselin et al. 1998), 2% in spotted seal (Delyamure et al. 1984), 41% in Baikal seal (Delyamure et al. 1982), 9% in bearded seal (Delyamure and Popov 1975), 24% in grey seals, 27% in Atlantic harbor seals, and 57% in harp seals (Gosselin et al. 1998). Intensity of *P. gymnurus* was reported as 35–120 worms in bearded seals (Delyamure and Popov 1975). In a systematic quantitative study of four species of Canadian seals, mean intensity of *P. gymnurus* was estimated as 139–896 (range: 37–3570) worms (Gosselin et al. 1998).

Prevalence of *P. hispidus* was 53% of ringed seals (Onderka 1989), 2 of 3 grey seals, and 2 of 7 ringed seals (Gosselin et al. 1998). Gosselin et al. (1998) estimated mean intensities of *P. hispidus* as 314 in grey seals and 1040 in ringed seals (range: 295–332 and 886–1196, respectively).

Species of *Parafilaroides* are reported in all age classes of hunted pinnipeds (Kontrimavichus and

Delyamure 1979; Onderka 1989; Gosselin et al. 1998). Onderka (1989) found that prevalence of *P. hispidus* in ringed seals increased with age (44% in seals ≤6 years to 71% in seals 7–13 years) but declined to 38% in seals > 13 years old. Hunted harp seals as young as 3 months old can be infected with *P. gymnurus* (J.-F. Gosselin, unpublished). Stranded pinnipeds are almost always young animals (young of the year or sexually immature adults) (Sweeney and Gilmartin 1974; Ridgway et al. 1975; Dierauf et al. 1985; Borgsteede et al. 1991; Claussen et al. 1991; Gage et al. 1993; Gerber et al. 1993), and infections with *Parafilaroides* spp. are commonly observed in these animals.

ENVIRONMENTAL LIMITATIONS. *Parafilaroides gymnurus* seems to have the widest distribution, with *P. decorus* apparently restricted to the Pacific coast of the United States (Dailey 1970; Dailey and Hill 1970; Dailey and Otto 1982). Apparently *P. decorus* L_1's die when subjected to cold temperatures found in northern California (Hill 1971). Larval *P. gymnurus* apparently survived in frozen lung tissue for 17 days at –20° C (J.-F. Gosselin, personal communiation). An unidentified species of *Parafilaroides* was reported from a Steller sea lion collected north of Vancouver Island, British Columbia (Margolis 1956), but infection may have been acquired elsewhere. The only known intermediate host, *Girella nigricans,* has a limited distribution, although other fish may be suitable hosts (Stroud and Dailey 1978). Gosselin et al. (1998) showed that ringed seals were more suitable hosts for *P. gymnurus* and *P. hispidus* than grey, harp, harbor, or bearded seals. Greater prevalence and maturity (females with larvae in utero) of *Parafilaroides* spp. in ringed seals compared to those from other seal species may relate to host physiology, diet, immune status, habitat, availability of infected intermediate hosts, transmission dynamics, or local environmental conditions. These factors remain to be investigated. The report of *P. gymnurus* in Lake Baikal seals indicates adaptation to a freshwater ecosystem (Delyamure et al. 1982).

CLINICAL SIGNS. Observations of pinnipeds infected with *Parafilaroides* spp. are made primarily on stranded animals undergoing rehabilitation or on naturally infected captive animals (Fleischman and Squire 1970; Migaki et al. 1971; Morales and Helmboldt 1971; Sweeney 1986). Attributing clinical signs to one parasite poses difficulties due to multiple infections including *O. circumlitus* and heartworm, *Acanthocheilonema spirocauda.* However, California sea lions apparently harbor only *P. decorus.* Clinical signs in sea lions vary from none to severe and include coughing, passing of mucus, and difficulty eating (Fleischman and Squire 1970; Ashizawa et al. 1978). In early or light infections, increased respiratory rate with a mild productive cough (Sweeney 1986) progresses to labored breathing (Migaki et al. 1971), vomiting, weight loss, and severe respiratory distress in advanced cases (Morales and Helmboldt 1971). Clinical signs may thus include anorexia, malaise, emaciation, dyspnea (as evidenced by flared nostrils and breathing through the mouth), bronchiospasm, and cough with expectoration of blood-flecked bronchial mucus. Upon auscultation of the thorax, rales, crackles, and wheezing sounds may be heard, although an absence of sounds may indicate total occlusion of the bronchi. Mucous membranes may be pale and cyanotic (Sweeney 1986).

PATHOLOGY AND PATHOGENESIS. Pathogenesis of *Parafilaroides* spp. has not been studied. Lesions have been described from hunted and stranded or captive animals. Severity of lesions depends on intensity of infections and host susceptibility. Onderka (1989) described minimal cellular inflammation around firm granulomatous nodules containing *P. hispidus* in hunted ringed seals. He thought a mild reaction indicated a parasite well adapted to its host. Suppuration and localized hemorrhage were seen around *P. gymnurus* in hunted ringed seals (Delyamure et al. 1980). In captured wild adult Australian sea lions, no gross lung lesions were observed, but histologic evidence of mild verminous pneumonia associated with *Parafilaroides* sp. was observed in small areas of the lungs (Nicholson and Fanning 1981). Adult and larval worms free in the lung parenchyma stimulated little inflammatory response. However, in some airways acute bronchitis and bronchopneumonia with increased mucous secretion, fibrinous exudate, and acute congestion of bronchial and alveolar vessels was observed around adult worms in alveolar ducts and sacs. The latter authors considered infections might predispose healthy animals to respiratory disease during times of stress.

Lesions attributed to *Parafilaroides* spp. in stranded pinnipeds or animals undergoing rehabilitation are well documented. Live adult worms in lung parenchyma appear to stimulate little inflammatory reaction in otherwise healthy animals. The inflammatory response during the early phase of infection is not described and requires experimental work; however, reactions to migrating nematodes are described in the liver, pulmonary arteries, and lymph nodes (Schumacher et al. 1990; Munro et al. 1992).

Verminous pneumonia due to *Parafilaroides* spp., often leading to death, is reported. Lesions include acute to chronic suppurative bronchitis, bronchiolitis, peribronchiolitis, mucoid bronchiolar obstruction, bronchopneumonia, pulmonary edema, multifocal atelectasis and emphysema, multiple microabcessation, and granuloma formation (Figs. 10.3, 10.4) (Dougherty and Herman 1947; Van den Broek and Wensvoort 1959; Fleischman and Squire 1970; Morales and Helmboldt 1971; Migaki et al. 1971; Sweeney and Gilmartin 1974; Stroud and Dailey 1978; Stroud and Roffe 1979; Van der Kamp 1987; Schumacher et al. 1990; Garner et al. 1997) and may largely be a response to the irritating presence of L1's (Fleischman and Squire 1970; Stroud and Dailey 1978; and others). Intra-alveolar hemorrhage also is reported (Fleischman and Squire 1970; Schumacher et al. 1990; Gulland et al. 1996). In a

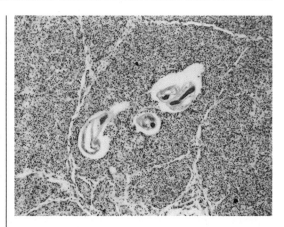

FIG. 10.3—Histologic section from a young elephant seal (*Mirounga angustirostris*) with pulmonary atelectasis and diffuse acute to subacute interstitial pneumonia showing *Parafilaroides* sp. within the parenchyma (Hematoxylin and eosin stain) (63X magnification). (Provided by Linda Lowenstine, University of California at Davis.)

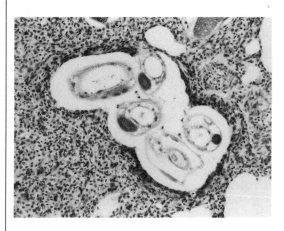

FIG. 10.4—Histologic section from a young elephant seal showing cellular reaction to immature *Parafilaroides* sp. within the parenchyma. (Hematoxylin and eosin stain) (130X magnification) (Provided by Linda Lowenstine, University of California at Davis.)

northern elephant seal, infection with *O. circumlitus* and *Parafilaroides* sp. likely triggered disseminated intravascular coagulation (Gulland et al. 1996).

Concurrent lungworm, heartworm, bacterial, or viral infections (such as phocine morbillivirus) may interfere with interpretation of pulmonary lesions (Breuer et al. 1988; Schumacher et al. 1990; Munro et al. 1992; Heide-J.rgensen et al. 1992). Various species of bacteria have been cultured from the lungs of animals with verminous pneumonia and multifocal microabscesses may form due to secondary bacterial infection (Flei-

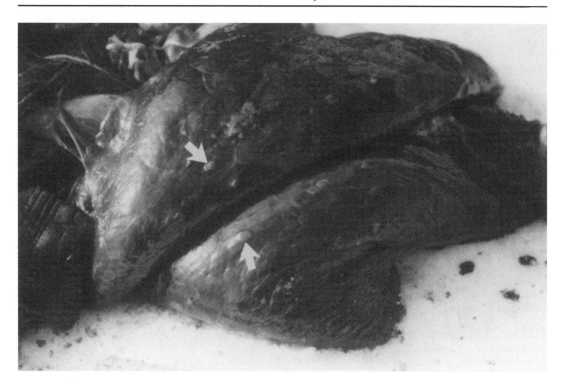

FIG. 10.5—Dorsal view of lungs from a harp seal (*Phoca groenlandica*). Arrows denote nodular lesions containing *Filaroides* (*Parafilaroides*) spp. (likely *P. gymnurus*). (Reprinted by permission National Research Council.)

schman and Squire 1970; Sweeney 1972; Sweeney and Gilmartin 1974; Claussen et al. 1991; Gulland et al. 1996). A mild to severe granulomatous reaction is commonly observed around dead, degenerating adult worms (Migaki et al. 1971 and others). A hypersensitivity reaction as described by Fleischman and Squire (1970) requires verification experimentally.

DIAGNOSIS. Adult specimens are described by Railliet (1899), Dougherty and Herman (1947), Mawson (1953), Delyamure (1955), Kontrimavichus and Delyamure (1979), Kennedy (1986), and Gosselin and Measures (1997). Adult worms are small; females are 5–90 mm long and 0.051–0.397 mm wide, and males are 3–37 mm long and 0.068–0.165 mm wide. Worms are in complex knots in tissue, often within nodular lesions (each nodule may contain one or more adults) (Fig. 10.5) (Gosselin et al. 1998). Due to their location and delicacy, worms are difficult to extract intact. Systematic slicing and examination of frozen lungs or compression of excised nodules using glass plates and a dissecting microscope may reveal infections (Gosselin et al. 1998). Dailey (1970) minced fresh lungs in seawater and allowed worms to migrate from tissues. Cutting around and mincing nodules visible on the surface of fresh lungs and placing them in a mild formalin solution (which stimulates activity) allows adult worms to be collected (M.D. Dailey, personal communication).

In live animals infection is determined by examination of feces or pulmonary/nasal mucus for L_1's (Dailey 1986). Eggs in utero are 49–68 μm long and 39–49 μm wide with a thin transparent shell. First-stage larvae are 220–304 μm long. Samples are examined using smears or suspension of feces in seawater (larvae can be washed and concentrated using centrifugation) followed by examination with a microscope. A modified Baermann apparatus can be used to collect larvae from a large quantity of feces (Bergeron et al. 1997b). Radiography is helpful in diagnosis of verminous pneumonia due to *P. decorus* (Ballarini 1974, Sweeney 1974). Haematologic and serum chemistry data for clinically healthy and sick pinnipeds with verminous pneumonia due to *P. decorus* or other lungworms is provided (Roletto 1993). Refer to the section on *O. circumlitus* for further details of larval identification.

IMMUNITY. *Parafilaroides* spp. is particularly prevalent in California sea lions < 2 years old (Sweeney and Gilmartin 1974) and harbor seals between 6 months and 2 years old (Van der Kamp 1987). Young animals may be more susceptible due to their poorly developed immune system or differences in diet. As young pinnipeds learn to feed independently postweaning, they initially eat invertebrates or easily caught small fish in shallow waters. Ingestion of a tide-pool fish found around sea lion rookeries may account for most infections in young California sea lions before they disperse (Dailey 1970). Dailey (1986) reported that infections may persist in pinnipeds 5 years in captivity. Gravid *P. decorus* were still present in lungs, and larvae were being passed in feces of California sea lions 1 year after being experimentally infected (Sweeney and Gilmartin 1974). These observations suggest that infections are not self-limiting, worms live a long time, and protective immunity may not develop.

CONTROL AND TREATMENT. Hubbard (1969) reported that fecal larval output of *P. decorus* ceased when California sea lions were treated with thiabendazole but resumed when treatment stopped. Gage et al. (1993) used ivermectin concurrently with dexamethasone. Dosage and duration of treatment is dependent on clinical signs and number of larvae seen in feces of sea lions infected with *P. decorus*. Refer to the section on *Otostrongylus circumlitus* for more information.

PUBLIC HEALTH CONCERNS. See section on *Otostrongylus circumlitus*.

MANAGEMENT IMPLICATIONS. *Parafilaroides* spp. can have serious implications including fatal verminous pneumonia in hosts immunocompromised by contaminants or other infectious agents, injury, or starvation (Sweeney and Gilmartin 1974; Ridgway et al. 1975; Stroud and Dailey 1978; Stroud and Roffe 1979; Joseph and Cornell 1986; Baker 1987, 1989; Breuer et al. 1988; Schumacher et al. 1990, Munro et al. 1992; Heide-J rgensen et al. 1992; Roletto 1993; Gage et al. 1993; Gulland et al. 1996; Garner et al. 1997). Captive California sea lions with subclinical infections can experience severe clinical disease when stressed during routine performances. Wild pinnipeds with moderate to severe infections may be less able to dive or forage efficiently, requiring longer recovery times at the surface, thereby increasing risk of predation. It has been postulated that *Parafilaroides* spp. may vector viral or bacterial infections such as *Brucella* spp. (Garner et al. 1997), calicivirus (Barlough et al. 1986; Smith et al. 1980), or morbillivirus (Breuer et al. 1988; Borgsteede et al. 1991; Heide-Jørgensen et al. 1992; Munro et al. 1992). This has not been confirmed.

LUNGWORMS OF CETACEANS

Pseudaliidae. The Pseudaliidae (Metastrongyloidea) include eight genera, seven of which are restricted to the Odontoceti: *Pseudalius* Dujardin, 1845; *Torynurus* Baylis and Daubney, 1925 (=*Irukanema* Yamaguti, 1951); *Pharurus* Leuckart, 1948 (=*Otophocaenurus* Skrjabin, 1942); *Stenurus* Dujardin, 1845; *Pseudostenurus* Yamaguti, 1951; *Skrjabinalius* Delyamure, 1942; and *Halocercus* Baylis and Daubney, 1925 (=*Delamurella* Gubanov, 1952) (Table 10.1). *Stenuroides* Gerichter, 1951 is found in the mongoose, *Herpestes ichneumon*. Species of *Halocercus* are found

TABLE 10.1—Pseudaliids in Odontoceti

Subfamily	Species	Host Range
Pseudaliinae	*Pseudalius inflexus* (Rudolphi, 1808) Schneider, 1866	Phocoenidae, Delphinidae
Stenurinae	*Torynurus convolutus* (Kuhn, 1829) Baylis and Daubney, 1925	Phocoenidae, Delphinidae
	T. dalli (Yamaguti, 1951) Delyamure, 1972	Phocoenidae
	Pharurus alatus (Leukart, 1848) Stiles and Hassall, 1905	Monodontidae
	P. pallasii (van Beneden, 1870) Arnold and Gaskin, 1975	Monodontidae
	P. asiaorientalis Petter and Pilleri, 1982	Phocoenidae
	Stenurus minor (Kuhn, 1829) Baylis and Daubney, 1925	Phocoenidae, Delphinidae
	S. globicephalae Baylis and Daubney, 1925	Delphinidae
	S. arctomarinus Delyamure and Kleinenberg, 1958	Monodontidae
	S. ovatus (Linstow, 1910) Baylis and Daubney, 1925	Delphinidae
	S. auditivus Hsu and Hoeppli, 1933	Phocoenidae, Delphinidae
	S. truei Machida, 1974	Delphinidae
	S. australis Sarmiento and Tantalean, 1991	Phocoenidae
	S. nanjingensis Tao, 1983	Phocoenidae
	S. yamaguti Kuramochi, Araki and Machida, 1990	Phocoenidae
	Pseudostenurus sunameri Yamaguti, 1951	Phocoenidae
	Skrjabinalius cryptocephalus Delyamure in Skrjabin, 1942	Delphinidae
	S. guevarai Gallego and Selva, 1979	Delphinidae
Halocercinae	*Halocercus delphini* Baylis and Daubney, 1925	Delphinidae
	H. taurica Delyamure in Skrjabin, 1942	Phocoenidae
	H. invaginatus (Quekett, 1841) Dougherty, 1943	Phocoenidae
	H. monoceris Webster, Neufeld and MacNeill, 1973	Monodontidae
	H. lagenorhynchi Baylis and Daubney, 1925	Delphinidae
	H. brasiliensis Lins de Almeida, 1933	Delphinidae
	H. dalli Yamaguti, 1951	Phocoenidae
	H. pingi Wu, 1929	Phocoenidae
	H. sunameri Yamaguti, 1951	Phocoenidae
	H. kirbyi Dougherty, 1944	Phocoenidae
	H. kleinenbergi Delyamure, 1951	Delphinidae
	H. hyperoodoni (Gubanov 1952) Anderson, 1978	Ziphiidae

within the pulmonary parenchyma, often with posterior extremities extending into the bronchioles or bronchi. *Pseudalius inflexus,* species of *Skrjabinalius,* a few species of *Stenurus,* and *Torynurus convolutus* are found in bronchi and bronchioles. Species of *Pharurus,* most species of *Stenurus, Pseudostenurus sunameri,* and occasionally *Torynurus convolutus* are found in the middle ear, eustachian tube, and cranial sinuses. Raga and Balbuena (1993) showed that 74% of *S. globicephalae* occurred in the cranial sinuses and 21% in the lungs, suggesting that the preferred site is the cranial sinuses. Pseudaliids found in the heart, pulmonary blood vessels, blowhole, or trachea are probably migrating to the lungs or migrating postmortem, or they may indicate aberrant locations in poorly adapted hosts. Infected odontocetes held in captivity often expel worms via the blowhole into their pool, on the edge of their pool, or into the face of their handlers! Presumably to avoid being expelled from the lungs during the rapid, forceful expiration characteristic of whales, some pseudaliids embed their cephalic extremity in the parenchyma or walls of bronchi or bronchioles (i.e., *Stenurus arctomarinus*). Others coil their body within parenchyma, leaving only the posterior extremity free in airways (i.e., *Halocercus kleinenbergi*), and some intertwine their anterior extremities in the parenchyma, forming complex knots that become encapsulated by host tissue (i.e., *Skrjabinalius* spp.). The latter are very difficult to extract intact. *Stenurus arctomarinus,* with perhaps a less secure form of attachment, can be expelled by infected beluga (*Delphinapterus leucas*) held captive at least 1 year (J.R. Boehm, personal communication).

LIFE HISTORY. Little is known of the life history of any of the pseudaliids, and consequently it is not possible to consider any particular species in detail in this review. However, it is instructive (and may stimulate further research) to consider possible life history strategies for those species where data are suggestive.

Metastrongyloids of terrestrial hosts are heteroxenous, and transmission involves gastropods and oligochaetes as intermediate hosts, except in a few metastrongyloid species for which intermediate hosts may be unnecessary (see Anderson 2000). Vertebrate intermediate hosts, such as fish, appear to be involved in transmission of metastrongyloids of pinnipeds (Dailey 1970; Bergeron et al. 1997a). Cetaceans are wholly aquatic and highly vagile, and some pelagic species spend their entire lives in deep water, rarely venturing near coastal areas. This poses unique transmission problems for parasites. Field data have not implicated intermediate hosts, but there are many reports of unidentified nematode larvae from fish (see Margolis and Arthur 1979; McDonald and Margolis 1995).

In studies involving large samples of odontocetes of all ages, data suggest that some pseudaliids are acquired postlactation, when calves begin to feed on invertebrate and vertebrate prey (Kleinenberg 1956; Geraci et al. 1978; Clausen and Andersen 1988; Reyes and Van Waerebeek 1995; Faulkner et al. 1998). This suggests that transmission is horizontal via the food chain. Vertical transmission via placenta or mammary [the latter occurs with the hookworm, *Uncinaria lucasi,* in northern fur seals (Olsen and Lyons 1965)] is a possible solution in the marine environment. Dailey et al. (1991) presented convincing evidence that transplacental transmission may occur in *Halocercus lagenorhynchi* of bottlenose dolphins *(Tursiops truncatus).* This is supported by the presence and, in some cases, high prevalence of *Halocercus* spp. in young porpoises and dolphins (Caldwell et al. 1968; Cowan and Walker 1979; Conlogue et al. 1985; Raga et al. 1989). First-stage larvae passed into the external environment may be infective to other cetaceans through contaminated water, aerosol, or vomitus (as seen with *Filaroides hirthi, Oslerus osleri,* and *Andersonstrongylus captivensis* in some terrestrial hosts (see Anderson 1992)), but this is probably unlikely as larvae would be easily dispersed and lost in the marine environment. However, Woodard et al. (1969) invoked this mode of transmission to account for an infection seen in a captive 21-year-old bottlenose dolphin born in captivity and presumably in contact with infected dolphins.

EPIZOOTIOLOGY

DISTRIBUTION. Pseudaliids are reported from odontocetes throughout the world (Table 10.2), but most work is done in the northern hemisphere, primarily with coastal or inshore populations.

HOST RANGE. Final hosts are odontocetes, including phocoenids (porpoises), delphinids (dolphins), monodontids (beluga, narwhal), and at least one ziphiid (beaked whale) (Tables 10.1, 10.2). Host range of pseudaliids requires careful study of the literature as some reports are based on histologic evidence only. Excluded from Table 10.2 are reports of unidentified species of *Stenurus, Halocercus,* and *Skrjabinalius.*

In the monodontids, two species of pseudaliids are unique to the beluga, one species is shared with the narwhal (*Monodon monoceros*), and one is unique to the narwhal but requires further research (Table 10.2). There is a rich fauna of pseudaliids in phocoenids and delphinids (Tables 10.1, 10.2). The only reported lungworm species in ziphiids is *Halocercus (=Delamurella) hyperoodoni,* reported originally from the northern bottle-nose whale, *Hyperoodon ampullatus* (Gubanov 1952, cited in Delyamure 1955, 276–280). However, this whale apparently is absent from the collection locality, the Sea of Okhotsk, and the host was probably Baird's beaked whale, *Berardius bairdi* (see Delyamure 1955; Tomilin 1957; Arnold and Gaskin 1975; Anderson 1978). *Halocercus* sp. is reported in a ziphiid, *Mesoplodon* sp., but requires confirmation (Moser and Rhinehart 1993). The apparent paucity of pseudaliids in ziphiids may be due to lack of study, differences in diet (most specialize on squid), and habitat (open sea, over deep water).

TABLE 10.2—Species of pseudaliid nematodes reported in odontocetes worldwide

Species	Host	Locality	Reference
Pseudalius inflexus	Phocoena phocoena, P. spinipinnis, Lagenorhynchus acutus	NW and NE Atlantic, SE Pacific	[1]Abeloos 1932, Andersen 1974, [2]Arnold and Gaskin 1975, [3]Balbuena et al. 1994, [4]Baylis 1932, [5]Baylis and Daubney 1925, [6]Brosens et al 1996, [7]Clausen and Andersen 1988, [8]Corcuera et al. 1995, [9]Dailey and Brownell 1972, [10]Delyamure 1955, [11]Dougherty 1943, [12]Geraci 1979, [13]Gibson and Harris 1979, Kastelein et al. 1990, [14]Kinze 1989, [15]Larsen 1995, [16]Raga et al. 1987a, 1989[17], Reyes and Van Waerebeek 1995, [18]Rogan and Berrow 1996, [19]Rokicki et al. 1997, [20]Stede 1994, [21]Wesenberg-Lund 1947
Torynurus convolutus	P. phocoena, L. acutus, Globicephala melas, G. macrorhynchus	NW and NE Atlantic, NW and NE Pacific	1–6, 9–14, 16–20, [22]Dailey and Stroud 1978, [23]Faulkner et al. 1998, Kontrimavichus et al. 1976, Margolis and Dailey 1972, [24]Scheffer and Slipp 1948, Sergeant 1962, [25]Stroud and Roffe 1979
T. dalli	Phocoenoides dalli	NW and NE Pacific	2, Dailey 1971, [26]Dailey and Walker 1978, Dailey 1988, [27]Kuramochi et al. 1990, [28]Machida 1974, [29]Yamaguti 1951
Pharurus alatus	Monondon monoceros	Canada (Baffin Island), Greenland	2, 4, 5, 9–11
P. pallasii	Delphinapterus leucas	NW Atlantic, NW and NE Pacific, Arctic Ocean, Hudson Bay, White, Kara and Barents Seas	2, 4, 5, 9, 11, Babero and Thomas 1960, Brodie 1971, Doan and Douglas 1953, [30]Delyamure and Kleinenberg 1958, Kenyon and Kenyon 1977, [31]Kleinenberg et al. 1964, [32]Kontrimavichus et al. 1976, [33]Martineau et al. 1986, [34]1988, [35]Measures et al. 1995, Wazura et al. 1986
P. asiaorientalis	Neophocaena phocaenoides	Yangtze R., China	Petter and Pilleri 1982
Stenurus minor	P. phocoena, P. dalli, P. spinipinnis, Delphinus delphis, Grampus griseus, Tursiops truncatus	NW, NE, and SW Atlantic, NW and SE Pacific, Arctic Ocean, Baltic, Azov and Black Seas	2, 4–20, 22, 23, 26, 31, 32, Johnston and Ridgway 1969 [36]Kleinenberg 1956, [37]Morales and 1969, Gomez 1993
S. nanjingensis	N. phocaenoides,	China	[38]Tao 1983
S. globicephalae	G. griseus, G. melas, G. macrorhynchus, L. acutus, Peponocephala electra, Pseudorca crassidens, Feresa attenuata	NW and NE Atlantic, SW and SE Pacific, Caribbean Sea	2, 5, 9, 11–13, 16, 21, 22, 37, [39]Abollo et al. 1998, Beverley-Burton 1978, Cannon 1977, Cowan 1967, Dollfus 1968, Forrester et al. 1980, Geraci 1978, Geraci et al. 1978, Kikuchi and Nakajima 1996, Mignucci-Giannoni et al. 1998, Odell et al. 1980, Parry et al. 1983, [40]Raga and Balbuena 1993, Yamaguti 1943
S. arctomarinus	D. leucas	Hudson Bay, Arctic Ocean, Barents and White Seas	2, 9, 25, 31, 35
S. ovatus	T. truncatus, Stenella coeruleoalba, Lagenodelphis hosei,	NE Atlantic, SW Pacific, Black, Mediterranean, and Adriatic Seas	4, 5, 9–11, 13, Baylis 1928, [41]Bowie 1984, Linstow 1910, McColl and Obendorf 1982, [42]Podesta et al. 1992, [43]Troncone et al. 1994
S. auditivus	N. phocaenoides,	China	Hsü and Hoeppli 1933
S. truei	P. dalli	NW Pacific	27, 28
S. australis	P. spinipinnis	SE Pacific	Sarmiento and Tantalean 1991, Torres et al. 1994
S. yamaguti	P. dalli	NW Pacific	27
Pseudostenurus sunameri	N. phocaenoides	Japan, China	29, 38
Skrjabinalius cryptocephalus	D. delphis, T. truncatus	SE Pacific, Black and Azov Seas	9–11, 32, 36, 41
S. guevarai	T. truncatus, D. delphis S. coeruleoalba	NE Atlantic, Adriatic Sea	16, 42, 43, Duignan et al. 1992, Gallego and Selva 1979, Raga and Carbonell 1985, Raga et al. 1987b
Halocercus delphini	D. delphis, T. truncatus, S. attenuata, S. longirostris, S. coeruleoalba	NE and SE Atlantic, Pacific Ocean, Mediterranean Sea	4, 5, 9–11, 13, 16, 39, 43, Dailey and Otto 1982, Dailey and Perrin 1973, Viale 1981, [44]Zam et al. 1971

TABLE 10.2   (*continued*)

Species	Host	Locality	Reference
H. taurica	*P. phocoena*	NW Atlantic, NW Pacific, Black and Azov Seas	2, 9, 10
H. monoceris	*M. monodon, D. leucas*	Canada (Quebec, Baffin Island)	35, Webster et al. 1973, MacNeill et al. 1975
H. lagenorhynchi	*Lagenorhynchus albirostris, D. delphis, T. truncatus, S. coeruleoalba*	NW, NE and SE Atlantic, Adriatic Sea, SW Pacific	4, 5, 9–11, 13, 44, Dailey et al. 1991, Johnston and Mawson 1941, Sweeney and Ridgway 1975, Woodard et al. 1969
H. invaginatus	*P. phocoena*	NW and NE Atlantic, NE Pacific, Baltic, Black, Azov and Barents Seas	2–4, 9–13, 15, 18, 19, 22, 24, 25, 32, 39, [45]Dougherty 1944, Moser and Rhinehart 1993, Smith and Threlfall 1973, Temirova and Usik 1971
H. brasiliensis	*Sotalia fluviatilis, Cephalorhynchus commersonii*	Brazil, Argentina, Colombia	9–11, 13, Greenwood and Taylor 1979, Lins de Almeida 1933, Santos et al. 1996
H. dalli	*P. dalli*	N Pacific	28, 29, Conlogue et al. 1985, Machida 1968
H. pingi	*N. phocaenoides, P. dalli*	China	4, 9, 11, Wu 1929
H. sunameri	*N. phocaenoides*	Japan	29
H. kleinenbergi	*D. delphis*	Black Sea, South Africa	9, 10, Harris 1982
H. hyperoodoni	*Berardius bairdii*	Sea of Okhotsk	9, Gubanov 1952 in Delyamure 1955
H. kirbyi	*P. dalli, P. phocoena*	California	9, 45

Lungworms are not reported from river dolphins (iniids, pontoporiids, platanistids) or sperm whales (physeterid, kogiids) (see Delyamure 1955; Tomilin 1957; Kontrimavichus et al. 1976). However, respiratory infections of unknown etiology, possibly due to a lungworm, are reported in the Amazon River dolphin or boto, *Inia geoffrensis* (Best and da Silva 1989). Reports of *Halocercus* sp. in *Inia geoffrensis, Stenurus* sp. in the pygmy sperm whale (*Kogia breviceps*), *Stenurus minor* in the beluga, *Halocercus* sp. in the melon-headed whale (*Peponocephala electra*), lungworms in the northern rightwhale dolphin (*Lissodelphis borealis*), *Halocercus* sp. in the humpbacked dolphin [*Sousa* sp. (*S. chinensis?*)], *Halocercus* sp. in the dusky dolphin (*Lagenorhynchus obscurus*), *Pseudostenurus* sp. in the harbor porpoise (*Phocoena phocoena*), and *Stenurus auditivus* in the false killer whale (*Pseudorca crassidens*) require verification (Delyamure 1955; Zam et al. 1971; Dailey and Brownell 1972; Smith and Threlfall 1973; Gibson and Harris 1979; Moser and Rhinehart 1993; Van Waerebeek et al. 1993). Interestingly, mysticetes do not appear to harbor any metastrongyloids (Delyamure 1955; Tomilin 1957; Cockrill 1960; Simpson and Gardner 1972), which may reflect their different evolutionary history, anatomy, diet, and behavior compared to odontocetes (Purves 1966; Yablokov et al. 1972; Gaskin 1976; Fordyce and Barnes 1994; Shimamura et al. 1997). With > 70 odontocetes known worldwide (some species being rare, endangered, or seldom seen) and most work involving stranded animals, there are likely many new species of pseudaliid yet to be discovered.

PREVALENCE AND INTENSITY. Most prevalence and intensity data are obtained from odontocetes that strand or die in fishing nets or traps (by-catch), with a few studies involving shooting or driving herds ashore or into nets. Efforts to examine thoroughly such animals and enumerate pseudaliid infections in a systematic manner vary enormously, and data should be evaluated with caution. In many cases intensity is not recorded as some lungworms are difficult to locate and remove intact from the lungs. Reports that appear to involve examination of histologic sections only are excluded from Table 10.3 as are unidentified species of pseudaliids.

One of the most frequently studied cetaceans is the harbor porpoise, for which there is much prevalence and some intensity data for the five pseudaliids found in this host (Table 10.3). *Pseudalius inflexus, T. convolutus,* and *H. invaginatus* frequently co-occur in harbor porpoises (Raga et al. 1989; Balbuena et al. 1994; Brosens et al. 1996; Rokicki et al. 1997). Young-of-the-year or neonate porpoises are generally not infected with pseudaliids, and prevalence increases with age, suggesting horizontal transmission through the food chain. This appears to be the case with most pseudaliids except *Halocercus* spp. Prevalence of *Halocercus* spp. in young-of-the-year harbor porpoises and Dall's porpoises (*Phocoenoides dalli*) is sometimes higher than in older animals, suggesting that transmission may be transplacental or transmammary (Conlogue et al. 1985; Raga et al. 1989).

Intensity data also suggest that some pseudaliid infections are retained for life (Delyamure 1955; Clausen and Andersen 1988; Faulkner et al. 1998). Intensities of some smaller pseudaliids such as *S. minor*

TABLE 10.3—Prevalence and intensity of pseudaliid infections in odontocetes

Parasite	Host	Prevalence (%)	Mean Intensity (Range)	Reference
Pseudalius inflexus	*P. phocoena*	34–97	20 (1–284) (5–114) (1–61)	[1]Arnold 1973, [2]Baker and Martin 1992, [3]Balbuena et al. 1994, [4]Brosens et al. 1996, [5]Clausen and Andersen 1988, [6]Raga et al. 1989, [7]Rogan and Berrow 1995, [8]Rokicki et al. 1997, Larsen 1995
Torynurus convolutus	*P. phocoena*	42–83	213 (1–1838) 144 (2–609) (2–2700) (4–436)	1–4, 6–8, [9]Dailey and Stroud 1978
T. dalli	*P. dalli*	75–100	nd[a]	Dailey and Walker 1978, [10]Machida 1974
	S. coeruleoalba	75	nd	Dailey 1988
Pharurus pallasii	*D. leucas*	85–88	up to 2100	Kenyon and Kenyon 1977, Martineau et al. 1985, 1986, 1988, [11]Measures unpublished data
Stenurus minor	*P. phocoena*	22–100	141 (24–302) 2362 (87–8920) (25–789) (145–1682)	2, 4–9, [12]Delyamure 1955, Faulkner et al. 1998, Larsen 1995, Rogan and Berrow 1996
S. globicephalae	*G. melas*	50–100	nd	[13]Abollo et al. 1998, Cowan 1967, Geraci et al. 1978
	L. acutus	67	up to 3300	Raga and Balbuena 1993
S. arctomarinus	*D. leucas*	44–71	1–540	11
S. ovatus	*T. truncatus*	4	nd	[14]Troncone et al. 1994
	S. coeruleoalba	4	nd	
S. truei	*P. dalli*	100	nd	10
S. australis	*P. spinipinnis*	91	1624 (1–5178)	Torres et al. 1994
Skrjabinalius cryptocephalus	*D. delphis*	17–40	(3–277)	12
S. guevarai	*S. coeruleoalba*	1–24	nd	14, Duignan et al. 1992
	T. truncatus	12	nd	
Halocercus delphini	*D. delphis*	18	nd	13
	S. attenuata	5–52	nd	[15]Zam et al. 1971, Cowan and Walker 1979, Dailey and Perrin 1973,
	S. longirostris	22–84	nd	
	S. coeruleoalba	20	nd	14
	T. truncatus	12	nd	14
H. taurica	*P. phocoena*	55	nd	1
H. invaginatus	*P. phocoena*	25–98	125 (1–1105)	1–3, 8, 9, 13
H. monoceris	*D. leucas*	29–88	4–12,500	11
H. lagenorhynchi	*T. truncatus*	78–79	nd	15, Woodard et al. 1969
H. brasiliensis	*S. fluviatilis*	13	7 (2–15)	Santos 1996
H. dalli	*P. dalli*	60–71	nd	10, Conlogue et al. 1985

[a]nd–not determined.

and *Halocercus* spp. can be very high (in the thousands) compared to the larger pseudaliids such as *P. inflexus* and *S. arctomarinus* (in the hundreds) (Table 10.3).

CLINICAL SIGNS. Few clinical signs are reported in infected odontocetes. Rattling or coughing sounds from the blowhole, expectoration of frothy mucus or mucopurulent exudate, or expelled worms are sometimes observed (Medway and Schryver 1973; MacNeill et al. 1975; Kastelein et al. 1990, 1997). Nonspecific signs such as anorexia and lethargy also are reported (Caldwell et al. 1968).

PATHOLOGY AND PATHOGENESIS. The pathogenesis of pseudaliid infections in odontocetes has not been studied. The literature contains many descriptions of lesions attributed to the presence of pseudaliids, primarily in the lungs of stranded or captive animals, but in many cases worms are not identified, or diagnosis is based on histologic sections.

Pseudaliids located in the cranial sinuses and middle ear provoke minor hemorrhage, mild to moderate nonsuppurative chronic inflammation, and thickening of the sinus mucosal lining, rarely purulent sinusitis (Delyamure 1955; Geraci 1979; Martineau et al. 1986; Geraci and St. Aubin 1986). No gross or microscopic lesions of auditory cranial nerves or penetration of the cranial vault by pseudaliids are observed (Dailey and Stroud 1978; Dailey and Walker 1978; Clausen and Andersen 1988; Faulkner et al. 1998). Geraci et al. (1978) reported *S. globicephalae* penetrating the round window of the inner ear of a stranded Atlantic whitesided dolphin (*Lagenorhynchus acutus*); however, this may indicate postmortem migration—no description of the associated histopathology was provided. Although it is suggested that pseudaliids may cause osseous lesions of the pterygoid sinuses (Dailey and Perrin 1973), such lesions are generally attributed to *Crassicauda grampicola,* which can co-occur with pseudaliids (Dailey and Walker 1978; Raga et al. 1982; Raga 1987; Faulkner et al. 1998). The reported "deafness" of harbor porpoises infected with large numbers of *Stenurus minor* in the middle ear has yet to be verified clinically (Delyamure 1955). Faulkner et al. (1998) reported *S. minor* in all harbor porpoises > 1 year old by-caught in gillnets. Mean intensity was over 2000 worms, but there was no apparent effect on body condition, suggesting infected porpoises were able to hunt effectively.

Verminous and bacterial pneumonia are common causes of mortality in small odontocetes (Sweeney and Ridgway 1975; Baker and Martin 1992; Brosens et al. 1996). The pathogenic effect of pulmonary pseudaliids is dependent on their location (bronchi, bronchioles, or parenchyma), intensity, species, and stage (larvae or adults), as well as various host factors (species, age, immune status) and the presence of other infectious agents. *Pseudalius inflexus, Torynurus convolutus, Stenurus ovatus,* and *Skrjabinalius* spp. can cause almost total occlusion of bronchi and bronchioles due to their physical presence (Delyamure 1955; McColl and Obendorf 1982; Clausen and Andersen 1988; Raga et al. 1987b; Baker and Martin 1992; Brosens et al. 1996). Lesions associated with these lungworms include acute suppurative bronchopneumonia, acute to chronic bronchitis, endobronchitis, peribronchitis, bronchiolitis, edema, focal areas of atelectasis, chronic interstitial pneumonia, hyperplasia and hypertrophy of the mucosal epithelium, and hypertrophy of peribronchiolar smooth muscle. Erosion of the bronchial epithelium is sometimes reported (Delyamure 1955; McColl and Obendorf 1982).

Pseudalius inflexus in the heart and pulmonary blood vessels of harbor porpoises causes endocarditis, vasculitis, and thrombosis that often is fatal (Andersen 1974; Geraci 1979; Howard et al. 1983; Baker and Martin 1992; Brosens et al. 1996). Deeply attached anterior extremities of pseudaliids such as *Skrjabinalius* spp. are bathed in mucopurulent material surrounded by a fibrous capsule, which may later calcify (Delyamure 1955; Bowie 1984; Raga et al. 1987b). Some adult pseudaliids (*T. convolutus, S. globicephalae*) stimulate no or little inflammatory response in bronchi or bronchioles (Cowan 1966, 1967; Dailey and Stroud 1978), but larvae in alveoli can cause a subacute purulent focal pneumonia (Dailey and Stroud 1978).

Pseudaliids found within pulmonary parenchyma, including species such as *H. brasiliensis, H. dalli, H. delphini, H. invaginatus, H. lagenorhynchi,* and *H. monoceris,* are particularly pathogenic. Lesions associated with these lungworms include mucopurulent bronchitis, peribronchitis, pneumonia, alveolar and interstitial edema, focal areas of emphysema and atelectasis, and hypertrophy of muscular sphincters of terminal bronchioles (Woodard et al. 1969; Hörning et al. 1971;

Temirova and Usik 1971; Migaki et al. 1971; Andersen 1974; Machida 1974; MacNeill et al. 1975; Dailey and Stroud 1978; Cowan and Walker 1979). Eroded bronchiolar and alveolar epithelium also is reported (Wu 1929; Migaki et al. 1971; Temirova and Usik 1971). In acute infections there may be intra-alveolar hemorrhage. In chronic infections, small pale subpleural nodules (Migaki et al. 1971; Temirova and Usik 1971; MacNeill et al. 1975; Conlogue et al. 1985) are visible evidence of a granulomatous reaction encapsulating worms that die, degenerate, and calcify. Testi and Pilleri (1969) provided a detailed description of the histopathology of lungworms in four common dolphins (*Delphinus delphis*). They suggested that larvae observed were likely *H. delphini,* but no adults were found, and six species of pseudaliid are reported from this host (Table 10.2).

Focal abscesses and areas of calcification commonly are associated with *H. invaginatus* (Dailey and Stroud 1978). Cowan and Walker (1979) report an acute suppurative reaction to adult *H. delphini* in bronchioles as well as marked inflammation and diffuse pneumonitis reaction to larvae in alveoli. Rupture of a dissecting aneurysm of the pulmonary trunk in a beluga may have been caused by lungworms (Martineau et al. 1986).

Severe secondary bacterial or viral infections can develop in association with pseudaliid infections, leading to abscessation and septicemia (MacNeill et al. 1975; Greenwood and Taylor 1979; McColl and Obendorf 1982; Clausen and Andersen 1988; Raga et al. 1987b; Baker and Martin 1992; Duignan et al. 1992). However, the role of lungworms in provoking secondary infections is not completely understood.

DIAGNOSIS. In live animals, swabs and smears are used to examine feces, mucus from the blowhole, or mucus expelled by trained animals for L_1's. Adult pseudaliids may be small (3.5–21 mm: *P. asiaorientalis, H. monoceris, T. dalli, P. alatus, S. truei,* or *S. yamaguti*) or large (62–293 mm: *P. inflexus, S. arctomarinus, H. lagenorhynchi,* or *H. kleinenbergi*). Other species are intermediate in size (14–96 mm: most species of *Stenurus* and *Halocercus, Pseudostenurus sunameri, Torynurus convolutus,* and species of *Skrjabinalius*). Morphology and morphometrics of some L_1's are provided (Delyamure 1955; Arnold and Gaskin 1975; Kontrimavichus et al. 1976). However, further study is required before pseudaliid larvae can be distinquished reliably, if possible, especially in multispecies infections.

IMMUNITY. There are few data on the immune response by odontocetes to pseudaliid infections. Prevalence and intensity data indicate that infections accumulate with age and are long-lived (Geraci et al. 1978; Clausen and Andersen 1988; Raga and Balbuena 1993). In contrast, initial infection of *S. minor* in harbor porpoises may stimulate protective immunity, which would serve to prevent further detrimental infections (Faulkner et al. 1998). Coevolution of pseudaliids and their hosts probably results in light infections posing no serious problem for healthy animals. However, contaminants (some of which are immunosuppressive), infectious diseases, stress of captivity, or stress prior to stranding may predispose odontocetes to severe pulmonary disease due to pseudaliid infections.

CONTROL AND TREATMENT. There is no practical control or treatment for lungworms in free-ranging odontocete populations. Naturally infected individuals brought into captivity or being rehabilitated can be treated with anthelminthics (Greenwood and Taylor 1978). However, the response to drug treatment is known for only a few species, and adverse reactions are reported (Spotte et al. 1979; Dierauf 1990; Kastelein et al. 1997). Supportive therapy for dehydration, stress, secondary bacterial infection, respiratory distress, and stimulation of expectoration of worms is recommended (Kastelein et al. 1990, 1997).

MANAGEMENT IMPLICATIONS. Marine mammal strandings have been observed by humans for hundreds of years. For explanations of marine mammal stranding events and reviews of possible causes, the reader is referred to Geraci (1978), Robson (1978), Sergeant (1982), Cordes (1982), Geraci and Lounsbury (1993), and Simmonds (1997). The pseudaliids, particularly those infecting the respiratory system and causing severe verminous bronchopneumonia, may cause sick infected individuals to strand. Pseudaliids in the auditory organs may be involved in strandings of single individuals, mother-calf pairs, or mass stranding if the herd leader is heavily infected (Delyamure 1955; Fraser 1966). However, effects of pseudaliids on functioning of the cranial sinus system of odontocetes with subsequent negative effects on diving performance, foraging, navigation, and body condition have not been demonstrated clinically (Geraci 1978; Clausen and Andersen 1988; Forrester 1992; Faulkner et al. 1998). Apparently healthy, small odontocetes collected by hunting or by-catch may carry large numbers of pseudaliids in the cranial sinuses or lungs with little or no pathologic consequence (Cowan 1966; Arnold 1973; Conlogue et al. 1985; Clausen and Andersen 1988; Faulkner et al. 1998). In the absence of empirical evidence, the role of pseudaliids in the phenomenon of odontocete stranding remains unresolved.

LITERATURE CITED
Abeloos, M. 1932. Sur des nématodes parasites des bronches du marsouin. *Bulletin Mensuel de la Société Linnéenne de Normandie,* 8 série, t.V No. 6:37–38.
Abollo, E., A. Lopez, C. Gestal, P. Benavente, and S. Pascual. 1998. Macroparasites in cetaceans stranded on the northwestern Spanish Atlantic coast. *Diseases of Aquatic Organisms* 32:227–231.
Andersen, S.H. 1974. A typical case history of the net-caught harbor porpoise, *Phocoena phocoena,* from Danish waters. *Aquatic Mammals* 2:1–6.
Anderson, R.C. 1978. *CIH keys to the nematode parasites of vertebrates.* No. 5, *Keys to genera of the superfamily*

Metastrongyloidea. Farnham Royal, Bucks, England: Commonwealth Agricultural Bureaux.
———. 2000. *Nematode parasites of vertebrates: Their development and transmission.* 2d ed. Cambridge: University Press, 650 pp.
Arnold, P.W. 1973. The lungworms (Metastrongyloidea, Pseudaliidae) of harbor porpoise (*Phocoena phocoena* L.). M.Sc. Thesis, University of Guelph, Guelph, Ontario.
Arnold, P.W., and D.E. Gaskin. 1975. Lungworms (Metastrongyloidea: Pseudaliidae) of harbor porpoise *Phocoena phocoena* (L. 1758). *Canadian Journal of Zoology* 53:713–735.
Ashizawa, H., T. Ezaki, Y. Arie, D. Nosaka, S. Tateyama, and K. Owada. 1978. Pathological findings on lungworm disease in California sea lions. *Bulletin of the Faculty of Agriculture, Miyazaki University* 25:287–295.
Babero, B.B., and L.J. Thomas. 1960. A record *of Pharurus oserkaiae* (Skrjabin, 1942) in an Alaskan whale. *The Journal of Parasitology* 46:726.
Baker, J.R. 1987. Causes of mortality and morbidity in wild juvenile and adult grey seals (*Halichoerus grypus*). *British Veterinary Journal* 143:203–220.
———. 1989. Natural causes of death in non-suckling grey seals (*Halichoerus grypus*). *The Veterinary Record* 125:500–503.
Baker, J.R., and A.R. Martin. 1992. Causes of mortality and parasites and incidental lesions in harbor porpoises (*Phocoena phocoena*) from British waters. *The Veterinary Record* 130:554–558.
Baker, J.R, and T.S. McCann. 1989. Pathology and bacteriology of adult male Antarctic fur seals, *Arctocephalus gazella,* dying at Bird Island, South Georgia. *British Veterinary Journal* 145:263–275.
Balbuena, J.R., P.E. Aspholm, K.I. Andersen, and A. Bjørge. 1994. Lung-worms (Nematoda: Pseudaliidae) of harbor porpoises (*Phocoena phocoena*) in Norwegian waters: Patterns of colonization. *Parasitology* 108:343–349.
Ballarini, G. 1974. Radiographic studies on healthy California sea lions (*Zalophus californianus*) and those with *Parafilaroides decorus.* *Folia Veterinaria Latina* 4:795–800.
Barlough, J.E., E.S. Berry, D.E. Skilling, and A.W. Smith. 1986. Sea lions, caliciviruses and the sea. *Avian/Exotic Practice* 3:8–20.
Baylis, H.A. 1928. Note on *Stenurus ovatus* (v. Linstow), a little-known lung-worm of Cetacea. *Annals and Magazine of Natural History* 10:464–6.
———. 1932. A list of worms parasitic in Cetacea. *Discovery Reports* 6:393–418.
Baylis, H.A., and R. Daubney. 1925. A revision of the lungworms of Cetacea. *Parasitology* 17:201–216.
Belopol'skaia, M.M. 1960. Helminth fauna of the harbor seal (*Phoca vitulina largha* Pall.) [In Russian]. *Vestnik Leningradskogo Universiteta* 3:113–121. [Canadian Translation of Fisheries and Aquatic Sciences, No. 5611.]
Bergeron, E. 1996. Ètude de la biologie d'*Otostrongylus circumlitus,* parasite des poumons des phoques annelés de l'arctique est-canadien. M.Sc. thesis, Université Laval, Québec, 78 pp.
Bergeron, E., L.N. Measures, and J. Huot. 1997a. Experimental transmission of *Otostongylus circumlitus* (Railliet, 1899) (Metastrongyloidea: Crenosomatidae), a lungworm of seals in eastern arctic Canada. *Canadian Journal of Zoology* 75:1364–1371.
———. 1997b. Lungworm (*Otostrongylus circumlitus*) infections in ringed seals (*Phoca hispida*) from eastern arctic Canada. *Canadian Journal of Fisheries and Aquatic Sciences* 54:2443–2448.
Best, R.C., and V.M.F. da Silva. 1989. Amazon River dolphin, boto *Inia geoffrensis* (de Blainville, 1817). In *Handbook*

of marine mammals. Vol. 4, *River dolphins and the larger toothed whales*. Ed. S.H. Ridgway and R. Harrison. London: Academic Press, pp. 1–23.

Beverley-Burton, M. 1978. Helminths of the alimentary tract from a stranded herd of the Atlantic white-sided dolphin, *Lagenorhynchus acutus*. *Journal of the Fisheries Reseach Board of Canada* 35:1356–1359.

Bird, A.F., and J. Bird. 1991. *The structure of nematodes*. San Diego: Academic Press, Inc., 316 pp.

Borgsteede, F.H.M., H.G.J. Bus, J.A.W. Verplanke, and W.P.J. Van der Burg. 1991. Endoparasitic helminths of the harbor seal, *Phoca vitulina*, in the Netherlands. *Netherlands Journal of Sea Research* 28:247–250.

Bowie, J.Y. 1984. Parasites from an Atlantic bottle-nose dolphin (*Tursiops truncatus*), and a revised checklist of parasites of this host. *New Zealand Journal of Zoology* 11:395–398.

Breuer, E.M., R.J. Hofmeister, R.H. Ernst, and F. Horchner. 1988. Pathologic-anatomic, histologic and parasitologic findings in harbor seals. *Zeitschrift fur Angewandte Zoologie* 75:139–145.

Brodie, P.F. 1971. A reconsideration of aspects of growth, reproduction, and behavior of the white whale (*Delphinapterus leucas*), with reference to the Cumberland Sound, Baffin Island, population. *Journal of the Fisheries Research Board of Canada* 28:1309–1318.

Brosens, L., T. Jauniaux, U. Siebert, H. Benke and F. Coignoul. 1996. Observations on the helminths of harbor porpoises (*Phocoena phocoena*) and common guillemots (*Uria aalge*) from the Belgian and German coasts. *The Veterinary Record* 139:254–257.

Caldwell, M.C., D.K. Caldwell, and S.G. Zam. 1968. Occurrence of the lung worm (*Halocercus* sp.) in Atlantic bottlenosed dolphins (*Tursiops truncatus*) as a husbandry problem. In *Proceedings of the Second Symposium on Diseases and Husbandry of Aquatic Mammals*. Ed. D.K. Caldwell and M.C. Caldwell, pp. 11-15.

Cannon, L.R.G. 1977. Some aspects of the biology of *Peponocephala electra* (Cetacea: Delphinidae). II. Parasites. *Australian Journal of Marine Freshwater Research* 28:717–722.

Clausen, B. 1978. Diseases and toxochemicals in the common seal in Denmark. *Riistatieteellisia Julkaisuja* 37:38–39.

Clausen, B., and S. Andersen. 1988. Evaluation of bycatch and health status of the harbor porpoise (*Phocoena phocoena*) in Danish waters. *Danish Review of Game Biology* 13:1–20.

Claussen, D., V. Strauss, S. Ising, M. Jager, T. Schnieder, and M. Stoye. 1991. The helminth fauna from the common seal (*Phoca vitulina vitulina*, Linné, 1758) of the Wadden Sea in Lower Saxony Part 2: Nematodes. *Journal of Veterinary Medicine B* 38:649–656.

Cockrill, W.R. 1960. Pathology of the cetacea. A veterinary study on whales—Part I and Part II. 116:133–144; 175–190.

Conlogue, G.J., J.A. Ogden, and W.J. Foreyt. 1985. Parasites of the Dall's porpoise (*Phocoenoides dalli* True). *Journal of Wildlife Diseases* 21:160–166.

Corcuera, J., F. Monzon, A. Aguilar, A. Borrell, and J.A. Raga. 1995. Life history data, organochlorine pollutants and parasites from eight Burmeister's porpoises, *Phocoena spinipinnis*, caught in northern Argentine waters. *Report of the International Whaling Commission*, Special Issue 16:365–372.

Cordes, D.O. 1982. The causes of whale strandings. *New Zealand Veterinary Journal* 30:21–24.

Cowan, D.F. 1966. Pathology of the pilot whale *Globicephala melaena*. l. *Archives of Pathology* 82:178–189.

———. 1967. Helminth parasites of the pilot whale *Globicephala melaena* (Traill 1809). *The Journal of Parasitology* 53:166–167.

Cowan, D.F., and W.A. Walker. 1979. Disease factors in *Stenella attenuata* and *Stenella longirostris* taken in the eastern tropical Pacific yellowfin tuna purse seine fishery. Southwest Fisheries Science, Report LJ-79-32C.

Dailey, M.D. 1970. The transmission of *Parafilaroides decorus* (Nematoda: Metastrongyloidea) in the California sea lion (*Zalophus californianus*). *Proceedings of The Helminthological Society of Washington*. 37:215–222.

———. 1971. Distribution of helminths in the Dall porpoise (*Phocoenoides dalli* True). *The Journal of Parasitology* 57:1348.

———. 1975. The distribution and intraspecific variation of helminth parasites in pinnipeds. *Rapport P.-v. Réunion Conseil International pour l`Exploration de la Mer* 169:338–352.

———. 1986. Parasitology—Basic considerations. In *Zoo and wild animal medicine*. Ed. M.E. Fowler). Philadelphia, PA: W.B. Saunders Company, pp. 781–784.

———. 1988. A survey of marine mammal metazoan parasites of the southern California coast with reference to potential research in Mexican populations. *VII Simposio Internationale Biologica Marinus*, pp. 87–93.

Dailey, M.D., and R.L. Brownell. 1972. A checklist of marine mammal parasites. In *Mammals of the sea: Biology and medicine*. Ed. S.H. Ridgway. Springfield, IL: Charles C. Thomas, pp. 528–589.

Dailey, M.D., and L.S. Fallace. 1989. Prevalence of parasites in a wild population of the Pacific harbor seal (*Phoca vitulina richardsi*) from Gray's Harbor, Washington. *Bulletin Southern California Academy of Science* 88:1–10.

Dailey, M.D., and B.L. Hill. 1970. A survey of metazoan parasites infecting the California (*Zalophus californianus*) and Steller (*Eumetopias jubatus*) sea lion. *Bulletin of the South California Academy of Science* 69:126–132.

Dailey, M.D., and K.A. Otto. 1982. Parasites as biological indicators of the distributions and diets of marine mammals common to the eastern Pacific. La Jolla, CA: Southwest Fisheries Center. NOAA/NMFS/SWFSC No. LJ-82-13C.

Dailey, M.D., and W.F. Perrin. 1973. Helminth parasites of porpoises of the genus *Stenella* in the eastern tropical Pacific, with descriptions of two new species: *Mastigonema stenellae* gen. et sp. n. (Nematoda: Spiruroidea) and *Zalophotrema pacificum* sp. n. (Trematoda: Digenea). *Fishery Bulletin* 71:455–471.

Dailey, M.D., and R. Stroud. 1978. Parasites and associated pathology observed in cetaceans stranded along the Oregon coast. *Journal of Wildlife Diseases* 14:503–511.

Dailey, M.D., and W.A. Walker. 1978. Parasitism as a factor in single strandings of southern California cetaceans. *The Journal of Parasitology* 64:593–596.

Dailey, M.D., M. Walsh, D. Odell, and T. Campbell. 1991. Evidence of prenatal infection in the bottlenose dolphin (*Tursiops truncatus*) with the lungworm *Halocercus lagenorhynchi* (Nematoda: Pseudaliidae). *Journal of Wildlife Diseases* 27:164–165.

de Bruyn, W.M. 1933. Contributions to the knowledge of *Strongylus circumlitus* Railliet from the lungs of seals: The new genus *Otostrongylus* [In Dutch]. *Zoolischer Anzeiger* 103:142–153. [Canadian Translation of Fisheries and Aquatic Science, No. 5583.]

Delyamure, S.L. 1955. *Helminthofauna of marine mammals (Ecology and Phylogeny)* [In Russian]. Ed. K.I. Skrjabin. Moscow: Izdatel'stvo Akademii Nauk SSR. [1968. Translated by Israel Program for Scientific Translations, Jerusalem, 522 pp.

Delyamure, S.L., and E.V. Alekseev. 1966. *Parafilaroides arcticus* n. sp. as parasites of the Chukotsk Sea ringed seal [In Russian]. *Problemy Parazitologii* 6:11–15. [1992. Canadian Translation of Fisheries and Aquatic Sciences, No. 5564,]

Delyamure, S.L., and S.E. Kleinenberg. 1958. New data on the helminthofauna of the white whale [In Russian]. *Bulletin of the Moscow Society of Naturalists* 63:25–32. [Canadian Translation of Fisheries and Aquatic Sciences, No. 5603, 13 pp.]

Delyamure, S.L., and V.N. Popov. 1975. A study of the helminth fauna of the bearded seal inhabiting the Sakhalin Bay [In Russian]. *Nauchye Doklady Vysshei Shkoly Biologicheskie Nauki* 10:7–10.

Delyamure, S.L., V.N. Popov, and A.N. Trashchenkov. 1980. Study of the helminth fauna of the seals of the Baltic Sea and Lake Ladoga [In Russian]. *Nauchnye Doklady Vysshei Shkoly, Biologicheski Nauki* 7:43–45. [1984. Canadian Translation of Fisheries and Aquatic Sciences, No. 5112.]

Delyamure, S.L., V.N. Popov, and E.S. Mikhalev. 1982. The helminth funa of *Pusa sibirica* [In Russian]. In *Morfofiziologicheskie i ekologicheskie issledovaniia baikalskoi nerpy*. Ed. V.D. Pastukhov. Nauka: Sibirskoe Otdelenie, Novosibirsk, USSR, pp. 99–122.

Delyamure, S.L., M.V. Yurakhno, V.N. Popov, L.M. Shults, and F.H. Fay. 1984. Helminthological comparison of subpopulations of Bering Sea spotted seals, *Phoca largha* Pallas. In *Soviet-American Cooperative Studies on Marine Mammals*. Vol.1, *Pinnipeds*. Ed. F.H. Fay and G.A. Fedoseev. NOAA Technical Report NMFS 12, pp. 61–65.

Dierauf, L.A. 1990. Marine mammal parasitology. In *CRC Handbook of marine mammal medicine: Health, disease and rehabilitation*. Ed. L.A. Dierauf. Boca Raton, FL: CRC Press, pp. 89–96.

Dierauf, L.A., D.J. Vandenbroek, J. Roletto, M. Koski, L. Amaya, and L.J. Gage. 1985. An epizootic of leptospirosis in California sea lions. *The American Veterinary Medical Association*. 187:1145–1148.

Doan, K.H., and C.W. Douglas. 1953. Beluga of the Churchill Region of Hudson Bay. Bulletin of the Fisheries Research Board of Canada, No. 98, 27 pp.

Dollfus, R.Ph. 1968. Nematodes des cétaces odontocetes (*Globicephalus* et *Tursiops*). *Bulletin de l'Institut des pêches maritimes du Maroc* 16:35–53.

Dougherty, E.C. 1943. Notes on the lungworms of porpoises and their occurrence on the California coast. *Proceedings of the Helminthological Society of Washington* 10:16–22.

———. 1944. The lungworms (Nematoda: Pseudaliidae) of the Odontoceti. Part. I. *Parasitology* 36:80–94.

———. 1946. The genus *Aelurostrongylus* Cameron, 1927 (Nematoda: Metastrongylidae), and its relatives: With descriptions of *Parafilaroides*, gen. nov., and *Angiostrongylus gubernaculus*, sp. nov. *Proceedings of the Helminthology Society of Washington* 13:16–26.

Dougherty, E.C., and C.M. Herman. 1947. New species of the genus *Parafilaroides* Dougherty, 1946 (Nematoda: Metastrongylidae), from sea-lions, with a list of the lungworms of the Pinnipedia. *Proceedings of the Helminthological Society of Washington* 14:77–87.

Duignan, P.J., J.R. Geraci, J.A. Raga, and N. Calzada. 1992. Pathology of morbillivirus infection in striped dolphins (*Stenella coeruleoalba*) from Valencia and Murcia, Spain. *Canadian Journal of Veterinary Research* 56:242–248.

Dungworth, D.L. 1985. The respiratory system. In *Pathology of domestic animals*. Ed. K.V.F. Jubb, P.C. Kennedy, and N. Palmer. Orlando, FL: Academic Press, Inc., pp. 413–556.

Dunn, J.L., and R.E. Wolke. 1976. *Dipetalonema spirocauda* infection in the Atlantic harbor seal (*Phoca vitulina concolor*). *Journal of Wildlife Diseases* 12:531–538.

Faulkner, J., L.N. Measures, and F.G. Whoriskey. 1998. *Stenurus minor* (Metastrongyloidea: Pseudaliidae) infections of the cranial sinuses of the harbor porpoise, *Phocoena phocoena*. *Canadian Journal of Zoology* 76:1209–1216.

Fleischman, R.W., and R.A. Squire. 1970. Verminous pneumonia in the California sea lion (*Zalophus californianus*). *Pathologica Veterinaria* 7:89–101.

Fordyce, R.W., and L.G. Barnes. 1994. The evolutionary history of whales and dolphins. *Annual Review of Earth Planet Sciences* 22:419–455.

Forrester, D.J. 1992. Whales and dolphins. In *Parasites and diseases of wild mammals of Florida*. Gainesville: University Press of Florida, pp. 218–250.

Forrester, D.J., D.K. Odell, N.P. Thompson and J.R. White. 1980. Morphometrics, parasites, and chlorinated hydrocarbon residues of pygmy killer whales from Florida. *Journal of Mammalogy* 61:356–360.

Fraser, F.C. 1966. Comments. In *Whales, dolphins and porpoises*. Ed. K.S. Norris. Berkeley and Los Angeles: University of California Press, p. 602.

Gage, L.J., J.A. Gerber, D.M. Smith, and L.E. Morgan. 1993. Rehabilitation and treatment success rate of California sea lions (*Zalophus californianus*) and northern fur seals (*Callorhinus ursinus*) stranded along the Central and Northern California coast, 1984–1990. *Journal of Zoo and Wildlife Medicine* 24:41–47.

Gallego, J., and J.M. Selva. 1979. *Skrjabinalius guevarai* n. sp. (Nematoda: Pseudaliidae), parasito pulmonar del delfin mular, *Tursiops truncatus* Montagu, 1821 (Cetacea: Delphinidae) en el Adriatico. *Revista Ibérica de Parasitologia* 39:203–208.

Garner, M.M., D.M. Lambourn, S.J. Jeffries, P.B. Hall, J.C. Rhyan, D.R. Ewalt, L.M. Polzin, and N.F. Cheville. 1997. Evidence of *Brucella* infection in *Parafilaroides* lungworms in a Pacific harbor seal (*Phoca vitulina richardsi*). *Journal of Veterinary Diagnostic Investigation* 9:298–303.

Gaskin, D.E. 1976. The evolution, zoogeography and ecology of Cetacea. *Oceanography and Marine Biology Annual Review* 14:247–346.

Geraci, J.R. 1978. The enigma of marine mammal strandings. *Oceanus* 21:38–47.

———. 1979. The role of parasites in marine mammal strandings along the New England coast. In *Biology of marine mammals: Insights through strandings*. Ed. J.R. Geraci and D.J. St. Aubin. U.S. Dept. of Commerce, NTIS Report PB-293-890, pp. 85–91.

Geraci, J.R., and D.J. St. Aubin. 1979. Stress and disease in the marine environment: Insights through strandings. In *Biology of marine mammals: Insights through strandings*. Ed. J.R. Geraci and D.J. St. Aubin. U.S. Dept. of Commerce, NTIS Report PB-293-890, pp. 223–233.

———. 1986. Effects of parasites on marine mammals. In *Proceedings of the Sixth International Congress of Parasitology*. Ed. M.J. Howell. Canberra: Australian Academy of Science, pp. 407–414.

Geraci, J.R., and V.J. Lounsbury. 1993. *Marine mammals ashore: A field guide for strandings*. Galveston: Texas A&M University Sea Grant College Program.

Geraci, J.R., S.A. Testaverde, D.J. St. Aubin, and T.H. Loop. 1978. A mass stranding of the Atlantic white-sided dolphin, *Lagenorhynchus acutus*: A study into pathobiology and life history. National Technical Information Service, PB-289-361.

Gerber, J.A., J. Roletto, L.E. Morgan, D.M. Smith, and L.J. Gage. 1993. Findings in pinnipeds stranded along the Central and Northern California coast, 1984–1990. *Journal of Wildlife Diseases* 29:423–433.

Gibson, D.I., and E.A. Harris. 1979. The helminth-parasites of cetaceans in the collection of the British Museum (Natural History). *Investigations on Cetacea* 10:309–324.

Gosselin, J.-F. and L.N. Measures. 1997. Redescription of *Filaroides (Parafilaroides) gymnurus* (Railliet, 1899) (Nematoda: Metastrongyloidea), with comments on other species in pinnipeds. *Canadian Journal of Zoology* 75:359–370.

Gosselin, J-F., L.N. Measures, and J. Huot. 1998. Lungworm (Nematoda: Metastrongyloidea) infections in Canadian phocids. *Canadian Journal of Fisheries and Aquatic Sciences* 55:825–834.

Greenwood, A.B., and D.C. Taylor. 1978. Clinical and pathological findings in dolphins in 1977. *Aquatic Mammals* 6:33–38.

———. 1979. Odontocete parasites—Some new host records. *Aquatic Mammals* 7:23–25.

Gulland, F.M.D., L. Werner, S. O`Neill, L.J. Lowenstine, J. Trupkiewitz, D. Smith, B. Royal, and I. Strubel. 1996. Baseline coagulation assay values for northern elephant seals (*Mirounga angustrirostris*), and disseminated intravascular coagulation in this species. *Journal of Wildlife Diseases* 32:536–540.

Gulland, F.M.D., K. Beckmen, K. Burek, L. Lowenstine, L. Werner, T. Spraker, M. Dailey, and E. Harris. 1997. Nematode (*Otostrongylus circumlitus*) infestation of northern elephant seals (*Mirounga angustirostris*) stranded along the central California coast. *Marine Mammal Science* 13:446–459.

Hanni, K.D., D.J. Long, R.E. Jones, P. Pyle, and L.E. Morgan. 1997. Sightings and strandings of Guadalupe fur seals in Central and Northern California, 1988–1995. *Journal of Mammalogy* 78:684–690.

Harris, A. 1982. The helminth parasites of the Cetacea (or "Parasitology" with a porpoise). *Parasitology* 85:71.

Heide-J̦rgensen, M.-P., T. Harkonen, R. Dietz, and P.M. Thompson. 1992. Retrospective of the 1988 European seal epizootic. *Diseases of Aquatic Organisms* 13:37–62.

Hill, B.L. 1971. Comparative morphology of *Parafilaroides decorus* (Nematoda: Metastrongyloidea) in the California and Steller sea lions. M.Sc. Thesis, California State College at Long Beach, Long Beach, CA.

Hörning, B., G. Pilleri, and F. Testi. 1971. Sulla presenza di nematodi del genere *Halocercus* in delfini *(Delphinus delphis* L.) del mare Adriatico. *La Nuova Veterinaria* 47:17–23.

Howard, E.B., J.O. Britt, Jr., and G. Matsumoto. 1983. Parasitic diseases. In *Pathobiology of marine mammal diseases,* vol. 1. Boca Raton, FL: CRC Press, Inc., pp. 119–232.

Hsü, H.F., and R. Hoeppli. 1933. On some parasitic nematodes collected in Amoy. *Peking Natural History Bulletin* 8:166–168.

Hubbard, R.C. 1969. Chemotherapy in captive marine mammals. *Bulletin of the Wildlife Disease Association* 5:218–230.

Johnson, D.G., and S.H. Ridgway. 1969. Parasitism in some marine mammals. *Journal of American Veterinary Medical Association* 155:1064–1072.

Joseph, B., and L.H. Cornell. 1986. Metastatic squamous cell carcinoma in a beached California sea lion (*Zalophus californianus*). *Journal of Wildlife Diseases* 22:281–283.

Johnston, T.H., and P.M. Mawson. 1941. Nematodes from Australian marine mammals. *Records of the South Australian Museum* 6:429–434.

Kastelein, R.A., M.J. Bakker and T. Dokter. 1990. The medical treatment of 3 stranded harbor porpoises (*Phocena phocoena*). *Aquatic Mammals* 15:181–202.

Kastelein, R.A., M.J. Bakker, and C. Staal. 1997. The rehabilitation and release of stranded harbor porpoises (*Phocoena phocoena*). In *The biology of the harbor porpoise.* Ed. A.J. Read, P.R. Wiepkema and P.E. Nachtigall. Woerden, The Netherlands: De Spil Publishers, pp. 9–61.

Kennedy, M.J. 1986. *Filaroides (Parafilaroides) hispidus* n. sp. (Nematoda: Metastrongyloidea) from the lungs of the ringed seal, *Phoca hispida* (Phocidae), from the Beaufort Sea, Canada. *Canadian Journal of Zoology* 64:1864–1868.

Kennedy, S., J.A. Smyth, P.F. Cush, P. Duignan, M. Platten, S.J. McCullough and G.M. Allan. 1989. Histologic and immunocytochemical studies of distemper in seals. *Veterinary Pathology* 26:97–103.

Kenyon, A.J., and B.J. Kenyon. 1977. Prevalence *of Pharurus pallasii* in the beluga whale (*Delphinapterus leucas*) of Churchill River basin, Manitoba. *Journal of Wildlife Diseases* 13:338–340.

Kikuchi, S., and M. Nakajima. 1996. Morphology of a pseudaliid nematode from the air sinus of a dolphin, *Peponocephala electra. Japanese Journal of Parasitology* 45:215–22l.

Kinze, C.C. 1989. On the reproduction, diet and parasitic burden of the harbor porpoise *Phocoena phocoena* in west Greenlandic waters. In *European Research on Cetaceans–3.* Ed. P.G.H. Evans and C. Smeenk. Proceedings of the Third Annual Conference of the European Cetacean Society, La Rochelle, France. Leiden, The Netherlands: European Cetacean Society, pp. 91–95.

Kleinenberg, S.E. 1956. *Mammals of the Black Sea and the Sea of Azov. Results of joint biological-commercial dolphin whaling studies* [In Russian]. Moscow: USSR Academy of Sciences Press. [1978. Fisheries and Marine Service Translation Series, No. 4319.]

Kleinenberg, S.E., A.V. Yablokov, B.M. Bel'kovich, and M.N. Tarasevich. 1964. Beluga (*Delphinapterus leucas*) investigation of the species. Academy of Sciences of the USSR. (in Russian). Translated by the Israel Program for Scientific Translations, Jerusalem. 1969.

Kontrimavichus, V.L., and S.L. Delyamure. 1979. Filaroids of domestic and wild animals. Fundamentals of Nematology. Volume 29. (In Russian). Translated for the US Dept. of Agriculture and National Science Foundation, Washington. 1985.

Kontrimavichus, V.L., and S.L. Delyamure, and S.N. Boev. 1976. *Metastrongyloids of domestic and wild animals* [In Russian]. Moscow: Academy of Sciences of the USSR, Nauka Publishers. [1985. Translated by Amerind Publishing Co. Pvt. Ltd., New Delhi. New Delhi: Oxonian Press Pvt. Ltd.]

Kurochkin, Y.V. 1975. Parasites of the Caspian seal *Pusa caspica. Rapport P.-v. Réunion Conseil International pour l`Exploration de la Mer* 169:363–365.

Kurochkin, Y.V., and V.I. Zablotsky. 1958. On the helminth fauna of the Caspian seal [In Russian]. *Trudy Astrakhanskogo Zapovednika* 1993. [Canadian Translation of Fisheries and Aquatic Sciences, No. 5587, pp. 337–343.]

Kuramochi, T., J. Araki and M. Machida. 1990. Pseudaliid nematodes from Dall's porpoise, *Phocoenoides dalli. Bulletin of the National Science Museum, Tokyo* 16:97–103.

Larsen, B.H. 1995. Parasites and pollutants in seven harbor porpoises (*Phocoena phocoena* L. 1758) from the Faroe Islands, 1987–1988. *Report of the International Whaling Commission,* Special Issue 16:223–230.

Lins de Almeida, J. 1933. Nouveau nématode parasite de cétacés du Brésil, *Halocerucs brasiliensis* n. sp. *Comptes Rendus de séances de la société de biologie et de ses filiales* 114:955–957.

Linstow, O. 1910. *Pseudalius ovatus* n. sp. *Zentralblatt für Bakteriologie und Parasitenkünde* 6:133–135.

Machida, M. 1968. Parasitic helminths of True`s porpoise. *Japanese Journal of Parasitology* 17:279–280.

———. 1974. Helminth parasites of the True`s porpoise, *Phocoenoides truei* Andrews. *Bulletin of the National Science Museum, Tokyo* 17:221–227.

MacNeill, A.C., J.L. Neufeld, and W.A. Webster. 1975. Pulmonary nematodiasis in a narwhal. *Canadian Veterinary Journal* 16:53–55.

Margolis, L. 1956. Parasitic helminths and arthropods from Pinnipedia of the Canadian Pacific coast. *Journal of the Fisheries Research Board of Canada* 13:489–505.

Margolis, L., and M.D. Dailey. 1972. Revised annotated list of parasites from sea mammals caught off the west coast of

North America. NOAA Technical Report NMFS SSRF-647.

Margolis, L., and J.R. Arthur. 1979. Synopsis of the parasites of the fishes of Canada. Bulletin of the Fisheries Research Board of Canada, No. 199, 269 pp.

Martineau, D., A. Lagacé, R. Massé, M. Morin, and P. Béland. 1985. Transitional cell carcinoma of the urinary bladder in a beluga whale (*Delphinapterus leucas*). *Canadian Veterinary Journal* 26:297–302.

Martineau, D., A. Lagacé, P. Béland, and C. Desjardins. 1986. Rupture of a dissecting aneurysm of the pulmonary trunk in a beluga whale (*Delphinapterus leucas*). *Journal of Wildlife Diseases* 22:289–294.

Martineau, D., A. Lagacé, P. Béland, R. Higgins, D. Armstrong, and L.R. Shugart. 1988. Pathology of stranded beluga whales (*Delphinapterus leucas*) from the St. Lawrence estuary, Québec, Canada. *Journal of Comparative Pathology* 98:287–311.

Mawson, P.M. 1953. Parasitic nematoda collected by the Australian national antarctic research expedition: Heard Island and MacQuarie Island, 1948–1951. *Parasitology* 43:291–297.

McColl, K.A., and D.L. Obendorf. 1982. Helminth parasites and associated pathology in stranded Fraser's dolphins, *Lagenodelphis hosei* (Fraser, 1956). *Aquatic Mammals* 9:30–34.

McDonald, T.E., and L. Margolis. 1995. Synopsis of the parasites of fishes of Canada: Supplement (1978–1993). Canadian Special Publication of Fisheries and Aquatic Sciences, No. 122, 265 pp.

Measures, L.N., and J.-F. Gosselin. 1994. Helminth parasites of ringed seal, *Phoca hispida*, from Northern Quebec, Canada. *Journal of the Helminthological Society of Washington* 61:240–244.

Measures, L.N., P. Béland, D. Martineau and S. De Guise. 1995. Helminths of an endangered population of belugas, *Delphinapterus leucas*, in the St. Lawrence estuary, Canada. *Canadian Journal of Zoology* 73:1402–1409.

Medway, W., and H.F. Schryver. 1973. Respiratory problems in captive small cetaceans. *Journal of the American Veterinary Medical Association* 163:571–573.

Menschel, E., B. Schiefer, and H. Kraft. 1966. Infestation with lungworms in seals (*Phoca vitulina* L.) under natural conditions [In German]. *Berliner und Münchener Tierärztliche Wochenschrift* 17:333–337. [Canadian Translation of Fisheries and Aquatic Sciences, No. 5633.]

Migaki, G., D. Van Dyke, and R.C. Hubbard. 1971. Some histopathological lesions caused by helminths in marine mammals. *Journal of Wildlife Diseases* 7:281–289.

Mignucci-Giannoni, A.M., E.P. Hoberg, D. Siegel-Causey, and E.H. Williams, Jr. 1998. Metazoan parasites and other symbionts of cetaceans in the Caribbean. *The Journal of Parasitology* 84:939–946.

Moesker, A. 1987. Treatment of infectious diseases in stranded harbor seals. *Aquatic Mammals* 13.2:57–60:

Morales, G.A., and C.F. Helmboldt. 1971. Verminous pneumonia in the California sea lion (*Zalophus californianus*). *Journal of Wildlife Diseases* 7:22–27.

Morales Vela, B., and L.D.O. Gomez. 1993. Varamiento de calderones *Globicephala macrorhynchus* (Cetacea: Delphinidae) en La Isla de Cozumel, Quintana Roo, Mexico. *Annales del Instituto de Biologia Universidad* 64:177–180.

Moser, M., and H. Rhinehart. 1993. The lungworm, *Halocercus* spp. (Nematoda: Pseudaliidae) in cetaceans from California. *Journal of Wildlife Diseases* 29:507–508.

Munro, R., H. Ross, C. Cornwell, and J. Gilmour. 1992. Disease conditions affecting common seals (*Phoca vitulina*) around the Scottish mainland, September–November 1988. *The Science of the Total Environment* 115:67–82.

Nicholson, A., and J.C. Fanning. 1981. Parasites and associated pathology of the respiratory tract of the Australian sea lion: *Neophoca cinerea*. In *Wildlife disease of the Pacific basin and other countries*. Ed. M.E. Fowler. Proceedings of the Fourth International Conference of the Wildlife Disease Association, Sydney, Australia, pp. 178–181.

Odell, D.K., E.D. Asper, J. Baucom and L.H. Cornell. 1980. A recurrent mass stranding of the false killer whale, *Pseudorca crassidens*, in Florida. *Fishery Bulletin* 78:171–177.

Olsen, O.W., and E.T. Lyons. 1965. Life cycle of *Uncinaria lucasi* Stiles, 1901 (Nematoda: Ancylostomatidae) of fur seals, *Callorhinus ursinus* Linn., on the Pribilof Islands, Alaska. *The Journal of Parasitology* 51:689–700.

Onderka, D.K. 1989. Prevalence and pathology of nematode infections in the lungs of ringed seals (*Phoca hispida*) of the western arctic of Canada. *Journal of Wildlife Diseases* 25:218–224.

Parry, K., M. Moore, and G. Hulland. 1983. Why do whales come ashore? *New Scientist* 97:716–717.

Petter, A.J., and G. Pilleri. 1982. *Pharurus asiaeorientalis* new species, metastrongylid nematode, parasite of *Neophocaena asiaeorientalis* (Phocoenidae, Cetacea). *Investigations on Cetacea* 13:141–148.

Podestà, M., L. Marsili, S. Focardi, M.T. Manfredi, W. Mignone, and C. Genchi. 1992. Ricerche patologiche, parassitologiche e sulla presenza di zenobiotici in *Stenella coeruleoalba* (Meyen, 1833)(Mammalia, Cetacea). *Atti della Società Italiana di Scienze Naturali e del Museo Civico di Storia Naturale di Milano* 133:101–112.

Popov, V.N. 1975. New data on the helminth fauna of the ribbon seal from the southern part of the Sea of Okhotsk [In Russian]. *Parazitologiya* 9:31–36. [Canadian Translation of Fisheries and Aquatic Sciences, No. 5614.]

Purves, P.E. 1966. Anatomy and physiology of the outer and middle ear in cetaceans. In *Whales, dolphins and porpoises*. Ed. K.S. Norris. Berkeley and Los Angeles: University of California Press, pp. 320–380.

Raga, J.A. 1987. Redescription de *Crassicauda grampicola* Johnston et Mawson, 1941, (Nematoda: Spirurida), parasite de *Grampus griseus* (Cuvier, 1812) (Cetacea: Delphinidae). *Vie Milieu* 37:215–219.

Raga, J.A., and J.A. Balbuena. 1993. Parasites of the long-finned pilot whale, *Globicephala melas* (Traill, 1809), in European waters. *Report of the International Whaling Commission*, Special Issue 14:391–406.

Raga, J.A., and E. Carbonell. 1985. New data about parasites on *Stenella coeruleoalba* (Meyen, 1833) (Cetacea: Delphinidae) in the western Mediterranean Sea. *Investigations on Cetacea* 17:207–213.

Raga, J.A., A. Casinos, S. Filella, and M.A. Raduan. 1982. Notes on cetaceans of the Iberian coasts. V. *Crassicauda grampicola* Johnson and Mawson, 1941, (Nematoda) cause of injuries in the pterygoids of some specimens of *Grampus griseus*. *Saugetierkundliche Mitteilungen* 30:315–318.

Raga, J.A., A.J. Petter, and R. Duguy. 1987a. Catalogue des parasites de Cétacés des collections du Musée Océanographique de la Rochelle. *Bulletin du Muséum National d'Histoire Naturelle, Paris*, 4 série, 9:159–168.

Raga, J.A., F. Abril, and P. Almor. 1987b. Skrjabinalius guevarai Gallego et Selva, 1979 (Nematoda: Pseudaliidae), a lungworm parasitizing dolphins (Cetacea: Delphinidae) in the Western Mediterranean Sea. *Rivista di Parassitologia* 4:27–32.

Raga, J.A., C.C. Kinze, J.A. Balbuena, T. Ortiz and M. Fernández. 1989. New data on helminth parasites of the harbor porpoise *Phocoena phocoena* in Danish waters. In

European research on cetaceans—3. Ed. P.G.H. Evans and C. Smeenk. Proceedings of the Third Annual Conference of the European Cetacean Society, La Rochelle, France. Leiden, The Netherlands: European Cetacean Society, pp. 88–90

Railliet, M.A. 1899. Sur quelques parasites rencontrés à l'autopsie d'un phoque (*Phoca vitulina* L.). *C.R. Société de Biologie, Paris* 6:128–130.

Reyes, J.C., and K. Van Waerebeek. 1995. Aspects of the biology of Burmeister's porpoise from Peru. In *Biology of the phocoenids.* Ed. A. Bjfrge and G.P. Donovan. *Report of the International Whaling Commission,* Special Issue 16:349–364.

Ridgway, S.H., J.R. Geraci, and W. Medway. 1975. Diseases of pinnipeds. *Rapport P.-v. Réunion Conseil International pour l'Exploration de la Mer* 169:327–337.

Robson, F.D. 1978. The way of the whale: Why they strand. *Journal of the American Cetacean Society* 12:4–11.

Rogan, E., and S.D. Berrow. 1995. The management of Irish waters as a whale and dolphin sanctuary. In *Whales, seals, fish and man.* Ed. A.S. Blix, L. Wallfe, and Ø. Ulltang. Amsterdam: Elsevier Science, pp. 671–681.

Rogan, E., and S.D. Berrow. 1996. A review of harbor porpoises, *Phocoena phocoena,* in Irish waters. *Report of the International Whaling Commission* 46:595–605.

Rokicki, J., B. Berland and J. Wróblewski. 1997. Helminths of the harbor porpoise, *Phocoena phocoena* (L.), in the southern Baltic. *Acta Parasitologica* 42:36–39.

Roletto, J. 1993. Hematology and serum chemistry values for clinically healthy and sick pinnipeds. *Journal of Zoo and Wildlife Medicine* 24:145–157.

Santos, C.P., K. Rohde, R. Ramos, A.P. Di Benedditto, and L. Capistrano. 1996. Helminths of cetaceans on the southeastern coast of Brazil. *Journal of the Helminthological Society of Washington* 63:149–152.

Sarmiento, L., and M. Tantalean. 1991. *Stenurus australis* n. sp. (Nematoda: Pseudaliidae) de *Phocoena spinipinnis* (Burmeister, 1865) (Cetacea: Phocoenidae) de Peru. *Publicaciones del Museo de Historia Natural UNMSM* 36:1–4.

Scheffer, V.B., and J.W. Slipp. 1948. The whales and dolphins of Washington State with a key to the cetaceans of the west coast of North America. *The American Midland Naturalist* 39:257–334.

Schroeder, R.J., C.A. Delli Quadri, R.W. McIntyre, and W.A. Walker. 1973. Marine mammal disease surveillance program in Los Angeles County. *Journal of American Veterinary Medical Association* 163:580–581.

Schumacher, U., H.-P. Horny, G. Heidemann, W. Schultz, and U. Welsch. 1990. Histopathological findings in harbor seals (*Phoca vitulina*) found dead on the German North Sea coast. *Journal of Comparative Pathology* 102:299–310.

Sergeant, D.E. 1962. The biology of the pilot or pothead whale *Globicephala melaena* (Traill) in Newfoundland waters. Bulletin of the Fisheries Research Board of Canada, No. 132, 83 pp.

———. 1982. Mass strandings of toothed whales (Odontoceti) as a population phenomenon. *Scientific Reports of the Whale Research Institute* 34:1–47.

Shimamura, M, H. Yasue, K. Ohshima, H. Abe, H. Kato, T. Kishiro, Mutsuo Goto, I. Munechika, and N. Okada. 1997. Molecular evidence from retroposons that whales form a clade within even-toed ungulates. *Nature* 388:666–670.

Simmonds, M.P. 1997. The meaning of cetacean strandings. *Bulletin de l'Institut Royal des Sciences Naturelles de Belgique* 67:29–34.

Simpson, J.G., and M.B. Gardner. 1972. Comparative microscopic anatomy of selected marine mammals. In *Mam-*

mals of the sea: Biology and medicine. Ed. S.H. Ridgway. Springfield, IL: Charles C. Thomas, pp. 298–413.

Skirnisson, K., and E. Olafsson. 1990. Parasites of seals in Icelandic waters, with special reference to the heartworm *Dipetalonema spirocauda* Leidy, 1858 and the sucking louse *Echinopthirius horridus* Olfers, 1916 [In Icelandic]. *Natturufraedingurinn* 60:93–102.

Skrjabin, K.I. 1933. *Kutassicaulus* n.g. nouveau représentant des nématodes de la sous-famille des Dictyocaulinae Skrjabin, 1933. *Annales de Parasitologie* 11:359–363.

Smith, A.W., D.E. Skilling, and R.J. Brown. 1980. Preliminary investigation of a possible lung worm (*Parafilaroides decorus*), fish (*Girella nigricans*), and marine mammal (*Callorhinus ursinus*) cycle for San Miquel Sea Lion Virus Type 5. *American Journal of Veterinary Research* 41:1846–1850.

Smith, F.R., and W. Threlfall. 1973. Helminths of some mammals from Newfoundland. *The American Midland Naturalist* 90:215–218.

Smith, T.G. 1987. The ringed seal (*Phoca hispida*) of the Canadian Western Arctic. *Canadian Bulletin of Fisheries and Aquatic Sciences* 216:1–81.

Smith, T.G., M.H. Hammill, D.W. Doidge, T. Cartier, and G. A. Sleno. 1979. Marine mammal studies in southeastern Baffin Island. Canadian Manuscript Report of Fisheries and Aquatic Sciences, No. 1552.

Spotte, S., C.W. Radcliffe, and J.L. Dunn. 1979. Notes on Commerson's dolphin (*Cephalorhynchus commersonii*) in captivity. *Cetology* 35:1–9.

Stede, M. 1994. On the cause of death of whales from the North Sea coast of Lower Saxony: The cause of whale strandings in this area [In German]. *Drosera* 94:7–19.

Stockdale, P.H.G., and T.J. Hulland. 1970. The pathogenesis, route of migration, and development of *Crenosoma vulpis* in the dog. *Pathologia Veterinaria* 7:28–42.

Stroud, R.K. and M.D. Dailey. 1978. Parasites and associated pathology observed in pinnipeds stranded along the Oregon coast. *Journal of Wildlife Diseases* 14:292–298.

Stroud, R.K., and T.J. Roffe. 1979. Causes of death in marine mammals stranded along the Oregon coast. *Journal of Wildlife Diseases* 15:91–97.

Sweeney, J.C. 1972. Management of pinniped diseases. In *American Association of Zoo Veterinarians Annual Proceedings,* Houston, Texas, pp. 141–171.

———. 1974. Procedures for clinical management of pinnipeds. *Journal of American Veterinary Medical Association* 165:811–814.

———. 1986. Clinical consideration of parasitic and noninfectious diseases. In *Zoo and wild animal medicine.* Ed. M.E. Fowler. Philadelphia, PA: W.B. Saunders Company, pp. 785–789.

Sweeney, J.C., and W.G. Gilmartin. 1974. Survey of diseases in free-living California sea lions. *Journal of Wildlife Diseases* 10:370–376.

Sweeney, J.C., and S.H. Ridgway. 1975. Common diseases of small cetaceans. *Journal of the American Veterinary Medical Association* 167:533–540.

Tao, J.-Y. 1983. A new species and a new Chinese record of nematodes from porpoise *Neophocaena phocaenoides. Sinica* 8:350–353.

Temirova, R.V., and V.D. Usik. 1971. Pathological and morphological changes in the lungs of *Phocoena phocoena* L. from the Azov and Black Seas due to parasitism by *Halocercus ponticus* Delamure, 1946) [In Russian]. *Materialy Nauchnykh Konferentsii Vsesoyuznogo Obshchestva Gel'mintologov* 22:256–260.

Testi, F., and G. Pilleri. 1969. Verminous pulmonitis induced by Nematoda (*Halocercus,* Pseudaliidae) in the dolphin (*Delphinus delphis* L.). *Investigations on Cetacea* 1:181–188.

Tomilin, A. G. 1957. *Mammals of the USSR and adjacent countries.* Vol. 9, *Cetacea.* [In Russian.] Moscow: Izdatel'stvo Akademi Nauk SSSR. [1967. Translated by the Israel Program for Scientific Translations, Jerusalem.]

Torres, P., P. Cortes, J.A. Oporto, L. Brieva, and R. Silva. 1994. The occurrence of *Stenurus australis* Tantalean and Sarmiento, 1991 (Nematoda: Metastrongyloidea) in the porpoise *Phocoena spinipinnis* (Burmeister, 1965) on the southern coast of Chile. *Memoire Instituto Oswaldo Cruz, Rio de Janeiro* 89:141–143.

Troncone, A., N. Zizzo, G. Colella, A. Perillo, M. T. Manfredi. 1994. Parassitosi dei delfini. Incidenza di infestazioni parassitarie in delfini "spiaggiati." *Obiettivi e Documenti Veterinari* 15:39–44.

Van den Broek, E. 1963. Mededelingen betreffende parasitologisch onderzoek bij de gewone zeehond, *Phoca vitulina* L. [In Dutch]. *Lutra* 5:22–30.

Van den Broek, E., and P. Wensvoort. 1959. On parasites of seals from the Dutch coastal waters and their pathogenity. *Säugetierkündliche Mitteilungen* 7:58–61.

Van der Kamp, J. S. 1987. Pulmonary diseases in seals—A histopathological review. *Aquatic Mammals* 13:122–124.

Van Haaften, J. L. 1982. Post-mortem findings in seals which died in nature [In Dutch]. *Tijdschrift voor Diergeneeskunde* 107:379–383.

Van Waerebeek, K., J.C. Reyes, and J. Alfaro. 1993. Helminth parasites and phoronts of dusky dolphins *Lagenorhynchus obscurus* (Gray, 1818) from Peru. *Aquatic Mammals* 19:159–169.

Vauk, G. 1973. Observations on seals (*Phoca vitulina*) on Helgoland [In German]. *Zjagdwiss* 19:117–121.

Viale, D. 1981. Lung pathology in stranded cetaceans on the Mediterranean coasts. *Aquatic Mammals* 8:96–100.

Wazura, K.W., J.T. Strong, C.L. Glenn, and A.O. Bush. 1986. Helminths of the beluga whale (*Delphinapterus leucas*) from the MacKenzie River Delta, Northwest Territories. *Journal of Wildlife Diseases* 22:440–442.

Webster, W.A., J.L. Neufeld, and A.C. MacNeill. 1973. *Halocercus monoceris* sp. n. (Nematoda: Metastrongyloidea) from the narwhal, *Monodon monoceros. Proceedings of the Helminthological Society of Washington* 40:255–258.

Wesenberg-Lund, E. 1947. On three parasitic nematodes from Cetacea. *Videnskabelige Meddelelser fra Dansk naturhistorisk Forening i K benhavn Bind* 110:17–30.

Woodard, J.C., S.G. Zam, D.K. Caldwell and M.C. Caldwell. 1969. Some parasitic diseases of dolphins. *Pathologia Veterinaria* 6:257–272.

Wu, H.W. 1929. On *Halocercus pingi* n. sp. a lung-worm from the porpoise, *Neomeris phocoenoides. The Journal of Parasitology* 15:276–279.

Yablokov, A.V., V.M. Bel'kovich, V.I. Borisov. 1972. Whales and dolphins. Part I and II. [In Russian.] Moscow: Izd-vo Nauka. [Translated for National Technical Information Service, Springfield, JPRS-62l50-1.]

Yamaguti, S. 1943. Mammalian Nematodes, IV. Pseudaliidae Railliet, 1916. *Japanese Journal of Zoology* 4:451–454.

———. 1951. Studies on the helminth fauna of Japan. Part 46. Nematodes of marine mammals. Arbeiten aus der Medizinischen FakultÑt Okayama. *Sonderabdruck* 7:295–308.

Yurakhno, M.V. 1972. Comparison of the helminth fauna of Chukchi and Bering populations of ringed seals [In Russian]. In *Theses of Works 5th All-Union Conference, Studies of Marine Mammals.* Part 2, *Makhachkala,* pp. 275–279.

Yurakhno, M.V., and V.N. Popov. 1976. Isolation of herds of Bering Sea ringed seal. *Soviet Journal of Ecology* 7:83–85.

Yurakhno, M.V., and A.S. Skrjabin. 1971. *Parafilaroides krascheninnikovi* sp. n. a parasite of the lungs of the ringed seal (*Pusa hispida krascheninnikovi* Naumov et Smirnov) [In Russian]. *Vestnik Zoologii* 5:32–36. [1992. Canadian Translation of Fisheries and Aquatic Sciences, No. 5563.]

Zam, S.G., D.K. Caldwell and M.C. Caldwell. 1971. Some endoparasites from small odontocete cetaceans collected in Florida and Georgia. *Cetology* 2:1–11.

Zimmerman, T. and W. Nebel. 1975. Diseases of seal in the area of the northern Friesean coast [In German]. *Deutsche Tierarztliche Wochenschrift* 82:233–235.

11

BAYLISASCARIS PROCYONIS AND RELATED SPECIES

KEVIN R. KAZACOS

Larva migrans (LM) refers to the prolonged migration and persistence of helminth larvae in the organs and tissues of humans and animals (Beaver 1969; Kazacos 1997). In these hosts, the larvae behave as they would in their natural intermediate or paratenic hosts, which are usually small mammals or birds. During their migration, the larvae may produce extensive tissue damage and inflammation, leading to diverse clinical disease. Larva migrans is separated clinically and pathologically into visceral (VLM), ocular (OLM), neural (NLM) and cutaneous larva migrans (CLM), based on the main organ systems involved (Kazacos 1997). A large number of helminth parasites of lower animals, particularly carnivores, are potential causes of larva migrans affecting the deeper tissues of man and other animals, that is, visceral, ocular, and neural larval migrans (Beaver 1969; Beaver et al. 1984; Kazacos 1991, 1996, 1997, 2000; Smyth 1995). These include various ascarids, hookworms, gnathostomes, *Spirometra*, *Alaria*, and others. Of these, the ascarids are the most important group, with *Toxocara* and *Baylisascaris* accounting for the majority of cases in humans and animals.

Baylisascaris procyonis, the common raccoon ascarid, is the most commonly recognized cause of clinical larva migrans in animals and affects a wide variety of wild and domestic species. Infection with *B. procyonis* is best known as a cause of fatal or severe neurologic disease (NLM, cerebrospinal nematodiasis), which has been seen in > 90 species of mammals and birds in North America. *Baylisascaris procyonis* is also an important zoonosis, producing damaging visceral, ocular, and neural laval migrans in humans. Infection has important health implications for free-ranging and captive wildlife, zoo animals, domestic animals, and human beings, on an individual as well as population basis. This chapter will focus on *B. procyonis* as a cause of animal and human disease, with some reference to other *Baylisascaris* species also capable of producing clinical larva migrans; it is dedicated to Drs. Jack D. Tiner and John F.A. Sprent, for their pioneering research on *Baylisascaris* larva migrans.

INTRODUCTION. The ascarids or large roundworms (Superfamily Ascaridoidea) are some of the most common and well-known parasites of mammals. Because of their large size, in heavy infections they may interfere with digestion and cause partial or complete obstruction of the small intestine, negatively affecting animal health. Those ascarids that undergo liver and lung migration in intermediate, paratenic or definitive hosts cause hepatic, pulmonary, and other migration-related damage, with further deleterious effects on the host. Those species whose larvae enter the central nervous system, including *B. procyonis* and relatives, produce some of the most devastating clinical diseases in animals and humans.

Ascaridoids are basically heteroxenous, and most species utilize intermediate or paratenic hosts in their life cycles (Anderson 2000). For ascaridoids of carnivores, these hosts are usually small vertebrates (rodents, rabbits, birds) in the food chain of the definitive host, and transmission is via predation or scavenging. The single most important factor in the success of ascaridoids of terrestrial animals is the marked resistance and longevity of their infective eggs in the environment, which ensures eventual transmission to susceptible hosts. In intermediate or paratenic hosts, larval ascarids commonly undergo somatic migration, entering various organs and tissues where they will become encapsulated and persist, for later transmission to carnivores (Sprent 1952a, 1953a,b; Tiner 1953a,b; Sprent et al. 1973; Sheppard and Kazacos 1997). Thus, ascarids of carnivores, and *B. procyonis* in particular, are excellent examples of helminths that produce larva migrans.

The remarkable disease-producing capability of *B. procyonis* in animals and humans is one of the most important aspects of ascaridoid biology to come to light in recent years. Strikingly nonspecific in their infection of animals, *B. procyonis* larvae undergo aggressive somatic migration in a broad assortment of potential intermediate hosts, in which most of the larvae become encapsulated in various internal organs and tissues. A small percentage of larvae enter the brain, where they produce marked traumatic damage and inflammation that often results in clinical central nervous system disease. *Baylisascaris procyonis* affects a wide variety of birds and mammals, including humans, and is receiving increased attention in North America and Europe. Other closely related ascarids (e.g., *B. columnaris* of skunks and *B. melis* of badgers) are also potential causes of clinical larva migrans in animals and humans.

ETIOLOGIC AGENT. *Baylisascaris procyonis* and relatives are large roundworms in the nematode Order Ascaridida, Superfamily Ascaridoidea. Members of the superfamily are mainly medium- to large-size worms possessing three lips that may be separated by interlabia (Hartwich 1974; Gibson 1983). The superfamily contains five families, with *Baylisascaris* and most other ascarids of terrestrial hosts included in the family Ascarididae (Anderson 2000). Within the Ascarididae, *Baylisascaris, Ascaris, Toxascaris, Parascaris,* and *Lagochilascaris* are in the subfamily Ascaridinae, and *Toxocara* and *Porrocaecum* are in the subfamily Toxocarinae.

The genus *Baylisascaris* was defined by Sprent (1968) to include several ascarids previously named as members of *Ascaris* or *Toxascaris,* but which possess cervical alae with cuticular bars reaching the surface of the cuticle, and characteristic pericloacal roughened areas (area rugosa) in the males (McIntosh 1939; Sprent 1952b, 1970; Hartwich 1962). Dorsal and subventral labial papillae are distinctly double, and males possess stout, uniform spicules, usually < 1 mm long, and discrete precloacal and postcloacal groups of papillae on the tail. The genus currently contains eight recognized (Table 11.1) and two provisional species (Sprent 1968, 1970).

Members of *Baylisascaris* occur primarily in carnivores (Table 11.1), with one species (*B. laevis*) occurring in rodents. Similar to other ascarids of terrestrial carnivores, transmission of most *Baylisascaris* species involves ingestion of larvae in small mammal intermediate hosts; direct infection by eggs also occurs for some species, particularly in young definitive hosts (Tiner 1952a, 1953a; Sprent 1953b; Sprent et al. 1973; Kazacos 1983b; Kazacos and Boyce 1989). *Baylisascaris laevis* of rodents is morphologically similar to *B. columnaris* and *B. procyonis,* and probably arose as a transmission "capture" derived from the heteroxenous forms occurring in carnivores (Berry 1985; Anderson 2000).

Baylisascaris procyonis was first reported (as *Ascaris columnaris*) from raccoons in the New York Zoological Park (McClure 1933) and on a fur farm in Minnesota (Olsen and Fenstermacher 1938). It was later described as a new species (*Ascaris procyonis*) from raccoons in Europe and subsequently included within *Baylisascaris* (Sprent 1968). Synonyms of *B. procyonis* include *A. columnaris* (Leidy 1856) in raccoons, *A. procyonis* (Stefanski and Zarnowski 1951), and *Toxascaris procyonis* (Stefanski and Zarnowski 1951; Sprehn and Haakh 1956). Common names of the parasite include raccoon ascarid, raccoon roundworm, and, in German, Waschbärenspulwurm.

Adult *B. procyonis* are large, tan-colored nematodes, the female reaching 20–22 cm long and the male 9–11 cm long (Hartwich 1962; Sprent 1968; Overstreet 1970; Gey 1998; K.R. Kazacos, unpublished.) Cervical alae are vestigial and inconspicuous, the vulva is located one-fourth to one-third the body length from the anterior end, and males possess pericloacal roughened areas (Sprent 1968; Overstreet 1970; Berry 1985; Averbeck et al. 1995). Morphological features have been examined by scanning electron microscopy (Kazacos and Turek 1982; Snyder 1989). The eggs of *B. procyonis* are ellipsoidal in shape, brown in color, contain a large single-celled embryo, and have a thick shell with a finely granular surface (Fig. 11.1a); they range in size from 63–88 x 50—70 µm, with most averaging 68–76 x 55–61 µm (Overstreet 1970; Kazacos and Turek 1983; Kazacos and Boyce 1989; Sakla et al. 1989; Miyashita 1993; Averbeck et al. 1995; Van Andel et al. 1995; Conboy 1996; Gey 1998).

LIFE HISTORY AND TRANSMISSION. Adult female worms in the small intestine of raccoons produce an estimated 115,000–179,000 eggs/worm/day, so that infected raccoons shed millions of eggs/day in their feces (Kazacos 1982; Snyder and Fitzgerald 1987). Naturally infected raccoons shed an average of 20,000–26,000 *B. procyonis* eggs/g feces, with higher shedding rates in juvenile raccoons than in adults (Kazacos 1982, 1983a; Snyder and Fitzgerald 1987). The highest reported shedding is 256,700 eggs/g feces (Kazacos 1983a). With adequate temperature and moisture, *B. procyonis* eggs can reach infectivity (second-stage larva) in 11–14 days (Sakla et al. 1989) (Fig. 11.1b) and can remain infective in the environment for years (Kazacos and Boyce 1989).

Young raccoons become infected by ingesting infective eggs, whereas older raccoons become infected by ingesting third-stage larvae (L_3's) in intermediate hosts, usually rodents (Fig. 11.2) (Tiner 1953a,b; Kazacos 1983a,b; Kazacos and Boyce 1989). Young raccoons become infected at an early age by ingesting eggs from their mother's contaminated teats or fur, from the contaminated den, or from raccoon latrines near their den. In young raccoons, larvae hatching from eggs enter the mucosa of the small intestine and develop there several weeks before reentering the intestinal lumen to mature, the worms reaching patency in 50–76 days (mean, 63). . In older raccoons, larvae from intermediate hosts develop to adults in the intestinal lumen, reaching patency in 32–38 days (mean, 35) (Kazacos 1983b; Kazacos and Boyce 1989). More extensive migration

TABLE 11.1—Recognized species of *Baylisascaris* [a]

Parasite	Primary Definitive Host(s)
B. procyonis (Stefanski and Zarnowski 1951)	Raccoons
B. columnaris (Leidy 1856)	Skunks
B. melis (Gedoelst 1920)	Badgers
B. devosi (Sprent 1952)	Martens, fishers
B. transfuga (Rudolphi 1819)	Bears
B. schroederi (McIntosh 1939)	Giant pandas
B. tasmaniensis (Sprent 1970)	Tasmanian devils, quolls, native "cats"
B. laevis (Leidy 1856)	Marmots, ground squirrels

[a]From Sprent (1968, 1970).

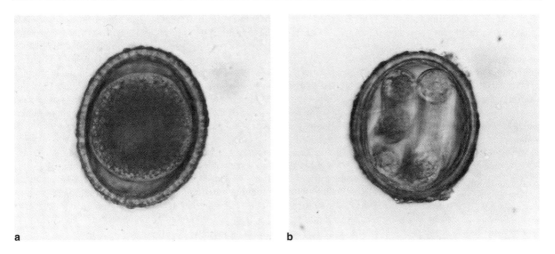

FIG. 11.1—**(a)** Undeveloped *Baylisascaris procyonis* egg from fresh raccoon feces. Note ellipsoidal shape, large single-celled embryo, and finely granular surface. **(b)** The other egg is infective and contains a second-stage larva. [Figure 1b reprinted from Kazacos (1983a) with the permission of Purdue Research Foundation.]

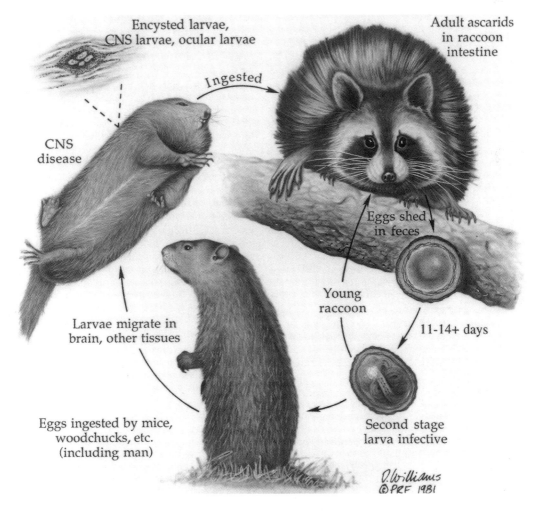

FIG. 11.2—Life cycle of *Baylisascaris procyonis*.

of *B. procyonis,* including somatic migration, does not appear to occur in raccoons, and although transmammary and transplacental transmission have not been investigated, based on the above their occurrence would be doubtful.

Tiner (1949, 1951, 1952a, 1953a,b) reported that *B. procyonis* larvae would produce fatal central nervous system disease in various experimentally infected rodents (white mice, house mice, cotton rats, hamsters, guinea pigs, gray squirrels). He also recovered similar larvae from the tissues of wild-caught fox squirrels and white-footed mice from raccoon-infested woodlots in Illinois (Tiner 1952a, 1953a). Based on counts of granulomas and larvae in wild-caught mice, Tiner (1954) estimated that 5% of *P. leucopus* mortalities in these woodlots were caused by *B. procyonis.* Since that time, *B. procyonis* has become well known as an important cause of morbidity and mortality in individuals and populations of small vertebrates sharing or frequenting the habitat of infected raccoons. *Baylisascaris* larvae have been recovered from numerous species of mammals and birds, most of which were suffering from clinical central nervous system disease (Kazacos and Boyce 1989; Sheppard 1995).

In intermediate hosts, *B. procyonis* larvae undergo aggressive somatic migration, similar to the larvae of several other carnivore ascarids (Sprent 1952a, 1955; Tiner 1953a,b). After ingestion, eggs hatch in the small intestine, and larvae quickly penetrate the intestinal wall and migrate through the liver to the lungs, presumably via the portal circulation and associated vascular channels. Pulmonary hemorrhages are evident by 12–48 hours postinfection, caused by larvae breaking out of capillaries in the lungs (Sprent 1952a, 1953b, 1955; Kazacos 1986). The larvae then enter the pulmonary veins, thereby gaining access to the left heart and systemic arterial circulation, which distributes them throughout the body but especially to the head and anterior carcass (Sprent 1952a, 1955; Tiner 1953b; Sheppard and Kazacos 1997). A few larvae probably migrate locally in the abdominal viscera after initial infection, and in the thoracic cavity once they reach the lungs; some others undergo tracheal migration, being swallowed and reentering the gastrointestinal tract. In white mice infected with *B. procyonis,* larvae enter the somatic tissues, eyes, and brain as early as 3 days postinfection (Tiner 1953b; Kazacos et al. 1985; Kazacos 1986), and clinical central nervous system disease is evident by 9–10 days postinfection (Tiner 1953a; Sheppard and Kazacos 1997). Larvae in visceral and somatic tissues become encapsulated in eosinophilic granulomas, where they will remain until ingested by raccoons. Host differences exist in the relative distribution and encapsulation of larvae in various tissues, but larvae entering the central nervous system of different hosts appear to be equally pathogenic (Tiner 1953a,b; Wirtz 1982; Sheppard and Kazacos 1997).

Larvae migrating in the brain produce traumatic damage and inflammation, resulting in progressive central nervous system disease, the onset and severity of which are dose related. The number of *B. procyonis* larvae entering the brain varies with animal species and dose and may be influenced by prior exposure or other factors (Kazacos and Boyce 1989; Sheppard and Kazacos 1997). A single *B. procyonis* larva in the brain of a mouse or small bird is usually fatal (Tiner 1953a,b; Sheppard and Kazacos 1997), and in natural cases one to five or more larvae are often recovered (Tiner 1953a; Armstrong et al. 1989; Van Andel et al. 1995; K.R. Kazacos, unpublished). In nature, the production of central nervous system disease in intermediate hosts has survival value for *B. procyonis,* because debilitation or death of intermediate hosts would result in increased transmission of *B. procyonis* back to raccoons, via predation or scavenging (Tiner 1953a,b; Kazacos and Boyce 1989; Sheppard and Kazacos 1997). Raccoons are opportunistic carnivores, so it is likely that increased pathogenicity of *B. procyonis* in intermediate hosts has been selected for over time.

Sources of *B. procyonis* infection for intermediate hosts include any areas or articles contaminated with the feces of feral or pet raccoons. In nature, most transmission to intermediate hosts occurs at raccoon latrines, preferred sites of raccoon defecation where their feces and *B. procyonis* eggs accumulate (Fig. 11.3) (Cooney 1989; Page 1998; Page et al. 1999). Raccoon latrines are found most often at the base of trees, in raised crotches of trees, and on large logs, stumps, rocks, tree limbs, and other horizontally oriented structures (Yeager and Rennels 1943; Stains 1956; Cooney 1989; Kazacos and Boyce 1989; Page 1998; Page et al. 1998). They are also found in barn lofts and garages and on woodpiles, decks, roofs, and other locations in the domestic environment (Kazacos et al. 1983; Kazacos and Boyce 1989). Large numbers of *B. procyonis* eggs occur at raccoon latrines, and these areas become important long-term sources of infection. As first alluded to by Tiner (1952a), there is mounting evidence that intermediate hosts, particularly granivorous rodents, become infected with *B. procyonis* by foraging for undigested seeds and other materials present in raccoon feces at latrines (Wirtz 1982; Kazacos and Boyce 1989; Sheppard and Kazacos 1997; Page 1998; Page et al. 1999). Recently, Page (1998) and Page et al. (1999) documented visitation to raccoon latrines by 16 species of mammals and 15 species of birds, with active foraging by white-footed mice (*Peromyscus leucopus*), eastern chipmunks (*Tamias striatus*), fox squirrels (*Sciurus niger*), opossums (*Didelphis virginiana*), white-breasted nuthatches (*Sitta carolinensis*), and hermit thrush (*Catharus guttatus*). Visitation by white-footed mice was significantly greater when corn, their most highly preferred seed type, was present in raccoon feces. Caching of raccoon feces by white-footed mice (Page 1998) and Allegheny woodrats (*Neotoma magister*) (McGowan 1993; K.R. Kazacos and S.A. Johnson, unpublished) has also been documented. Such behavior and subsequent infection with *B. procyonis* have been linked to extirpation of *N. magister* from parts of its

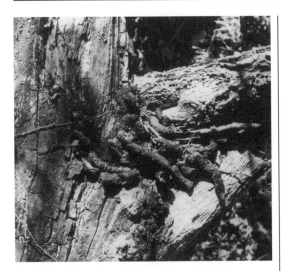

FIG. 11.3—Raccoon latrine on a log in an Indiana woodlot. The raccoon feces contain corn fragments and seeds, and are in various stages of weathering/decomposition.

northeastern range (McGowan 1993). Animals could also become infected while investigating a latrine site, or indirectly through grooming, after having become contaminated at a latrine (Sheppard and Kazacos 1997; Page et al. 1999).

Infection with *B. procyonis* has also been linked to the use of straw, hay, feed, and enclosures contaminated by wild raccoons (Richardson et al. 1980; Kazacos et al. 1982a, 1983, 1986; Armstrong et al. 1989; Sanford 1991; Van Andel et al. 1995; Campbell et al. 1997; Pessier et al. 1997; C.L. Eng and K.R. Kazacos, unpublished; A.M. Lennox and K.R. Kazacos, unpublished; J.C. Martin, unpublished), and cages or enclosures previously used to house raccoons (Schueler 1973; Church et al. 1975; Koch and Rapp 1981; Reed et al. 1981; Larson and Greve 1983; Myers et al. 1983; Dixon et al. 1988; Medway et al. 1989; Fitzgerald et al. 1991; Coates et al. 1995; Garlick et al. 1996; K.R. Kazacos, unpublished; M.A. Nieves et al., unpublished). In zoos, raccoon latrines in open exhibits or on the tops of "roundhouse" enclosures, and contaminated logs or tree limbs placed into exhibits have resulted in infections with *B. procyonis* (Armstrong et al. 1989; Kazacos and Boyce 1989; Stringfield and Sedgwick 1997; K.R. Kazacos, unpublished). An extensive outbreak involving *B. columnaris* infection in three species of marmosets and tamarins was linked to two infected skunks kept in the same exhibit, presumably to make it more "natural" (Huntress and Spraker 1985; K.R. Kazacos and P.L. Wolff, unpublished). Marmosets and tamarins spend much time on the ground foraging, which could lead to infection with *Baylisascaris* (Pessier et al. 1997). At least ten cases of fatal or severe central nervous system disease due to *B. pro-*

cyonis have occurred in young children following contact with contaminated areas or articles in the domestic environment.

EPIDEMIOLOGY

Distribution and Prevalence of *B. procyonis* in Raccoons. *Baylisascaris procyonis* is indigenous in raccoons in North America, Europe, and parts of Asia. In North America, it is more common in the midwestern and northeastern United States and along the west coast, where prevalences reach 68%–82% (Kazacos and Boyce 1989) (Table 11.2). The annual prevalence of *B. procyonis* appears to be stable in endemic areas (Table 11.3). In Wisconsin, the prevalence of *B. procyonis* decreases from south to north (75% in the southern half versus 18% in the northern quarter) and correlates with relative raccoon abundance (Amundson and Marquenski 1986). Interestingly, the prevalence of *B. procyonis* also decreases from northern to southern United States, so that the parasite is less common or absent in raccoons in the deep south (Table 11.2). In the southeast, *B. procyonis* appears to be found primarily in mountainous areas, not in the coastal regions or on coastal islands, an exception being south coastal Texas (Kerr et al. 1997). Its farthest known southeastern distribution is central Georgia (Babero and Shepperson 1958). It is important to note that local prevalences of *B. procyonis* may vary, so it is unwise to discount its occurrence in a particular area until an adequate sample of raccoons has been examined. Also, with the influx or translocation of infected raccoons (Lotze and Anderson 1979; Schaffer et al. 1981) and/or changes in their population density, prevalence in an area may change over time. Although *B. procyonis* was not found in east or central Texas by Chandler (1942) or Schaffer et al. (1981), it was identified recently in raccoons in east Texas and south coastal Texas (Table 11.2). Limited data are available on the occurence of *B. procyonis* in other southwestern states, and no data are available from the Rocky Mountain states.

Raccoons are native to North and Central America (Lotze and Anderson 1979) but have been introduced elsewhere, taking *B. procyonis* with them. Raccoons have become well established in major areas of Europe and Asia, following their escape or release decades ago. For example, it is estimated that > 100,000 wild raccoons occur in Germany (C. Bauer, personal communication, 1991), with a prevalence of *B. procyonis* infection of 71% (Gey 1998). The increase in raccoons in Europe has been accompanied by *B. procyonis*–induced larva migrans in various species, including humans (Kelly and Innes 1966; Koch and Rapp 1981; Küchle et al. 1993), the extent of which deserves further investigation. Over 20,000 raccoons have been imported into Japan as pets since 1977, and many have escaped and now inhabit wild areas of central Honshu and Hokkaido. Recently, *B. procyonis* was found in raccoons in Japan (Table 11.2) (Miyashita 1993). Even

TABLE 11.2—Geographic distribution, prevalence, and intensity of intestinal *Baylisascaris procyonis* in raccoons (*Procyon lotor*)

Geographic Location	No. Examined	Percent Infected	Intensity: Mean (Range)	Reference/Source
1. United States: Midwest				
Illinois	6	4 of 6	27 (2–71)	Leigh 1940
Central Illinois	1	1 of 1	~120	Tiner 1952a
Central Illinois/Wisconsin	na[a]	na	na	Tiner 1953a
Southern Illinois	36	64	na	Barnstable and Dyer 1974
NE Illinois (Chicago)	26	42	21 (1–101)	Pigage et al. 1983
Illinois	310	82	52 (1–328)	Snyder and Fitzgerald 1985
Illinois	100	86	52 (1–241)	Snyder and Fitzgerald 1987
Southern Illinois	60	5	na	Birch et al. 1994
Indiana	25	28	na	Robinson et al. 1957
Central Indiana	4	3 of 4	na	Reed et al. 1981
Indiana	95[b]	20	na	Jacobson et al. 1982
	218[c]	29	na	Jacobson et al. 1982
Indiana:	1425	72	na	Kazacos and Boyce 1989
1982 sample	391	74	43 (1–283)	Kazacos, unpub.
NW Indiana	219[c]	15	na	Cooney 1989
Iowa	1	1 of 1	(quite abundant)	Morgan and Waller 1940
Iowa	10	20	na	Waller 1940
Iowa	24[c] and 22[c]	13 and 73	na	Greve 1985
Iowa	25[b]	48	na	Hill et al. 1991
Kansas	na	na	na	Lindquist 1978
NE Kansas:	128	44	(1–263)	Robel et al. 1989
Fort Riley	36	33	14 (1–124)	Robel et al. 1989
Rural Manhattan	92	75	21 (1–263)	Robel et al. 1989
Eastern Kansas	8	5 of 8	na	Ball et al. 1998
Michigan	256	0	na	Stuewer 1943
Michigan, Wisconsin, and Ohio	25	32	(1–18)	R.L. Rausch, unpub. (1944–48); in Hoberg and McGee 1982
SE Michigan	33	58	27 (1–110)	Schultz 1962
Michigan	1	1 of 1	na	Thomas 1988
Minnesota	1	1 of 1	(numerous)	Olsen and Fenstermacher 1938
Minnesota	1	0	na	Larson and Scharf 1975
Minnesota:	163	61	na	S.A. Schmit, G.A. Averbeck, and B.E. Stromberg, unpub.na
Twin Cities Metro Area	109	66	na	S.A. Schmit, G.A. Averbeck, and B.E. Stromberg, unpub.
Nebraska	4	3 of 4	na	Armstrong et al. 1989
Southern Ohio	1	1 of 1	na	Rausch 1946
Central Ohio	28	25	na	Dubey 1982
Ohio and Northern West Virginia	10	20	3 (?–5)	Schaffer et al. 1981
South Dakota	250	12	na (?–46)	Boddicker and Progulske 1968
Wisconsin:	213	51	na (1–241)	Amundson and Marquenski 1986
Southern 1/2	114	75	48	Amundson and Marquenski 1986
Northern 1/2	99	23	28	Amundson and Marquenski 1986
2. United States: Northeast/Middle Atlantic				
Connecticut	1	1 of 1	(1321)	Carlson and Nielsen 1984
Maryland	19	5	(many)	Habermann et al. 1958
Maryland	304[b]	30	na	K.R. Kazacos and N.P. Garner, unpub.
New Jersey	21[b]	24	na	LoGiudice 1995
	137[c]	34	na	LoGiudice 1995
New York (New York City)	1	1 of 1	(10)	McClure 1933
New York (New York City)	na	+++[d]	na	Herman 1939
Eastern New York	2	2 of 2	389 (141–636)	Stone 1983
Western New York	429	68	48 (1–480)	Ermer and Fodge 1986
Southern New York (Ithaca)	277[b]	20 (4–42)	na	Kidder et al. 1989
SE New York (Long Island)	49[c]	39	na	Feigley 1992
SE Pennsylvania	1	1 of 1	5	Dubey et al. 1992
Washington, DC	23	35	na	Tecec 1987
	21[c]	52	na	Tecec 1987

TABLE 11.2 *(continued)*

Geographic Location	No. Examined	Percent Infected	Intensity: Mean (Range)	Reference/Source
3. United States: Southeast				
Alabama	371	0	na	Johnson 1970
Arkansas	30	0	na	Richardson et al. 1992
Florida	19	0	na	Harkema and Miller 1964
Central Florida	51	0	na	Schaffer et al. 1981
Southern Florida (Miami)	90	0	na	K.R. Kazacos et al., unpub. [1997]
Central Georgia	6	+++	na	Babero and Shepperson 1958
Eastern Georgia (Ossabaw Is.)	100	0	na	Jordan and Hayes 1959
Georgia	22	0	na	Harkema and Miller 1964
Northern Georgia	110	1	na	V.F. Nettles, unpub. [1976–77] in Kazacos and Boyce 1989
Northern Georgia/ Western North Carolina	23	0	na	Schaffer et al. 1981
SE Georgia	10	0	na	Schaffer et al. 1981
Eastern Georgia (St.Cath.Is.)	32	0	na	Price and Harman 1983
Western Kentucky	70	30	(?–61)	Cole and Shoop 1987
North Carolina:				
Coastal	61	0	na	Harkema and Miller 1964
Inland	148	0	na	Harkema and Miller 1964
SE North Carolina	10	0	na	Schaffer et al. 1981
South Carolina (Cape Is.)	16	0	na	Harkema and Miller 1962
South Carolina:				
Cape Island	17	0	na	Harkema and Miller 1964
Coastal	16	0	na	Harkema and Miller 1964
Inland	31	0	na	Harkema and Miller 1964
South Carolina	128	0	na	Yabsley and Noblet 1999
Tennessee	253	8	(1–221)	Bafundo et al. 1980
NE Tennessee/Virginia	20	0	na	Schaffer et al. 1981
NW Tennessee/ SW Kentucky	145	3	(?–83)	Smith et al. 1985
Virginia	6	0	na	Harkema and Miller 1964
Western Virginia	7	5 of 7	(17–93)	Jacobson et al. 1976
Eastern Virginia (coastal)	10	0	na	Schaffer et al. 1981
Virginia:				
Eastern	38	0	na	Jones and McGinnes 1983
Western (mountains)	34	56	16 (?–129)	Jones and McGinnes 1983
4. United States: West/Southwest				
Southern California	na	+++	na	Voge 1956
Southern California	na	+++	na	Overstreet 1970
Northern California	12	67	na	Goldberg et al. 1993
Northern California	26	58	na	Park et al. 1998
Northern California	56	70 (52 and 18[b])	(1–tremendous nos.)	W.J. Murray et al., unpub. [1999]
Northern California (coastal)	15	100	na	W.J. Murray et al., unpub. [1998]
Western Nevada	1[c]	1 of 1	na	G.N. Cooper and R.D. Anderson, unpub.
Oklahoma	1	1 of 1	(large nos.)	Campbell et al. 1997
Oregon	1	0	na	Senger and Neiland 1955
Eastern Texas	13	0	na	Chandler 1942
Central Texas	37	0	na	Schaffer et al. 1981
Eastern Texas	62[b]	23	na	S,C, Waring and D.D. Dingley, unpub.; in Kazacos and Boyce 1989
Southern Texas (coastal)	33	70	6 (1–28)	Kerr et al. 1997
SW Washington	29	3	1	McNeil and Krogsdale 1953
Washington	62	79	na	W.J. Foreyt, unpub. [1998]
5. Canada				
SW British Columbia	82	61	27 (1–226)	Ching et al. 2000
Nova Scotia	219	8	na	Anderson and Mills 1991
Nova Scotia	236	7	(1–46)	Smith 1992
Nova Scotia	491	7	na	J.K. Mills, unpub. [1993]
Ontario	na	+++	na	Sprent 1968
Ontario (Toronto)	23	43	(numerous)	Cranfield et al. 1984
Southern Ontario (Guelph)	41	51	(1–40)	Berry 1985
Prince Edward Island	50	2	na	G.A. Conboy, unpub. [1998]
Quebec	21	57	(?–86)	Mackay et al. 1995
Southern Saskatchewan	31	0	na	Hoberg and McGee 1982

(continued)

TABLE 11.2 (*continued*)

Geographic Location	No. Examined	Percent Infected	Intensity: Mean (Range)	Reference/Source
6. Germany				
Brandenburg	41	0	na	Lux and Priemer 1995
Hessen	185	71	(1–232)	Gey 1998
7. Poland	1	1 of 1	50	Stefanski and Zarnowski 1951
8. Czech and Slovak Rep.	1	1 of 1	2	Tenora et al. 1991
	1	1 of 1	28	Tenora and Stanek 1990
9. Japan	291[b]	27	na	Miyashita 1993
Zoos (n=21)	178[b]	40	na	Miyashita 1993
Animal dealers (n=6)	37[b]	8	na	Miyashita 1993
Pets	39[b]	8	na	Miyashita 1993
Wild	37[b]	0	na	Miyashita 1993

[a]na = not available
[b]Examination of raccoon feces for eggs.
[c]Examination of raccoon feces from latrines for eggs.
[d]+++ = positive, no numbers given.

TABLE 11.3—Prevalence of *Baylisascaris procyonis* in raccoons in Indiana, 1981-1986 [a]

Year	No. Examined	Percent Infected
1981	157	72
1982	391	74
1983	145	68
1984	259	73
1985	308	72
1986	165	67
Total	1425	72

[a]Animals collected in November and December.

though no cases of *B. procyonis*–induced larva migrans have been reported from Japan, its occurrence there can be predicted with certainty based on what is known from North America and Europe. *Baylisascaris procyonis* was also recovered from a kinkajou (*Potos flavus*) in Colombia (Overstreet 1970), thereby extending the geographical range of the parasite into South America. The parasite may occur in raccoons in Central America and in other procyonids in the Americas, although this has not been studied.

Prevalence and Intensity of *B. procyonis* in Raccoons. In areas where *B. procyonis* is common in raccoons, it has much higher prevalence in juvenile raccoons (> 90%) than in adults (37%–55%). Average parasite intensity ranges from 43 to 52 worms, with juvenile raccoons having a higher mean intensity (48–62, range 1–480) than adult raccoons (12–22, range 1–257) (Table 11.4) (Snyder and Fitzgerald 1985; Ermer and Fodge 1986; K.R. Kazacos, unpublished). The highest reported worm numbers (636 and 1321) occurred in juvenile raccoons that died of intestinal obstruction due to *B. procyonis,* with resulting starvation and emaciation (Stone 1983; Carlson and Nielsen 1984). The age distribution of *B. procyonis* correlates with what is known

about the life cycle (Fig. 11.2), namely that young raccoons in their first season are susceptible to egg infection, whereas adult raccoons become infected via intermediate hosts (Kazacos 1983b; Kazacos and Boyce 1989). Thus, the parasite appears to be recruited into the raccoon population mainly through the young, which have higher worm burdens and prevalence of infection. Age resistance and/or intestinal immunity with self-cure may also contribute to the lower prevalence of *B. procyonis* in older raccoons.

There is mounting evidence that *B. procyonis* may undergo a yearly cycle in raccoons in temperate regions, with self-cure occurring in winter months (January-February). New infections are recruited into the raccoon population in late spring and summer, and the overall prevalence peaks in the fall (September-November) (Schultz 1962; Smith et al. 1985; Kidder et al. 1989; K.R. Kazacos, unpublished). Based on necropsies, Schultz (1962) first found *B. procyonis* in 3-month-old raccoons, with highest intensities at 5–6 months of age (September-October). Kidder et al. (1989) examined raccoon fecal samples from July 1986 to May 1987 and found the highest prevalence of patency (42%) in September-November, vs. 6% in December-August; this correlated with higher prevalences in both juvenile (61%) and adult (23%) raccoons in September-November as compared to the rest of the year (10% and 4%, respectively). Based on necropsies, Smith et al. (1985) in Kentucky/Tennessee, K.R. Kazacos (unpublished) in Indiana, and M.W. Dryden (unpublished) in Kansas have identified sharp declines in the prevalence of *B. procyonis* in raccoons in winter, occurring suddenly in January-February in Indiana and Kansas. As suggested by LoGiudice (1995), this sudden loss of worms may be related to the dramatic reduction in food intake by raccoons at this time of year in northern temperate regions, leading to as much as 50% reduction in their body weight (Folk et al. 1968) and negatively impacting worm survival.

TABLE 11.4—Prevalence of *Baylisascaris procyonis* in raccoons in Indiana, November-December 1982

Age/Sex Class (no.)	No. (% Infected)	Parasite Intensity +/- SE	Range
All animals (391)	289 (74)	42.6 +/- 2.6	1–283
Juvenile male (125)	113 (90)	49.3 +/- 4.6[a]	1–283
Juvenile female (139)	129 (93)	47.4 +/- 3.9[a]	1–256
Juvenile (male+female) (264)	242 (92)[b]	48.3 +/- 3.0[ac]	1–283
Adult male (71)	29 (41)	14.9 +/- 3.9	1–81
Adult female (56)	18 (32)	13.0 +/- 3.7	1–56
Adult (male+female) (127)	47 (37)[b]	14.2 +/- 2.8[c]	1–81
Male (juvenile+adult) (196)	142 (73)	42.05 +/- 3.91	1–283
Female (juvenile+adult) (195)	147 (75)	43.04 +/- 3.55	1–256

[a] Based on 108 juvenile males and 124 juvenile females.
[b,c] Significantly different (P < 0.0001); one way ANOVA (F=8.54; df=3, 278).

TABLE 11.5—Intestinal *Baylisascaris procyonis* in nonraccoon hosts

Host	Geographic Location	Natural (N) or Experimental (E)	Number Infected	Intensity: Mean (Range)	Reference/Source
Potos flavus	Colombia	N	na[a]	(13)	Overstreet 1970
	Indiana	N	2	(20–25+)	K.R. Kazacos, unpub.
Bassaricyon gabbii	na	na	1	1	Overstreet 1970
Canis familiaris	Iowa	N	2	(2–3)	Greve and O'Brien 1989
	Missouri	N	2	13 (na)	G.A. Averbeck et al. 1995 and unpub.
	Indiana	N	12	8 (3–13)[b]	K.R. Kazacos, unpub.
	Michigan	N	7+5[c]	2 (1–3)[d]	D.D. Bowman, unpub.
	Japan	E	1/3[e]	6	Miyashita 1993
		E	3/4[f]	(4–5)	Miyashita 1993
Didelphis virginiana	Georgia	E	0/1[e]	na	V.F. Nettles, unpub.; in Kazacos and Boyce 1989
		E	1/1[f]	13	

[a] na = not available.
[b] Based on ten dogs.
[c] Probable infections; based on single fecal exam.
[d] Based on four dogs.
[e] Fed infective eggs.
[f] Fed third-stage larvae.

Host Range of Adult *B. procyonis*. *Baylisascaris procyonis* is restricted primarily to raccoons but has also been found in related procyonids (kinkajous) and other hosts (Table 11.5). Intestinal infections could be expected to occur in coatimundis (*Nasua* spp.) and ringtails (*Bassariscus* spp.). Over two dozen cases of patent *B. procyonis* infection have been identified in domestic dogs (*Canis familiaris*) from the midwestern United States (Table 11.5). In several of these, *B. procyonis* occurred as a mixed infection with *Toxocara canis* and other helminths. It is not known how these dogs became infected with *B. procyonis*, however, 1 of 3 dogs fed infective eggs and 3 of 4 dogs fed L$_3$'s from mice developed intestinal *B. procyonis* infections; no infections were seen in cats fed eggs or larvae (Miyashita 1993). The biological relationship of *B. procyonis* in dogs is particularly interesting when one considers that several dogs have died from severe neural larva migrans due to this parasite (Snyder 1983;

Thomas 1988; Rudmann et al. 1996). Whether dogs with patent infections also have larvae in their somatic tissues is not known. Because of their indiscriminate defecation habits, dogs infected with *B. procyonis* would produce more widespread contamination with eggs, posing a particular zoonotic threat. It is likely that canine infection with adult *B. procyonis* is more common and widespread than is currently known.

Partial or complete development of *B. procyonis* probably takes place in other hosts, but the extent is unknown and not easily determined. Berry (1985) showed limited cross-transmission of *B. procyonis* to skunks, but found no genetic evidence that this occurred in nature. The author has anecdotal reports of patent *Baylisascaris* infections naturally occurring in opossums. This is supported by experimental evidence of a patent infection in a young opossum fed mice containing *B. procyonis* larvae (V.F. Nettles, unpublished: cited in Kazacos and Boyce 1989).

Environmental Limitations. In most areas where raccoons occur, there should be no environmental limitations on the presence of *B. procyonis,* although conditions for optimal egg development and survival will vary based on temperature and humidity. *Baylisascaris procyonis* eggs become infective in 11–14 days at 22°C–25° C and 100% humidity (Sakla et al. 1989), similar to eggs of *B. columnaris* (11–16 d) (Berry 1985). Under natural conditions, with cooler and/or fluctuating temperatures, egg development will be slower and will take several weeks to months. For example, *B. procyonis* eggs deposited in spring in Indiana do not develop until ambient temperatures increase, at which time the eggs embryonate slowly and later reach infectivity (K.R. Kazacos, unpublished). Under sufficiently warm but fluctuating temperatures (*e.g.,* cooler nights), most eggs should reach infectivity in 3–4+ weeks.

Embryonated *B. procyonis* eggs stored 9–12 years at 4° C retained their infectivity and central nervous system pathogenicity for mice (Lindquist 1978; W.D. Lindquist, personal communication in Kazacos et al. 1982b). Given adequate moisture, embryonated eggs will last years in the soil, including through harsh winters (Kazacos 1986, 1991; Kazacos and Boyce 1989). Conditions of extreme heat and dryness, as occur in barn lofts and attics in summer months, will kill *B. procyonis* eggs by desiccation, probably in a few weeks or months (Kazacos and Boyce 1989).

It is doubtful that the lack of *B. procyonis* in the deep southeastern United States is based on environmental limitations, since *Toxocara* and other ascarids do very well there. Rather, it is probably a result of the parasite's absence in raccoons colonizing those areas or its failure to establish due to inadequate host/parasite densities. With current high raccoon densities, translocation of raccoons by hunting clubs, pet owners, and others could introduce *B. procyonis* into new areas, where it could establish and pose a threat to indigenous birds and mammals, including humans (Kazacos and Boyce 1989).

Host Range for Clinical Neural Larva Migrans Caused by *B. procyonis* and Relatives. Few other parasites are as indiscriminate as *B. procyonis* in causing neurologic disease in wild, zoo, and domestic animals as well as human beings (Table 11.6). As would be expected, the geographic distribution of animals and humans clinically affected by *B. procyonis* parallels the occurrence and prevalence of the parasite in raccoons in different areas. Wherever raccoons occur or are introduced, the potential exists for disease caused by *B. procyonis,* a situation that should be taken very seriously.

Susceptibility to *Baylisascaris* larva migrans varies among animal groups and species (Wirtz 1982; Sheppard and Kazacos 1997). Animal groups particularly susceptible to *Baylisascaris* NLM include rodents, rabbits, primates, and birds, based on the number of cases and species affected (Table 11.6). Some animal groups and species are only marginally susceptible, with limited migration occurring in the intestinal wall or viscera; others appear to be resistant (Kazacos and Boyce 1989). For example, no cases of *B. procyonis* NLM have been documented in opossums, which are commonly exposed through foraging at raccoon latrines (Page 1998; Page et al. 1999), or in adult domestic livestock or zoo hoofstock, which are commonly exposed through contaminated hay. Very limited or no migration was seen in sheep, goats, and swine experimentally infected with *B. procyonis* (Dubey 1982; Snyder 1983; Kazacos and Kazacos 1984). No cases have been documented in cats or raptors, which eat rodents possibly contaminated with eggs and/or containing L_3's. Shrews (*Blarina brevicauda*) are resistant to experimental infection with *B. procyonis,* at dosages much higher than are lethal to mice (Sheppard 1996; K.R. Kazacos et al., unpublished); the reasons for this resistance are unclear, but may include unique or potent gastrointestinal enzymes and failure of egg hatching or larval survival. Unless complete necropsies are performed, including a thorough examination of the brain in all cases of central nervous system disease, then apparent species limitations to *Baylisascaris* infection should be regarded with caution.

Special circumstances, including prior exposure, concurrent infections (Sheppard and Kazacos 1997), and hormone fluctuations during pregnancy, may also influence infection. Although ruminants appear to be poorly susceptible to infection, a newborn lamb was diagnosed with *Baylisascaris* NLM and could only have been infected prenatally (Anderson 1999). It is hypothesized that pregnancy hormones increased the susceptibility of the ewe to infection and/or stimulated larval migration, with resultant transplacental transmission of larvae to the fetus. Reminiscent of *Toxocara canis* transmission in dogs, but previously unrecognized for *Baylisascaris,* this finding has important potential health implications for other pregnant mammals, including women.

The susceptibility of poikilothermic vertebrates and invertebrates to *Baylisascaris* is for the most part unknown, but infection would not be expected based on typical host stimuli necessary for larval hatching and migration. Berry (1985) was unable to infect northern leopard frogs (*Rana pipiens*), earthworms (*Eudrilus eugenioe*), cockroaches (*Blatta orientalis*), or African crickets (*Acheata domesticus*) with *B. columnaris,* or northern leopard frogs or African crickets with *B. procyonis,* by feeding infective eggs. However, even though egg hatching apparently doesn't occur, invertebrates could possibly serve as paratenic hosts for *Baylisascaris* eggs recently ingested from raccoon or skunk feces.

In much of the geographic range of *B. procyonis,* skunks infected with *B. columnaris* and, in more limited areas, badgers infected with *B. melis* also are found. Both of these parasites are potential causes of clinical NLM (Kazacos and Boyce 1989); however, based on differences in definitive host ecology,

TABLE 11.6—Host range for clinical neural larva migrans (cerebrospinal nematodiasis) caused by *Baylisascaris procyonis* **(Bp) and** *B. columnaris* **(Bc)**

Host	Geographic Location	Parasite[a]	Natural (N) or Experimental (E)	Number Affected[b]	Reference/Source[c]
O. Rodentia					
Mus musculus	Illinois	Bp	N	Several	Tiner 1949, 1953a
	Illinois	Bp	E	3/3	Tiner 1952a
Mus musculus (white,lab)	Illinois	Bp	E	12/12; 15/21; 8/9	Tiner 1949, 1952a, 1953a
	Illinois	Bc	E	3/9; 7/11	Tiner 1952a, 1953a
	Australia	Bc	E	4/9; 12/32; [2/9][d] [1/5][d]	Sprent 1953a, 1955
	Minnesota	Bc	E	54/70	Clark et al. 1969
	Indiana	Bc	E	0/12	Boyce et al. 1988b
	Missouri	Bp	E	6/6	Lindquist 1978
	Indiana	Bp	E	25/25	Kazacos 1981
	Ohio	Bp	E	66/66	Dubey 1982
	Indiana	Bp	E	10/10	Wirtz 1982
	Indiana	Bp	E	12/12	Boyce et al. 1988b
	Japan	Bp	E	70/75	Miyashita 1993
	Indiana	Bp	E	24/25	Garrison 1996
	Indiana	Bp	E	28/30	Sheppard and Kazacos 1997
Peromyscus leucopus	Illinois	Bp	N	[1][d]	Tiner 1953a,b, 1954
	Illinois	Bp	E	na; 7/10	Tiner 1949, 1953a
	Illinois	Bc	E	0/6; 1/4	Tiner 1953a
	Indiana	Bp	E	17/30	Sheppard and Kazacos 1997
	Indiana	Bp	N	1+[1][d]	Sheppard and Kazacos 1997 and unpub.[c]
	Indiana	Bp	N/E	10/46	Page 1998
Peromyscus maniculatus	California	Bp/Bc	N	1	R.H. Evans, unpub.
Peromyscus boylei	California	Bp/Bc	N	1	R.H. Evans, unpub.
Chaetodipus californicus	California	Bp/Bc	N	1	R.H. Evans, unpub.
Reithrodontomys megalotis	Indiana	Bp	E	3/3	Sheppard 1996
Zapus hudsonius	Indiana	Bp	E	1/1	Sheppard 1996
Microtus pennsylvanicus	Indiana	Bp	E	29/30	Sheppard 1996
	Ontario	Bc	E	[8][d]	Berry 1985
Microtus ochrogaster	Indiana	Bp	E	3/4	Sheppard 1996
Mesocricetus auratus	Illinois	Bp	E	na	Tiner 1949
	Indiana	Bp	E	32/32	Kazacos 1981
	Indiana	Bp	E	23/23	Wirtz 1982
Thomomys bottae	California	Bp	N	2	R.H. Evans, unpub.
	California	Bp/Bc	N	2	K.R. Kazacos and F.H. Dunker, unpub.
Neotoma magister	New York	Bp	N/E	10/10	McGowan 1993
	New Jersey	Bp	N/E	1	K. LoGiudice, unpub.
	Indiana	Bp	N	1	K.R. Kazacos and S.A. Johnson, unpub.
	Pennsylvania	Bp	N	1	J. Wright et al., unpub.
	Indiana	Bp	E	26/26	K.R. Kazacos, unpub.
Neotoma fuscipes	California	Bp/Bc	N	2	R.H. Evans, unpub.
Sigmodon hispidus	Illinois	Bp	E	6/6; 7/8; 3/3	Tiner 1949, 1952a, 1953a
	Illinois	Bc	E	0/4	Tiner 1952a
Rattus norvegicus (white,lab)	New Jersey	Bp	E	[2/3][d]	Tiner 1954
	Indiana	Bp	E	12/19	Wirtz 1982
Tamias striatus	Indiana	Bp/Bc	N	1	K.R. Kazacos and S.A. Johnson, unpub.
	Indiana	Bp	E	1	K.R. Kazacos, unpub.; in Kazacos and Boyce 1989

(continued)

TABLE 11.6 *(continued)*

Host	Geographic Location	Parasite[a]	Natural (N) or Experimental (E)	Number Affected[b]	Reference/Source[c]
Sciurus carolinensis	Illinois	Bp	E	4/6	Tiner 1949, 1952a, 1953a
	Indiana	Bp	E	10/10	Wirtz 1982
	Indiana	Bp	N	3	K.R. Kazacos, unpub.
	Washington	Bp	N	11/16	Tseng 1997
Sciurus niger	Indiana	Bp/Bc	N	2	K.R. Kazacos, unpub.
	California	Bp/Bc	N	5	Stringfield and Sedgwick 1997, and unpub.
Sciurus granatensis	Maryland	Bp	N	1	Schueler 1973
Sciurus sp. (*griseus* or *carolinensis*)	California	Bp	N	2	R.H. Evans, unpub.
Tamiasciurus douglasii	Br. Columbia	Bp	N	1	Coates et al. 1995
Spermophilus tridecemlineatus	Illinois	Bp/Bc	N	28	Fritz et al. 1968
	Illinois	Bp/Bc	N	1	Pigage et al. 1983
	Illinois	Bp/Bc	N	1	J.I. Everitt and S.E. McDonald, unpub.
Spermophilus beecheyi	California	Bp/Bc	N	8	R.H. Evans, unpub.
	California	Bp/Bc	N	1	C.E. Stringfield and C.J. Sedgwick, unpub.
Cavia porcellus	Illinois	Bp	E	na	Tiner 1949, 1953b
	Pennsylvania	Bp	E	na	Donnelly et al. 1989
	Missouri	Bp	N	30/50	Van Andel et al. 1995
	Nova Scotia	Bp	N	2	Craig et al. 1995
Chinchilla lanigera	Pennsylvania	Bp/Bc	N	6	Richter and Kradel 1964
	Ontario	Bp	N	100	Sanford 1991
Cynomys ludovicianus	Iowa	Bp	N	na	Greve 1985
	New York/ Wisconsin	Bp	N	3/52	Dixon et al. 1988
	Illinois	Bp	N	1	K.R. Kazacos, unpub.
Ondatra zibethicus	New York	Bp/Bc	N	4	W.B. Stone, unpub.
Marmota monax	Pennsylvania	Bp/Bc	N	4/4	Richter and Kradel 1964
	Connecticut	Bp/Bc	N	na	Swerczek and Helmboldt 1970
	Connecticut	Bc	E	1/5; [4/5][d]	Swerczek and Helmboldt 1970
	Virginia	Bp	N	3/3	Jacobson et al. 1976
	New York	Bp/Bc	N	6	Fleming and Caslick 1978
	New York	Bp/Bc	N	5/5	Fleming et al. 1979
	Indiana	Bp/Bc	N	3	Kazacos et al. 1981a; and K.R. Kazacos, unpub.
	New York	Bp/Bc	N	12/12	Roth et al. 1982
	Iowa	Bp/Bc	N	na	Greve 1985
	Indiana	Bp	E	3/3	K.R. Kazacos, unpub.
Myocastor coypus	Michigan	Bp/Bc	N	20/35	Dade et al. 1977
	Germany	Bp	N	65	Koch and Rapp 1981
Erethizon dorsatum	Pennsylvania	Bp	N	3	Medway et al. 1989
	Indiana	Bp	N	2	Fitzgerald et al. 1991
	New York	Bp/Bc	N	2	W.B. Stone, unpub.
Castor canadensis	Ireland	Bp/Bm	N	na	Kelly and Innes 1966
	New York	Bp/Bc	N	2	W.B. Stone, unpub.
Dolichotis patagonum	Illinois	Bp	N	4	K.R. Kazacos et al., unpub.
Hydrochaeris hydrochaeris	Illinois	Bp	N	1	K.R. Kazacos et al., unpub.

(continued)

TABLE 11.6 (*continued*)

Host	Geographic Location	Parasite[a]	Natural (N) or Experimental (E)	Number Affected[b]	Reference/Source[c]
O. Lagomorpha					
Sylvilagus floridanus	Illinois	Bp	E	na	J.D. Tiner, unpub., in Tiner 1954
	Illinois	Bp/Bc	N	1	Ferris et al. 1960
	Virginia	Bp	N	16/60	Nettles et al. 1975
	Connecticut	Bp/Bc	N	1	Church et al. 1975
	Virginia	Bp	N	18/72	Jacobson et al. 1976
	Virginia	Bp	E	1/1	Jacobson et al. 1976
	Iowa	Bp/Bc	N	na	Greve 1985
	Indiana/Illinois	Bp/Bc	N	3	K.R. Kazacos, unpub.
	Illinois	Bp/Bc	N	1	R.H. Evans, unpub.
Sylvilagus audubonii	California	Bp/Bc	N	3	R.H. Evans, unpub.
Oryctolagus cuniculus	Illinois	Bp	E	na	J.D. Tiner, unpub.; in Tiner 1954
	Connecticut	Bp	N	Several	Church et al. 1975
	Connecticut	Bc	E	3/4	Church et al. 1975
	Michigan	Bp/Bc	N	80	Dade et al. 1975
	Indiana	Bp	N	25	Kazacos et al. 1983
	Iowa	Bp	N	na	Greve 1985
	Indiana	Bp	N	3	K.R. Kazacos, unpub.; in Boyce et al. 1988a
	Indiana	Bp	N	15	Kazacos and Kazacos 1988b
	Indiana	Bp	E	1/1	Boyce et al. 1989
	Ontario	Bp	N	na	P. Lautenslager and S.E. Sanford, unpub.; in Sanford 1991
	Washington	Bp	N	4	Deeb and DiGiacomo 1994
	Illinois	Bp	N	2	K.R. Kazacos, unpub.
	Illinois	Bp	N	6	L.J. Hardy, unpub.
	Illinois	Bp	N	4	P.J. Didier, unpub.
	Illinois	Bp/Bc	N	2	R.H. Evans, unpub.
	Indiana	Bp/Bc	N	6	K.R. Kazacos, unpub.
	Indiana	Bp/Bc	N	3	N.A.Q. Mehdi, unpub.
	Indiana	Bp	N	1	D.D. Harrington, unpub.
	New York	Bp	N	3	L. Roth, unpub.
	New York	Bp	N	2	W.B. Stone, unpub.
O. Carnivora					
Vulpes vulpes	Iowa	Bp	N	4/4	Larson and Greve 1983
Canis familiaris	Illinois	Bp	E	3/5	Snyder 1983
	Michigan	Bp	N	1	Thomas 1988
	Indiana	Bp	N	1	Rudmann et al. 1996
Taxidea taxus	California	Bp	N	1	R.H. Evans, unpub.
Enhydra lutris nereis	California	Bp	N	1	N.J. Thomas et al., unpub.
Mustela putorius furo	Indiana	Bp	E	3/4	Kazacos 1981; Kazacos and Kazacos 1988a
Mustela nivalis	Indiana	Bp	E	1	K.R. Kazacos, unpub.
O. Primates					
Varecia variegata variegata	Oklahoma	Bp	N	2	Campbell et al. 1997
	Rhode Island	Bp	N	4/6	J.C. Martin, unpub.
	Tennessee	Bp	N	3	S.J. Barrett, unpub.
Varecia variegata rubra	Rhode Island	Bp	N	2/3	J.C. Martin, unpub.
Mirza coquereli	California	Bp	N	1	K.R. Kazacos and F.H. Dunker, unpub.
Callithrix geoffroyi	Texas	Bc	N	3	Huntress and Spraker 1985
	Illinois/Texas	Bc	N	1	K.R. Kazacos and P.L. Wolff, unpub.
Saguinus nigricollis	Texas	Bc	N	1	Huntress and Spraker 1985

TABLE 11.6 (*continued*)

Host	Geographic Location	Parasite[a]	Natural (N) or Experimental (E)	Number Affected[b]	Reference/Source[c]
Saguinus midas	Texas	Bc	N	1	Huntress and Spraker 1985
Leontopithecus rosalia chrysomelas	Maryland	Bp	N	2	Pessier et al. 1997
	California	<u>Bp</u>/Bc	N	3	Stringfield and Sedgwick 1997; Pessier et al. 1997
Saimiri sciureus	Indiana	Bp	E	4/4	Kazacos et al. 1981b
Macaca fascicularis	Indiana	Bp	E	4/4	Kazacos et al. 1984b, 1985
Hylobates lar	Kansas	Bp	N	1	Ball et al. 1998
Ateles sp.	Maryland	Bp	N	1	Garlick et al. 1996
Cercopithecus neglectus	Indiana	Bp	N	2	C.L. Eng and K.R. Kazacos, unpub.
Homo sapiens	Missouri	<u>Bp</u>/Bc	N	1[e]	Anderson et al. 1975
	Pennsylvania	Bp	N	1	Huff et al. 1984
	Illinois	Bp	N	1	Fox et al. 1985
	New York	Bp	N	1[e]	Cunningham et al. 1994
	California	Bp	N	1	Rowley et al. 2000
	California	Bp	N	1[e]	Park et al. 2000
	California	Bp	N	1	W.A. Kennedy et al., unpub.
	Michigan	Bp	N	1[e]	J.M. Proos et al., unpub.
	Illinois	Bp	N	1[e]	M.B. Mets et al., unpub.
	Minnesota	Bp	N	2[e]	C.L. Moertel et al., unpub.
O. Marsupialia					
Macropus rufus	Michigan	Bp	N	11/20	Agnew et al. 1994
O. Artiodactyla					
Ovis aries	Idaho	<u>Bp</u>/Bc/Bm	N	1/3	Anderson 1999
O. Galliformes					
Gallus gallus	Indiana	Bp	N	622	Richardson et al. 1980
(domesticated)	Indiana	Bp	E	17/50	Kazacos and Wirtz 1983
Colinus virginianus	Indiana	Bp	N	85/85	Reed et al. 1981
	Iowa	Bp	N	na	Greve 1985
	Kansas	<u>Bp</u>/Bc	N	1	Williams et al. 1997
Callipepla californica	California	<u>Bp</u>/Bc	N	4	R.H. Evans, unpub.
Alectoris chukar	Maryland	<u>Bp</u>/Bc	N	1/30	Sass and Gorgacz 1978
Bonasa umbellus	New York	<u>Bp</u>/Bc	N	3	W.B. Stone, unpub.
Phasianus colchicus	Wisconsin	Bp	N	200-400	Kazacos et al. 1986
Alectura lathami	Indiana/Missouri	Bp	N	1	Kazacos et al. 1982a
Meleagris gallopavo	New York	<u>Bp</u>/Bc	N	2	W.B. Stone, unpub.
O. Columbiformes					
Columba livia	Oregon	<u>Bp</u>/Bc	N	10/45	Helfer and Dickinson 1976
	Illinois	<u>Bp</u>/Bc	N	1	Evans and Tangredi 1985
	Br.Columbia	Bp	N	2	Coates et al. 1995
	Nebraska	Bp	N	>15	V. Rinne and E.W. Pendleton, unpub.
Zenaida macroura	New York	<u>Bp</u>/Bc	N	2	Evans and Tangredi 1985
	Illinois	<u>Bp</u>/Bc	N	>25	C.U. Meteyer et al., unpub.
	California	Bp, <u>Bp</u>/Bc	N	9	R.H. Evans, unpub.

(continued)

TABLE 11.6 (*continued*)

Host	Geographic Location	Parasite[a]	Natural (N) or Experimental (E)	Number Affected[b]	Reference/Source[c]
O. Passeriformes					
Passer domesticus	California	Bp	N	2	R.H. Evans, unpub.
Psaltriparus minimus	California	Bp	N	3	R.H. Evans, unpub.
Serinus canarius	California	Bp/Bc	N	2	B.C. Barr, unpub.
Carpodacus mexicanus	California	Bp/Bc	N	2	R.H. Evans, unpub.
Pipilo maculatus	California	Bp/Bc	N	1	R.H. Evans, unpub.
Toxostoma redivivum	California	Bp/Bc	N	2	R.H. Evans, unpub.
Turdus migratorius	Illinois	Bp/Bc	N	1	Evans and Tangredi 1985
Cyanocitta cristata	Illinois	Bp/Bc	N	2	Evans and Tangredi 1985
Aphelocoma californica	California	Bp/Bc	N	2	R.H. Evans, unpub.
Mimus polyglottos	California	Bp/Bc	N	7	R.H. Evans, unpub.
Sturnus vulgaris	California	Bp/Bc	N	1	R.H. Evans, unpub.
Corvus brachyrhynchos	New York	Bp/Bc	N	1	B.P. Tangredi and K.R. Kazacos, unpub.
O. Psittaciformes					
Melopsittacus undulatus	California	Bp/Bc	N	10	B.C. Barr et al., unpub.
Nymphicus hollandicus	Iowa	Bp	N	3	Myers et al. 1983
Eolophus roseicapillus	California	Bp/Bc	N	3	Stringfield and Sedgwick 1997
Ara ararauna	Nebraska	Bp	N	3/4	Armstrong et al. 1989 and unpub.
Ara macao	Nebraska	Bp	N	3/4	Armstrong et al. 1989
	Iowa	Bp	N	2	M.A. Nieves et al., unpub.
Ara ararauna x *A. macao*	Nebraska	Bp	N	2/2	Armstrong et al. 1989
Amazona aestiva aestiva	California	Bp/Bc	N	1	B.C. Barr, unpub.
Amazona ochrocephala oratrix	Indiana	Bp	N	2	A.M. Lennox and K.R. Kazacos, unpub.
Aratinga acuticaudata	Indiana	Bp	N	5	A.M. Lennox and K.R. Kazacos, unpub.
Aratinga canicularis	Indiana	Bp	N	1	A.M. Lennox and K.R. Kazacos, unpub.
Aratinga solstitialis	Indiana	Bp	N	2	A.M. Lennox and K.R. Kazacos, unpub.
O. Strigiformes					
Tyto alba	California	Bp/Bc	N	1	R.H. Evans, unpub.
O. Ciconiiformes					
Nycticorax nycticorax	California	Bp	N	2	R.H. Evans, unpub.
O. Charadriiformes					
Calidris alba	California	Bp/Bc	N	1	R.H. Evans, unpub.
O. Anseriformes					
Anas platyrhynchos	California	Bp/Bc	N	2	R.H. Evans, unpub.
(domesticated)	Indiana	Bp	E	8/21	Wirtz 1982

(*continued*)

TABLE 11.6 *(continued)*

Host	Geographic Location	Parasite[a]	Natural (N) or Experimental (E)	Number Affected[b]	Reference/Source[c]
O. Casuariiformes					
Dromaius novaehollandiae	Indiana	Bc	N	2	Winterfield and Thacker 1978; Kazacos et al. 1982b
	Indiana	Bp	N	2	Kazacos et al. 1991
	Ontario	Bp/			
	Kansas	Bp/Bc	N	2/4	Suedmeyer et al. 1996
	Michigan	Bp	N	1	D.W. Agnew and K.R. Kazacos, unpub.
	Kansas, Missouri, Nebraska, New York	Bp	N	>15	K.R. Kazacos, unpub.
	California	Bp/Bc	N	1	L.W. Woods, unpub.
O. Struthioniformes					
Struthio camelus	Indiana	Bp	N	1	Kazacos et al. 1991

Probable *Baylisascaris* NLM, based on characteristic histopathologic lesions, clinical signs, and history of exposure, but larvae not found in histologic sections:

Host	Geographic Location	Parasite[a]	Natural (N) or Experimental (E)	Number Affected[b]	Reference/Source[c]
O. Rodentia					
Neotoma magister	New York	Bp	N/E	1	McGowan 1993
Sciurus carolinensis	Indiana	Bp	N	2	K.R. Kazacos, unpub.
	Washington	Bp	N	4	Tseng 1997
O. Lagomorpha					
Sylvilagus floridanus	Indiana	Bp/Bc	N	1	K.R. Kazacos, unpub.
Sylvilagus audubonii	California	Bp/Bc	N	2	C.E. Stringfield and C.J. Sedgwick, unpub.
Oryctolagus cuniculus	Indiana	Bp	N	2	K.R. Kazacos, unpub.
O. Primates					
Homo sapiens	Oregon	Bp	N	1	M. Lahr and R.D. Jansen, unpub.; in Cunningham et al. 1994
O. Marsupialia					
Bettongia penicillata	California	Bp/Bc	N	1	J.E. Wynne, unpub.
O. Chiroptera					
Pteropus giganteus	California	Bp/Bc	N	1	Stringfield and Sedgwick 1997
O. Galliformes					
Pavo cristatus	Nebraska	Bp/Bc	N	1	Armstrong et al. 1989
O. Psittaciformes					
Agapornis sp.	California	Bp/Bc	N	1	B.C. Barr, unpub.
O. Casuariiformes					
Dromaius novaehollandiae	Oklahoma	Bp	N	3	Campbell et al. 1997

Probable *Baylisascaris* NLM, based on clinical signs and history of exposure, but unproven because animals survived or were lost to follow-up:

Host	Geographic Location	Parasite[a]	Natural (N) or Experimental (E)	Number Affected[b]	Reference/Source[c]
O. Marsupialia					
Petrogale xanthopus	California	Bp/Bc	N	2	Stringfield and Sedgwick 1997
O. Primates					
Leontopithecus rosalia chrysomelas	California	Bp/Bc	N	2	Stringfield and Sedgwick 1997
O. Psittaciformes					
Calyptorhynchus magnificus	California	Bp/Bc	N	1	Stringfield and Sedgwick 1997
Rhynchopsitta pachyrhyncha	California	Bp/Bc	N	1	Stringfield and Sedgwick 1997

(continued)

TABLE 11.6 (*continued*)

Host	Geographic Location	Parasite[a]	Natural (N) or Experimental (E)	Number Affected[b]	Reference/Source[c]
O. Casuariiformes					
Dromaius novaehollandiae	Indiana	Bp	N	2	K.R. Kazacos, unpub.
O. Rheiformes					
Rhea americana	Indiana	Bp	N	2	K.R. Kazacos, unpub.

Baylisascaris larva migrans (VLM, OLM) identified, without recognition of concurrent NLM or clinical CNS disease:

Host	Geographic Location	Parasite[a]	Natural (N) or Experimental (E)	Number Affected[b]	Reference/Source[c]
O. Rodentia					
Mus musculus (white, lab)	Great Britain	Bc	E	2/2	Goodey and Cameron 1923
	Australia	Bc	E	4/5	Sprent 1953a
Peromyscus leucopus	Illinois	Bp/Bc	N	13/67	Tiner 1953a, 1954
	Indiana	Bp/Bc	N	111/487	Page 1998
	Indiana	Bp	N/E	13/46	Page 1998
Sciurus carolinensis	Illinois	Bp	E	2/6	Tiner 1952a
	Indiana	Bp	N	3	K.R. Kazacos, unpub.
Sciurus niger	Illinois	Bp	N	8/12	Tiner 1951, 1953a
Castor canadensis	Kansas	Bp/Bc	N	1	McKown et al. 1995
O. Primates					
Homo sapiens	Kentucky	Bp	N	1	Raymond et al. 1978
	Michigan	Bp/Bc	N	1	Raymond et al. 1978
	Wisconsin	Bp/Bc	N	1	Williams et al. 1988
	California	Bp	N	1	Goldberg et al. 1993
	Germany	Bp	N	1	Küchle et al. 1993
	Massachusetts	Bp/Bc	N	1	Boschetti and Kasznica 1995

[a]Bp/Bc: species could not be determined (Bp or Bc); Bp/Bc: species involved most likely *B. procyonis;*
Bm: possible *B. melis.*
[b]na = not available
[c]Unpublished cases have been confirmed by the author, with information and data on file at Purdue University.
[d]Positive for *Baylisascaris* NLM, but without clinical central nervous system disease
[e]Positive for *Baylisascaris* NLM based on serology.

defecation habits, other epidemiologic factors, and larval pathogenicity, their role in this syndrome is considerably less than that of *B. procyonis.* Since the third-stage larvae of these parasites are very difficult or impossible to differentiate, especially in histologic sections, species determination in cases and outbreaks often is based on epidemiologic findings, which indicate exposure to raccoon or skunk feces. In situations where both raccoons and skunks occur and epidemiologic studies are not done, a specific identification beyond *Baylisascaris* sp. cannot be made (although one or the other species might be considered more likely based on relative host abundance). In all but two cases and outbreaks where epidemiologic studies were done, *B. procyonis* was determined to be the parasite involved (Table 11.6), clearly indicating that the raccoon ascarid is the most likely cause of this disease syndrome.

CLINICAL SIGNS. Except in very heavy infections with intestinal obstruction, raccoons infected with *B. procyonis* appear clinically normal with no outward signs of infection. Similarly, other species with

Baylisascaris larva migrans usually are asymptomatic if no larvae enter the brain. At high infecting dosages, individuals may become dull and anorexic, with dyspnea and increased respiratory rates 2–5 days postinfection, due to hemorrhagic pneumonitis from pulmonary migration (Kazacos et al. 1981b; Donnelly et al. 1989; Kazacos 1997). The severity and progression of central nervous system disease in NLM depends on the number of eggs ingested, the number of larvae entering the brain, the location and extent of migration damage and inflammation in the brain, and the size of the brain. Thus, clinical disease will vary from mild, insidious, slowly progressive central nervous system disease with subtle clinical signs to acute, fulminating, rapidly progressive central nervous system disease with marked clinical signs. Although larvae enter the somatic tissues, eyes, and brain of some species as early as 3 days postinfection, clinical central nervous system disease is not usually apparent before 9–10 days postinfection, and in many cases not until 2–4+ weeks postinfection, due to the lag time in causing central nervous system damage and inflammation (Kazacos 1997; Sheppard and Kazacos 1997). If the larvae leave the brain or

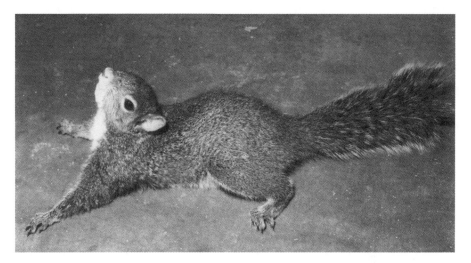

FIG. 11.4—Gray squirrel with encephalitis due to *Baylisascaris procyonis,* showing arching of the head and neck, and extensor rigidity of forelegs. [Reprinted from Kazacos (1983a) with permission of Purdue Research Foundation.]

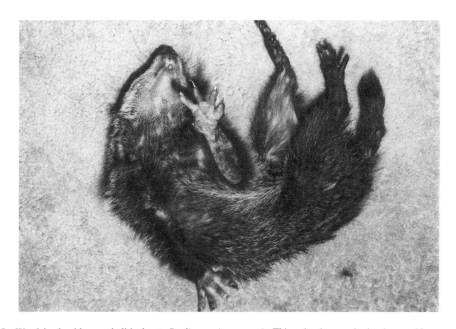

FIG. 11.5—Woodchuck with encephalitis due to *Baylisascaris procyonis.* This animal was submitted as a rabies suspect because of ataxia, circling, and loss of fear of humans.

become encapsulated, clinical signs can stabilize, and the animal can survive and function with variable central nervous system deficits.

Initial clinical signs in rodents and other small mammals include depression, lethargy, or nervousness; rough hair coat; tremors in the front paws; slight head and/or body tilts; and circling or jumping when disturbed. These signs progress to various combinations of severe head and/or body tilts, ataxia, continuous circling, leaning, falling over, opisthotonos, lateral recumbency, rolling around the longitudinal axis, coma, and death (Kazacos and Boyce 1989; Sheppard and Kazacos 1997). Other clinical signs include "stargazing," slow arching of the head and neck, blindness, nystagmus, various degrees of motor weakness or posterior paresis, hypotonia or extensor rigidity, and paddling movements while recumbent (Figs. 11.4, 11.5) (Kazacos and Boyce 1989; Sheppard and Kazacos 1997; references in Table 11.6).

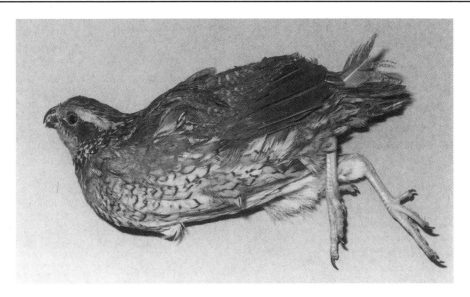

FIG. 11.6—Northern bobwhite with encephalitis due to *Baylisascaris procyonis,* from an outbreak linked to pet raccoons (Reed et al. 1981). Note lateral recumbency, torticollis, and extensor rigidity.

Monkeys experimentally infected with *B. procyonis* became less vocal, their activity declined, and they began to have problems with manual dexterity, with increasing difficulty grasping and handling food, climbing, and traversing the cage floor. These signs progressed rapidly to marked ataxia, loss of balance, inability to maintain an upright posture or to grasp food, torticollis, truncal ataxia, swaying and bobbing of the head, intention tremors of the head and forelimbs, and head pressing. Two monkeys became narcoleptic and a third had nondirected, unsolicited vocalizations. Finally, they became semicomatose and recumbent on the cage floor, with opisthotonos, extensor rigidity, and nystagmus, and were unresponsive to touching or prodding (Kazacos et al. 1981b). Many of these clinical signs and a similar progression were seen in marmosets, lemurs, a gibbon, and human infants infected with *Baylisascaris* (Huff et al. 1984; Fox et al. 1985; Huntress and Spraker 1985; Kazacos 1996, 2000; Campbell et al. 1997; Ball et al. 1998). Mildly affected primates suffered only subtle forelimb tremors (C.L. Eng and K.R. Kazacos, unpublished) or had slight head tilt and ataxia (Pessier et al. 1997).

Clinical signs in birds include ruffled feathers, disorientation, head tremors, torticollis, poor grip reflexes, incoordination, loss of balance, walking in circles, falling, rolling, inability to fly or loss of flight control, blindness, recumbency, extensor rigidity, and paralysis of one or both wings or legs (Fig. 11.6) (Richardson et al. 1980; Reed et al. 1981; Coates et al. 1995; references in Table 11.6). Clinically affected ratites exhibit varying degrees of incoordination, loss of equilibrium and balance, muscle weakness, wobbling, and progressive ataxia. They typically stagger, walk in circles,

assume a wide, splay-legged stance with their head extended downward for balance, and walk rapidly backward, stumbling and falling; eventually they are unable to stand or walk and become increasingly emaciated (Kazacos et al. 1991; Kwiecien et al. 1993; Suedmeyer et al. 1996).

PATHOLOGY AND PATHOGENESIS. Somatic migration of *Baylisascaris* larvae causes mechanical damage and tissue necrosis and provokes vigorous inflammatory reactions. The principal pathologic alterations are those of eosinophilic and granulomatous inflammation, which may occur in a variety of organs and tissues, including the liver, lungs, heart, brain, and eyes. The most important lesions are in the brain and consist of focal to diffuse meningoencephalitis, necrosis, and spongiosis. Inflammatory reactions are directed against larval excretory-secretory antigens, which consist of enzymes, cuticular proteins, and metabolic wastes released by the larvae during migration. Eosinophils are a major component of host reactions, and toxic eosinophil proteins released in the tissues probably contribute to pathologic changes and clinical signs (Hamann et al. 1989; Kazacos and Boyce 1989; Kazacos 1996, 1997; C.L. Moertel et al., unpublished). A key factor in the pathogenesis of *Baylisascaris* NLM is the large size attained by the larvae, which when combined with their aggressive migration, results in considerable damage to the central nervous system. *Baylisascaris procyonis* L_2's are ~300 μm long (275–310 μm) when they hatch from ingested eggs (Berry 1985; Sakla et al. 1989). The larvae grow rapidly following infection, reaching a length of 1058 μm (range, 625–1429 μm) at 10 days postinfection, 1573 μm (range, 1319–1888 μm) at 15 days postinfection, and 1750 μm (range, 1450–1850 μm) at 31 days postinfection (Tiner 1953b; Goldberg et al. 1993). Most *B. procyonis* larvae recovered from clinical cases are 1500–1900 μm long and 60–80 μm in greatest width (Kazacos 1997).

Early migration of *Baylisascaris* larvae through the liver and lungs and subsequent migration in other organs and tissues produce traumatic damage and inflammation. Rabbits naturally infected with *B. procyonis* had acute hemorrhagic tracks in the liver associated with focal necrosis and hepatitis. Also noted were multifocal eosinophilic myocarditis and myositis, with associated myofiber loss and fibrosis, interstitial pneumonitis, and focal nephritis. Inflammatory infiltrates consisted of eosinophils, macrophages, lymphocytes, and plasma cells (Kazacos et al. 1983). Similar lesions and others were seen in monkeys experimentally infected with *B. procyonis* (Kazacos et al. 1981b). The severe hepatic pathology associated with liver trapping of larvae in *Toxocara* infections has not been seen with *Baylisascaris,* reflecting differences in migration, antigenicity, and/or host responses between the two parasites (Kazacos 1997). *Baylisascaris* larvae migrate quickly through the liver and lungs, and the liver is not a major site of larval accumulation, before or after somatic migration.

Pulmonary migration of *Baylisascaris* can produce considerable lung damage, and in heavy infections clinical signs of verminous pneumonitis are noted within 2–5 days postinfection (Goodey and Cameron 1923; Sprent 1952a, 1953b, 1955; Kazacos et al. 1981b; Donnelly et al. 1989). Petechial and ecchymotic hemorrhages are evident in the lungs within 12–48 hours postinfection (Fig. 11.7), and within another day or two the lungs are often uniformly dark red. The hemorrhage subsides and is replaced by acute neutrophilic then eosinophilic inflammation (Kazacos 1997). Using bronchopulmonary lavage cytology to assess pulmonary migration of *B. procyonis* in mice, Wyand-Ouellette et al. (1983) saw a marked increase in erythrocytes on day 1, peaking on days 2–3 at up to 130X controls, and returning to normal by days 7–8. This was followed by a biphasic nucleated cell (leukocyte) response, which peaked on days 3 and 8, at 7–9X control mice; the early peak was due to neutrophils (210X control) and macrophages (3X control) and the latter peak to eosinophils (209X control) and macrophages (4X control). In affected lungs, alveolar septa are thickened by congestion, edema, and cellular infiltrates, and hemosiderosis develops in areas of resolving hemorrhage.

Following migration in extraneural tissues, larvae become encapsulated in well-circumscribed eosinophilic granulomas, usually 1–2 mm in diameter (Figs. 11.8, 11.9). Larval granulomas are often visible grossly (Fig. 11.8) and are found in many organs and tissues, including the liver, lungs, heart, diaphragm, pancreas, spleen, kidneys, mesentery, mesenteric

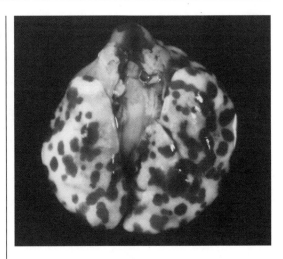

FIG. 11.7—Multifocal, coalescing hemorrhages in the lungs of a lab mouse, due to pulmonary migration of *Baylisascaris columnaris* larvae; 2 days postinfection with eggs.

lymph nodes, intestinal wall, skeletal muscles, brain, and eyes (Sprent 1952a; Kazacos et al. 1981b; Kazacos 1996, 1997). The development and distribution of *B. procyonis* larval granulomas varies with host species, which is an important consideration during necropsy examinations for this infection (Sheppard and Kazacos 1997). Tiner (1953a) found that gray squirrels had numerous larval granulomas primarily in the thorax, in the wall of the caval veins, heart, lungs, diaphragm, and intercostal muscles; the author has also noted this distribution in infected squirrels (K.R. Kazacos, unpublished). Naturally infected rabbits (*O. cuniculus*) had granulomas in the heart, lungs, diaphragm, liver, mesentery, intestine, and skeletal muscles (Kazacos et al. 1983; K.R. Kazacos, unpublished). In experimentally infected rats, most granulomas were in the wall of the intestine, with some in the heart and diaphragm (Wirtz 1982). Naturally infected woodchucks, lemurs, and marmosets (with *B. columnaris*) had numerous larval granulomas along the intestinal tract, in addition to other locations (Richter and Kradel 1964; Jacobson et al. 1976; Fleming and Caslick 1978; Huntress and Spraker 1985; K.R. Kazacos and P.L. Wolff, unpublished; K.R. Kazacos, unpublished). In children, granulomas were numerous in the heart, lungs, and mesentery; and in experimentally infected monkeys, they were abundant in these tissues as well as the anterior somatic musculature, diaphragm, and tissues of the head and neck (Kazacos et al. 1981b; Huff et al. 1984; Fox et al. 1985). Different species may react differently to *Baylisascaris* larvae, and host reactions may also be affected by prior infection. For example, previously unexposed *Mus musculus* showed a strong tendency to develop large granulomas, which were prominent in the heart (Fig. 11.8), diaphragm, body wall, and ante-

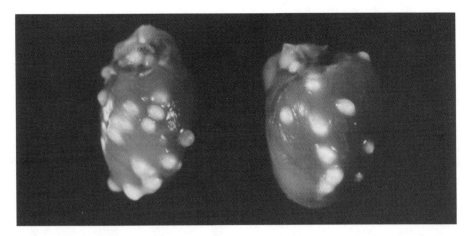

FIG. 11.8—Larval granulomas in the hearts of lab mice infected with *Baylisascaris columnaris;* 15 days postinfection. Similar granulomas develop in *B. procyonis* infections.

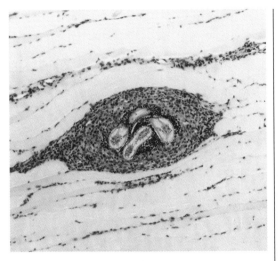

FIG. 11.9—*Baylisascaris procyonis* larval granuloma in skeletal muscle of a hamster. The larva is in a central pool of eosinophils. [Reprinted from Kazacos (1983a) with permission of Purdue Research Foundation.]

rior body musculature, but not along the gastrointestinal tract. In *P. leucopus,* granulomas were few, very small, rarely noted grossly, and found primarily in the heart and along the gastrointestinal tract. The large granulomas in *M. musculus* were characterized by a marked inflammatory reaction and contained significantly more eosinophils, whereas those in *P. leucopus* lacked an intense response and consisted primarily of macrophages (Sheppard and Kazacos 1997).

Unlike mammals, avian species infected with *Baylisascaris* typically lack gross lesions at necropsy, and histopathologic alterations are usually confined to the brain (Kazacos and Boyce 1989). Wirtz (1982) saw no gross larval granulomas in experimentally infected chickens and ducks and found only a single granuloma histologically, in an extrinsic ocular muscle. Solitary larval granulomas also were noted histologically in the lungs of a naturally infected brush turkey and bobwhite (Kazacos et al. 1982a; Williams et al. 1997). The comparative lack of gross lesions and paucity of larval granulomas in avian species with *Baylisascaris* NLM has been documented in various natural cases and outbreaks (Richardson et al. 1980; Reed et al. 1981; Myers et al. 1983; Evans and Tangredi 1985; Armstrong et al. 1989; Kazacos et al. 1991; Kwiecien et al. 1993).

In most clinical cases involving birds, including large ratites, few or no larvae are found in visceral or somatic tissues, even though 1–3 larvae are found in the brain. Thus, most avian cases appear to involve low-level infections, with a higher probability of larval migration to the brain; however, much higher infection levels are occasionally documented. For example, in a recent outbreak involving massive infection in a mixed collection of parrots and conures (Table 11.6), 17–150 (mean, 87) *B. procyonis* larvae were recovered from the brains and 47–285 (mean, 173) larvae from the viscera and carcasses of six birds dying from acute, severe central nervous system disease (A.M. Lennox and K.R. Kazacos, unpublished); interestingly, no gross lesions or larval granulomas were noted.

The most important pathological alterations due to *Baylisascaris* are in the brain. Gross lesions include hemorrhagic foci and tracks, congestion, swelling and softening, and cerebellar herniation. The leptomeninges may be congested and/or thickened and discolored (Sprent 1955; Kazacos et al. 1981b; Huff et al. 1984; Fox et al. 1985; Kazacos 1997). Early histopathologic lesions consist of focal migration tracks, with tissue disruption, hemorrhage, necrosis, and spongiosis, with a few inflammatory cells

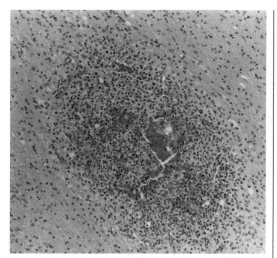

FIG. 11.10—Hemorrhagic migration track in the cerebral white matter of a squirrel monkey with *Baylisascaris procyonis* encephalitis, showing microcavitation, hemorrhage, necrosis, and influx of macrophages and other leukocytes. [Reprinted from Kazacos et al. (1981b) with permission of *JAVMA*.]

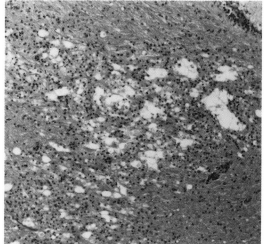

FIG. 11.11—Cerebellar peduncle of a rabbit with *Baylisascaris procyonis* encephalitis, showing extensive necrosis and inflammation. [Reprinted from Kazacos et al. (1983) with permission of *JAVMA*.]

(Kazacos 1997). Migration tracks may be found in any portion of the brain and spinal cord, but are especially important in critical areas such as the cerebellum, midbrain, and medulla. Migration tracks quickly become infiltrated with inflammatory cells, primarily macrophages in the early stages, followed by eosinophils, lymphocytes, and plasma cells (Fig. 11.10). As the reaction progresses, perivascular cuffing becomes prominent, especially adjacent to areas of inflammation in the neuropil, and there is more extensive spongiosis and cavitation (Figs. 11.11–11.13). Depending on the numbers of larvae present, central nervous system lesions may be focal or diffuse and may extend to the leptomeninges. Lesions in heavy infections are typically more extensive and severe. Other central nervous system lesions include neuronal degeneration, swelling and degeneration of axons, demyelination, and prominent gliosis (Kazacos 1997). Larvae may be seen within migration tracks and areas of inflammation and necrosis (Fig. 11.14); however, they are also commonly found in normal-appearing neuropil away from obvious lesions, indicating their active migration in the central nervous system at the time of fixation. Encapsulation of larvae in the central nervous system lags far behind encapsulation in other tissues, resulting in prolonged larval migration in this site. If the animal survives long enough, however, encapsulation eventually occurs, and larvae become walled off in sharply demarcated foci of granulomatous inflammation. These foci resemble the granulomas in other tissues but are usually walled off by gliosis rather than fibrosis (Kazacos 1997). Eosinophilic deposits

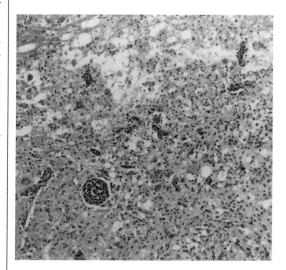

FIG. 11.12—Cerebrum of a rabbit with *Baylisascaris procyonis* encephalitis, showing extensive spongiosis, microcavitation, necrosis, swollen and degenerating axons, infiltration by inflammatory cells, and perivascular cuffing.

[Splendore-Hoeppli (SH) substance] may be prominent in areas of necrotic eosinophils, in migration tracks, and within granulomas adjacent to larvae. Immunofluorescence studies of fatal *Baylisascaris* infections in children indicated that these SH deposits consist of extracellular eosinophil major basic protein, originating from extensive eosinophil degranulation in the tissues (Hamann et al. 1989). Recently, two children with

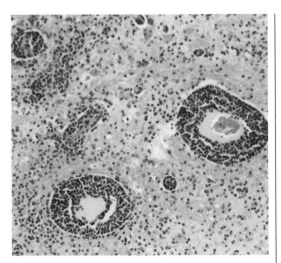

FIG. 11.13—Cerebrum of a ferret with *Baylisascaris procyonis* encephalitis, showing prominent perivascular cuffing with leukocytes.

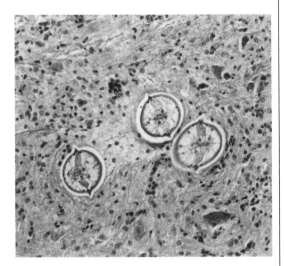

FIG. 11.14—Cross sections of *Baylisascaris procyonis* larva migrating in the cerebellar peduncle of a chicken with encephalitis (Richardson et al. 1980).

severe *Baylisascaris* NLM were found to have measurable levels of interleukin 5, eosinophil-derived neurotoxin, and major basic protein in their cerbrospinal fluid (C.L. Moertel et al., unpublished).

Different species of *Baylisascaris* vary in their central nervous system pathogenicity, based on differences in somatic migration and invasion of the brain, larval aggressiveness in the central nervous system, and the ability of the host to wall them off. *Baylisascaris procyonis* and *B. melis* are the most pathogenic, followed by *B. columnaris* and the others (Kazacos and Boyce 1989). *Baylisascaris procyonis* is clearly more pathogenic than *B. columnaris,* requiring fewer infective eggs ingested and fewer larvae in the brain to cause the same or worse clinical disease. A single *B. procyonis* larva in the brain of a mouse is usually fatal, whereas five to six or more *B. columnaris* larvae in the brain aren't necessarily fatal, even when central nervous system signs are present (Sprent 1952a, 1955; Tiner 1953a,b; Clark et al. 1969; Sheppard and Kazacos 1997). Clinical signs appear much earlier and progress much more quickly in mice infected with *B. procyonis* than with *B. columnaris.* In addition, *B. columnaris* larvae in the brain have a greater tendency to settle down and become encapsulated than do larvae of *B. procyonis* (Tiner 1953a,b; Sprent 1955; Clark et al. 1969). The author has confirmed these differences on several occasions, indicating the much greater pathogenicity of *B. procyonis* over *B. columnaris.* However, at sufficient dosages, *B. columnaris* has the ability to produce clinically significant NLM (Table 11.6) and should be treated with the same precautions as *B. procyonis* and *B. melis.*

In mice concurrently infected with eastern encephalitis or Colorado tick fever virus, migrating *B. columnaris* larvae induced mortality at rates considerably higher than those produced by virus or larvae alone or the sum of mortalities of each agent alone (Clark et al. 1969). The authors postulated that when sufficient migrating larvae breached the blood-brain barrier, it allowed increased amounts of virus to spill into susceptible neural tissue. Whether this pathogenic interaction occurs between *Baylisascaris* larvae and these or other neurotropic agents in natural populations is unknown.

Ocular larva migrans was seen in mice, hamsters, gray squirrels, woodchucks, and two species of monkeys experimentally infected with *B. procyonis* (Kazacos et al. 1984b, 1985); in rabbits and woodchucks experimentally infected with *B. columnaris* (Swerczek and Helmboldt 1970; Church et al. 1975); and in psittacines with naturally occurring *B. procyonis* infections (A.M. Lennox and K.R. Kazacos, unpublished). Ocular larva migrans due to *Baylisascaris* is an important disease in humans, in which *B. procyonis* has been identified as the primary cause of the large nematode variant of diffuse unilateral subacute neuroretinitis (DUSN) (Gass and Braunstein 1983; Kazacos et al. 1984a,b, 1985; Goldberg et al. 1993). Ocular disease due to *Baylisascaris* is manifested as unilateral loss of vision, usually seen in patients with no symptoms of visceral or neural larva migrans; this reflects the lower numbers of larvae typically present in patients with OLM and chance migration of a single larva into the eye (Kazacos 1997). In heavy primary infections, OLM may be seen in conjunction with NLM (Rowely et al. 2000; Park et al., 2000). In experimentally infected monkeys, *B. procyonis* larvae reached the eye as early as 7 days postinfection (Kazacos et al. 1984b, 1985). Larvae produce migration tracks in the retina and stimulate inflammatory reactions primarily involving the retina, choroid, and vitreous. Early histopathologic lesions consist of retinal disruption, nuclear pyknosis, and hyperplasia and migration of the pigment epithelium. These progress to intense eosinophilic retinitis, with necrosis, vasculitis, vitritis, choroiditis, and abundant eosinophilic hyaline material (SH substance). In addition to producing these migration-related lesions, *Baylisascaris* larvae become walled off in granulomatous masses in the retina and choroid (Kazacos et al. 1984b, 1985; Kazacos 1997).

DIAGNOSIS. *Baylisascaris* infections in raccoons are diagnosed by finding ascarids in the small intestine at necropsy, or passed in the feces spontaneously or following anthelmintic treatment. Patent infections are diagnosed by finding characteristic *Baylisascaris* eggs in the feces. Differentiation of adults of several *Baylisascaris* species, including *B. procyonis* and *B. columnaris,* is difficult or impossible because of similarities and overlap of morphological characters. Although various morphological features have been described for separating *B. procyonis* from *B. columnaris,* including the shape of lip denticles, male pericloacal rough areas, and male tail (Tiner 1952a,b; Hartwich 1962; Sprent 1968), Berry (1985) concluded that these and other characters were variable enough that the two species could not be distinguished morphologically.

Distinct biological differences exist in the migration, development, and pathogenicity of *B. procyonis* and *B. columnaris* larvae in intermediate hosts (Sprent 1952a, 1955; Tiner 1952a, 1953a,b; Berry 1985; Sheppard and Kazacos 1997). In addition, Berry (1985) described morphological differences between the third-stage larvae of each parasite at 10 days, as well as electrophoretic differences in alleles for 6-phosphogluconate dehydrogenase. These data indicate that these parasites are closely related but distinct species. Although limited experimental cross-transmission of *B. procyonis* and *B. columnaris* between raccoons and skunks was possible, Berry (1985) found no evidence that cross-infection or hybridization by or of these parasites occurs in nature. Based on the apparent genetic isolation of these two species, in geographic areas where both parasites occur, the most useful criterion for separating them appears to be host (procyonid versus mephitid). The application of molecular genetic techniques should help answer the question of relatedness among these and other *Baylisascaris* species (Nadler 1992; Nadler and Hudspeth 2000).

Diagnosis of *Baylisascaris* larva migrans is based on clinical signs, a history of exposure, antemortem labratory findings (including serology, cytology, imagery, and examination of cerebrospinal fluids), postmortem gross and histopathologic lesions, and recovery and/or identification of larvae at necropsy, in biopsies, or in or from affected eyes (Huff et al. 1984; Kazacos et al. 1984a,b, 1985; Fox et al. 1985; Kazacos 1991, 1996, 1997, 2000; Goldberg et al. 1993). Of these, only iden-

tification of larvae in/from the tissues is confirmatory, although positive serology would be indicative of infection.

Prior to the mid-1980s, when *Baylisascaris* NLM was becoming widely recognized and better considered and sought by diagnosticians, many cases of NLM were misdiagnosed clinically. Most individuals exhibiting abnormal behavior were submitted as rabies suspects (Fig. 11.5) (Richter and Kradel 1964; Fleming and Caslick 1978; Kazacos et al. 1981a; Roth et al. 1982), despite the fact that the species involved (woodchucks, squirrels, rabbits, birds) were less likely candidates for rabies. The diagnostic focus on rabies in these cases masked the widespread occurrence of *Baylisascaris* NLM, because typically the entire head or brain was sent for rabies diagnosis, leaving no central nervous system tissues for examination for other possible causes. With the widespread occurrence of *Baylisascaris* NLM documented by our laboratory and others, this situation has changed, so that *Baylisascaris* NLM is now at or near the top of the differential list for central nervous system disease in these and related species. Of course, other possible causes of central nervous system disease, including rabies, must still be considered and appropriate samples taken, along with appropriate specimens for *Baylisascaris* NLM. Although clinical signs of NLM are nonspecific, in common target species they are still highly suggestive, especially in conjunction with compatible diagnostic findings and history.

Other possible causes of central nervous system disease in these animals would include protozoal (e.g., toxoplasmosis, sarcocystosis, free-living amebae), bacterial, or viral encephalitis, fungal infections, other migratory helminth larvae (e.g., *Alaria* mesocercariae, spargana, gnathostomes, filariids), helminth egg–induced encephalitis (e.g., *Dendritobilharzia* in waterfowl), aberrant migration of dipteran larvae (*Cuterebra* and others), as well as pesticide toxicoses and trauma. Causes of eosinophilic meningitis and meningoencephalitis are more limited and include migratory helminths, certain fungal agents, and some neoplasms and other noninfectious causes (Kuberski 1979; Weller and Liu 1993; Connor et al. 1997). Causes of eosinophilia are more diverse and include various other helminth infections, certain deep mycoses and bacterial infections, various allergies and hypersensitivities, myeloproliferative and neoplastic diseases, and some other conditions (Weller 1992). Multisystem granulomas also characterize some other diseases, including certain bacterial and deep mycotic infections (Connor et al. 1997; Kazacos 1997).

An important clinical and diagnostic finding in *Baylisascaris* NLM is eosinophilic pleocytosis of the cerebrospinal fluid, particularly in animals or humans with concurrent peripheral eosinophilia and progressive central nervous system disease. Eosinophil numbers appear to be higher in the cerebrospinal fluid during acute disease, and their levels would be related to the degree of central nervous system damage and eosinophilic inflammation caused by migrating larvae. Since some other migratory helminths and pathologic conditions could cause eosinophilic pleocytosis, this finding is most useful in patients with typical clinical signs and a history and/or evidence of exposure. Antemortem imaging techniques, including computed tomography (CT) and magnetic resonance imaging (MRI), may yield important information on the location, severity, and progression of central nervous system lesions (Huff et al. 1984; Fox et al. 1985; Cunningham et al. 1994; Ball et al. 1998; Rowley et al. 2000). For example, MRI revealed diffuse white matter disease with deep periventricular involvement in children with severe *Baylisascaris* NLM (Rowley et al. 2000; Park et al., 2000), and a large, focal lesion in the frontal cortex of a gibbon with NLM (Ball et al. 1998). Important findings in *Baylisascaris* OLM/ DUSN include compatible lesions on ophthalmoscopy, eosinophils on intraocular cytology, positive serum and/or intraocular antibody levels, and intraocular larvae with characteristics of *B. procyonis* (Kazacos 1991, 1997; Goldberg et al. 1993).

Serologic methods, including indirect immunofluorescence, ELISA, and Western blotting, have been developed for *Baylisascaris* and applied primarily to human cases (Huff et al. 1984; Fox et al. 1985; Goldberg et al. 1993; Cunningham et al. 1994; Rowley et al. 2000; K.R. Kazacos, unpublished). Immunofluorescence assays use frozen sections of *B. procyonis* third-stage larvae, whereas ELISA and Western blotting use excretory-secretory antigens produced by larvae maintained in vitro (Boyce et al. 1988a,b, 1989). Children strongly positive for *Baylisascaris* antibodies in serum and cerebrospinal fluid were negative for *Toxocara* by ELISA, indicating that the two infections can be distinguished serologically. It was also possible to detect antibodies to *Baylisascaris* in experimentally and naturally infected rabbits, mice, and monkeys by Western blotting, but other than these studies, serologic testing has not been applied to nonhuman species. Development of similar serologic methods for other species is possible but would require animal species-specific reagents. The serologic diagnosis of *Baylisascaris* was possible only to genus (Boyce et al. 1988a,b, 1989). Thus, identification of the particular species of *Baylisascaris* involved in cases or outbreaks is best determined epidemiologically through an assessment of probable exposure.

Histopathologic lesions of *Baylisascaris* migration in the brain (i.e., eosinophilic meningoencephalitis, necrosis, spongiosis, cavitation) are characteristic and highly suggestive of this infection, particularly in typical target species. However, finding or isolating the larvae is important for confirmation. Routine histopathology may fail to detect larvae, particularly in low-level infections. In such cases, the likelihood of finding larvae is increased if numerous blocks and slides are examined and if suspect lesions are step or serially sectioned. The sensitivity of histopathology for detecting larvae in the central nervous system is increased in heavier infections; in two human cases larvae were identified in brain biopsies (Rowley et al. 2000; W.A. Kennedy et al., unpublished). In most cases, the majority of larvae occur in extraneural tissues, where they produce migration-related lesions and granulomas, which should be correlated with central nervous system findings. It is very important to thoroughly examine other organs and tissues for larval granulomas from which *Baylisascaris* larvae can be isolated by dissection or digestion, or identified using histopathology. Particular attention should be paid to the heart, lungs, and associated vessels, anterior somatic musculature, and the gastrointestinal tract, especially the mesentery and wall of the small and large intestines. For example, in a recent case involving a black-and-white ruffed lemur with central nervous system disease, the author isolated 2 larvae from the brain, 2 from the skeletal muscles of the head, 17 from the heart and lungs, and 118 from the intestinal wall. If characteristic lesions without larvae are seen in the brain, identification of larvae in other tissues gives strong support to *Baylisascaris* as a probable cause of the central nervous system lesions and clinical disease.

Considering the drawbacks of histopathology, larval isolation methods are more efficient and useful for detecting *Baylisascaris* larvae in the brain and other tissues, particularly in low-level infections. The best methods for isolating *Baylisascaris* larvae from the brain of affected hosts are brain squash, artificial digestion, and the Baermann technique. Of these, we usually use brain squash or digestion because there is less chance of missing or losing the larvae, especially in low-level infections. The Baermann technique will usually work but has some inherent problems, as described below. Digestion methods are also very useful for isolating larvae from other organs and tissues, even when granulomas are not readily apparent. Since other diseases must also be considered and sought in clinical cases, a good approach is to combine histopathology with one of these other methods. For example, several slices of brain may be taken for histopathology and the remainder processed for larvae; right and left halves of the brain may be examined by the respective methods; or, if sufficient numbers of affected animals are available, the whole brain of representative animals may be processed for larvae. These decisions are made by the diagnostician based on the particular situation and the differential list for the particular species. Each of the larval isolation methods can be performed with conventional laboratory equipment and is described in detail below. The brain is first removed with scissors or using a Stryker or hacksaw. The spinal cord of rodents and small birds is easily removed by ejection, using water pressure (Meikle and Martin 1981; Sheppard and Kazacos 1997), while that of larger animals is removed by laminectomy, using a Stryker saw, bone rongeurs, or other means.

Brain Squash. The brain or spinal cord to be examined is first rinsed with saline or water by squirt bottle to remove any bone chips that may be present. This is done over a Petri dish or beaker that is also examined for larvae. Approximately 1-g pieces of brain or spinal cord are placed on round glass plates (12.7 mm diameter) and minced with fine forceps, second (top) plates are added, and the tissue is flattened to the periphery using steady hand pressure. We often separate the brain into right and left cerebral hemispheres, cerebellum, and midbrain-medulla and process each separately. The brain of a mouse or small bird or half the brain of a slightly larger animal can be processed on one to three plates. If small pieces of bone are present, they will prevent the tissue from being squashed and must first be removed by separating the plates. The squashed brain is examined using a dissecting microscope with bottom-transmitted light and 10–15X magnification. A fiberoptic light source works best, since it will transmit light through the brain tissue better than a standard light. When the light is adjusted properly, the larvae will refract the light and appear bright in the brain tissue, making them easier to find. It is important to examine the plate systematically and thoroughly, usually in two directions. This is aided by dividing the plate into numbered quadrants using a fine marker (Sharpie, Vis-a-Vis). When larvae are found, they are circled with the marker. Areas of inflammatory cell infiltration can also be seen, as focal, irregular, dark grainy areas, best noted in the clearer neuropil. When the exam is complete, any larvae present are isolated by carefully separating the plates, scraping and rinsing the tissue from the positive quadrant or half (both plates) into a Petri dish (100 x 20 mm) of saline, further mixing and macerating it with forceps, and examining it using an inverted or dissecting microscope until the larvae are found. An inverted microscope with a scanning objective (2.5–3.5X) works best since one can see "under" the debris. The dish is gently swirled in a circular motion to bring any larvae present into the center for easier detection. Larvae are removed with a Pasteur pipette to a small dish of saline and either placed on microscope slides for immediate identification or fixed in hot (65°C–70° C) fixative for later identification and storage. Appropriate fixatives include hot AFA (alcohol:formalin:acetic acid), 70% ethanol, or 5% or 10% formalin in saline, with long-term storage in glycerin-alcohol (9:1, 70% ethanol:glycerin). Fixatives are best heated using two beakers set up as a double boiler, on a hot plate on low heat, with the center (fixative) beaker capped with aluminum foil. We usually remove the larvae to a glass vial, draw off most of the saline under a dissecting microscope, then fill the vial with hot fixative. If necessary, larvae for microscopic examination can be cleared with phenol-alcohol or glycerin.

The advantage of this method is that it is nearly foolproof, assuming the squash is done properly and examined well; even if only a single larva is present, it will be found. The most common errors are using too much tissue, so that the squash isn't thin enough, and not doing a systematic, thorough search. Very dark areas of brain are harder to see through without a bright light and demand greater attention and a thin squash. The larvae can be lost in trying to retrieve them from the plates; however, since all the material is present, it can be comminuted and reexamined until they are found or processed further by digestion (see below). The main disadvantage of this method is that it is tedious and time-consuming when used on large brains (> 8–10 g), because many 1-g squashes must be examined. In such cases, we usually process the brain by digestion.

Artificial Digestion. The brain or other tissue is weighed, cut into pieces with scissors, then either pulverized in a small (100 ml) beaker (brain), finely minced with scissors, or comminuted in a Waring blender in warm (37° C) artificial digestive fluid (1% pepsin- 1% HCl-0.85% saline). Brain samples are thoroughly pulverized using a metal spatula (75 x 17 mm) to mash the brain pieces against the side of the beaker; other tissues are finely minced with scissors. Warm digestive fluid is then used to rinse the brain or other tissue into a flask for digestion. If a blender is used, the cut-up tissue is blended in warm digestive fluid. Prior to examination of the gastrointestinal tract, it is first opened along its length and all ingesta is removed and washed off to remove undigestible material and any confounding intestinal nematodes. We recommend using small glass blender jars (Eberbach #8470, 450 ml) with screw lids, filled about one-third with fluid. We also recommend using 3–4-second pulses until the tissue is comminuted to small bits. After processing, the samples are poured and rinsed into Erlenmeyer flasks at a final concentration of 20 ml digestive fluid per gram of tissue. The flasks are placed in a shaking incubator or oscillatory shaker at 37° C and 180–200 rpm or on a magnetic stirrer on low speed 2–2.5 hours. The digests are then coarsely filtered and rinsed through a single layer of cheesecloth into tall conical beer glasses (350–400 ml) (preferred) or graduated cylinders (250–500 ml), which are then filled with cold saline or water and allowed to stand 20–30 minutes for larvae to settle. If the digest is too large for two or three glasses, it is first sedimented in the flask (propped at an angle in a wire basket), drawn down to 400–600 ml by vacuum aspiration, and filtered into the glasses. Cold saline or tap water is used for all rinsing and filling, as it aids in flotation of lipids and fine debris. After sedimentation in the glasses, the surface ("floating") layer and two-thirds of the supernatant are removed by vacuum aspiration, and the glasses are refilled with cold saline or tap water and allowed to sediment again. This process may be repeated several times. The sediment is agitated and suspended in the remaining liquid, poured and rinsed into a Petri dish, and examined for larvae using a dissecting or inverted microscope. The dish is gently swirled to bring any larvae into the center. Larvae are removed and fixed as described previously.

This method is easy to perform and is very effective in recovering *Baylisascaris* larvae from different tissues (Fig. 11.15). Brain does not digest well, so it is

lung, or other tissue. Just prior to loading the sample, the funnel is filled with warm (37° C) saline (preferred) or water to a level that will cover the sample, mesh, and cheesecloth. The funnel can also be filled with artificial digestive fluid (see above) as a combined method. The pulverized brain or minced tissue is scooped onto the cheesecloth, which is folded into the funnel to prevent wicking of liquid over the side. The funnel is allowed to stand undisturbed several hours or overnight (if overnight, use saline), preferably in a 37° C incubator. Stimulated by the warmth, the larvae migrate out of the tissue and down through the cheesecloth and mesh, then gravitate into the stem of the funnel. Later, the clamp is opened and fluid is drawn off into one or several 50-ml centrifuge tubes and gently centrifuged several minutes or allowed to stand 15–20 minutes. About two-thirds of the supernatant is removed by vacuum aspiration, and the sediment is resuspended in the remaining fluid, poured and rinsed into a Petri dish, and examined for larvae as described previously. In the case of cloudy samples, a saline wash step can be added.

The advantage of the Baermann technique is its ease of use. The disadvantage is that not all larvae may come down, so that in low infections, false negative results may be obtained (Richardson et al. 1980; Kazacos and Wirtz 1983). We have found that larvae can become trapped in the brain sludge on the cheesecloth, so that for negative samples it is a good idea to stir this material well and rerun the Baermann (Fox et al. 1985). Alternatively, one can remove the brain material to a Petri dish, macerate it further, and examine it thoroughly with an inverted microscope. The material may also be processed further by digestion (see above). Because of these limitations, we prefer brain squashes and digestion for the detection or recovery of *Baylisascaris* larvae.

Identification of *Baylisascaris* L₃'s is based on morphologic characteristics of larvae recovered from tissues or seen in histopathologic sections. Other nematode larvae besides *Baylisascaris* may be seen in or recovered from the tissues of animals, especially wild species, although brain infection with other nematodes is much less frequent. The morphology of *B. procyonis* L₃'s has been described in detail (Berry 1985; Bowman 1987; Donnelly et al. 1989), and their histologic identification by Kazacos (1986, 1997) and Bowman (1987). Histologic features of other ascarid and helminth larvae are described by Nichols (1956a,b), Chitwood and Lichtenfels (1972), Binford and Connor (1976), Bowman (1987), Connor et al. (1997), and Gutierrez (2000). *Baylisascaris procyonis* larvae are stout, 1500–1900 µm x 60–80 µm, with a smoothly rounded anterior end and three partially differentiated lips (Figs. 11.15, 11.16). Large, single lateral alae commence halfway between the anterior end and the nerve ring and extend to near the tip of the tail, and the cuticle has prominent transverse striations. The esophagus is clavate, strongyliform, ends in a pyriform bulb, and is ~13%–15% of the body length (Figs. 11.15, 11.16). The excretory cell nucleus is large (~20 µm), ovoid,

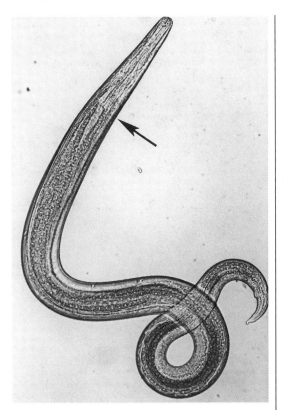

FIG. 11.15—*Baylisascaris procyonis* larva recovered by artificial digestion from the carcass of a conure with encephalitis. Note overall shape and proportions, smoothly rounded anterior end, sharply flexed tail tip, length of esophagus (arrow at esophageal-intestinal junction), prominent intestine, and transverse cuticular striations (seen at bend in midbody).

important to pulverize it thoroughly before digestion. Stock 1% HCl-0.85% saline can be stored in an incubator, and pepsin added (1 g/100 ml, on magnetic stirrer) just prior to use. Care should be taken to avoid blending the tissue for too long, or the larvae may be damaged. However, even if larvae are damaged (e.g., cut in half), the pieces are often recovered later. Digestion for 2 hours is usually sufficient, and overdigestion (> 3 hours) should be avoided, as larvae may be killed and digested. For sedimentation and later processing of larvae in Petri dishes, saline is preferred over water, which will eventually cause osmotic damage.

Baermann Technique. A Baermann funnel is a small- to medium-sized (4–5-inch diameter) glass funnel with a piece of tubing and a clamp on the stem; a piece of wire mesh is cut to fit the top third of the funnel and is used to support a double thickness piece of cheesecloth and the sample during processing. The Baermann funnel can be used on pulverized brain, finely minced

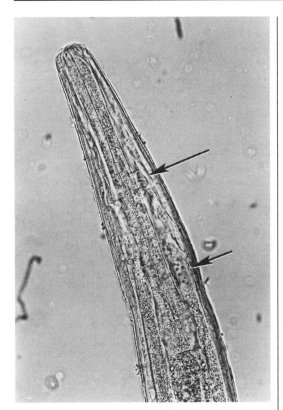

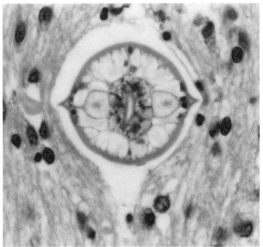

FIG. 11.17—Cross section through midbody/midintestinal region of a *Baylisascaris procyonis* larva in the brain of a ferret, showing characteristic diagnostic features. Note prominent, single lateral alae; large, centrally-located, laterally-compressed intestine with open lumen and microvillous border; and lateral excretory columns which are smaller than intestine, roughly triangular in shape, slightly dissimilar in size, and with prominent canaliculi. In histologic sections, larvae usually measure 60–70 μm in greatest width.

FIG. 11.16—Esophageal region of *Baylisascaris procyonis* larva recovered by the Baermann technique from the brain of a chicken with encephalitis (Richardson et al. 1980). Note partially differentiated lips, clavate strongyliform esophagus, nerve ring (long arrow), and large excretory cell nucleus (short arrow).

and seen in the left side (dorsal view) or right side (ventral view) of the excretory commissure near the esophageal bulb (Fig. 11.16). The intestine has a patent lumen, and the cells contain abundant granules. The tail tapers gradually from anus to tip, which is flexed sharply dorsad and ends in a tiny knob (Fig. 11.15) (Berry 1985; Bowman 1987; Donnelly et al. 1989; K.R. Kazacos, unpublished).

Histologically, the characteristic features of *Baylisascaris* larvae are best seen in transverse sections through the midbody/midintestinal region (Fig. 11.17) (Kazacos 1997). The larvae are usually 60–70 μm in greatest width and have prominent, single lateral alae, strongly pointed and flexed dorsad. The large, centrally located intestine has an open lumen and is laterally compressed in the mid to posterior regions; six to nine low columnar cells are usually visible, each with a thin microvillous border and numerous cytoplasmic granules. The intestine is flanked by prominent lateral cords supporting the lateral excretory columns, which are smaller than the intestine, roughly triangular in shape,

slightly dissimilar in size, and with prominent central canaliculi. Three hypodermal nuclei are usually visible in the lateral cords, just below the cuticle. The shape and relative prominence of the excretory columns and intestine change as one progresses posteriorly from esophagus to anus (Fig. 11.18) (Kazacos 1997). The same structures can usually be seen in longitudinal or tangential sections, although they may be more difficult to identify (Suedmeyer et al. 1996).

IMMUNITY. It is likely that raccoons develop age resistance and/or intestinal immunity following infection with *B. procyonis*. This, combined with self-cure of intestinal infections, probably accounts for the lower prevalence of *B. procyonis* in adult raccoons.

It is well known that intermediate hosts infected with *B. procyonis* larvae develop strong antibody and inflammatory cell responses, directed at excretory-secretory antigens given off by the migrating parasites. The strong antibody responses form the basis for immunodiagnostic tests (immunofluorescence, ELISA, Western blotting) used for this infection (Fox et al. 1985; Boyce et al. 1988a,b, 1989; Goldberg et al. 1993; Cunningham et al. 1994). *Baylisascaris* also stimulates strong blood and tissue eosinophil levels, another indication that the parasite induces a strong T-helper type 2 cell response (Sheppard and Kazacos 1997). As might be expected, host species appear to

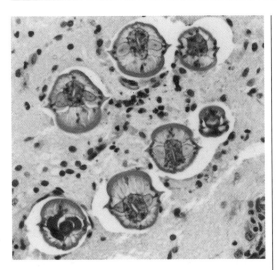

FIG. 11.18—Cross sections of a *Baylisascaris procyonis* larva in the brain of a squirrel monkey, showing changes in the shape and relative prominence of the excretory columns and intestine at different levels of the larva. The larva is coiled vertically from lower left to lower right and is sectioned at the following levels: (lower left) posterior esophagus at excretory commissure, showing excretory cell nucleus; (upper left and middle, lower second and third) midintestinal region, with upper middle section near midbody; (upper right) posterior intestinal region, beyond ends of excretory columns; (lower right) intestinorectal valve. [Reprinted from Kazacos (1983a) with permission of Purdue Research Foundation.]

vary in their specific responses to infection (Sheppard and Kazacos 1997).

Whether immune responses to *Baylisascaris* larvae in intermediate hosts are protective or not is less well known; some protective effect seems possible, especially in previously infected animals in which central nervous system invasion hasn't occurred. Reinfection of such animals might trigger immune responses directed at preventing infection or slowing down and walling off the larvae. This will continue to be difficult to test experimentally, because animals infected with *B. procyonis* often die from central nervous system disease (Boyce et al. 1988a,b, 1989). The only findings that may support this possibility come from a large epizootic of *Baylisascaris* NLM in rabbits in Michigan, in which only young or recently introduced rabbits were clinically affected. No disease developed in older breeder rabbits that had been on the farm for an extended period, suggesting that there was previous contact with the parasite and an acquired immunity (Dade et al. 1975). Whether this was indeed the case or not is unknown, and the question of protective immunity in *Baylisascaris* infections needs further study.

OTHER SPECIES OF *BAYLISASCARIS*. Several other species of *Baylisascaris*, including *B. melis* of

badgers, *B. devosi* of fisher and marten, *B. transfuga* of bears, and *B. tasmaniensis* of marsupial carnivores, are potential causes of larva migrans disease if enough eggs are ingested. All four species undergo somatic migration in rodents, but with variations in larval growth, migratory behavior, and distribution of larvae to somatic and visceral tissues, as compared to *B. procyonis* and *B. columnaris* (Sprent 1952a, 1953a,b, 1955; Tiner 1953a,b; Sprent et al. 1973). Similar to *B. procyonis* and *B. columnaris*, *B. melis* larvae grow considerably and, in addition to invading other tissues and organs, enter the brain to cause NLM. *Baylisascaris melis* produced central nervous system disease in laboratory mice, deer mice (*P. maniculatus artemisiae*), ground squirrels (*Citellus armatus*), and rabbits (Tiner 1953a,b; Boyce et al. 1988b; K.R. Kazocos, unpublished) and entered the eyes of mice, producing OLM (K.R. Kazacos, unpublished). As pointed out by Tiner (1953a), *B. melis* is probably responsible for naturally occurring clinical NLM in ground squirrels and other rodents which share the habitat of badgers and constitute their normal food supply.

The larvae of the other species are smaller and/or grow more slowly and are distributed primarily to the anterior carcass musculature (*B. devosi*) and intestinal wall or mesentery (*B. transfuga, B. tasmaniensis*) of mice (Sprent 1952a, 1953a,b, 1955; Sprent et al. 1973). Although a few larvae also entered the brain, central nervous system disease was absent or rare with *B. devosi* and was not caused by *B. transfuga* or *B. tasmaniensis*. However, other research indicates that *B. transfuga* can produce clinical NLM as well as OLM in some infected mice (Papini and Casarosa 1994; Papini et al. 1996). Although they are potential causes of larva migrans disease in animals and humans, *B. transfuga, B. devosi*, and *B. tasmaniensis* are much less pathogenic than the other three *Baylisascaris* species discussed. Because of their much greater disease-producing capabilities, *B. procyonis, B. melis*, and *B. columnaris* are clearly the most dangerous members of this group and should be handled with the greatest precautions.

TREATMENT

Definitive Hosts. Many of the common anthelmintics used to treat ascarids in dogs, cats, and other species are effective against adult *Baylisascaris* in raccoons, skunks, dogs, and bears. We have successfully treated *B. procyonis*–infected raccoons with the following drugs (dosage x treatment day other than one): piperazine citrate (120–240 mg/kg), pyrantel pamoate (6–10 mg/kg), and fenbendazole (50–100 mg/kg x 3–5 days) (Kazacos et al. 1982a; Kazacos 1986); follow-up treatments are recommended to ensure removal of all worms. The following anthelmintics were 100% effective against *B. procyonis* in raccoons when fed in small amounts of moist cat food: pyrantel pamoate (20 mg/kg), ivermectin (1 mg/kg), moxidectin

(1 mg/kg), albendazole (50 mg/kg x 3 days), fenbenda-zole (50 mg/kg x 3 days), and flubendazole (22 mg/kg x 3 days) (Bauer and Gey 1995). Intramuscular iver-mectin cleared *B. procyonis* from 11 of 12 raccoons, but 1 animal continued to shed eggs following treat-ment at 2 mg/kg (Hill et al. 1991).

Raccoons and skunks kept in captivity for any reason should be examined regularly (by fecal flotation) and strategically dewormed for *Baylisascaris,* in order to prevent or decrease environmental contamination with eggs and possible transmission to humans and other species (Kazacos and Boyce 1989). Newly acquired raccoons and skunks should be quarantined and dewormed immediately, with at least two follow-up treatments at 14-day intervals to ensure elimination of all developing worms. Young raccoons and skunks pose a particular threat because they have a higher preva-lence of infection and are often acquired during the prepatent period (50–76 days for *B. procyonis,* via eggs), when they will be false-negative by fecal exam (Kazacos 1983b). These individuals can be fecal-negative many weeks, then suddenly begin shedding large numbers of eggs, resulting in extensive contami-nation. Thus, strategic deworming of young raccoons and skunks should be started at ~5–6 weeks of age and repeated on a regular basis (e.g., every 2 weeks for five or six treatments). It is recommended that all captive raccoons and skunks be housed away from other species, in clean dedicated cages or enclosures that can be decontaminated if necessary. Placing young rac-coons or skunks in egg-contaminated cages or feeding raccoons and skunks meat from wild animals (rodents, rabbits, birds) can result in *Baylisascaris* infection (Kazacos and Boyce 1989). Based on the minimum known prepatent period of *Baylisascaris* in raccoons and skunks (32 days for *B. procyonis,* via larvae), once infections are eliminated, strategic deworming at monthly intervals should prevent future environmental contamination with eggs (Kazacos and Boyce 1989; Bauer and Gey 1995).

Intermediate Hosts (Neural and Ocular Larva Migrans). With or without treatment, NLM due to *Baylisascaris* carries a guarded to poor prognosis. The efficacy of anthelmintic treatment of NLM depends on drug pharmacokinetics and activity against larvae in the central nervous system; clinical efficacy also depends on the level and duration of central nervous system infection and the extent of central nervous sys-tem damage at the time of treatment. Treatment of early, low-level central nervous system infection appears possible, using larvicidal drugs which effec-tively cross the blood-brain barrier; presently, the best candidates appear to be albendazole and diethylcarba-mazine (see below). Unfortunately, *Baylisascaris* NLM usually is not considered or diagnosed until central nervous system signs are pronounced, and extensive, irreparable central nervous system damage has already occurred; anthelmintic treatment at this stage is usually ineffective. Killing larvae in the central nervous system

carries the added risk of exacerbating inflammatory reactions, due to the release of larval antigens (Kazacos and Boyce 1989). Controlling parasite-induced inflam-mation in the central nervous system with corticos-teroids, and supportive maintenance of the patient are both very important. Any anthelmintic treatments should be started as early as possible, because larvae in early migration in extraneural sites are more amenable to treatment than after they have entered the central nervous system. Possible drugs for such treatment include albendazole, mebendazole, fenbendazole, thi-abendazole, diethylcarbamazine, and levamisole.

Baylisascaris procyonis larvae enter the brain of mice as early as 3 days postinfection, and clinical cen-tral nervous system disease develops by 9–10 days postinfection (Tiner 1953a,b; Kazacos 1986; Sheppard and Kazacos 1997). Mice infected with 100 *B. procyo-nis* eggs and treated daily 1–10 days postinfection with albendazole (25 mg/kg), mebendazole (25 mg/kg), or thiabendazole (500 mg/kg) were protected 100%, 80%, and 80%, respectively, from development of central nervous system disease (Miyashita 1993). When treat-ment was 1–3 days postinfection only, central nervous system protection declined to 40%, 20%, and 20%. Several other anthelmintics had lower efficacy. Mice infected with 250 *B. procyonis* eggs and treated daily 1–10, 3–10, and 7–10 days postinfection with albenda-zole (50 mg/kg) +/- prednisone (1 mg/kg) were pro-tected 100%, 95%, and 75%, respectively, from central nervous system disease (Garrison 1996). Mice treated similarly with diethylcarbamazine (100 mg/kg) +/- prednisone were protected at 100%, 100%, and 45%, respectively. In these experiments, inclusion of steroids did not significantly improve treatment efficacy.

Gradual improvement was seen in two black-and-white ruffed lemurs with probable *Baylisascaris* NLM at the Nashville Zoo, following extended treatment with albendazole (5 mg/kg 3 times per day for alternat-ing 2-week periods and rest over 4 months) (S.J. Bar-rett, unpublished). The slowly progressing central nervous system disease was arrested after the first 2-week course, and the animals gradually improved, relearning some motor skills. These animals probably had low-level infections, as evidenced by their mild signs and low cerebrospinal fluid eosinophilia, making them good candidates for treatment. A California infant with *Baylisascaris* NLM was treated with albendazole (40 mg/kg x 28 days) and steroids (methylpred-nisolone, 20 mg/kg/day), but without obvious clinical improvement, probably due to the extent of central nervous system damage (Park et al., 2000).

Because of its efficacy against a variety of other par-asites, ivermectin has received considerable attention for the treatment of *Baylisascaris* NLM. Unfortunately, ivermectin does not cross the blood-brain barrier well and has proved unsuccessful in all treatment attempts of which the author is aware. The following animals and humans with clinical NLM, when treated with ivermectin at the dosages indicated, failed to improve, continued to deteriorate, and died or were euthanized, with living larvae subsequently recovered from the brain: rabbits (600 μg/kg) (Deeb and DiGiacomo 1994); gray squirrels (200 μg/kg every 2 weeks for three treatments) (Tseng 1997); rock doves and a Douglas squirrel (300 μg/kg) (Coates et al. 1995); macaws (400 μg/kg) (Armstrong et al. 1989); emus (200 μg/kg) (Suedmeyer et al. 1996); marmosets (100 μg/kg) (Huntress and Spraker 1985); and a child (175 μg/kg, total dose 1.5 mg) (Cunningham et al. 1994). Similarly, treatment of clinically affected rabbits with thiabendazole (25 mg/kg x 28 days) or tetramisole (8 mg/kg) (Dade et al. 1975), marmosets with fenbendazole (10 mg/kg x 10 days) (Huntress and Spraker 1985), and two children with thiabendazole (50 mg/kg x 6–7 days) (Fox et al. 1985; Cunningham et al. 1994) was unsuccessful.

Although there is a general lack of effective anthelmintic therapy for clinical NLM due to *Baylisascaris* (except for early treatment as noted above), several anthelmintics show great promise as preventatives for this infection. Currently, the best candidates are the pyrantel compounds, pyrantel tartrate and pyrantel pamoate, which prevent initial infection and thus subsequent central nervous system disease due to *Baylisascaris*. When administered continuously in the feed, pyrantel tartrate (Banminth, Pfizer) is a well-known preventative for *Ascaris suum* migration in swine. Experimentally infected mice given pyrantel tartrate at 0.25% and 0.5% and pyrantel pamoate at 0.2% concentration in their feed were fully protected against *B. procyonis* infection and central nervous system disease, which proved 100% fatal to untreated mice (Lindquist 1978). As pointed out by Kazacos and Boyce (1989, Addendum 1995) and Suedmeyer et al. (1996), pyrantel tartrate for swine could be formulated directly into ratite or other feed, or the pelleted formulation (Strongid C for horses) could be added as a top dressing; all would constitute extralabel usages of these drugs. Because of their high efficacy, acceptance, and ease of use, pyrantel drugs are recommended for prevention of *Baylisascaris* larval infection in mammals and birds. They should be used whenever animals are exposed to known or potentially contaminated environments, particularly on premises with an ongoing problem, where the sources of infection cannot be identified or effectively decontaminated. Pyrantel tartrate pellets (Strongid C) were well accepted by emus at the Kansas City Zoological Gardens, whereas acceptance of oral ivermectin was inconsistent (Suedmeyer et al. 1996). Pyrantel tartrate pellets are also being fed to lemurs and other species at various zoos in the United States.

Periodic treatment with ivermectin has also been used in an effort to kill *Baylisascaris* larvae in preneural migration, but with less consistent results. Miyashita (1993) found that only 20% of mice treated daily 1–10 days postinfection with ivermectin (1 mg/kg) were protected from central nervous system disease. In an outbreak of *Baylisascaris* encephalitis in emus, all remaining birds were placed on ivermectin (200 μg/kg) per os every 2 months. However, when an additional emu developed central nervous system disease 2 months later, the regimen was increased to monthly treatment, and no subsequent clinical cases were seen (Kwiecien et al. 1993). In another outbreak, three emus were treated with ivermectin (200 μg/kg per os) every 20–30 days, and all remained clinically normal for a year, whereupon one developed progressive central nervous system disease and was euthanized. The remaining two emus were then treated with ivermectin weekly and, a year later, were put on pyrantel tartrate pellets (50 mg/kg) in their feed (Suedmeyer et al. 1996).

Cases of OLM and DUSN due to *Baylisascaris* in humans have been successfully treated using laser photocoagulation to destroy the intraretinal larvae, thus preventing further migration damage (Raymond et al. 1978; Williams et al. 1988; Goldberg et al. 1993; Küchle et al. 1993). Visual improvement following treatment depends on the location and extent of intraocular damage and on successful resolution of intraocular inflammation using corticosteroids. The efficacy of oral anthelmintics against intraocular *Baylisascaris* larvae has not been evaluated.

PREVENTION AND CONTROL. Considering the seriousness of *Baylisascaris* infection in animals and humans, as well as the lack of effective treatment for NLM, prevention of infection with *Baylisascaris* is of utmost importance. The three key elements for preventing and controlling *Baylisascaris* infections in animals and humans are (1) reducing environmental contamination with infective eggs, (2) preventing contact with contaminated areas or articles, and (3) educating people about these parasites as causes of animal and human disease. These approaches are interrelated and should be carried out in concert as part of a comprehensive prevention and control program.

Reducing environmental contamination with eggs in an area can only be accomplished by treating, removing, or relocating infected raccoons and skunks. Keeping raccoons and skunks as pets should be strongly discouraged, especially in households with young children. Pet permittees and those involved in wildlife rehabilitation should have adequate knowledge of *Baylisascaris* and other zoonotic diseases or be provided such information. Anthelmintic treatment of raccoons and skunks kept as pets or for other reasons is readily accomplished but must be done adequately and properly (see above) in order to prevent contamination.

Feral raccoons and skunks are much more difficult to deal with and are involved in the majority of *Baylisascaris* infections. Feral raccoons and skunks can be a considerable nuisance in and around zoos and other animal facilities, on farms, and in the suburban domestic environment, where they are responsible for widespread fecal contamination. The excellent climbing ability of raccoons and the fact that they will establish latrines in elevated locations poses a particular problem for zoos using roundhouse enclosures, especially in or near wooded areas. It should theoretically be possible to use baits containing anthelmintics to deworm feral raccoons and skunks in an area, similar to the use of baits for rabies vaccination of wildlife or the bait treatment of *Echinococcus* in foxes in Europe. The timing, frequency, and logistics of such treatments, as well as their effectiveness in decreasing prevalence of *Baylisascaris* in local populations, are not well known, although some encouraging results were seen in a recent study. LoGiudice (1995) baited raccoons with piperazine at two sites in central New Jersey and saw a significant reduction in egg-positive scats in latrines at one of the sites post-baiting, whereas positive scats increased at one of two control sites (the other treatment and control sites showed no differences). Although there was a significant overall reduction in positive scats at the treatment sites as compared to control sites, it was impossible to identify the contributions of individual animals at latrines. Two of three scats which contained a fluorescent marker (indicating bait consumption) also had adult *Baylisascaris* present, indicating successful treatment. Because too few raccoons were trapped and examined for eggs, nothing could be stated as to the effects of anthelmintic baiting on prevalence of the parasite. Additional studies are needed to better assess the usefulness of baiting for control of *Baylisascaris* in wild populations. With the very high population densities of feral raccoons and skunks in many suburban areas, as well as the likelihood of reinfection, this approach could prove costly and time-consuming and still have questionable effectiveness, especially if attempted on too large a scale. Depending on the situation, however, it may be advantageous to deworm a stable, localized resident population on a regular basis as part of overall control efforts, combined with latrine cleanup and decontamination. It is also very important to discourage people from intentionally feeding feral raccoons and to control other food sources (pet food, garbage) which serve to maintain high populations. This would not only help stabilize local raccoon populations but could also reduce the establishment of new latrine sites and levels of fecal contamination in the domestic environment.

The other, more straightforward method of dealing with this problem is through depopulation and removal of raccoons and skunks. This has the advantage of immediately reducing new environmental contamination in an area and is also best combined with latrine cleanup and decontamination. Trapped animals may be relocated to distant sites (thereby making them someone else's problem), or euthanized. Many suburban zoos have ongoing wildlife control programs in an effort to reduce and control nuisance wildlife and their diseases. The main impediments to such approaches are not technological or logistical, but political and social, primarily objections from animal rights and related groups (Stringfield and Sedgwick 1997). However, there is no question but that this is the most direct and effective method of reducing environmental contamination and transmission of *Baylisascaris* to all

species, and it must be considered seriously wherever this disease problem occurs.

Dealing with contaminated areas is more problematic, because of the marked resistance of *Baylisascaris* eggs. Once in the environment, the eggs can survive for years. Eggs are resistant to all common disinfectants, including bleach, although certain solvent mixtures will kill them. Thus, small areas of contamination on resistant surfaces can be treated with 1:1 xylene:ethanol after most organic material has been removed (Kazacos and Boyce 1989). Treatment with 20% bleach (1% sodium hypochlorite) will remove the outer protein coat, making the eggs nonadherent and able to be washed away, but will not kill them. Chemical treatments which kill eggs are generally not practical for use in the environment (Kazacos and Boyce 1989; Kazacos 1991). Desiccants such as sodium borate broadcast onto latrine sites at a sufficient rate might hasten egg death, but this has not been studied.

Heat is by far the best method of killing *Baylisascaris* eggs. Boiling water, a propane flame gun, steam cleaner, autoclave, burning straw, or other means can be used for small or large areas of contaminated soil or concrete, metal cages, enclosures, holding pens, and contaminated tools and utensils (Kazacos and Boyce 1989; Kazacos 1991, 2000). Direct flame from a propane gun is the most effective method for destroying eggs. Our laboratory routinely uses such a device (VT 3-30 Red Dragon Vapor Torch; Flame Engineering, LaCrosse, Kansas) to decontaminate live traps, cages, and enclosures that have held *Baylisascaris*-infected raccoons or skunks. This method has also been used to decontaminate concrete-floored animal rooms, kennel runs, and raccoon latrine sites in zoos and around homes (Pegg 1977; Abdelrasoul and Fowler 1979; Kazacos and Boyce 1989; Kazacos 1991; K.R. Kazacos, unpublished). Surface soil can be flamed, broken up, and turned over several times with a shovel or rake and reflamed each time to ensure decontamination. Obviously, appropriate care should be taken when using this method, particularly in or around buildings and other flammable materials.

For heavily contaminated areas, it may be desirable to remove and discard the top several inches of soil and replace it; this may be combined with heat treatment of the area (e.g., with a flame gun). Dried raccoon feces and other contaminated material (hay, straw, leaves) in exhibits or buildings should be carefully removed and properly disposed of (e.g., by incineration). Residual material in buildings can then be treated with steam or boiling water or removed using a canister-type vacuum cleaner containing a disposable filter bag. Personnel cleaning contaminated areas should wear disposable coveralls, rubber gloves, washable rubber boots, and a particulate face mask to prevent the inhalation or ingestion of any eggs and fecal fungi stirred up in dust (Kazacos and Boyce 1989). When finished, disposable items should be incinerated, autoclaved, or otherwise properly disposed of. The presence of eggs in soil or environmental debris, as well as the effectiveness of their destruction or removal, can be assessed using centrifugal sedimentation-flotation methods on detergent-washed samples (Kazacos 1983c).

It is important to prevent contact with known or suspected contaminated areas or articles until they can be properly assessed and effectively decontaminated, or removed or destroyed. This would include cages or enclosures which previously housed raccoons or skunks, areas or articles contaminated by feral animals, and raccoon latrine sites in and around the domestic or zoo environment. Care should be taken to prevent raccoon fecal contamination of hay, straw, and feed, and contaminated materials should not be used. Fallen timber, large tree limbs, and rocks from the wild should be carefully inspected, washed, and heat-treated before use in animal enclosures or exhibits.

Education of individuals and groups about the health hazards associated with *Baylisascaris* is perhaps the most important aspect of prevention and control (Kazacos 1991). Efforts should be made to inform a wide spectrum of people about these parasites, including wildlife biologists, natural resources personnel, animal care directors and staff, wildlife rehabilitators, animal damage control officers, public health personnel, veterinarians, physicians, and the general public. The diseases caused by *Baylisascaris* are preventable through simple, straightforward measures, but these will not be taken unless people understand and appreciate the problem.

PUBLIC HEALTH CONCERNS. Extensive opportunities exist for contact and infection of human beings with *Baylisascaris,* especially *B. procyonis* from raccoons. Raccoons are extremely common and well adapted to coexistence with human beings in urban, suburban, and rural environments. Some of the highest recorded densities of raccoons are from suburban residential areas, particularly in and around wooded parks and neighborhoods; in these areas, humans are very likely to encounter raccoon fecal contamination (Hoffman and Gottschang 1977; Greve 1985; Kidder 1990; Rosatte et al. 1991; Feigley 1992; W.J. Murray et al., unpublished; Park et al. 2000). Because of their engaging qualities, raccoons are often encouraged through feeding to frequent peoples' yards and homes, where they will establish latrine sites. In addition, raccoons and skunks are frequently kept as pets, increasing the likelihood of human contact and infection with *Baylisascaris.*

Human infection with *Baylisascaris* was anticipated in the 1960s (Beaver 1969), based on experiments done in rodents by Tiner (1951, 1952a, 1953a,b) and Sprent (1951, 1952a, 1955). The zoonotic importance of *B. procyonis* was indicated by Kazacos and associates in the 1980s, based on epidemiologic studies of infected animals and experimental infection of subhuman primates and other species (see Kazacos 1981, 1983a, 1986, 1991; Kazacos et al. 1981b, 1984a,b, 1985; Kazacos and Boyce 1989). Human deaths caused by *B.*

procyonis were first documented in children in 1984–85 (Huff et al. 1984; Fox et al. 1985), at which time the parasite was also implicated as a cause of human OLM (Kazacos et al. 1984a,b, 1985). To date, there have been documented fatalities from *Baylisascaris* NLM in infants in Pennsylvania (Huff et al. 1984), Illinois (Fox et al. 1985), and Minnesota (C.L. Moertel et al., unpublished), and cases of severe, disabling central nervous system disease in infants in New York (Cunningham et al. 1994), Michigan (J.M. Proos et al., unpublished), Illinois (M.B. Mets et al., unpublished), Minnesota (C.L. Moertel et al., unpublished), and California (Rowley et al. 2000; Park et al. 2000), with a probable case in Missouri (Anderson et al. 1975). The parasite also produced central nervous system disease in a 21-year-old man in Oregon (cited in Cunningham et al. 1994) and a 17-year-old boy in California (W.A. Kennedy et al., unpublished) and was considered the cause of death from an eosinophilic intracardiac mass in a 10-year-old boy in Massachusetts (Boschetti and Kasznica 1995). *Baylisascaris* infection was demonstrated serologically in clinically normal individuals in New York (Cunningham et al. 1994) and Germany (Conraths et al. 1996), indicating that asymptomatic, low-level infection also takes place. In cases involving infants, infection was linked to contact with raccoon feces in open fireplaces in the home, coming from raccoons living in the chimneys (Huff et al. 1984), chewing on pieces of bark from contaminated firewood brought into the home (Fox et al. 1985), and geophagia at or near raccoon latrines in the domestic environment (Cunningham et al. 1994; M.B. Mets et al., unpublished; C.L. Moertel et al., unpublished; Park et al. 2000).

In humans, *Baylisascaris* more commonly causes clinical OLM, with dozens of cases now recognized in North America and Europe (Gass and Braunstein 1983; Kazacos et al. 1984a,b, 1985; Kazacos 1991, 1997, unpublished; Goldberg et al. 1993; Küchle et al. 1993). Large nematode larvae were documented in human eyes as early as 1952 in the United States (Parsons 1952) and 1961 in Europe (Schrott 1961), and seven cases were assembled by Gass and Braunstein (1983) in their further description of DUSN, but the etiology was not determined. *Baylisascaris procyonis* was suggested as the probable cause, based on the pathogenesis of *B. procyonis* in animals and the compatible size, geographic location, and pathogenesis of the larvae in these patients; in addition, one of the patients had known raccoon contact (Kazacos et al. 1984a,b, 1985). With additional, well-documented cases linked morphometrically and serologically to *Baylisascaris* infection and raccoon exposure (Goldberg et al. 1993; Küchle et al. 1993), *B. procyonis* is now recognized as an important cause of human OLM and the primary cause of the large nematode variant of DUSN.

The fact that OLM and DUSN are usually related to low-level infection further indicates that human infection with *Baylisascaris* is probably common. Many more people will contract low-level infections than heavy infections, and unless the larvae migrate to the eye or brain in sufficient numbers, these individuals will not develop clinically significant disease. Similar to infections with *Toxocara canis,* most human infections with *Baylisascaris* are probably asymptomatic. These cases would be characterized only by low serum antibody titer, with or without mild eosinophilia, and without signs of visceral, ocular, or neural larva migrans (Kazacos 1991, 1997; Cunningham et al. 1994; Conraths et al. 1996).

At the other end of the spectrum, infants 1–4 years old are at greatest risk of heavy infection with *Baylisascaris* because of their poor hygiene and propensity for pica and geophagia. Special attention should be paid to this age group and other children in order to prevent life-threatening infections with these parasites (Kazacos 2000). Children should be kept away from known or potentially contaminated areas and taught to recognize and avoid raccoon latrines they may encounter in the environment. They should also be monitored closely to prevent pica and geophagia and taught to wash their hands regularly, especially after contact with outdoor areas or animals and prior to eating.

DOMESTIC ANIMAL HEALTH CONCERNS. Ample opportunities exist for contact and infection of domestic animals with *Baylisascaris,* especially *B. procyonis.* Fatal central nervous system disease due to *B. procyonis* has been seen in pet dogs, rabbits, porcupines, and psittacines, as well as farm-raised rabbits, chinchillas, poultry, quail, pheasants, and ratites (Table 11.6). *Baylisascaris* appears to have only limited migration in large domestic livestock (Dubey 1982; Snyder 1983; Kazacos and Kazacos 1984), except perhaps during pregnancy; the only known case involved a lamb with transplacentally acquired infection (Anderson 1999). Infection of domestic animals is commonly associated with keeping raccoons on the premises, using cages or enclosures that previously held raccoons, using contaminated hay, straw, or feed, and exposure to fecal contamination from feral raccoons (Kazacos and Boyce 1989).

Two fatalities in hunting dogs were linked to wild-caught raccoons kept on the premises for training purposes (Thomas 1988; Rudmann et al. 1996). Many dogs, especially puppies, are coprophagic and will ingest raccoon feces they encounter in the domestic environment or surrounding woods. This could result in fatal central nervous system disease, or in some cases patent intestinal infection with *B. procyonis* (Greve and O'Brien 1989; Miyashita 1993; Averbeck et al. 1995; D.D. Bowman, unpublished; K.R. Kazacos, unpublished). In the largest outbreak of NLM recorded to date, 622 chickens died over a 7-week period, following the use of raccoon feces–contaminated straw litter in a poultry facility (Richardson et al. 1980). In another case, 100% mortality occurred in 85 bobwhite quail placed in a 12 x 24 foot dirt pen previously used to house three young pet raccoons (Reed et al. 1981).

Over a 3-month period, these raccoons contaminated the pen with over 155,500,000 *B. procyonis* eggs, even though they were shedding at a low rate (1300–5400 eggs/g feces, mean 2800/g) (Kazacos 1982). In a recent dramatic outbreak, 10 pet psittacines in a mixed collection were killed acutely by massive *B. procyonis* infection acquired from contaminated feed. Feral raccoons had contaminated a stored seed mixture kept in a bin in the owner's garage (A.M. Lennox and K.R. Kazacos, unpublished). These examples graphically illustrate the health hazard posed by *B. procyonis* to a variety of domestic and farm-raised animals.

MANAGEMENT IMPLICATIONS. Without management and control of raccoon and skunk populations in an area or particular situation, it would be very difficult or impossible to reduce or eliminate potential transmission of *Baylisascaris.* It is well established that wildlife populations can increase to the point of serious nuisance, particularly in urban and suburban areas, with damage to buildings and vegetation, predation on domestic and zoo animals, widespread fecal contamination, and transmission of infectious and parasitic diseases. Raccoons and skunks are foremost examples of this problem, and in addition to causing property damage and other losses, pose the real threat of *Baylisascaris* transmission to animals and humans in an area.

An excellent example of the problems and management implications associated with nuisance wildlife and *Baylisascaris* was recently described by Stringfield and Sedgwick (1997) at the Los Angeles Zoo. What they depict is not unlike the situation at many other suburban zoos, and much can be learned from it: "The Los Angeles Zoo sits in the middle of Griffith Park, which is a large wild area. Previous nonmanagement of pests had allowed the zoo to become overrun with these animals, and problems had reached epidemic proportions in 1995. Coyotes living in the zoo were hunting gerenuk and flamingos, skunks were everywhere, and raccoons had free-roam of the zoo. In the past 3 yr at the Los Angeles Zoo, we have seen numerous cases of central nervous system disease secondary to *Baylisascaris*". A change in zoo management brought an immediate and aggressive, multifaceted response to these problems. This included trapping and removal of the resident raccoon, skunk, and coyote populations, repairing gaps in the perimeter fence to prevent future influx, trimming trees and overhanging foliage, installing wire mesh along the bottoms of exhibits to prevent animal access, repairing garbage bins, rehabilitating contaminated exhibits, and instituting ongoing surveillance and control measures, coupled with a program of staff education. Although the scope of the task was daunting, with thoughtful planning and implementation the program was successful, and nuisance wildlife and *Baylisascaris* transmission to zoo animals were both brought under control.

A second example involves the impact of *Baylisascaris* on indigenous wildlife, including threatened and endangered species, following introduction of the parasites and/or increases in raccoon or skunk populations in an area. The Allegheny woodrat (*Neotoma magister*) was extirpated from New York state and Connecticut and continues to decline in other parts of its northeastern range. In the Hudson Highlands region of New York, declines were linked to an increase in the raccoon population and to NLM caused by *Baylisascaris*. In Mohonk Preserve, New Paltz, New York, abnormal behavior was documented in various animals including gray squirrels and deer mice found circling or unable to climb (Smiley and Huth 1986). Ward Stone, Associate Wildlife Pathologist for the state, suggested *B. procyonis* NLM as the probable cause and also hypothesized its role in the extirpation of woodrats from the preserve between 1959 and 1977. Previously, Smiley (1977a,b) had astutely noted declines in the woodrat population as well as increases in the raccoon population and wondered if the two were related. Sighting a raccoon at Mohonk was a rarity from 1923 to 1932, but by the end of 1949 and subsequently they were abundant (Smiley 1977a).

The New York Department of Environmental Conservation (DEC) began surveying historic woodrat sites in 1978 and noted marked declines in the species, which became extirpated from the state in 1987. The DEC undertook release studies at Mohonk in 1991, which indicated that *B. procyonis* was the likely cause of extirpation of *N. magister* from the region, in combination with other factors (McGowan 1993). The steep rock and boulder talus slopes preferred by woodrats are also very attractive to raccoons, which use them for den and latrine sites. Uninfected woodrats from West Virginia released into these areas, as well as their offspring, died of *Baylisascaris* NLM, which was documented in all 11 woodrats recovered and examined; 4 woodrats had exhibited abnormal behavior when livetrapped (McGowan 1993). In addition, *Baylisascaris* NLM was identified recently in Allegheny woodrats in southern Indiana (K.R. Kazacos and S.A. Johnson, unpublished) and southcentral Pennsylvania (J. Wright et al., unpublished), and in a woodrat released in New Jersey (K. LoGiudice, unpublished). In New York and Indiana, the caching of raccoon feces by woodrats also was documented, indicating a direct behavioral link to *B. procyonis* infection in this species. The plight of the Allegheny woodrat demonstrates that *Baylisascaris* can have a significant impact on indigenous wildlife. Because of *Baylisascaris,* the reintroduction and/or long-term survival of particular animal species may be difficult or impossible without management of raccoon and skunk populations in an area.

LITERATURE CITED

Abdelrasoul, K., and M. Fowler. 1979. Epidemiology of ascarid infection in captive carnivores. *Proceedings of the American Association of Zoo Veterinarians* pp. 105–106a.

Agnew, D.W., K.R. Kazacos, G.L. Watson, B. Yamini, R. Barbiers, and R. D. Garrison. 1994. Neural larva migrans due to *Baylisascaris procyonis* in red kangaroos. *Proceedings of the American Association of Veterinary Parasitologists* 39:68.

Amundson, T., and S. Marquenski. 1986. *Baylisascaris procyonis* in Wisconsin raccoons. Madison, WI: Wisconsin Department of Natural Resources, 7 pp.

Anderson, B.C. 1999. Congenital *Baylisascaris* sp. larval migrans in a newborn lamb. *The Journal of Parasitology* 85:128–129.

Anderson, D.C., R. Greenwood, M. Fishman, and I.G. Kagan. 1975. Acute infantile hemiplegia with cerebrospinal fluid eosinophilic pleocytosis: An unusual case of visceral larva migrans. *Journal of Pediatrics* 86:247–249.

Anderson, R.C. 2000. *Nematode parasites of vertebrates: Their development and transmission,* 2nd ed. Wallingford, UK: CAB International, 650 pp.

Anderson, S.B., and J. Mills. 1991. Occurrence of the raccoon roundworm (*Baylisascaris procyonis*) in raccoons in Nova Scotia. Technical Note No. 67. Kentville: Nova Scotia Department of Lands and Forests, 2 pp.

Armstrong, D.L., R.J. Montali, A.R. Doster, and K.R. Kazacos. 1989. Cerebrospinal nematodiasis in macaws due to *Baylisascaris procyonis*. *Journal of Zoo and Wildlife Medicine* 20:354–359.

Averbeck, G.A., J.A. Vanek, B.E. Stromberg, and J.R. Laursen. 1995. Differentiation of *Baylisascaris* species, *Toxocara canis,* and *Toxascaris leonina* infections in dogs. *Compendium on Continuing Education for the Practicing Veterinarian* 17:475–478, 511.

Babero, B.B., and J.R. Shepperson. 1958. Some helminths of raccoons in Georgia. *The Journal of Parasitology* 44:519.

Bafundo, K.W., W.E. Wilhelm, and M.L. Kennedy. 1980. Geographic variation in helminth parasites from the digestive tract of Tennessee raccoons, *Procyon lotor. The Journal of Parasitology* 66:134–139.

Ball, R.L., M. Dryden, S. Wilson, and J. Veatch. 1998. Cerebrospinal nematodiasis in a white-handed gibbon (*Hylobates lar*) due to *Baylisascaris* sp. *Journal of Zoo and Wildlife Medicine* 29:221–224.

Barnstable, R.W., and W.G. Dyer. 1974. Gastrointestinal helminths of the raccoon, *Procyon lotor,* in southern Illinois. *Transactions of the Illinois State Academy of Science* 67:451–460.

Bauer, C., and A. Gey. 1995. Efficacy of six anthelmintics against luminal stages of *Baylisascaris procyonis* in naturally infected raccoons (*Procyon lotor*). *Veterinary Parasitology* 60:155–159.

Beaver, P.C. 1969. The nature of visceral larva migrans. *The Journal of Parasitology* 55:3–12.

Beaver, P.C., R.C. Jung, and E.W. Cupp. 1984. *Clinical parasitology,* 9th ed. Philadelphia, PA: Lea and Febiger, 825 pp.

Berry, J.F. 1985. Phylogenetic relationship between *Baylisascaris* spp. Sprent, 1968 (Nematoda: Ascarididae) from skunks, raccoons and groundhogs in southern Ontario. M.S Thesis. University of Guelph, Guelph, Ontario, 99 pp.

Binford, C.H., and D.H. Connor. 1976. *Pathology of tropical and extraordinary diseases.* Washington, DC: Armed Forces Institute of Pathology, 696 pp.

Birch, G.L., G.A. Feldhamer, and W.G. Dyer. 1994. Helminths of the gastrointestinal tract of raccoons in southern Illinois with management implications of *Baylisascaris procyonis* occurrence. *Transactions of the Illinois State Academy of Science* 87:165–170.

Boddicker, M.L., and D.R. Progulske. 1968. Helminth parasites of raccoon in South Dakota. *Proceedings of the South Dakota Academy of Science* 47:161–166.

Boschetti, A., and J. Kasznica. 1995. Visceral larva migrans induced eosinophilic cardiac pseudotumor: A cause of sudden death in a child. *Journal of Forensic Sciences* 40:1097–1099.

Bowman, D.D. 1987. Diagnostic morphology of four larval ascaridoid nematodes that may cause visceral larva migrans: *Toxascaris leonina, Baylisascaris procyonis, Lagochilascaris sprenti,* and *Hexametra leidyi. The Journal of Parasitology* 73:1198–1215.

Boyce, W.M., B.A. Branstetter, and K.R. Kazacos. 1988a. In vitro culture of *Baylisascaris procyonis* and initial analysis of larval excretory-secretory antigens. *Proceedings of the Helminthological Society of Washington* 55:15–18.

———. 1988b. Comparative analysis of larval excretory-secretory antigens of *Baylisascaris procyonis, Toxocara canis* and *Ascaris suum* by western blotting and enzyme immunoassay. *International Journal for Parasitology* 18:109–113.

Boyce, W.M., D.J. Asai, J.K. Wilder, and K.R. Kazacos. 1989. Physicochemical characterization and monoclonal and polyclonal antibody recognition of *Baylisascaris procyonis* larval excretory-secretory antigens. *The Journal of Parasitology* 75: 540–548.

Campbell, G.A., J. P. Hoover, W.C. Russell, and J.E. Breazile. 1997. Naturally occurring cerebral nematodiasis due to *Baylisascaris* larval migration in two black-and-white ruffed lemurs (*Varecia variegata variegata*) and suspected cases in three emus (*Dromaius novaehollandiae*). *Journal of Zoo and Wildlife Medicine* 28:204–207.

Carlson, M.S., and S.W. Nielsen. 1984. Jejunal obstruction due to *Baylisascaris procyonis* in a raccoon. *Journal of the American Veterinary Medical Association* 185:1396–1397.

Chandler, A.C. 1942. The helminths of raccoons in east Texas. *The Journal of Parasitology* 28:255–268.

Ching, H.L., B.J. Leighton, and C. Stephen. 2000. Intestinal paarasites of raccoons (*Procyon lotor*) from southwest British Columbia. *Canadian Journal of Veterinary Research* 64:107–111.

Chitwood, M., and J.R. Lichtenfels. 1972. Identification of parasitic metazoa in tissue sections. *Experimental Parasitology* 32:407–519.

Church, E.M., D.S. Wyand, and D.H. Lein. 1975. Experimentally induced cerebrospinal nematodiasis in rabbits (*Oryctolagus cuniculus*). *American Journal of Veterinary Research* 36:331–335.

Clark, G.M., C.B. Philip, and L. Fadness. 1969. Observations on the effect in mice of concurrent infections with migratory *Ascaris columnaris* larvae and certain neurotropic arboviruses. *Folia Parasitologica* 16:67–73.

Coates, J.W., J. Siegert, V.A. Bowes, and D.G. Steer. 1995. Encephalitic nematodiasis in a Douglas squirrel and a rock dove ascribed to *Baylisascaris procyonis. Canadian Veterinary Journal* 36:566–569.

Cole, R.A., and W.L. Shoop. 1987. Helminths of the raccoon (*Procyon lotor*) in western Kentucky. *The Journal of Parasitology* 73:762–768.

Conboy, G. 1996. Diagnostic parasitology. *Canadian Veterinary Journal* 37:181–182.

Connor, D.H., F.W. Chandler, D.A. Schwartz, H.J. Manz, and E E. Lack. 1997. *Pathology of infectious diseases.* Stamford, CT: Appleton and Lange, 1707 pp.

Conraths, F.J., C. Bauer, J. Cseke, and H. Laube. 1996. Arbeitsplatzbedingte Infektionen des Menschen mit dem Waschbärspulwurm *Baylisascaris procyonis* [In German]. *Arbeitsmedizin Sozialmedizin Umweltmedizin* 31:13–17.

Cooney, T.A. 1989. Environmental contamination with *Baylisascaris procyonis* in an urban park. M.S. Thesis, Purdue University, West Lafayette, IN, 125 pp.

Craig, S.J., G.A. Conboy, and P.E. Hanna. 1995. *Baylisascaris* sp. infection in a guinea pig. *Laboratory Animal Science* 45:312–314.

Cranfield, M.R., I.K. Barker, K.G. Mehren, and W.A. Rapley. 1984. Canine distemper in wild raccoons (*Procyon lotor*)

at the metropolitan Toronto Zoo. *Canadian Veterinary Journal* 25:63–66.

Cunningham, C.K., K.R. Kazacos, J.A. McMillan, J.A. Lucas, J.B. McAuley, E.J. Wozniak, and L.B. Weiner. 1994. Diagnosis and management of *Baylisascaris procyonis* infection in an infant with nonfatal meningoencephalitis. *Clinical Infectious Diseases* 18:868–872.

Dade, A.W., J.F. Williams, D.L. Whitenack, and C.S.F. Williams. 1975. An epizootic of cerebral nematodiasis in rabbits due to *Ascaris columnaris. Laboratory Animal Science* 25:65–69.

Dade, A.W., J.F. Williams, A.L. Trapp, and W.H. Ball Jr. 1977. Cerebral nematodiasis in captive nutria. *Journal of the American Veterinary Medical Association* 171:885–886.

Deeb, B.J., and R.F. DiGiacomo. 1994. Cerebral larva migrans caused by *Baylisascaris* sp. in pet rabbits. *Journal of the American Veterinary Medical Association* 205:1744–1747.

Dixon, D., G.R. Reinhard, K.R. Kazacos, and C. Arriaga. 1988. Cerebrospinal nematodiasis in prairie dogs from a research facility. *Journal of the American Veterinary Medical Association* 193:251–253.

Donnelly, J.J., A.A. Sakla, M. Khatami, and J.H. Rockey. 1989. *Baylisascaris procyonis* (Stefanski and Zarnowski, 1951) Ascarididae: Nematoda. II. Third stage larvae, morphogenesis and migratory behaviour. *Assiut Veterinary Medical Journal* 21:77–85.

Dubey, J.P. 1982. *Baylisascaris procyonis* and eimerian infections in raccoons. *Journal of the American Veterinary Medical Association* 181: 1292–1294.

Dubey, J.P., A.N. Hamir, C.A. Hanlon, and C.E. Rupprecht. 1992. Prevalence of *Toxoplasma gondii* infection in raccoons. *Journal of the American Veterinary Medical Association* 200:534–536.

Ermer, E.M., and J.A. Fodge. 1986. Occurrence of the raccoon roundworm in raccoons in western New York. *New York Fish and Game Journal* 33:58–61.

Evans, R.H., and B. Tangredi. 1985. Cerebrospinal nematodiasis in free-ranging birds. *Journal of the American Veterinary Medical Association* 187:1213–1214.

Feigley, H.P. 1992. The ecology of the raccoon in suburban Long Island, N.Y., and its relation to soil contamination with *Baylisascaris procyonis* ova. Ph.D. Thesis, State University of New York College of Environmental Science and Forestry, Syracuse, 139 pp.

Ferris, D.H., R.D. Lord Jr., P.D. Beamer, and T.E. Fritz. 1960. A new disease in Illinois cottontails. *The Journal of Wildlife Management* 24:179–184.

Fitzgerald, S.D., M.R. White, and K.R. Kazacos. 1991. Encephalitis in two porcupines due to *Baylisascaris* larval migration. *Journal of Veterinary Diagnostic Investigation* 3:359–362.

Fleming, W.J., and J.W. Caslick. 1978. Rabies and cerebrospinal nematodiasis in woodchucks (*Marmota monax*) from New York. *Cornell Veterinarian* 68:391–395.

Fleming, W.J., J.R. Georgi, and J.W. Caslick. 1979. Parasites of the woodchuck (*Marmota monax*) in central New York. *Proceedings of the Helminthological Society of Washington* 46:115–127.

Folk, G.E., Jr., K.B. Coady, and M.A. Folk. 1968. Physiological observations on raccoons in winter. *Proceedings of the Iowa Academy of Science* 75:301–305.

Fox, A.S., K.R. Kazacos, N.S. Gould, P.T. Heydemann, C. Thomas, and K. M. Boyer. 1985. Fatal eosinophilic meningoencephalitis and visceral larva migrans caused by the raccoon ascarid *Baylisascaris procyonis. New England Journal of Medicine* 312:1619–1623.

Fritz, T.E., D.E. Smith, and R.J. Flynn. 1968. A central nervous system disorder in ground squirrels (*Citellus tridecemlineatus*) associated with visceral larva migrans.

Journal of the American Veterinary Medical Association 153:841–844.

Garlick, D.S., L.C. Marcus, M. Pokras, and S.H. Schelling. 1996. *Baylisascaris* larva migrans in a spider monkey (*Ateles* sp.). *Journal of Medical Primatology* 25:133–136.

Garrison, R.D. 1996. Evaluation of anthelmintic and corticosteroid treatment in protecting mice (*Mus musculus*) from neural larva migrans due to *Baylisascaris procyonis*. M.S. Thesis, Purdue University, West Lafayette, IN, 102 pp.

Gass, J.D.M., and R.A. Braunstein. 1983. Further observations concerning the diffuse unilateral subacute neuroretinitis syndrome. *Archives of Ophthalmology* 101:1689–1697.

Gey, A.B. 1998. Synopsis der Parasitenfauna des Waschbären (*Procyon lotor*) unter Berücksichtigung von Befunden aus Hessen. Dissertation, Fachbereich Veterinärmedizin, Justus Liebig Universität, Giesen, Germany, 203 pp.

Gibson, D.I. 1983. The systematics of ascaridoid nematodes—A current assessment. In *Concepts in nematode systematics.* Ed. A.R. Stone, H.M. Platt, and L.F. Khalil. New York: Academic Press, pp. 321–338.

Goldberg, M.A., K.R. Kazacos, W.M. Boyce, E. Ai, and B. Katz. 1993. Diffuse unilateral subacute neuroretinitis. Morphometric, serologic, and epidemiologic support for *Baylisascaris* as a causative agent. *Ophthalmology* 100:1695–1701.

Goodey, T., and T.W.M. Cameron. 1923. Observations on the morphology and life history of *Ascaris columnaris* Leidy, a nematode parasite of the skunk. *Journal of Helminthology* 1:1–8.

Greve, J.H. 1985. Raccoon ascarids pose public health threat. *Iowa State University Veterinarian* 47:13–14.

Greve, J.H., and S.E. O'Brien. 1989. Adult *Baylisascaris* infections in two dogs. *Companion Animal Practice* 19:41–43.

Gutierrez, Y. 2000. *Diagnostic pathology of parasitic infections with clinical correlations,* 2nd ed. New York: Oxford University Press, 769 pp.

Habermann, R.T., C.M. Herman, and F.P. Williams, Jr. 1958. Distemper in raccoons and foxes suspected of having rabies. *Journal of the American Veterinary Medical Association* 132:31–35.

Hamann, K.J., G.M. Kephart, K.R. Kazacos, and G.J. Gleich. 1989. Immunofluorescent localization of eosinophil granule major basic protein in fatal human cases of *Baylisascaris procyonis* infection. *American Journal of Tropical Medicine and Hygiene* 40:291–297.

Harkema, R., and G.C. Miller. 1962. Helminths of *Procyon lotor solutus* from Cape Island, South Carolina. *The Journal of Parasitology* 48:333–335.

———. 1964. Helminth parasites of the raccoon, *Procyon lotor,* in the southeastern United States. *The Journal of Parasitology* 50:60–66.

Hartwich, G. 1962. Über den Waschbärenspulwurm *Ascaris procyonis* Stefanski et Zarnowski 1951, und seine stellung im system der Ascaroidea (Nematoda)[In German]. *Ceskoslovenská parasitologie* 9:239–256.

———. 1974. Keys to genera of the Ascaridoidea. *CIH keys to the nematode parasites of vertebrates,* no. 2. Ed. R.C. Anderson, A.G. Chabaud, and S. Willmott. Farnham Royal, England: Commonwealth Agricultural Bureaux, 15 pp.

Helfer, D.H., and E.O. Dickinson. 1976. Parasitic encephalitis in pigeons. *Avian Diseases* 20:209–210.

Herman, C.M. 1939. Parasites obtained from animals in the collection of the New York Zoological Park during 1938. *Zoologica (New York)* 24:481–485.

Hill, R.E. Jr., J.J. Zimmerman, J.H. Greve, and G.W. Beran. 1991. Use of ivermectin against several nematodes in

naturally infected raccoons (*Procyon lotor*). *Journal of Zoo and Wildlife Medicine* 22:417–420.

Hoberg, E.P., and S.G. McGee. 1982. Helminth parasitism in raccoons, *Procyon lotor hirtus* Nelson and Goldman, in Saskatchewan. *Canadian Journal of Zoology* 60:53–57.

Hoffman, C.O., and J.L. Gottschang. 1977. Numbers, distribution, and movements of a raccoon population in a suburban residential community. *Journal of Mammalogy* 58:623–636.

Huff, D.S., R.C. Neafie, M.J. Binder, G.A. De León, L.W. Brown, and K.R. Kazacos. 1984. The first fatal *Baylisascaris* infection in humans: An infant with eosinophilic meningoencephalitis. *Pediatric Pathology* 2:345–352.

Huntress, S.L., and T. Spraker. 1985. *Baylisascaris* infection in the marmoset. *Proceedings of the American Association of Zoo Veterinarians,* p. 78.

Jacobson, H.A., P.F. Scanlon, V.F. Nettles, and W.R. Davidson. 1976. Epizootiology of an outbreak of cerebrospinal nematodiasis in cottontail rabbits and woodchucks. *Journal of Wildlife Diseases* 12:357–360.

Jacobson, J.E., K.R. Kazacos, and F.H. Montague, Jr. 1982. Prevalence of eggs of *Baylisascaris procyonis* (Nematoda:Ascaroidea) in raccoon scats from an urban and a rural community. *Journal of Wildlife Diseases* 18:461–464.

Johnson, S.A. 1970. Biology of the raccoon (*Procyon lotor varius*), Nelson and Goldman in Alabama. Bulletin No. 402. Auburn, AL: Auburn University Agricultural Experiment Station, 148 pp.

Jones, E.J., and B.S. McGinnes. 1983. Distribution of adult *Baylisascaris procyonis* in raccoons from Virginia. *The Journal of Parasitology* 69:653.

Jordan, H.E., and F.A. Hayes. 1959. Gastrointestinal helminths of raccoons (*Procyon lotor*) from Ossabaw Island, Georgia. *The Journal of Parasitology* 45:249–252.

Kazacos, E.A., and K.R. Kazacos. 1988a. Pathogenesis and pathology of experimental baylisascariasis in ferrets. *Proceedings of the American Society of Parasitologists* 63:60.

Kazacos, K.R. 1981. Animal and public health implications of the nematode genus *Baylisascaris*. *Proceedings of the American Association of Veterinary Parasitologists* 26:21.

———. 1982. Contaminative ability of *Baylisascaris procyonis* infected raccoons in an outbreak of cerebrospinal nematodiasis. *Proceedings of the Helminthological Society of Washington* 49:155–157.

———. 1983a. Raccoon roundworms (*Baylisascaris procyonis*). A cause of animal and human disease. Bulletin No. 422. West Lafayette, IN: Purdue University Agricultural Experiment Station, 25 pp.

———. 1983b. Life cycle studies on *Baylisascaris procyonis* in raccoons. *Proceedings of the Conference of Research Workers in Animal Diseases* 64:24.

———. 1983c. Improved method for recovering ascarid and other helminth eggs from soil associated with epizootics and during survey studies. *American Journal of Veterinary Research* 44:896–900.

———. 1986. Raccoon ascarids as a cause of larva migrans. *Parasitology Today* 2:253–255.

———. 1991. Visceral and ocular larva migrans. *Seminars in Veterinary Medicine and Surgery (Small Animal)* 6:227–235.

———. 1996. Baylisascariasis. In *Rudolph's pediatrics,* 20th ed. Ed. A.M. Rudolph, J.I.E. Hoffman, and C.D. Rudolph. Stamford, CT: Appleton and Lange, pp. 716–717.

———. 1997. Visceral, ocular, and neural larva migrans. In *Pathology of infectious diseases,* vol. 2. Ed. D.H. Connor, F.W. Chandler, D.A. Schwartz, H.J. Manz, and E.E.

Lack. Stamford, CT: Appleton and Lange, pp. 1459–1473.

———. 2000. Protecting children from helminthic zoonoses. *Contemporary Pediatrics* 17(Supplement): 1–24.

Kazacos, K.R., and W.M. Boyce. 1989. *Baylisascaris* larva migrans. *Journal of the American Veterinary Medical Association* 195:894–903. Addendum. 1995. In *Zoonosis updates from the Journal of the American Veterinary Medical Association*, 2nd ed. Shaumburg, IL: American Veterinary Medical Association, pp. 29–30.

Kazacos, K.R., and E.A. Kazacos. 1984. Experimental infection of domestic swine with *Baylisascaris procyonis* from raccoons. *American Journal of Veterinary Research* 45:1114–1121.

———. 1988b. Diagnostic exercise: Neuromuscular condition in rabbits. *Laboratory Animal Science* 38:187–189.

Kazacos, K.R., and J.J. Turek. 1982. Scanning electron microscopy of the labia of *Baylisascaris procyonis* (Nematoda). *The Journal of Parasitology* 68:634–641.

———. 1983. Scanning electron microscopy of the eggs of *Baylisascaris procyonis, B. transfuga,* and *Parascaris equorum,* and their comparison with *Toxocara canis* and *Ascaris suum. Proceedings of the Helminthological Society of Washington* 50:36–42.

Kazacos, K.R., and W.L. Wirtz. 1983. Experimental cerebrospinal nematodiasis due to *Baylisascaris procyonis* in chickens. *Avian Diseases* 27:55–65.

Kazacos, K.R., G.O. Appel, and H.L. Thacker. 1981a. Cerebrospinal nematodiasis in a woodchuck suspected of having rabies. *Journal of the American Veterinary Medical Association* 179:1102–1104.

Kazacos, K.R., W.L. Wirtz, P.P. Burger, and C.S. Christmas. 1981b. Raccoon ascarid larvae as a cause of fatal central nervous system disease in subhuman primates. *Journal of the American Veterinary Medical Association* 179:1089–1094.

Kazacos, K.R., E.A. Kazacos, J.A. Render, and H.L. Thacker. 1982a. Cerebrospinal nematodiasis and visceral larva migrans in an Australian (Latham's) brush turkey. *Journal of the American Veterinary Medical Association* 181:1295–1298.

Kazacos, K.R., R.W. Winterfield, and H.L. Thacker. 1982b. Etiology and epidemiology of verminous encephalitis in an emu. *Avian Diseases* 26:389–391.

Kazacos, K.R., W.M. Reed, E.A. Kazacos, and H.L. Thacker. 1983. Fatal cerebrospinal disease caused by *Baylisascaris procyonis* in domestic rabbits. *Journal of the American Veterinary Medical Association* 183:967–971.

Kazacos, K.R., W.A. Vestre, E.A. Kazacos, and L.A. Raymond. 1984a. Diffuse unilateral subacute neuroretinitis syndrome: Probable cause. *Archives of Ophthalmology* 102:967–968.

Kazacos, K.R., W.A. Vestre, and E.A. Kazacos. 1984b. Raccoon ascarid larvae (*Baylisascaris procyonis*) as a cause of ocular larva migrans. *Investigative Ophthalmology and Visual Science* 25:1177–1183.

Kazacos, K.R., L.A. Raymond, E.A. Kazacos, and W.A. Vestre. 1985. The raccoon ascarid. A probable cause of human ocular larva migrans. *Ophthalmology* 92:1735–1743.

Kazacos, K.R., W.M. Reed, and H.L. Thacker. 1986. Cerebrospinal nematodiasis in pheasants. *Journal of the American Veterinary Medical Association* 189:1353–1354.

Kazacos, K.R., S.D. Fitzgerald, and W.M. Reed. 1991. *Baylisascaris procyonis* as a cause of cerebrospinal nematodiasis in ratites. *Journal of Zoo and Wildlife Medicine* 22:460–465.

Kelly, W.R., and J.R.M. Innes. 1966. Cerebrospinal nematodiasis with focal encephalomalacia as a cause of paralysis

of beavers (*Castor canadensis*) in the Dublin Zoological Gardens. *British Veterinary Journal* 122:285–287.

Kerr, C. L., S. E. Henke, and D. B. Pence. 1997. Baylisascariasis in raccoons from southern coastal Texas. *Journal of Wildlife Diseases* 33:653–655.

Kidder, J.D. 1990. Density and distribution of an urban/suburban raccoon population and the prevalence of patent *Baylisascaris procyonis* infection. M.S. Thesis, Cornell University, Ithaca, NY, 81 pp.

Kidder, J.D., S.E. Wade, M.E. Richmond, and S.J. Schwager. 1989. Prevalence of patent *Baylisascaris procyonis* infection in raccoons (*Procyon lotor*) in Ithaca, New York. *The Journal of Parasitology* 75:870–874.

Koch, F., and J. Rapp. 1981 . Zerebrale Nematodiasis bei Sumpfbibern (*Myocastor coypus*)—verursacht durch Larven von *Baylisascaris* (Nematoda). *Berliner und Münchener Tierärztliche Wochenschrift* 94:111–114.

Kuberski, T. 1979. Eosinophils in the cerebrospinal fluid. *Annals of Internal Medicine* 91:70–75.

Küchle, M., H.L.J. Knorr, S. Medenblik-Frysch, A. Weber, C. Bauer, and G.O.H. Naumann. 1993. Diffuse unilateral subacute neuroretinitis syndrome in a German most likely caused by the raccoon roundworm, *Baylisascaris procyonis. Graefe's Archive for Clinical and Experimental Ophthalmology* 231:48–51.

Kwiecien, J.M., D.A. Smith, D.W. Key, J. Swinton, and L. Smith-Maxie. 1993. Encephalitis attributed to larval migration of *Baylisascaris* species in emus. *Canadian Veterinary Journal* 34:176–178.

Larson, D.J., and J.H. Greve. 1983. Encephalitis caused by *Baylisascaris* migration in a silver fox. *Journal of the American Veterinary Medical Association* 183:1274–1275.

Larson, O.R., and W.C. Scharf. 1975. New helminth records from Minnesota mammals. *Proceedings of the Helminthological Society of Washington* 42:174–175.

Leidy, J. 1856. A synopsis of entozoa and some of their ectocongeners observed by the author. *Proceedings of the Academy of Natural Sciences Philadelphia* 8:42–58.

Leigh, W.H. 1940. Preliminary studies on parasites of upland game birds and fur-bearing mammals in Illinois. *Bulletin of the Illinois Natural History Survey* 21:185–194.

Lindquist, W.D. 1978. *Baylisascaris procyonis* for testing anthelmintics against migratory ascarids. *American Journal of Veterinary Research* 39:1868–1869.

LoGiudice, K. 1995. Control of *Baylisascaris procyonis* (Nematoda) in raccoons (*Procyon lotor*) through the use of anthelmintic baits: A potential method for reducing mortality in the Allegheny woodrat (*Neotoma floridana magister*). M.S. Thesis, Rutgers University, New Brunswick, NJ, 78 pp.

Lotze, J.-H., and S. Anderson. 1979. *Procyon lotor.* Mammalian Species no. 119. American Society of Mammalogists,8pp.

Lux, E., and J. Priemer. 1995. Zur Parasitierung wildlebender Waschbären unter dem Aspekt ihrer nordamerikanischen. *Verhandlungsbericht Erkrankungen der Zootiere* 37:429–434.

Mackay, A., J. Robitaille, S. Messier, and A. Villeneuve. 1995. *Baylisascaris* chez le raton laveur au Québec: possibilité, de zoonose. *Le Médecin Vétérinaire du Québec* 25:102–105.

McClure, G.W. 1933. Nematode parasites of mammals. From specimens collected in the New York Zoological Park, 1931. *Zoologica (New York)* 15:29–47.

McGowan, E.M. 1993. Experimental release and fate study of the Allegheny woodrat (*Neotoma magister*). New York Federal Aid Project W-166-E; E-1, Job No. VIII-7. Albany: New York State Department of Environmental Conservation, 15 pp.

McIntosh, A. 1939. A new nematode, *Ascaris schroederi,* from a giant panda, *Ailuropoda melanoleuca. Zoologica (New York)* 24:355–357.

McKown, R.D., J.K. Veatch, R.J. Robel, and S.J. Upton. 1995. Endoparasites of beaver (*Castor canadensis*) from Kansas. *Journal of the Helminthological Society of Washington.* 62:89–93.

McNeil, C.W., and J.T. Krogsdale. 1953. Parasites of raccoons in southwest Washington. *Journal of Mammalogy* 34:123–124.

Medway, W., D.L. Skand, and C.F. Sarver. 1989. Neurologic signs in American porcupines (*Erethizon dorsatum*) infected with *Baylisascaris* and *Toxoplasma. Journal of Zoo and Wildlife Medicine* 20:207–211.

Meikle, A.D.S., and A.H. Martin. 1981. A rapid method for removal of the spinal cord. *Stain Technology* 56:235–237.

Miyashita, M. 1993. Prevalence of *Baylisascaris procyonis* in raccoons in Japan and experimental infections of the worm to laboratory animals [In Japanese]. *Journal of Urban Living and Health Association* 37:137–151.

Morgan, B.B., and E.F. Waller. 1940. Severe parasitism in a raccoon, (*Procyon lotor lotor* Linnaeus). *Transactions of the American Microscopical Society* 59:523–527.

Myers, R.K., W.E. Monroe, and J.H. Greve. 1983. Cerebrospinal nematodiasis in a cockatiel. *Journal of the American Veterinary Medical Association* 183:1089–1090.

Nadler, S.A. 1992. Phylogeny of some ascaridoid nematodes, inferred from comparison of 18S and 28S rRNA sequences. *Molecular Biology and Evolution* 9:932–944.

Nadler, S.A., and D.S.S. Hudspeth. 2000. Phylogeny of the Ascariodoidea (Nematoda: Ascaridida) based on three genes and morphology: Hypotheses of structural and sequence evolution. *Journal of Parasitology* 86:380–393.

Nettles, V.F., W.R. Davidson, S.K. Fisk, and H.A. Jacobson. 1975. An epizootic of cerebrospinal nematodiasis in cottontail rabbits. *Journal of the American Veterinary Medical Association* 167:600–602.

Nichols, R.L. 1956a. The etiology of visceral larva migrans. I. Diagnostic morphology of infective second-stage *Toxocara* larvae. *The Journal of Parasitology* 42:349–362.

———. 1956b. The etiology of visceral larva migrans. II. Comparative larval morphology of *Ascaris lumbricoides, Necator americanus, Strongyloides stercoralis,* and *Ancylostoma caninum. The Journal of Parasitology* 42:363–399.

Olsen, O.W., and R. Fenstermacher. 1938. The raccoon, a new host of *Ascaris columnaris* Leidy, 1856 (Nematoda:Ascaridae). *Proceedings of the Helminthological Society of Washington* 5:20.

Overstreet, R.M. 1970. *Baylisascaris procyonis* (Stefanski and Zarnowski, 1951) from the kinkajou, *Potos flavus,* in Colombia. *Proceedings of the Helminthological Society of Washington* 37:192–195.

Page, L.K. 1998. Ecology and transmission dynamics of *Baylisascaris procyonis.* Ph.D. Thesis, Purdue University, West Lafayette, IN, 138 pp.

Page, L.K., R.K. Swihart, and K.R. Kazacos. 1998. Raccoon latrine structure and its potential role in transmission of *Baylisascaris procyonis* to vertebrates. *American Midland Naturalist* 140:180–185.

———. 1999. Implications of raccoon latrines in the epizootiology of baylisascariasis. *Journal of Wildlife Diseases* 35:474–480.

Papini, R., and L. Casarosa. 1994. A report on the pathology of *Baylisascaris transfuga* (Ascarididae: Nematoda) for mice. *Revue de Medecine Veterinaire* 145:949–952.

Papini, R., G. Renzoni, S. LoPiccolo, and L. Casarosa. 1996. Ocular larva migrans and histopathological lesions in mice experimentally infected with *Baylisascaris transfuga* embryonated eggs. *Veterinary Parasitology* 61:315–320.

Park, C., D.J. Levee, S. Gilbreath, R. Parman, L. Frazer, R. Kaufman, and W.J. Murray. 1998. A survey of the prevalence of the raccoon ascarid, *Baylisascaris procyonis,* in a geographically defined population of suburban and urban raccoons. *Proceedings of the American Society for Microbiology* 98:547.

Park, S.Y., C. Glaser, W.J. Murray, K.R. Kazacos, H.R. Rowley, D. Frederick, and N. Bass. Raccoon roundworm (*Baylisascaris procyonis*) encephalitis: Case report and field investigation. *Pediatrics.* 106:E56.

Parsons, H.E. 1952. Nematode chorioretinitis. Report of a case, with photographs of a viable worm. *Archives of Ophthalmology* 47:799–800.

Pegg, E.J. 1977. A new approach to the control of *Toxocara canis* and other parasitic ova on concrete-floored kennel runs. *British Veterinary Journal* 133:427–431.

Pessier, A.P., C. Stringfield, J. Tragle, H.J. Holshuh, D.K. Nichols, and R.J. Montali. 1997. Cerebrospinal nematodiasis due to *Baylisascaris* sp. in golden-headed lion tamarins (*Leontopithecus chrysomelas*): Implications for management. *Proceedings of the American Association of Zoo Veterinarians,* pp. 245–247.

Pigage, J.C., H.K. Pigage, and K.S. Todd, Jr. 1983. Intestinal parasites of mammals from Willowbrook Wildlife Haven: A survey with implications for management. *Proceedings of the National Wildlife Rehabilitation Association* 2:174–184.

Price, R.L., and D.M. Harman. 1983. Helminths from the raccoon, *Procyon lotor litoreus* Nelson and Goldman 1930, on St. Catherines Island, Georgia. *Proceedings of the Helminthological Society of Washington* 50:343–344.

Rausch, R. 1946. The raccoon, a new host for *Microphallus* sp., with additional notes on *M. ovatus* from turtles. *The Journal of Parasitology* 32:208–209.

Raymond, L.A., Y. Gutierrez, L.E. Strong, A.H. Wander, R. Buten, and D. Cordan. 1978. Living retinal nematode (filarial-like) destroyed with photocoagulation. *Ophthalmology* 85:944–949.

Reed, W.M., K.R. Kazacos, A.S. Dhillon, R.W. Winterfield, and H.L. Thacker. 1981. Cerebrospinal nematodiasis in bobwhite quail. *Avian Diseases* 25:1039–1046.

Richardson, D.J., W.B. Owen, and D.E. Snyder. 1992. Helminth parasites of the raccoon (*Procyon lotor*) from north-central Arkansas. *The Journal of Parasitology* 78:163–166.

Richardson, J.A., K.R. Kazacos, H.L. Thacker, A.S. Dhillon, and R.W. Winterfield. 1980. Verminous encephalitis in commercial chickens. *Avian Diseases* 24:498–503.

Richter, C.B., and D.C. Kradel. 1964. Cerebrospinal nematodosis in Pennsylvania groundhogs (*Marmota monax*). *American Journal of Veterinary Research* 25:1230–1235.

Robel, R.J., N.A. Barnes, and S.J. Upton. 1989. Gastrointestinal helminths and protozoa from two raccoon populations in Kansas. *The Journal of Parasitology* 75:1000–1003.

Robinson, V.B., J.W. Newberne, and D.M. Brooks. 1957. Distemper in the American raccoon (*Procyon lotor*). *Journal of the American Veterinary Medical Association* 131:276–278.

Rosatte, RC., M.J. Powers, and C.D. MacInnes. 1991. Ecology of urban skunks, raccoons and foxes in metropolitan Toronto. In *Wildlife conservation in metropolitan environments.* Ed. L.W. Adams and D.L. Leedy. Columbia, MD: National Institute of Urban Wildlife, pp. 31–38.

Roth, L., M.E. Georgi, J.M. King, and B.C. Tennant. 1982. Parasitic encephalitis due to *Baylisascaris* sp. in wild and captive woodchucks (*Marmota monax*). *Veterinary Pathology* 19:658–662.

Rowley, H.A., R.M. Uht, K.R. Kazacos, J. Sakanari, W.V. Wheaton, A.J. Barkovich, and A.W. Bollen. 2000. Radiological-pathological findings in raccoon roundworm (*Baylisascaris procyonis*) encephalitis. *American Journal of Neuroradiology* 21:415–420.

Rudmann, D.G., K.R. Kazacos, S.T. Storandt, D.L. Harris, and E.B. Janovitz. 1996. *Baylisascaris procyonis* larva migrans in a puppy: A case report and update for the veterinarian. *Journal of the American Animal Hospital Association* 32:73–76.

Sakla, A.A., J.J. Donnelly, M. Khatami, and J.H. Rockey. 1989. *Baylisascaris procyonis* (Stefanski and Zarnowski, 1951) Ascarididae: Nematoda. I. Embryonic development and morphogenesis of second stage larvae. *Assiut Veterinary Medical Journal* 21:68–76.

Sanford, S.E. 1991. Cerebrospinal nematodiasis caused by *Baylisascaris procyonis* in chinchillas. *Journal of Veterinary Diagnostic Investigation* 3:77–79.

Sass, B., and E.J. Gorgacz. 1978. Cerebral nematodiasis in a chukar partridge. *Journal of the American Veterinary Medical Association* 173:1248–1249.

Schaffer, G.D., W.R. Davidson, V.F. Nettles, and E.A. Rollor III. 1981. Helminth parasites of translocated raccoons (*Procyon lotor*) in the southeastern United States. *Journal of Wildlife Diseases* 17:217–227.

Schrott, E.R. 1961. Parasitäre Netzhauterkrankung durch Askaris. *Verhandlungen der Österreichischen Ophthalmologischen Gesellschaft* 6:160–165.

Schueler, R.L. 1973. Cerebral nematodiasis in a red squirrel. *Journal of Wildlife Diseases* 9:58–60.

Schultz, A.L. 1962. A survey of parasites of the raccoon (*Procyon lotor*) in southeastern Michigan. M.S. Thesis, The University of Michigan, Ann Arbor, MI, 42 pp.

Senger, C.M., and K.A. Neiland. 1955. Helminth parasites of some fur-bearers of Oregon. *The Journal of Parasitology* 41:637–638.

Sheppard, C.H. 1995. Susceptibility of *Peromyscus leucopus* (white-footed mouse) and *Mus musculus* (albino mouse) to infection with *Baylisascaris procyonis*. M.S. Thesis, Purdue University, West Lafayette, IN, 108 pp.

———. 1996. Verhalten und Pathogenität der Larven von *Baylisascaris procyonis* Stefanski und Zarnowski, 1951 (Ascarididae) in verschiedenen Mäusearten. Dissertation, Doctor Medicinae Veterinariae, Tierärztliche Hochschule Hannover, Hannover, Germany, 100 pp.

Sheppard, C.H., and K.R. Kazacos. 1997 . Susceptibility of *Peromyscus leucopus* and *Mus musculus* to infection with *Baylisascaris procyonis*. *The Journal of Parasitology* 83:1104–1111.

Smiley, D. 1977a. Research report—Raccoon. New Paltz, NY: Mohonk Preserve, Daniel Smiley Research Center, 19 pp.

———. 1977b. Research report—Cave (Wood) Rat. New Paltz, NY: Mohonk Preserve, Daniel Smiley Research Center, 5 pp.

Smiley, D., and P.C. Huth. 1986. "Crazy" animals. Natural Science Note No. 115. New Paltz, NY: Mohonk Preserve, Daniel Smiley Research Center, 2 pp.

Smith, R.A., M.L. Kennedy, and W.E. Wilhelm. 1985. Helminth parasites of the raccoon (*Procyon lotor*) from Tennessee and Kentucky. *The Journal of Parasitology* 71:599–603.

Smith, S.L. 1992. The presence of the raccoon roundworm, *Baylisascaris procyonis* in *Procyon lotor* in Nova Scotia. Senior Honors Thesis, Acadia University, Wolfville, Nova Scotia, 12 pp.

Smyth, J.D. 1995. Rare, new and emerging helminth zoonoses. *Advances in Parasitology* 36: 1–45.

Snyder, D.E. 1983. The prevalence, cross-transmissibility to domestic animals and adult structure of *Baylisascaris procyonis* (Nematoda) from Illinois raccoons (*Procyon lotor*). Ph.D. Thesis, University of Illinois at Urbana-Champaign, Urbana, IL, 233 pp.

———. 1989. Scanning electron microscopic observations of adult *Baylisascaris procyonis* (Nematoda). *International Journal for Parasitology* 19:571–574.

Snyder, D.E., and P.R. Fitzgerald. 1985. The relationship of *Baylisascaris procyonis* to Illinois raccoons (*Procyon lotor*). *The Journal of Parasitology* 71:596–598.

———. 1987. Contaminative potential, egg prevalence, and intensity of *Baylisascaris procyonis*-infected raccoons (*Procyon lotor*) from Illinois, with a comparison to worm intensity. *Proceedings of the Helminthological Society of Washington* 54:141–145.

Sprehn, C., and U. Haakh. 1956. Zur Morphologie des Waschbärenspulwurmes und seiner Stellung im System. *Zeitschrift für angewandte Zoologie* 1:95–102.

Sprent, J.F.A. 1951. On the migratory behavior of the larvae of various *Ascaris* species in mice. *The Journal of Parasitology* 37(Supplement): 21.

———. 1952a. On the migratory behavior of the larvae of various *Ascaris* species in white mice. I. Distribution of larvae in tissues. *Journal of Infectious Diseases* 90:165–176.

———. 1952b. On an Ascaris parasite of the fisher and marten, *Ascaris devosi* sp. nov. *Proceedings of the Helminthological Society of Washington* 19:27–37.

———. 1953a. On the migratory behavior of the larvae of various *Ascaris* species in white mice. II. Longevity of encapsulated larvae and their resistance to freezing and putrefaction. *Journal of Infectious Diseases* 92:114–117.

———. 1953b. On the life history of *Ascaris devosi* and its development in the white mouse and the domestic ferret. *Parasitology* 42:244–258.

———. 1955. On the invasion of the central nervous system by nematodes. II. Invasion of the nervous system in ascariasis. *Parasitology* 45:41–55.

———. 1968. Notes on *Ascaris* and *Toxascaris,* with a definition of *Baylisascaris* gen.nov. *Parasitology* 58:185–198.

———. 1970. *Baylisascaris tasmaniensis* sp.nov. in marsupial carnivores: Heirloom or souvenir? *Parasitology* 61:75–86.

Sprent, J.F.A., J. Lamina, and A. McKeown. 1973. Observations on migratory behaviour and development of *Baylisascaris tasmaniensis*. *Parasitology* 67:67–83.

Stains, H.J. 1956. The raccoon in Kansas. *Miscellaneous Publications of the Museum of Natural History, University of Kansas*, 10:1–76.

Stefanski, W., and E. Zarnowski. 1951. *Ascaris procyonis* n. sp. z jelita szopa (*Procyon lotor* L.) *Ascaris procyonis* n. sp. provenant de l'intestin de *Procyon lotor* L. *Annales Musei Zoologici Polonici* 14:199–202.

Stone, W.B. 1983. Intestinal obstruction in raccoons caused by the ascarid *Baylisascaris procyonis*. *New York Fish and Game Journal* 30:117–118.

Stringfield, C.E., and C.J. Sedgwick. 1997. Baylisascaris: A zoo-wide experience. *Proceedings of the American Association of Zoo Veterinarians*, pp. 73–77.

Stuewer, F.W. 1943. Raccoons: Their habits and management in Michigan. *Ecological Monographs* 13:204–257.

Suedmeyer, W.K., A. Bermudez, and K.R. Kazacos. 1996. Cerebellar nematodiasis in an emu (*Dromaius novaehollandiae*). *Journal of Zoo and Wildlife Medicine* 27:544–549.

Swerczek, T.W., and C.F. Helmboldt. 1970. Cerebrospinal nematodiasis in groundhogs (*Marmota monax*). *Journal of the American Veterinary Medical Association* 157:671–674.

Tecec, T.G. 1987. Occurrence of *Baylisascaris procyonis* in raccoon populations on military installations in the Washington, DC, area. *Military Medicine* 152:83–84.

Tenora, F., and M. Stanek. 1990. Scanning electron microscopy of *Toxascaris procyonis* Stefanski et Zarnowski, 1951 (Nematoda). *Helminthologia* 27:73–77.

Tenora, F., M. Hönigová, and M. Stanek. 1991. Interesting findings of two species of Ascaridata (Nematoda)—Parasites of carnivora in Czech and Slovak Federative Republic. *Helminthologia* 28:131–135.

Thomas, J.S. 1988. Encephalomyelitis in a dog caused by *Baylisascaris* infection. *Veterinary Pathology* 25:94–95.

Tiner, J.D. 1949. Preliminary observations on the life history of *Ascaris columnaris*. *The Journal of Parasitology* 35(Supplement): 13.

———. 1951. Observations on larval carnivore ascarids in rodents. *The Journal of Parasitology* 37(Supplement): 21–22.

———. 1952a. A study of the epidemiology of ascarid nematodes in carnivores and rodents. Ph.D. Thesis, University of Illinois, Urbana, IL, 130 pp.

———. 1952b. Speciation in the genus *Ascaris:* Additional experimental and morphological data. *The Journal of Parasitology* 38(Supplement): 27.

———. 1953a. Fatalities in rodents caused by larval *Ascaris* in the central nervous system. *Journal of Mammalogy* 34:153–167.

———. 1953b. The migration, distribution in the brain, and growth of ascarid larvae in rodents. *Journal of Infectious Diseases* 92:105–113.

———. 1954. The fraction of *Peromyscus leucopus* fatalities caused by raccoon ascarid larvae. *Journal of Mammalogy* 35:589–592.

Tseng, F.S. 1997. Baylisascaris in squirrels. *Proceedings of the North American Veterinary Conference*, pp. 817–818.

Van Andel, R.A., C.L. Franklin, C. Besch-Williford, L.K. Riley, RR. Hook, Jr., and K.R. Kazacos. 1995. Cerebrospinal larva migrans due to *Baylisascaris procyonis* in a guinea pig colony. *Laboratory Animal Science* 45:27–30.

Voge, M. 1956. A list of nematode parasites from California mammals. *American Midland Naturalist* 56:423–429.

Waller, E.F. 1940. Infectious gastroenteritis in raccoons (*Procyon lotor*). *Journal of the American Veterinary Medical Association* 96:266–268.

Weller, P.F. 1992. Eosinophilic syndromes. In *Cecil textbook of medicine,* 19th ed., vol. 1. Ed. J.B. Wyngaarden, L.H. Smith, Jr., and J.C. Bennett. Philadelphia, PA: W.B. Saunders Co., pp. 965–967.

Weller, P.F., and L.X. Liu. 1993. Eosinophilic meningitis. *Seminars in Neurology* 13:161–168.

Williams, C.K., R.D. McKown, J.K. Veatch, and R.D. Applegate. 1997. *Baylisascaris* sp. found in a wild northern bobwhite (*Colinus virginianus*). *Journal of Wildlife Diseases* 33:158–160.

Williams, G.A., T.M. Aaberg, and S.S. Dudley. 1988. Perimacular photocoagulation of presumed *Baylisascaris procyonis* in diffuse unilateral subacute neuroretinitis. *In Laser photocoagulation of retinal disease.* Ed. K.A. Gitter, H. Schatz, L.A. Yannuzzi, and H.R. McDonald. San Francisco, CA: Pacific Medical Press, pp. 275–280.

Winterfield, R.W., and H.L. Thacker. 1978. Verminous encephalitis in the emu. *Avian Diseases* 22:336–339.

Wirtz, W.L. 1982. Cerebrospinal nematodiasis due to the raccoon ascarid, *Baylisascaris procyonis*. M.S. Thesis, Purdue University, West Lafayette, IN, 90 pp.

Wyand-Ouellette, W.K., K.R. Kazacos, and D.B. DeNicola. 1983. Assessment of pulmonary migration of ascarids (*Baylisascaris, Ascaris*) by bronchopulmonary lavage. *Proceedings of the American Association of Veterinary Parasitologists* 28:24.

Yabsley, M.J., and G.P. Noblet. 1999. Nematodes and acanthocephalans of raccoons (*Procyon lotor*), with a new geographical record for *Centrorhynchus conspectus* (Acanthocephala) in South Carolina, USA. *Journal of the Helminthological Society of Washington* 66:111–114.

Yeager, L.E., and R.G. Rennels. 1943. Fur yield and autumn foods of the raccoon in Illinois river bottom lands. *The Journal of Wildlife Management* 7:45–60.

12

FILARIOID NEMATODES

ROY C. ANDERSON

INTRODUCTION. Filarioid nematodes are highly specialized parasites of tissues and tissue spaces of vertebrates other than fishes. Most produce modified first-stage larvae called microfilariae that enter blood or lodge in the skin of the definitive host, where they are available to arthropods that ingest blood and serve as intermediate hosts and vectors. In the intermediate host microfilariae develop to infective third-stage larvae that move to the mouthparts of the vector. Larvae leave the vector when it is feeding on the host. These larvae generally invade the puncture wound made by the vector when it is feeding on the definitive host. In ticks that remain attached to the host, larvae may leave by way of salivary secretions. In the definitive host larvae develop to adulthood after undergoing two molts and then migrate to a specific site where they produce microfilariae which reach the blood or skin.

If vectors of a filarioid have broad feeding preferences, infective larvae can be transmitted to a variety of vertebrates other than those to which they are adapted. Most transmission of this type is probably harmless because larvae that leave the vector when it is feeding will not invade the tissues if the host is unsuitable or, if they do, they perish shortly thereafter. In some instances, however, larvae may develop to a more advanced stage but eventually become encapsulated and destroyed by the host's defense mechanisms (e.g., subcutaneous *Dirofilaria* spp.).

On the other hand, some filarioids are not highly host specific. *Brugia malayi* in southeast Asia, for example, can be found in humans, monkeys, felids, canids, viverrids, and pangolins. It can be transmitted experimentally to lorises, rats, and jirds. This species is very well adapted to wild animals in the tropics and is not associated with disease in them. Although developing normally to the adult stage and producing microfilariae in humans, it provokes inflammation in the lymphatics that, in chronic infections, can lead to elephantiasis. Evidently, humans are not as well adapted to *B. malayi* as are the wild animal reservoirs.

Another zoonotic filarioid, *Brugia pahangi,* is well adapted to canids, felids, monkeys, and some other mammals in southeast Asia. In humans, however, it fails to produce microfilariae and provokes a strong allergic reaction in the host ("tropical eosinophilia"). Elaeophorosis provides an excellent example of a filarioid perfectly adapted to one host species, but highly pathogenic in related hosts. *Elaeophora schneideri,* the arterial nematode of mule deer (*Odocoileus hemionus hemionus*) and black-tailed deer (*Odocoileus h. columbianus*) of western North America, is clinically silent in these hosts to which it is perfectly adapted. In elk/wapiti (*Cervus elaphus*), moose (*Alces alces),* sheep, and goats, however, which acquire infective larvae from biting Tabanidae that have fed on infected deer, the parasite provokes vascular abnormalities or allergic reactions. Thus, the parasite develops in the new host as it does in the usual natural host, but subtle variations in behavior combined with inappropriate host responses lead to severe disease (cf. parelaphostrongylosis).

There are few other examples of filarioids known to cause disease in wild mammals. The heartworm, *Dirofilaria immitis,* of dogs can be transmitted to wild canids, felids, and mustelids and has the potential to be a pathogen in these new hosts. Reports of *Setaria cervi* in the central nervous system of deer are worth a mention in view of the proven neurotropism of *Setaria digitata* of cattle. Two species of *Pelecitus* found in leg joints of their host appear capable of causing arthritis. Finally, recent studies of lymphatic filarioids in wild rodents have revealed skin and eye lesions associated with the microfilariae, which inhabit the skin of the host.

ETIOLOGIC AGENTS

***Elaeophora schneideri* Wehr and Dikmans, 1935: Elaeophorosis.** Members of the genus *Elaeophora* Railliet and Henry, 1912 occur in the arteries of ruminants. *Elaeophora schneideri* of cervids in North America is the only species studied intensively, and excellent reviews have been published (Hibler and Adcock 1971; Hibler and Prestwood 1981; Pence 1991).

Elaeophora schneideri are rather robust worms with markedly tapered extremities (Fig. 12.1). Adult females are 60–120 mm in length and 0.6–0.9 mm in width; males are 55–85 mm in length and 0.4–0.9mm in width. Worms tend to coil probably as an adaptation to holding themselves in the arteries of their hosts. The tail in both sexes ends in a terminal cone-shaped protuberance and two lateroventral, tongue-like appendages.

342

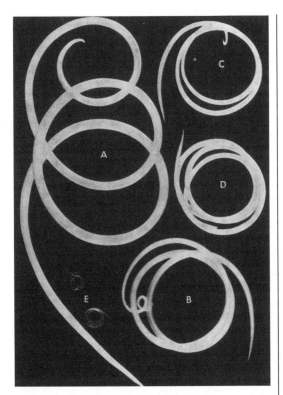

FIG. 12.1—*Elaeophora schneideri* from the arteries of deer and elk. (**A**) sexually mature gravid female from a deer; (**B**) sexually mature male from deer; (**C, D**) sexually immature fifth-stage male and female from a blind elk, and (**E**) late fourth-stage male and female from a blind elk. (4X magnification) [After Hibler, C.P., and J.L. Adcock (1971) with permission of Iowa State University Press]

Elaeophora schneideri was first described from domestic sheep and mule deer (Wehr and Dikmans 1935). Worms in two sheep from New Mexico were found in the "carotid artery in the parotid gland region, from the posterior aorta in the iliac region, and from the mesenteric arteries." Specimens from a deer in Utah were "obtained from cut surfaces of the head . . . approximately 24 hours after it had been killed and the head removed."

Kemper (1938) found *E. schneideri* in domestic sheep in New Mexico with "filarial dermatitis" (or "sore-head") and foot lesions associated with microfilariae of *E. schneideri*. Davis and Kemper (1951) described in detail the histopathologic features of cutaneous lesions in sheep in New Mexico, which they attributed to the presence of microfilariae of *E. schneideri*. Douglas et al. (1954) reported filarial dermatitis in sheep in California and Oregon, which they attributed to an allergic reaction. In 1954, Smith et al. reported filarial dermatitis sheep in Nebraska, which they attributed to the presence of microfilariae. Jensen

and Seghetti (1955) described in considerable detail the lesions in sheep and attributed various lesions, including those in the nasal and oral mucosae and the cornea, to microfilariae. They reported for the first time arterial damage associated with adult *E. schneideri*.

In the meantime, *E. schneideri* was reported in deer in California (Herman 1945; Longhurst et al. 1952) and British Columbia (Cowan 1946). Douglas et al. (1954) pointed out that filarial dermatitis was not reported in deer infected with *E. schneideri* in Arizona, British Columbia, California, Colorado, and Utah.

During roughly the same period that filarial dermatitis was being reported and studied in sheep in the western United States, reports of blind elk (or wapiti) were accumulating, beginning with Rush (1932) and Mills (1936) with cases from Yellowstone National Park. Other reports came from Arizona (White 1957–1959; Gallizioli 1963) and Wyoming (Howe and Hepworth 1964). The latter also reported necrosis of the nose and tips of the ears in a blind elk. Davis et al. (1965) reported brain lesions in three blind elk from Arizona.

Adcock et al. (1965), in a preliminary communication, reported lesions in the eyes, optic nerves, and brains of blind elk, and they discovered *E. schneideri* in this host for the first time. In 1969 Adcock and Hibler reported that lesions in elk, including blindness, were not the result of reaction to microfilariae, but of vascular changes impairing cephalic arterial circulation leading to ischemic necrosis. These changes were directly related to the presence of adult *E. schneideri* in the arteries. This classic discovery opened up new research that finally elucidated the details of the biology of *E. schneideri* and its relationship to mule deer and elk (Hibler et al. 1969, 1970, 1971, 1974).

As Pence (1991) noted, elaeophorosis is a complex disease. In recent years there have been relatively few reports of the disease in elk and moose. This should not be interpreted as evidence that the disease has disappeared or is now of little consequence. Prevalence of the disease is presumably related to the density of reservoir hosts and susceptible alternate hosts (e.g., moose, elk) as well as the abundance of tabanid vectors, all of which can be highly variable from 1 year to the next. In particular, tabanid populations can be affected by unpredictable weather patterns, and this could temporarily restrict transmission for varying periods of time.

LIFE HISTORY. *Elaeophora schneideri* is found mainly in the common carotid arteries and the internal maxillary arteries but has also been reported in the heart, thoracic and abdominal aortas, and femoral and digital arteries (Hibler and Prestwood 1981). It can probably occur in any artery large enough to accommodate the adult worm. Microfilariae are found in capillaries of the skin of the forehead and face. They have been found in the mucous membranes of the head and in the skin of the lower legs in sheep.

The parasite is transmitted by horseflies (Tabanidae; Diptera) of the genera *Hybomitra* and *Tabanus* (see

TABLE 12.1—Intermediate hosts (vectors) of *Elaeophora schneideri* (from Pence 1991)

Area/Study	Species	Reference
Gila National Forest, New Mexico	*Hybomitra laticornis, H. phaenops, H. tetrica rubilata Tabanus abditus, T. eurycerus, T. gilanus Silvius quadrivittatus*	Clark and Hibler 1973
Northern California	*Hybomitra procyon Tabanus monsensis*	Anderson and Weinmann 1972
Vermejo Ranch, New Mexico	*Hybomitra aatos Tabanus punctifer, T. subsimilis, T. stoni*	Davies 1979
South Island, South Carolina	*Tabanus lineola hinettus, T. nigrovittatus*	Couvillion et al. 1984
Central Montana	*Hybomitra rupestris, H. tetrica, H. osburni*	Espinosa 1987

Table 12.1 from Pence 1991). In the Gila National Forest in New Mexico horseflies were found only at elevations above 6000 feet (1829 m) and were most numerous at about 7000 feet (2134 m) (Hibler and Adcock 1971). They were active from 0900 to 1700 hours, with maximum activity from 1100 to 1400 hours at temperatures of 90° F–100° F (32°C–38° C) and humidity < 10%. They were less active on cool cloudy, humid days or in windy conditions. Flies feed mainly on the forehead and face of deer and elk, and engorgement requires about 3 minutes.

In the Gila National Forest, horseflies emerged about the last week in May and reached peak numbers during the hot, dry month of June (Hibler et al. 1969). They disappeared almost completely with the advent of summer rains, which began the first week of July. This was generally true throughout the enzootic areas and helped to explain why infections in elk calves generally occurred during the second and third weeks of life (Hibler et al. 1969).

Hybomitra laticornis constituted 90% of infected flies collected in the Gila National Forest (Hibler et al. 1969, 1971) and is considered the main vector (Clark and Hibler 1973). Horseflies, mainly *H. laticornis,* in the Sacramento Mountains of the Lincoln National Forest in southeastern New Mexico, peaked about the third week in June, and high numbers persisted for 2–3 weeks (Pence 1991). The population size of the flies is much greater in dry than in wet years. *Hybomitra aatos* was the most commonly infected fly in the Vermejo Ranch, New Mexico, (Davies 1979) and Espinosa (1987) incriminated three tabanids in southwestern Montana (Table 12.1).

Prevalences of infected larvae in horseflies were high but variable, depending on the locality of study. Hibler et al. (1971) reported 20% and Clark (1972) 15% in the Gila National Forest. Davies (1979) reported 10% in Vermejo Ranch, New Mexico, and Espinosa (1987) reported 0.8% in Montana.

In eastern North America third-stage larvae occurred in only 31 of 10,540 (0.3%) of *Tabanus lineola hinellus* collected in South Island, South Carolina (Couvillion et al. 1984). Only two larvae were found in 9543 *T. nigrovittatus* and none in *Chrysops* spp. and two other species of *Hybomitra*. Intensity of larvae in flies in the Gila National Forest was 17.4 (1–181) (Hibler et al. 1971). Intensity in infected flies collected in South Carolina was 14 (1–64) (Couvillion et al. 1984).

Microfilariae invaded the fat body lining the abdomen of horseflies and grew into first-stage larvae (Hibler et al. 1971; Hibler and Metzger 1974). When about 350–400 μm in length, larvae left the fat body and continued development to the third stage in the hemocoel. Infective larvae were 3.29–5.03 mm in length and could readily be identified to sex by the structure of the genital primordia. The tail of the infective larva had a posterior, cone-shaped projection and a pair of lateral, tongue-like structures. Neither the time required for development to the infective stage nor the time of the two molts has been determined. Larvae eventually migrated to the head and mouthparts of the fly.

The precise behavior of larvae in mule deer, the usual host, is still not fully understood, and some parts of the following account require confirmation. Information is based on examination of experimentally infected deer and sheep, and necropsy findings of other deer and sheep (Hibler et al. 1969, 1970, 1974; Hibler and Metzger 1974). It is believed infective larvae remain at the subcutaneous site of entry 6–12 hours and then enter the venous system and are carried to the heart and lungs, where they enter the arterial system. The infective larvae of *E. schneideri* are enormous compared to those of other filarioids, and perhaps the large size is related to the need to maintain themselves in arteries with a rapid blood flow. It is not known how larvae entered the carotid or cephalic arterial system, but they eventually reached the leptomeningeal arteries, where they rapidly grew into immature adults 10–13 mm in length in about 2 weeks. In 3.5–4 weeks nematodes (18–20 mm in length) moved into the carotids, where they matured in about 4.5 months. The prepatent period was about 5.5 months, although skin-inhabiting microfilariae were difficult to demonstrate by biopsy until some time after that (in mid-December and early January in deer infected in June).

HOSTS AND GEOGRAPHIC DISTRIBUTION

MULE DEER AND BLACK-TAILED DEER. Mule and black-tailed deer in western North America are well-adapted hosts of *E. schneideri*. The parasite has been

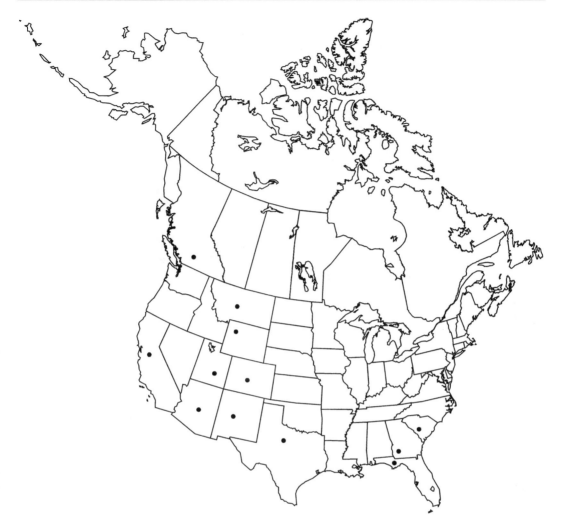

FIG. 12.2—States and provinces where *Elaeophora schneideri* has been reported in North America. Western reports refer almost totally to *Odocoileus hemionus*. Case reports in the southeastern states (Florida, Georgia, South Carolina) refer to *Odocoileus virginianus* and are probably the result of introductions of infected deer from western regions.

found in deer in Utah, Colorado, New Mexico, Arizona, Texas, California, Montana, Wyoming, and British Columbia. Prevalences in mule deer are often high. Hibler et al. (1969) noted that nearly all mule deer in certain areas of southwestern, western, and northern New Mexico were infected. Hibler and Adcock (1971) reported prevalences of 19%–58% in mule deer in Arizona, 4%–57% in Colorado, 60%–100% in New Mexico, and 4%–44% in California (Fig. 12.2). Weinmann et al. (1973) found 78% of black-tailed deer infected in California. Pence and Gray (1981) reported 100% prevalence in northwest Texas.

WHITE-TAILED DEER. *Elaeophora schneideri* is not as common in white-tailed deer as it is in mule deer. Hibler et al. (1969) reported infections in 13% of 15 white-

tailed deer in contrast to 59% of 46 mule deer in the same region in Arizona. Prestwood and Ridgeway (1972) found infected white-tailed deer in the southern Atlantic and Gulf coastal plain of Florida, Georgia, and South Carolina, but prevalences ranged from only 2% to 10%. Waid et al. (1984) found only 9% of 89 white-tailed deer infected in the central Texas hill country. It has been suggested that *E. schneideri* was introduced into the southeastern United States in recent times, perhaps by interstate movement of animals from enzootic areas in the west to eastern regions (Prestwood and Ridgeway 1972; Pence 1991). The parasite has evidently not spread significantly in eastern North America.

ELK (WAPITI) AND MOOSE. Infected elk have been reported in Arizona, New Mexico, Colorado, and

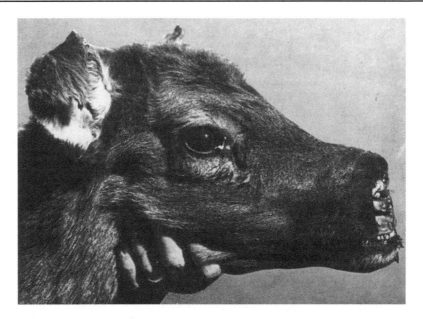

FIG. 12.3—Blind elk calf, 5 months old, showing dry gangrene of the ear tips and extensive necrosis of the muzzle and nostrils [After Hibler C.P. and J.L. Adcock (1971) with permission of Iowa State University Press].

Wyoming. Hibler and Adcock (1971) reported infection in 88% of 42 elk from the Sitgreaves National Forest in Arizona. In the Gila National Forest in New Mexico, 93% of 15 elk were infected, and in southwestern Colorado 12% of 100 were infected. Four infected moose have been found in Montana (Worley et al. 1972, Worley 1975) and 2 from Colorado (Madden et al. 1991).

SHEEP. It was estimated in 1971 that *E. schneideri* occurred in about 1% of domestic sheep in New Mexico, Arizona, and Colorado. Pence and Grey (1981) reported the nematode in three of nine Barbary sheep (*Ammotragus lervia*) in northwestern Texas.

SIKA DEER (*CERVUS NIPPON*). Robinson et al. (1978) reported lesions in Sika deer on game farms in Texas.

CLINICAL SIGNS. Clinical signs generally are absent in mule and black-tailed deer. Obstruction of a coronary artery in an experimentally infected white-tailed deer fawn caused death (Titche et al. 1979). Clinical signs (Figs. 12.3, 12.4) in elk are striking and include bilateral blindness, usually without opacity of the ocular refractive media ("clear-eyed blindness") (Hibler and Adcock 1971). Other signs include circling, ataxia, nystagmus, necrosis of the muzzle and nostrils, dry gangrene of the ear tips, abnormal antler growth, and emaciation. Clinical signs are seen mainly in calves and yearlings. Clinical signs in two moose included blindness, circling, staggering, and ataxia (Worley et al. 1972, Madden et al. 1991).

Domestic sheep infected with small numbers of larvae may develop severe brain damage, blindness, and death (C.P. Hibler, personal communication). Chronic signs in domestic sheep consist of a dermatitis with tissue proliferation involving skin in the region of the pole and sometimes extending forward over the face to the nostrils and lips (Kemper 1938). Numerous small abscesses were produced in the skin. Similar lesions occurred on the abdomen and feet. Lesions are obviously aggravated by rubbing and scratching with the feet. *Elaeophora schneideri* is highly pathogenic in goats, and more than ten nematodes can result in severe brain damage and associated signs of disease (C.P. Hibler, personal communication).

PATHOLOGY AND PATHOGENESIS

MULE AND BLACK-TAILED DEER. There are no major pathologic changes associated with the presence of *E. schneideri* in these hosts, although Hibler and Adcock (1971) reported dead and mineralized adults, thrombosis and fibrous intimal sclerosis in carotid and internal maxillary arteries, and chronic granulomatous dermatitis associated with microfilariae in the skin of the forehead.

WHITE-TAILED DEER. Titche et al. (1979) infected fawns, and one died because of coronary obstruction caused by *E. schneideri*. Plaque-like lesions were observed on the internal lining of carotids, as were subintimal thickening and proliferation of fibrous tissue in vessel walls; the changes were considered minor,

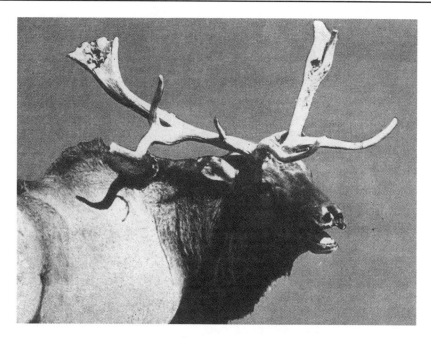

FIG. 12.4—Blind mature bull elk kept alive in captivity since calfhood. Note the malformed antlers, cropped ear, and healed muzzle. [After Hibler, C.P. and J.L. Adcock (1971) with permission of Iowa State University Press].

however. Couvillion et al. (1986) reported intimal thickening, disruption of the internal elastic lamina, and verminous thrombosis in cephalic arteries with *E. schneideri*. Microfilariae caused focal necrosis and fibrosis in the myocardium. In addition, 11 of 14 deer had oral food impaction, mainly sublingual, which might have been related to the presence of *E. schneideri,* but the observations were inconclusive.

ELK. The pathology and pathogenesis in elk have been described in detail by Adcock and Hibler (1969) and Hibler and Adcock (1971) in classic papers. In this host the disease mainly affects ". . . the cephalic arterial system resulting in circulatory impairment which produces secondary ischemic damage in the brain, eyes, optic nerves, ears, muzzle, and other tissues of the head . . ." (including the growing antlers) (Hibler and Adcock 1971). "Blindness and other clinical features and death are attributed to lesions in these secondarily affected structures." The disease can affect all age groups of elk and be fatal in a few weeks or several months.

Larvae and adult nematodes occur mainly in the cephalic arteries from the ascending aorta and the common brachiocephalic trunk to small leptomeningeal arteries and small arteries supplying the eyes and optic nerves. Microfilariae are present mainly in smaller arteries as well as in arterioles and capillaries of the brain, eyes, optic nerve, and skin of the head. The presence of various stages of the nematodes in the arteries provokes intimal damage due to mechanical irritation,

consisting of swelling, degeneration, and loss of the endothelium, followed by the buildup of plasma protein on, or within, the intima (Fig. 12.5). As the process advances, thrombosis, inflammatory infiltration of the intima, and fibroblastic intimal proliferation eventually results in occlusion of the vessel (Fig. 12.6). Arteriolar and capillary changes caused by microfilariae are similar to those induced by larvae and adult nematodes (i.e., thrombosis, endothelium proliferation, degeneration and inflammation of vessel walls, and the formation of granulomas).

Vascular occlusion results in ischemic necrosis in the cerebral cortex, basal nuclei, thalamus, hippocampus, lateral geniculate bodies, and cerebellum. Blindness is the result of damage in the occipital cortex and lateral geniculate bodies or of ischemic lesions in the retina, choroid, and optic nerve caused by larval and adult nematodes in arteries. Microfilariae in arterioles and capillaries of the retina and uveal tract may also contribute to blindness. Bilateral lesions in the optic nerves also occur, with axonal swelling, slight loss of myelin, and gliosis. Changes (infarction) have also been reported in the optic nerve.

SHEEP (INCLUDING BARBARY), GOATS, AND SIKA DEER. Arterial lesions are uncommon in sheep, goats, and Sika deer. However, the skin lesions seen in infected animals are apparently the result of host reaction to the presence of microfilariae, which induces a hypersensitivity (Jensen and Seghetti 1955; Robinson et al. 1978). As indicated earlier, small numbers of

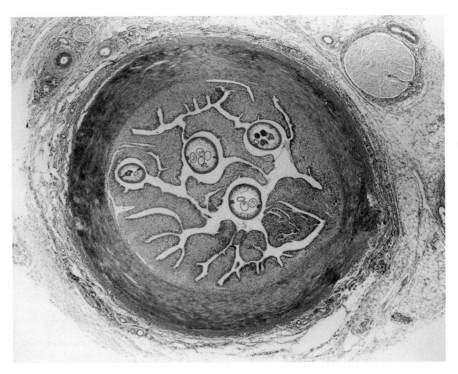

FIG. 12.5—Artery of elk showing fibroblastic intimate proliferation around sections of *Elaeophora schneideri*. Note multiple villous projections extending into the lumen. Hematoxylin and eosin stain (60× magnification). (Photo by C.P. Hibler.)

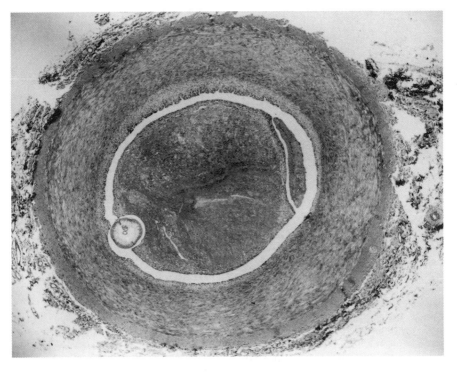

FIG. 12.6—Artery with organized thrombus and single sections of *Elaeophora schneideri*. Hematoxylin and eosin stain (60× magnification). (Photo by C.P. Hibler.)

nematodes are highly pathogenic in kids and can result in early brain damage (C.P. Hibler, personal communication).

DIAGNOSIS. In deer of the genus *Odocoileus,* diagnosis can be made by skin biopsy of the pole, forehead, and face. Hibler and Adcock (1971) recommended removing a piece of skin 2.5 cm² that is then divided to provide a piece for sectioning and another for soaking in saline (at 24°C–26°C) to release microfilariae. Diagnosis in other ungulates can be made by the characteristic clinical signs of elaeophorosis. It may be extremely difficult or impossible to locate microfilariae in skin lesions associated with infection in sheep. Elk may die before microfilariae have built up in the skin of the head, and it is unlikely that searching for microfilariae would be helpful in diagnosis.

CONTROL AND TREATMENT. *The Merck Veterinary Manual* (1991) recommends piperazine salt at 100 mg/lb (220 mg/k) body weight for noncerebral aspects of the disease in domestic animals.

MANAGEMENT IMPLICATIONS. The translocation of reservoir hosts (especially O. *hemionus*) should take into account the possiblility of transporting elaeophorosis to new localities where suitable vectors exist. Also, the possible impact of the disease should be considered when introducing susceptible animals into enzootic areas.

Dirofilaria immitis (Leidy 1856): Dirofilariosis. Members of the genus *Dirofilaria* are long, rather robust filarioids that, except for *D. immitis,* the heartworm of dogs, occur in subcutaneous tissues of carnivores and primates. Microfilariae are long with tapered tails, are unsheathed, and occur in the blood. Intermediate hosts of most species studied (*corynodes, immitis, magnilarvatum, repens, striata, tenuis*) are mosquitoes, but *D. ursi* of bears develops in Simuliidae (for review see Anderson 2000). Microfilariae develop in primary cells of the Malpighian tubules of the mosquito vector.

Subcutaneous *Dirofilaria* spp. are not regarded as significant pathogens of their definitive hosts. *Dirofilaria immitis* is, however, a significant pathogen of dogs. It has been reported fairly commonly in wild canids and sporadically in various other wild and caged mammals (Abraham 1988).

Species of *Dirofilaria* are occasionally transmitted to humans exposed to vectors, and immature *D. immitis* have been reported in the heart and lungs of humans (Boreham 1988; Gutierrez et al. 1996). Subcutaneous species of the genus have been reported in tumors and abscesses in subcutaneous tissues associated with the eye, upper lip, and breast. In North America these worms probably belong to *D. tenuis* of raccoons, *D. ursi* of bears, *D. subdermata* of porcupines, and *D. striata* of felids (e.g., *Lynx*) (Orihel and Beaver 1965; Gutierrez 1983; Orihel and Isbey 1990). In Europe most human cases of subcutaneous *Dirofilaria* refer to

D. repens of dogs (Pampiglione et al. 1995). Heartworm is readily distinguished from most subcutaneous *Dirofilaria* in cross section, because it has a smooth cuticle, whereas other members of the genus have longitudinal ridges (Anderson 1952; Faust 1957; Beaver and Orihel 1965).

A brief summary of the biology of *D. immitis* is given below because it has the potential to be a significant pathogen of wild canids, in which it behaves presumably as in *Canis familiaris.*

LIFE HISTORY. Adults occur in the right ventricle, pulmonary artery, right atrium, and the vena cava of dogs. Rarely, it occurs in other locations. Microfilariae occur in the blood. Vectors found infected in the field include *Culex annulirostris* and *Aedes polynesiensis* in French Oceania (Rosen 1954), *A. fijiensis, A. polynesiensis, A. pseudoscutellaris, C. annulirostris,* and *C. fatigens* in Fiji (Symes 1960), and *A. trivittatus* in Iowa, in the United States (Christenson 1977). Numerous species of *Aedes, Culex,* and *Mansonia* have been experimentally infected (Kartman 1957; Lok 1988).

Microfilariae are 290 ± 20 µm in length (Webber and Hawking 1955) or 300 ± 15 µm (Taylor 1960). In *A. trivittatus* in Iowa the first molt occurred in 7–8 days and the second in 10–11 days postinfection at 26.5° C (Christenson 1977). Infective larvae were 0.82–1.12 mm in length with three short, knob-like swellings (Yen et al. 1982).

Orihel (1961) examined dogs 5–278 days postinfection. Larvae occurred in subcutaneous tissues and muscles for the first 80 days and in the heart in 90 days. The third and fourth molts took place in tissues in 9–12 and 60–70 days, respectively. Lichtenfels et al. (1985) reported that in dogs the third molt occurred within 3 days and that fourth-stage larvae were 1.5 mm long 3–6 days postinfection. The fourth molt took place 50–58 days postinfection, when worms were 12.0–14.8 mm long.

Kotani and Powers (1982) found 93% of larvae near the site of inoculation in dogs and in the abdomen 3 days postinfection. On day 21, 87% of larvae were from the abdomen and 8% from the thorax. After day 21, larvae in the abdomen decreased to 46%, and by day 41, 41% of larvae were from the thorax. Young adults were first found in the heart and pulmonary arteries 70 days postinfection. The precise route taken by worms to reach the heart is still not fully understood but presumably involves the veins or lymphatics. The observations of Kotani and Powers (1982) might indicate worms move to the body cavity, where they would have access to the thoracic duct.

The prepatent period is 6–9 months (Bancroft 1904; Webber and Hawking 1955; Newton 1957; Orihel 1961). Christenson (1977) allowed infected *A. trivittatus* to engorge on a dog that developed a patent infection about 210 days later. *Dirofilaria immitis* apparently behaves similarly in domestic cats and ferrets (*Putorius putorius*); the latter are useful experimental hosts (Supakorndej et al. 1994).

TABLE 12.2—Prevalence and distribution of *Dirofilaria immitis* in wild canids

Host	Common Name	Location	Prevalence	Reference
Canis familiaris dingo	Dingo	Australia	18/32	Starr and Mulley 1988
Canis latrans	Coyote	Texas	3/13	Thornton et al. 1974
		Kansas, Colorado	11/133	Graham 1975
		Iowa	8/220	Franson et al. 1976
		Louisiana	41/71	Crowell et al. 1978
		Georgia	8/17	Holzman et al. 1992
		Indiana	1/8	Kazacos and Edberg 1979
		Texas	9/150	Pence and Meinzer 1979
		California	43/115	Weinmann and Garcia 1980
		Texas, Louisiana	17/24	Custer and Pence 1981
		California	33/193	Acevedo and Theis 1982
		New Hampshire	8/204	Agostine and Jones 1982
		Connecticut	1/4	Agostine and Jones 1982
		Arkansas	127/193	King and Bohring 1984
Canis rufus	Red wolf	Texas, Louisiana	8/8	Custer and Pence 1981
C. latrans χ *C. rufus*	Hybrid	Texas, Louisiana	38/46	Custer and Pence 1981
Urocyon cinereoargenteus	Gray fox	Louisiana	1/20	Crowell et al. 1978
		Indiana	3/18	Kazacos and Edberg 1979
		Arkansas	3/163	King and Bohring 1984
		Alabama, Georgia	0/149	Simmons et al. 1980
		Illinois	3/267	Dyer and Klimstra 1982
		Connecticut	1/1	Carlson and Nielson 1983
Vulpes fulva	Red fox	Louisiana	5/31	Crowell et al. 1978
		Indiana	1/8	Kazacos and Edberg 1979
		Illinois	8/225	Hubert et al. 1980
		Illinois	5/145	Dyer and Klimstra 1981
		Arkansas	1/26	King and Bohring 1984
		Australia	6/68	Mulley and Starr 1984

TABLE 12.3—Sporadic infections of *Dirofilaria immitis* in non-canid hosts

Host	Common Name	Location	Reference
Nyctereates procyonoides	Raccoon dog	Japan	Kagei et al. 1983
Phoca vitulina	Harbor seal	USA	Medway and Wieland 1975
Zalophus californianus	California sea lion	USA	White 1975
Castor canadensis	Beaver	USA	Foil and Orihel 1975
Mustela putorius	Ferret	USA	Miller and Merton 1982
			Parrott et al.1984
Aelurus fulgens	Red panda	USA	Harwell and Craig 1981
		Japan	Narushima et al. 1984
Ursus armericanus	Black bear	USA	Johnson 1975
			Crum et al. 1978
Gulo gulo	Wolverine	USA	Williams and Dade 1976
Neofelis neburosa	Clouded leopard	Japan	Okada et al. 1983

HOSTS AND GEOGRAPHIC DISTRIBUTION. *Dirofilaria immitis* is a cosmopolitan parasite of dogs in warmer parts of the world. For example, it is common in the United States, but occurs in Canada only in a few southern locations. In addition, the species has been found in various wild canid hosts (Table 12.2) and sporadically in a few other wild species, usually animals kept as pets or in zoos (Table 12.3).

Microfilariaemias may develop in dogs, cats, red wolves (*Canis rufus*), coyotes (*Canis latrans*), gray fox (*Urocyon cinereoargenteus*), red fox (*Vulpes vulpes*), California sea lion (*Zalophus californianus*), wolverine (*Gulo gulo*), and ferrets. Ferrets may prove to be useful experimental hosts (Supakorndej et al. 1994).

CLINICAL SIGNS. Clinical signs are reported mainly in dogs and cats. In dogs signs include coughing, decreased tolerance to activity, and weight loss as well as dyspnea, fever, and ascites. Numerous worms in the right atrium and vena cava can cause sudden weakness and death. In cats, anorexia, coughing, lethargy, respiratory difficulties, vomiting, weight loss, and sudden death are reported (Atwell 1988).

PATHOLOGY AND PATHOGENESIS. Worms impede blood flow and cause endarteritis, subintimal proliferation of smooth muscle cells, and rugose and villous protrusions into the lumen. The effect of these lesions, in conjunction with obstructing fibrosis, is development of pulmonary hypertension and secondary right heart enlargement. The kidney may exhibit glomerulonephritis and hemosiderosis of the convoluted tubules. There may also be enlarged hepatic venules and centerlobular necrosis (*The Merck Veterinary Man-*

ual 1991). For an exhaustive treatment of pathology and pathogenesis the reader is referred to Sutton (1988).

DIAGNOSIS. The standard method of diagnosis is to identify microfilariae in the blood, taking care to distinguish them from those of *D. repens* and *Dipetalonema reconditum.* In silent infections, screening by serologic tests (ELISA for adult *D. immitis* antigen) can be carried out. Occult infections can be diagnosed by radiographic findings including evidence of enlargement of the main pulmonary artery and the right ventricle, with perivascular parenchymal pattern, with a caudal lobar artery distribution (*The Merck Veterinary Manual* 1991). Also M-mode echocardiographic evidence of adults in the right atrium with movement into the right ventricle is considered pathognomic.

CONTROL AND TREATMENT. Thiacotarsamide is the adulticide commonly used in dogs but is potentially toxic (*The Merck Veterinary Manual* 1991). Microfilaricidal treatment should follow adulticidal treatment within 3–6 weeks. Dithiazamine iodine is the only approved microfilaricide. Milbemycin oxime, fenthion, and levamisole also are used.

MANAGEMENT IMPLICATIONS. Dogs in contact with infected wild canids are at some risk and visa versa. Those translocating domesticated canids as well as wild canids (e.g., wolves) should consider the possiblility that heartworm may be introduced to new localities and the negative impacts of such introductions.

Setaria cervi (**Rudolphi 1819**): **Setariosis.** Members of the genus *Setaria* are large, slender worms that occur normally free in the abdominal and thoracic cavities of artiodactyles, hyracoids, and equines. Sheathed microfilariae occur in the blood, and known vectors are mosquitoes and stable flies. *Setaria digitata* (Linstow, 1906) of Asian cattle invades the central nervous system of horses, sheep, and goats, resulting in neurologic disease (Innes and Shoho 1953; Ishii et al. 1953; Itagaki and Taniaguchi 1954; Innes and Pillai 1955; Shoho and Nair 1960); it has recently been shown that *Setaria marshalli* (Boulanger, 1921) of cattle in Japan is transmitted prenatally (Fujii et al. 1995). *Setaria marshalli* was not detected in cattle older than 2 years, thus prenatal infection probably is usual. *Setaria cervi,* in deer, deserves a brief mention because it has been reported from the central nervous system.

LIFE HISTORY. Adults occur in the abdominal and thoracic cavities. They also may occur on the meninges (Lubimov 1945, 1948, 1959; Shol' 1964) often associated with *Elaphostrongylus cervi* Cameron, 1931 (Metastrongyloidea). The significance of the worms in the central nervous system is unknown.

The only known vector is the stable fly, *Haematobia stimulans* (see Osipov 1966). Microfilariae (205–231

μm in length) developed in the fat body of *H. stimulans* in the southern Altai of the former USSR. The second molt occurred in 11 days, and in 12 days larvae left the fat body and grew for 5 to 11 days in the hemocoel (Osipov 1966). Infective larvae were 1.65–2.32 mm in length. The prepatent period was 224–235 days, and infections lasted 1.5 years.

HOSTS AND GEOGRAPHIC DISTRIBUTION. This species is reported in Cervidae (*Alces alces, Capreolus capreolus, Cervus axis, C. dama, C. elaphus, C. nippon, Muntiacus muntjak*) in Asia and Europe.

CLINICAL SIGNS. Neurologic signs in infected deer may be related to concurrent infections with *Elaphostrongylus cervi.* Pathologic changes have not been described.

MANAGEMENT IMPLICATIONS. The neurologic effects of *S. cervi* in deer should be distinguished from those caused by the neurotropic metastrongyloid *Elaphostrongylus cervi.*

Pelecitus scapiceps (**Leidy 1886**): **Pelecitosis** **Synonym:** *Dirofilaria scapiceps.*

Members of the genus *Pelecitus* Railliet and Henry are mainly parasites of birds. However, *P. scapiceps* and *P. roemeri* occur in mammals. Species of the genus occupy sites associated with the limb joints, especially of the legs and feet of the host. Current information generally is restricted to life history and host distribution.

LIFE HISTORY. Adult worms occur mainly in connective tissue surrounding tendons of ankles of hind legs; rarely in muscle fascia near the knee joint. Microfilariae occur in blood and are 262–300 μm in length with a loose sheath. In Ontario, Canada, the following Culicidae are known vectors–*Aedes canadensis, A. euedes, A. excrucians, A. provocans, A. punctor, A. stimulans/ fitchii, A. vexans,* and *Mansonia perturbans* (Bartlett 1984a). *Aedes aegypti* is a suitable experimental host. Transmission occurred in July and August. Microfilariae invaded the fat body of the mosquito and developed within syncytia with hypertrophied adipocyte nuclei. At 26° C larvae reached the infective stage in 10–12 days (Bartlett 1984a).

Development to subadults took place in the subcutaneous tissues of the definitive host. The exact site of development was related to the point of entry of the infective larvae. Third and fourth molts occurred 6 and 12 days postinoculation. Subadults then migrated through subcutaneous tissues and reached the ankles as early as 16 days postinfection. The prepatent period was 137–234 days, and the microfilariaemia was nonperiodic (Bartlett 1984b).

HOSTS AND DISTRIBUTION. The species is found in lagomorphs in North America, namely snowshoe hare (*Lepus americanus*) (62%), eastern cottontail rabbit (*Sylvilagus floridanus*) (27%), European hare (*Lepus capensis)* (4%), and European wild rabbit (*Oryctolagus cuniculus*) (13% domestic rabbits and experimental infections) (Bartlett 1983).

PATHOLOGY AND PATHOGENESIS. Clinical signs have not been reported. In *S. floridanus,* tendons and tendon sheaths occupied by nematodes appeared consistently normal, and all worms were adults. Microfilariaemias were generally high in cottontail rabbits. In snowshoe hares a chronic proliferation synovitis characterized by fibrous exudate, hyperplasia and hypertrophy of the intima and inflammatory cells (mainly lymphoctyes and plasma cells), and infiltration of the intimal and fibrous layers of the synovial sheath led to encapsulation of nematodes and often their death. Microfilariae become trapped in the capsule around worms, and few or no microfilariae were detected in the blood of hares (Bartlett 1984c). Although *P. scapiceps* can be maintained in populations of snowshoe hares, this host is considered subnormal. It is hypothesized that this is a parasite that spread from rabbits to hares in fairly recent times.

Pelecitus roemeri (Linstow 1905): Pelecitosis.
Synonym: *Dirofilaria roemeri.*

LIFE HISTORY. The parasites occur in subcutaneous and intermuscular tissues of the knee of various marsupials. The microfilariae occur in blood and have closely fitting sheaths (179–220 µm in length) (Spratt 1972b). Intermediate hosts are Tabanidae (i.e., *Dasybasis hebes, D. acutipalpis, D. circumdata, D. dubiosa, D. moretonensis, D. neobasalis, D. oculata, Mesomyia fuliginosa, Scaptra testaceomaculata, Tabanus australicus, T. pallipennis, T. particaecus, T. parvicallosus, T. strangmenii,* and *T. townsvilli*) (see Spratt 1972c, 1974).

Microfilariae in flies developed in the abdominal fat body to infective larvae 1.9–2.7 mm in length in ~10–11 days. The most important vector was apparently *D. hebes,* and maximum levels of larvae appear in these flies under natural conditions in April. The prepatent period in wallaroos was 256–272 days, and microfilariae established a diurnal subperiodicity (Spratt 1972a, 1975).

HOSTS AND GEOGRAPHIC DISTRIBUTION. This species is found in Australian macropodid marsupials including eastern grey kangaroo (*Macropus giganteus),* eastern wallaroo *(M. robustus),* red-necked wallaby *(Wallabia. rufogrisea),* and red kangaroo (*Megaleia rufa).* The wallaroo is regarded as the most suitable host and the red kangaroo as a secondary reservoir; microfilariaemias do not develop in the other hosts (Spratt 1972a, 1974, 1975).

PATHOLOGY AND PATHOGENESIS. Clinical signs have not been reported; however, male and female worms were found in vascular, fibrous capsules surrounding the sartorius muscle of wallaroos 149–150 days

postinoculation (Spratt 1972a, 1975). Tissue surrounding worms contained small lymphocytes, plasma cells, macrophages, and a few degranulated mast cells in a laminated fibrous capsule. In the less suitable red kangaroo, many capsules contained flattened oval pellets of varying sizes and hardness. Dead and degenerate worms were observed in fibrous capsules in loose fascia between the skin and muscle immediately distal to the femur or tibial joint. Many microfilariae were trapped in aggregations of eosinophils and macrophages in thick-walled capsules; the microfilariaemia is of brief duration in the red kangaroo but prolonged in the wallaroo.

MANAGEMENT IMPLICATIONS. The location of the parasite in the legs is probably not an important factor in the commercial use of the flesh of the animals.

Monanema martini [Bain, Bartlett, and Petit 1986]:
Monanemosis
Synonym: *Monanema nilotica* Bain, Petit and Gueye, 1983 (not El Bihari Hussein and Muller, 1983).

LIFE HISTORY. *Monanema martini* occurs in African murid rodents, *Arvicanthis niloticus* and *Lemniscomys striatus.* Adults are found in lymphatics of the wall of the colon, and rarely in the cecum. The sheathed microfilariae inhabit cutaneous lymphatic vessels, mainly of the ears. Intermediate hosts are hexapod larvae of ixodid ticks (*Hyalomma truncatum, Rhipicephalus sanquineus, R. turanicus*) (Petit et al. 1988). Microfilariae ingested by larval ticks invaded and developed in the epidermis of the tick. The infective stage appeared during the molt of the tick to the nymphal stage, which took place in 11 days at 26° C (Petit et al. 1988).

Experimentally, *Meriones unguiculatus* was infected by inoculating larvae subcutaneously, but *L. striatus* was a much more suitable host, and the recovery rate of worms was 50% in contrast to the 20% in the former host. Infective larvae were found in the peripheral lymphatic vessels 6 hours postinoculation, and in 5 days the worms were found in the lumbar and mesenteric lymph nodes. The third and fourth molts occurred at 10 and 21 days postinoculation, respectively. By the final molt, most worms were in the lymphatic vessels of the colon (Wanji et al. 1990).

The microfiladermias (microfilariae in the skin) that developed in experimentally infected *L. striatus* reached their peaks 6 to 9 months postinoculation. Intensity of microfilariae in skin of the ears was positively related to the number of infective larvae inoculated. The microfiladermia tended to remain constant for more than 8 months (Wanji et al. 1994).

PATHOLOGY AND PATHOGENESIS. Adult worms in lymphatic vessels of the colon and cecum were associated with inflammatory lesions in the surrounding tissues. There were lymphoid hyperplasia of the Peyer's patches, infiltrations of mast cells, and dilation of lymphatic vessels. Hyperplasia of the mesothelial lining of the mesentery was noted (Vuong et al. 1991). Microfilariae in the lumen of lymphatic capillaries were normally concentrated in the dermis of the ear. Lesions generally developed around microfilariae in the form of foreign body granulomas. Blood capillaries were dilated, and infiltration of mast cells was observed, as well as necrosis of dermal connective tissue (Vuong et al. 1986, 1991). Lesions were irregularly distributed in the ear and were sometimes severe. Corneal lesions were reported in *A. niloticus* and chorioretinal atrophy in *L. striatus*. Interstitial nodules and keratitis were observed in infected *A. niloticus* and stromal lesions in infected *L. striatus* (Aimard et al. 1993). The lesions are believed to resemble those seen in humans with onchocerciasis (*O. volvulus*).

DIAGNOSIS. Small pieces of skin from the ears should be soaked in saline, which causes the microfilariae to leave the tissues and move into the saline, where they can be studied microscopically.

Cercopithifilaria johnstoni (Mackerras 1954): Cercopithifilariosis

LIFE HISTORY. *Cercopithifilaria johnstoni* occurs in subcutaneous connective tissues of Australian rodents and marsupials. The microfilariae are sheathed and inhabit the lymphatic vessels of the skin, mainly the ears. Microfilariae are associated with ocular lesions in the host. The intermediate hosts are ixodid ticks, mainly *Ixodes trichosura* but also *I. facialis, I. holocyclus,* and *I. tasmani.* (Spratt and Haycock 1988).

Development occurs after engorged ticks leave the definitive host and during ecdysis from larva to nymph or from nymph to adult (Spratt and Haycock 1988). Transmission to *Rattus fuscipes* occurred in summer and winter and was associated with peaks of larvae and/or nymphal ticks on the animals. *Rattus fuscipes* was infected by inoculation of infective larvae or by allowing infected ticks to feed on the host. The prepatent period was ~3 months, and the microfiladermia persisted more than 25 months.

HOSTS AND GEOGRAPHIC DISTRIBUTION. The parasite occurs in the following animals in Australia: Muridae (*Rattus fuscipes, R. lutriolus, Uromys candimaculatus*); Marsupialia, Paramelidae (*Perameles gunni, P. nasuta, Isoodon macrourus, I. obsulus*); Petauridae (*Petauroides volans*); and Dasyuridae (*Sarcophilus harrisii*).

CLINICAL SIGNS. None reported that can be attributed conclusively to *C. johnstoni.*

PATHOLOGY AND PATHOGENESIS. The parasite induces skin and ocular lesions in infected animals (Vuong et al. 1993). Microfilariae live in lymphatic vessels, and their exit gives rise to localized inflammatory reactions resulting in fibrosis. Microfilariae were found in the limbus, cornea, eye lids, and the stroma of the mucosal region of the eye lid. They were inside and outside lymphatic vessels. Inflammation was most pronounced in the limbus, with dilation of lymphatics and blood vessels, vascularization, and infiltration of melanophages and mast cells. Acute inflammatory lesions of the limbus frequently spread to the periphery of the cornea. Corneal fibrosis was mild to severe in the various animals examined.

DIAGNOSIS. Small pieces of skin from the ears can be soaked in saline, which will cause the microfilariae to leave the tissue and move into the saline where they can be observed microscopically.

MANAGEMENT IMPLICATIONS. The eye lesions resemble those associated with human onchocerciasis, and the parasite may be useful in drug testing.

LITERATURE CITED

Elaeophorosis
Adcock, J.L., C.P. Hibler. 1969. Vascular and neuroophthalmic pathology of elaeophorosis in elk. *Pathologia Veterinaria* 6:185–213.
Adcock, J.L., C.P. Hibler, Y. Abdelbaki, and R.W. Davis. 1965. Elaeophorosis in elk (*Cervus canadensis*). *Bulletin of the Wildlife Disease Association* 1:48.
Anderson, J.Z., and C.J. Weinmann. 1972. The population dynamics, parity profiles, and infection rates of tabanid vectors of *Elaeophora schneideri* (Filariidae). *Proceedings of the 14th International Congress of Entomology,* Canberra, Australia.
Clark, G.G. 1972. The role of horse flies (Diptera: Tabanidae) in the transmission of *Elaeophora schneideri* Wehr and Dikmans, 1935, in the Gila National Forest, New Mexico. Ph.D. Dissertation, Colorado State University, Fort Collins, 169 pp.
Clark, G.G., and C.P. Hibler. 1973. Horse flies and *Elaeophora schneideri* in the Gila National Forest, New Mexico. *Journal of Wildlife Diseases* 9:21–25.
Couvillion, C.E., V.F. Nettles, C.A. Rawlings, and R.L. Joyner. 1986. Elaeophorosis in white-tailed deer: Pathology of the natural disease and its relation to oral food impactions. *Journal of Wildlife Diseases* 22:214–223.
Couvillion, C.E., D.C. Sheppard, V.F. Nettles, and O.M. Bannaga. 1984. Intermediate hosts of *Elaeophora schneideri* Wehr and Dikmans, 1935 on South Island, South Carolina. *Journal of Wildlife Diseases* 20:59–61.
Cowan, I.M. 1946. Parasites, diseases, and anomalies of the Columbian black-tailed deer (*Odocoileus hemionus columbianus*) (Richardson) in British Columbia. *Canadian Journal of Research* 24:71–103.
Davies, R.B. 1979. The ecology of *Elaeophora schneideri* in Vermejo Park, New Mexico. Ph.D. Dissertation, Colorado State University, Fort Collins, 216 pp.
Davis, C.L., and H.E. Kemper. 1951. The histopathologic diagnosis of filarial dermatosis in sheep. *Journal of the American Veterinary Medical Association* 118:103–106.
Davis, R.W., Y.Z. Abdelbaki, and J.L. Adcock. 1965. Investigation of diseases of elk. Completion Report, Federal Aid Project. No. W-78-R-9. Work Plan No. 3. Job No. 2. Phoenix: Arizona Game and Fish Department.
Douglas, J.R., D.R. Cordy, and G.M. Spurlock. 1954. *Elaeophora schneideri* Wehr and Dikmans, 1935 (Nematoda: Filarioidea) in California sheep. *Cornell Veterinarian* 44:252.

Espinosa, R.H. 1987. Tabanid vectors of the arterial nematode, *Elaeophora schneideri* in southwestern Montana. M.S. Thesis, Montana State University, Bozeman, MT, 58 pp.

Gallizioli, S. 1963. Investigation of diseases of elk. Job Completion Report. Federal Aid Project No. W-78-R-7. Work Plan No. 3, Job No. 2. Phoenix: Arizona Game and Fish Department.

Herman, C.M. 1945. Some worm parasites of deer in California. *California Fish and Game* 31:201–208.

Hibler, C.P., and J.L. Adcock. 1968. Redescription of *Elaeophora schneideri* Wehr and Dikmans, 1935 (Nematoda: Filarioidea). *The Journal of Parasitology* 54:1095–1098.

———. 1971. Elaeophorosis. In *Parasitic diseases of wild mammals.* Ed. J.W. Davis and R.C. Anderson. Ames: Iowa State University Press, pp. 263–278.

Hibler, C.P., and C.J. Metzger. 1974. Morphology of the larval stages of *Elaeophora schneideri* in the intermediate hosts with some observations on their pathogenesis in the abnormal definitive hosts. *Journal of Wildlife Diseases* 10:361–369.

Hibler, C.P., and A.K. Prestwood. 1981. Filarial nematodes of white-tailed deer. In *Disease and parasites of white-tailed deer.* Ed. W.R. Davidson, F.A. Hayes, V. Nettles, and F.E. Kellogg. Miscellaneous Publication. Tallahassee, FL: Tall Timbers Research Station, pp. 351–362.

Hibler, C.P., J.L. Adcock, R.W. Davis, and Y.Z. Adbelbaki. 1969. Elaeophorosis in deer and elk in the Gila National Forest, New Mexico. *Bulletin of the Wildlife Diseases Association* 5:27–30.

Hibler, C.P., J.L. Adcock, G.H. Gates, and R. White. 1970. Experimental infection of domestic sheep and mule deer with *Elaeophora schneideri. Journal of Wildlife Diseases* 6:110–111.

Hibler, C.P., G.H. Gates, R. White, and B.R. Donaldson. 1971. Observations on horse flies infected with larvae of *Elaeophora schneideri. Journal of Wildlife Diseases* 7:45–45.

Hibler, C.P., G.H. Gates, and B.R. Donaldson. 1974. Experimental infection of immature mule deer with *Elaeophora schneideri. Journal of Wildlife Diseases* 10:44–46.

Howe, D.L., and W.G. Hepworth. 1964. Diagnosis of diseases in mammals and birds. Job Completion Report. Federal Aid Project No. FW-3-R-11. Work Plan No. 1, Job No. 1 W. Cheyenne: Wyoming Game and Fish Commission.

Jensen, L., and L. Seghetti. 1955. Elaeophorosis in sheep. *Journal of the American Veterinary Medical Association* 130:220–224.

Kemper, H.E. 1938. Filarial dermatosis of sheep. *North American Veterinarian* 19:36–41.

Longhurst, W.M., A.S. Leopold, and R.F. Dasmann. 1952. A survey of California deer herds. Game Bulletin 6. Sacramento: California Department of Fish and Game.

Madden, D.J., T.R. Spraker, and W.J. Adrian. 1991. *Elaeophora schneideri* in moose (*Alces alces*) from Colorado. *Journal of Wildlife Diseases* 27:340–341.

The Merck Veterinary Manual. 1991. Rahway, NJ: Merck and Company, Inc.

Mills, H.B. 1936. Observations on Yellowstone elk. *Journal of Mammalogy* 17:250–253.

Pence, D.B. 1991. Elaeophorosis in wild ruminants. *Bulletin of the Society for Vector Ecology* 16:149–160.

Pence, D.B., and G. G. Gray. 1981. Elaeophorosis in Barbary sheep and mule deer from the Texas Panhandle. *Journal of Wildlife Diseases* 17:49–56.

Prestwood, A.K., and T.R. Ridgeway. 1972. Elaeophorosis in white-tailed deer of the southeastern USA: Case report and distribution. *Journal of Wildlife Diseases* 8:233–236.

Robinson, R.M., L.P. Jones, T.J. Galvin, and G.M. Harwell. 1978. Elaeophorosis in Sika deer in Texas. *Journal of Wildlife Diseases* 14:137–141.

Rush, N.M. 1932. Northern Yellowstone elk study. Montana Fish and Game Commission, pp. 1–131.

Smith, H.C., V.E. Lovell, and R.F. Reppert. 1954. Filarial dermatosis in sheep. *North American Veterinarian* 35:588–589.

Titche, A.R., A.K. Prestwood, and C.P. Hibler. 1979. Experimental infections of white-tailed deer with *Elaeophora schneideri. Journal of Wildlife Diseases* 15:273–280.

Waid, D.D., R.J. Warren, and D.B. Pence. 1984. *Elaeophora schneideri* Wehr and Dikmans, 1935 in white-tailed deer from the Edwards plateau of Texas. *Journal of Wildlife Diseases* 20:342–345.

Wehr, E.E., and G. Dikmans. 1935. New nematodes (Filarioidae) from North American ruminants. *Zoological Anzeiger* 110:202–208.

Weinmann, C.J., J.R. Anderson, W.M. Longhurst, and G. Connolly. 1973. Filarial worms of Columbian black-tailed deer in California. 1. Observations in the vertebrate host. *Journal of Wildlife Diseases* 9:213–220.

White, R.W. 1957–1959. Diseases of elk. Job Completion Report. Federal Aid Project. No. W-78-R-1 to 3. Work Plan No. 3, Job No. 2. Phoenix: Arizona Game and Fish Department.

Worley, D.E. 1975. Observations on the epizootiology and distribution of *Elaeophora schneideri* in Montana ruminants. *Journal of Wildlife Diseases* 11:486–488.

Worley, D.E., C.K. Anderson, and K.R. Greer. 1972. Elaeophorosis in moose from Montana. *Journal of Wildlife Diseases* 8:242–244.

Dirofilariosis

Abraham, D. 1988. Biology of *Dirofilaria immitis.* In *Dirofilariasis.* Ed. P.F.L. Boreham and R.B. Atwell. Boca Raton, FL: CRC Press Inc., pp. 29–46.

Acevedo, R.A., and J.H. Theis. 1982. Prevalence of heartworm (*Dirofilaria immitis* Leidy) in coyotes from five northern California counties. *American Journal of Tropical Medicine and Hygiene* 31:968–972.

Agostine, J.C., and G.S. Jones. 1982. Heartworm (*Dirofilaria immitis*) in coyotes (*Canis latrans*) in New England. *Journal of Wildlife Diseases* 18:343–345.

Anderson, R.C. 1952. Description and relationship of *Dirofilaria ursi* Yamaguti, 1941 and a review of the genus *Dirofilaria* Railliet and Henry, 1911. *Transactions of the Royal Canadian Institute* 29:35–65.

———. 2000. Nematode Parasites of Vertebrates, their Development and Transmission, 2nd ed. Wallingford, UK: CAB International, Wallingford, Oxon, UK, 650 pp.

Atwell, R.B. 1988. Clinical signs and diagnosis of canine dirofilariasis. In *Dirofilariasis.* Ed. P.F.L. Boreham and R.B. Atwell. Boca Raton, FL: CRC Press Inc., pp. 61–97.

Bancroft, T.L. 1904. Some further observations of the life history of *Filaria immitis* Leidy. *British Medical Journal* 1:822–823.

Beaver, P.C., and T.C. Orihel. 1965. Human infections with filariae of animals in the United States. *American Society of Tropical Medicine and Hygiene* 14:1010–1029.

Boreham, P.F.L. 1988. Dirofilariasis in man. In *Dirofilariasis.* Ed. P.F.L. Boreham and R.B. Atwell. Boca Raton, FL: CRC Press Inc., pp. 218–226.

Carlson, B.L., and S.W. Nielson. 1983. *Dirofilaria immitis* infection in a gray fox. *Journal of the American Veterinary Medical Association* 183:1275–1276.

Christenson, B.M. 1977. Laboratory studies on the development and transmission of *Dirofilaria immitis* by *Aedes trivittatus.* Mosquito News 37:367–372.

Crowell, W.A., T.R. Klei, D.I. Hall, N.K. Smith, and J.D. Newsom. 1978. Occurrence of *Dirofilaria immitis* and associated pathology in coyotes and foxes from Louisiana. *Proceedings of the Heartworm Symposium.*

Ed. G.F. Otto. Bonner Springs, KS: Veterinary Medicine Publications, pp. 10–13.

Crum, J.M., V.F. Nettles, and W.R. Davidson. 1978. Studies on endoparasites of the black bear (*Ursus americanus*) in the southeastern United States. *Journal of Wildlife Diseases* 14:178–186.

Custer, J.W., and D.B. Pence. 1981. Dirofilariasis in wild canids from the Gulf coastal prairies of Texas and Louisiana, USA. *Veterinary Parasitology* 8:71–82.

Dyer, W.G., and W.D. Klimstra. 1981. Dirofilariasis in *Vulpes vulpes* from southern Illinois. *Transactions of the Illinois Academy of Sciences* 74:143–145.

———. 1982. *Dirofilaria immitis* in *Urocyon cinereoargenteus*. *Transactions of the Illinois Academy of Sciences* 75:81–83.

Faust, E.C. 1957. Human infection with *Dirofilaria*. *Zeitschrift für Tropenmedizin und Parasitologie* 8:59–68.

Foil, L., and T.C. Orihel. 1975. *Dirofilaria immitis* (Leidy, 1856) in the beaver, *Castor canadensis*. *The Journal of Parasitology* 61:433.

Franson, J.C., R.D. Jorgenson, and E.K. Boggess. 1976. Dirofilariasis in Iowa coyotes. *Journal of Wildlife Diseases* 12:165–166.

Graham, J.M. 1975. Filariasis in coyotes from Kansas and Colorado. *The Journal of Parasitology* 6:513–516.

Gutierrez, Y. 1983 Diagnostic characterisation of *Dirofilaria subdermata* in cross sections. *Canadian Journal of Zoology* 61:2097–2103.

Gutierrez, Y., M.D. Catallaer, and D.L. Wicker. 1996. Extrapulmonary *Dirofilaria immitis* like infections in the western hemisphere. *The American Journal of Surgical Pathology* 20:299–305.

Harwell, G., and T.M. Craig. 1981. Dirofilariasis in a red panda. *Journal of American Veterinary Medical Association* 179:1258.

Holzman, S., M.J. Conroy, and W.R. Davidson. 1992. Diseases, parasites and survival of coyotes in south-central Georgia. *Journal of Wildlife Diseases* 28:572–580.

Hubert, G.F., Jr., T.J. Kick, and R.D. Andrews. 1980. *Dirofilaria immitis* in red foxes in Illinois. *Journal of Wildlife Diseases* 16:229–232.

Johnson, C.A. 1975. *Ursus americanus* (black bear) a new host for *Dirofilaria immitis*. *The Journal of Parasitology* 61:940.

Kagei, N., H. Shiomi, H. Sugaya, and H. Akiyama. 1983. On the helminths from raccoon dogs in Japan. *Japanese Journal of Parasitology* 32:367–369.

Kartman, L. 1957. The vectors of canine filariasis: A review with special reference to factors influencing susceptibility. *Publicaç es Avulsas. Revista Brasileira de Malariologia e Doenças Tropicaes* No. 5, pp. 1–41.

Kazacos, K.R., and E.O. Edberg. 1979. *Dirofilaria immitis* infection in foxes and coyotes in Indiana. *Journal of the American Veterinary Medical Association* 175:909–910.

King, A.W., and A.M. Bohring. 1984. The incidence of heartworm *Dirofilaria immitis* (Filarioidea), in the wild canids of Northern Arkansas. *Southwestern Naturalist* 29:89–92.

Kotani, T., and K.G. Powers. 1982 Developmental stages of *Dirofilaria immitis* in the dog. *American Journal of Veterinary Research* 43:2199–2206.

Lichtenfels, J.R., P.A. Pilitt, T. Kotani, and K.G. Power. 1985. Morphogenesis of developmental stages of *Dirofilaria immitis* (Nematoda) in the dog. *Proceedings of the Helminthological Society of Washington* 52:98–113.

Lok, J.B. 1988. *Dirofilaria* sp.: Taxonomy and distribution. In *Dirofilariasis*. Ed. P.F.L. Boreham and R.B. Atwell. Boca Raton, FL: CRC Press Inc., pp. 1–28.

Miller, W.R., and D.A. Merton. 1982. Dirofilariasis in a ferret. *Journal of American Veterinary Medical Association* 180:1103–1104.

Medway, W., and T.C. Wieland. 1975. *Dirofilaria immitis* infection in a harbour seal. *Journal of American Veterinary Medical Association* 167: 549–550.

The Merck Veterinary Manual. 1991. Rahway, NJ: Merck and Company, Inc.

Mulley, R.C.S., and T.W. Starr. 1984. *Dirofilaria immitis* in red foxes (*Vulpes vulpes*) in an endemic area near Sydney, Australia. *Journal of Wildlife Diseases* 20:152–153.

Narushima, E., F. Hashizaki, N. Kokno, M. Saito, K. Tanabe, M. Hayasaki, and I. Ohishi. 1984. *Dirofilaria immitis* infections in lesser pandas (*Aelurus fulgens*) in Japan. *Japanese Journal of Parasitology* 33:475–481.

Newton, W.L. 1957. Experimental transmission of the dog heartworm, *Dirofilaria immitis*, by *Anopheles quadrimaculatus*. *The Journal of Parasitology* 43:589.

Okada, R., S. Imai, and T. Ishii. 1983. Clouded leopard, *Neofelis neburosa*, new host for *Dirofilaria immitis*. *Japanese Journal of Veterinary Science* 45:849–851.

Orihel, T.C. 1961 Morphology of the larval stages of *Dirofilaria immitis* in the dog. *The Journal of Parasitology* 47:251–262.

Orihel, T.C., and P.C. Beaver. 1965. Morphology and relationship of *Dirofilaria tenuis* and *Dirofilaria conjunctivae*. *American Journal of Tropical Medicine and Hygiene* 14:1030–1043.

Orihel, T.C., and E.K.J. Isbey. 1990. *Dirofilaria striata* infection in a North Carolina child. *American Journal of Tropical Medicine and Hygiene* 42:124–126.

Pampiglione, S., G. Canestri, S.G. Trothia, and F. Rivasi. 1995. Human dirofilariasis due to *Dirofilaria* (*Nochtiella*) *repens:* A review of world literature. *Parassitologia* 37:149–193.

Parrott, T.Y., E.C. Greiner, and J.D. Parrott. 1984. *Dirofilaria immitis* infections in three ferrets. *Journal of American Veterinary Medical Association* 184:582–583.

Pence, D.B., and W.P. Meinzer. 1979. Helminth parasitism in the coyote *Canis latrans* from the rolling plains of Texas. *International Journal of Parasitology* 9:339–344.

Rosen, L. 1954. Observations on *Dirofilaria immitis* in French Oceania. *Annals of Tropical Medicine and Parasitology* 48:318–328.

Simmons, J.M., W.S. Nicholson, E.P. Hill, and D.B. Briggs. 1980. Occurrence of *Dirofilaria immitis* in gray fox (*Urocyon cinereoargenteus*) in Alabama and Georgia. *Journal of Wildlife Diseases* 16:225–228.

Starr, T.W., and R.C. Mulley. 1988. *Dirofilaria immitis* in the dingo in a tropical region of the Northern Territory, Australia. *Journal of Wildlife Diseases* 24:164–165.

Supakorndej, P., J.W. McCall, and J.J. Jung. 1994. Early migration and development of *Dirofilaria immitis* in the ferret, *Mustela putorius furo*. *Journal of Parasitology* 80:237–244.

Sutton, R.H. 1988. Pathology and pathogenesis of dirofilariasis. In *Dirofilariasis*. Ed. P.F.L. Boreham and R.B. Atwell. Boca Raton, FL: CRC Press Inc., pp. 99–132.

Symes, C.B. 1960. A note on *Dirofilaria immitis* and its vectors in Fiji. *Journal of Helminthology* 34:39–42.

Taylor, A.E.R. 1960 The development of *Dirofilaria immitis* in the mosquito *Aedes aegypti*. *Journal of Helminthology* 34:27–38.

Thornton, J.E., R.R. Bill, and M.J. Reardon. 1974. Internal parasites of coyotes in southern Texas. *Journal of Wildlife Diseases* 10:232–236.

Webber, W.A.F., and F. Hawking. 1955 . Experimental maintenance of *Dirofilaria repens* and *D. immitis* in dogs. *Experimental Parasitology* 4:143–164.

Weinmann, C.J., and R. Garcia. 1980. Coyotes and canine heartworm in California. *Journal of Wildlife Diseases* 16:217–221.

White, G.L. 1975. *Dirofilaria immitis* and heartworm disease in the California sea lion. *Journal of Zoological Animal Medicine* 6:23.

Williams, J.F., and A.W. Dade. 1976. *Dirofilaria immitis* infection in a wolverine. *The Journal of Parasitology* 62:174–175.

Yen, P.K.F., V. Zaman, and J.W. Mak. 1982. Identification of some common infective larvae in Malaysia. *Journal of Helminthology* 56:69–80.

Setariosis

Fujii, T., T. Hayashi, A. Ishimoto, S. Takahashi, H. Asano, and T. Kato. 1995. Prenatal infection with *Setaria marshalli* (Boulenger, 1921) in cattle. *Veterinary Parasitology* 56:303–309.

Innes, J.R.M., and C.P. Pillai. 1955. Kumri—So called lumbar paralysis—Of horses in Ceylon (India and Burma) and its identification with cerebrospinal nematodiasis. *British Veterinary Journal* 111:223–235.

Innes, J.R.M., and C. Shoho. 1953. Cerebrospinal nematodiasis. Focal encephalomyelomata of animals caused by nematodes (*Setaria digitata*), a disease which may occur in man. *Archives of Neurology and Psychiatry* 70:325–349.

Ishii, S., A. Yagima, Y. Sugawa, T. Ishiwara, T. Ogata, and Y. Hashiguchi. 1953. The experimental reproduction of so called lumbar paralysis—Epizootic cerebrospinal nematodiasis in goats in Japan. *British Veterinary Journal* 107:160–167.

Itagaki, S., and M. Taniaguchi. 1954. Pathogenicity of *S. digitata* in domestic animals (sheep, goats, and horses) and its life cycle [In Japanese]. *Japanese Journal of Sanitary Zoology IV* Special Number Commemorating the 70th Birthday of Dr. H. Kobayashi.

Lubimov, M.P. 1945. New worm diseases of the brain of deer with unossified antlers [In Russian]. *Sbornik nauchno-issledovatel'skikh rabot Laboratoriyi panto-vogo olenvodstva Ministerstva sovkhozov SSSR* 1:225–232.

———. 1948. New helminths of the brain of maral deer [In Russian]. *Trudi Gel'minthologicheskoi Laboratorii* 1:198–201.

———. 1959. The season dynamics of elaphostrongylosis and setariosis in *Cervus elaphus maral. Trudy Gel'minthologicheskoi Laboratorii* 9:155–156.

Osipov, A.N. 1966. Life cycle of *Setaria altaica* (Rajewskaja, 1928), a parasite of the brain of Siberian deer. *Doklady Akademii Nauk SSSR* 168:247–248.

Shoho, C., and V.K. Nair. 1960 Studies on cerebrospinal nematodiasis in Ceylon 7. Experimental production of cerebrospinal nematodiasis by the inoculation of infective larvae of *Setaria digitata* into susceptible goats. *Ceylon Veterinary Journal* 8:2–12.

Shol', A.V. 1964. Diagnosis of *Setaria* infections in deer [In Russian]. In *Parasites of farm animals in Kazakhstan*, vol. 31. Ed. S.N. Boev. Alma Ata: Izdatel Akademii Nauk Kazakhstan SSR, pp. 101–103.

Pelecitosis

Bartlett, C.M. 1983. Zoogeography and taxonomy of *Dirofilaria scapiceps* (Leidy, 1886) and *D. uniformis* Price, 1957 (Nematoda: Filarioidea) of lagomorphs in North America. *Canadian Journal of Zoology* 61:1011–1022.

———. 1984a. Development of *Dirofilaria scapiceps* (Leidy, 1886) (Nematoda: Filarioidea) in *Aedes* spp. and *Mansonia perturbans* (Walker) and responses of mosquitoes to infection. *Canadian Journal of Zoology* 62:112–129.

———. 1984b. Development of *Dirofilaria scapiceps* (Leidy, 1886) (Nematoda: Filarioidea) in lagomorphs. *Canadian Journal of Zoology* 62:965–979.

———. 1984c. Pathology and epizootiology of *Dirofilaria scapiceps* (Leidy, 1886) (Nematoda: Filarioidea) in *Syvilagus floridanus* (J.A. Allen) and *Lepus americanus* Erxleben. *Journal of Wildlife Diseases* 20:197–206.

Spratt, D.M. 1972a. Aspects of the life-history of *Dirofilaria roemeri* in naturally and experimentally infected kangaroos, wallaroos, and wallabies. *International Journal for Parasitology* 2:139–156.

———. 1972b. Histological morphology of adult *Dirofilaria roemeri* and anatomy of the microfilaria. *International Journal for Parasitology* 2:193–200.

———. 1972c. Natural occurrence, histopathology, and developmental stages of *Dirofilaria roemeri* in the intermediate host. *International Journal for Parasitology* 2:201–208.

———. 1974. Comparative epidemiology of *Dirofilaria roemeri* infection in two regions of Queensland. *International Journal for Parasitology* 4:481–488.

———. 1975. Further studies of *Dirofilaria roemeri* (Nematoda: Filarioidea) in naturally and experimentally infected Macropodidae. *International Journal for Parasitology* 5:561–564.

Monanemosis and Cercopithfilariosis

Aimard, L., S. Wanji, P.N. Vuong, G. Petit, and O. Bain. 1993. Ophthalmological study of the lesions induced by the filarial worm with dermal microfilariae, *Monanema martini. Current Eye Research* 12:885–891.

Bain, O., C.M. Bartlett, and G. Petit. 1986. Une filaire de muridés africains dan la paroi du colon, *Monanema martini* n.sp. *Annales de Parasitologie Humaine et Compareé* 61:465–472.

Petit, G., O. Bain, C. Carrat, and F. de Marval. 1988. Developpement de la filaire *Monanema martini* dans l'epiderme des tiquis Ixodidae. *Annales de Parasitologie Humaine et Compareé* 63:54–63.

Spratt, D.M., and P. Haycock. 1988. Aspects of the life history of *Cercopithifilaria johnstoni* (Nematoda: Filarioidea). *International Journal for Parasitology* 18:1087–1092.

Vuong, P.N., O. Bain, G. Petit, and A.C. Chabaud. 1986. Etude anatomo-pathologique de lésion cutanées et oculaires de ronqeurs infestés par *Monanema* spp. Intérét pour l'études de l'onchocercose humaine. *Annales de Parasitologie Humaine et Compareé* 61:311–320.

Vuong, P.N., S. Wanji, L. Sakka, S. Klager, and O. Bain. 1991. The murid filaria *Monanema martini:* A model for onchocerciasis. Part 1. Description of lesions. *Annales de Parasitologie Humaine et Compareé* 66:109–120.

Vuong, P.N., D. Spratt, L. Wanji, L. Aimard, and O. Bain. 1993. Onchocerca-like lesions induced by the filarioid nematode *Cercopithifilaria johnstoni* in its natural hosts and in the laboratory rat. *Annales de Parasitologie Humaine et Compareé* 68:176–181.

Wanji, S.J., J.C. Cabaret, J.C. Gantier, N. Bonnand, and O. Bain. 1990. The fate of the filaria *Monanema martini* in two rodent hosts: Recovery rate, migration and localization. *Annales de Parasitologie Humaine et Compareé* 65:80–88.

Wanji, S.J., J.C. Gantier, G. Petit, J. Rapp, and O. Bain. 1994. *Monanema martini* in its murid hosts: Microfiladermia related to infective larvae and adult filariae. *Tropical Medicine and Parasitology* 45:107–111.

13

DIOCTOPHYMATOSIS

LENA N. MEASURES

Dioctophyme renale (Goeze 1782).

Classification: Nematoda: Dioctophymatoidea: Dioctophymatidae.

Synonyms: *Ascaris renales* Goeze, 1782; *Ascaris visceralis* Gmelin, 1790; *Ascaris renalis* Gmelin, 1790; *Strongylus gigas* Rudolphi, 1802*; Eustrongylus gigas* (Rudolphi, 1802) Diesing, 1851*; Mirandonema intestinalis* (Kreis, 1945) Anderson and Bain, 1982; *Dioctophyma renale* (Goeze, 1782).

Common Name: Giant kidney worm

Dioctophyme renale (Goeze 1782), or giant kidney worm, is a parasitic nematode found in the kidney of carnivores, particularly mustelids and canids. Other mammals including humans can also be infected. It occurs aberrantly in the peritoneal cavity, especially in canids, and rarely in other organs or tissues. Distribution includes North and South America, Europe, the former USSR, the Middle East, and central and eastern Asia. Since Karmanova's (1959, 1960, 1961, 1962) work, including a translation of Karmanova (1968) in 1985, and Fyvie's (1971) review, additional research has contributed to our understanding of the biology and epizootiology of this roundworm parasite, especially in North America, where mink (*Mustela vison*) is the common definitive host.

Although giant kidney worm was known since 1583, it was first described from specimens found in the kidney of a dog by Goeze in 1782. After some debate on the use of *Dioctophyme* Collet-Meygret, 1802 and *Dioctophyma* Bosc, 1803, the International Commission on Zoological Nomenclature (1989) ruled on the application of Tollitt (1987) that the giant kidney worm be named *Dioctophyme renale.*

Adult worms are extremely large, females can be up to 103 cm long and 6–12 mm wide and males up to 35 cm long and 3–5 mm wide (Fig. 13.1). Worms tend to be smaller in mink (28–60 cm for females and 11–30 cm for males) than worms from canids. When alive, adults are blood-red in color.

LIFE HISTORY. Adult *D. renale* reside in the kidney, usually the right kidney, where adult females deposit eggs that are passed with urine into the aquatic environment. Fertilized eggs of *D. renale* in urine sediment are oval, contain two cells, are 73–83 µm long,

45–47 µm wide, brownish-yellow, and thick-shelled with a mammillated (pitted) surface except at the two poles (Fig. 13.2). First-stage larvae develop in eggs in about 35 days at 20° C (Mace and Anderson 1975) after which they are infective to the aquatic oligochaete, *Lumbriculus variegatus* (Muller 1774), which is the intermediate host (Karmanova 1959, 1960, 1962; Mace and Anderson 1975). First-stage larvae develop and molt to the second stage on day 50 and to the infective third stage on day 100 at 20° C in the ventral blood vessel *of L. variegatus* (Mace and Anderson 1975). Third-stage larvae retain the cuticles of the first and second stages.

Infective third-stage larvae in oligochaetes can infect mink directly or may infect suitable paratenic hosts such as fish or frogs, which then infect the final host when ingested (Mace and Anderson 1975; Measures and Anderson 1985) (Fig. 13.2). Third-stage larvae do not develop or grow in paratenic hosts; they invade various tissues, encapsulating mostly within abdominal muscles, the wall of the stomach, and mesenteries of fish and frogs (Woodhead 1950; Hallberg 1953; Karmanova 1961; Mace and Anderson 1975). Karmanova (1968) counted 1 to 12 larvae in various species of fish. Mace and Anderson (1975) examined 4 species of frogs (*Rana catesbeiana, R. clamitans melanota, R. septentrionalis, R. pipens*) and found 5.6% of 504 infected with a mean intensity of 1.6 larvae. Measures and Anderson (1985) observed larvae predominantly in the hypaxial musculature of pumpkinseed fish (*Lepomis gibbosus*), at prevalences of 5%–23%, with a mean intensity of 1–2 larvae per fish.

Third-stage larvae in intermediate or paratenic hosts eaten by mink penetrated the wall of the stomach, where a molt occurred 5 days postexposure (Mace and Anderson 1975). Lesions in the liver suggest larvae pass through the liver prior to entering the right kidney or abdominal cavity. Fifty days postexposure, one larva or young adult (9.0 cm long, with a patent vulva but incompletely developed reproductive system) was located in the peritoneal cavity of a mink (Mace and Anderson 1975). Eggs deposited by adult females in the abdominal cavity cannot exit from the host; however, those deposited in the kidney are passed with urine through the ureter, which usually remains functional. The prepatent period, as determined by eggs in the urine, is 135 days in dogs and 154 days in mink (Karmanova 1968; Mace and Anderson 1975). Adult

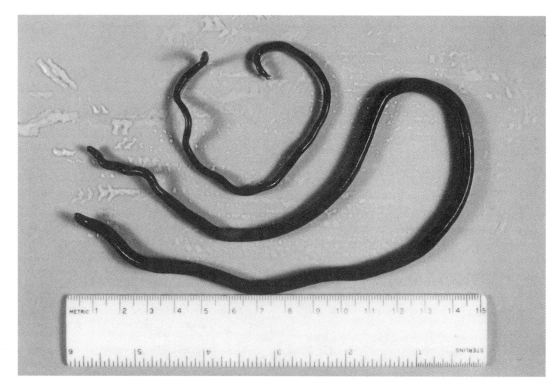

FIG. 13.1—Adult female (below) and male (above) *Dioctophyme renale* (Goeze, 1782).

worms were found in the kidney of experimentally infected ferrets (*Mustela putorius*) examined at 108, 134, and 155 days postexposure (Woodhead 1950; Measures and Anderson 1985). The longevity of *D. renale* as well as the patent period in the final host is unknown; however, Karmanova (1968) indicated that worms may live 3 to 5 years in the definitive host.

EPIZOOTIOLOGY

Distribution. *Dioctophyme renale* has been reported from Canada, the United States, Mexico, Brazil, Paraguay, Argentina, France, Holland, Germany, Bulgaria, Romania, Italy, Poland, the former USSR, Iran, Afghanistan, India, Vietnam, Thailand, China, and Japan. It may have been Holarctic in origin, spreading to other parts of the world by translocation of infected hosts (especially dogs) or by feeding infected fish from enzootic areas to susceptible animals. The only known intermediate host, *L. variegatus,* belongs to the Holarctic family Lumbriculidae and has been introduced to the southern hemisphere (Africa, Australia, New Zealand) (Brinkhurst and Jamieson 1971). *Dioctophyme renale* has been commonly reported in animals (especially dogs) from South America; however, the reported absence of lumbriculids in South America

(Brinkhurst and Jamieson 1971) may indicate that other oligochaetes can serve as intermediate hosts.

Host Range. Final hosts include Mustelidae: mink, short-tailed weasel (*Mustela erminea*), long-tailed weasel (*M. frenata*), Siberian weasel (*M. sibirica*), European polecat or ferret (*M. putorius*), marten (*Martes americana*), river otters (*Lutra canadensis, L. lutra* and *L. longicaudis*), wolverine (*Gulo gulo*), little grison (*Galictis cuja*); Canidae: coyote (*Canis latrans*), golden jackal (*C. aureus*), timber wolf (*C. lupus*), red wolf (*C. rufus*), domestic dog (*C. familaris*), maned wolf (*Chrysocyon brachyurus*), red fox (*Vulpes vulpes*), gray fox (*Urocyon cinereoargenteus*), bush dog (*Speothos venaticus*), raccoon *dog (Nyctereutes procyonoides)*; and Procyonidae: raccoon (*Procyon lotor*) and coati (*Nasua nasua*). Occasional hosts include cattle, horses, swine, and humans. Popov and Taikov (1985) reported *D. renale* from the Caspian seal (*Phoca caspica*). Reports from other mammal hosts such as domestic cat (*Felis catus*), wildcat (*F. silvestris*), cheetah (*Acinonyx jubatus*), brown bear (*Ursus arctos*), phocid seals (*Phoca* sp.), rat (*Rattus norvegicus*), and mongoose (species not given) (Karmanova 1968; Mace 1976a) and reports from Africa and Australia, as indicated in Karmanova (1968), are equivocal and require verification.

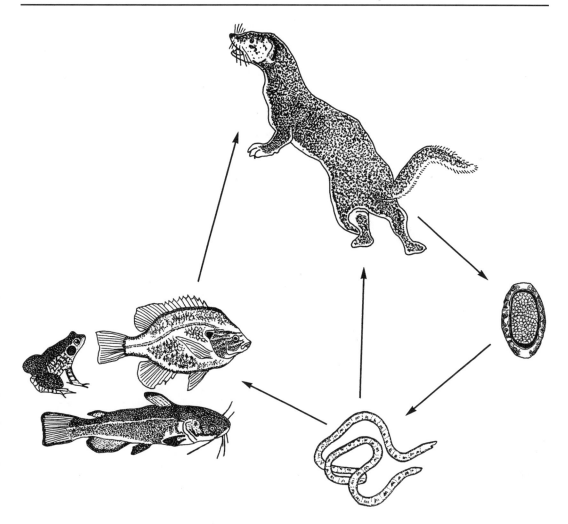

FIG. 13.2—Life cycle of *Dioctophyme renale* (Goeze, 1782) in North America (definitive host—mink; intermediate host—aquatic oligochaete; paratenic hosts—fish, frogs).

Paratenic hosts include Ranidae: frogs (*Rana cates-beiana, R. clamitans melanota, R. septentrionalis, R. ridibunda*) and Pisces: fresh-water fish [Acipenseridae (*Pseudoscaphirynchus kaufmanni*); Ictaluridae (*Ictalurus nebulosus, I. melas*); Esocidae (*Esox lucius*); Cyprinidae (*Leuciscus idus, Aspius aspius, Rutilus rutilus, Chalcalburnus chalcoides, Pelecus cultratus, Barbus branchicephalus, Gobio gobio, Alburnoides taeniatus*); Percidae (*Perca fluviatilis*); Siluridae (*Silurus glanis*); Poeciliidae (*Gambusia affinis*); Centrarchidae (*Lepomis gibbosus, L. cyanellus, Micropterus salmoides*)] (see Karmanova 1961, 1968; Mace and Anderson 1975; Measures and Anderson 1985; A.K. Prestwood unpublished).

Intermediate hosts are aquatic oligochaetes, with only one species, *Lumbriculus variegatus,* being found naturally infected with larval *D. renale* as well as being

a suitable experimental host (Karmanova 1959, 1960, 1962; Mace and Anderson 1975). The observation by Woodhead (1950) that branchiobdellid oligochaetes parasitic on crayfish are intermediate hosts has been discredited (Chitwood and Chitwood 1950; Mace and Anderson 1975).

Prevalence and Intensity. While *D. renale* is widely distributed, it only occurs in localized enzootic areas where prevalence among hosts varies from year to year. For example, in the Parry Sound area of Ontario, Canada, 24%–50% of trapped mink (depending on year of collection) were infected (Fyvie 1971). Fyvie further reported *D. renale* in 1.5% of weasels (*Mustela* sp.), 2.2% of otters, 1% of timber wolves, 0.9% of coyotes, and 18% of mink examined throughout Ontario (over 6500 animals comprising 12 species were examined). In the Washago area of Ontario ~50% of mink were infected (Mace and Anderson 1975). Seville and Addison (1995) reported 2% of 405 marten from Ontario were infected with *D. renale* or had evidence of previous infections (right kidney destroyed, leaving a fibrous capsule). They also reported 37% of mink from Parry Sound and 17% of mink from Ft. Francis infected. In other Canadian wildlife, *D. renale* was found in 1 of 25 wolves examined from southwestern Quebec (McNeill and Rau 1984), in none of 98 wolves and 1 of 75 coyotes from Alberta (Holmes and Podesta 1968), and 3 of 246 mink from Manitoba (Crichton and Urban 1970). In the United States, recorded prevalences include 2.5%–8.6% in wild mink from Michigan (Woodhead and McNeil 1939; Sealander 1943), 2.5% of 120 mink from North Carolina, 1 raccoon (Miller and Harkema 1964; Harkema and Miller 1964), 13 of 16 coyotes from California (Brunetti 1959; Beaver and Theis 1979), and 0.2% of 1185 mink from North Dakota (Jorde 1980). In Central and South America, gray fox from Mexico (Pineda-Lopez 1984), 2 little grisons from Brazil (Barros et al. 1990), and captive and wild maned wolves from Brazil and Argentina (see Costa and Lima 1988; Estevez et al. 1993) were infected. Most of the latter are case reports with little or no data on prevalence or intensity in wild populations. In Europe, dogs, ranched foxes, and other domestic animals are more commonly infected than wildlife (see Karmanova 1968). Prevalence in dogs ranged from 4% to 66% depending on locality. Golden jackals (7 of 20) and wolves from northern Iran also were infected (Sadighian and Amini 1967). There are numerous case reports of infections in domestic dogs in North and South America and from the Old World (see Ehrenford and Snodgrass 1955; Osborne et al. 1969; Celerin and McMullen 1981; Eslami and Mohebali 1988; Le Riche et al. 1988; Costa et al. 1990).

Infections with the giant kidney worm may involve a single worm, single sex infections, or both sexes of worms. Mean intensity in wild mink in Ontario was 2.7 with 54% of infected mink having male and female worms (Mace and Anderson 1975). Infections may involve only the kidney (86%), only the abdominal cavity (6%), or both locations in the same infected individual (7%) (Fyvie 1971). Less than 1% of infections in mink involve both kidneys. Intensities in dogs may be much greater than in mink—27 adult worms (13 in the abdomen and 14 in the right kidney) in an infected dog in Iran (Sadighian and Amini 1967) and 42 worms (20 in the abdomen and 22 in the right kidney) in another infected dog (Karmanova 1968). Rare infections have involved the mammary gland, uterus, ovaries, urinary bladder, inguinal subcutaneous tissues, and stomach of mink and dogs (Fyvie 1971; Samuell et al. 1990; Miranda et al. 1992; Mattos and Pinheiro 1994) and subcutaneous tissues and thoracic wall of humans (Beaver and Theis 1979; Beaver and Khamboonruang 1984; Gutierrez et al. 1989).

Environmental Limitations. Development of eggs in the external environment and development of larvae in the oligochaete host are temperature dependent (Mace and Anderson 1975). First-stage larvae develop within 15–102 days when eggs are kept in well-oxygenated, fresh water and incubated between 14° C and 30° C. Eggs do not survive desiccation, freezing, or high temperatures (Lukasiak 1930, Mace and Anderson 1975). Eggs incubated 60 days at 6° C or 10° C did not develop (cell division not apparent) but resumed development when the temperature was increased to 14° C (Mace and Anderson 1975). Larvated eggs do not survive desiccation or freezing, as evidenced by their inability to infect oligochaetes after such treatment. Third-stage larvae develop within 70 to 159 days when infected oligochaetes are incubated between 15° C and 30° C (Mace and Anderson 1975). The development rate of larvae in oligochaetes was slower when there were multiple infections (more than four larvae). No host reaction was observed around larvae within the ventral blood vessel of infected oligochaetes. It is unknown whether the behaviour of infected oligochaetes is altered by the presence of larval *D. renale*.

The longevity of encapsulated third-stage larval *D. renale* in fish and frogs has not been studied, but larvae likely remain alive and infectious for years. Given that eggs of *D. renale* are freezing intolerant, transmission to oligochaetes in temperate climates likely occurs only from spring to fall with subsequent development being restricted to the summer months when water temperatures are greater than 14° C. Once water temperatures attain 20° C, eggs develop in the external environment, and third-stage larvae develop in oligochaetes within ~140 days under ideal conditions. Transmission to fish may occur at any time of the year but is probably restricted to when fish are feeding intensely (spring to end of fall). Mink remain active during winter when fish often are an important component of their diet (Sealander 1943; Wilson 1954; Gerell 1967). If transmission to fish then mink is favorable, a period of 154 days is required before infections in mink are patent, thus completing the life cycle within 1 year [Karmanova (1968) estimated 8.5 to 9 months]. In southern Ontario, Canada eggs of *D. renale* freshly deposited in the external environment in April can develop and infect oligochaetes in which larvae develop to the infective stage during summer. Subsequent infection of fish or frogs by consumption of infected oligochaetes may occur as early as October. If mink acquire infections from infected paratenic hosts during fall or early winter, infections may become patent the following spring (April). In southern latitudes, such as South America, transmission likely occurs year-round.

CLINICAL SIGNS. During experimental infections mink become agitated shortly after being fed infective larvae, and violent vomition occurs within 30 minutes of infection and lasts up to an hour, presumably due to larvae invading the stomach wall (Mace and Anderson 1975). Vomition has also been observed in ferrets and dogs (Hallberg 1953; Karmanova 1968; Measures and Anderson 1985). Clinical signs and symptoms may not be apparent, but when present may include hematuria, pyuria, weakness, reluctance to walk, increased frequency of urination, anorexia, convulsions, anemia, ascites, renal and abdominal colic, weight loss, irritability, polydipsia, depression, micturition, proteinuria, and uremia (Karmanova 1968; Osborne et al. 1969; Mace and Anderson 1975; Measures and Anderson 1985).

PATHOLOGY AND PATHOGENESIS. In mink, infection of the kidney by *D. renale* results in almost total destruction of the renal parenchyma—atropy and fibrosis of renal tubules, periglomerular fibrosis, and connective tissue infiltration of interstitial tissue—leaving a thickened kidney capsule (Fig. 13.3) containing parasites bathed in a sanguinopurulent fluid containing red blood cells, leucocytes, parasite eggs, degenerating cells, and calcified debris. In 45%–70% of cases in mink a "staghorn" bone formation develops in the dorsal wall of the kidney capsule (McNeil 1948; Mace 1976b). Bone formation, renal calculi, or calci-

fication of necrotic tissue has been observed in other wild mink (Hallberg 1953; Fyvie 1971), experimentally infected mink (Mace and Anderson 1975) and ferrets (Woodhead 1950; Measures and Anderson 1985), and naturally infected dogs and coyotes (Brunetti 1959; McLeod 1967; Osborne et al. 1969). Usually the ureter is functional, but in some cases worms within the kidney pelvis may block the ureter, resulting in hydronephrosis. Destruction of the right kidney may result in compensatory hypertrophy of the left kidney.

Experimental infection involving a dose of 28 *D. renale* larvae caused death of mink, with hemorrhage of the stomach wall 24 hours postexposure (Mace and Anderson 1975). Such massive infections probably are rare in wild mink, given reported mean intensities of 1–2 larvae in fish and 2.7 larvae in mink. Larvae within the stomach wall 5 days postexposure were surrounded by red blood cells, fibroblasts, lymphocytes, and a layer of fibrous connective tissue (Mace and Anderson 1975). Migrating worms caused chronic persistent hepatitis (mainly in the right lobes of the liver) and proliferative chronic inflammatory reactions on the peritoneum. A matrix of fibrin, fibrous connective tissue, eggs of *D. renale,* giant cells, macrophages, lymphocytes, neutrophils, and plasma cells in the mesothelium

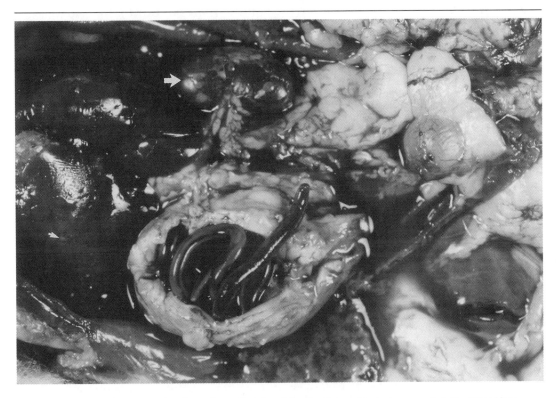

FIG. 13.3—Opened abdominal cavity of experimentally infected ferret with two *Dioctophyme renale* in the right kidney 133 days postexposure. Uninfected left kidney is indicated by a large arrow (*top*). Small arrow (*left*) indicates lesion on liver capsule caused by migrating worms.

was observed histologically in mink and experimentally infected ferrets (Mace 1976b; Measures and Anderson 1985). Chronic hemorrhagic peritonitis with perforated mesenteries, adhesions, hepatic necrosis, abdominal fluid containing blood, fibrin, *D. renale* eggs and cellular debris, hydronephrosis, pyonephrosis, hemorrhagic pyelitis, and chronic pyelonephritis have been observed in dogs (Smits et al. 1965; McLeod 1967; Osborne et al. 1969; Coppo and Brehm 1983).

The migratory route of larval *D. renale* from the stomach to the right kidney has been the subject of various theories (Hallberg 1953; Karmanova 1968; Mace and Anderson 1975). Larvae may penetrate the duodenal wall, entering the abdominal cavity prior to entering the right kidney as adults (Hallberg 1953). Alternatively, larvae may penetrate the stomach wall, passing through the liver and abdominal cavity prior to entering the right kidney as adults (Karmanova 1968; Mace and Anderson 1975). As only adult worms have been observed in the kidney, it is believed that it is the adult stage which penetrates the kidney. The migratory route may be influenced by host anatomy. In mink the stomach, right lobe of the liver, first loop of the duodenum, and right kidney are in close proximity, and Hallberg (1953) and Mace and Anderson (1975) postulated that this may account for 85% of infections in mink involving the right kidney. In dogs these organs (stomach, first loop of the duodenum, right lobe of the liver, and right kidney) are less intimate, and Hallberg (1953) believed that this may account for greater percentages of *D. renale* in the abdominal cavity in dogs compared to mink.

DIAGNOSIS. The presence of large, blood-red nematodes in the kidney or abdominal cavity at necropsy is usually diagnostic for *D. renale* (Fig.13.3). The characteristic eggs of *D. renale* (may be unfertilized in the case of infections involving only female worms) in the urine, in ascitic fluid (caused by worms in the abdomen), or worms passed in the urine also are diagnostic (Fig.13.2; see Life History section). Intestinal helminths passed in the stool should be distinguished from those passed in urine. Infections, particularly of the kidney, also can be detected using palpation, laparotomy, aspiration of eggs in fluid from the kidney or abdominal cavity (paracentesis), and x-ray, but apparently not using sonography (see Narvaez et al. 1994). Tuur et al. (1987) cautioned that so-called Liesegang rings in the kidney of humans not be confused with eggs of *D. renale*. Larvae similar to third-stage larval *D. renale* have been described histologically from subcutaneous nodules in humans (Beaver and Theis 1979; Beaver and Khamboonruang 1984; Gutierrez et al. 1989). Identification of larval *D. renale,* particularly histologically, is problematic as they could be confused with larval *Eustrongylides* spp. Fourth-stage larval *D. renale* have not been adequately described. Karmanova (1968, p. 73) gave a brief description of fourth-stage larvae, but no drawings

were provided nor was the location of larvae given. She indicated that the third molt occurred in the liver and the fourth molt in the body cavity of the final host (Karmanova 1968, p. 82). Mace and Anderson (1975) observed a molt in the stomach of mink 5 days postexposure. Measures (1988a,b) described third-stage and fourth-stage *Eustrongylides tubifex* and indicated how to distinquish these larvae from third-stage *D. renale.*

IMMUNITY. No data exist on whether hosts develop immunity to *D. renale.* However, natural and experimental infections suggest that hosts are infected only once (Hallberg 1953). In infections involving more than one worm, worms are always at the same stage of development (Hallberg 1953; Mace and Anderson 1975).

CONTROL AND TREATMENT. The only possible control is to avoid consumption of raw fish and frogs, especially in areas known to be enzootic for *D. renale.* Treatment usually is initiated when clinical signs reveal infection of the kidney. Some drugs may help alleviate pain or facilitate the expulsion of worms from the kidney (Vibe 1985; Chen and Liu 1988). Nephrectomy is frequently performed in infected dogs.

PUBLIC HEALTH CONCERNS. According to Beaver and Theis (1979) 13 unequivocal cases of dioctophymatosis in humans have been documented. Additional cases have been reported (Beaver and Theis 1979; Beaver and Khamboonruang 1984; Vibe 1985; Chen and Liu 1988; Gutierrez et al. 1989, Narvaez et al. 1994); however, larvae resembling *D. renale* in histologic sections need to be distinquished from larval *Eustrongylides* spp. Both *Dioctophyme* and *Eustrongylides* are transmitted to humans by the consumption of raw or poorly cooked fish containing infective larvae. Although most fish destined for human consumption are eviscerated, the discovery of third-stage larval *D. renale* in the hypaxial musculature of sport fish such as pumpkinseed or bass (centrachids) indicates the potential risk for consumers of these fish (Measures and Anderson 1985).

DOMESTIC ANIMAL HEALTH CONCERNS. Domestic animals such as dogs or farmed furbearers such as mink and fox are at risk if fed raw fish or frogs containing infective *D. renale.* Adequate cooking or freezing of infected food will eliminate this risk. Other domestic animals may be at risk if infected oligochaetes are ingested with water. Fencing around water sources known to harbor infected oligochaetes or provision of filtered water may prevent infection.

MANAGEMENT IMPLICATIONS. Although *D. renale* is widely distributed, it is locally abundant only in certain enzootic areas. Dry, arid areas that neither favor the intermediate host nor have abundant fish or fish-eating mammals can be expected to have lower prevalences of this parasite compared to humid, water-rich areas (Jorde 1980). Translocation of infected dogs, other canids, or mustelids to areas where the intermediate host and potential paratenic hosts are present should be avoided. Despite complete destruction of the right kidney, hosts such as mink can survive infections as long as one kidney remains functional and disease free and there are no severe lesions caused by migrating worms or worms resident in the abdomen. Dead worms were resorbed in two mink (Mace and Anderson 1975). Seville and Addison (1995) observed six trapped marten with evidence of previous infection with *D. renale*—an empty fibrous capsule was all that remained of the right kidney, while the left kidney was hypertrophied. Similar observations have been made with regard to infected dogs (see Osborne et al. 1969). Thus, infected hosts survive unilateral kidney infections, but involvement of both kidneys is fatal. Worms free in the abdominal cavity can lead to peritonitis and damage of other tissues, occasionally with a fatal outcome. Data on significance of mortality due to *D. renale* in wild mustelid populations, however, are lacking.

LITERATURE CITED

Anderson, R.C., and O. Bain. 1982. Keys to genera of the superfamilies Rhabditoidea, Dioctophymatoidea, Trichinelloidea and Muspiceoidea, no. 9. In *CIH keys to the nematode parasites of vertebrates*. Ed. R.C. Anderson, A.G. Chabaud and S. Willmott. Wallingford, UK: CAB International, pp. 15–16.

Barros, D.M., M.L. Lorini, and V.G. Persson. 1990. Dioctophymosis in the little grison (*Galictis cuja*). *Journal of Wildlife Diseases* 26:538–539.

Beaver, P.C. and C. Khamboonruang. 1984. *Dioctophyma*-like larval nematode in a subcutaneous nodule from man in northern Thailand. *American Journal of Tropical Medicine and Hygiene* 33:1032–1034.

Beaver, P.C., and J.H. Theis. 1979. Dioctophymatid larval nematode in a subcutaneous nodule from man in California. *American Journal of Tropical Medicine and Hygiene* 28:206–212.

Brinkhurst, R.O., and B.G.M. Jamieson. 1971. *Aquatic oligochaeta of the world*. Toronto: University of Toronto Press.

Brunetti, O.A. 1959. Occurrence of the giant kidney worm, *Dioctophyma renale*, in the coyote of California. *California Fish and Game* 45:351–352.

Celerin, A.J., and M.E. McMullen. 1981. Giant kidney worm in a dog. *Journal of the American Veterinary Medical Association* 179:245–246.

Chen, H.C., and G.H. Liu. 1988. Report of a case of *Dioctophyma renale* infection. *Chinese Journal of Parasitology and Parasitic Diseases* 6:237.

Chitwood, B.G., and M.B. Chitwood. 1950. *Introduction to nematology*. Baltimore, MD: University Park Press.

Coppo, J.A., and J.J. Brehm. 1983. Canine dioctophymosis in the north east of Argentine. *Revista do Instituto de Medicina Tropical de Sao Paulo* 25:259–262.

Costa, H.M. de A., and W. dos S. Lima. 1988. Occurrence of *Dioctophyme renale* (Goeze, 1782) in Minas Gerais state. *Arquivo Brasileiro de Medicina Veterinaria e Zootecnia* 40:243–244.

Costa, J.O., W. dos S. Lima, M.P. Guimaraes, and E.N.M. Lima. 1990. Endo- and ectoparasites of dogs from Vitoria County, Espirito Santo, Brazil. *Arquivo Brasileiro de Medicina Veterinariae Zootecnia* 42:451–452.

Crichton, V.J., and R.E. Urban. 1970. *Dioctophyme renale* (Goeze, 1782) (Nematoda: Dioctophymata) in Manitoba mink. *Canadian Journal of Zoology* 48:591–592.

Ehrenford, F.A., and T.B. Snodgrass. 1955. Incidence of canine dioctophymiasis (giant kidney worm infection) with a summary of cases in North America. *Journal of the American Veterinary Medical Association* 126:415–417.

Eslami, A., and M. Mohebali. 1988. Parasitisme des chiens de bergers et implications en sante. *Bulletin de la Société de Pathologie exotique* 81:94–96.

Estevez, J.O., E.G. Maubecin, and R.E. Mentzel. 1993. Finding of *Dioctophyma (Dioctophyme) renale* in a maned wolf (*Chrysocyon brachyurus*) and its treatment by nephrectomy. *Correo Veterinario* 159:11–12.

Fyvie, A. l971. *Dioctophyma renale*. In *Parasitic diseases of wild mammals*. Ed. J.W. Davis and R.C. Anderson. Ames: The Iowa State University Press, pp. 258–262.

Gerell, R. 1967. Food selection in relation to habitat in mink (*Mustela vison* Schreber) in Sweden. *Oikos* 18:233–246.

Gutierrez, Y., M. Cohen, and C.N. Machicao. 1989. *Dioctophyme* larva in the subcutaneous tissues of a woman in Ohio. *American Journal of Surgical Pathology* 13:800–802.

Hallberg, C.W. 1953. *Dioctophyma renale* (Goeze, 1782). A study of the migration routes to the kidneys of mammals and resultant pathology. *Transactions of the American Microscopical Society* 72:351–63.

Harkema, R., and G.C. Miller. 1964. Helminth parasites of the raccoon, *Procyon lotor,* in the southeastern United States. *The Journal of Parasitology* 50:60–66.

Holmes, J.C., and R. Podesta. 1968. The helminths of wolves and coyotes from the forested regions of Alberta. *Canadian Journal of Zoology* 46:1193–1204.

International Commission on Zoological Nomenclature. 1989. Opinion 1552. *Bulletin of Zoological Nomenclature* 46:199–200.

Jorde, D.G. 1980. Occurrence of *Dioctophyma renale* (Goeze, 1782) in mink from North Dakota. *Journal of Wildlife Diseases* 16:381–382.

Karmanova, E.M. 1959. The life-cycle of the nematode, *Dioctophyme renale* [In Russian]. *Doklady Akademii Nauk SSSR* 127:1317–1319.

_____. 1960. The life-cycle of the nematode, *Dioctophyme renale* (Goeze, 1782) parasitic in the kidneys of carnivorous animals and man [In Russian]. *Doklady Akademii Nauk SSSR* 132:1219–1221.

_____. 1961. The first report of *Dioctophyme renale* larvae in fish of the USSR [In Russian]. *Trudy Gel'mintologicheskoi Laboratorii, Akademiya Nauk SSSR* 11:118–121.

_____. 1962. The life-cycle of *Dioctophyme renale* in its intermediate and definitive hosts [In Russian]. *Trudy Gel'mintologicheskoi Laboratorii, Akademiya Nauk SSSR* 12:27–36.

_____. 1968. Dioctophymidea of animals and man and diseases caused by them. *Fundamentals of nematology*, vol. 20. Academy of Sciences of the USSR. [1985. Translation by U.S. Department of Agriculture. New Delhi: Amerind Publishing Co., 383 pp.]

Le Riche, P.D., A.K. Soe, Q. Alemzada, and L. Sharifi. 1988. Parasites of dogs in Kabul, Afghanistan. *British Veterinary Journal* 144:370–373.

Lukasiak, J. 1930. *Eustrongylus gigas* (Rud.) [In Russian]. *Archives of the Biological Society of Science and Letters, Warsaw* 3:1–100.

Mace, T.F. 1976a. Bibliography of giant kidney worm *Dioctophyma renale* (Goeze, 1782) (Nematoda: Dioctophymatoidea). *Wildlife Disease* No. 69.

Mace, T.F. 1976b. Lesions in mink (*Mustela vison*) infected with giant kidney worm (*Dioctophyma renale*). *Journal of Wildlife Diseases* 12:88–92.

Mace, T.F., and R.C. Anderson. 1975. Development of the giant kidney worm, *Dioctophyma renale* (Goeze, 1782) (Nematoda: Dioctophymatoidea). *Canadian Journal of Zoology* 53:1552–1568.

Mattos Junior, D.G., and J. Pinheiro. 1994. *Dioctophyma renale* (Goeze, 1782) in subcutaneous tissues of the inguinal regional of a dog. *Arquivo Brasileiro de Medicina Veterinariae Zootecnia* 46:301–302.

McLeod, J.A. 1967. *Dioctophyma renale* infections in Manitoba. *Canadian Journal of Zoology* 45:505–508.

McNeil, C.W. 1948. Pathological changes in the kidney of mink due to infection with *Dioctophyma renale* (Goeze, 1782), the giant kidney worm of mammals. *Transactions of the American Microscopical Society* 67:257–261.

McNeill, M.A., and M.E. Rau. 1984. Helminths of wolves (*Canis lupus* L.) from southwestern Quebec. *Canadian Journal of Zoology* 62:1659–1660.

Measures, L.N. 1988a. The development of *Eustrongylides tubifex* (Nematoda: Dioctophymatoidea) in oligochaetes. *The Journal of Parasitology* 74:294–304.

———. 1988b. Epizootiology, pathology, and description of *Eustrongylides tubifex* (Nematoda: Dioctophymatoidea) in fish. *Canadian Journal of Zoology* 66:2212–2222.

Measures, L.N., and R.C. Anderson. 1985. Centrarchid fish as paratenic hosts of the giant kidney worm, *Dioctophyma renale* (Goeze, 1782) in Ontario, Canada. *Journal of Wildlife Diseases* 21:11–19.

Miller, G.C., and R. Harkema. 1964. Studies on helminths of North Carolina vertebrates. V. Parasites of the mink, *Mustela vison* Schreber. *The Journal of Parasitology* 50:717–720.

Miranda, M.A., R.N.M. Benigno, G.R. Galvao, and S.A.L. de Oliveira. 1992. *Dioctophyme renale* (Goeze, 1782): localizacao ectopicae alta intensidade parasitaria em *Canis familiaris* do Para-Brasil. *Arquivo Brasileiro de Medicina Veterinariae Zootecnia* 44:151–153.

Narvaez, J.A., L.P. Turell, J. Serra, and F. Hidalgo. 1994. Hyperdense renal cystic lesions caused by *Dioctophyma renale*. *American Journal of Roentgenology* 163:997–998.

Osborne, C.A., J.B. Stevens, G.F. Hanlon, E. Rosin, and W.J. Bemrick. 1969. *Dioctophyma renale* in the dog. *Journal of the American Veterinary Medical Association* 155:605–620.

Pineda-Lopez, R. 1984. First report of *Dioctophyme renale* (Nematoda: Dioctophymatidae) in Tabasco, Mexico. *Anales del Instituto de Biologia, Zoologia, Universidad Nacional Autonoma de Mexico* 55:307–310.

Popov, V.N., and I.M. Taikov. 1985. The discovery of the nematode *Dioctophyme renale* in the Caspian seal. *Vestnik Zoologii* 1985(5): 7.

Sadighian, A., and F. Amini. 1967. *Dioctophyma renale* (Goeze, 1782) Stiles, 1901 in stray dogs and jackals in Shahsavar Area, Caspian Region, Iran. *The Journal of Parasitology* 53:561.

Samuell, C.A., L.A. Fusé, and C. A. San Romé. 1990. Un caso de *Dioctophyme renale* en glandula mamaria de perra. *Revisita de Medicina Veterinaria (Buenos Aires)* 71:162–164.

Sealander, J.A. 1943. Winter food habits of mink in southern Michigan. *The Journal of Wildlife Management* 7:411–417.

Seville, R.S., and E.M. Addison. 1995. Nongastrointestinal helminths in marten (*Martes americana*) from Ontario, Canada. *Journal of Wildlife Diseases* 31:529–533.

Smits, G.M., W. Disdorp, A.C. Rijpstra, and N.H. Swellengrebel. 1965. *Dioctophyma renale* in a dog in the Netherlands. *Tropical and Geographical Medicine* 17:162–168.

Tollitt, M.E. 1987. Case 2604 *Dioctophyme* Collet-Meygret, 1802 (Nematoda): Proposed confirmation of spelling (CIOMS Case No. 7). *Bulletin of Zoological Nomenclature* 44:237–239.

Tuur, S.M., A.M. Nelson, D.W. Gibson, R.C. Neafie, F.B. Johnson, F.K. Mostofi, and D.H. Connor. 1987. Liesegang rings in tissue. How to distinquish Liesegang rings from the giant kidney worm, *Dioctophyma renale*. *American Journal of Surgical Pathology* 11:598–605.

Vibe, P.P. 1985. Invasion of man with *Dioctophyme renale*. *Meditsinskaja Parazitologija i Parazitarnye Bolezni* 1:83–84.

Wilson, K.A. 1954. The role of mink and otter as muskrat predators in northeastern North Carolina. *The Journal of Wildlife Management* 18:199–207.

Woodhead, A.E. 1950. Life history cycle of the giant kidney worm, *Dioctophyma renale* (Nematoda), of man and many other mammals. *Transactions of the American Microscopical Society* 69:21–46.

Woodhead, A.E., and C.W. McNeil. 1939. *Dioctophyme renale*, the giant kidney worm occurring in mink, from the southern counties of Michigan. *The Journal of Parasitology* 25:23.

14

HEPATIC CAPILLARIASIS

DAVID M. SPRATT AND GRANT R. SINGLETON

INTRODUCTION. *Calodium hepaticum* (Bancroft 1893) Moravec 1982 (syn. *Hepaticola hepatica* Bancroft 1893, syn. *Capillaria hepatica* (Bancroft 1893) Travassos 1915) is a nematode parasite of vertebrates belonging to the superfamily Trichinelloidea, subfamily Capillariinae (Anderson and Bain 1982). It is cosmopolitan in its distribution and has been recorded in Africa, Asia, Australia, Europe, India and North, Central and South America.

Calodium hepaticum is catholic in its host spectrum, although primarily a parasite of the hepatic parenchyma of rodents belonging to the genera *Actomys, Akodon, Apodemus, Arvicanthis, Arvicola, Bandicota, Castor, Citellus, Clethrionomys, Cricetomys, Cricetulus, Cynomys, Dasymys, Ellobius, Geomys, Gerbillus, Lemmus, Lemniscomys, Marmota, Microtus, Mus, Myopotamus, Napeozapus, Neotoma, Ondatra, Otomys, Peromyscus, Rattus, Sciurus, Sigmodon, Suncus, Synaptomys, Tatera,* and *Thomomys* (Hall 1916; Weidman 1917, 1925; Yokogawa 1920; Cram 1928; Price 1931; Dikmans 1932; Chitwood 1934; Harkema 1936; Luttermoser 1936, 1938b; Herman 1939; Ameel 1942; Penn 1942; Brown and Roy 1943; Firlotte 1948; Read 1949; Vogelsang and Espin 1949; Calero et al. 1950; Meyer and Reilly 1950; Davis 1951; Doran 1955; Lubinsky 1956, 1957; Wantland et al. 1956; Skrjabin et al. 1957; Freeman 1958; Freeman and Wright 1960; Pavlov 1960; Layne 1963, 1968; Layne and Griffo 1961; Rausch 1961; Fisher 1963; Lubinsky et al. 1971; Ishimoto 1974; Reynolds and Gavutis 1975; Brown et al. 1975a,b; Herman 1981; Koval'chuk and Bonina 1981; Chineme and Ibrahim 1984; Borucinska and Nielsen 1993). Studies generally have found a high prevalence of infection of *C. hepaticum* in field populations of rats of the genus *Rattus* (Fielding 1927; Momma 1930; Price and Chitwood 1931; Luttermoser 1936; Seo et al. 1964; Waddell 1969; Galvão 1976, 1981; Farhang-Azad 1977a; Liat et al. 1977; Farhang-Azad and Schlitter 1978; Chaiyabutr 1979; Conlogue et al. 1979; Sinniah et al. 1979; Chieffi et al. 1981; Markus and Yeo cited in Cheetham and Markus 1983; Saenong 1984; Childs et al. 1988; Singleton et al. 1991). However, *C. hepaticum* has been recorded in marsupials (Schmidt 1975), lagomorphs (Nicoll 1911; Suda 1928; Ward 1934; Hörning 1974; Kutzer and Frey 1976; Gevrey and Chirol 1978), insectivores (Solomon and Handley 1971; Brander et al. 1990), artiodactyls (Foster and Johnson 1939; Barrett and Chalmers 1972;

Partington and Montali 1986), perissodactyls (Nation and Dies 1978; Monroe 1984), carnivores (Wright 1930; Vianna 1954; Smit 1960; Layne and Winegarner 1971; Stokes 1973; Wobeser and Rock 1973; Rao et al. 1975; Crowell et al. 1978; LeBlanc et al. 1983; Brander et al.1990), and primates (Troisier et al. 1928; Foster and Johnson 1939; Caballero and Grocot 1952; Kumar et al. 1983) including man (Dive et al. 1924; MacArthur 1924; Otto et al. 1954; Turhan et al. 1954; Ewing and Tilden 1956; Ward and Dent 1959; Kallichurum and Elsdon-Dew 1961; Romero and Biagi 1962; Piazza et al. 1963; Cislagi and Radice 1970; Pampiglione and Concini 1970; Slais and Sterba 1972; Slais 1973; Galvão 1979; Vargas et al. 1979; Attah et al. 1983; Johnson et al. 1989; Berger et al. 1990; Choe et al. 1993). Some of the records of infection in vertebrate animal hosts other than rodents come from zoos where control of rodents, especially of *Rattus* spp., is an ongoing challenge (see Weidman 1917, 1925; Chitwood 1934; Schmidt 1975, Partington and Montali 1986).

LIFE HISTORY. The life cycle of *C. hepaticum* is direct; no intermediate hosts are required (Fig. 14.1). Following ingestion by the host of embryonated eggs containing first-stage larvae, hatching of the larva occurs in the small intestine (Wright 1961) or cecum (Luttermoser 1938b; Solomon and Soulsby 1973; Zahner et al. 1976). Larvae penetrate the cecal wall and migrate via the mesenteric and portal veins to the liver (Fülleborn 1925; Nishigori 1925; Vogel 1930; Luttermoser 1938b), which is reached in about 2 days (Freeman and Wright 1960; Wright 1961). All molts occur in the liver; L_1 to L_2 at 3–4 days, L_2 to L_3 at 4–5 days and L_3 to L_4 at 7–9 days postinfection (Wright 1961). The nematodes grow rapidly, and L_4 molt to L_5 males and females at 18 and 20 days postinfection, respectively (Wright 1961). Adults are enclosed in multinucleate cytoplasmic masses originating from cells of the liver and presumably feed on the cytoplasm surrounding their anterior ends (Wright 1974). Females move through a syncytium of host cells in sinuous tracts, depositing clusters of uncleaved eggs that become encapsulated by host tissue (Luttermoser 1938a,b; Pavlov 1955). Time to first appearance of eggs in the liver varies: in mice it is reported to be 18 days (Luttermoser 1938b), 21 days (Pavlov 1955; Freeman and Wright 1960; Wright 1961) or 23 days (Shimatani

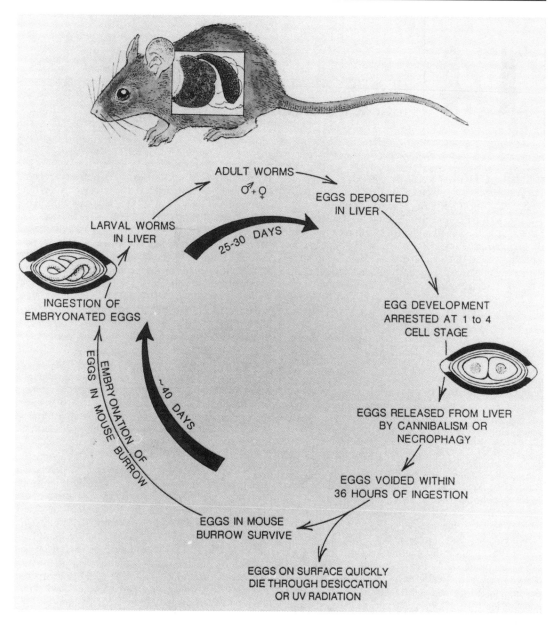

FIG. 14.1—The life cycle of *Calodium hepaticum.*

1961); in rats 21–33 days (Fülleborn 1925; Nishigori 1925; Luttermoser 1938b; Lee 1964); and in multimammate rats, *Mastomys natalensis,* 20 days (Zahner et al. 1976). However, massive infection of multimammate rats with about 50,000 eggs produced retardation of development and delayed the appearance of eggs in the liver by about 2 days (Lämmler et al. 1974). In this host, the dynamics and duration of egg production were dependent upon the infective dose: maximum egg production was between 60 and 72 days in animals infected with 50 eggs, 36–48 days in those infected with 300 eggs, and about 30 days in those infected with 800 eggs (Zahner et al. 1976). The time of death and subsequent degeneration of adult worms in the liver has been reported to vary between 26 and 72 days (Fülleborn 1925; Luttermoser 1938b; Pavlov 1955; Freeman and Wright 1960; Wright 1961; Lee 1964; Waddell 1969; Lämmler et al. 1974). During this time and subsequently, the eggs become progressively entrapped in fibrotic tissue.

The life cycle of *C. hepaticum* is unique among helminths of mammals (Fig. 14.1). Eggs of other hepatic helminths are shed into the environment via the bile duct, intestine, and feces. However, eggs of *C. hepaticum* cannot be liberated from the infected living host in this manner because of the fibrotic reaction (Bancroft 1893; Fülleborn 1924). They are liberated only by ingestion and subsequent digestion of the infected liver by another invertebrate or vertebrate animal (Freeman and Wright 1960; Wright 1961; Herman 1981). In rodents, the eggs are thought to be liberated via cannibalism (intraspecific predation or necrophagy), predation by vertebrates, or natural death and decomposition possibly assisted by scavenging invertebrates (Momma 1930; Luttermoser 1938b; Freeman and Wright 1960; Layne 1968; Mobedi and Arfaa 1971; Farhang-Azad 1977a,b; Conlogue et al. 1979; Herman 1981). If insects and other scavenging invertebrates play an effective role in this life cycle in nature, it is essential that they either distribute eggs to an environment suitable for egg embryonation or that they themselves provide that environment.

Infected liver ingested by rodents is digested, and the eggs are released into the environment with the feces of the animal. Spratt and Singleton (1986) reported that most eggs were passed in the feces of mice within 40 hours of ingestion. These eggs contained uncleaved embryos or embryos at the 2–4-cell stage of cleavage and were unchanged from those in the original infected liver (see also El Nassery et al. 1991). They are not embryonated and thus not infective to any animal. Eggs require a period of time in the environment to undergo the critical embryonation phase, the change from the early cleavage stage blastocyst (0–8 cells) to a fully formed nematode larva inside the egg shell. Viable eggs generally do not result from decaying livers (Shorb 1931; Luttermoser 1938a; Pavlov 1955; Spratt and Singleton 1986). Eggs are susceptible to desiccation (Bancroft 1893; Johnston 1918). Moisture and oxygen appear critical for embryonation, and temperature governs the rate of embryonation. This takes ~5–7 weeks at 25° C and is arrested < 10° C (Luttermoser 1938a; Pavlov 1955; Wright 1961; Spratt and Singleton 1986). Eggs are hardy and can withstand temperatures below freezing for considerable time periods (Wright 1961; El Nassery et al. 1991). They remain viable for lengthy periods (> 1 year) provided, it is thought, they are maintained in a moist environment with oxygen. Nevertheless, eggs of *C. hepaticum* have remained viable underground 3 years in experimental enclosures in the Mallee Region of Victoria, Australia, at soil water values ranging from 10% to 24% through a vertical distance of 0.5 m. There is no evidence that transmission of *C. hepaticum* can occur by transseminal, transplacental or transmammary routes (Spratt and Singleton 1986). We consider that transmission of *C. hepaticum* in mice in Australia is a consequence of ingestion of embryonated eggs with soil particles during the grooming behavior observed in mice of all ages in the moist, warm environment of the mouse burrow.

EPIZOOTIOLOGY

Prevalence and Intensity. *Calodium hepaticum* is primarily a parasite of the hepatic parenchyma of rodents (Table 14.1). In general, the highest prevalences of infection occurred in commensal populations of the Norway rat (*R. norvegicus*) (Table 14.1). In this host prevalence was > 55% in 12 of 15 studies and > 75% in 7 of those studies. The parasite has been recorded often in commensal populations of the black rat (*R. rattus*), but prevalence generally has been < 10% and not > 60%.

Most instances of *C. hepaticum* infection in non-rodent mammals occur where these animals have been living in close association with infected populations of *R. norvegicus*. This is particularly so in zoological parks. For example, 7 of 18 dik dik (*Madoqua kirkii*) were infected with *C. hepaticum* at the National Zoological Park, Washington DC, where infected *R. norvegicus* were found throughout the zoo grounds (Partington and Montali 1986). On the other hand, Crowell et al. (1978) reported *C. hepaticum* in histological sections of 21 of 71 coyotes (*Canis latrans*) trapped in Louisiana, but found no evidence of infection in the livers of red foxes (*Vulpes fulva*) and grey foxes (*Urocyon cineroargenteus*) from the same areas. These authors were unable to interpret these unexpected findings because extensive surveys of rodents for *C. hepaticum* had not been reported from Louisiana.

There are few reports on the intensity of infection of *C. hepaticum* in field populations of mammals because (1) living adult worms are long, thread-like, and very difficult to dissect from sinuous tracts in the liver without rupturing, making quantification difficult; (2) adult worms generally die, are walled off inside the liver within 60 days, and are gradually destroyed; and (3) egg counts, although feasible (see Wright 1961; Singleton et al. 1995), are extremely labor intensive and time-consuming, requiring homogenization of the liver, digestion of the homogenate, sieving through a 150-μm sieve, and counts using a compound microscope and a McMaster slide. The correlation between number of eggs in the liver and number of adult nematodes present is unknown.

Epizootiology in Natural Habitats. Several studies in different countries have examined the epizootiology of *C. hepaticum* infection in small mammals in natural habitats (Pavlov 1955; Freeman and Wright 1960; Layne and Griffo 1961; Layne 1968; Solomon and Handley 1971; Herman 1981). In the Voronezh Reserve in the former USSR, Pavlov (1955) considered floodplain habitat was most suitable for development of eggs and, as the habitat of the red-backed vole (*Clethrionomys glareolus*) and the striped field mouse (*Apodemus agrarius*), was responsible for the highest prevalence of infection occurring in these hosts. Freeman and Wright (1960) found that prevalence of infection with *C. hepaticum* was not correlated with predation but varied

TABLE 14.1—Geographic location, habitat type and prevalence of infection of *Calodium hepaticum* in wild rodents

Host	Number Examined	Prevalence (% Infected)	Habitat Type	Geographic Location	Reference
Apodemus agrarius	282	0.3	Agricultural	Novosibirsk, Russia	Koval'chuk and Bonina 1981
Arvicola terrestris	262	33.0	Agricultural	Novosibirsk, Russia	Koval'chuk and Bonina 1981
Bandicota indica	7	14.3	Agricultural	Peninsular Malaysia	Liat et al. 1977[a]
Clethrionomys gapperi	142	2.8	Native forest	Ontario, Canada	Freeman and Wright 1960
Melomys cervinipes	86	1.0	Native rainforest	North Queensland, Australia	Singleton et al. 1991
Microtus pennsylvanicus	Not given	Not given	Native forest	Ontario, Canada	Freeman and Wright 1960
M. oeconomus	33	3	Agricultural	Novosibirsk, Russia	Koval'chuk and Bonina 1981
Mus domesticus	(i) 335 (ii)(a) 658 (b) 2764	5.4 24.6 Nil	Urban (a) Urban (b) Rural	Maryland, USA Eastern Australia	Childs et al. 1988 Singleton et al. 1991
Napaeozapus insignis	Not given	Not given	Native forest	Ontario, Canada	Freeman and Wright 1960
Ondatra zibethicus	Not given	Not given	Native forest	Ontario, Canada	Freeman and Wright 1960
Peromyscus maniculatus	769 341	9.4 80.0	Native forest Native forests on islands	Ontario, Canada British Columbia, Canada	Freeman and Wright 1960 Herman 1981
Peromyscus floridanus	723	2.9	Native forest	Florida, USA	Layne and Griffo 1961
P. gossypinus	270	6.3	Scrub and forest	Florida, USA	Layne 1968[b]
Praomys albipes	118	0.9	Urban	Shao Province, Ethiopia	Farhang-Azad and Schlitter 1978
Rattus annandalei	145	26.2	Agricultural and urban	Peninsular Malaysia	Sinniah et al. 1979
R. argentiventer	74 205 147 240	18 6.3 50.3 0.8	Agricultural Agricultural and urban Rice fields Rural and urban	Peninsular Malaysia Peninsular Malaysia West Java, Indonesia Indonesian Archipelago	Liat et al. 1977 Sinniah et al. 1979 Saenong 1984 Brown et al. 1975b
R. bartelsii	220	2.7	Rural and urban	Indonesian Archipelago	Brown et al. 1975b
R. edwardsi	1	100.0	Rural and urban	Indonesian Archipelago	Brown et al. 1975b
R. exulans	455 3182	5.9 0.2	Agricultural and urban Rural and urban	Peninsula Malaysia Indonesian Archipelago	Sinniah et al. 1979 Brown et al. 1975b
R. fuscipes	80	1	Native rainforest	North Queensland, Australia	Singleton et al. 1991
R. hellwaldi	20	15.0	Rural and urban	Indonesian Archipelago	Brown et al. 1975b
R. hoffmanni	209	0.5	Rural and urban	Indonesian Archipelago	Brown et al. 1975b
R. jalorensis	92	15.2	Agricultural and urban	Peninsular Malaysia	Sinniah et al. 1979
R. marmosurus	66	1.5	Rural and urban	Indonesian Archipelago	Brown et al. 1975b
R. musschenbroekii	4	25.0	Rural and urban	Indonesian Archipelago	Brown et al. 1975b
R. niviventer	83	2.4	Rural and urban	Indonesian Archipelago	Brown et al. 1975b

(continued)

TABLE 14.1   *(continued)*

Host	Number Examined	Prevalence (% Infected)	Habitat Type	Geographic Location	Reference
R. norvegicus	614	8.5	Urban	Townsville, Australia	Fielding 1927
	2500	85.6	Urban	Baltimore, MD, USA	Luttermoser 1936
	200	73.5	Urban (zoo)	New York, USA	Herman 1939
	731	94.1	Urban	Baltimore, MD, USA	Davis 1951
	325	88.0	Urban-University campus	Soeul, South Korea	Seo et al. 1964
	240	79.0	Urban	Brisbane, Australia	Waddell 1969
	138	56.5	Urban	Salvador, Brazil	Galvão 1976
	845	75.0	Urban (zoo)	Baltimore, MD, USA	Farhang-Azad 1977
	26	30.8	Urban	Peninsular Malaysia	Liat et al. 1977
	138	42.0	Urban	Bangkok, Thailand	Chaiyabutr 1979
	86	82.0	Urban	Hartford, CT, USA	Conlogue et al. 1979
	430	9.8	Agricultural and urban	Peninsular Malaysia	Sinniah et al. 1979
	191	56.5	Urban	São Paulo, Brazil	Chieffi et al. 1981
	340	87.4	Urban	Baltimore, MD, USA	Childs et al. 1988
	138	21.0	Urban	Alexandria, Egypt	El Nassery et al. 1991
	43	60.5	Urban	Eastern Australia	Singleton et al. 1991
R. rattus	1157	5.4	Urban	Townsville, Australia	Fielding 1927
	308	6.2	Urban	Shao Province, Ethiopia	Farhang-Azad and Schlitter 1978
	27	7.4	Urban	Bangkok, Thailand	Chaiyabutr 1979
	14	8.6	Urban	São Paulo, Brazil	Chieffi et al. 1981
	235	58.0	Urban	Witwatersrand, South Africa	Cheetham and Markus 1983
	20	15.0	Urban	Alexandria, Egypt	El Nassery et al. 1991
	152	46.0	Urban	Eastern Australia	Singleton et al. 1991
R. r. diardii	235	4.3	Urban	Peninsula Malaysia	Liat et al. 1977
	931	24.3	Agricultural and urban	Peninsular Malaysia	Sinniah et al. 1979
	812	0.6	Rural and urban	Indonesian Archipelago	Brown et al. 1975b
R. r. palelae	926	0.1	Rural and urban	Indonesian Archipelago	Brown et al. 1975b
R. sabanus	13	15.4	Rural and urban	Indonesian Archipelago	Brown et al. 1975b
R. tiomanicus	213	26.3	Agricultural	Peninsula Malaysia	Liat et al. 1977
Sigmodon hispidus	428	10.5	Scrub and forest	Florida, USA	Layne 1968
Suncus murinus	74	16.0		West Java, Indonesia	Brown et al. 1975a
	766	0.0		Central Sulawesi, Indonesia	Brown et al. 1975a
Synaptomys cooperi	Not given	Not given	Native forest	Ontario, Canada	Freeman and Wright 1960
Uromys caudimaculatus	21	24	Native rainforest	North Queensland, Australia	Singleton et al. 1991

[a]Also 11 species of forest rodents and 1 flying squirrel in Peninsular Malaysia; prevalences were less than 8% (Liat et al. 1977).

[b]Also results from North American rodents on one further species, *Sciurus niger,* and on seven studies of *Rattus norvegicus* not shown in this table (Layne 1968).

directly with host density in a population of deer mice (*Peromyscus maniculatus*) in Algonquin Park, Canada. The winter nest under the snow was considered the primary focus of infection. Most eggs were thought to be released in late winter when food reserves were depleted and starvation and cannibalism most intense. These authors considered that the eggs could survive in the winter nest because in the laboratory they withstood temperatures of at least –15° C for 60 days and subsequently embryonated. In contrast to *P. maniculatus,* the source of infection in the southern red-backed vole (*Clethrionomys gapperi*) in the same study area was thought to be carnivore feces and/or contact with *P. maniculatus.* This was based on the higher prevalence of metacestode infection in *C. gapperi* (4.2%) as compared to *P. maniculatus* (0.8%).

In contrast to this study, Layne and Griffo (1961) could offer no satisfactory explanation for the occurrence of *C. hepaticum* infection in the Florida deer mouse (*Peromyscus floridanus*) in restricted and xeric habitats in peninsular Florida. Similarly, Layne (1968) found no evidence of communal nesting or of cannibalism in *P. floridanus,* the cotton mouse (*P. gossypinus*), or the cotton rat (*Sigmodon hispidus*) in Florida and concluded that the more likely method of dissemination of eggs was interspecific predation, rather than intraspecific predation or necrophagy as postulated for *P. maniculatus* in northern Ontario (Freeman and Wright 1960) and for *R. norvegicus* in the Baltimore Zoo (Farhang-Azad 1977b).

Solomon and Handley (1971) assessed the occurrence and distribution of *C. hepaticum* in small mammals in the southern Appalachian mountains and proposed the existence of primary and secondary foci of infection, involving both host and habitat, in the maintenance of natural infections. Those species which were primarily vegetarian were uninfected, while those which were at least partially carnivorous or omnivorous, especially those living in cliff habitats, were most frequently infected. The parasite was maintained and highest prevalence of infection occurred in two species, *P. maniculatus* and the eastern wood rat (*Neotoma floridana*), where close contact occurred in rocky habitats.

Herman (1981) concluded that competition among scavengers (shrews and carabid beetles) for mouse carcasses plus the distribution of predators, rather than a varying intensity of cannibalism, best accounted for the distribution and abundance of *C. hepaticum* in populations of *P. maniculatus* on an island in the Barkley Sound region of British Columbia, Canada. Lowest prevalence of infection occurred on islands with abundant scavengers, and he considered that these competed with deer mice for carcasses, thus removing ova of *C. hepaticum* from the pool of embryonating eggs in the environment. The high prevalence of infection in deer mice on islands, compared to mainland North America (Freeman and Wright 1960; Layne 1968; Lubinsky et al. 1971; Solomon and Handley 1971) was attributed to increased necrophagy as a consequence of the increased availability of mouse carcasses. Interspecific predators played no direct role in the distribution of the parasite in island populations.

Borucinska et al. (1997) reported that the severity and character of hepatic lesions in their experimental studies in muskrats (*Ondatra zibethicus*) were similar to those reported in wild muskrats (Borucinska and Nielsen 1993) but at the milder end of the spectrum. They concluded that hepatic capillariasis was unlikely to contribute significantly to mortality in populations of wild muskrats, although it may predispose sick animals to predation. Nevertheless, the degree of egg viability both at the time of mortality in muskrats and in chronic infections would ensure that muskrats

served as a natural reservoir of *C. hepaticum* infection in the environment.

Epizootiology in Commensal Habitats. Other studies have examined the epizootiology of *C. hepaticum* in commensal habitats (Farhang-Azad 1977b; Childs et al. 1988; Singleton et al. 1991). Childs et al. (1988) studied the occurrence of *C. hepaticum* in four species of rodents in different residential and parkland habitats of Baltimore, Maryland. There was a high prevalence and intensity of infection of *C. hepaticum* in *R. norvegicus* that increased with body weight in animals trapped in residential areas and with relative density of rats. A low prevalence of infection occurred in the house mouse (*Mus musculus = M. domesticus*) in residential sites, and there was a correlation between prevalence and estimated density. Infection was not found in meadow voles (*Microtus pennsylvanicus*) or in white-footed deer mice (*P. leucopus*), although natural infections may occur in these host species (see Freeman and Wright 1960; Solomon and Handley 1971). It was concluded that transmission of *C. hepaticum* was more intense in residential areas than in parklands. Interspecific interactions (e.g., predation by cats), as well as intraspecific mechanisms, were suggested as having a role in egg dissemination in urban environments (Childs et al. 1988). *Calodium hepaticum* was widely distributed and prevalent in three introduced rodents (*M. domesticus, R. rattus,* and *R. norvegicus*) over the Melbourne and Metropolitan Board of Works farm (10,850 ha) at Werribee, Australia, where much of the habitat had been modified to function as a land filtration system for industrial and human waste (Singleton et al. 1991). However, infection was not detected in cattle, sheep, goats, the European rabbit (*Oryctolagus cuniculus*), cats (*Felis catus*), a red fox (*Vulpes vulpes*), or fat-tailed dunnarts (*Sminthopsis crassicaudata,* Marsupialia) from the same farm.

CLINICAL SIGNS. Clinical signs of infection, particularly hepatomegaly and splenomegaly, have been reported in experimental infection of mice, multimammate rats, the Plains rat (*Pseudomys australis*), and muskrats with *C. hepaticum* (Luttermoser 1939b; Lämmler et al. 1974; Zahner et al. 1976; Spratt and Singleton 1986; Borucinska et al. 1997), but generally not in rats (Luttermoser 1938b; Spratt and Singleton 1986) or in marsupial brushtail possums (*Trichosurus vulpecula*) (Spratt and Singleton 1986). Clinical signs in mice appeared as early as 5 days postinfection and death occurred 8–11 days postinfection in animals dosed with 100 embryonated eggs (Spratt and Singleton 1986). Sudden death occurred in muskrats 25–39 days after inoculation of 17,000 embryonated eggs into the stomach, although not in multimammate rats dosed perorally with a larger number of embryonated eggs per kilogram of body weight (Vollerthun et al. 1974). We are not aware of reports of clinical signs in animals naturally infected with *C. hepaticum.*

PATHOLOGY AND PATHOGENESIS. The pathological changes in naturally and experimentally infected animals have been well documented (Bancroft 1893; Fülleborn 1925; Nishigori 1925; Höppli 1925; Luttermoser 1938b; Foster and Johnson 1939; Gupta and Ranhawa 1960; Vollerthun et al. 1974; Winkelmann 1974; El Nassery et al. 1991; Borucinska et al. 1997). Host response commenced with a polymorphonuclear leucocytic perivascular infiltration of the liver tissue (Bancroft 1893; Nishigori 1925; Höppli 1925; Lee 1964; El Nassery et al. 1991). Granuloma formation commenced early, with mononuclear cells, giant cells, and polymorphonuclear cells, predominantly eosinophils, appearing (Höppli 1925; Luttermoser 1938b; Ward and Dent 1959; Gupta and Ranhawa 1960; Smit 1960; Calle 1961; Zahner and Rudolph 1980; El Nassery et al. 1991) as a consequence of an immune response to egg antigen (Solomon and Soulsby 1973; Raybourne and Solomon 1984). Borucinska et al. (1997) described periportal inflammatory lesions in muskrats experimentally infected with *C. hepaticum,* a feature consistent with a persistent immune response. Encapsulation by connective tissue ensued, and at a later stage calcification occurred, with dead parasites in the center of lesions. In humans, chimpanzees (*Pan satyrus*), and rabbits the eggs of *C. hepaticum* undergo mineralization and destruction by giant cells during chronic disease, and there is pronounced parasite-induced hepatic fibrosis or cirrhosis. In rats, house mice, the Plains rat, brushtail possums, and muskrats the eggs are not destroyed (Lämmler et al. 1974; Spratt and Singleton 1986; El Nassery et al. 1991; Borucinska et al. 1997). In studies with multimammate rats, Lämmler et al. (1974) demonstrated that the injurious effects of *C. hepaticum* infection were not constrained to the phase of oviposition by the female worm. Enzyme studies indicated persistence of liver damage in the chronic phase of the disease, which might be more damaging than that which occurs at earlier stages of infection.

In multimammate rats and muskrats, maximum mortality, elevated liver enzymes, and leukocytosis occurred around 30 days postinfection (Lämmler et al. 1974; Borucinska et al. 1997). Acute mortality caused by liver damage induced by parasite metabolites, parasite migration and oviposition, and inflammatory mediators released by host cells in the liver, with maximum eosinophilia, aspartate aminotransferase, and alanine aminotransferase values occurring 21–28 days postinfection, has been reported in multimammate rats, specific pathogen-free rabbits, and muskrats (Vollerthun et al. 1974; Winkelmann 1974; Borucinska et al. 1997). However, in experimental studies in the laboratory, changes were not observed in most clinical parameters including total protein albumin, blood urea nitrogen, total bilirubin, direct and indirect bilirubin, lactic dehydrogenase, alkaline phosphatase, hematocrit, and hemoglobin (Vollerthun et al. 1974; Winkelmann 1974; Borucinska et al. 1997).

Lämmler et al. (1974) and Vollerthun et al. (1974) identified an acute and a chronic phase in multimammate rats infected with *C. hepaticum.* Disorder of the liver cells was detected initially in the first week postinfection through activated glutamic dehydrogenase, even when infection was induced with x-irradiated embryonated eggs (sterile nematodes). Serum glutamic oxalacetic transaminase, glutamic pyruvic transaminase, lactic dehydrogenase, and sorbitol dehydrogenase were elevated in the second and third weeks, indicating loss of function and integrity of liver cells associated with focal changes and possible mechanical damage due to migrating juveniles. As well, cytotoxic effects of metabolites from growth, molting, and maturation occurred during this acute phase of infection. A second disorder in liver cells was detected at the end of the prepatent period through a second peak of activated glutamic dehydrogenase at 23 days postinfection and through maximum values of other liver enzymes at this time. The prolonged and constant elevation of enzymes indicated continuing liver damage in this chronic phase, without indication of repair. A gradual decrease in serum cholinesterase and serum alkaline phosphatase demonstrated progressive exhaustion of liver parenchyma during patency, due to cirrhosis. The high number of eggs in the parenchyma and their metabolites, or egg antigen, may have pathophysiological consequences. Similarly, the presence of dead eggs and the death and degeneration of adult worms are additional pathogenic factors. The pronounced decrease in cholinesterase activity commencing with the fourth week of infection corresponded with the reduction of liver parenchyma and its replacement by eggs. The persistent increase of activated glutamic dehydrogenase suggested a cytotoxic effect, which may be the reason for the persistent liver damage seen in multimammate rats (Lämmler et al. 1974; Vollerthun et al. 1974; Zahner et al. 1981). True cirrhosis of the liver has been reported in rabbits (Suda 1928), humans (Otto et al. 1954; Pereira and Franca 1983), and heavily infected house mice (Luttermoser 1938a). We have observed it in heavily infected house mice and in the Plains rat. However, there are reports of the livers of monkeys and peccaries (Foster and Johnson 1939) and of rats (Luttermoser 1938a) healing without development of cirrhosis, something we have observed in the bush rat (*R. fuscipes*) and the brushtail possum. El Nassery and El-Nazar (1991) demonstrated that the metabolites of the migrating larvae, adult worms, and eggs of *C. hepaticum* impair cell-mediated immunity.

DIAGNOSIS. Eggs of *C. hepaticum* are retained in the liver of the host and not released from the host until death. Starry fur, lethargy, hepatomegaly, and splenomegaly may be apparent in small animals (less than rat-size) heavily infected with this parasite; however, such clinical signs are uncommon in larger animal species, and infection cannot be diagnosed other than by biopsy or postmortem examination. Boruicinska et al. (1997) studied *C. hepaticum* infection in experimentally infected muskrats and concluded that laboratory evaluation of hepatic functions and differential counts of white blood cells would be insufficient to diagnose hepatic capillariasis in wild populations.

Infection in adult humans often is asymptomatic and is diagnosed only after death due to other causes (Slais 1973; Johnson et al. 1989). Diagnosis generally is based upon the location of the parasite in the liver and the morphological appearance, generally of eggs but occasionally of adult worms, in histological sections following death or as a result of a biopsy examination. Infected children generally exhibit chronic fever, hepatomegaly, pronounced eosinophilia, and hyperglobulinemia (Otto et al. 1954; Cochrane et al. 1957; Cislagi and Radice 1970; Silverman et al. 1973; Berger et al. 1990). This syndrome has been known to be pathognomic for visceral larva migrans in humans, a condition normally associated with the larval stages of ascaridoid nematodes of animals (Cochrane et al. 1957; Silverman et al. 1973; Slais 1974; Kumar et al. 1985). This suggests that some cases of human hepatic capillariasis may have been incorrectly diagnosed in the past.

IMMUNITY. Solomon and Soulsby (1973) demonstrated that granuloma formation to eggs of *C. hepaticum* had an immunological basis and that the cell composition of the granuloma (initially mononuclear cells around eggs, leading to formation of granulomatous lesions characterized by macrophages and lymphocytes, followed by infiltration of eosinophils) suggested that a cell-mediated component was involved as part of the specific response. These authors also suggested that, unlike the schistosome egg granuloma in the lung, a foreign-body reaction was not a major component of the *C. hepaticum* egg granuloma in the liver. Raybourne et al. (1974) found agglutinating and homocytotropic antibodies but no precipitating antibodies in mice with primary and secondary granulomas (sensitize-challenge). Subsequently, they demonstrated conclusively that at least two classes of circulating antibody, IgM and IgG, were present, and there was a delayed dermal reactivity during granuloma formation to eggs of *C. hepaticum* in the liver of mice (Raybourne and Solomon 1975). Immunoglobulin M persisted at considerable levels 7 weeks in response to primary granuloma formation; however, prior sensitization with eggs of *C. hepaticum* altered the peripheral antibody response substantially during formation of secondary liver granulomas. Fractionation of soluble egg antigens produced two major protein peaks that, in addition to unfractionated antigen, were able to sensitize mice to produce larger granulomas in the liver (Raybourne and Solomon 1984). Granuloma size was related to the amount of antigen used to sensitize mice, and antibody response in infected mice was directed primarily toward the high molecular weight components (Raybourne and Solomon 1984).

In mice, titers of humoral antibodies demonstrable by immunoprecipitation and hemagglutination were low (Raybourne et al. 1974), but a substantial humoral

antibody response was detected in multimammate rats (Lämmler et al. 1974). Using soluble egg antigen extracted from unembryonated eggs, antibodies were detected as early as 15 days after infection. Thus, antigens produced by late larval and early adult nematodes are important in the humoral response. There was a peak response at the end of the prepatent period, followed by a continuous decline. El Nassery et al. (1991) reported maximal titers of antibodies to worms in white mice in weeks 5 and 6 postinfection and to eggs in weeks 11 to 14 postinfection, using an indirect fluorescent antibody test (IFAT). Lee (1964) reported a relative increase in the beta-globulin fraction of serum of rabbits infected with *C. hepaticum*. Localization of antigen on the inner membrane of the egg shell in frozen sections of unembryonated eggs of *C. hepaticum* was detected by IFAT (Kim et al. 1985). Immunoglobulin G titers (range 16–1024) detected by IFAT increased rapidly up to 3 weeks postinfection, were maintained until 5 weeks, decreased gradually from 7–9 weeks, and thereafter returned to normal by 13 weeks postinfection. Mean titers were higher in white rats receiving 2000 embryonated eggs than in those receiving a dose of 200 eggs. Lee et al. (1985) detected antibodies to *C. hepaticum* by micro-ELISA using soluble antigen from embryonated eggs. Absorbance values increased up to 3 weeks postinfection, were maintained until 5 weeks and thereafter decreased, with most sera returned to normal by 13 weeks postinfection. Mean absorbance values were greater in white rats receiving 2000 embryonated eggs than in those receiving a dose of 200 eggs.

The relatively low prevalence of human hepatic capillariasis in contrast to its high prevalence and wide dissemination among other animals prompted Nascimoto and Sadigursky (1986) to determine the potential of spurious (inoculation of unembryonated eggs) infection to protect against true infection (inoculation of embryonated eggs). These authors demonstrated that the humoral immunity produced by spurious infection in mice did not have any protective potential against a true infection by *C. hepaticum*.

MANAGEMENT IMPLICATIONS. *Rattus norvegicus* and *R. rattus* are the principal reservoir species for *C. hepaticum* infection in zoological gardens and fauna parks. In the presence of either of these species, house mice are likely to become infected and become an important carrier of the parasite because of their greater ability to infiltrate buildings such as nocturnal houses and food storage and preparation areas. The non-rodent species which have the greatest risk of infection are those which come into contact with the burrows of these commensal rodents. Maintenance of a moist substrate increases the survival of eggs of *C. hepaticum* and therefore increases the risk of infection.

Control of commensal rodent populations is the best management strategy. In our experience at one zoological garden, complete eradication of rodents was not possible, especially in the nocturnal house where native small mammal species were maintained on a peat moss and potting mix substrate. In combination with a rodent control campaign, transmission of the disease was effectively minimized by using a drier substrate and by regularly removing and replacing that substrate. Consequently, even in zoos and fauna parks, the potential for infection of non-rodent hosts with *C. hepaticum* is habitat dependent. However, we have little knowledge of the impact of such infection on non-rodent hosts.

PUBLIC HEALTH CONCERNS. Cases of human hepatic capillariasis have been recorded in Brazil, Czechoslovakia, India, Italy, Korea, Mexico, Nigeria, South Africa, Switzerland, Turkey, the United States, and Yugoslavia. However, diagnostic methods are imprecise. There are more than 300 species in the subfamily Capillariinae, and members parasitize all classes of vertebrates (fishes, amphibians, reptiles, birds, and mammals); consequently, species other than *C. hepaticum* may have been responsible for some of these human infections. Severe infection occurs mainly in children aged 1–5 years, some known to be prodigious eaters of soil (Cochrane et al. 1957; Cislagi and Radice 1970; Slais 1973; Berger et al. 1990). These patients generally exhibit chronic fever, hepatomegaly, pronounced eosinophilia, and hyperglobulinemia (Otto et al. 1954; Cochrane et al. 1957; Cislagi and Radice 1970; Silverman et al. 1973; Berger et al. 1990).

Calodium hepaticum has never been recorded in humans in Australia, although this nematode parasite was described originally from introduced rodents (*Rattus* spp.) in Brisbane, Queensland, more than a century ago (Bancroft 1893). It was reported also in both Sydney (Johnston 1918) and Townsville early this century (Fielding 1927) and currently is widespread in introduced rodents, particularly *Rattus* spp., in large towns and cities in eastern Australia (Singleton et al. 1991).

Successful chemotherapeutic treatment for *C. hepaticum* infection has been reported in Norway rats (Waddell 1969), in multimammate rats (Lämmler and Grüner 1976), in mice (Cheetham and Markus 1983; Markus and Cheetham 1985) and in acutely ill young and adult humans (Cochrane et al. 1957; Cochrane and Skinstad 1960; Calle 1961; Silverman et al. 1973; Pereira and Franca 1983; Misic et al. 1986). Spurious infections, with eggs of *C. hepaticum* being passed in feces, may occur in humans following ingestion of unembryonated eggs in the cooked livers of infected animals (Wright 1931; Vogel 1932; Sandground 1933; Faust and Martinez 1935; Foster and Johnson 1939; Brosius et al. 1948; McQuown 1950, 1954).

It is perhaps not surprising that the majority of cases of human hepatic capillariasis have been reported from the developed world. The importance of *C. hepaticum* as a zoonosis probably has been underestimated because of confusion with visceral larva migrans and because diagnosis of infection generally has been dependent upon biopsy of liver or postmortem exami-

nation (see Lämmler et al. 1974). Such underestimation is particularly likely to be the case in third world countries in tropical and subtropical regions where the full suite of requirements for transmission—high density rodent and human populations, moist soil and poor hygiene—occur commonly. The ubiquitous nature of this nematode parasite prompted Solomon and Soulsby (1973) to suggest that light infections in humans may be involved in the etiology of eosinophilia of undetermined origin, frequently reported throughout the world. Similarly, Borucinska et al. (1997) suggested that *C. hepaticum* may be a poorly diagnosed cause of other parasitic syndromes of man and animals including visceral larva migrans (Kumar et al. 1985), tropical eosinophilia (Gupta and Ranhawa 1960), and helminthic anaphylactic syndrome (Odujno 1970).

BIOCONTROL. In Australia, *C. hepaticum* is known primarily from populations of the three recently introduced murids, the Norway rat, the black rat, and the house mouse, and only in the urban environments of towns situated close to the coast (Singleton 1985; Spratt and Singleton 1986, Singleton et al. 1991). In addition, eggs believed to be those of *C. hepaticum* have been observed in histological sections of the livers of three native murids, the bush rat, the fawn-footed Melomys (*Melomys cervinipes*), and the white-tailed rat (*Uromys caudimaculatus*), in the rainforests of the Atherton tablelands in far north Queensland (Spratt and Singleton 1986; Singleton et al. 1991). In the laboratory, *C. hepaticum* was infective to the bush rat, the Plains rat, and the brushtail possum (Spratt and Singleton 1986). All of the evidence available from parasitological and wildlife disease studies in the field in Australia during the past three decades and from the literature in Australia during the past century points to a natural, ecological, exclusion of this parasite from native mammals, with the possible exception of those in tropical rainforests. The most urbanized of Australian native mammals, the brushtail possum, and the most infamous of Australia's vertebrate pests, the European rabbit, which are both susceptible to infection, appear not to come in contact with embryonated eggs of *C. hepaticum* in Australia. The lesions produced in the liver of the host by this parasite are conspicuous and simply would not have been overlooked by parasitologists and veterinarians working with free-ranging and captive wildlife.

On this basis, we undertook to determine the potential of *C. hepaticum* as a bioagent in the control of house mouse plagues in the cereal-growing regions of southeastern Australia. The studies of Johnston (1918) demonstrated that *C. hepaticum* eggs can neither survive in water in sunlight nor survive desiccation. We postulated that transmission of *C. hepaticum* in the cereal-growing region would be restricted to the mouse burrow, because that was where the requirements essential for embryonation and survival of eggs would be met, and demonstrated survival of eggs in soils of the wheat belt at temperatures and moisture contents of mouse burrows (Singleton and Spratt 1987).

Experimental studies in the laboratory demonstrated that the pathogenicity of *C. hepaticum* infection in mated female BALB/c mice dosed with 50 eggs was manifest by a reduction of productivity over a 90-day period (Singleton and Spratt 1986). There was a significant delay in the production of second litters, a reduction in the number of young weaned/litter, and pronounced reductions in the number of live young produced/female/90 days and in the number of young weaned/female/90 days.

Comment is warranted on the value of models when examining the interaction between host and parasite populations in natural populations. Models were developed to assist in the evaluation of the potential of *C. hepaticum* to control populations of house mice and reduce the severity of plagues (McCallum and Singleton 1989; Singleton and McCallum 1990). The parasite life cycle operates on a timescale similar to that of the host because of the requirement of death of the host for transmission to occur. The models demonstrated that the destabilizing effects of parasite transmission on host death and parasite depression of fecundity induced cycles in mouse populations unless the carrying capacity of mice was close to the threshold for parasite maintenance. Thus, *C. hepaticum* was unlikely to be a suitable organism for classical biological control but could be used as a tactical agent provided it was introduced into mouse populations as early as possible in the developmental period of an outbreak (McCallum and Singleton 1989; Singleton and McCallum 1990).

The hypothesis that infection with *C. hepaticum* would regulate populations of house mice around an equilibrium density significantly lower than that of uninfected house mice was then tested in enclosures in the wheat belt of southeastern Australia by assessing changes in mouse abundance and the relationship between mortality and host abundance in three treatment and three control populations (Barker et al. 1991). An unknown regulating factor(s) masked any effect of *C. hepaticum* and caused density-dependent mortality in both control and treatment populations. Transmission occurred throughout the 18-month study, but strong seasonal trends in transmission further confounded the test.

Further modeling using the age structure of mouse and parasite populations suggested that the requirement of host death for transmission slowed parasite increase unless an initial release killed substantial numbers of hosts, thereby assisting the parasite to reproduce (McCallum 1992, 1995). With addition of seasonal mouse reproduction and death, the model demonstrated that the pulse in death of mice, which occurs annually in spring in southern Australia when densities are moderate to high, assisted the spread of *C. hepaticum*.

Only field experiments can determine transmission rates and threshold population levels. Hence, a replicated, 2-year, field investigation on seven sites was conducted to examine the effect of *C. hepaticum* on

populations of wild mice on the Darling Downs in southeastern Queensland (Singleton et al. 1995). The parasite was released successfully on three occasions at three different stages of mouse population dynamics. Release in winter into a low-density, nonbreeding population resulted in significantly lower survival of mice for 4 months on treated compared to untreated sites, particularly of young mice (< 72 mm long) 2 months after release. However, there was poor survival of mice on untreated sites after this period, and population abundance was similar to that on treated sites. Subsequently, breeding commenced, but *C. hepaticum* had no measurable effect on mouse population dynamics. This was attributed to (1) the parasite having no effect on breeding mice, (2) minimal transmission, and (3) the parasite having a diminishing effect on survival. The apparent lack of transmission was thought due to a combination of low population density, the transient nature of the mouse population, and predominantly dry weather for 6 months after release.

A second release into a breeding, medium-density population increasing rapidly in abundance was made (Singleton et al. 1995). Less than 2% of the population was affected during this release. Transmission occurred at a low rate, and *C. hepaticum* persisted 4.5 months. At this time a third release was made to increase the proportion of mice infected, to follow the effect of the parasite on an overwintering population and to assess the demographic effects during the next breeding season. This release was compromised by a synchronous, widespread, and rapid decline in mouse densities from > 500 ha^{-1} to < 1 ha^{-1}. It was concluded that *C. hepaticum* would not limit mouse populations if released into a low-density population during a long dry period on the Darling Downs and that much more knowledge of the factors influencing survival and transmission of the parasite under field conditions was required (Singleton et al. 1995).

Another manipulative field experiment was conducted in southern Australia, in a markedly different geoclimatic zone and some 1500 km from the Darling Downs (Singleton and Chambers 1996). The parasite was released in early spring into a breeding, medium-density population increasing rapidly in abundance. There were two noticeable changes from the previous study. First, both embryonated and unembryonated eggs of *C. hepaticum* were used to infect the host population in an effort to increase the transmission rate of the parasite. Second, the zone of treatment was increased to 16 km^2 to reduce the effect of mice migrating from adjacent high density populations. Approximately 40,000 mice were treated on four sites, representing 5%–7% of the population. A month later, a further 20,000 mice were infected to increase the prevalence of infection to ~10%. Two months after the release approximately 30% of the mouse population was infected, and although the parasite persisted for the duration of the 12-month study, there was a significant reduction in prevalence of *C. hepaticum* with time. The parasite reduced host survival by 5%–10%

but had only a minimal effect on the breeding of mice and on the rate of growth of their populations. As with the previous study in Queensland, very dry conditions followed the release, and although we had sustained transmission of the parasite, it was too slow to significantly limit the growth of a rapidly increasing mouse population.

This series of experiments in Australia underlined that models are a valuable tool to assist interpretation of laboratory or field studies. The modeling focused effort on key population parameters that enable assessment of the impact of parasites on survival or fecundity of individual hosts in terms of the impact of a disease on the host population as a whole (McCallum 1995). For example, if parasites are aggregated in natural host communities, as often occurs with helminths (Crofton 1971; Anderson 1978; Keymer 1982), the average fecundity of a population with a particular mean parasite burden will be much greater than that of an individual with that parasite burden. Because most parasites will be in relatively few females, the fecundity of most of that population will not be affected. For this reason, laboratory experiments on individuals may overestimate the impact of the parasite on a population (McCallum 1995).

LITERATURE CITED

Ameel, D. 1942. Two larval cestodes from the muskrat. *Transactions of the American Microscopical Society* 69:267–271.

Anderson, R.C., and O. Bain. 1982. Keys to genera of the superfamilies Rhabditoidea, Dioctophymatoidea, Trichinelloidea and Muspiceoidea, no. 9. In *CIH Keys to the Nematode Parasites of Vertebrates*. Wallingford, UK: CAB International, pp. 1–26.

Anderson, R.M. 1978. The regulation of host population growth by parasitic species. *Parasitology* 76:119–157.

Attah, E.B., S. Nagarajan, E.N. Obineche, and S.C. Gera. 1983. Hepatic capillariasis. *American Journal of Clinical Pathology* 79:127–130.

Bancroft, T.L. 1893. On the whipworm of the rat's liver. *Journal of the Proceedings of the Royal Society of New South Wales* 27:86–90.

Barker, S.C., G.R. Singleton, and D.M. Spratt. 1991. Can the nematode *Capillaria hepatica* regulate abundance in wild house mice? Results of enclosure experiments in southeastern Australia. *Parasitology* 103:439–449.

Barrett, M.W., and G.A. Chalmers. 1972. *Capillaria hepatica* (Nematoda: Trichuridae) in a pronghorn antelope *(Antilocapra americana)* in Alberta. *Journal of Wildlife Diseases* 8:332–334.

Berger, T., A. Degremont, J.O. Gebbers, and O. Tonz. 1990. Hepatic capillariasis in a 1-year-old child. *European Journal of Pediatrics* 149:333–336.

Borucinska, J., and S.W. Nielsen. 1993. Hepatic capillariasis in muskrats *(Ondatra zibethicus)*. *Journal of Wildlife Diseases* 29:518–520.

Borucinska, J.D., H.J. Van Kruiningen, J.N. Caira, and A.E. Garmendia. 1997. Clinicopathological features and histopathology of experimental hepatic capillariasis in muskrats *(Ondatra zibethicus)*. *Journal of Wildlife Diseases* 33:122–130.

Brander, P., T. Denzler, and M. Henzi. 1990. *Capillaria hepatica* bei einem Hund und einem Igel. *Schweizer Archiv für Tierheilkunde* 132:365–370.

Brosius, O.T., E.E. Thomas, and B. Brosius 1948. *Capillaria hepatica:* A case report. *Transactions of the Royal Society of Tropical Medicine and Hygiene* 42:95–97.

Brown, J.H., and G.D. Roy 1943. The Richardson ground squirrel, *Citellus richardsonii* Sabine, in southern Alberta, its importance and control. *Scientific Agriculture (Review of Agronomy in Canada)* 24:176–197.

Brown, R.J., W.P. Carney, J.H. Cross, and J.S. Saroso 1975a. *Capillaria* hepatitis in the Indonesian house shrew *Suncus murinus*. *Southeast Asian Journal of Tropical Medicine and Public Health* 6:599–601.

Brown, R.J., W.P. Carney, P.F.D. Van Peenen, J.H. Cross, and J.S. Saroso 1975b. Capillariasis in wild rats of Indonesia. *Southeast Asian Journal of Tropical Medicine and Public Health* 6:219–222.

Caballero, Y.C.E., and R.G. Grocott 1952. Nota sobre la presencia de *Capillaria hepatica* en un mono araña *(Ateles geoffroyi vellerosus)* de México. *Anales del Instituto Biologia Universidad de México* 23:211–215.

Calero M.C.P., O. Oritzo, and L. De Souza 1950. Helminths in rats from Panama City and suburbs. *Journal of Parasitology* 36:426.

Calle, S. 1961. Parasitism by *Capillaria hepatica*. *Pediatrics* 27:648–655

Chaiyabutr, N. 1979. Hepatic capillariasis in *Rattus norvegicus*. *Journal of the Science Society of Thailand* 5:48–50.

Cheetham, R.F., and M.B. Markus. 1983. Effects of drugs on experimental hepatic capillariasis in mice. *South African Journal of Science* 79:470.

Chieffi, P.P., R.M.D.S. Dias, A.C.S. Mangini, D.M.A. Grispino, and M.A.D. Pacheco 1981. *Capillaria hepatica* in rats trapped in the municipality of S.o Paulo, SP, Brazil [In Portugese]. *Revista do Instituto de Medicina Tropical de S.o Paulo* 23:143–146.

Childs, J.E., G.E. Glass, and G.W. Korch Jr. 1988. The comparative epizootiology of *Capillaria hepatica* (Nematoda) in urban rodents from different habitats of Baltimore, Maryland. *Canadian Journal of Zoology* 66:2769–2775.

Chineme, C., and M.A. Ibrahim 1984. Hepatic capillariasis in African giant rats *(Cricetomys gambianus* Waterhouse). *Journal of Wildlife Diseases* 20:341–342.

Chitwood, B.G. 1934. *Capillaria hepatica* from the liver of *Castor canadensis canadensis*. *Proceedings of the Helminthological Society of Washington* 1:10.

Choe, G., H.S. Lee, J.K. Seo, J. Chai, S. Lee, K.S. Eom, and J.E.G. Chi. 1993. Hepatic capillariasis: First case report in the Republic of Korea. *American Journal of Tropical Medicine and Hygiene* 48:610–625.

Cislagi, F., and C. Radice 1970. Infection by *Capillaria hepatica*. First case report in Italy. *Helvetica Pediatrica Acta* 25: 647–654.

Cochrane, J.C., and E.E. Skinstad. 1960. *Capillaria hepatica* in man—Follow-up of a case. *South African Medical Journal* 34:21–22.

Cochrane, J.C., L. Sagorin, and J.C. Wilcocks. 1957. *Capillaria hepatica* infection in man. *South African Medical Journal* 31:751–755.

Conlogue, G., W. Foreyt, M. Adess, and H. Levine. 1979. *Capillaria hepatica* (Bancroft) in select rat populations of Hartford, Connecticut, with possible public health implications. *The Journal of Parasitology* 65:105–108.

Cram, E.B. 1928. A note on parasites of rats *(Rattus norvegicus* and *Rattus norvegicus albus)*. *The Journal of Parasitology* 15:72.

Crofton, H.D. 1971. A quantitative approach to parasitism. *Parasitology* 62:179–194.

Crowell, W.A., T.R. Klei, D.I. Hall, N.K. Smith, and J.D. Newsom 1978. *Capillaria hepatica* infection in coyotes of Louisiana. *Journal of the American Veterinary Medical Association* 173:1171–1172.

Davis, D.E. 1951. The relation between the level of population and prevalence of *Leptospira, Salmonella* and *Capillaria* in Norway rats. *Ecology* 32:465–468.

Dikmans, G. 1932. The pocket gopher, *Thomomys fosor*, a new host of the nematode *Capillaria hepatica. Journal of Parasitology* 19:83.

Dive, G.H., H.M. Lafrenais, and W.P. MacArthur. 1924. A case of deposition of the eggs of *Hepaticola hepatica* in the human liver with a note on the identity of the eggs. *Journal of the Royal Army Medical Corp* 43:1–4.

Doran, D.J. 1955. A catalogue of the protozoa and helminths of North American rodents. III. Nematoda. *American Midland Naturalist* 53:162–175.

El Nassery, S.F., W.M. El-Gebali, and N.Y. Oweiss 1991. *Capillaria hepatica:* An experimental study of infection in white mice. *Journal of the Egyptian Society of Parasitology* 21:467–480.

El Nassery, S.M.F., and S.Y.A. El-Nazar 1991. Depressed membrane interleukin-1 activity of macrophage in mice infected with *Capillaria hepatica. Journal of the Medical Research Institute* 12(4)(Supplement): 261–278.

Ewing, G.M., and H. Tilden. 1956. *Capillaria hepatica* : Report of a fourth case of true human infestation. *Journal of Pediatrics* 48:341–348.

Farhang-Azad, A. 1977a. Ecology of *Capillaria hepatica* (Bancroft, 1893) (Nematoda). I. Dynamics of infection among Norway rat populations of the Baltimore Zoo, Baltimore, Maryland. *Journal of Parasitology* 63:117–122.

————. 1977b. Ecology of *Capillaria hepatica* (Bancroft, 1893) (Nematoda). II. Egg-releasing mechanisms and transmission. *Journal of Parasitology* 63:701–706.

Farhang-Azad, A., and D.A. Schlitter 1978. *Capillaria hepatica* in small mammals collected from Shoa province, Ethiopia. *Journal of Wildlife Diseases* 14:358–361.

Faust, E.C., and W.H. Martinez 1935. Nematode eggs in the faeces of individuals from the Chagres River, Panama. *Journal of Parasitology* 21:332–336.

Fielding, J.W. 1927. Observations on rodents and their parasites. *Journal and Proceedings of the Royal Society of New South Wales* 61:123–129.

Firlotte, W.R. 1948. A survey of the parasites of the brown Norway rat. *Canadian Journal of Comparative Medicine* 1:187–191.

Fisher, R.L. 1963. *Capillaria hepatica* from the rock vole in New York. *Journal of Parasitology* 49:450.

Foster, A.O., and C.M. Johnson 1939. Explanation for occurrence of *Capillaria hepatica* ova in human faeces suggested by finding of three hosts used as food. *Transactions of the Royal Society of Tropical Medicine and Hygiene* 32:639–644.

Freeman, R.S. 1958. On the epizootiology of *Capillaria hepatica* (Bancroft, 1893) in Algonquin Park, Ontaro. *Journal of Parasitology* 44(Supplement): 33.

Freeman, R.S., and K.A. Wright. 1960. Factors concerned with the epizootiology of *Capillaria hepatica* (Bancroft, 1893) (Nematoda) in a population of *Peromyscus maniculatus* in Algonquin Park, Canada. *Journal of Parasitology* 46:373–382.

Fülleborn, F. 1924. Über den Infectionsweg bei *Hepaticola hepatica. Archiv für Schiffs- und Tropen-Hygiene* 28:48–61.

————. 1925. Über den Infektionsweg bei *Hepaticola hepatica. Archiv für Schiffs- und Tropen-Hygiene* 28:48–61.

Galvão, A. 1976. (*Capillaria hepatica:* Incidence in rats from Salvador, Bahia, and preliminary immunopathological data [In Portuguese]. *Revista da Sociedade Brasiliera de Medicina Tropical* 10:333–338.

Galvão, V.A. 1979. An attempt to diagnose *Capillaria hepatica* infection in man [In Portuguese]. *Revista do Instituto Medicina Tropical de São Paulo* 21:231–236.

————.1981. Studies on *Capillaria hepatica:* An evaluation of its role as a human parasite [In Portugese]. *Memórias do Instituto Oswaldo Cruz* 76:415–433.

Gevrey, J., and C. Chirol 1978. A propos d'un cas de capillariose à *Capillaria hepatica* observé dans un élevage de lapins croisés garenne. *Revue de Médicine Vétérinaire* 129:1019–1026.

Gupta, I.M., and H.S. Ranhawa. 1960. Pathological changes in the liver of wild rats due to *C.hepatica,* with a note on its probable human occurrence in India. *Indian Journal of Medical Research* 48:565–570.

Hall, M.C. 1916. Nematode parasites of mammals of the orders Rodentia, Lagomorpha and Hyracoidea. *Proceedings of the United States National Museum* 50:1–258.

Harkema, R. 1936. The parasites of North Carolina rodents. *Ecological Monographs* 6:152–232.

Herman, C.M. 1939. A parasitological survey of wild rats in the New York Zoological Park. *Zoologica* 24:305–308.

Herman, T.B. 1981. *Capillaria hepatica* (Nematoda) in insular populations of the deer mouse *Peromyscus maniculatus:* Cannibalism or competition for carcasses? *Canadian Journal of Zoology* 59:776–784.

Höppli, R. 1925. Die histologischen Veränderungen in der Rattenleber bei Infektion mit *Hepaticola hepatica* (Bancroft, 1893) Hall, 1916. *Zeitschrifts für Infektionskrankheiten, parasitäre Krankheiten u. Hygiene der Haustiere* 27:199–206.

Hörning, B. 1974. Zur Kenntnis der Parasitenfauna des Wildkaninchens der St.-Peters-Insel. *Schweizer Archiv für Tierheilkunde* 116:99–101.

Ishimoto, Y. 1974. Studies on helminths of voles in Hokkaido. I. Taxonomical study. *Japanese Journal of Veterinary Research* 22:1–12.

Johnston, T.H. 1918. Notes on certain entozoa of rats and mice, together with a catalogue of the internal parasites recorded as occurring in rodents in Australia. *Proceedings of the Royal Society of Queensland* 30:53–78.

Kallichurum, S., and R. Elsdon-Dew. 1961. *Capillaria* in man. A case report. *South African Medical Journal* 35:860–861.

Keymer, A.E. 1982. Density-dependent mechanisms in the regulation of intestinal helminth populations. *Parasitology* 84:573–587.

Kim, D.-U., K.-S. Eom, and H.-J. Rim 1985. Indirect fluorescent antibody test on the sectioned egg antigen of *Capillaria hepatica* in the liver of white rat. *Korea University Medical Journal* 22(1): 173–184.

Koval'chuk, E.S., and O.M. Bonina 1981. A focus of *Hepaticola hepatica* infection in the Barabin lowlands [In Russian]. In *Biologicheskie problemy priorodnoi ochagovosti boleznei.* Ed. A.A. Maksimov. Novosibirsk, USSR: "Nauka" Sibirskoe Otdelenie, pp. 152–156.

Kumar, V., W. DeMeurichy, A.M. Delahaye, and J. Mortelmans. 1983. Tissue dwelling capillarid nematode infections in the fauna of Zoological Garden, Antwerp. *Acta Zoologica et Pathologica Antverpiensia* 77:87–95.

Kumar, V., J. Brandt, and J. Mortelmans. 1985. Hepatic capillariasis may simulate the syndrome of visceral larva migrans, an analysis. *Annals de la Société Belge de Mèdicine Tropicale* 65:101–104.

Kutzer, E., and H. Frey 1976. Die Parasiten der Feldhasen (*Lepus europaeus*) in Österreich. *Berliner und Münchener Tierärztliche Wochenschrift* 89:480–483.

Lämmler, G., and D. Grüner 1976. Zur Wirksamkeit von Anthelminthika gegen *Capillaria hepatica.* Berliner und Münchener Tierärztliche Wochenschrift 89: 222–225; 229–233.

Lämmler, G., H. Zahner, R. Vollerthun, and R. Rudolph 1974. Egg production and host reaction in *Capillaria hepatica* infection of *Mastomys natalensis.* In *Parasitic zoonoses. Clinical and experimental studies.* Ed. E.J.L. Soulsby. New York: Academic Press. Inc., pp. 327–341.

Layne, J.N. 1963. A study of the parasites of the Florida mouse, *Peromyscus floridanus,* in relation to host and environmental factors. *Tulane Studies in Zoology* 11:1–27.

——. 1968. Host and ecological relationships of the parasitic helminth *Capillaria hepatica* in Florida mammals. *Zoologica (New York)* 53:107–123.

Layne, J.N., and J.V. Griffo Jr. 1961. Incidence of *Capillaaria hepatica* in populations of the Florida deer mouse, *Peromyscus floridanus.* *The Journal of Parasitology* 47:31–37.

Layne, J.N., and C.E. Winegarner 1971. Occurrence of *Capillaria hepatica* (Nematoda: Trichuridae) in the spotted skunk in Florida. *Journal of Wildlife Diseases* 7:256–257.

LeBlanc, P., B. Fagin, and B.A. Kulwich 1983. *Capillaria hepatica* infection: Incidental finding in a dog with renal insufficiency. *Canine Practice* 10:12–14.

Lee, C.W. 1964. *Capillaria hepatica.* The experimental studies on *Capillaria hepatica. Korean Journal of Parasitology* 2:3–80.

Lee, K.-Y., K.-S. Eom, and H.-J. Rim. 1985. Micro-ELISA test in *Capillaria hepatica* of white rat using soluble egg antigen. *Korea University Medical Journal* 22(3): 33–44.

Liat, L.B., Y.L. Fong, and M. Krishnasamy 1977. *Capillaria hepatica* infection of wild rodents in Peninsular Malaysia. *Southeast Asian Journal of Tropical Medicine and Public Health* 8:354–358.

Lubinsky, G. 1956. On the probable presence of parasitic liver cirrhosis in Canada. *Canadian Journal of Comparative Medicine* 20:457–465.

——. 1957. List of helminths from Alberta rodents. *Canadian Journal of Zoology* 35:623–627.

Lubinsky, G., B.R. Jacobsen, and R.W. Baron 1971. Wildlife foci of *Capillaria hepatica* infections in Manitoba. *Canadian Journal of Zoology* 49:1201–1202.

Luttermoser, G.W. 1936. A helminthological survey of Baltimore house rats (*Rattus norvegicus*). *American Journal of Hygiene* 24:350–360.

——. 1938a. Factors influencing the development and viability of eggs of *Capillaria hepatica. American Journal of Hygiene* 27:457–465.

——. 1938b. An experimental study of *Capillaria hepatica* in the rat and the mouse. *American Journal of Hygiene* 27:321–340.

MacArthur, W.P. 1924. A case of infestation of the human liver with *Hepaticola hepatica* (Bancroft, 1893) Hall 1916; with sections from the liver. *Proceedings of the Royal Society of Medicine (Section of Tropical Diseases and Parasitology)* 17:83–84.

Markus, M.B., and R.F. Cheetham. 1985. Chemotherapy for *Capillaria hepatica* infection. *Journal of Antimicrobial Chemotherapy* 15:79–791.

McCallum, H.I. 1992. Evaluation of a nematode (*Capillaria hepatica* Bancroft, 1893) as a control agent for populations of house mice (*Mus musculus domesticus* Schwartz and Schwartz, 1943). *Revue Scientifique et Technique Office International des Epizooties* 12:83–93.

——. 1995. Modelling host-parasite interactions to help plan and interpret field studies. *Wildlife Research* 22:21–29.

McCallum, H.I., and G.R. Singleton 1989. Models to assess the potential of *Capillaria hepatica* to control outbreaks of house mice. *Parasitology* 98:425–437.

McQuown, A.L. 1950. *Capillaria hepatica:* Report of genuine and spurious cases. *American Journal of Tropical Medicine* 30:761–767.

——. 1954. *Capillaria hepatica. American Journal of Clinical Pathology* 24:448–452.

Meyer, M.C., and J.R. Reilly 1950. Parasites of muskrats in Maine. *American Midland Naturalist* 44:467–477.

Misic, S., G. Kokai, and V. Perisic. 1986. *Capillaria hepatica* infection in a two-year-old child. Proceedings of the 6th International Congress of Parasitology, Brisbane, Queensland, Australia, S8, C22, p. 995.

Mobedi, I., and F. Arfaa. 1971. Probable role of ground beetles in the transmission of *Capillaria hepatica. Journal of Parasitology* 57:1144–1145.

Momma, K. 1930. Notes on modes of rat infestation with *Hepaticola hepatica. Annals of Tropical Medicine and Parasitology* 24: 109–113.

Monroe, G.A. 1984. Pyloric stenosis in a yearling with an incidental finding of *Capillaria hepatica* in the liver. *Equine Veterinary Journal* 16:221–222.

Nascimoto, I., and M. Sadigursky 1986. *Capillaria hepatica:* Some immunopathological aspects of spurious infection and true infection [In Portuguese]. *Revista da Sociedade Brasiliera de Medicina Tropical* 19:21–25.

Nation, P.N., and K.H. Dies 1978. *Capillaria hepatica* in a horse. *Canadian Veterinary Journal* 19:315–316.

Nicoll, W. 1911. On a unique pathological condition in a hare. Proceedings of the Zoological Society of London, September 1911, pp. 674–676.

Nishigori, M. 1925. On the life history of *Hepaticola hepatica. Journal of the Formosan Medical Association (2nd Report)* 247:3–4.

Odujno, E.O. 1970. Helminthic anaphylactic syndrome (HAS) in children. *Pathologia Microbiologica* 35:220–223.

Otto, G.F., M. Berthrong, R.E. Appleby, J.C. Rawlins, and O. Wilbur. 1954. Eosinophilia and hepatomegaly due to *Capillaria hepatica* infection. *Bulletin of the Johns Hopkins Hospital* 94:319–336.

Pampiglione, S., and C. Concini 1970. Primo caso capillariouse epatica osservata nell' oumo in Italia. *Parassitologia* 12:125–134.

Partington, C., and R.J. Montali 1986. *Capillaria hepatica* in Kirk's dik dik, *Madoqua kirkii. Journal of Zoo Animal Medicine* 17:123–129.

Pavlov, A.V. 1955. Biology of the nematode *Hepaticola hepatica* and features of the epizootiology of the disease caused by it [In Russian]. [Cited in Skrjabin K.E., N.P. Shikhobalova, and I.V. Orlov. 1957. *Essentials of nematology.* Vol. 6, Trichocephalidae and Capillariidae of animals and man and the diseases caused by them. Academy of Sciences of the USSR.] [Translated 1970. Israel Program for Scientific Translations, Jerusalem.]

——. 1960. Morphology of *Hepaticola hepatica* in the black beaver and its position in the system of nematodes [In Russian]. *Trudy Voronezhskogo gosudarstvennogo zapovednika* 9:215–220.

Penn, G.H. 1942. Parasitological survey of Louisiana muskrats. *Journal of Parasitology* 28:348–349.

Pereira, V.G., and L.C.M. Franca. 1983. Successful treatment of *Capillaria hepatica* infection in an acutely ill adult. *American Journal of Tropical Medicine and Hygiene* 32:1272–1274.

Piazza, R., M.O.A. Corréa, and R.N. Fleury. 1963. Sôbre um caso de infestação humana por *Capillaria hepatica. Revista do Instituto de Medicine Tropical de São Paulo* 5:37–41.

Price, E.W. 1931. *Hepaticola hepatica* in liver of *Ondatra zibethica. The Journal of Parasitology* 18:51.

Price, E.W., and B.G. Chitwood 1931. Incidence of internal parasites in wild rats in Washington. *The Journal of Parasitology* 18:55.

Rao, R.R., M.R. Marathe, T.B. Nair, and S.D. Gangoli 1975. *Capillaria hepatica* in a mongrel dog. *Indian Veterinary Journal* 52:393–394.

Rausch, R. 1961. Notes on the occurrence of *Capillaria hepatica* (Bancroft, 1893). *Proceedings of the Helminthological Society of Washington* 28:17–18.

Raybourne, R., and G.B. Solomon. 1975. *Capillaria hepatica:* Granuloma formation to eggs III. Anti-immunoglobulin augmentation and reagin activity in mice. *Experimental Parasitology* 38:87–95.

———. 1984. Granulomatous hypersensitivity and antibody production in response to antigens of *Capillaria hepatica* eggs. *International Journal for Parasitology* 14:371–375.

Raybourne, R., G.B. Solomon, and E.J.L. Soulsby 1974. *Capillaria hepatica:* Granuloma formation to eggs II. Peripheral immunological responses. *Experimental Parasitology* 36:244–252.

Read, C.P. 1949. Studies on North American helminths of the genus *Capillaria* Zeder, 1800 (Nematoda). I. Capillarids from mammals. *Journal of Parasitology* 35:223–230.

Reynolds, W.A., and G. Gavutis 1975. *Capillaria hepatica* in a groundhog (*Marmota monax*). *Journal of Wildlife Diseases* 11:13.

Romero, G.M, and F. Biagi 1962. Eosinofilia elevada con manifestationes viscerales. Primer caso de infeccion por *Capillaria hepatica* en México. *Boletín médico del Hospital infantil, México* 19:473.

Saenong, T.H.S.A. 1984. (Penelitan *Capillaria hepatica* pada *Rattus argentiventer* di daerah Cakung [In Indonesian]. MSc. Thesis, University of Jakarta.

Sandground, J.H. 1933. Parasitic nematodes from East Africa and Southern Rhodesia. *Bulletin of the Museum of Comparative Zoology (Harvard)* 15:263–293.

Schmidt, V. 1975. Causes of death in kangaroos [In German]. In *Verhandlungsbericht des XVII Internationalen Symposiums über die Erkrankungen der Zootiere, Tunis, 4–8 June, 1975.* Berlin, Germany: Akademie-Verlag, pp. 321–325.

Seo, B.S., H.J. Rim, C.W. Lee, and J.S. Woo. 1964. Studies on the parasitic helminths of Korea II. Parasites of the rat, *Rattus norvegicus* Erxl. in Seoul, with the description of *Capillaria hepatica* (Bancroft, 1893) Travassos, (1915). *Korean Journal of Parasitology* 2:55–62.

Shimatani, T. 1961. Studies on the ecology of *Capillaria hepatica* eggs [In Japanese]. *Journal of Kyoto Prefectural Medical University* 64:1063–1083.

Shorb, D.A. 1931. Experimental infestation of white rats with *Hepaticola hepatica. Journal of Parasitology* 17:151–154.

Silverman, N.H., J.S. Katz, and S.E. Levin. 1973. *Capillaria hepatica* infestation in a child. *South African Medical Journal* 47:219–221.

Singleton, G.R. 1985. Population dynamics of *Mus musculus* and its parasites in Mallee Wheatlands in Victoria during and after a drought. *Australian Wildlife Research* 12:437–445.

Singleton, G.R., and L.K. Chambers. 1996. A manipulative field experiment to examine the effect of *Capillaria hepatica* (Nematoda) on wild mouse populations in southern Australia. *International Journal for Parasitology* 26:383–398.

Singleton, G.R., and H.I. McCallum. 1990 The potential of *Capillaria hepatica* to control mouse plagues. *Parasitology Today* 6:190–192.

Singleton, G.R., and D.M. Spratt. 1986. The effects of *Capillaria hepatica* (Nematoda) on natality and survival to weaning in BALB/c mice. *Australian Journal of Zoology* 34:677–681.

Singleton, G.R., L.K. Chambers, and D.M. Spratt 1995. An experimental field study to examine whether *Capillaria hepatica* (Nematoda) can limit house mouse populations in eastern Australia. *Wildlife Research* 21:31–53.

Singleton, G.R., D.M. Spratt, S.C. Barker, and P.F. Hodgson 1991. The geographic distribution and host range of *Capillaria hepatica* (Bancroft) (Nematoda) in Australia. *International Journal for Parasitology* 21:945–957.

Sinniah B., M. Singh, and K. Anuar 1979. Preliminary survey of *Capillaria hepatica* (Bancroft, 1893) in Malaysia. *Journal of Helminthology* 53:147–152.

Skrjabin K.E., N.P. Shikhobalova, and I.V. Orlov 1957. *Essentials of nematology.* Vol. 6, *Trichocephalidae and Capillariidae of animals and man and the diseases caused by them.* Academy of Sciences of the USSR. [Translated 1970. Israel Program for Scientific Translations, Jerusalem.)

Slais, J. 1973. The finding and identification of solitary *Capillaria hepatica* (Bancroft, 1893) in man from Europe. *Folia Parasitologica (Praha)* 20:149–161.

———. 1974. Notes on the differentiation of *Capillaria hepatica* and visceral larva migrans. *Folia Parasitologica (Praha)* 21:95.

Slais, J., and J. Sterba 1972. Solitary liver granulomas in man caused by *Capillaria hepatica* (Bancroft, 1893) in Czechoslovakia. *Folia Parasitologica (Praha)* 19:373–374.

Smit, J.D. 1960. *Capillaria hepatica* infestation in a dog. *Onderstepoort Journal of Veterinary Research* 28:473–478.

Solomon, G.B., and C.O. Handley Jr. 1971. *Capillaria hepatica* (Bancroft, 1893) in Appalachian mammals. *The Journal of Parasitology* 57:1142–1144.

Solomon, G.B., and E.J.L. Soulsby 1973. Granuloma formation to *Capillaria hepatica* eggs. 1. Descriptive definition. *Experimental Parasitology* 33:458–467.

Spratt, D.M., and G.R. Singleton. 1986. Studies on the life cycle, infectivity and clinical effects of *Capillaria hepatica* (Bancroft) (Nematoda) in mice, *Mus musculus. Australian Journal of Zoology* 34: 663–675.

———. 1987. Experimental embryonation and survival of eggs of *Capillaria hepatica* (Nematoda) under mouse burrow conditions in cereal-growing soils. *Australia Journal of Zoology* 35: 337–341.

Stokes, R. 1973. *Capillaria hepatica* in a dog. *Australian Veterinary Journal* 49: 109.

Suda, A. 1928. On liver cirrhosis in the rabbit caused by *Hepaticola hepatica. Journal of the Medical Association of Aichi.* 35(1).

Troisier, J., R. Deschiens, H. Limousin, and M. Delorme 1928. L'infestation du chimpanzee par un nématode du genre *Hepaticola. Les Annales de l'Institute Pasteur* 42:827–841.

Turhan, B., E.K. Unat, M. Ynermar, and C. Sumer 1954. Insan karacigerinde: *Capillaria hepatica* (Bancroft, 1893) Travassos, 1915. *Mikrobiologi dergisi* 7:149–159.

Vargas, G., H. Lopez, R. Victoria, and G. Hernandez 1979. *Capillaria hepatica.* Report of the 2nd case found in the Mexican Republic. *Boletín médico del Hospital infantil, México* 36:909–917.

Vianna, Y.L. 1954. Sôbre un caso de capilariose hepática em canino do Rio de Janeiro. *Veterinária, Rio de Janeiro* 8:3–19.

Vogel, H. 1930. Über die Organotropie von *Hepaticola hepatica. Zeitschrift für Parasitenkunde* 2:502–505.

———. 1932. Beiträge vor Epidemiologie der Schistosomiasis in Liberia und Französisch-Guinea. *Archives für Schiffs- und Tropenkrankheiten* 35:108–135.

Vogelsang, E.G., and J. Espin 1949. Dos nuevos huespedes para *Capillaria hepatica* (Bancroft, 1893) Travassos 1915; nutria (*Myopotamus coypus*) y el raton mochilero (*Akodon venezuelensis*). *Revista de medicina veterinaria y parasitologia, Caracas* 8:73–78.

Vollerthun, R., G. Lämmler, and J. Schuster 1974. *Capillaria hepatica*—Infecktion der *Mastomys natalensis:* Veränderungen des Enymaktivitäten im Serum. *Zeitschrift der Parasitenkunde* 44:43–58.

Waddell, A.H. 1969. Methyridine in the treatment of experimental *Capillaria hepatica* infection in the rat. *Annals of Tropical Medicine and Parasitology* 63:63–65.

Wantland, W.W., H.M. Kemple, G.R. Beers, and K.E. Dye 1956. *Cysticercus fasciolaris* and *Capillaria hepatica* in *Rattus norvegicus*. *Transactions of the Illinois Academy of Science* 49: 177–181.

Ward, J.W. 1934. A study of some parasites of central Oklahoma. *The Biologist* 15:83–84.

Ward, R.L., and J.H. Dent. 1959. *Capillaria hepatica* infection in a child. *Bulletin of the Tulane Medical Faculty* 19:27–33.

Weidman, F. 1917. Dr. Weidman's report. In H. Fox. 1916. Annual Report of the Zoological Society of Philadelphia, pp. 33–40.

_____. 1925. Hepaticoliasis, a frequent and sometimes fatal verminous infestation of the livers of rats and other rodents. *The Journal of Parasitology* 12:19–25.

Winkelmann, J. 1974. Infektiosität und Pathogenität von *Capillaria hepatica* (Bancroft 1893) in SPF-Kaninchen. Doktorgrades Dissertation, zur Erlangung des Justus Liebig-Universität Gießen, Gießen, Germany, pp. 51–64. [Cited in J.D. Borucinska, H.J. Van Kruiningen, J.N. Caira, and A.E. Garmendia. 1997. Clinicopathological features and histopathology of experimental hepatic capillariasis in muskrats (*Ondatra zibethicus*). *Journal of Wildlife Diseases* 33:122–130.]

Wobeser, G., and T.W. Rock. 1973. *Capillaria hepatica* (Nematoda: Trichuridae) in a coyote (*Canis latrans*). *Journal of Wildlife Diseases* 9:225–226.

Wright, H.E. 1931. Further observations on the incidence of *Hepaticola*(*Capillaria*) *hepatica* ova in human faeces. *American Journal of Tropical Medicine* 18:329–330.

Wright, K.A. 1961. Observations on the life cycle of *Capillaria hepatica* (Bancroft, 1893) with a description of the adult. *Canadian Journal of Zoology* 39:167–182.

_____. 1974. The feeding site and probable feeding mechanism of the parasitic nematode *Capillaria hepatica*. *Canadian Journal of Zoology* 52:1215–1220.

Wright, W.H. 1930. *Capillaria hepatica* in dogs. *The Journal of Parasitology* 17:54–55.

Yokogawa, S. 1920. A new nematode from the rat. *The Journal of Parasitology* 7:29–33.

Zahner, H., and R. Rudolph 1980. *Capillaria hepatica*—Infektionen der *Mastomys natalensis:* Pathologische Veränderungen der Leber und Milz mit embryonierten und röntgenattenuierten Eisern. *Zentralblatt Veterinärmedizin B* 27:85–101.

Zahner, H., G. Bruckmann, H. Schmidt, G. Lämmler, and E. Geyer 1976. *Capillaria hepatica*—Infektion der *Mastomys natalensis:* Zur Entwicklung, Eiproduktion und Wirtsreaktion. *Zeitschrift der Parasitenkunde* 49:41–61.

Zahner, H., H. Schmidt, G. Lämmler, and E. Geyer. 1981. Empfindlichkeit embryonierter *Capillaria hepatica* Eier gegen Röntgenstrahlen sowie Serum-GLDH-Aktivität und Antiköpertiter bei *Mastomys natalensis* nach Infektion mit unbestrahlten bzw. röntgenbestrahlten Eiern. *Zeitschrift der Parasitenkunde* 65:107–116.

15

TRICHINELLA SPP. AND TRICHINELLOSIS

TERRY A. DICK AND EDOARDO POZIO

INTRODUCTION. The association of nematodes in the genus *Trichinella* with mammals and birds is unique among animal parasitic associations, because (1) there are at least 150 host species (Campbell 1983a); (2) most isolates recovered from wild animals infect a wide range of experimental, wild, and semidomestic hosts; and (3) isolates are widely distributed, extending from the Arctic to the tropics, including Oceania.

From its first discovery in a human cadaver, trichinellosis has been associated with humans, pork, and rats (Campbell 1983b). For more than a century, the genus *Trichinella* was considered monospecific, since only *Trichinella spiralis* was recognized (Dick 1983a). However, differences in infectivity in experimental animals (primarily mice, rats, and hamsters, but also swine), size of worms, biochemistry, and longevity of infections in the gut and muscle were reported (Dick 1983a). There was little doubt that there were different isolates, ecotypes, subspecies, or species. The ability to survive freezing clearly was a key attribute of the circumpolar *Trichinella,* as was the ability of other isolates to survive in decomposing carrion from other regions of the world. There have been numerous intellectual controversies surrounding this genus, including encysted larvae considered a free-living stage (Madsen 1974), the number of molts prior to the muscle stage, whether or not muscle larvae are neotenic, and current views on speciation and factors causing speciation.

Dick (1983b) proposed a subspecies status for at least four of the major forms until more information accumulated and also suggested that local populations are likely genetically different as their biological characteristics (phenotypes) varied in the same experimental host. The original taxonomy was influenced by the epidemiology of trichinellosis. It was generally considered a pathogen of domestic pigs and synanthropic rats; however, it was known that *Trichinella* occurred in Arctic animals, an unlikely place for both rats and swine (Rausch 1970). After *Trichinella* isolated from wildlife was passaged in experimental hosts, it differed in infectivity and pathogenicity from worms collected from domestic pigs and passaged in experimental animals (especially rats) and in pigs (Nelson 1970; Rausch 1970). In 1972, Britov and Boev (1972) described two new species: *T. nativa* and *T. nelsoni.* This work was based on breeding experiments between isolates of *Trichinella* from sylvatic and domestic animals collected in the Palearctic region and South Africa. In the same year, another Russian scientist discovered and described *T. pseudospiralis,* which was characterized by a larval stage that did not induce cyst formation in host striated muscle. In fact, *T. pseudospiralis* does not cause modification of the muscular cell into a nurse cell as do the other species in the genus (Garkavi 1972). The description of these new species generated a debate on their taxonomic validity because there was (1) a lack of morphological differences among these supposed species, (2) a lack of host specificity as observed for many other parasites, (3) controversy surrounding single breeding pair experiments and the definition of a species, and (4) a lack of type isolates for each species, except for *T. pseudospiralis.* In addition, variation in biological characteristics, such as infection levels between wild and experimental hosts, and genotypic and phenotypic variation among current recognized species, remains unresolved. Some of this variation is undoubtedly related to geographical differences (reviewed by Dick 1983a).

RECOVERY AND IDENTIFICATION. The simplest method to recover larvae of *Trichinella* spp. is to compress pieces of striated muscle (preferably from the tongue, diaphragm, or intercostals of mammals) between glass slides or with the aid of a trichinoscope and then view them with a dissecting microscope. Another method is the digestion of muscle tissue in 1% HCl/pepsin solution at 37° C for several hours followed by filtering the digest through a final metal screen of number 80 mesh (CE Syler). Larvae recovered by this method are usually reported as larvae per gram (larvae/g) muscle tissue. While cysts of most *Trichinella* spp. are easily recognized, the nonencysting smaller larvae of *T. pseudospiralis* are more difficult to find. Adult *Trichinella* are generally short-lived in the intestine of most hosts (10–12 days from ingestion of cysts), but adults, associated with mucous and epithelium, can be observed with the aid of a microscope. By contrast, adult *T. pseudospiralis* live much longer in the intestine of experimentally infected birds, but few studies have searched for adults in the intestine of wild birds.

Identification of isolates of *Trichinella* spp. has come a long way since 11 biological characteristics were reviewed by Dick (1983a). Most of these traits

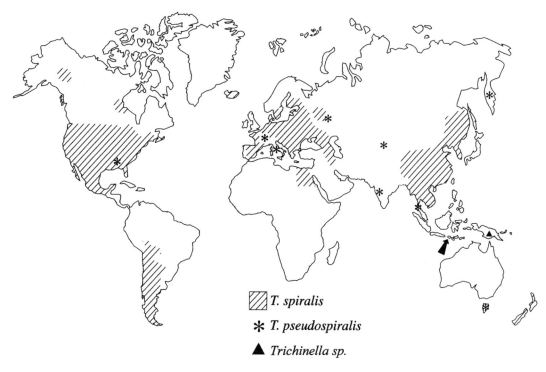

FIG. 15.1—Distribution of *Trichinella spiralis,* and *Trichinella pseudospiralis,* and *Trichinella* sp. throughout the world, based on data from the International Trichinella Reference Center. Arrow shows the island of Bali where *Trichinella* is widespread in domestic pigs. Distribution of these species is probably underestimated.

show remarkable variation and confound species designation. Interestingly, the erection of species followed closely the application of biochemical techniques (Flockhart et al. 1982; Mydynski and Dick 1985; Pozio 1987; La Rosa et al. 1992), molecular biology (Curran et al. 1985; Klassen et al. 1986; Zarlenga et al. 1991), and PCR (polymerase chain reaction) technology (Dick et al. 1992; Bandi et al. 1995) to discriminate among individual larvae. These techniques permitted investigators of *Trichinella* isolates to go beyond morphology and pathogenicity. Recent screening of sera from wild animals is showing promise (Zarnke et al. 1997).

Establishment of the International Trichinella Reference Center (ITRC) in 1989 in Italy has resulted in collection and storage of large numbers of isolates used in comparative studies (Pozio et al. 1989a). Allozyme analysis of 152 isolates from various host species and geographical regions identified eight phenotypes, four corresponding to the species previously described, and four apparently new taxonomic entities (La Rosa et al. 1992). Pozio et al. (1992a) recognized the same eight phenotypes during study of seven biological and two environmental characters of 40 other isolates. On the basis of biochemical, biological, and environmental characters, the taxonomy of the genus *Trichinella* was reviewed. The four species previously reported from Russian authors were considered valid, and a new

species, *T. britovi,* was described. Because few isolates were examined for each of the other three phenotypes, they were given nonspecific ranks of *Trichinella* T5, T6, and T8 (Pozio et al. 1992b). Genotypic analysis of eight phenotypes described by La Rosa et al. (1992) showed significant differences and supported the presence of five sibling species (Bandi et al. 1995, Cuperlovic 1996, Wu et al. 1998). The main characteristics of these species are described below.

Trichinella spiralis is the etiological agent of domestic and sylvatic trichinellosis found on most continents. The cosmopolitan distribution of this species is probably due to passive introduction with domestic pigs and synanthropic rats (Fig. 15.1). Furthermore, this parasite has been transmitted from domestic animals to wildlife and now is considered a parasite of sylvatic carnivores and omnivores.

Trichinella nativa is the etiological agent of sylvatic trichinellosis in frigid zones of the Holarctic region (Fig. 15.2). The main hosts are carnivorous mammals. Its presence in domestic and sylvatic swine is very rare. The main biological characteristic of muscle larvae in carnivore muscle is their resistance to freezing for several years. There are no reports of this species in synanthropic rats.

Trichinella britovi (synonym *T. nelsoni* Britov and Boev 1972, in part) is the etiological agent of sylvatic

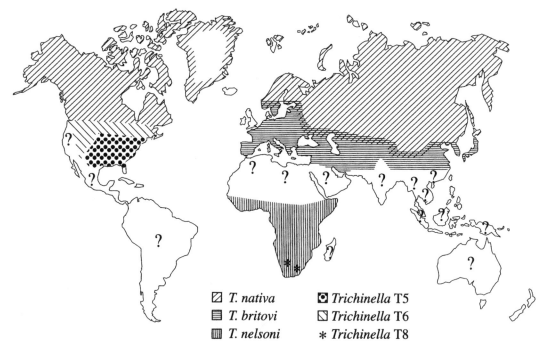

FIG. 15.2—Distribution of sylvatic species and genotypes *Trichinella* throughout the world; based on data from the International Trichinella Reference Center. '?' indicates a lack of information on species and genotypes of *Trichinella* in wildlife. In Eurasia, between the -4° C and -6° C isotherm in January, both *T. nativa* and *T. britovi* are present in wildlife.

trichinellosis in temperate areas of Eurasia (Fig. 15.2). The main hosts are carnivorous mammals. Its presence in domestic and sylvatic swine and in synanthropic rats is rare. This parasite can infect domestic pigs but is not able to maintain a domestic cycle.

Trichinella nelsoni is the etiological agent of sylvatic trichinellosis in Africa south of the Sahara (Fig. 15.2). This parasite seems to be restricted to carnivores from preserves and parks.

Trichinella pseudospiralis differs the most from other species in the genus (Fig. 15.1). It has a cosmopolitan distribution, likely because of its broad host range, which includes marsupials, and its capacity to infect experimental bird hosts such as raptors (Saumier et al. 1986), gulls, and galliformes (Bober and Dick 1983; T.A. Dick, unpublished).

LIFE HISTORY OF THE SYLVATIC CYCLE.

Trichinellosis is primarily a disease of sylvatic carnivores with cannibalistic and scavenger behavior. All warm-blooded animals can be infected; however, the spread and maintenance of trichinellosis in nature relies on ingestion of muscle larvae from one individual by another, that is, from carnivore to carnivore (Fig. 15.3). Herbivores and omnivores may acquire the parasite but are less important in its transmission. The sylvatic cycle involves transmission of *Trichinella*

among wildlife, either by ingestion of infected prey or fresh, frozen, or decomposing carcasses. Infective larvae can survive several weeks in decomposing caracasses (Madsen 1974; T.A. Dick and E. Pozio, unpublished). Human activity influences the distribution of *Trichinella* in Arctic regions (C.M.O. Kapel, personal communication), particularly the behavior of hunters leaving carcasses of carnivores in the environment. A concentration of *Trichinella* infections in fisher and marten (Dick et al. 1986) was likely associated with consumption of many carcasses that were placed in the area as baits to attract black bears (for purposes of hunting). Interestingly, not all isolates resisted freezing, suggesting that carcass sources other than wildlife might be involved.

ARCTIC REGIONS/*T.NATIVA*.

Trichinellosis in arctic mammals was discovered in 1934 (Rausch 1970). Subsequently, several authors recognized high prevalence of infection among carnivores from Canada, Alaska, Greenland, the Svalbard islands, and Siberia. *Trichinella* strains from arctic mammals showed biological features different from those of domestic strains from pigs (Rausch 1970; Dick and Belosevic 1978; Belosevic and Dick 1979; Belosevic and Dick 1980, Chadee and Dick 1982; Dick 1983b,c). The main characters of strains from frigid zones are (1) low or no

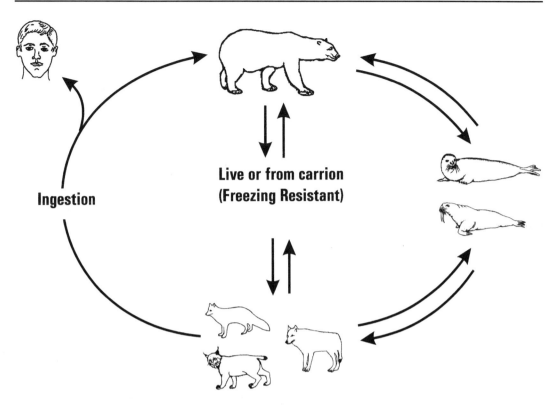

FIG. 15.3—Transmission cycle of sylvatic *Trichinella* in Arctic regions. Ability to withstand freezing in carrion is a key characteristic since it ensures survival of infective larvae until they are consumed by carrion feeders and scavenging animals.

infectivity to laboratory rats, mice, and domestic pigs (Pozio et al. 1992a; Kapel et al. 1998), (2) high resistance of muscle larvae to freezing when they are in muscle tissue of carnivores (i.e., > 4 years in an arctic fox (Kapel et al. 1999), 3 years in polar bear, 5 years in experimentally infected raccoons (T.A. Dick, unpublished), and 34 months in grizzly bear [(Worley et al. 1986) (Table 15.1)], and (3) a thick capsule formed rapidly around the muscle larvae by the nurse cell (Pozio et al. 1992a).

Although there are differences among Arctic isolates there is also a high degree of predictability among some isolates. Dick (1983b) reported on four isolates of *Trichinella* from arctic fox recovered in 1980 with varying reproductive capacity indices (RCIs). Annual passages of four arctic fox isolates from 1980 to 1998 in experimental mouse hosts has seen the RCI values stay remarkably constant within and among isolates (T.A. Dick, unpublished). In North America all isolates recovered from carnivorous mammals from Arctic and north temperate regions and exhibiting freezing resistance are infective to mice (T.A. Dick, unpublished).

The list of mammals found naturally infected in Arctic and north temperate regions is impressive: ursidae (3 species), felidae (4 species), canidae (6 species), mustelidae (6 species), phocidae (1 species), otaridae (1 species), sciuridae (3 species), cricetidae (4 species), castoridae (1 species), and leporidae (1 species) (Tables 15.2 and 15.3). *Trichinella nativa* has been identified from 7 species from North America and 14 species from Eurasia (Tables 15.2 and 15.3); but *T. spiralis* is also reported from animals near human settlements in the Arctic, from brown bear in Alaska (E. Pozio, unpublished), and from polar bear in Canada. There are also reports of human trichinellosis from consumption of bear or walrus meat (MacLean et al. 1992), but the species is not known. Polar bears are a key component in the transmission of *Trichinella* in the Arctic (Born and Henriksen 1990) with prevalences as high as 60% from Baffin Island (T.A. Dick, unpublished) and 23% from Greenland. Prevalence increases with increasing age of bears: 7.7% in 1-year-old animals, 11.7% in animals 2–6 years, 36.1% in animals 7–10 years, and 62.2% in animals > 10 years (Henriksen et al. 1994). The main source of *Trichinella* infection for polar bears and most Arctic predators is cannibalism or scavenging carcasses of arctic foxes and sled dogs. The importance of the polar bear as reservoir of *T. nativa* is increased by the survival of larvae in bears for several years. By contrast, *T. nativa* were detected in 0.6% of 571 brown bear (the key host) from Kamchatka at up to 100 larvae/g and 29.7% of wolverine (Britov 1997).

TABLE 15.1—Resistance to freezing of different species and genotypes of *Trichinella* in muscles from several hosts

Trichinella Species or Genotype	Host	Temperature below Zero	Time of Survival of Freezing	Reference
T. nativa	Arctic fox	−18° C	4 years	Kapel et al. 1999
	Arctic fox	−18° C	12–14 months	Chadee and Dick 1982
	Arctic fox	−18° C	3 years	T.A. Dick, unpublished
	Polar bear	−18° C	5 years	T.A. Dick, unpublished
	Polar bear	−18° C	6 months	Chadee and Dick 1982
	Raccoon[a]	−18° C	30–270 days	Dick 1983c
	Laboratory mice	−10° C	8–22 days	Pozio et al. 1994a
Trichinella T6	Grizzly bear	−6.5 to −20° C	34 months	Worley et al. 1986
	Laboratory mice	−10° C	5–13 days	Pozio et al. 1994a
T. britovi	Wolf	−20° C	6 months	Pozio et al. 1989b
	Fox	−15° C	11 months	E. Pozio, unpublished
	Wild boar	−20° C	3 weeks	E. Pozio, unpublished
	Laboratory mice	−10° C	4–7 days	Pozio et al. 1994a
Trichinella T5	Laboratory mice	−10° C	12–108 hours	Pozio et al. 1994a
T. spiralis	Laboratory mice	−10° C	12–48 hours	Pozio et al. 1994a
T. nelsoni	Laboratory mice	−10° C	no survival	Pozio et al. 1994a
T. pseudospiralis	Laboratory mice	−10° C	no survival	Pozio et al. 1994a

[a] Experimental infection from frozen arctic fox carcasses to raccoons and then refrozen.

Arctic foxes are also a key species in transmission in the Arctic as they are usually associated with large predators and carrion and frequently are found close to settlements. In arctic fox from Greenland, overall prevalence is 6% with a geographical variation from 0% to 35% (Kapel et al. 1996). All infected foxes originated from only two of eight districts investigated. The average age was higher in infected animals, and the infection averaged 38 larvae/g (range 0.1–148). Infection is related to composition of the surrounding fauna and the hunting practices of the traditional Inuit culture (Kapel et al. 1996). Prevalence of *Trichinella* in arctic fox from Victoria Island was 30% (T.A. Dick, unpublished). European lynx are also important hosts; Oksanen et al. (1998) detected *Trichinella* in 40.4% of 132 animals and found the prevalence in lynx was correlated with the density of raccoon dogs *(Nyctereutes procyonoides)*.

The southern limit of *T. nativa* distribution in Eurasia is the isotherm −5° C in January in Eurasia. A similar physical barrier probably occurs in North America; however, another phenotype, *Trichinella* T6, occurs in wild carnivores in North America along the Rocky Mountains and in Pennsylvania, south of the isotherm −5° C in January. It is strongly related to *T. nativa*, as supported by breeding experiments (Britov 1995), but differs by three unique marker allozymes (Pozio et al. 1992b), the RAPD (random amplified polymorphic DNA) pattern (Bandi et al. 1995), and PCR-RFLP (polymerase chain reaction–restriction fragment length polymorphism) pattern (Wu et al. 1999). Muscle larvae of *Trichinella* T6 can survive freezing for a long period (Worley et al. 1986). *Trichinella* T6 larvae are identified from 13 animals in Montana, Idaho, and Pennsylvania (E. Pozio, unpublished) (Table 15.2). Dick et al. (1986) recovered several isolates from fisher and marten that are likely related to T6. This phenotype is

likely present in southern regions of Canada and in other northern regions of United States. From a survey of 4773 individuals of 19 species in central and northwestern Ontario, Canada, *Trichinella* was found in 83 fisher (4.6%) and 68 marten (3.4%) (Dick et al. 1986). Dick and Leonard (1979) and Poole et al. (1983) also reported *Trichinella* from fisher (1.2%) and marten (1.0%), respectively, from Manitoba.

Although species status needs to be confirmed, numerous isolates have been tested from central and western Canada using RFLPs. Thiessen (1987) evaluated 21 isolates of *Trichinella* using a DNA probe developed from *T. spiralis* (Klassen et al. 1986). Thiessen (1987) found the probe hybridized to 3 isolates from domestic pigs and 2 from black bears from the United States, but not to isolates from the 4 arctic foxes, 1 marten, and 1 wolverine collected from Canada; 1 gray fox from Pennsylvania; and *T. pseudospiralis*. In addition RFLPs of the 5 that hybridized are identical, suggesting these isolates are *T. spiralis*. Two of these isolates are identified as *T. spiralis* by allozymes and by the ITRC (La Rosa et al. 1992; Pozio et al. 1992b). Of 15 sylvatic isolates from wild animals digested with five endonucleases, 9 differed from each other with respect to their RFLPs. Of 4 arctic fox isolates, 2 showed identical RFLP patterns, and 2 showed similar patterns for most enzymes but differed when Cla 1 was used. Three marten isolates have similar RFLPs, while 1 from South Indian Lake in northern Manitoba (Canada) and 1 from southern Ontario showed a second pattern. Both fisher isolates from Canada have a unique RFLP pattern. The remaining isolates from wolverine and a polar bear (both from Canada) and from a gray fox and a black bear (both from Pennsylvania, United States) each had unique RFLPs. Subsequently, the gray fox and the black bear isolates were identified as *Trichinella* T6 and

TABLE 15.2—Hosts and country of origin for *Trichinella* species and genotypes[a]

Trichinella Species or Genotype/ Host	No. of Isolates	Country of Origin
T. spiralis		
Rattus norvegicus, Brown rat	3	Estonia, New Zealand, The Netherlands
Alopex lagopus, Blue fox (from a farm)	3	Estonia
Vulpes vulpes, Red fox	22	Bulgaria, Croatia, France, Germany, Italy, Poland, Russia, Spain
Canis lupus, Wolf	1	Spain
Canis familiaris, Domestic dog	3	China, Egypt, Spain
Felis concolor, Mountain lion	2	Argentina
Felis domestica, Domestic cat	3	France, Great Britain (old isolate), United States (Illinois)
Felis silvestris, Wild cat	1	Spain
Lynx rufus, Bobcat	1	United States (Montana)
Ursus americanus, Black bear	1	United States (Pennsylvania)
Ursus arctos, Brown bear	1	Alaska
Equus caballus, Horse	6	Canada, Mexico, Poland, Romania, Serbia
Sus scrofa, Domestic pig and wild boar	177	Argentina, Austria, Byelorussia, Bulgaria, Chile, China, Denmark (old isolate), Egypt, Finland, France, Germany, Hungary, Ireland (old isolate), Kazakhstan, Lithuania, Poland, Romania, Russia, Spain, Sweden, Thailand, United States (Indiana, Maryland, New Hampshire, Pennsylvania), Yugoslavia
Homo sapiens, Man	9	Canada, Italy, Lithuania, Poland, Thailand, United States
T. nativa		
Rattus norvegicus, Brown rat	1	Russia
Alopex lagopus, Blue fox	3	Canada, Estonia
Vulpes corsac, Corsac fox	1	Kazakhstan
Vulpes vulpes, Red fox	13	Canada, Estonia, Finland, Kazakhstan, Norway, Sweden
Felis euptilura, Far eastern forest cat	1	Russia
Felis domestica, Domestic cat	1	China
Martes americana, Marten	1	Alaska
Lynx lynx, Lynx	4	Estonia
Panthera tigris, Tiger	1	Russia
Canis aureus, Jackal	3	Kazakhstan
Canis lupus, Wolf	15	Canada, Estonia, Russia
Canis familiaris, Domestic dog	6	China, Greenland, Kazakhstan
Nyctereutes procyonoides, Raccoon dog	6	Estonia, Finland, Russia
Ursus arctos, Brown bear	2	Estonia
Ursus maritimus, Polar bear	12	Alaska, Canada, Greenland, Norway (Svalbard Islands)
Sus scrofa, Wild boar	2	Estonia
T. britovi		
Homo sapiens, Man	2	France, Italy
Felis silvestris, Wild cat	3	Italy, Kazakhstan
Felis domestica, Domestic cat	4	Italy
Lynx lynx, Lynx	5	Estonia, Switzerland
Martes foina, Beech marten	1	Italy
Meles meles, Badger	1	Italy
Vulpes vulpes, Red fox	104	Bulgaria, France, Germany, Italy, Kazakhstan, Norway, Poland, Slovak Republic, Spain, Sweden, Switzerland, The Netherlands
Nyctereutes procyonoides, Raccoon dog	8	Estonia, Japan
Rattus rattus, Black rat	1	Italy
Rattus norvegicus, Brown rat	5	Italy
Canis aureus, Jackal	4	Kazakhstan
Canis lupus, wolf	26	Estonia, Italy, Spain
Canis familiaris, Domestic dog	4	Italy
Ursus arctos, Brown bear	3	Italy, Slovakian Republic
Ursus thibetanus japonicus, Black bear	1	Japan
Sus scrofa, Wild boar and domestic pig	49	Byelorussia, Croatia, Estonia, Italy, Lithuania, Macedonia, Slovak Republic, Spain
Equus caballus, Horse	2	Former Yugoslavia
T. nelsoni		
Crocuta crocuta, Spotted hyena	4	Kenya, Tanzania
Phacochoerus aethiopicus, Wart hog	1	Tanzania
Panthera leo, Lion	4	South Africa, Tanzania
Panthera pardus, Leopard	1	Tanzania
Otocyon megalotis, Bat-eared fox	1	Tanzania
Acinonyx jubatus, Cheetah	1	Tanzania
Hyaena hyaena, Striped hyena	1	Tanzania

(continued)

TABLE 15.2 *(continued)*

Trichinella Species or Genotype/ Host	No. of Isolates	Country of Origin
T. pseudospiralis		
Homo sapiens, Man	1	Thailand
Nyctereutes procyonoides, Raccoon dog	1	Krasnodar
Sus scrofa, Wild boar	1	Papua New Guinea
Sus scrofa, Domestic pig	1	Russia (Kamchatka)
Aquila rapax, Eagle	1	Kazakhstan
Dasyurus maculatus, Spotted-tailed quolls	1	Tasmania
Strix aluco, Tawny owl	1	Italy
Athene noctua, Little owl	1	Italy
Coragypus atratus, Black vulture	1	United States (Alabama)
Trichinella T5		
Homo sapiens, Man	1	France[b]
Ursus americanus, Black bear	4	United States (Pennsylvania)
Procyon lotor, Racoon	5	United States (Illinois)
Vulpes vulpes, Red fox	3	United States (Illinois)
Felis rufus, Bobcat	1	United States (Georgia)
Canis latrans, Coyote	2	United States (Indiana)
Trichinella T6		
Ursus arctos, Grizzly bear	3	United States (Montana)
Gulo gulo, Wolverine	2	United States (Montana)
Felis concolor, Mountain lion	3	United States (Idaho, Montana)
Canis lupus, Gray wolf	1	United States (Montana)
Urocyon cinereoargenteus, Grey fox	1	United States (Pennsylvania)
Martes pennanti, Fisher	1	United States (Montana)
Ursus americanus, Black bear	2	United States (Montana)
Trichinella T8		
Crocuta crocuta, Spotted hyena	1	South Africa
Panthera leo, Lion	2	Namibia, South Africa

[a]From 1986 to 1998, 583 isolates collected worldwide were identified at the species or genotype level at the International *Trichinella* Reference Center, Italy (E. Pozio, unpublished).
[b]Horse meat imported from United States (Connecticut).

Trichinella T5 by La Rosa et al. (1992). From the formula $F = 2N_{xy}/N_x + N_y$ (Nei and Li 1979), the F values for *T. spiralis* (isolate from domestic pig), *T. nativa* (isolate from an arctic fox), and *T. pseudospiralis* (Garkavi's strain) are about 0.20, with a range of 0.14–0.27. Among the wild animal isolates, six groups representing 11 isolates had the greatest similarity to *T. nativa* (F values ranged from 0.95 to 0.99), while 4 isolates from arctic fox, gray fox, and black bear showed the greatest difference from *T. nativa*, with F values ranging from 0.56 to 0.89. Interestingly, arctic and gray fox isolate combinations were the highest (F = 0.89; F= 0.79; and AF3-PF, F= 0.79). Minchella et al. (1989), La Rosa et al. (1992), and Wu et al. (1999) also report biochemical and molecular variation of some isolates from wild animals in North America. Although more work needs to be done on *Trichinella* concerning species status and their distributions within North America, it appears that genotypic and phenotypic variations are high and that some of this variation may relate to host species and/or geographical origin (Thiessen 1987; Wu et al. l999).

The distribution of *Trichinella* in North America is interesting due to the largely intact boreal region and the extensive wild game populations in the Rocky Mountains. A number of multispecies surveys have been conducted since the last major review of *Trichinella* in North America. Smith and Snowdon

(1988) reported *Trichinella* in 41 of 1567 arctic foxes, 3 of 96 red foxes, 5 of 63 wolves, 1 of 211 coyotes, 1 of 119 raccoons, 1 of 31 lynx, 1 of 127 bobcats, and 3 of 10 dogs. Dies and Gunson (1984) reported *Trichinella* from 32 of 57 cougars and 1 of 35 grizzly bears in Alberta, Canada. Bourque (1985) examined 11 species for *Trichinella* in southwestern Quebec, Canada, and reported that only 2 of 29 red foxes and 1 of 56 marten were infected. Recently, human cases have been traced to eating cougar jerky (Dworkin et al. 1996). In western North America and the Rocky Mountain region, *Trichinella* spp. is reported from Alaskan polar bears (Weyermann et al. 1993), lynx with prevalences of 4%–59% and 0.27–2.35 larvae/g (Zarnke et al. 1995), black and grizzly bear with a prevalence of 15.6% and an average of 35.6 ± 69.1 larvae/g (Worley et al. 1991), and gray wolf (Worley et al. 1990). Large-scale serological screening of wildlife by Zarnke et al. (1997) determined exposure to *Trichinella* in 878 grizzly bears from 1973 to 1987. They concluded that differences in the number of positive sera by region (ranging from 5% to 83%) may relate to feeding patterns.

TEMPERATE NEARCTIC REGION/ *TRICHINELLA SPP.* In comparison with the Palearctic region, there are very few reports of trichinellosis in wildlife from

TABLE 15.3—Hosts infected with *Trichinella* larvae in regions in addition to those in Table 15.2[a]

Host	Country

Arctic and Subarctic Areas of Holarctic Region
(probably *T. nativa* or *Trichinella* T6 in areas of Southern Canada and Northern USA)[b]

Host	Country
Lesser shrew, *Sorex minutus*	Siberia
Common shrew, *Sorex minutus*	Siberia
Shrew, *Sorex minutus*	Canada
White-footed deer mouse, *Peromyscus maniculatus*	Canada
Striped field mouse, *Apodemus agrarius*	Siberia
Red squirrel, *Tamiasciurus hudsonicus*	Alaska, Canada
Squirrel, *Sciurus vulgaris*	Russia (Chukotskiy Peninsula)
Long-tailed susliks (scientific name unknown)	Russia (Uelen, Bering Strait)
Narrow-skulled susliks (scientific name unknown)	Russia (Uelen, Bering Strait)
Brown lemming, *Lemmus sibiricus*	Alaska
Ground squirrel, *Citellus undulatus*	Alaska, Canada
Red-backed vole, *Clethrionomys rutilus*	Alaska
Vole, *Microtus gregalis*	Alaska
Muskrat, *Ondata zibethica*	Alaska
Beaver, *Castor canadensis*	Alaska
Varying hare, *Lepus americanus*	Alaska
Wildcat, *Felis sylvestris*	Russia
Bobcat, *Lynx rufus*	Canada
Skunk, *Mephitis mephitis*	Canada
Weasel, *Mustela frenata*	Canada
Ermine, *Mustela erminia*	Alaska, Kamchatka, Siberia
Siberian ferret, *Mustela sibiricus*	Russia
Weasel, *Mustela nivalis*	Alaska
Marten, *Martens americana*	Canada
Sable, *Martes zibellina*	Kamchatka
Marten, *Martes martes*	Karelia
Coyote, *Canis latrans*	Canada
White whales, *Delphinapterus leucas*	Alaska, Greenland
Walrus, *Odobenus rosmarus*	Alaska, Canada, Norway, Greenland, Russia (Chukotskiy Peninsula)
Bearded seal, *Erignathus barbatus*	Alaska, Greenland
Ringed seal, *Phoca hispida*	Alaska, Greenland
Greenland seal, *Phoca groenlandica*	Russia
Fared seal, *Eumetopias jubatus*	Russia
Reindeer, *Rangifer tarandus*	Russia

Temperate Areas of the Nearctic Region
(probably *Trichinella* T5 or *Trichinella* T6)[b]

Host	Country
White-footed mouse, *Peromyscus leucopus*	United States (Illinois)
Beaver, *Castor canadensis*	United States (Iowa)
Fox squirrel, *Sciurus niger*	United States (Iowa)
Muskrat, *Ondatra zibethicus*	United States (Iowa, Ohio)
Opossum, *Didelphis marsupialis*	United States (Iowa, Virginia)
Striped skunk, *Mephitis mephitis*	United States (Idaho, Iowa, Louisiana, Maryland, Montana, North Dakota, Wyoming)
Mink, *Mustela vison*	United States (Iowa)
Weasel, *Mustela rixosa*	United States (Iowa)
Weasel, *Mustela frenata*	United States (Virginia)
Fisher, *Martes pennanti*	United States (Idaho, Montana, Wyoming)
Marten, *Martes americana*	United States (Idaho, Montana, Wyoming)
Spotted skunk, *Spilogale interrupta*	United States (Iowa, Virginia)
Badger, *Taxidae taxus*	United States (Iowa)
Wolverine, *Gulo gulo*	United States (Iowa)

Temperate Areas of the Palearctic Region
(probably *T. britovi*)[b]

Host	Country
Lesser shrew, *Sorex minutus*	Poland (Bialowieza Forest)
Common shrew, *Sorex araneus*	Poland (Bialowieza Forest)
Common shrew, *Sorex caecutiens*	Poland (Bialowieza Forest)
Water shrews, *Neomys fodiens*	Poland (Bialowieza Forest)
Common moles, *Talpa europea*	Poland (Bialowieza Forest)
Hedgehog, *Erinaceus europeus*	Ukraine
Afghan hedgehog, *Hemiechinus megalotis*	Afghanistan
Yellow-necked mouse, *Apodemus flavicollis*	Poland (Bialowieza Forest), Ukraine
Striped field mouse, *Apodemus agrarius*	Ukraine
Harvest mouse, *Micromys minutus*	Poland (Bialowieza Forest)
Muskrat, *Ondatra zibethicus*	Belgium
Polecat, *Mustela putorius*	Former Yugoslavia
Marten, *Martes martes*	Switzerland

(continued)

TABLE 15.3 *(continued)*

Host	Country
Mongoose, *Hepestes auropunctatus*	Afghanistan
Wild teddy cat, *Paradoxurus hermaphroditus*	India
Wild civet cat, *Viverricula indica*	India
Common genet, *Genetta genetta*	Spain
Hyena, *Hyaena hyaena*	Iran
Ethiopic Region **(probably *T. nelsoni*)**	
Soft-furred rat, *Praomys natalensis*	South Africa
Bush pig, *Potamochoerus porcus*	Ethiopia, Kenya, Senegal, Tanzania
Serval, *Felis serval*	Kenya
Wild dog, *Lycaon pictus*	Kenya
Stripped jackal, *Canis adustus*	Kenya, Senegal
Black-backed jackal, *Canis mesomelas*	Namibia, South Africa, Tanzania
Domestic dog, *Canis familiaris*	Kenya
Man, *Homo sapiens*	Ethiopia, Kenya, Senegal, Tanzania
Southeast Asia and Oceania **(probably *T. spiralis*)**	
Black rat, *Rattus rattus*	Hawaii
Little rat, *Rattus exulans*	Hawaii
Wild squirrel (the scientific name is unknown)	Thailand
Mongoose, *Herpestes javanicus*	Hawaii
Wild hog (the scientific name is unknown)	Hawaii
Domestic pig, *Sus scrofa*	Malaysia (Bali), New Zealand
Black bear, *Ursus thibetanus*	Thailand
Jackal, *Canis aureus*	Thailand
Neotropic Region **(probably *T. spiralis*)**	
Rodent, *Graomys griseoflavus*	Argentina
Armadillo, *Chaetophractus villosus*	Argentina
Fox, *Pseudolopex gracilis*	Argentina
Nonencapsulating *Trichichella*	
Pomarine jaeger, *Stercorarius pomarinus*	Alaska
Horn-owl, *Bubo virginianus*	United States (Iowa)
Buzzard, *Buteo buteo*	Spain
Cooper's hawk, *Accipiter cooperi*	United States (California)
Marsh harrier, *Circus aeruginous*	Tasmania
Masked owl, *Tyto novahollandiae*	Tasmania
Rook, *Corvus frigileus*	Kazakhstan
Indian mole rat, *Bandicota bengalensis*	India
Tasmanian devils, *Sarcophilus harrisii*	Tasmania
Eastern quolls, *Dasyurus viverrinus*	Tasmania
Brush-tailed possums, *Trichosurus vulpecula*	Tasmania
Corsac fox, *Vulpes corsac*	Kazakhstan

[a]Parasites are not identified to species or genotype.
[b]Some of these hosts could be also infected with *T. spiralis.*

temperate areas of the Nearctic region, and very few strains are identified to species or phenotype. The first infections were reported in three (6.6%) black bears from New York (King et al. 1960). Infected black bears were also discovered in Pennsylvania, Vermont, West Virginia, New England, and Minnesota (Zimmermann 1970; Schultz 1970; Schad et al. 1986; Stromberg and Prouty 1987). In Iowa, Zimmermann et al. (1962) and Zimmermann and Hubbard (1969) found *Trichinella* larvae in mink, red fox, gray fox, opossum (*Didelphis marsupialis*), raccoon (*Procyon lotor*), striped skunk (*Mephitis mephitis*), spotted skunk (*Spilogale interrupt*), coyote (*Canis latrans*), badger (*Taxidae taxus*), beaver, weasel (*Mustela rixosa*), wolverine, fox squirrel (*Sciurus niger*), and muskrat. Thirteen percent of

raccoons from Kentucky were infected (Cole and Shoop 1987). Mountains lions, with 0.2–115.4 larvae/g, and infected bobcats are reported from Arizona and South Dakota (Schitoskey and Linder 1981; LeCount and Zimmermann 1986). *Trichinella* parasites were also reported in wildlife from Colorado, Maryland, North Dakota, Ohio, and Illinois. In this last state, Martin et al. (1968) found *Trichinella* larvae in the white-footed mouse (*Peromyscus leucopus*). Synder (1987) reported prevalences of 1.3% from 380 raccoons, 10% of 20 coyotes, and 5% of 20 foxes. All these reports are concerned with the presence of larvae in muscle samples, but no information is available on their species or phenotype. We can speculate that parasites observed in the above reported hosts could belong to *T. spiralis.*

However, in the northern states (Vermont, New England, North Dakota, Minnesota) as well as in Colorado, which is located in the Rocky Mountains, the sylvatic phenotype could be *Trichinella* T6. About 32 isolates from the United States have been identified as *Trichinella* T5, from black bears from Pennsylvania; raccoons, coyotes, and red foxes from Illinois; a mink, red foxes, coyotes and raccoons from Indiana; a bobcat (*Felis rufus*) from Georgia; and a domestic horse from Connecticut (Minchella et al. 1989; Pozio et al. 1992b; Snyder et al. 1993; Yao et al. 1997; E. Pozio, unpublished).

A summary of transmission of *Trichinella* spp. from Arctic and temperate regions of North America reveals some differences. Primary hosts appear to differ among geographical regions. Bears are important in parts of eastern United States and New Brunswick as well as throughout the Rocky Mountains, Arctic regions of Canada, and Alaska. Interestingly, few infected black bear have been found in Newfoundland and Labrador (Butler and Khan 1992), Ontario (Dick et al. 1986), or the prairie region of Canada (T.A. Dick, unpublished). However, it should be noted that Addison et al.(1979) found 1.7% of 59 black bears infected in Ontario, including those frequenting garbage dumps, and Duffy et al. (1994) reported *Trichinella* in 0.4% of black bear from New Brunswick. Raccoons appear unimportant hosts in central and western Canada (Dick 1983c; Dick et al. 1986; T.A. Dick, unpublished) but are important in parts of the United States. Foxes are an important host in temperate regions with large urban communities and large tracts of agricultural lands as well as in the Arctic. By contrast, small furbearers such as marten, and perhaps fisher, appear important in transmission in areas with large tracts of relatively intact forest lands (especially the boreal region). In the Rocky Mountains cougar, bear, and perhaps marten are important hosts.

TEMPERATE PALEARCTIC REGION/*T. BRITOVI*.
Trichinellosis was reported from red foxes in Germany in 1919 (Lehmensick 1970); today it is known from 23 mammalian hosts (Table 15.3). Initially the parasite was identified as *T. nelsoni* (Britov and Boev 1972) but was renamed *T. britovi* by Pozio et al. (1992a). Epidemiological studies indicate its northern limit is isotherm -6° C (Shaikenov and Boev 1983; Shaikenov 1992; Pozio et al. 1996a, Pozio 1998). *Trichinella nativa* and *T. britovi* are sympatric in sylvatic animals between isotherm -6° C and -5° C in January (Pozio et al. 1995, 1998) (Fig. 15.2). *Trichinella britovi* also is widespread in wildlife from Asiatic countries (Armenia, Azerbaijan, Georgia, Iran, Kazakhstan, Kyrgyzstan, Tadzhikistan, Turkmenistan, and Uzbekistan). Unidentified *Trichinella* larvae occur in wildlife from Afghanistan, India, Israel, and Turkey. The southern limits are unknown, but are thought to be north of the Sahara in Africa and the Arabian peninsula. Western and eastern limits are the Iberian Peninsula and Japan

(Pozio et al. 1996a). Distribution is unknown for India and southeastern Asia, including the temperate regions of China.

Distribution of *T. britovi* in western Europe is influenced by humans, fragmented ecosystems, and concentration of carnivores in remote wilderness areas, national parks, and mountain regions (Pozio et al. 1996a). Red fox living at 400–500 m above sea level are the most common host of *T. britovi* in central and southern Europe, but it is also reported from fox in the Netherlands (van der Giessen et al. 1998). High moisture and low temperatures in the mountains, plus an ability to survive freezing, enhance its survival in carrion (Pozio et al. 1996b; E. Pozio, unpublished). *Trichinella britovi* is found in raccoon dogs in Finland, the Baltic republics, and Russia and at low levels in wild boar (Pozio et al. 1992a). Pozio et al. (1996a) report it from Japan in Japanese black bear (*Ursus thibetanus japonicus*) and raccoon dogs.

Prevalence of *T. britovi* is low in sylvatic and domestic swine (Kapel et al. 1998) and in synanthropic rats (Pozio et al. 1992a). Prevalences in wild boar range from 0.0002%–0.003% in France, to 0%–0.006% in Italy, to 0.08%–0.48% in the Extremadura region of Spain, with the highest prevalences occurring above 500 m elevation. Although there are few reports of *T. britovi* in domestic animals, it can infect domestics and humans when (1) domestic animals are pastured in remote wild areas, (2) domestic animals are fed the remains of sylvatic animals, and (3) humans consume raw game. Domestic animals are a "dead end" for the sylvatic cycle of *T. britovi,* but human infections are reported from Spain, France, and Italy following consumption of wild boar, domestic pig, fox, and horse meat.

ETHIOPIC REGION/*T. NELSONI?* *Trichinella* spp. was first discovered in Africa south of the Sahara in 1959, in humans from Kenya who had eaten bushpig (*Potamochoerus porcus*) (Nelson 1970). Nelson and coworkers conducted numerous epidemiological studies on wildlife of Kenya. Further outbreaks in humans occurred in Kenya, Tanzania, Senegal, and Ethiopia. In each case the source of infection was bushpig or warthog (*Phacochoerus aethiopicus*). Spotted hyena (*Crocuta crocuta*) is the main reservoir (43.5%) (0.5–31 larvae/g in the diaphragm), but larvae were also found in five other species of carnivores (Table 15.3). Of several thousand rodents examined from Kruger National Park, South Arica, 1 *Praomys natalenisis* (as well as 2 dogs) was infected (Young and Kruger 1967). Warthogs and 4 large carnivore species from Namibia, Senegal, South Africa, Tanzania, and Zaire were infected (Pozio et al. 1994b). *Trichinella nelsoni* was identified in 1 of 6 bat-eared foxes (*Otocyon megalotis*), 1 of 5 cheetahs (*Acinonyx jubatus*), 1 of 3 leopards, 3 of 24 lions, and 3 of 13 spotted hyenas from the Serengeti National Park (Tanzania) (Pozio et al. 1997a). Six larvae/g of masseter were found in the spotted hyena, 0.5 larvae/g in the cheetah, and 2 larvae/g in the lion.

Trichinella from wildlife in Kenya have low infectivity to pigs and laboratory rats (Nelson 1970). It also seems to have low pathogenicity. In a human outbreak in Kenya, abdominal disorders and diarrhea were found in patients with > 3000 larvae/g and only patients with > 4000 larvae/g died (Nelson 1970). Patients from Tanzania with 5560–6530 larvae/g (the highest ever recorded from humans) survived the infection.

The taxonomy and biology of *T. nelsoni* is complex, as polymorphisms of three isolates are correlated with geographical origin (La Rosa et al. 1994). *Trichinella nelsoni sensu stricto* was described, and a new isolate from a spotted hyena of South Africa was identified as *Trichinella* T8 (Pozio et al. 1992a), but T8 is similar to *T. britovi* from Europe. *Trichinella* T8's presence in South Africa is an enigma, but perhaps it was introduced with domestic animals. Low levels of *T. nelsoni* in sylvatic suidae are also enigmatic, but may relate to religious and cultural practices in Africa south of the Sahara.

SOUTHEAST ASIA AND OCEANIA/*T.SPIRALIS?*
There are very few reports of encapsulated *Trichinella* larvae in wildlife from these geographical areas. In Thailand, larvae from wild boars, black bears (*Ursus thibetanus*), a jackal (*C. aureus*), and a wild squirrel (scientific name unknown), as well as from several domestic pigs, were sources of infection for humans (Khamboonruang 1991). Three human isolates and one pig isolate from Thailand were identified as *T. spiralis*. In New Zealand, synanthropic brown rats and domestic cats harbored *T. spiralis*. There were no infections reported in New Zealand wildlife, domestic animals, or humans as of 1997 (Fairley 1996; J.R.H. Andrews, personal communication), but Buncic (1997) reported *Trichinella* from the domestic pig. In the Hawaiian Islands, larvae, probably *T. spiralis,* were found in brown rat, black rat, little rat (*Rattus exulans*), mongoose (*Herpestes javanicus*), and wild hog (Alicata 1970). A wild pig was the source of infection for humans (Barrett-Conner et al. 1976).

CENTRAL AND SOUTH AMERICA/*T. SPIRALIS.*
Sylvatic trichinellosis in wildlife from the region is very rare, and *T. spiralis* appears to be the only species present. We can speculate that it was introduced by synanthropic rodents and domestic animals during the colonization from Europe. In Argentina and Chile, where domestic trichinellosis is widespread in synanthropic rodents, domestic pigs, domestic dogs, and cats, infection has been detected only in a fox (*Pseudolopex gracilis*), armadillo (*Chaetophractus villosus*), and a sylvatic rodent (*Graomys griseoflavus*), even though thousands of wild animals have been examined (Minoprio et al. 1967). All three infected animals were from Argentina. Isolates of *Trichinella* from two mountain lions and a fox (unknown species) from Argentina were identified as *T. spiralis* (E. Pozio, unpublished).

WORLDWIDE/*T.PSEUDOSPIRALIS.*
The wide host range (birds, marsupialia, rodentia, carnivora, artiodactyla, and primates), biochemical and molecular characteristics, and lack of the nurse cell suggest that *T. pseudospiralis* is ancestral in the genus. This nonencapsulating species was described in a raccoon dog from the Krasnodar region of Caucasus (Garkavi 1972). For several years, the original host species was confused with the raccoon, a North American mammal not present in the Caucasus (Capo and Despommier 1996). Wheeldon et al. (1983) reported *T. pseudospiralis* from a young male Cooper's hawk (*Accipiter cooperi*) in northern California, based on histological evidence. This parasite was also identified in a rook (*Corvus frugilegus*), eagle (*Aquila rapax*), and corsac fox (*Vulpes corsacae*) from Kazakhstan; an Indian mole rat (*Bandicota bengalensis*) from India (Shaikenov and Boev 1983); Tasmanian devils (*Sarcophilus harrisii*), spotted-tailed quolls (*Dasyurus maculatus*), eastern quolls (*D. viverrinus*), brush-tailed possums (*Trichosurus vulpecula*), a marsh harrier (*Circus aeruginous*), and a masked owl (*Tyto novahollandiae*) from Tasmania (Obendorf et al. 1990; Obendorf and Clarke 1992); a black vulture (*Coragypus atratus*) from Alabama (Lindsay et al. 1995); a human from Tasmania (Andrews et al. 1995); wild pig and humans from Thailand (Jongwutiwes et al. 1998); two nocturnal birds of prey from central Italy and wild pig from Papua New Guinea (Pozio et al. 1999); and a wild boar and humans from France (E. Pozio, unpublished). *Trichinella pseudospiralis* also was found in domestic pigs raised in open pasture from the Caucasus, Tula, and Kamchatka regions of Russia (Pozio et al. 1997b) and in humans in Kamchatka (Britov 1997).

Currently only a single species of this parasite is recognized, but intraspecific genetic variability related to geographical origin is reported (Zarlenga et al. 1996). Detection by trichinoscope is difficult due to the small size of larvae and lack of a cyst; thus, it may be missed in routine epidemiological surveys of wildlife. Given the protected status of many species of birds, it is unlikely that the extent of the range of hosts will ever be known.

Recently, larvae of a nonencapsulated *Trichinella* have been detected in a wild pig from Papua New Guinea. Preliminary molecular, morphological, and biological studies suggest that these larvae belong to a new genotype (E. Pozio, unpublished).

DOMESTIC TRICHINELLOSIS/*T.SPIRALIS.*
Trichinellosis in domestic pigs, dogs, cats, horses, and synanthropic rats occurs in several countries in the world (Fig. 15.4). The etiological agent is *T. spiralis.* Endemic areas are present in Europe (Bulgaria,

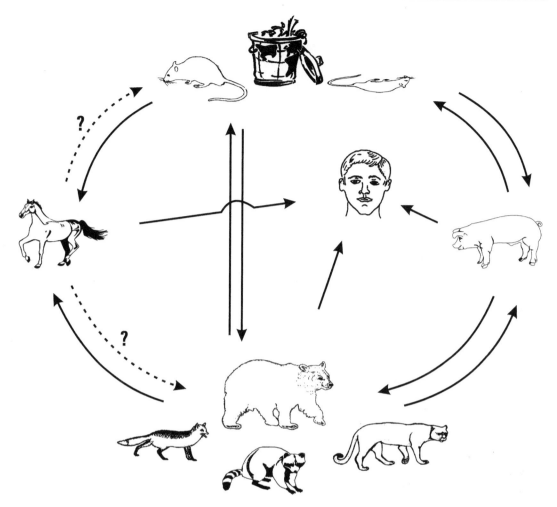

FIG. 15.4—Transmission cycle of sylvatic and domestic animals in temperate regions. Carrion plays a key role, with evidence that domestic animals can be infected with sylvatic forms, such as *T. britovi,* and wildlife can be infected with *T. spiralis* from domestic animals and/or rats.

Byelorussia, Finland, the former Yugoslavia, Lithuania, Poland, Romania, Russia, Spain, Ukraine), Africa (Egypt), Asia (Cambodia, China, Thailand, Vietnam, Laos), North America (Mexico), and South America (Argentina, Chile). However, this is only the tip of the iceberg, as it is probably more widespread with a low prevalence in several other countries. The relationship between sylvatic and domestic life cycles has been clearly shown in Pennsylvania (Schad et al. 1987) and New Jersey (Dame et al. 1987; Murrell et al. 1987) and is evidenced by *T. spiralis* in black bears in Pennsylvania, a coyote in Indiana, wild boars in New Hampshire (Worley et al. 1994), and a raccoon, opossum, and skunk in New Jersy. A similar epidemiological picture occurs in temperate areas of Europe and Asia where *T. spiralis* can be now considered a common parasite in wildlife. In the sylvatic ecosystem where both *T. spi-*

ralis and *T. britovi* cycles exist, wild boars were infected with both species (Pozio et al. 1997c). In frigid zones of the Holarctic region, *T. spiralis* has been detected only in domestic pigs, synanthropic rats, and sylvatic animals living near human settlements. This suggests that *T. spiralis* cannot be transmitted among wildlife living in frigid zones, because muscle larvae do not survive freezing. Recent social changes and wars in eastern Europe and Asia have seen trichinellosis increase as large farming units are replaced by small farms, contacts between sylvatic and domestic cycles increase, and meat inspection declines (Pozio et al. 1998).

PATHOLOGY. There are very few observations on the pathological role of *Trichinella* parasites in wildlife. However, there is good experimental data suggesting that hosts are affected, even at low infection levels (Minchella et al. 1994). The intensity in wildlife is generally very low (range 0.1–10 larvae/g in preferential muscles); > 50–100 larvae/g is exceptional. In fox populations in Italy the average intensity was 0.1 to 25 larvae/g; however, a young fox infected with both *T. britovi* and scabies harbored 1215 larvae/g in the masseter. *Trichinella britovi* infection in wild boar is very rare and occurs at 0.2–16 larvae/g; however, a boar with an old gunshot wound harbored 120 larvae/g in the diaphragm (E. Pozio, unpublished). These two examples suggest that immune status of the host plays an important role in controlling the level of infection. According to Nelson (1970), an old lion with a heavy *Trichinella* infection showed signs of chronic disease; however, the relationship was circumstantial.

Diarrhea, sloughing of gut epithelium, and local hemorrhaging occur in the intestines of experimentally infected domestic and laboratory animals. The median lethal dose (LD50) in mice with different isolates indicates different levels of virulence correlated with infective dose and time to complete calcification of the cysts (T.A. Dick, unpublished). The effects of *Trichinella* on the behavior of laboratory animals and birds are well documented (Minchella et al. 1994). Two sylvatic isolates of *Trichinella* (T5 genotype) and *T. spiralis* modified mouse behavior by influencing exploratory activity (time to emerge from cage, time spent inside cage, and number of rears), and the effects were dose dependent (200 larvae/host showed no difference in behavior, while 500 larvae/host did). Similarly, complete cessation of activity, as measured by number of revolutions on an activity wheel, is directly correlated with infection dose, peak intestinal pathology, and invasive stage into striated muscle (T.A. Dick, unpublished). Uninfected male CFLP mice are less likely to mount and copulate with infected females of the same strain (Edwards and Barnard 1987). Furthermore, infected females are more likely to avoid or respond aggressively to attempts to mount by males. Porier et al. (1995) found that *T. nativa* had a much greater effect on mouse behavior than did *T. pseudospiralis*. They attributed this to the ability of *T. pseudospiralis* to modulate the immune response and suggested that the variation noted in diel behavior may affect transmission to a certain type of host. A captive American kestrel (*Falco sparverius*) experimentally infected with *T. pseudospiralis* had reduced reproductive success (delayed onset of egg laying, lower laying success, fewer eggs, greater egg breakage and embryo mortality) (Saumier et al. 1986, 1988). Mild behavioral changes occurred in the first 5 days postinfection, corresponding with the intestinal phase, but the most severe effects were noted during the muscle phase, persisting 5 weeks. Clinical signs included reduced exercising and flying, elevated perching and preening, and more time spent walking and floor perching.

Although most of the reports of the effects of trichinellosis are from laboratory animal studies or ani-

mals held under controlled conditions, there is good evidence that *Trichinella* infections, even at relatively low infection doses (50–100 larvae/host), induce sufficient pathophysiology to cause behavioral changes that could enhance predation and alter reproductive success. The lowered locomotor activity during the intestinal phase has little effect on transmission because infective larvae are not yet present. However, during the muscle invasive phase, it likely enhances transmission of the parasite as some of the earliest larvae are infective by the end of this phase.

Domestic animals tolerate high levels of infection and show very few clinical signs (fever, loss of appetite, arrest of growth in young animals). No pathology is reported from infected cow, ram, or reindeer. Only doses in the range of 100,000 larvae induce severe pathological change and death in swine. Young animals appear to be less tolerant to the infection than adults. Females of sylvatic isolates produce fewer larvae and are less pathogenic than *T. spiralis* (Pozio et al. 1992a). Swine and rats are naturally resistant to sylvatic species (except *T. pseudospiralis*), and few adults develop in the gut and few newborn larvae establish in muscles (Pozio et al. 1992b). In addition, muscle larvae that establish are rapidly destroyed. In contrast, larvae of sylvatic species can survive in muscles of carnivores for a long period of time. Infecting larvae of *T. nativa* were collected from muscles of a polar bear caught in nature in the Svalbard islands (Norway) and held in captivity more than 20 years (Kumar et al. 1990).

Since horses (wild and domestic) are occasionally a source of human infection, experimental infections in horses are reported. Infection of 5000–50,000 *T. spiralis* larvae produced no major clinical signs, but one horse had raised rectal temperature, and two horses infected with 50,000 larvae had stiff hindlegs (Soule et al. 1989). Naturally infected horses with 600 larvae/g in the tongue also showed no clinical signs (E. Pozio, unpublished). Worm numbers decline rapidly after infection, and horses are *Trichinella*-free in several months (Soule et al. 1989).

CONCLUSIONS. While the knowledge of *Trichinella* species complexes and epizootiology of trichinellosis has advanced significantly in recent years, there are several questions that need to be addressed. Specific primers for the development of a sensitive polymerase chain reaction (PCR) that allows identification of single larvae of *Trichinella* at the species and genotype level are needed. Much is known about host primary and secondary responses to *T. spiralis* in laboratory animals, but less is known about the response in genetically undefined wild animals. More experimental infections are needed in natural hosts to clearly understand the biological variation and its significance in transmission. Antigenic properties of various species and isolates as well as effects on mucosal and systemic immunity need further study. Perhaps this will help us understand if the host immune system has a major role in selection, hence speciation, and how this may relate to transmission of *Trichinella* spp. Furthermore, as the specificity of serological methods improve, screening of large natural populations of animals and birds may be possible.

Other potential ecological isolating mechanisms need further study (e.g., the importance of fragmented ecosystems on genotypic variation). The importance of local host foci and small isolated populations of a species in a fragmented ecosystem on parasite phenotypic/genotypic variation needs further investigation. This has significance for local adaptations to a specific host and/or homogenization of the gene pool and may begin to explain genetic and biological variation among isolates and species.

Better methods to investigate gene flow among genotypes are necessary to establish if gene flow is restricted. These markers must be species, population, and individual specific. Molecular methods may also allow correlations among various quantitative biological traits and molecular markers. The distribution of different genotypes, particularly those in Africa, Central and South America, Canada, the United States, Southeast Asia, and India, need to be mapped. This will help sort out sylvatic and domestic transmission patterns.

As ecosytems become more fragmented and human-wildlife interactions intensify, a clear understanding of what constitutes a truly natural distribution of *Trichinella* genotypes and species is needed. For example, foxes frequently are reported as harboring *Trichinella,* but they are one of few predators that adapt well to human habitation and are still numerous in many parts of the world. This may reflect the new reality of urban *Trichinella* transmission, but may not be the basis of its historical ecology. Furthermore, in some parts of the world we see intense interaction between land users (farming and recreation) and wildlands; while in others we see rejuvenation of wildlands, increasing small carnivorous mammal populations, and increased interactions of these populations with humans and their domestic animals. When social unrest and change is added to this ecological "brew," trichinellosis from wildlife sources will appear sporadically in human populations.

Regardless of the number of species that are eventually described and the new transmission patterns that will undoubtedly develop, Campbell (1983b) quite aptly places *Trichinella* in a worldwide context as follows: given the impressive list of host species infected ". . . it would be rash to allege that any mammalian species is fully refractory to the infection." We would extend that statement to include birds. It is quite apparent from the perspective of wildlife biology and public health that *Trichinella* will be around for a long time and that the knowledge of its transmission dynamics will continue to evolve.

LITERATURE CITED

Addison, E.M., M.J. Pybus, and H.J. Reitveld. 1979. Helminth and arthropod parasites of black bear, *Ursus americanus,* in central Ontario. *Canadian Journal of Zoology* 56:2122–2126.

Alicata, J. 1970. Trichinosis in the Pacific Islands and adjacent areas. In *Trichinosis in man and animals.* Ed. S.E. Gould. Springfield, IL: C.C. Thomas Publisher, pp. 465–472.

Andrews, J.R.H., C. Bandi, E. Pozio, M.G. Gomez Morales, R. Ainsworth, and D. Abernethy. 1995. Identification of *Trichinella* from a human case using amplified polymorphic DNA. *American Journal of Tropical Medicine and Hygiene* 53:185–188.

Bandi, C, G. La Rosa, M.G. Bardin, G. Damiani, S. Comincini, L. Tasciotti, and E. Pozio. 1995. Random amplified polymorphic DNA fingerprints of the eight taxa of *Trichinella* and their comparison with allozyme analysis. *Parasitology* 110:401–407.

Barrett-Conner, E., C.F. Davis, R.N. Hamburger, and I. Kagan. 1976. An epidemic of trichinosis after ingestion of wild pig in Hawaii. *Journal of Infectious Diseases* 133:473–477.

Belosevic, M., and T.A. Dick. 1979. *Trichinella spiralis:* Comparison of stages in host immune intestine with those of an arctic *Trichinella* sp. *Experimental Parasitology* 48:432–446.

———. 1980. *Trichinella spiralis:* Comparison with an Arctic isolate. *Experimental Parasitology* 49:266–276.

Bober, C.M., and T.A. Dick. 1983. A comparison of the biological characteristics of *Trichinella* var. *pseudospiralis* between mice and bird hosts. *Canadian Journal of Zoology* 61:2110–2119.

Born, E.W., and S.A. Henriksen. 1990. Prevalence of *Trichinella* sp. in polar bears (*Ursus maritimus*) from northeastern Greenland. *Polar Research* 8:313–316.

Bourque, M. 1985. A survey of *Trichinella spiralis* in wild carnivores in southwestern Quebec. *Canadian Veterinary Journal* 26:203–204.

Britov, V.A. 1995. Trichinellosis problem in the Primorsk region [In Russian]. Vladivostok: Veterinary Scientific Research Institute of the Far East, Primorsk Branch, 51 pp.

———. 1997. Trichinellosis in Kamchatka. *Wiadomosci Parazytologiczne* 43:287–288.

Britov, V.A., and S.N. Boev. 1972. Taxonomic rank of various strains of *Trichinella* and their circulation in nature [In Russian]. *Vestnik Akademii Nauk KSSR* 28:27–32.

Buncic, S. 1997. A case of a pig infested with *Trichinella spiralis. Surveillance* 24:8.

Butler, C.E. and R.A. Khan. 1992. Prevalence of *Trichinella spiralis* in black bears (*Ursus americanus*) from Newfoundland and Labrador, Canada. *Journal of Wildlife Diseases* 28:474–475.

Campbell, W.C. 1983a. Epidemiology I: Modes of transmission. In *Trichinella and trichinosis.* Ed. W.C. Campbell. New York: Plenum Press, pp. 425–444.

———. 1983b. Historical introduction. In *Trichinella and trichinosis.* Ed. W.C. Campbell. New York: Plenum Press, pp. 1–30.

Capo, V., and D.D. Despommier. 1996. Clinical aspects of infection with *Trichinella* spp. *Clinical Microbiology Reviews* 9:47–54.

Chadee, K.C., and T.A. Dick. 1982. Biological characteristics and host influence on a geographical isolate of *Trichinella* (Wolverine: 55 00 N, 100 00 W, 1979). *The Journal of Parasitology* 68:451–456.

Cole, R.A. and W. Shoop. 1987. Helminths of the raccoon (*Procyon lotor*) in western Kentucky. *The Journal of Parasitology* 73:762–768.

Cuperlovic, K. 1996. Trichinellosis. The state of the art. *Mikrobiologia (Zemun)* 33:139–152.

Curran, J., D. L.Baillei, and J.M. Webster. 1985. Use of genomic DNA restriction fragment length differences to identify nematode species. *Parasitology* 90:137–144.

Dame, J.B., K.D. Murrell, D.E. Worley, and G.A. Schad. 1987. *Trichinella spiralis:* Genetic evidence for synanthropic subspecies in sylvatic hosts. *Experimental Parasitology* 64:195–203.

Dick, T.A. 1983a. Species and intraspecific variation. In *Trichinella and trichinosis.* Ed. W.C.Campbell. New York: Plenum Press, pp. 31–73.

———. 1983b. The species problem in *Trichinella.* In *Concepts in nematode systematics.* Ed. A.R Stone, H.M. Platt, and L.F. Khalil. New York: Academic Press, pp. 351–360.

———. 1983c. Infectivity of isolates of *Trichinella* and the ability of an arctic isolate to survive freezing temperatures in the raccoon, *Procyon lotor,* under experimental conditions. *Journal of Wildlife Diseases* 19:333–336.

Dick, T.A., and M. Belosevic. 1978. Observations on a *Trichinella spiralis* isolate from a polar bear. *The Journal of Parasitology* 64:1143–1145.

Dick, T.A., and R.D. Leonard. 1979. Helminth parasites of fisher *Martes pennanti* (Erxleben) from Manitoba, Canada. *Journal of Wildlife Diseases* 15:409–412.

Dick, T.A., B. Kingscote, M.A. Strickland, and C.E. Douglas. 1986. Sylvatic trichinosis in Ontario, Canada. *Journal of Wildlife Diseases* 22:42–47.

Dick, T.A., M. Lu, T. deVos, and K. Ma. 1992. The use of the polymerase chain reaction to identify procine isolates of *Trichinella. The Journal of Parasitology* 78:145–148.

Dies, K.H and J.R. Gunson. 1984. Prevalence and distribution of larvae of *Trichinella* spp. in cougars, *Felis concolor* L., and grizzly bears, *Ursus arctos* L., in Alberta. *Journal of Wildlife Diseases* 20:242–244.

Duffy, M.S., T.A. Greaves, and M.D.B. Burt. 1994. Helminths of black bear, *Ursus americanus,* in New Brunswick. *The Journal of Parasitology* 80:478–480.

Dworkin, M.S., H.R. Gamble, D.S. Zarlenga, and P.O. Tennican. 1996. Outbreak of trichinellosis associated with eating cougar jerky. *Journal of Infectious Diseases* 174:663–666.

Edwards, J.C., and C.J. Barnard. 1987. The effects of *Trichinella* infection on intersexual interactions between mice. *Animal Behaviour* 37:533–540.

Fairley, R. 1996. Infectious agents and parasites of New Zealand pigs transmissible to humans. *Surveillance* 23:17–18.

Flockhart, H.A., S.E. Harrison, and A.R. Dobinson. 1982. Enzyme polymorphism in *Trichinella. Transactions of the Royal Society of Tropical Medicine and Hygiene* 76:541–545.

Garkavi, B.L. 1972. Species of *Trichinella* isolates from wild animals [In Russian]. *Veterinariya* 10:90–91.

Henriksen, S.A., E.W. Born, and L. Eiersted. 1994. Infections with *Trichinella* in polar bears (*Ursus maritimus*) in Greenland: Prevalence according to age and sex. In *Trichinellosis.* Proceedings of the 8th International Conference on Trichinellosis. Ed. C.W. Campbell, E. Pozio, F. Bruschi. Rome: Instituto Superiore di Sanita Press, pp. 565–568.

Jongwutiwes, S., N. Chantachum, P. Kraivichian, P. Siriyasatien, C. Putaporntip, A. Tamburrini, G. La Rosa, C. Sreesunpasirikul, P. Yingyourd, and E. Pozio. 1998. First outbreak of human trichinellosis caused by *Trichinella pseudospiralis. Clinical Infectious Diseases* 26:111–115.

Kapel, C.M.O., S.A. Henriksen, T.B. Berg, and P. Nansen. 1996. Epidemiologic and zoogeographic studies on *Trichinella nativa* in arctic fox, *Alopex lagopus,* in Greenland. *Journal of Helmithological Society of Washington* 63:226–232.

Kapel, C.M.O., E. Pozio, L. Sacchi, and P. Prestrud. 1999. Freeze tolerance, morphology, +RAPD-PCR identification of *Trichinella nativa*–infected arctic foxes. *The Journal of Parasitology.* 85:144–147.

Kapel, C.M.O., P. Webster, P. Lind, E. Pozio, S.A. Henriksen, K.D. Murrell, and P. Nansen. 1998. *Trichinella spiralis, Trichinella britovi,* and *Trichinella nativa:* Infectivity, muscle larvae distribution and antibody response after experimental infection of pigs. *Parasitology Research* 84:264–271.

Khamboonruang, C. 1991. The present status of trichinellosis in Thailand. *The Southeast Asian Journal of Tropical Medicine and Public Health* 22:312–315.

King, J.J., H.C. Black, and O.H. Hewitt. 1960. Pathology, parasitology and hematology of the black bear in New York. *New York Fish Game Journal* 7:99–111.

Klassen, G.R., J.P. Thiessen, and T.A. Dick. 1986. Strain specific 1.7 kilobase repetitive deoxyribonuclease acid sequence family in *Trichinella spiralis. Molecular and Biochemical Parasitology* 21:227–233.

Kumar, V., E. Pozio, J. De Borchgrave, J. Mortelmans, and W. De Meurichy. 1990. Characterization of a *Trichinella* isolate from polar bear. *Annales de la Societe Belge de Medicine Tropicale* 70:131–135.

La Rosa, G., L. Tasciotti, and E. Pozio. 1994. DNA repetitive probes for the characterization and identification of *Trichinella* parasites. In *Trichinellosis.* Proceedings of the 8th International Conference on Trichinellosis. Ed. C.W. Campbell, E. Pozio, F. Bruschi. Rome: Instituto Superiore di Sanita Press, pp. 89–94.

La Rosa, G., E. Pozio, P. Rossi, and K.D. Murrell. 1992. Allozyme analysis of *Trichinella* isolates from various host species and geographic regions. *The Journal of Parasitology* 78:641–646.

LeCount, A.L. and W.J. Zimmermann. 1986. Trichinosis in mountain lions in Arizona. *Journal of Wildlife Diseases* 22:432–434.

Lehmensick, R. 1970. Inspection of pork and control of trichinosis in Germany. In *Trichinosis in man and animals.* Ed. S.E. Gould. Springfield, IL: C.C. Thomas Publisher, pp. 437–448.

Lindsay, D.S., D.S. Zarlenga, H.R. Gamble, F. Al-Yaman, P.C. Smith, and B.L. Blagburn. 1995. Isolation and characterization of *Trichinella pseudospiralis* Garkavi, 1972 from a black vulture (*Coragyps atratus*). *The Journal of Parasitology* 81:920–923.

MacLean, J.D., L. Poirier, T.W. Gyorkos, J.F. Proulx, J. Bourgeault, A. Corriveau, S. Illisituk, and M. Staudt. 1992. Epidemiologic and serologic definition of primary and secondary trichinosis in the Arctic. *Journal of Infectious Diseases* 165:908–912.

Madsen, H. 1974. The principles of the epidemiology of trichinelliasis with a new view on the life cycle. In *Trichinellosis.* Ed. C.W. Kim. New York: Intext, pp. 615–638.

Martin, R.J., P.R. Schnurrenberger, F.L. Anderson, and C.K. Hsu. 1968. Prevalence of *Trichinella spiralis* in wild animals on two Illinois swine farms. *The Journal of Parasitology* 54:108–111.

Minchella, D.J., B.A. Branstetter, and K.R. Kazacos. 1989. Molecular characterization of sylvatic isolates of *Trichinella spiralis. The Journal of Parasitology* 75:388–392.

Minchella, D., A.R. Eddings and S.T. Neel. 1994. Genetic, phenotypic and behavioural variation in North American sylvatic isolates of *Trichinella. The Journal of Parasitology* 80:696–704.

Minoprio, J.L., H. Naves, and D. Abdon. 1967. Factores ecologicos que determina la trichiniasis silvestre en el Oeste de San Luis y Este de Mendoza. *Anales de Sociedad Cientifica Argentina* 183:19–30.

Murrell, K.D., F. Stringfellow, J.B. Dame, D.A. Leiby, C. Duffy, and G.A. Schad. 1987. *Trichinella spiralis* in an agricultural ecosystem. II. Evidence for natural transmission of *Trichinella spiralis* from domestic swine to wildlife. *The Journal of Parasitology* 73:103–109.

Mydynski, L.J., and T.A. Dick. 1985. The use of enzyme polymorphisms to identify genetic differences in the genus *Trichinella. The Journal of Parasitology* 71:671–677.

Nei, M., and W.-H. Li. 1979. Mathematical model for studying genetic variation in terms of restriction endonucleases. *Proceedings of National Academy of Sciences, USA* 76:5269–5273.

Nelson, G.S. 1970. Trichinosis in Africa. In *Trichinosis in man and animals.* Ed. S.E. Gould. Springfield, IL: C.C. Thomas Publisher, pp. 473–492.

Obendorf, D.L., and K.P. Clarke. 1992. *Trichinella pseudospiralis* infections in free-living Tasmanian birds. *Proceedings of the Helminthological Society of Washington* 59:144–147.

Obendorf, D.L., J.H. Handlinger, R.M. Mason, K.P. Clarke, A.J. Forman, P.T. Hooper, S.J. Smith, and M. Holdsworth. 1990. *Trichinella pseudospiralis* in Tasmanian wildlife. *Australian Veterinary Journal* 67:108–110.

Oksanen, A., E. Lindgren, and P. Tunkari. 1998. Epidemiology of trichinellosis in lynx in Finland. *Journal of Helminthology* 72:47–53.

Poole, B.C., K. Chadee, and T.A. Dick. 1983. Helminth parasites of pine marten, *Martes americana* (Turton), from Manitoba, Canada. *Journal of Wildlife Diseases* 19:10–13.

Porier, S.R, M.E. Rau, and X. Yang. 1995. Diel locomotory activity of deer mice (*Peromyscus maniculatus*) infected with *Trichinella nativa*, or *Trichinella pseudospiralis. Canadian Journal of Zoology* 73:1323–1334.

Pozio, E. 1987. Isoenzymatic typing of 23 *Trichinella* isolates. *Tropical Medicine and Parasitology* 38:111–116.

———. 1998. Trichinellosis in the European Union: Epidemiology, ecology and economic impact. *Parasitology Today* 14:35–38.

Pozio, E., G. La Rosa, and P. Rossi. 1989a. *Trichinella* Reference Centre. *Parasitology Today* 5:169–170.

Pozio, E., G. La Rosa , P. Rossi, and R. Fico. 1989b. Survival of *Trichinella* muscle larvae in frozen wolf carcasses in Italy. *The Journal of Parasitology* 75:472–473.

Pozio, E., G. La Rosa, K.D. Murrell, and J.R. Lichtenfels. 1992a. Taxonomic revision of the genus *Trichinella. The Journal of Parasitology* 78:654–659.

Pozio, E., G. La Rosa, P. Rossi, and K.D. Murrell. 1992b. Biological characterizations of *Trichinella* isolates from various host species and geographic regions. *The Journal of Parasitology* 78:647–653.

Pozio, E., G. La Rosa, and M. Amati. 1994a. Factors influencing the resistance of *Trichinella* muscle larvae to freezing. In *Trichinellosis.* Proceedings of the 8th International Conference on Trichinellosis. Ed. C.W. Campbell, E. Pozio, and F. Bruschi. Rome: Instituto Superiore di Sanita Press, pp. 173–178.

Pozio, E., A. Verster, L. Braack, D. De Meneghi and G. La Rosa. 1994b. Trichinellosis south of the Sahara. In *Trichinellosis.* Proceedings of the 8th International Conference on Trichinellosis. Ed. C.W. Campbell, E. Pozio, F. Bruschi. Rome: Instituto Superiore di Sanita Press, pp. 527–532.

Pozio, E., C. Bandi, G. La Rosa, T. Jarvis, I. Miller, and C.M. Kapel. 1995. Concurrent infection with sibling *Trichinella* species in a natural host. *International Journal for Parasitology* 25:1247–1250.

Pozio, E., G. La Rosa, T. Yamaguchi, and S. Saito. 1996a. *Trichinella britovi* from Japan. *The Journal of Parasitology* 82:847–849.

Pozio, E., G. La Rosa, F.J. Serrano, J. Barrat, and L. Rossi. 1996b. Environmental and human influence on the ecology of *Trichinella spiralis* and *Trichinella britovi* in Western Europe. *Parasitology* 113:527–533.

Pozio, E., D. De Meneghi, M.E. Roelke-Parker, and G. La Rosa. 1997a. *Trichinella nelsoni* in carnivores from the Serengeti ecosystem, Tanzania. *The Journal of Parasitology* 83:1195–1198.

Pozio, E., S. Jongwutiwes, G. La Rosa, P. Kraivichian, N. Chantachum, A. Tamburrini, P. Siriyasatein, C. Sreesunpasirigul, and P. Yingyourd. 1997b. Pork as source of *Trichinella pseudospiralis* infection for humans in Thailand. In *Trichinellosis.* Proceedings of the 9th International Conference on Trichinellosis. Ed. G. Ortega-Pierres, R. Gamble, F. van Knapen, and D. Wakelin. Mexico, D.F. Mexico: Centro de Investigacion y de Estudios Avanzados IPN, pp. 525–530.

Pozio, E., F.J. Serrano, G. La Rosa, D. Reina, E. Perez-Martin, and I. Navarrete. 1997c. Evidence of potential gene flow in *Trichinella spiralis* and in *Trichinella britovi* in Nature. *The Journal of Parasitology* 83:163–166.

Pozio, E., I. Miller, T. Jarvis, C.M.O . Kapel, and G. La Rosa. 1998. Distribution of sylvatic species of *Trichinella* in Estonia according to climate zones. *The Journal of Parasitology* 84:193–195.

Pozio, E., M. Goffredo, R. Fico, C.M.O. Kapel, and G. La Rosa. 1999. *Trichinella pseudospiralis* in sedentary night-birds of prey from Central Italy. *The Journal of Parasitology.* 85:759–761.

Rausch, R.L. 1970. Trichinosis in the Arctic. In *Trichinosis in man and animals.* Ed. S.E. Gould. Springfield, IL: C.C. Thomas Publisher, pp. 348–373.

Saumier, M.D., M.E. Rau, and D.M. Bird. 1986. The effect of *Trichinella pseudospiralis* infection on the reproductive success of captive American kestrels (*Falco sparverius*). Canadian Journal of Zoology 64: 2133–2125.

———. 1988. The influence of *Trichinella pseudospiralis* infection on the behaviour of captive, nonbreeeding American Kestrels (*Falco sparverius*). *Canadian Journal of Zoology* 66:1685–1692.

Schad, G.A., D.A. Leiby, C.H. Duffy, K.D. Murrell, and G.L. Alt. 1986. *Trichinella spiralis* in the black bear (*Ursus americanus*) of Pennsylvania: Distribution and intensity of infection. *Journal of Wildlife Diseases* 22:36–41.

Schad, G.A., C.H. Duffy, D.A. Leiby, K.D. Murrell and E.W. Zirkle. 1987. *Trichinella spiralis* in an agricultural ecosystem: Transmission under natural and experimentally modified on-farm conditions. *The Journal of Parasitology* 73:95–102.

Schitoskey, E.C., and R.L. Linder. 1981. Helminths of South Dakota bobcats. *Proceedings of the South Dakota Academy of Science* 60:135–141.

Schultz, M.G. 1970. Reservoirs of *Trichinella spiralis* in nature and its routes of transmission to man. *The Journal of Parasitology* 56:309.

Shaikenov, B.S. 1992. Ecological border of distribution of *Trichinella nativa* Britov and Boev 1972 and *T. nelsoni* Britov and Boev 1972. *Wiadomosci Parazytologiczne* 38:85–91.

Shaikenov, B.S., and S.N. Boev. 1983. Distribution of *Trichinella* species in the old world. *Wiadomosci Parazytologiczne* 29:595–608.

Smith, H.J., and K.E. Snowdon. 1988. Sylvatic trichinosis in Canada. *Canadian Journal Veterinary Research* 52:488–489.

Snyder, D.E. 1987. Prevalence and intensity of *Trichinella spiralis* infection in Illinois wildlife. *The Journal of Parasitology* 73:874–875.

Snyder, D.E., D.S. Zarlenga, G. La Rosa, and E. Pozio. 1993. Biochemical, biological and genetic characteristics of a sylvatic isolate of *Trichinella. The Journal of Parasitology* 79:347–352.

Soule, C., J. Dupouy-Camet, P. Georges, T. Ancelle, J.P. Gillet, J. Vasssaire, A. Delvigne, and E. Plateau. 1989. Experimental trichinellosis in horses; biological and parasitological evaluation. *Veterinary Parasitology* 32:19–36.

Stromberg, B.E., and S.M. Prouty. 1987. Prevalence of trichinellosis in the north-central United States. *Proceedings of the Helminthological Society of Washington* 54:231–232.

Thiessen, J.P. 1987. Genetic characterization of *Trichinella spiralis* isolates by analysis of repetitive DNA. M.S. Thesis, University of Manitoba, Winnipeg, 140 pp.

Van der Giessen, J.W.B., Y. Rombout, H. Franchimount, G. LaRosa, and E. Pozio. 1998. *Trichinella britovi* in foxes from the Netherlands. *The Journal of Parasitology* 84:1065–1068.

Weyermann, D., D.E. Worley, and F.M. Seesee. 1993. Survey of *Trichinella nativa* in Alaskan polar bears, *Ursus maritimus. Helminthologia (Bratislava)* 30:143–145.

Wheeldon, E.B., T.A. Dick, and T.A. Schulz. 1983. First report of *Trichinella spiralis* var. *pseudospiralis* in North America. *The Journal of Parasitology* 69:781–782.

Worley, D.E., F.M. Seesee and R.H. Espinosa. 1991. Prevalence and geographic distribution of *Trichinella spiralis* infection in hunter-killed bears in Montana, USA. *Helminthologia (Bratislava)* 28:53–55.

Worley, D.E., D.S. Zarlenga, and F.M. Seesee. 1990. Freezing resistance of a *Trichinella spiralis nativa* isolate from a gray wolf, *Canis lupus,* in Montana (USA) with observations on genetic and biological characteristics of the biotype. *Journal of the Helminthological Society of Washington* 57:57–60.

Worley, D.E., F.M. Seesee, R.H. Espinosa, and M.C. Sterner. 1986. Survival of sylvatic *Trichinella spiralis* isolates in frozen tissue and processed meat products. *Journal of American Veterinary Association* 189:1047–1049.

Worley, D.E., F.M. Seesee, D.S. Zarlenga, and K.D. Murrell. 1994. Attempts to eradicate trichinellosis from a wild boar population in a private game park (USA). In *Trichinellosis.* Proceedings of the 8th International Conference on Trichinellosis. Ed. W.C. Campbell, E. Pozio, and F. Bruschi. Rome: Instituto Superiore di Sanita Press, pp. 611–616.

Wu, Z., I. Nagano, and Y. Takahashi. 1998. Detection of *Trichinella* with polymerase chain reaction (PCR) primers constructed using sequences of random amplified polymorphic DNA (RAPD) or sequences of complementary DNA encoding excretory-secretory (E-S) glycoproteins. *Parasitology* 117:173–183.

Wu, Z., I. Nagano, E. Pozio, and Y. Takahashi. 1999. Polymerase chain reaction-restriction fragment length polymorphism (PCR-RFLP) for the identification of *Trichinella* isolates. *Parasitology* 118:212–218.

Yao, C., A.K. Prestwood, and R.A. McGraw. 1997. *Trichinella spiralis* (T1) and *Trichinella* T5: A comparison using animal infectivity and molecular biology techniques. *The Journal of Parasitology* 83:88–95.

Young, E., and S.P. Kruger. 1967. *Trichinella spiralis* (Owen, 1835) Railliet, 1895 infestation of wild carnivores and rodents in South Africa. *Journal of South Africa Veterinary Medical Association* 38:441–443.

Zarlenga, D.S., R.A. Aschenbrenner, and J.R. Lichtenfels. 1996. Variations in microsatellite sequences provide evidence for population differences and multiple ribosomal gene repeats within *Trichinella pseudospiralis. The Journal of Parasitology* 82:534–538.

Zarlenga, D.S., F. Al-Yaman, D.J. Minchella, and G. La Rosa. 1991. A repetitive DNA probe specific for a North American sylvatic genotype of *Trichinella. Molecular and Biochemical Parasitology* 48:131–138.

Zarnke, R.L., A.A. Gajadhar, G.B. Tiffin, and M. Ver-Hoef. 1995. Prevalence of *Trichinella nativa* in lynx (*Felix lynx*) from Alaska, 1988–1993. *Journal of Wildlife Diseases* 31:314–318.

Zarnke, R.L., R. Gamble, R.A. Heckert, and J. Ver-Hoef. 1997. Serological survey for *Trichinella* spp. in grizzly bears in Alaska. *Journal of Wildlife Diseases* 33:474–479.

Zimmermann, W.J. 1970. The epizootiology of trichiniasis in wildlife. *Journal of Wildlife Diseases* 6:329–334.

Zimmermann, W.J., and E.D. Hubbard. 1969. Trichiniasis in wildlife in Iowa. *American Journal of Epidemiology* 90:84–92.

Zimmermann, W.J., E.D. Hubbard, L.H. Schwarte, and H.E. Biester. 1962. *Trichinella spiralis* in Iowa wildlife during the years 1953–1961. *The Journal of Parasitology* 48:429–432.

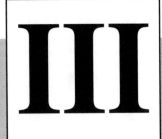

PART

PROTOZOANS

16

ENTERIC PROTOZOANS

AMEBIASIS, BALANTIDIASIS, AND ENTERIC TRICHOMONIASIS

A. ALAN KOCAN

INTRODUCTION. Enteric protozoan parasites that are infective for mammals include the pathogenic amoebae *Entamoeba histolytica*, the ciliate *Balantidium coli*, flagellated organisms such as *Giardia* spp. and *Trichomonas* spp., and Apicomplexan (Coccidia) parasites of the genera *Cyclospora, Eimeria, Isospora,* and *Cryptosporidium.*

ENTAMOEBA HISTOLYTICA (AMEBIASIS), AND *BALANTIDIUM COLI* (BALANTIDIASIS)

Etiologic Agent(s). Intestinal and luminal infections caused by the amoebae *Entamoeba histolytica* and the ciliate *Balantidium coli* occur frequently in human beings throughout the world. On a global scale, *E. histolytica* infections are the third most common cause of parasite-induced death in humans (Martinez-Paloma 1987, 1993). The existence and perhaps importance of enteric amoebic

and ciliate infections in wild mammals lies in the fact that many nonhuman primates and a few other mammalian species are also susceptible to infection with these organisms. At a time when human access to both captive and free-ranging populations of nonhuman primates is increasing and when captive situations strive for release of these animals back into indigenous habitats, diseases, especially those that may be contracted from humans and maintained within the semicaptive population, become increasingly more significant.

Epizootiology and Pathology. The pathogenic amoeba *E. histolytica* is one of at least six species of amoebae that infect the intestinal tract of man, nonhuman primates, and occasionally canines. Old World and New World monkeys are susceptible to *E. histolytica* infections, as are the Great Apes (Swenson 1993). Different strains of *E. histolytica* are recognized, each of which may vary in virulence (Mirelman 1987). Additionally, host susceptibility, nutritional status, and various stress factors also appear to play a role in virulence. Virulence is recognized when amoebae invade the gut mucosa. Affected individuals show signs of weakness, anorexia, dehydration, and severe diarrhea. Extraintestinal lesions resulting from invasion of the liver,

397

lungs, and central nervous system can also occur, creating a more complicated and serious condition. Nonclinical intestinal infections with *E. coli* and *E. bovis* have been reported in captive white-tailed deer (Kingston 1981).

In early invasive intestinal amebiasis, edema, hyperemia, and mucosal thickening occur. Invasion begins in the interglandular epithelium. The initial ulceration is superficial, with cell infiltration being minimal. Ulcers then deepen and progress superficially, producing typical "flask ulcers" extending through the mucosa and muscularis mucosa into the submucosa. Lysis of inflammatory cells may be involved in the focal necrosis seen in the mucosa. Connective tissue proliferation or scar tissue formation is usually not seen.

Extraintestinal lesions, especially liver lesions, occur in ~2% of adult humans with *E. histolytica* infections, with slightly higher percentages in epidemic situations. Invasion of the liver occurs as amoebae enter via the portal system from intestinal ulcerations. Early stages of liver involvement are characterized by acute cellular infiltration. Neutrophils and histocytes are generally associated with the periphery of the lesion. As the lesions progress, necrosis increases, macrophages and epitheloid cells replace leukocytes, and granulomas develop.

Balantidium coli infections appear to be common in captive primate colonies, with the highest prevalence in gorillas (Swenson 1993). Many *B. coli* enteric infections appear to be noninvasive and, in reality, studies have not proven that invasion of intact mucosa is possible. However, once past the epithelial barrier, invasion is easily accomplished. In many nonhuman primates, disease is often self-limiting without intervention or following treatment for concurrent pathogens including bacterial and helminth organisms. Disease, especially in gorillas, can progress rapidly from loose stools to hemorrhage and death (Janssen and Bush 1990). Pathogenesis in *B. coli* infections is similar to that of invasive forms of *E. histolytica,* although no extraintestinal involvement occurs (Zaman 1993).

Treatment. Metronidazole (Flagyl) is the drug of choice for enteric *E. histolytica* infections at 750 mg t.i.d. orally, 5 to 10 d. Diiodohydroxyquin (Diodoquin) (650 mg t.i.d. orally, 20 d) is often used in conjunction with Metronidazole. Hepatic lesions are best treated with Metronidazole (750 mg t.i.d. for 5–10 days). Complete cure is not always achieved in either enteric or hepatic infections. Treatment of *B. coli* infections usually involves tetracycline [15 mg/kg t.i.d. (young) or 500–1000 mg t.i.d. (adults) for 10–14 days] or Iodoquinol (Amebaquin) [12–16 mg/kg t.i.d. orally (young) or 650 mg t.i.d. (adults) for 14–21 days]. Metronidazole (Flagyl) is effective but often difficult to administer. In most, if not all, *B. coli* infections, other pathogens must be considered since the ability of the organism to invade intact mucosa may be limited. An exception may be in gorillas, where once mucosal integrity is compromised by other pathogens the disease may be more likely to develop.

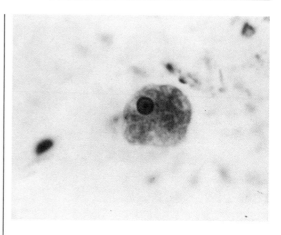

FIG. 16.1—Uninucleate trophozoite of *Entamoeba histolytica.* Note concentration of chromatin material along the nuclear membrane.

Diagnosis. As in all enteric protozoan pathogens, diagnosis is accomplished by microscopic detection of trophozoites or cysts in fresh fecal samples. Direct, wet-mount preparations are useful, but concentration procedures are usually required to detect organisms. In suspected *E. histolytica* cases, repeat examination of at least three consecutive samples is required to increase the likelihood of detection. Differentiation from nonpathogenic species is essential (Fig. 16.1). Serologic evaluation, especially indirect hemagglutination (IHA) is useful in detecting invasive conditions, although titers remain for extended periods following such infections. Latex agglutination and immunofluorescence evaluations are most useful in detecting acute invasive infections. Detection of *B. coli* infections by demonstration of either motile trophozoites or cyst stages is accomplished by either wet-mount preparations or following concentration procedures (Fig. 16.2). In *B. coli* infections, care must be taken since the prevalence of this organism in many situations is sufficiently high in asymptomatic carriers to require that the pathogenesis of the diarrhea and related signs be carefully evaluated.

Public Health and Domestic Animal Significance. Although enteric invasive *E. histolytica* infections occur in nonhuman primates, humans should be considered the main reservoirs and source of infection. *Balantidium coli* should also be considered as primarily a human parasite, although the prevalence is usually low. In addition to a high prevalence of infection in some nonhuman primate colonies, hogs are also known to have a high prevalence of *B. coli* infection. Hogs harbor both *B. coli* and *B. suis;* the former is infectious for humans and the latter, often more prevalent, is not.

As a general rule, both *E. histolytica* and *B. coli* enteric infections in nonhuman primates and other mammals should be considered as originating from human sources. Feces-contaminated food sources such

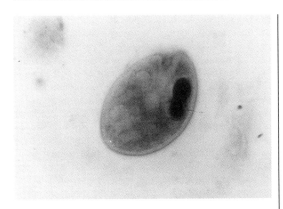

FIG. 16.2—Trophozoite of the ciliate, *Balantidium coli.* Note the prominent cytostome, cilia, and macronucleus.

as fruits and vegetables and contaminated water sources, either contaminated in the field or through handling food with contaminated hands, are the most common initial points of contamination. Once established, infections can be maintained within primate colonies and between individuals. Infections can also be maintained and spread by aerosolizaton of infectious stages during cleaning and pressure-spraying of facilities as well as during cleaning, sanitizing, and handling cages and food or water pans.

***TRICHOMONAS* SPP. (ENTERIC TRICHOMONIASIS).** Flagellated organisms belong to the subphylum Sarcomastigophora and the superclass Mastigophora. They are characterized by having one or more flagella (some may also possess pseudopodia and produce cysts), and they multiply by longitudinal binary fission. There are two classes in this subphylum, the Phytomastigophorasida and the Zoomastigophora. The Zoomastigophora is further divided into two groups, the hemoflagellates (*Trypanosoma* and *Leishmania*), which live in the blood, lymph, and tissues, and all other flagellates including the genera *Giardia* and *Trichomonas,* whose members inhabit the intestine and other tissues.

Of the trichomonads of medical importance, only a few species have a proven pathogenic potential for mammals. In general, trichomonads that inhabit the intestinal tract of mammals appear to be commensal, while those species that are known to be pathogenic inhabit other locations within the host. Although enteric trichomonad parasites of wild mammals have not been studied in depth, little or no information is available that indicates a pathogenic potential for any of the species reported. Captive white-tailed deer have been reported to harbor nonclinical enteric infections with *Tetratrichomonas* sp. (Kingston 1981). An extensive review of trichomonads is available in BonDurant and Honigberg (1994).

LITERATURE CITED
BonDurant, R.H. and B.M. Honigberg. 1994. Trichomonads of veterinary importance. In *Parasitic protozoa,* vol 9. Ed. J.P. Kreier. New York: Academic Press, pp. 11–118.
Janssen, D.L. and R.M. Bush. 1990. Review of medical literature of great apes in the 1980's. *Zoo Biology* 9:123.
Kingston, N. 1981. Protozoan parasites. In *Diseases and parasites of white-tailed deer.* Ed. W.R. Davidson, F.A. Hayes, V.F. Nettles, and F.E. Kellogg. Tallahassee, FL: Tall Timbers Research Station, pp. 193–236.
Martinez-Paloma, A. 1987. The pathogenesis of amoebiasis. *Parasitology Today* 3:111–118.
———. 1993. Parasitic amoebas in the intestinal tract. In *Parasitic protozoa,* vol. 3. Ed. J.P. Kreier and J.R. Baker. New York: Academic Press, pp. 65–141.
Mirelman, D. 1987. Effect of culture conditions and bacterial associates on the zymodemes of *Entamoeba histolytica. Parasitology Today* 3:37–43.
Swenson, R.B. 1993. Protozoal parasites of great apes. In *Zoo and wildlife animal medicine.* Vol. 3, *Current therapy.* Ed. M.E. Fowler. Philadelphia, PA: W.B. Saunders Co., pp. 353–355.
Zaman, V. 1993. *Balantidium coli.* In *Parasitic protozoa,* vol 3. Ed. J.P. Kreier and J.R. Baker. New York: Academic Press, pp. 43–63.

GIARDIA AND GIARDIASIS

MERLE E. OLSON AND ANDRE G. BURET

INTRODUCTION. *Giardia* is a flagellated binucleate protozoan parasite that colonizes the intestine of mammals, birds, reptiles, and amphibians. The first reported observation of the parasite is credited to Anton van Leeuwenhoek who described the organism after examination of his own diarrheic feces in 1681 (Adam 1991; Meyer 1990; Wolfe 1992). *Giardia* cysts have been identified in 2,000-year-old human paleofecal specimens from Israel and Tennessee, indicating that the parasite was present in both the Old and New Worlds in ancient periods (Faulkner et al. 1989). *Giardia* was once believed to be a commensal microorganism of the small intestine, but during the later half of this century, physicians, veterinarians, and parasitologists have recognized that this parasite is a significant pathogen. Today it is known as the most common human intestinal parasite worldwide (Adam 1991). Backpackers, campers, and wilderness explorers are familiar with giardiasis as this organism often contaminates backcountry lakes and streams. Wildlife has been implicated as the source of human infections and as a result giardiasis is also called "beaver fever" in North America.

ETIOLOGIC AGENT. *Giardia* is a protozoan parasite that belongs to the subphylum Sarcomastigophora (vesicular nucleus, flagella, no spore formation), the superclass Mastigophora (one or more flagella, asexual reproduction by longitudinal binary fission, no sexual reproduction), the class Zoomastigophorea (no chromatophores, one or more flagella), the order Diplomonadida (four pairs of flagella, two nuclei, no mitochondria, no Golgi, cyst, free living or parasitic), and the family Hexamitida (bilaterally symmetrical, oval in shape with duplication of organelles). *Giardia* may be the most primitive eukaryote based upon its small-subunit rRNA sequences (Sogin et al. 1989).

Giardia species were traditionally assigned on the basis of host specificity, and older literature has used names such as *G. cati* (from cats), *G. bovis* (cattle), or *G. canis* (dogs) (Wolfe 1992). In 1952 Felice proposed to differentiate three species of *Giardia* based on trophozoite morphology and the shape of the median bodies, two distinctive intracellular structures that can be easily preserved and visualized using standard cytological procedures (Felice 1952):

(1) *Giardia duodenalis* (synonymous with *G. lamblia* and *G. intestinalis*) parasitizes humans and other vertebrates and has clawhammer-shaped median bodies within a pear-shaped trophozoite (11 to 16 µm long and 5 to 9 µm wide). *Giardia* recovered from humans is often referred to as *Giardia lamblia,* but the same species of *Giardia* isolated from nonhuman sources is referred to as *Giardia duodenalis* (Mahbubani et al 1992). As this nomenclature suggests that there is something unique about human-derived *Girardia* isolates, it has been proposed that *Giardia duodenalis* be used to describe this species complex (Thompson et al. 2000).

(2) The slightly rounded *Giardia muris* (~10 µm long and 7 µm wide) trophozoites can be found in rodents (and possibly some birds and reptiles) and contain two small spherical median bodies.

(3) *Giardia agilis* trophozoites colonize the intestine of amphibians and are long and narrow (20–30 µm x 4.5 µm) with long teardrop shaped median bodies.

This classification does not address the considerable phenotypic and genotypic homogenity and minor heterogeneity within *G. duodenalis* (Thompson and Melani 1993). *Giardia psittaci* (from parakeets) and *Giardia ardeae* (from great herons and straw-necked ibis) have been proposed as possible new species based on their morphological characteristics, including the absence of an anterior ventrolateral flange or the presence of a single caudal flagellum, respectively (Table 16.1, Fig. 16.4) (Erlandsen and Bemrick 1987; Erlandsen et al. 1990; McRoberts et al. 1996). Another feature of most *G. duodenalis* isolates is that they can be maintained and grown in culture, while this has not been achieved with *G. muris* (Adam 1991; Wolfe 1992). In an attempt to identify pathogenic vs. nonpathogenic *G. duodenalis* strains and/or to distinguish animal from human isolates, ongoing research efforts make extensive use of antigenic comparisons, isoenzyme determinations, DNA fingerprinting, and other molecular techniques to further characterize *Giardia* species (Stranden et al. 1990; Upcroft et al. 1990; Nash 1992; Mahbubani et al. 1992; Bruderer et al. 1993; Thompson and Melani 1993; Chen et al. 1994; Meloni et al. 1995; Ey et al. 1996; Monis et al. 1996; Ey et al. 1997; Hopkins et al. 1997; Homan et al. 1998; Monis et al. 1998; Van Keulen et al. 1998).

Research data available today indicate that there is considerable genetic diversity within *G. duodenalis* populations and that isolates from humans and many mammalian species fall into two major genetic assemblages (reviewed by Thompson et al. 2000). Assemblage A consists of isolates from humans, livestock, cats, dogs, beavers, and nonhuman primates. Assemblage B includes a genetically diverse group of predominantly human isolates, but also isolates from nonhuman primates, dogs, beavers, chinchilla and rats (Thompson et al. 1999). Through the use of polymerase chain reaction (PCR), *G. duodenalis* isolates exhibiting a limited host range (dog, cat, cattle, muskrat) have also been identified (Ey et al. 1997; Hopkins et al. 1997; Monis et al. 1998; Van Keulen et al. 1998; Thompson et al. 2000). This suggests that some isolates have become adapted to a particular host species, but these isolates may or may not infect other species. Molecular analysis of *Giardia* isolates suggests that strains from animal origin often cannot be

TABLE 16.1—Morphological features of *Giardia*

Species	Host	Morphological Features
Giardia duodenalis	Dog, cats, ruminants, wild mammals	Trophozoites: length = 11–16 µm, width = 5–9 µm, Cyst: 6–10 µm long and elliptical. Trophozoites have a pyriform body. Two clawhammer-shaped median bodies.
Giardia muris	Mice, small rodents	Trophozoites: length = 10 µm, width = 7 µm, Cyst: 6–10 µm long and elliptical. Trophozoites have a short body with a large adhesive disc. It has small, round median bodies.
Giardia agilis	Amphibians	Trophozoites: length = 20 µm, width = 4.5 µm, Cyst: 6–10 µm long and elliptical. Trophozoites have a long narrow body, a short adhesive disc, and long club-shaped median bodies.
Giardia ardeae	Great blue heron	Pleomorphic median body (clawhammer to oval), caudal flagellum on right and rudimentary on left (as viewed dorsally). Same size as *G. duodenalis*
Giardia psittaci	Parakeets	Lacked ventrolateral flange, clawhammer-shaped median body. Same size as *G. duodenalis.*

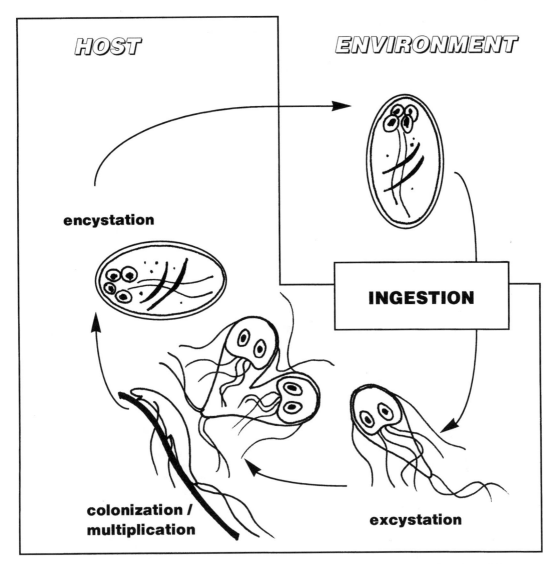

FIG. 16.3—Life cycle of the parasite *Giardia* sp. with two stages, the trophozoites that colonize the intestine, and the cysts which are passed in the feces.

distinguished from human isolates, and there is no evidence to support the hypothesis that *G. duodenalis* pathogenicity may be strain dependent (Meloni et al. 1995; Ey et al. 1996, 1997; Thompson et al. 1999).

LIFE HISTORY. *Giardia* has a simple, direct, life cycle (Fig. 16.3). The infection is obtained by ingestion of the quadrinucleate cysts. Cysts resist gastric juices and excyst within the duodenum, each releasing two trophozoites that multiply by binary fission and colonize the entire small intestine. Trophozoites adhere to the intestinal epithelium by means of a ventral adhesive

disk but do not invade the mucosal tissue. Trophozoites encyst in the ileum and large intestine, and the cysts are passed in the feces. These cysts are resistant to the environment and remain infective for months in cold water or damp, cool environments (see Epizootiology section).

MORPHOLOGY. *Giardia* trophozoites are binucleate organisms with four pairs of flagella and a ventral adhesive disc (Figs. 16.4, 16.5). The median bodies used in taxonomy are a pair of organelles found in the anterior half (*G. agilis*) or close to the center of the

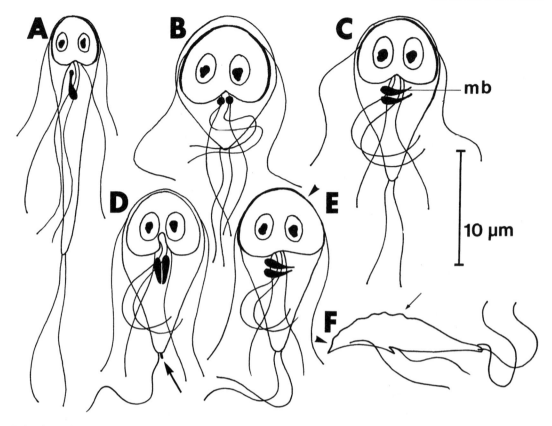

FIG. 16.4—Diagrammatic representation of ventral (A–E) and lateral (F) views of *Giardia* species recognized to date. (**A**) *G. agilis* from amphibians, with its characteristic elongated morphology and tear-drop shaped median bodies. (**B**) *G. muris*, circular in shape, has spherical median bodies. (**C**) *G. duodenalis*, which infects humans and animals, has pear-shaped trophozoites and contains "claw hammer" median bodies orientated perpendicular to the long axis of the organism. (**D**) *G. ardea* (found in herons) resembles *G. duodenalis* but is characterized by an absent or rudimentary left caudal flagellum (large arrow), a deep indented notch in the ventral adhesive disc, and median bodies that lie parallel to the longitudinal axis of the trophozoite. (**E**) and (**F**) *G. psittaci.* Unlike in other *Giardia* species, the ventral lateral flange is absent at the anterolateral border of the adhesive disc (arrowhead), and the dorsal surface possesses characteristic protrusions (small arrow). (mb = median bodies)

organism. The cysts are elliptic in shape and approximately 6–10 μm long and 4–6 μm wide. Under light microscopy, two or four nuclei, ventral disc components, and axonemes of flagella can often be recognized within chemically stained cysts (Fig. 16.7). Transmission electron microscopy (Fig.16.5) and scanning (Fig.16.6) have permitted recognition of detailed internal and external structures of the trophozoite and cyst as reviewed by Meyer (1994).

EPIZOOTIOLOGY

Distribution, Host Range, and Prevalence. *Giardia lamblia* is an ubiquitous intestinal pathogen (Adam 1991; Wolfe 1992). Prevalences (Tables 16.2–16.5) are often underestimated because of the low sensitivity of current parasite detection methods and the intermittent nature of cyst excretion during a *G. duodenalis* infection. Humans (Adam 1991; Wolfe 1992), dogs (Collins 1987; Hahn et al. 1988; Lewis 1988; Sykes and Fox 1989; Tonks et al. 1991; Barr and Bowman 1994), cats (Belosevic et al. 1984; Kirkpatrick and Farrell 1984; Kirkpatrick 1986; Collins 1987; Tonks et al. 1991; Barr and Bowman 1994), and several wildlife species (Davis and Hibler 1979; Roach et al. 1993) are described as the predominant hosts. Approximately 1%–25% of domestic dogs and cats are infected with *Giardia* throughout the world.

Recent studies have also identified domestic livestock (e.g., cattle, sheep, pigs, horses) as common hosts for this parasite (Kirkpatrick 1989; Buret et al. 1990c; Taylor et al. 1993; Xiao et al. 1993, 1994a,b; Xiao 1994; Xiao and Herd 1994; Olson et al. 1997a). *Giardia* infections in calves and sheep have been reported throughout the world including in Canada, Britain, the United States, Switzerland, Austria, Czechoslovakia, South Africa, and India, with prevalence varying from 1% to 100%. Calves and lambs are infected within 4 days of birth, and the infection persists several

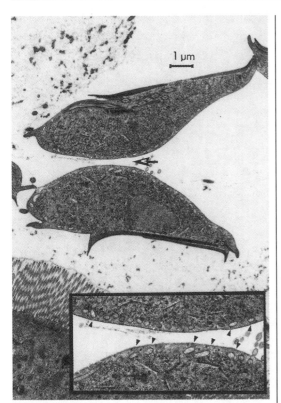

FIG. 16.5—Transmission electron micrograph of *Giardia duodenalis* trophozoites in the small intestine of a Mongolian gerbil (*Merlones unguiculatus*). Inset: Illustration of the dorsal vesicles (arrowheads) containing secretory-excretory products with unknown pathogenic functions.

months (Xiao 1994; Olson et al. 1997a; O'Handley et al. 1999). Recent reports suggest that giardiasis in swine may reach high prevalence in some farms, but the significance and overall prevalence of the disease in the porcine industry need to be established in more depth (Xiao 1994). In general, prevalence is lower in adults. In females, excretion of *Giardia* cysts often increases during periparturient periods (Xiao et al. 1994b).

High prevalence in some species of birds has lead to public health concerns as birds are highly mobile, aggregate around water, and often have close association with humans (e.g., parakeets) (Erlandsen and Bembrick 1987; Upcroft et al. 1997; Graczyk et al. 1998).

Most wild mammals can be infected with *Giardia* (Tables 16.3–16.5). Prevalence may vary from very low to 100%. *Giardia* has been identified in many zoo animals, presumably due to confinement and the ease of disease transmission. The common occurrence of giardiasis in carnivores and in coprophagic animals may reflect foodborne infection and autoinfection. *Giardia muris* has been identified in mice and voles but *G. duodenalis* is the species that apparently infects most other wild mammals. The authors believe that in many cases

wild animals may be infected from environmental contamination by feces of human and/or domestic animal origin.

The probability of contracting giardiasis from drinking water is difficult to predict with accuracy. Indeed, the level of water contamination with *Giardia* cysts varies with location, season, and time of day. Potential for waterborne infection depends upon the concentration, viability, and virulence of cysts in the water (Wallis 1994). Processed drinking water, raw municipal water, and backcountry streams and lakes all may contain infective *Giardia* cysts (Roach et al. 1993; Wallis 1994). Numbers of cysts in raw and processed drinking water samples can exceed 1000 cysts/l, while sewage samples may contain more than 88,000 cysts/l (Wallis et al. 1996). Clearly *Giardia* cysts are much more prevalent than *Cryptosporidium* oocysts in water and sewage (Table 16.6). Sewage effluent produced by human and domestic animals represents a serious source of contamination for wild animal species. Several outbreaks of giardiasis have been reported in Canada and the United States (Wallis 1994). It is probable that the true prevalence of waterborne giardiasis is greatly underestimated because a number of infection cases may remain asymptomatic and because symptomatic cases may not be diagnosed or reported.

Transmission. Ingestion of as few as ten cysts has led to infections in humans and animals (Adam 1991; Wolfe 1992). The risk of *Giardia* infection is enhanced with high population density, poor hygiene, and certain feeding behaviors. Infection rates are high in areas of large human and animal populations partly because of the increased opportunity for direct or indirect disease transmission. Prevalence of giardiasis is highest in the young, which are immunologically naive and more prone to ingestion of fecal matter. There is also increased susceptibility in a host with inadequate maternal passive immune transfer, concurrent disease, stress, or inadequate nutrition or in one that is otherwise immunocompromised (Perlmutter et al. 1985; Farthing 1994). Highest risks of contracting a *Giardia* infection occur in developing countries and disadvantaged societies (Islam 1990; Meloni et al. 1993; Farthing 1994). Together, these observations indicate that *Giardia* is a parasite that may be easily transmitted between animal species and that infected animals may play the role of reservoirs for human disease (Davis and Hibler 1979; Bemrick 1984; Woo 1984; Swabby et al. 1988; Kasprzak and Pawlowski 1989).

Fecal-oral transmission of *Giardia* is common both in animals and humans (Adam 1991; Wolfe 1992; Zajac 1992; Barr and Bowman 1994; Farthing 1994). High prevalence of giardiasis in children from day-care centers has been often reported (Adam 1991). Similarly, animals in close confinement may be exposed to large numbers of infective cysts in fecal material, increasing the likelihood of disease transmission. Coprophagia, which is common in animals, is a significant route for autoinfection and amplifies disease spread within a population.

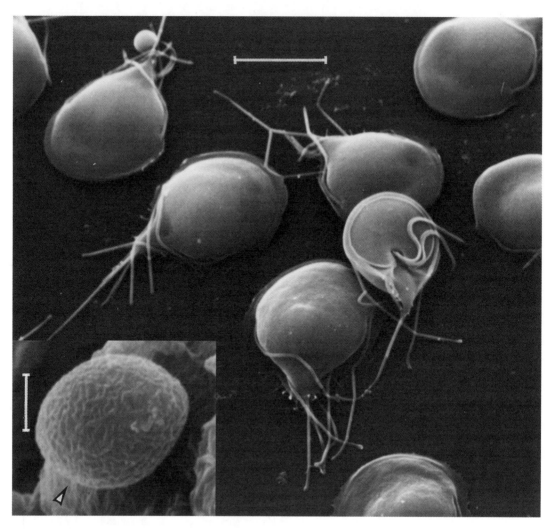

FIG. 16.6—Scanning electron micrographs of *G. muris* trophozoites adhering to a plastic substrate and of a *G. duodenalis* cyst (arrowhead) in the ileal lumen of a cat (inset). (Bars = 5 μm)

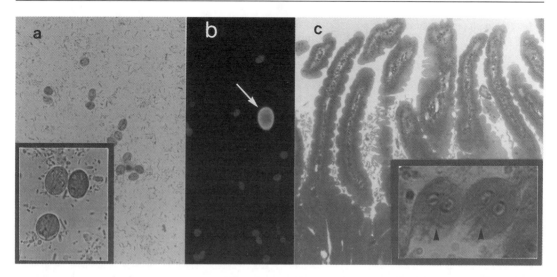

FIG. 16.7—*Giardia* sp. Cysts as seen with light microscopy stained (**a**) with Lugol's iodine or (**b, arrow**) with a fluorescently labelled monoclonal antibody. Smaller *Cryptosporidium* oocysts can be stained on the same sample, using a separate antibody. (**c**) High numbers of *Giardia* trophozoites are visible between the villi of a duodenal biopsy stained with basic fuchsin and methylene blue. Some trophozoites harbor characteristic claw-hammer–shaped median bodies (inset, arrowheads).

TABLE 16.2—Prevalence of giardiasis in companion and food mammals

Species	Location	Prevalence (%)	References
Puppies	US	36	Zajac 1992, Barr et al. 1994, Hahn et al. 1988
Dogs	US	10	Zajac 1992, Barr et al. 1994, Hahn et al. 1988
	Canada	10	Lewis 1988
	England	15.5–29	Sykes and Fox 1989
Cats	US	1–11	Kirkpatrick and Farrell 1984, Kirkpatrick 1986, Hahn et al. 1988, Zajac 1992, Barr et al. 1994,
Parakeets	US	65–70	Erlandsen and Bembrick 1987
Calves	US	89	Xiao 1994, Xiao et al. 1994b
	Canada	23–73	Buret et al. 1990c, Olson et al 1997a, 1997c
Lambs	US	82	Xiao et al. 1994a
	Canada	34	Buret et al. 1990c, Olson et al 1997a
	England	69	Taylor et al. 1993
Pigs	Europe	44	Xiao 1994
	Canada	10	Olson et al 1997a
	US	7	Xiao 1994
Goats	Europe	50	Xiao 1994
Horses	Canada	20	Olson et al. 1997a
Foals	US	32	Xiao 1994, Xiao and Herd 1994

TABLE 16.3—*Giardia* in rodents and lagomorphs

Name	Latin Name	Location	Prevalence (%)	Reference
Beaver	*Castor canadensis*	Alberta	3, 4	Wallis et al. 1984, 1986
		New England	17	Erlandsen and Bemrick 1987
		Washington	10.5, 24	Pacha et al. 1985
		Colorado	18, 47	Davis and Hibler 1979, Monzinga and Hibler 1987
		Yukon	14	Roach et al. 1993
Muskrat	*Ondatra zibethicus*	Colorado	83, 100	Davis and Hibler 1979, Swabby et al. 1988
		New Jersey	70	Kirkpatrick and Benson 1987
		Washington	51, 83	Pacha et al. 1985
		Yukon	25	Roach et al. 1993
Porcupine	*Erethizon dorsatum*	Poland	33	Peisert et al. 1988
Water vole	*Microtus richardsoni*	Washington	100	Pacha et al. 1987
Red-backed vole	*Clethrionomys gapperi*	Alberta	86, 95	Wallis et al. 1984, 1986
Heather vole	*Phenacomys intermedius*	Alberta	50	Wallis et al. 1984
Meadow vole	*Microtus pennsylvanicus*	Alberta	75, 33	Wallis et al. 1984, 1986
		Ontario	99	Grant and Woo 1978
Norway rat	*Rattus norvegicus*	Ontario	100	Grant and Woo 1978
Long-tailed vole	*Microdus longicaudus*	Alberta	33	Wallis et al. 1984
		Ontario	98	Grant and Woo 1978
		Washington	100	Pacha et al. 1987
Deer mouse	*Peromyscus maniculatus*	Alberta	10	Wallis et al. 1984
		Ontario	98	Grant and Woo 1978
Gerbil	*Meriones ungiculatus*	Quebec	?	Belosevic et al. 1983
Pouched rat	*Cricetomys gambianus*	Poland	?	Majewska and Kasprzak 1990
Wood rat	*Neotoma cinerea*	Alberta	7	Wallis et al. 1986
Cuis	*Galean musteloides*	Poland	?	Majewska and Kasprzak 1990
Chinchilla	*Chinchilla laniger*	Georgia	21	Shelton 1954
		Colorado	100	Davis and Hibler 1979
Guinea pig	*Cavia porcellus*	US	?	Vetterling 1976
Hamster	*Mesocricetus auratus*	US	?	Wagner 1987
Rabbits	*Oryctolagus cuniculus*	US	?	Pakes 1974

Disease outbreaks of epidemic proportions have most often been attributed to waterborne transmission (Craun 1986). Contamination of water with human effluent and/or infected animal feces can lead to widespread infections in both humans and animals (Weniger et al. 1983; Craun 1986; Gradus 1989; LeChevallier et al. 1991; Roach et al. 1993). Water mammals such as beavers have been implicated in a number of waterborne infections (LeChavallier et al. 1991); however, these observations have become subjects of controversy and other animals appear more likely to contaminate water supplies. Indeed, attempts at controlling waterborne infections by eliminating water mammals have been largely unsuccessful, implying that in a number of waterborne outbreaks, water mammals are probably not the source of infection. As *Giardia* cysts

TABLE 16.4—*Giardia* in primates

Common Name	Latin Name	Location	Prevalence (%)	Reference
Arabian sacred baboon	*Papio hamadryas arabicus*	Saudi Arabia	39	Nasher 1988
Squirrel monkey	*Saimiri sciureus sciureus*	California	33–70	Hamlen and Lawrence 1994
Chimpanzee	*Chimpansee triglodytes*	Poland	25	Peisert et al. 1985
Marmoset	*Callithrix agentata*	Poland	100	Peisert et al. 1985
Slow loris	*Nycticebus coucang*	Poland	?	Majewska and Kasprzak 1990
Lesser slow loris	*Nycticebus pygmaeus*	Poland	?	Majewska and Kasprzak 1990
Siamang	*Symphalangus syndactylus*	Poland	?	Majewska and Kasprzak 1990
Grivet monkey	*Cercopithecus aethiops*	Chile	?	Gorman et al. 1986
Gorillas	*Gorilla gorilla*	Missouri	?	US Public Health Service, 1979; World Health Organization 1979
Orangutans	*Pongo pygaemus*	Missouri	?	US Public Health Service, 1979; World Health Organization 1979
Gibbons	*Hylobates spp*	Missouri	?	US Public Health Service, 1979; World Health Organization 1979
Rhesus monkey	*Macca mulatta*	Maryland	0.3	Reardon and Rininger 1968

TABLE 16.5—*Giardia* in wild hoofed animals and carnivores

Common Name	Latin Name	Location	Prevalence (%)	Reference
Dall sheep	*Ovis dalli*	Yukon	40	Roach et al. 1993
Camel	*Camelus bactrianus*	Chile	?	Gorman et al. 1986
Giraffe	*Giraffa camelopardalis*	Chile	?	Gorman et al. 1986
Muskox	*Ovibus moschatus*	NW Territories	20	M.E. Olson, unpubl.
Elk	*Cervus canadensis*	Washington	3	Pacha et al. 1987
Llama	*Lama glama*	Wisconsin	?	Kiorpes et al. 1987
Wolves	*Canis lupus*	Yukon	33	Roach et al. 1993
Coyote	*Canis latrans*	Yukon	75	Roach et al. 1993
European wild cat	*Felis silvestris*	Poland	33	Peisert et al. 1985
Serval	*Felis serval*	Poland	14	Peisert et al. 1985
Cougar	*Felis concolor*	Chile	?	Gorman et al. 1986
		Canada	90	M.E. Olson, unpubl.
Leopard	*Panthera pardus*	Thailand	2	Patton and Rabinowitz 1994
Grizzly bear	*Ursus arctos*	Yukon	100	Roach et al. 1993
Harbour seal	*Phoca vitulina*	E. Canada	25	Measures and Olson 1999
Harp seal	*Phoca grenlandica*	E. Canada	50	Measures and Olson 1999
Grey seal	*Halichoerus grypus*	E. Canada	25	Measures and Olson 1999
Ring seal	*Phoca hispida*	NW Territories	20	Olson et al. 1997d

TABLE 16.6—*Giardia* sp. and *Cryptosporidium* sp. in Canadian water and sewage samples (from Wallis et al. 1996)

Sample Type	Number of Samples	*Giardia* (% positive)	*Cryptosporidium* (% positive)
Raw drinking water	1173	245 (20.9%)	53 (4.5%)
Treated drinking water	423	77 (18.2%)	15 (3.6%)
Raw sewage	164	119 (72.6%)	10 (6.1%)
Total samples	1760	441 (25.1%)	78 (4.4%)

may survive in water for several months, the source of contamination is sometimes difficult to ascertain. Nevertheless, the feces of domestic animals such as cattle, sheep, horses, and swine have a tremendous potential to contaminate water (Craun 1986). Therefore, during waterborne outbreaks, humans and domestic livestock, as well as wildlife, must be considered as potential sources of infection.

Foodborne infections in humans have been associated with inappropriate food handling or with washing food with contaminated water (Adam 1991; Wolfe 1992). Carnivorous animals may be susceptible to foodborne infection when they ingest infected prey. Feed-like cereal grains may also be contaminated by feces from animals, such as small rodents, and hence become a potential source of *Giardia* infection.

Environmental Limitations. *Giardia* trophozoites do not survive in the environment. In contrast, *Giardia* cysts are resistant to some environmental factors while highly susceptible to others (Olson et al. 1999b). They are able to survive for long periods of time in waters that contain low concentrations of bacteria and organic contaminants. Laboratory observations suggest that high concentrations of bacteria in the surrounding environment lead to cyst degradation (Jakubowski 1990). Optimal temperatures for cyst survival in water range between 4° C and 8° C (Jakubowski 1990). This corresponds to the temperatures found in mountain streams where the prevalence of *Giardia* cysts is high. Extended freezing and temperatures above 20° C are detrimental to cysts (Bingham et al. 1979; Jakubowski 1990; Olson et al. 1999b). Boiling destroys *Giardia* cysts instantaneously. Desiccation and ultraviolet irradiation inactivate cysts within 24 hours (Bingham et al. 1979). *Giardia* cysts are degraded within weeks in feces and soil (Olson et al. 1999b).

The potential for waterborne giardiasis in humans and animals has forced major modifications on the water treatment industry. *Giardia* cysts may be removed by filtration or by chemical treatment (Bingham et al. 1979; Jakubowski 1990). Large-scale water processing technologies use diatomaceous earth, sand, and coagulation systems; while small-volume filtration systems employ cartridge filters made of ceramics, polycarbonate paper, or yarn-wound cotton (Jakubowski 1990; Wallis 1994). When used appropriately, the latter can remove > 99% of *Giardia* cysts from a contaminated water sample (Jakubowski 1990). The downfall of using filter cartridges is that malfunctions that would require filter replacement are often difficult to detect.

Water chlorination systems typically used to control bacterial pathogens are usually ineffective against *Giardia* cysts. Indeed, high concentrations of chlorine, warmer water temperatures, and long contact times are necessary for chlorine to inactivate these cysts (Wallis et al. 1993). Chloramine is an effective giardiacidal agent, but it too requires high concentrations and extended contact times. Ozone is a highly effective anti-*Giardia* agent that is not influenced by temperature. Unfortunately, water treatment facilities using ozone are expensive to install. Finally, iodine solutions used by backpackers have shown empirical efficacy in inactivating *Giardia* cysts, but detailed studies on the effects of these products have yet to be conducted.

The published literature contains little information about the effects of chemical disinfectants on *Giardia* within fecal waste (Zajac 1992; Wallis 1994). Organic iodine, tincture of iodine, chlorine, and bleach (hypochlorite) are all effective in destroying cysts. Several manufacturers of phenol, quaternary ammonium salt, and halogen disinfectants claim efficacy against fecal *Giardia* cysts, but scientific evidence to substantiate these claims is often lacking. At any rate, prolonged contact times (15 to 30 minutes) should be employed to ensure inactivation of fecal cysts.

CLINICAL SIGNS. Infection with *Giardia* can cause diarrhea or remain asymptomatic. Young animals are most likely to develop clinical symptoms. Clinical signs of giardiasis include acute or chronic diarrhea, abdominal pain, dehydration, body weight loss or reduction in body weight gain, and failure to thrive (Adam 1991; Wolfe 1992; Zajac 1992; Barr and Bowman 1994; Farthing 1994). Fatal infections have been reported in chinchillas and, more recently, in birds (Shelton 1954; Forshaw et al. 1992; Upcroft et al. 1997). Giardiasis in cattle and sheep may induce diarrhea and weight loss, but most infections in ruminants appear to be asymptomatic (Kirkpatrick 1989; Taylor et al. 1993; Xiao 1994; Olson et al. 1995). A recent study demonstrated that while experimentally infected lambs may pass feces with abnormal consistency compared to controls, they do not develop severe diarrhea (Olson et al. 1995). This study showed for the first time that giardiasis is an economically important disease in ruminants as it caused reduced rate of body weight gain, impaired feed efficiency and lower carcass weight. Dogs and cats may be asymptomatic carriers of the infection or show signs of diarrhea (Collins 1987; Tonks et al. 1991; Barr and Bowman 1994). Allergic disease and urticaria have been associated with giardiasis in humans, horses, and birds (Adam 1991; Di Prisco et al. 1993), leading to the speculation that this disease may be responsible for cases of atopy in other animals such as dogs, cats, and parakeets in which infection is common. However, the clinical assessment of symptoms directly resulting from giardiasis is often confounded by a number of other factors, such as concurrent infections, nutritional deficiencies, or stress.

PATHOLOGY AND PATHOGENESIS. The small intestine colonized with *Giardia* is commonly filled with mucus and fluid and shows impaired activity of digestive enzymes (disaccharidases, lipases, amylase, proteases) (Buret et al. 1990a, 1991; Buret 1994; Faubert and Belosevic 1990). Clinical malabsorption in giardiasis has been associated with severe villus atrophy and crypt hyperplasia in some cases and with normal histology in others (Farthing 1994; Buret et al. 1990a, 1991; Buret 1994; Faubert and Belosevic 1990). Accumulation of polymorphonuclear leucocytes or eosinophils does usually not occur in giardiasis, but proliferation of intraepithelial lymphocytes and mucosal mast cells has been described during the clearance phase of the infection (Gillin and Ferguson 1984; Hardin et al. 1997). While the mechanisms responsible for symptoms in giardiasis remain incompletely understood, recent studies in laboratory animals have provided insights into the pathophysiology of the disease. When *Giardia* trophozoites colonize the small intestine, they cause a diffuse reduction in the height of the microvilli and therefore a generalized loss of absorptive surface area (Buret et al. 1990a,b, 1991, 1992). This reduction in membrane surface area leads to the malabsorption of glucose, electrolytes, and water and

TABLE 16.7—Methods for the diagnosis of giardiasis

Sample	Method	Comments	Reference
Feces	Fecal smear, direct examination	Inexpensive, insensitive	Zajac 1992, Barr et al. 1994, Burke 1977.
	Fecal smear, iodine or trichrome stain	Inexpensive, cysts may be hidden in debris	Zajac 1992, Barr et al. 1994, Burke 1977
	Sucrose gradient flotation, iodine stain	Removes debris, inexpensive	Buret et al. 1990c
	Zinc sulfate flotation, iodine stain.	Removes debris, inexpensive	Zajac 1992, Barr et al. 1994, Burke 1977
	Flotation, immunofluorescent antibody stain	Accurate, more sensitive, more expensive	Zajac 1992, Barr et al. 1994, Olson et al. 1997a
	Fecal *Giardia* antigens by enzyme linked immunosorbant assay (ELISA)	Rapid, accurate, expensive, not qualitative	Isaac-Renton 1991, Chappell and Matson 1992
Duodenal fluid	String test	Inaccurate, cannot be used in animals	Adam 1991, Barr et al. 1994
Duodenal biopsy	Direct examination or Giemsa stained	Accurate, requires endoscopy	Adam 1991, Burke 1977
Serum	ELISA for anti-*Giardia* antibodies (IgM, IgG, IgA)	Only works in chronic giardiasis, useful for seroprevalence.	Adam 1991, Isaac-Renton 1991
Skin test	Immunoreactivity to *Giardia* proteins injected intradermally	Never tried in animals, may only be useful for chronic giardiasis, invasive	Di Prisco et al. 1993
Histology	Demonstration of *Giardia* trophozoites in fixed tissue	Good for biopsy specimens and for postmortem examination, invasive	Buret et al. 1990c

impairs digestion by reducing disaccharidase activity. Increased intestinal motility has been observed in experimentally infected animals (Deselliers et al. 1997). In summary, *Giardia* infections lead to intestinal malabsorption, maldigestion, and hypermotility, which are responsible, at least in part, for the diarrhea seen in this disease. Finally, Hardin et al. (1997) recently demonstrated that giardiasis causes an increase in intestinal macromolecular uptake associated with intestinal and cutaneous mast cell hyperplasia. These findings suggest that allergic symptoms observed during or after *Giardia* infections may result from host sensitization to food and/or parasite proteins.

The role played in pathogenesis by *Giardia* excretory-secretory products, like those contained in the vesicles lining the dorsum of trophozoites (Fig. 16.5), has yet to be established. Similarly, host factors appear to be responsible, at least in part, for the mucosal abnormalities associated with giardiasis, but the mechanisms and mediators of these events remain unknown (Buret 1994).

DIAGNOSIS. Diagnosis of giardiasis is achieved by the detection of trophozoites, cysts or *Giardia* antigens in feces or in the intestine, and/or by demonstration of a specific immune response in the host (Table 16.7).

Fecal Samples. Evaluation of fecal samples is ideally suited as a non-invasive method to demonstrate the presence of the parasite in a host. The relatively low

probability for a single stool specimen to demonstrate the presence of *Giardia* cysts (50%–70%) is due to difficult detection of the parasite and the intermittent fecal shedding of cysts (Burke 1977). Stool samples can be examined fresh or fixed in 10% neutral buffered formalin or polyvinyl alcohol. Fixation may interfere with some commercial immuofluorescent stains. Trophozoites are infrequently observed and usually only in the very lose stools that may be associated with heavy infections. Fecal smears can be chemically (e.g., Lugol's iodine [Fig. 16.7], trichrome, iron haematoxylin) or immunofluorescently stained to differentiate the cysts from other fecal material (Buret et al. 1990c; Zajac 1992; Barr and Bowman 1994; Olson et al. 1997a). In order to increase the sensitivity and to remove background interference, cysts can be concentrated using zinc sulphate, formalin ethyl acetate or sucrose prior to staining (Adam 1991; Zajac 1992; Barr and Bowman 1994; Buret et al. 1990c; Olson et al. 1997a). Fecal flotation solutions should have a maximal specific gravity of 1.18 g/mm^3 as the hypertonic saturated sugar or salt solutions commonly used for parasite concentration may induce cyst distortion. A certain degree of technical expertise is required from the microscopist to appropriately recognize this parasite. Immunofluorescent stains (Giardi-a-Glo, Waterborne, New Orleans, LA; Meridian, Cincinnati OH; Giardia-Celisa, Techlab, Blacksburg, VA) greatly enhances the accuracy, sensitivity and speed of sample analysis but requires an epifluorescent microscope (Olson et al. 1997a). In summary, the microscopic

TABLE 16.8—Procedure for concentration and staining of fecal samples for *Giardia* spp. and *Cryptosporidium* spp.

Fecal clarification and concentration:
The fecal sample is combined with PBS (1:1) and shaken to give a homogenous suspension. Approximately 4 g of the feces and PBS mixture is weighed and filtered through gauze (Four Ply, NuGauze, Johnson and Johnson, Montreal, PQ). The sample is compressed to yield ~ 7 ml of filtrate, which is layered over 7 ml of 1 M sucrose solution (specific gravity 1.18 g/mm³) and is centrifuged 5 minutes at 800 g on a fixed rotor centrifuge in order to concentrate the cysts and oocysts at the sucrose/water interface. The water layer (upper layer) and the interface are removed and centrifuged 5 minutes at 800 g to concentrate the particulate material and cysts/oocysts. The supernatant is decanted and discarded and the pellet is resuspended to a volume of 1 ml.

Fecal staining:
The fecal concentrate can be stained with 1:1 parts of Lugol iodine and examined directly on a light microscope at 100X and 400X. Alternatively, the concentrate can be stained with a FITC monoclonal antibody. A 15 µl sample of the suspension is spotted and spread over a glass slide and air-dried at ambient temperature. Slides are dip-fixed with acetone, then rinsed with PBS and allowed to air dry. The spots are reacted with 20 ml of either FITC-labeled mouse monoclonal antibody against *Giardia* cysts or *Cryptosporidium* oocysts (Giardi-a-Glo or Crypt-o-Glo, Waterborne, Inc., New Orleans). Slides are placed in a humidity chamber 30 minutes at room temperature, then rinsed with PBS and air dried. Slides are then prepared for viewing by applying mounting medium (Aqua-poly/mount, Polysciences, Warrington, PA) and a cover slip. The entire smear is viewed at 200X and 400X magnifications by epifluorescence microscopy. Positive control samples (provided by Waterborne, Inc., New Orleans) are run with test samples.

methods used to diagnose *Giardia* are fairly laborious and success of the procedure depends on the skill of the microscopist. ELISA test kits (Prospect T, Alexon Inc., Sunnyvale, CA; Giardia-Celisa [above]), which detect *Giardia* antigens in feces have been developed and are effective in providing a rapid, accurate diagnosis without the use of a microscope (Chappell and Matson 1992). These kits are well-suited for diagnostic laboratories and animal clinics, but they are expensive and do not provide information on the number of cysts per gram of feces. To date, the method to demonstrate and quantitate fecal *Giardia* cysts (as well as *Cryptosporidium* oocysts) with the highest benefit/cost ratio is to perform a sucrose gradient flotation followed by immunofluorescent staining and analysis by light microscopy (Table 16.8).

Duodenal Samples. In humans, duodenal samples can be obtained by having the patient swallow a string or capsule on a string, letting it pass into the duodenum and then recovering the trophozoite-studded string (Entero-test, Hedeco, Palo Alto, CA). Of course, this method is impractical for animals as they may bite and sever the recovery string. Duodenal biopsies may be obtained during endoscopic examination of larger monogastric mammals. Duodenal samples can be stained (e.g., Giemsa stain) or examined directly for the presence of trophozoites. However, the invasive nature, the equipment costs/availability and the duration of the procedure makes it impractical as routine diagnostic methodology.

Serum Samples. Serological testing is useful for epidemiological and, immunologic studies but has limited value as a diagnostic tool. Indeed, it is difficult to differentiate between actively infected animals and those that have cleared the infection. Moreover, weak serum immune response has been observed in *Giardia*-infected animals (Faubert 1996; Olson et al. 1996).

Postmortem Samples. The autolytic changes that occur in the intestine rapidly after death dislodge the trophozoites from the mucosal surface. Following death, immediate fixation of the tissue is necessary to demonstrate the trophozoites *in situ*. Carnoy's fixation followed by plastic embedding and staining (Lee's methylene blue and basic fuchsin) yields quality morphological features of the parasite and host (Fig. 16.7). This procedure stains the median bodies assisting in *Giardia* species determination (Buret 1990c).

Environmental Detection. Methods for detection of *Giardia* cysts in water have been developed to assist in the study of suspected waterborne disease outbreaks, for the evaluation of drinking water treatment processes, and to monitor water quality in urban, rural and wilderness environments. To assess the presence of waterborne parasitic cysts (*Giardia*) and oocysts (*Cryptosporidium*) in water samples helps determine the impact of human and animal effluent on water quality, which in turn provides useful information towards risk assessment for human and animal infections. Several methods for the environmental detection of *Giardia* cysts have been proposed, with various degrees of efficiency and convenience (Hibler 1988; Wallis 1994). These include the use of polymerase chain reaction (PCR) to detect Giardia DNA and the ELISA system developed for the detection of *Giardia* coproantigens (Mahbubani et al. 1992; Thompson et al. 1993). Isolation of waterborne parasites can be accomplished by passage of a large amount of water through a filter, which can be processed to recover the cysts (Table 16.9). Cysts are concentrated and enumerated using a method similar to that used for the demonstration of *Giardia* cysts in fecal samples. This method is used routinely for cyst recovery from environmental samples but the detection of cysts in the filter lacks sensitivity (1%–5%). Raw sewage samples can be processed for *Giardia* detection like fecal samples.

IMMUNITY AND VACCINATION. Infection with *Giardia* induces cellular immunity as represented by proliferation of intra-epithelial lymphocytes and mast cells. Also, *Giardia*-specific IgA is produced in the infected small intestine and milk (reviewed by Faubert

TABLE 16.9—Procedure for collection and analysis of water samples for *Giardia* spp. cysts and *Cryptosporidium* spp. oocysts

Equipment:
The basic equipment consists of a filter housing, a water meter, and connecting hoses and fittings. This is described in Standard Methods for Examination of Water and Wastewater, APHA 1989. A good quality wound filter made of polypropylene, rayon, or cotton will work.

Sampling:
Sampling for *Giardia* cysts and *Cryptosporidium* oocysts is accomplished by filtering the water through a 25 cm woven cotton fiber cartridge filter with a porosity of 1 μm. Influent water is passed through a pressure-reducing valve maintaining pressures below 100 kPa. Water leaving this valve is passed directly to the filter housing containing the filter cartridge. The volume of water passing through the filter is recorded using a flow meter. Depending on the situation, 100 to 15,000 liters of water may be passed through the filter.

Filter analysis:
The filter is then removed, cut from the core with a razor knife, and placed in a plastic wash tub containing 500–1000 ml water, 3 drops of Tween 80, and 0.5 g of SDS. The fibers are hand washed until they are completely white. Washings are centrifuged 6 minutes at 725 X g in swinging buckets. Pellets are resuspended in 25 ml of PBS.

Staining:
Giardia cysts and *Cryptosporidium* oocysts can then be demonstrated and counted as described above for fecal samples.

Sample shipment:
Filters may be shipped in coolers with ice packs by surface or air transport. If rapid shipment is not possible (< 48 hr) filters may be preserved by soaking in 4% formalin solution.

1996). Trophozoites can be killed by both IgG and IgM in the presence of complement (Faubert 1996). However, levels of circulating immunoglobulins in *Giardia*-infected hosts may be similar to the levels measured in non-infected hosts (Wright et al. 1977; Faubert 1996; Yanke et al. 1998). The inability of the host to be strongly immunostimulated may be due to the intraluminal and non-invasive nature of the parasite. Chronic infections are common in both humans and animals (Perlmutter et al. 1985; Farthing 1994). Yet, the particularly severe clinical signs reported in immunocompromised hosts infected with *Giardia* (Perlmutter et al. 1985; Farthing 1994), the observation that infection becomes chronic in athymic animals (Stevens et al. 1978), and the lower prevalence of infection and diarrhea in individuals repeatedly exposed to *Giardia* (Smith 1984; Faubert 1996) further support the significance of specific immunity in the clearance of the infection. Taken together, these observations have provided a rational basis for the development of an anti-*Giardia* vaccine (Olson et al. 1999a). Immunization with a polyvalent vaccine provides protection to animals against subsequent challenge with *Giardia* cysts or trophozoites (Olson et al. 1996, 1997b, 1999a). Moreover, vaccination has yielded promising results in

dogs and cats (Olson et al. 1996, 1997b) suggesting that immunization may be used to prevent giardiasis in other animal species. Whether immunotherapy may be used to treat chronic giardiasis warrants further study. In addition to therapeutic benefits there is a sound rationale for an anti-*Giardia* vaccine to minimize trophozoite colonization and fecal cysts in animals acting as a zoonotic reservoirs.

TREATMENT. Most commonly, the rationale for treatment in giardiasis is to eliminate the clinical signs that may be associated with the infection. However, asymptomatic animals colonized with the parasite may also require treatment, as *Giardia* infections may lead to an increase susceptibility to other diseases and/or reduced weight gain and feed conversion (Olson et al. 1995). In addition, infected animals that are in direct contact with humans or their environment should be treated (e.g., pets, zoo animals, etc.) (US Public Health Service 1979). Many drugs are available for the treatment of giardiasis in animals and man (Table 16.10). Successful therapy usually requires continued treatment for 3 to 10 days. In animals, reinfection frequently occurs unless infective cysts are eliminated from the environment. This implies a thorough cleaning and disinfection where feasible, as well as ensuring that water and feed are not contaminated by feces. Obviously, full cyst eradication cannot be achieved in the environment of most animals. The development of an effective and cost efficient method of treatment of giardiasis in farm and companion animals is important as these animals may be reservoirs of infection in humans and wildlife. Effective chemotherapeutic agents include nitroimidazoles (metronidazole, tinidazole), quinacrine, furazolidone and as demonstrated most recently, benzimidazoles (fenbendazole, albendazole) and ionophores (salinomycin). Nitroimidazoles such as metronidazole, tinidazole and ipronidazole have proven to be effective in the treatment of giardiasis in people and some companion animals (Goldman 1980; Davidson 1984). These drugs act by interfering with electron transport in the parasite. It is often difficult to get animals to take metronidazole as it has an unpleasant metallic taste (Goldman 1980; Davidson 1984). In addition, the undesirable side effects and toxicology data of nitroimidazoles make these compounds unattractive for the treatment of giardiasis. Indeed, metronidazole therapy in dogs has resulted in moderate to severe intestinal and neurological disease (Dow et al. 1989; Finch et al. 1992; Zajac 1992). Metronidazole is also a mutagen and teratogen (Goldman 1980). Nitrofurans such as furazolidone have been used in the treatment of giardiasis in humans and animals. Furazolidone acts by inhibiting the parasite's anaerobic respiration. It is less effective than metronidazole and is carcinogenic. Resistance of *Giardia* to both metronidazole and furazolidone has been reported (Townson et al. 1992; Upcroft and Upcroft 1993). Quinacrine is an antimalarial drug that is effective in the treatment of

TABLE 16.10—Chemotherapeutic agents for treating giardiasis

Species	Agent	Dosage	Duration	Reference
Human	Quinacrine	6 mg/kg, p.o.	3X daily for 5 days	Adam 1991
	Metronidazole	15 mg/kg, p.o.	3X daily for 5 days	Adam 1991
	Tinidazole	50 mg/kg, p.o.	Single dose	Adam 1991
	Furazolidone	8 mg/kg, p.o.	4X daily for 10 days	Adam 1991
	Albendazole	200 mg/kg, p.o.	1X daily for 5–10 days	Adam 1991
Dogs/cats	Quinacrine	6.6 mg/kg, p.o.	2X daily for 5 days	Zajac 1992
	Metronidazole	10-25 mg/kg, p.o.	2X daily for 5 days	Zajac 1992
	Furazolidone	4 mg/kg, p.o.	2X daily for 7 days	Zajac 1992
	Albendazole	25 mg/kg, p.o.	2X daily for 3–5 days	Barr et al. 1994
	Fenbendazole	50 mg/kg, p.o.	1X daily for 3–5 days	Barr et al. 1994
Horses	Metronidazole	5 mg/kg	3X daily for 10 days	Kirkpatrick 1989
Calves	Albendazole	20 mg/kg	1X daily for 5 days	Xiao and Herd 1996
	Fenbendazole	5 mg/kg	1X daily for 3 days	O'Handley et al. 1997
		0.8mg/kg	1X daily for 6 days	O'Handley et al. 1997

giardiasis in humans and animals (Adam 1991). An additional benefit of quinacrine is its ability to inactivate *Giardia* cysts which results in the passage of nonviable fecal cysts during therapy. Several benzimidazoles have been demonstrated to be highly effective for treatment of giardiasis in humans and dogs (Adam 1991; Wolfe 1992; Barr et al. 1993; Morgan et al. 1993; Barr et al. 1994). It is believed that benzimidazoles selectively inhibit polymerization of tubulin which is a major component of the *Giardia* cytoskeleton (Chavaz et al. 1992; Morgan et al. 1993; Oxberry et al. 1994). Albendazole has been shown to cause ultrastructural alterations to the ventral adhesive disk of *Giardia* trophozoites. Combined, these observations suggest that benzimidazoles affect structural proteins (Chavaz et al. 1992). Benzimidazoles *in vitro* were found to be 50 times more effective than metronidazole (Morgan et al. 1993). Both albendazole and fenbendazole have been shown to effectively eliminate *Giardia* from dogs (Barr et al. 1993; Barr et al. 1994). High doses of albendazole and fenbendazole were shown to reduce or eliminate *Giardia* cyst excretion in naturally infected calves (Xiao and Herd 1996). O'Handley et al. (1997) demonstrated that a ruminant *Giardia* isolate was highly susceptible to fenbendazole *in vitro* (0.024 µg/ml) and in significantly smaller doses than those recommended for effective treatment in calves. Albendazole has been shown to cause weight loss, blood dyscrasias and bone marrow cellular depletion in chronically treated dogs (Barr et al. 1993, 1994). Moreover, albendazole has also been shown to be toxic to embryos and teratogenic in cattle and dogs (Barr et al. 1993; Wetzel 1985). Resistance of *Giardia* spp to fenbendazole and albendazole has not be demonstrated (Morgan et al. 1993; Upcroft and Upcroft 1993; O'Handley et al. 1997). The side-effects of with some benzimidazoles have not been observed with fenbendazole therapy.

Our laboratory is currently screening drugs commonly used in food animals for their efficacy in controlling giardiasis. Laboratory and field studies have identified that certain ionophores (e.g., salinomycin) exhibit anti-*Giardia* properties (Olson et al. 1994;

McAllister 1996). To date, the major limitations in using ionophores extensively are their toxic side-effects. Further research is required to identify effective giardiacidal chemotherapeutic agents that have few side-effects.

PUBLIC HEALTH CONCERNS. Similarities in morphology, protein characteristics, and DNA have been demonstrated among *Giardia* isolated from animals and humans (Thompson et al. 1988; Capon et al. 1989; Kasprzak and Pawlowski 1989; De Jonckheere et al. 1990; Majewska et al. 1993; Thompson et al. 1988; Meloni et al. 1995; Ey et al. 1996). A number of clinical reports and transmission studies suggest that giardiasis is a zoonotic disease (Rendtorff 1954; US Public Health Service 1979; Cribb and Spracklin 1986; Majewska 1994). There are two reports of humans experimentally infected with *Giardia* from animal sources (Davis and Hibler 1979; Majewska 1994). Thus, wild animals as well as companion and food animals could potentially infect humans either through waterborne transmission or direct contact with contaminated feces. This justifies the concern that infected wild and domestic animals may contaminate surface and ground waters, which in turn may drain into municipal water reservoirs. Indeed, an outbreak of waterborne giardiasis in humans has been attributed to pasture run-off leading to drinking water contamination (Weniger et al. 1983). In 1979, a report from the World Health Organization recommended that giardiasis should be recognized as a zoonotic disease (World Health Organization 1979). Almost 20 years later our understanding of the role of animals in human infections is still incomplete, and considerable research is required to make appropriate risk assessments.

DOMESTIC ANIMAL CONCERNS. It is clear that *Giardia* is highly prevalent in both companion animals and domestic food animals (Barr and Bowman 1994; Xiao 1994; Olson et al. 1997a). Wild animals may also be infected by direct contact with domestic animals

(Woo and Patterson 1986) or following drinking of water contaminated by agricultural effluent. Indeed, infections in wild animals may reflect the degree of environmental contamination by domestic animals and humans. This is supported by the observation that beavers in the remote wilderness areas of the Yukon Territory were not infected while *Giardia* cysts were observed in Yukon beavers that were in contact with humans and domestic animals (Roach et al. 1993). Companion animals (e.g., dogs, horses) frequently accompany humans into parks and wilderness areas thereby exposing wildlife to *Giardia* cysts in their feces. Eleven 11% of canine fecal samples collected from parks are positive for *Giardia* (Grimason et al. 1993). Cattle, sheep and horses frequently share grazing areas with wild mammals. As up to 100% of some domestic animal species can be excreting *Giardia* cysts, wildlife can be easily infected by direct contact with fecal material or by waterborne transmission. With expanding agricultural production, the management of food animal fecal waste has become an environmental concern and wildlife may become a victim of pressures to produce more food. Every effort must be made to prevent domestic animals from contamination of water with *Giardia* cysts and from deposition of fecal matter in wilderness areas.

MANAGEMENT IMPLICATIONS. Treatment and prevention of *Giardia* infections in domestic and zoo animals is necessary as it causes clinical disease (diarrhea, allergies), affects performance and is a potential zoonotic disease. The disease in domestic animals and zoo animals can be controlled by use of chemotherapeutic agents and vaccination in conjunction with containment and disinfection. In the past, wild animals suspected of shedding *Giardia* cysts (e.g., beavers) have been eliminated to prevent or stop waterborne outbreaks of giardiasis in humans. The benefits of this practise have not been scientifically demonstrated. Often, wildlife is incriminated in waterborne outbreaks and elimination of wildlife associated with a watershed is easy and inexpensive (yet ineffective) solution to a complex and difficult problem. Once a population of wild mammals is infected with this parasite it would be virtually impossible to eliminate it. The disease is present in many wild species without obvious clinical signs but because of the infection they may be susceptible to other diseases or starvation. As the disease is not treatable in wildlife, it is critical that there is minimal exposure to *Giardia* contaminated effluent from humans and domestic animals. The prevalence of *Giardia* in some wild animal species should be monitored to evaluate any changes in infection levels that may reflect environmental contamination of the habitat and the overall health of the species.

Giardia is a ubiquitous parasite that does not respect host species barriers and carries serious potential for zoonotic transmission. Animal infections are often blamed on human activity and are frequently impli-

cated in endemic outbreaks of human giardiasis. As a result, this parasite is the ongoing topic of considerable environmental interest, particularly in the area of water contamination. *Giardia* can infect animals and humans worldwide, and high prevalence has been reported in temperate climates as well as in developing countries. This protozoan can cause moderate to severe enteric disease, but infected hosts may also remain asymptomatic. Giardiasis is highly prevalent in most wild and domestic animals in which it may negatively affect health and performance. Over the past decade the vast majority of research has been directed toward understanding this disease in humans. The impact of *Giardia* infections in animals must be further explored.

LITERATURE CITED

Adam, R.D. 1991. The Biology of *Giardia* spp. *Microbiology Reviews* 55:706–732.

Barr, S.C., and D.D. Bowman. 1994. Giardiasis in dogs and cats. *The Compendium on Continuing Education for the Practicing Veterinarian* 16:603–611.

Barr, S.C., D.D. Bowman, and R.L. Heller. 1994. Efficacy of fenbendazole against giardiasis in dogs. *American Journal of Veterinary Research* 55:988–989.

Barr, S.C., D.D. Bowman, R.L. Heller, and H.N. Erb. 1993. Efficacy of albendazole against giardiasis in dogs. *American Journal of Veterinary Research* 54:926–928.

Belosevic, M., G.M. Faubert, J.D. MacLean, C. Law, and N.A. Croll. 1983. *Giardia lamblia* infections in Mongolian gerbils: An animal model. *Journal of Infectious Diseases* 147:222–226.

Belosevic, M., G.M. Faubert, R.R. Guy, and J.D. MacLean. 1984. Observations on natural and experimental infections with *Giardia* isolated from cats. *Canadian Journal of Comparative Medicine* 48:241–244.

Bemrick, W.J. 1984. Some prospectives on transmission of giardiasis. In Giardia *and Giardiasis*. Ed. S.L. Erlandsen and E.A. Meyers. New York:Plenum, pp. 379–400.

Bingham, A.K., E.L. Jarroll, and E.A. Meyer. 1979. *Giardia* sp.: Physical factors of excystation in vitro, and excystation vs eosin exclusion as determination of viability. *Experimental Parasitology* 47:284–291.

Bruderer, T., P. Papanastosiou, R. Castro, and P. Kohler. 1993. Variant cysteine-rich surface proteins of *Giardia* isolates from human and animal services. *Infection and Immunity* 61:2937–2944.

Buret, A. 1994. Pathogenesis: How does *Giardia* cause disease? In *Giardia,* from molecules to disease. Ed. R.C.A. Thompson, J.A. Reynoldson, and A.J. Lymbery. Wallingford, UK: CAB International, pp. 293–315.

Buret, A., D.G. Gall, and M.E. Olson. 1990a. Effects of murine giardiasis on growth, intestinal morphology and disaccharidase activity. *The Journal of Parasitology* 76:403–409.

Buret, A., D.G. Gall, P.N. Nation, and M.E. Olson. 1990b. Intestinal protozoa and epithelial kinetics, structure and function. *Parasitology Today* 6:375–380.

Buret, A., N. Denhollander, P.M. Wallis, D. Befus, and M.E. Olson. 1990c. Zoonotic potential of domestic ruminants. *Journal of Infectious Diseases* 162:231–238.

Buret, A., D.G. Gall, and M.E. Olson. 1991. Growth, activities of enzymes in the small intestine and ultrastructure of microvillus brush border in gerbils infected with *Giardia lamblia*. *Parasitology Research* 77:109–114.

Buret, A., J.A. Hardin, M.E. Olson, and D.G. Gall. 1992. Pathophysiology of small intestinal malabsorption in gerbils infected with *Giardia lamblia. Gastroenterology* 103:506–513.

Burke, J.A. 1977. The clinical and laboratory diagnosis of giardiasis. *CRC Critical Reviews in Clininical Laboratory Science* 7:373–391.

Capon, A.G., J.A. Upcroft, F.L. Boreham, L.E. Cottis, and P.G. Bundesen. 1989. Similarities of *Giardia* antigens derived from human and animal origin. *International Journal of Parasitology* 19:91–98.

Chappell, C.L., and C.C. Matson. 1992. *Giardia* antigen detection in patients with chronic gastrointestinal disturbances. *Journal of Family Practice* 35:49–53

Chavaz, B., M. Espinosa-Cantellano, R.C. Rivera, A. Ramiraz, and A. Martinez-Palomo. 1992. Effects of albendazole on *Entamoeba histolytica* and *Giardia lamblia* trophozoites. *Archives of Medical Research* 23:63–67.

Chen, N., J.A. Upcroft, and P. Upcroft. 1994. Physical map of a 2 Mb chromosome of the intestinal protozoan parasite *Giardia duodenalis. Chromosome Research* 2:307–313.

Collins, G.H. 1987. Diagnosis and prevalence of *Giardia* spp. in dogs and cats. *Australian Veterinary Journal* 64:89–90.

Craun, G.F. 1986. Waterborne outbreaks in the United States 1965–1984. *Lancet* 1986:513–514.

Cribb, A.E., and D. Spracklin. 1986. Giardiasis in a home. *Canadian Veterinary Journal* 27:169.

Davidson, R.A. 1984. Issues in clinical parasitology: The treatment of giardiasis. *American Journal Gastroenterology* 79:256–261.

Davis, R.B., and C.P. Hibler. 1979. Animal reservoirs and cross species transmission of *Giardia*. In *Waterborne transmission of giardiasis*. Ed. W. Jakubowski and J.C. Hoff. EPA-600/9-79/001. Cincinnati, OH: US Enviromental Protection Agency, pp. 104–126.

De Jonckheere, J.F., A.C. Majewska, and W. Kasprzak. 1990. *Giardia* isolates from primates and rodents display the same molecular polymorphism as human isolates. *Molecular and Biochemical Parasitology* 39:23–28.

Deselliers, L.P., D.T.M. Tan, L.B. Scott, and M.E. Olson. 1997. The effect of giardiasis on intestinal motility. *Digestive Diseases and Science* 42:2411–2419.

Di Prisco, M.C., I. Hagel, N.R. Lynch, N. Alvarez, and R. Lopez. 1993. Possible relationship between allergic disease and infection by *Giardia lamblia. Annals of Allergy* 70:210–213.

Dow, S.W., R.A. LeCouteur, M.L. Poss, and D. Beadleston. 1989. Central nervous system toxicosis associated with metronidazole treatment of dogs: five cases (1984–1987). *Journal of the American Veterinary Medical Association* 195:365–368.

Erlandsen, S.L., W.J. Bemrick, C.L. Wells, D.E. Feely, L. Knudson, S.R. Campbell, H. Van Keulen, and E.L. Jarroll. 1990. Axenic culture and characterization of *Giardia ardeae* from the great blue heron. *The Journal of Parasitology* 76:717–724.

Ey, P.L., T. Bruderer, C. Werli, and P. Kohler. 1996. Comparison of genetic groups determined by molecular and immunological analysis of *Giardia* isolated from animals and humans in Switzerland and Australia. *Parasitology Research* 82:52–60.

Ey, P.L., M. Mansouri, J. Kulda, E. Nohynkova, P.T. Monis, R.H. Andrews, and G. Mayrhofer. 1997. Genetic analysis of *Giardia* from hoofed farm animals reveals artiodactyl-specific and potentially zoonotic genotypes. *Journal of Eukaryotic Microbiology* 44:626–635.

Erlandsen, S.L., and W.J. Bemrick. 1987. SEM evidence for a new species, *Giardia psittaci. The Journal of Parasitology* 73:623–629.

Faulkner, C.T., S. Patton, and S.S. Johnson. 1989. Prehistoric parasitism in Tennessee: Evidence from the analysis of

desiccated fecal material collected from Big Bone Cave, Van Buren County, Tennessee. *The Journal of Parasitology* 75:461–463.

Farthing, M.J.G. 1994. Giardiasis as a disease. In *Giardia: From molecules to disease.* Ed. R.C.A. Thompson, J.A. Reynoldson, and A.J. Lymbery. Wallingford, UK: CAB International, pp. 15–37.

Faubert, G.M. 1996. The immune response to *Giardia. Parasitology Today* 12:140–145.

Faubert, G.M., and M. Belosevic. 1990. Animal models for *Giardia duodenalis* type organisms. In *Human parasite diseases.* Vol. 3, *Giardiasis.* Ed. E.A. Meyer. Amsterdam: Elsevier, pp. 77–90.

Felice, F.P. 1952. Studies on the cytology and life history of *Giardia* from the laboratory rat. *University of California Publications in Zoology* 57:53–146.

Finch, R., M. Moore, and D. Roen. 1992. A warning to clinicians: Metronidazole neurotoxicity in a dog. *Progess in Veterinary Neurology* 2:307–309.

Forshaw, D., D.G. Palmer, S.A. Halse, R.M. Hopkins, and R.C.A. Thompson. 1992. *Giardia* infection in straw-necked ibis (*Threskiornis spinicollis*). *Veterinary Record* 131:267–268.

Gillin J., and A. Ferguson. 1984. Changes in the small intestinal mucosa in giardiasis. In *Giardia and giardiasis.* Ed. S.L. Erlandsen and E.A. Meyer. New York: Plenum Press, pp. 163–183.

Goldman, P. 1980. Drug therapy, metronidazole. *New England Journal of Medicine* 303:1212–1218.

Gorman, T.R., V. Riveros, H.A. Alcaino, D.R. Salas, and E.R. Thiermann. 1986. Helminthiasis and toxoplasmosis among mammals at the Santiago zoo. *Journal of American Veterinary Medical Association* 189:1068–1070.

Graczyk T.K., R. Fayer, J.M. Trout, E.J. Lewis, C.A. Farley, I. Sulaiman, and A.A. Lal. 1998. *Giardia* sp. cysts and *Cryptosporidium parvum* oocysts in the feces of migratory Canada geese (*Branta canadensis*). *Journal of Applied and Environmental Microbiology* 64:2736–2738.

Gradus, M.S. 1989. Water quality and waterborne protozoa. *Clinical Microbiology News* 11:121–125.

Grant, D.R., and P.T.K. Woo. 1978. Comparative studies of *Giardia* in small mammals in southern Ontario. Prevalence and identity of the parasites with taxonomic discussion of the genus. *Canadian Journal Zoology* 56:1348–1359.

Grimason A.M., H.V. Smith, J.F.W. Parker, M.H. Jackson, P.G. Smith, and R.W.A. Girdwood. 1993. Occurrence of *Giardia* sp. cysts and *Cryptosporidium* oocysts from public parks in the west of Scotland. *Epidemiology and Infection* 110:641–645.

Hahn, N.E., C.A. Glaser, D.W. Hird, and D. C. Hirsh. 1988. Prevalence of *Giardia* in the feces of pups. *Journal American Veterinary Medical Association* 192:1428–1429.

Hamlen, H.J., and J.M. Lawrence. 1994. Giardiasis in laboratory-housed squirrel monkeys: A retrospective study. *Laboratory Animal Science* 44:235–239.

Hardin, J.A., A.G. Buret, M.E. Olson, and D.G. Gall. 1997. Mast cell hyperplasia and increased macromoler uptake in an animal model of giardiasis. *The Journal of Parasitology* 83:908–912.

Hibler, C.P. 1988. Analysis of municipal water samples for cysts of *Giardia*. In *Advances in Giardia research.* Ed. P.M. Wallis and B.R. Hammond. Calgary: University of Calgary Press, pp. 237–245.

Homan W. L., M. Gilsing, H. Bentala, L. Limper, and F. Knapen. 1998. Characterization of *Giardia duodenalis* by polymerase-chain-reaction fingerprinting. *Parasitology Research* 84:707–714.

Hopkins, R.M., B.P. Meloni B., D.M. Groth, J.D. Wetherall, J.A. Reynoldson, and R.C.A. Thompson. 1997. Ribosomal RNA sequencing reveals differences between genotypes of *Giardia* isolates recovered from humans and dogs living in the same locality. *The Journal of Parasitology* 83:44–51.

Isaac-Renton, J.L. 1991. Immunological methods of diagnosis in Giardiasis: An overview. *Annals of Clinical and Laboratory Science* 21:116–122.

Islam, A. 1990. Giardiasis in developing countries. In *Giardiasis.* Ed. E.A. Meyer. Amsterdam: Elsevier, pp. 235–266.

Jakubowski, W. 1990. The control of *Giardia* in water supplies. In *Giardiasis.* Ed. E.A. Meyer. Amsterdam: Elsever, pp. 336–353.

Kasprzak, W. and Z. Pawlowski. 1989. Zoonotic aspects of giardiasis: A review. *Veterinary Parasitology* 32:101–108.

Kirkpatrick, C.E. 1986. Feline giardiasis: A review. *Journal of Small Animal Practise* 27:69–80.

———. 1989. Giardiasis in large animals. *The Compendium on Continuing Education for the Practicing Veterinarian* 11:80–84.

Kirkpatrick, C.E., and C.E. Benson. 1987. Presence of *Giardia* spp. and absence of *Salmonella* spp. in New Jersey muskrats. *Applied and Environmental Microbiology* 53:1790–1792.

Kirkpatrick, C.E., and J.P. Farrell. 1984. Feline giardiasis: Observations on natural and induced infections. *American Journal Veterinary Research* 45:2182–2188.

Kiorpes, A.L., C.E. Kirkpatrick, and D.D. Bowman. 1987. Isolation of *Giardia* from a llama and from sheep. *Canadian Journal of Veterinary Research* 51:277–280.

LeChevallier, M.W., W.D. Norton, and R.G. Lee. 1991. Occurrence of *Giardia* and *Cryptosporidium* spp. in surface water supplies. *Applied and Environmental Microbiology* 57:2610–2616.

Lewis P.D. 1988. Prevalence of *Giardia* sp. in dogs from Alberta. In *Advances in Giardia research.* Ed. P.M. Wallis and B.R. Hammond. Calgary: University of Calgary Press, pp. 61–64.

Mahbubani, M.H., A.K. Bej, M.H. Perlin, F.W. Schaefer, W. Jakubowski, and W. Atlas. 1992. Differentiation of *Giardia duodenalis* from other species by using polymerase chain reaction and gene probes. *Journal of Clinical Microbiology* 30:74–78.

Majewska, A.C. 1994. Successful experimental infections of a human volunteer and Mongolian gerbils with *Giardia* of animal origin. *Transactions of Royal Society of Tropical Medicine and Hygiene* 88:360–362.

Majewska, A.C., and W. Kasprzak. 1990. Axenic isolation of *Giardia* strains from primates and rodents. *Veterinary Parasitology* 35:169–174.

Majewska, A.C., W. Kasprzak, and E. Kaczmarek. 1993. Comparative morphology of *Giardia* trophozoites from man and animals. *Acta Protozoologica* 32:191–197.

McAllister, T.A., C.B. Annett, M.E. Olson, D.M. Morck, and K.-J. Cheng. 1996. Effect of salinomycin on giardiasis and coccidiosis in growing lambs. *Journal of Animal Science* 74:2896–2903.

McRoberts, K.M., B.P. Melani, U.M. Morgan, R. Marano, N. Binz, S.L. Erlandsen, S.A. Halse, and R.C.A. Thompson. 1996. Morphological and molecular characterization of *Giardia* isolated from the straw-necked ibis (*Threskiornis spinicollis*) in western Australia. *The Journal of Parasitology* 82:711–718.

Measures, L.N., and M.E. Olson. 1999. Giardiasis in pinnipeds from eastern Canada. *Journal of Wildlife Diseases* 35:779–782.

Meloni, B., P., R.C.A. Thompson, R.M. Hopkins, J.A. Reynodson, and M. Gracey. 1993. The prevalence of *Giardia* and other intestinal parasites in children, dogs and cats from aboriginal communities in the Kimberley. *Medical Journal of Australia* 158:157–159.

Meloni B.P., A.J. Lymbery, and R.C. Thompson. 1995. Genetic characterization of isolates of *Giardia duodenalis* by enzyme electrophoresis: Implications for reproductive biology, population structure, taxonomy and epidemiology. *The Journal of Parasitology* 81:368–383.

Meyer, E.A. 1990. Taxonomy and nomenclature. In *Giardiasis.* Ed. A.A. Meyer. Amsterdam: Elsevier, pp. 51–60.

———. 1994. *Giardia* as an organism. In Giardia: *From Molecules to Disease.* Ed. R.C.A. Thompson, J.A. Reynoldson, and A.J. Lymbery. Wallingford, UK: CAB International, pp. 3–13.

Monis, P.T., G. Mayrhofer, R.H. Andrews, W.L. Homan, L. Limper, and P.L. Ey. 1996. Molecular genetic analysis of *Giardia intestinalis* isolates at the glutamate dehydrogenase locus. *Parasitology* 112:1–12.

Monis, P.T., R.H. Andrews, G. MAyrhofer, G. MacKrill, J. Kulda, J.L. Isaac-Renton, and P.L. Ey. 1998. Novel linages of *Giardia intestinalis* identified by genetic analysis of organisms isolated from dogs in Australia. *Parasitology* 116:7–19.

Monzingo, D.L., Jr., and C.P. Hibler. 1987. Prevalence of *Giardia* sp. in a beaver colony and the resulting environmental contamination. *Journal of Wildlife Diseases* 23:576–585.

Morgan, U.M., J.A. Reynoldson, and R.C.A. Thompson. 1993. Activities of several benzimidazoles and tublin inhibitors against *Giardia* spp. in vitro. *Antimicrobial Agents and Chemotherapy* 37:328–331.

Nash, T.E. 1992 Surface antigen variability and variation in *Giardia lamblia. Parasitology Today* 8: 229–234.

Nasher A.K. 1988. Zoonotic parasite infections of the Arabian sacred baboon *Papio hamadryas arabicus* in Asir province, Saudi Arabia. *Annales de Parasitologie Humaine et Comparée* 63:448–454.

O'Handley, R.M., M.E. Olson, T.A. McAllister, D.W. Morck, M. Jelinski, G. Royan, and K.-J. Cheng. 1997. The efficacy of fenbendazole in the treatment of giardiasis in calves. *American Journal of Veterinary Research* 58:384–388.

O'Handley, R.M., C. Cockwill , T.A. McAllister, M. Jelinski, D.W. Morck, and M.E. Olson. 1999. Duration of naturally acquired giardiosis and cryptosporidiosis in dairy calves and their association with diarrhea. *American Journal of Veterinary Medical Association* 214:391–396.

Olson M.E., A.D. Griffith, D. and W. Morck. 1994. In vitro evaluation of anticoccidial agents for *Giardia lamblia.* In Giardia: *From molecules to disease.* Ed. R.C.A. Thompson, J.A. Reynoldson, and A.J. Lybery. Wallingford, UK: CAB International, p. 367.

Olson, M.E., T.A. McAllister, L. Deselliers, D.W. Morck, A.G. Buret, K.J. Cheng, and H. Ceri. 1995. The effect of giardiasis on production in a ruminant model. *American Journal of Veterinary Research* 56:1470–1474.

Olson, M.E., D.W. Morck, and H. Ceri. 1996. The efficacy of a *Giardia lamblia* vaccine in kittens. *Canadian Journal of Veterinary Research* 60:249–256.

Olson, M.E., C. Thorlakson, L.P. Deselliers, T.A. McAllister, and D. W. Morck. 1997a. *Giardia* and *Cryptosporidium* in Canadian farm animals. *Veterinary Parasitology* 68:375–381.

Olson, M.E., D.W. Morck, and H. Ceri. 1997b. The efficacy of a *Giardia* vaccine in puppies. *Canadian Veterinary Journal* 38:777–779.

Olson, M.E., N.J. Guselle, R. O'Handley, T.A. McAllister, M.D. Jelinski, and D.W. Morck. 1997c. *Giardia* and *Cryptosporidium* in British Columbia dairy calves. *Canadian Veterinary Journal* 38:703–706.

Olson, M.E., P.D. Roach, M. Stabler, and W. Chan. 1997d. *Giardia* in ringed seals (*Phoca hispida*) in the western arctic. *Journal of Wildlife Diseases* 58:384–388.

Olson, M.E., H. Ceri, and D.W. Morck. 2000. *Giardia* vaccination. *Parasitology Today* 16:212–217.

Olson, M.E., J. Goh, M. Phillips, N. Guselle, and T.A. McAllister 1999. *Giardia* cysts and *Cryptosporidium* oocyst survival in water, soil and cattle feces. *Journal of Environmental Quality* 28:1991–1996.

Oxberry, M.F., R.C.A. Thompson, and J.A. Reynoldson. 1994. Evaluation of the effect of albendazole and metronidazole on the ultrastructure of *Giardia duodenalis, Trichomonas vaginalis* and *Spironucleus muris* using transmission electron microscopy. *International Journal of Parasitology* 24:695–703.

Pacha, R.E., G.W. Clark, and E.A. Williams. 1985. Occurrence of *Campylobacter jejuni* and *Giardia* species in muskrat. *Applied and Environmental Microbiology* 50:177–178.

Pacha, R.E., G.W. Clark, E.A. Williams, A.M. Carter, J.J. Scheffelmaier, and P. Debusschere. 1987. Small rodents and other mammals associated with mountain meadows as reservoirs of *Giardia* and *Campylobacter. Applied and Environmental Microbiology* 53:1574–1579.

Pakes, S.P. 1974. Protozoal diseases. In *The biology of the laboratory rabbit.* Ed. S.H. Weisbroth, R.E. Flatt, and A.L. Kraus. New York: Academic Press, pp. 263–286.

Patton S.A., and R. Rabinowitz. 1994. Parasites of wild *Fedidae* in Thailand. A coprological survey. *Journal of Wildlife Diseases* 30:72–475.

Peisert, W., A. Taborski, Z. Pawlowski, A. Karlewiczow, and M. Zdun. 1985. *Giardia* infection in animals in Poznan zoo. *Veterinary Parasitology* 13:183–186.

Perlmutter, D.H., A.M. Leichtner, H. Goldman, and H.S. Winter. 1985. Chronic diarrhea associated with hypogammaglobulinemia and enteropathy in infants and children. *Digestive Diseases and Science* 30:1149–1155.

Reardon, L.V., and B.F. Rininger. 1968. A survey of parasites in laboratory primates. *Laboratory Animal Care* 18:577–580.

Rendtorff, R.C. 1954. The experimental transmission of human intestinal protozoan parasites. *Giardia lamblia* cysts given in capsules. *American Journal of Hygiene* 60:327–338.

Roach, P.D., M.E. Olson, G. Whitley, and P.M. Wallis. 1993. Waterborne *Giardia* cysts and *Cryptosporidium* oocysts in Yukon, Canada. *Applied and Environmental Microbiology* 59:67–73.

Shelton, G.C. 1954. Giardiasis in the chinchilla. *American Journal of Veterinary Research* 15:71–78.

Smith P.D. 1984. Human immune responses to *G. lambli.* In *Giardia and giardiasis.* Ed. S.L. Erlandsen and E.A. Meyer. New York: Plenum Press, pp. 201–218.

Sogin, M.L., J.H. Gunderson, H.J. Elwood, R.A. Alonso, and D.A. Peattie. 1989. Phylogenetic meaning of the Kingdom concept: An unusual ribosomal RNA from *Giardia lamblia. Science* 243:75–77.

Stevens, D.P., D.M. Frank, and A.F. Mahmond. 1978. Thymus dependency of host resistance to *Giardia muris* infection: Studies in nude mice. *Journal of Immunology* 120:680–682.

Stranden, A.M., J. Eckert, and P. Kohler. 1990. Electrophoretic characterization of *Giardia* isolated from humans, cattle, sheep, and a dog in Switzerland. *The Journal of Parasitology* 76:660–668.

Swabby, K.D., C.P. Hibler, and N. WEgrzyn. 1988. Infection of Mongolian gerbils with *Giardia* from human and animal species. In *Advances in* Giardia *research.* Ed. P.M. Wallis and B.R. Hammond. Calgary: University of Calgary Press, pp. 75–77.

Sykes, J.T., and M.T. Fox. 1989. Patterns of infection with *Giardia* in dogs in London. *Transactions of the Royal Society of Tropical Medicine and Hygiene* 83:239–240.

Taylor, M.A., J. Catchpole, R.N. Marshall, and J. Green. 1993. Giardiasis in lambs at pasture. *Veterinary Record* 133:131–133.

Thompson, R.C.A., and B.P. Melani. 1993. Molecular variation in *Giardia* and its implications. *Acta Tropica* 53:167–184.

Thompson, R.C.A., B.P. Meloni, and A.J. Lymbery. 1988. Humans and cats have genetically identical forms of *Giardia:* Evidence of a zoonotic relationship. *Medical Journal of Australia* 148:207–209.

Thompson, R.C.A., J.A. Reynoldson, A.H.W. Mendis. 1993. *Giardia* and giardiasis. *Advances in Parasitology* 32:71–160.

Thompson, R.C.A., R.M. Hopkins, and W.L. Homan. 2000. Nomenclature and genetic groupings of *Giardia* infecting mammals. *Parasitology Today* 16:210–213.

Tonks, M.C., T.J. Brown, and G. Ionas. 1991. *Giardia* infection of cats and dogs in New Zealand. *New Zealand Veterinary Journal* 39:33–34.

Townson, S.M., H. Laqua, P. Upcroft, P.F.L. Boreham, and J.A. Upcroft. 1992. Induction of metronidazole and furazolidone resistance in *Giardia. Transactions of the Royal Society of Tropical Medicine and Hygiene* 86:521–522.

Upcroft, J.A., and P. Upcroft. 1993. Drug resistance and *Giardia. Parasitology Today* 9:187–190.

Upcroft, J.A., P.A. McDonnell, A.N. Gallagher, N. Chen, and P. Upcroft. 1997. Lethal *Giardia* from a wild caught sulphur-crested cockatoo (*Cacatua galerita*) established in vitro chronically infects mice. *Parasitology* 114:407–412.

Upcroft, P., R. Mitchell, and P.F.L. Boreham. 1990. DNA fingerprinting of the intestinal parasite *Giardia duodenalis* with the M13 phase genome. *International Journal of Parasitology* 20:319–323.

US Public Health Service. 1979. Giardiasis in apes and zoo attendants, Kansas City, Missouri. In *CDC Veterinary public health notes.* Atlanta: Public Health Service, US Department of Health, Education and Welfare, pp. 7–8.

Van Keulen, H., D. E. Feely, P. T. Macechko, E. L. Jarroll, and S. L. Erlandsen. 1998. The sequence of Giardia small subunit rRNA shows that voles and muskrats are parasitized by a unique species *Giardia microti. The Journal of Parasitology* 84:294–300.

Vetterling, J.M. 1976. Protozoan Parasites. In *The biology of the guinea pig.* Ed. J.E. Wagner and P.M. Manning. New York: Academic Press, pp. 171–172.

Wagner, J.E. 1987. Parasitic diseases. In *Laboratory hamsters.* Ed. G.L. van Hoosier and C.W. McPherson. New York: Academic Press, pp. 135–156.

Wallis, P.M. 1994. Abiotic transmission—Is water really significant? In Giardia: *From molecules to disease.* Ed. R.C.A. Thompson and J.A. Lymbery. Wallingford, UK: CAB International, pp. 99–122.

Wallis, P.M., J.M. Buchanan-Mappin, G.M. Faubert, and M. Belosevic. 1984. Reservoirs of *Giardia* in southwestern Alberta. *Journal of Wildlife Diseases* 20:279–283.

Wallis, P.M., R.M. Zammuto, and J.M. Buchanan-Mappin. 1986. Cysts of *Giardia* and surface waters in southwestern Alberta. *Journal of Wildlife Diseases* 22:115–118.

Wallis, P.M., W.J. Robertson, P.D. Roach, and M.J. Wallis. 1993. *Giardia* and *Cryptosporidium* in Canadian water supplies. In *Disinfection dilemma: Microbiological control vs by-products.* Ed. W.J. Robertson, R. Tobin, K. Kjartanson. Proceedings of the 5th National Conference on Drinking Water, Winnipeg, 1992. Washington, DC: American Public Health Association, pp. 165–185.

Wallis, P.M., S.L. Erlanson, J.L. Isaac-Renton, M.E. Olson, W.J. Robertson, and H. VanKeulen. 1996. Prevalence of *Giardia* cysts and *Cryptosporidium* oocysts and characterization of *Giardia* spp. isolated from drinking water in Canada. *Applied and Environmental Microbiology* 62:2789–2797.

Weniger, B.G., M.J. Blaser, J. Gedrose, E.C. Lippy, and D.D. Juranek. 1983. An outbreak of waterborne giardiasis associated with heavy water runoff due to warm weather and volcanic ashfall. *American Journal of Public Health* 73:868–872.

Wetzel, H. 1985. Use of albendazole in pregnant cows. Field studies on its safety in usage. *Zentralblatt fuer Veterinaermedizin* 32:375–394.

Wolfe, M.S. 1992. Giardiasis. *Clinical Microbiological Reviews* 5:93–100.

Woo, P.T.K. 1984. Evidence for animal reservoirs and transmission of *Giardia* infection between animal species. In *Giardia and Giardiasis*. Ed. S.L. Erlandsen and E.A. Meyers. New York: Plenum, pp. 341–364.

Woo, P.T.K., and W.B. Patterson. 1986. *Giardia lamblia* in children in day-care centres in southern Ontario, Canada and susceptability of animals to *G. lamblia*. *Transactions of the Royal Society of Tropical Medicine and Hygiene* 80:56–59.

World Health Organization. 1979. Parasitic zoonoses. Report of a WHO Expert Committee with the Participation of FAO Technical Report Series No. 637. Geneva: World Health Organization.

Wright, S.G., A.M. Tomkins, and D.S. Ridley. 1977. Giardiasis: Clinical and therapeutic aspects. *Gut* 18:343–350.

Xiao, L. 1994. *Giardia* infection in farm animals. *Parasitology Today* 10:436–438.

Xiao, L., and R.P Herd. 1994. Epidemology of equine *Cryptosporidium* and *Giardia* infections. *Equine Veterinary Journal* 26:14–17.

———. 1996. Efficacy of albendazole and fenbendazole against *Giardia* infection in cattle. *Veterinary Parasitology* 61:165–170.

Xiao, L., R.P. Herd, and D.M. Rings. 1993. Infection patterns of *Cryptosporidium* and *Giardia* in calves. *Veterinary Parasitology* 51:41–48.

Xiao, L., R.P. Herd, and G.L. Bowman. 1994a. Prevalence of *Cryptosporidium* and *Giardia* infections on two Ohio farms with different management systems. *Veterinary Parasitology* 52:331–336.

Xiao, L., R.P. Herd, and K.E. McClure. 1994b. Periparturient rise in the excretion of *Giardia* sp. cysts and *Cryptosporidium parvum* oocysts as a source of infection for lambs. *The Journal of Parasitology* 80:55–59.

Yanke, S.J., H. Ceri, T.A. McAllister, D.W. Morck, and M.E. Olson. 1998. Serum immune response to *Giardia duodenalis* in experimentally infected lambs. *Veterinary Parasitology* 75:9–19.

Zajac, A.M. 1992. Giardiasis. *The Compendium on Continuing Education for the Practicing Veterinarians* 14:604–611.

CYCLOSPORA, EIMERIA, ISOSPORA, AND CRYPTOSPORIDIUM SPP.

DONALD W. DUSZYNSKI AND STEVE J. UPTON

INTRODUCTION. Coccidia are exceptionally common protist parasites of both vertebrates and, to a lesser extent, invertebrates. Every vertebrate species that ever has been examined intensively, over a broad geographic range, has been found to have at least one coccidian species unique to it and may have as many as five, ten, or more species. They also may have addi-tional coccidia shared with close relatives (congenerics, sometimes confamilials) and/or with sympatrics. The history of the development of our knowledge about coccidian parasites of wild mammals is long and tangled and has been reviewed by Levine (1973a,b), Joyner (1985), and Long and Joyner (1996). Suffice it to say that the coccidia were among the very first protozoans ever visualized when Antonie van Leeuwenhoek saw what surely were the oocysts of *Eimeria stiedai* in the bile of a rabbit in 1674 (see Wenyon 1926; Dobell 1932).

In this review, we limit our coverage to the coccidia of wild mammals that have direct (homoxenous) life cycles; reproduce both asexually (merogony) and sexually (gamogony) within the epithelial or endothelial cells of the gastrointestinal tract or related structures (e.g., bile duct, renal tubular epithelium, etc.) of their host; and produce as an end product, a resistant propagule, the oocyst, which leaves the host, usually via the feces. By far, the majority of coccidia with these characteristics are placed taxonomically into four genera contained in two families: Eimeriidae (*Cyclospora, Eimeria, Isospora*) and Cryptosporidiidae (*Cryptosporidium*). The taxonomy of the coccidia is reviewed below.

Before proceeding, we must distinguish between *infection* by coccidia and *coccidiosis*. Most wild mammals examined are found to be infected with coccidian parasites at one or more times during their life, and some (e.g, wild rabbits, some squirrels) may be infected during their entire lives with several species that constantly cycle through them. Given this ubiquitous nature of the coccidia, it is likely that most probably are harmless under natural, wild conditions. It is only when hosts are brought together in groups, enhancing transmission via their rapid, direct life cycles, that some species cause disease. As a result, coccidiosis is recognized as a major health hazard only during intensive husbandry of domestic animals, in wild animals that are in captivity (i.e., zoos, breeding or research facilities), in wild animal populations when habitat is lost and crowding occurs, or in wild animal species that have great reproductive potential and are protected by laws so that their populations increase inordinately (e.g., kangaroos in Australia); the latter two conditions are the result of human intervention or perturbation.

By searching the relevant literature, we can gain a sense of the prevalence of this disease (coccidiosis) in wild mammals. For those who study disease processes, one of the logical outlets to publish their findings is the *Journal of Wildlife Diseases,* which started publication in 1965. From 1965 to 1996, the *JournaL of Wildlife Diseases* published 2830 articles, abstracts, and case reports on wildlife diseases and > 50 lengthy articles as part of their microfiche series. During these 32 years, 27–117 articles were published each year (mean = 90 articles/year). In 5 years (1965, 1968, 1972, 1976, 1982) no articles appeared on coccidia, and in 7 additional years (1971, 1978, 1979, 1981, 1987, 1989, 1995) no articles mentioned coccidia in mammals; in all years, only 76 articles (2.7%) reported coccidia in wild animals, but only 39 (1.3%) covered topics dealing with mammalian infections with coccidia, 32 with *Eimeria* and *Isospora* spp., and 7 with *Cryptosporidium* spp.

Of the 32 articles addressing *Eimeria* and/or *Isospora* infections in mammals, 16 were simple surveys from bison (2), coyotes (2), deer (1), foxes (2), gophers (1), monkeys (1), mouflons (1), opossums (2), and rabbits (4); 9 were descriptions/redescriptions of oocysts; 4 documented experimental transmission of oocysts in deer (2), pigs (1), and squirrels (1); and only 3 reported pathological processes: 1 in wild rabbits (death during captivity, cause unknown), another in a camel (death in a zoo animal with clinical intestinal coccidiosis), and the third in two captive wombats (pathology demonstrated histologically during heavy infection in juvenile animals; one animal died, see below).

Of the seven articles that identified *Cryptosporidium* infections in deer, foxes, opossums (experimental infection), primates, raccoons, rabbits, rodents (voles), and ruminants, only Heuschele et al. (1986) suggested a cause and effect relationship between the presence of *Cryptosporidium* sp. and clinical disease (diarrhea) in 52 of 183 (28%) neonatal captive ruminants and in 2 of 86 (2%) captive primates. Thus, it seems clear that pathogenicity of coccidian parasites in wild mammals may be overestimated, and coccidiosis appears, in most cases, to be a disease due to human intervention.

CLASSIFICATION. The protistan phylum Apicomplexa Levine, 1970 comprises a large, heterogeneous assemblage of obligate, intracellular parasites consisting of five major groups: coccidia, gregarines haemogregarines, piroplasms, and malarial organisms. Members of this phylum are characterized further by having an apical complex typically composed of one or more polar rings, rhoptries, micronemes, and often a conoid. Subpellicular microtubules and micropores are also a common feature of this group. Three classes currently are recognized, based primarily on the presence and structure of a cone-shaped organelle, the conoid, located within the anterior end of one or more stages of the organism. The coccidia are placed in the class Conoidasida (Levine 1988), which is typified by the presence of a complete conoid consisting of a hollow, truncate cone.

The Conoidasida has two subclasses, Gregarinasina Dufour, 1828 and Coccidiasina Leukart, 1879. The gregarines are large, are generally homoxenous, and occur commonly in the digestive tract or body cavity of invertebrates or lower chordates; mature gamonts of most species are extracellular, with their apical ends often modified into attachment organelles called mucrons or epimerites. The coccidia have gamonts that usually develop intracellularly. A mucron or epimerite is lacking and, though some species are found in inverte-

brates, most tend to infect vertebrates. Life cycles may be either homoxenous or heteroxenous.

Four orders within the coccidia are distinguished by the presence or absence of various sexual and asexual stages. The order Eucoccidiorida (Léger and Duboscq 1910) is the largest, and members all possess merogony, gamogony, and sporogony. Suborders are recognized by the number of microgametes produced and whether or not gametes associate in syzygy prior to fertilization. The suborder Eimeriorina (Léger 1911) is typified by coccidia that lack syzygy, produce microgametocytes with many flagellated, motile microgametes, and possess a stationary rather than motile zygote. Two families, the Eimeriidae (Minchin 1903) and Cryptosporidiidae (Léger 1911), contain members that often parasitize enteric sites in mammals.

Eimeriids are homoxenous or facultatively heteroxenous, with merogony, gamogony, and formation of oocysts occurring within the same host. Oocysts leave the host via the feces and are unsporulated; sporogony occurs outside the host. The most speciose genus is *Eimeria* Schneider, 1875, which contains > 1700 named species. The genus *Isospora* Schneider, 1881 also is well represented with > 350 species. The genus *Cyclospora* Schneider, 1881 has fewer than 20 named species but has generated significant interest in recent years because at least 1 species appears to be a common parasite of humans. The three genera are distinguished by the structure of their sporulated oocysts: those of *Eimeria* spp. possess four sporocysts, each with two sporozoites (Fig. 16.8, c-c[1]); those of *Cyclospora* possess two sporocysts, each with two sporozoites (Fig. 16.8, a-a[1]); and those of *Isospora* spp. have two sporocysts, each with four sporozoites (Fig. 16.8, d-d[1]).

Cryptosporidids contain a single genus, *Cryptosporidium*. All known species are homoxenous, and development occurs just under the host cell membrane rather than deep within it. Thus, the parasites appear, at first, to develop extracellularly on the lumenal surface of host cells. All developmental stages possess a unique feeder organelle, at the interface between parasite and host cell. This organelle appears to consist of a desmosome-like junction and ribosomal-studded foldings of the parasite cytoplasm. Their microgametes are unusual among coccidia because they lack flagella. Oocysts sporulate endogenously, but when sporulated, they lack sporocysts and contain four naked sporozoites (Fig. 16.8, b-b[1]).

Since the oocyst is the stage that leaves the host, usually in the feces, it is the structure most readily available to the practitioner who wants to identify the coccidian species, in most cases without having to kill the host. Thus, about 98% of the coccidian species known from mammals are characterized only from this one life-cycle stage, the sporulated oocyst. Although Levine (1962) once calculated there could be at least 2,654,736 structurally different sporulated oocysts (and hence structurally different species) in the *Eimeria* alone, in reality it doesn't work that way. In some

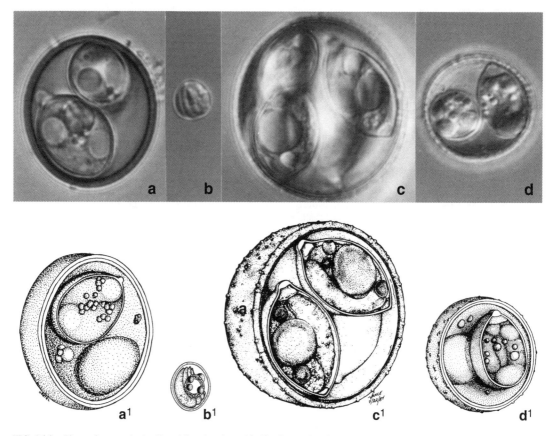

FIG. 16.8—Photomicrographs (a–d) and line drawings (a¹–d¹) of sporulated oocysts of the four genera discussed in this chapter. (**a, a¹**) *Cyclospora angimuriensis* Ford, Duszynski & McAllister, 1990 from *Chaetodipus hispidus.*(**b, b¹**) *Cryptosporidium parvum* Tyzzer, 1912 from humans. (**c, c¹**) *Eimeria parastiedica* Duszynski, 1985 from *Neurotrichus gibbsi.* (**d, d¹**) *Isospora brevicauda* Hertel & Duszynski, 1987 from *Blarina brevicauda.* Figures were chosen to show the variability in size and shape (*C. parvum,* for example, is ~7.0 (μm long) of oocysts within and between the two families of coccidia discussed in this chapter and some of the key structural features of sporulated oocysts noted in Figure 16.9 a–d.

cases, oocysts from unrelated host species look very nearly identical in size and structure and cannot be reliably differentiated by morphology and size alone (Joyner 1982). In other instances, a single coccidian species may produce oocysts that vary greatly in size (40%) and appearance (Duszynski 1971; Parker and Duszynski 1986; Gardner and Duszynski 1990). In truth, sporulated oocysts of *Eimeria, Isospora,* and *Cyclospora* have a limited number of structural characters, and those of *Cryptosporidium* even fewer. Unfortunately, the fewer the number of morphological characteristics, the more bothersome the species problem becomes, and within the Eimeriidae and Cryptosporidiidae, it is difficult to delimit what is a species to everyone's satisfaction. Thus, if the taxonomy of these groups is to be useful for higher level examination (systematic, phylogenetic, zoogeographic, host specificity, and other studies), the *taxonomic procedure* followed in collecting oocysts and documenting new species should be consistent and should follow the intent, if not the letter, of the International Code of Zoological Nomenclature (Ride et al. 1985); after all, the value of any classification scheme, from the species to all higher taxonomic categories, rests on the foundation of the species description.

Lom and Arthur (1989) recognized a serious deficiency in the way myxosporean species were described, and in an attempt to standardize the effort of workers in the field, they published "A Guideline for the Preparation of Species Descriptions in Myxosporea." They pointed out the many difficulties created for later workers by published descriptions of poor quality and emphasized that such practice, "ridicules taxonomic research in this group in the eyes of other parasitologists." Similarly, Duszynski and Wilber (1997) emphasized greater precision in the description of new coccidian species when only the sporulated oocyst was available and tried to set minimal guidelines for proper description of coccidian oocysts.

LABORATORY METHODS

Saving and Storing Oocysts. Oocysts must be kept properly to remain viable so that their structural integrity remains intact until they are studied. Oocysts from most mammalian hosts keep best when fresh feces are placed into 2%–2.5% aqueous (w/v) potassium dichromate ($K_2Cr_2O_7$) in a 1:5 ratio of feces to $K_2Cr_2O_7$ (by volume). In field collections, either snap-cap or screw-cap 16–25-ml vials work well, but one should not fill the vial all the way to the top; leave a layer of air between the top of the feces-dichromate mixture and the cap to allow the oocysts some atmospheric oxygen. Unfortunately, other solutions for feces [e.g., 2% (v/v) aqueous sulfuric acid (see Wash et al. 1985) or common laboratory fixatives for oocysts (see Duszynski and Gardner 1991)] are unsatisfactory either for keeping oocysts viable or for preserving them as types.

Handling and Processing Oocysts. Upon return to the laboratory, the fecal-dichromate mixture should be placed into a petri dish, the fecal pellets broken, and the fecal material spread out in the dish and covered (Duszynski and Conder 1977). The petri dishes generally should be maintained at room temperature (20°C–23° C) 7–10 days, which will allow any oocysts present to sporulate. It has been our experience that fecal-dichromate mixtures should not be refrigerated prior to the sporulation process as this seems to interfere with sporulation success. In most species, the mixture can be washed from the petri dish with clean 2% $K_2Cr_2O_7$ into a screw-cap jar (baby food jars work well) after ~7–10 days, then put into a standard refrigerator (4°C–7° C) until examination. Oocysts processed in this way can remain viable, or at least structurally intact, in the refrigerator 3–4 years for some species. However, it is probably best to study and document the structure of sporulated oocysts as soon as possible after they are sporulated.

Sporulated oocysts are best separated from the dichromate-fecal mixture by suspending an aliquot (1–3 ml) from the sample in 12–14 ml of modified Sheather's (Sheather 1923) sugar flotation solution (500 g sucrose, 350 ml tap water, 5 ml phenol) via centrifugation (5 minutes at 1500 rpm [= 225 g]). It is best to use only number 1, 18 mm^2, coverslips on top of the 15-ml centrifuge tubes (those with a smooth, beaded edge work best) as this reduces the surface area that needs to be scanned for oocysts. After centrifugation, lift the coverglass carefully from the centrifuge tube, place onto a glass slide, and set aside for 5–10 minutes; this allows the sugar along the edges of the coverglass to harden and minimizes movement of the oocysts during observation, measurement, and photography. The coverglass should be scanned systematically (100–400X) until oocysts are located. Measuring and detailing the structure of sporulated oocysts should always be done using an oil immersion objective (Neofluar and Nomarski optics are both useful). Apochromatic lenses are superior to achromats, and the higher the numerical aperture on the objective lens, the more accurate will be the measurements.

Species Differentiation. We suggest that those interested in making accurate identifications of oocysts found in the feces of wild mammals carefully follow the guidelines proposed by Duszynski and Wilber (1997). First, make sure that the host has been reliably identified and that as much ecological information as possible is noted. Whenever possible, deposit the actual host specimen from which the new species was described (= symbiotype; see Frey et al. 1992 and Brooks 1993) into an appropriate, accredited museum. Next, use only sporulated oocysts for mensural data, being careful to identify all of the quantitative and qualitative features of the oocysts and sporocysts (Fig. 16.9, a-d). Finally, be sure that the published manuscript includes at least one photomicrograph of a sporulated oocyst and the accredited museum accession number, in addition to the composite line drawing.

Those who describe new coccidian species based only on the structure of sporulated oocysts should be aware that at least some host groups (e.g., ground squirrels) have coccidia that are not always strictly host specific (Duszynski 1986; Wilber et al. 1998). In addition, many species (e.g., *E. nieschulzi, E. arizonensis*) occur naturally over large geographic ranges especially when hosts (e.g., *Rattus*) are introduced from continent to continent through human activities or when individuals in a specious host genus (e.g., *Peromyscus*) have contiguous ranges across a continent. Thus, finding oocysts in a new host species or new geographic locality may not be sufficient to warrant creation of a new species.

Archiving Oocysts and Host Specimens. The cornerstone of taxonomy is the type specimen, which is intended to be unchanging and objective, whereas the limits of the nominal species are recognized to be subjective and transient. The type specimen serves as the anchor for the name, and to some extent, it *is* the name (Mayr et al. 1953). Without the type specimen, some contend there is no "species." Coccidia present problems when it comes to collecting type specimens for two major reasons: (1) their endogenous stages are intracellular, transient, difficult to collect, and impossible to identify under field conditions; and (2) no standardized methods have been developed to permanently preserve oocysts. Unlike other parasites (arthropods, helminths) that stay on/in the host for lengthy periods and easily can be preserved and deposited into museums for later retrieval, coccidian oocysts preserve poorly (Duszynski and Gardner 1991). Thus, historically, those who have described new coccidian species have done so based on quantitative and qualitative observations of the oocyst, on the host species and its locality, and by using a drawing as the type specimen. Although it may seem obvious that drawings are cartoons subject to author interpretation, this tradition

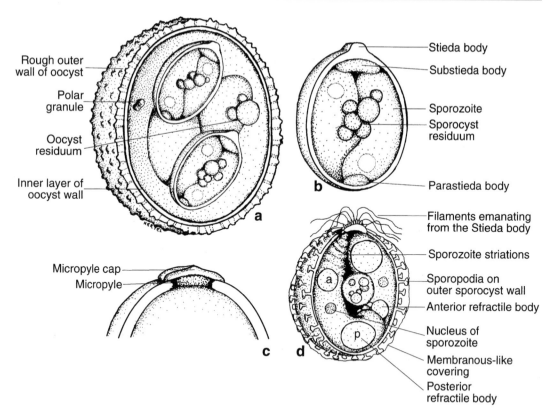

FIG. 16.9—Line drawings of the parts of (hypothetical) sporulated oocysts/sporocysts (*Cyclospora, Cryptosporidium, Eimeria, Isospora*). (a) A completely sporulated oocyst of an *Eimeria* sp. showing major structural features with four sporocysts, each with two sporozoites. (b) A sporulated sporocyst of an *Eimeria* sp. showing the major structural features, including two sporozoites. (c) The end of an oocyst showing micropyle and micropyle cap present in some oocysts, especially those of ruminants. (d) Another sporulated sporocyst showing a variety of structural features, some of which may be present on the sporocysts of different coccidia species.

among coccidian taxonomists has, unfortunately, persisted to the present. Bandoni and Duszynski (1988) criticized the lack of a type specimen tradition in coccidian systematic treatments and suggested that, at the very least, phototypes be deposited in accredited museums. The concept of phototypes, originally proposed by Kellerman (1912, see Frizzell 1933) was not new, but it has taken a long time for coccidian taxonomists to accept it.

Similarly, the traditional concept is that the coccidia are usually host specific. However, if one looks at many of the original descriptions of coccidia, the hosts are either haphazardly or incidently identified, some only by common names. This historical omission undermines the entire concept of host specificity. In an attempt to begin to correct the inadequacy of linking the name of a new coccidian species to an actual host species, Frey et al. (1992) suggested that parasitologists deposit specimens (symbiotypes) of hosts into museums from which type specimens of new parasite species are collected and identified. They correctly pointed out that whether one emphasizes microevolutionary (e.g., Price 1980) or macroevolutionary (e.g., Brooks and McLennan 1993) aspects of parasite evolutionary biology, much of the context of parasite evolution involves the hosts in which they live. Brooks (1993) extended the symbiotype concept by suggesting that parasitologists deposit voucher specimens of all host species examined in the course of survey or inventory studies, including purely ecological field studies. His argument, especially that documenting the case of our lack of knowledge about the parasites of "*Rana pipiens*," is compelling (no hosts deposited, numerous parasite species described, and now the host "species" is recognized as a clade of 27 or more extant and recently extinct species). Thus, the deposition of symbiotype host specimens into accredited museums is central to all parasitology if we are to develop a meaningful conceptual framework for our discipline.

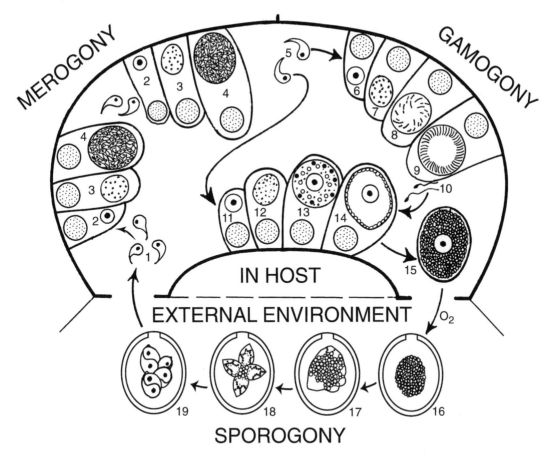

FIG. 16.10—Line drawing showing the major steps in the endogenous and exogenous development of a "typical" coccidia life cycle (*Cyclospora, Eimeria, Isospora;* somewhat modified in *Cryptosporidium,* see text and Fig. 16.11). (**1**) Sporozoites released from sporocysts/oocysts. (**2**) Sporozoite penetrates host enterocyte and rounds up. (**3**) Mitotic nuclear division in the meront. (**4**) Merozoite formation. (**5**) Last generation of merozoites penetrate other enterocytes to begin gamogony. (**6**) Merozoite rounds up in the first stage of developing into a microgametocyte. (**7**) Mitosis. (**8**) Microgametogenesis. (**9**) Mature microgametocyte with fully formed microgametes around the periphery. (**10**) Flagellated microgametes leave host enterocyte to penetrate another enterocyte with a fully developed macrogamete. (**11**) Merozoite rounds up in the first stage of developing into a macrogametocyte. (**12**) Early macrogamont. (**13**) Production of wall-forming bodies in the developing macrogamete. (**14**) Mature macrogamete. (**15**) After fertilization occurs and the 2N condition is restored, the unsporulated oocyst leaves the host enterocyte and enters the lumen of the gut. (**16**) Unsporulated oocyst, containing the sporoplasm of the next generation, leaves the host in the feces. (**17**) Meiosis takes place, and the sporocysts begin to form. (**18**) The pyramid stage of sporocyst development. (**19**) After the last mitotic division of the nuclei, sporozoite formation within each sporocyst is completed, resulting in the sporulated oocyst, the transmission propagule that is infective to the next host.

FAMILY EIMERIIDAE

Life History. Known life cycles of eimerian and isosporan species from mammals are all homoxenous and all go through three developmental stages: merogony (asexual)→gamogony (sexual)→sporogony (spore formation). The first two stages occur within the epithelial or endothelial cells of the gastrointestinal tract or related structures (e.g., bile duct) of the host. The end product of gamogony, which results from fertilization, is a resistant oocyst, the only stage in the cycle to leave the host, usually via the feces. The details of this developmental cycle follow (see Fig. 16.10).

SPORULATED OOCYST. When ingested by an appropriate host (Fig. 16.10, nos. 19–1), the sporozoites within the sporocysts within the oocyst must first excyst before infection can proceed. If the oocyst has a micropyle and micropyle cap, these structures are somehow altered and made permeable, presumably by digestive processes of the stomach and/or upper digestive tract (Wang 1982). If the oocyst does not have a micropyle, then the oocyst wall must be breached or broken. This process has been documented in chickens, where the crop and ventriculus rupture oocysts and free sporocysts, but in mammals it apparently is a combination of digestive and proteolytic enzymes that accomplishes this task (Kheysin 1967). The key to excystation is getting the sporocysts into contact with pancreatic enzymes, trypsin, bile, and/or bile salts (Kheysin 1967; Wang 1982).

EXCYSTATION OF SPOROZOITES. The details of excystation from sporocysts have been studied in vitro, but only in relatively few species when compared to the total number of described species from mammals (Box et al. 1980; Duszynski et al. 1981). Sporozoites excyst from sporocysts by two distinctly different methods, each related to sporocyst structure (presence or absence of a Stieda body). In *Eimeria* and *Isospora* spp. with sporocysts and Stieda bodies, the Stieda body disappears when exposed to digestive enzymes, the sub-Stieda body, if present, either pops out of the sporocyst or is digested in situ, and the sporozoites exit the sporocyst through a hole created by dissolution of these structures. Those species that possess a sub-Stieda body all excyst quite rapidly, whereas those with only a Stieda body excyst more slowly (for reveiws see Speer and Duszynski 1975; Speer et al. 1976; Duszynski et al. 1977). In species in which the sporocyst lacks a Stieda body, the sporocyst wall consists of four curved plates; digestive enzymes act upon the junction between two apposing plates, causing collapse of the sporocyst during which sporozoites are released randomly (Speer et al. 1973, 1976; Box et al. 1980). This method of excystation has been seen in *Isospora* spp. from canids (Speer et al. 1973), felids (Duszynski and Speer 1976), and primates (Duszynski and File 1974; Duszynski and Speer 1976), as well as in *Toxoplasma gondii* from cats (Christie et al. 1978) and *Sarcocystis* sp. from birds (Box et al. 1980). Unfortunately, it is not yet known whether those *Eimeria* spp. with sporocysts that lack Stieda bodies excyst in a similar manner.

PENETRATION OF HOST CELLS. Once the sporozoites are free within the intestinal milieu (Fig. 16.10, no. 1) they must penetrate a host cell to continue development. This is where the organelles of the apical complex (rhoptries, conoid, micronemes, etc.) come into play. Host cell invasion involves a sequential series of complicated steps that include recognition of and attachment to host cell surface components, formation of a tight moving junction that progressively envelops the sporozoite, discharge of microneme and rhoptry contents to facilitate entry into the host cell, formation and maintenance of a parasitophorous vacuole membrane, resealing the host cell membrane, and exocytosis of dense granules (for reviews see Chobotar and Scholtyseck 1982; Doran 1982; Sam-Yellowe 1996). Once safely inside its parasitophorous vacuole within

the host cell, the sporozoite is ready to initiate merogony (asexual multiple fission).

MEROGONY. Before beginning nuclear division, the sporozoite usually develops into a spheroid stage, the uninuclear meront (Fig. 16.10, no. 2). As the meront grows, its nucleus divides (Fig. 16.10, no. 3). Eventually, cytokinesis occurs, forming merozoites (Fig. 16.10, no. 4), the number of which corresponds to the number of nuclei in the mature meront. In some species, nuclear division occurs before the spheroid stage develops, and the multinucleate meront maintains its elongate, sporozoite-like shape (Chobotar and Scholtyseck 1982). As few as two or as many as 100,000 merozoites can be formed by each sporozoite, depending upon the species (Kheysin 1967). Once the merozoites are mature, they leave their host cell, killing it in the process. Each merozoite then seeks to penetrate a new epithelial cell within which to undergo another merogonous process (Fig. 16.10, repeat nos. 2-4). The general consensus is that each eimerian and isosporan species has a genetically programmed, specific number of merogonous generations characteristic for that species. For example, *Eimeria separata* from *Rattus* and *E. bovis* from *Bos* each have two merogonous generations (Roudabush 1937; Hammond et al. 1963), whereas *E. nieschulzi,* also from *Rattus,* and *E. utahensis* from *Dipodomys* have four merogonous stages (Marquardt 1966; Ernst and Chobotar 1978). Whatever the number, these developmental stages result in tremendous biological magnification of the parasite.

GAMOGONY. After a specific number of merogonous generations, the merozoites (Fig. 16.10, no. 5) that enter host cells develop not into additional meronts, but into gamonts. Most of the last generation merozoites develop into macrogametocytes (macrogamonts) to form uninucleate macrogametes (Fig. 16.10, nos. 11-14). The other last generation merozoites develop into microgametocytes, each of which will undergo multiple fission to produce many motile, biflagellated microgametes (Fig. 16.10, nos. 6-9). These leave the cells in which they developed (Fig. 16.10, no. 10) and seek out and penetrate cells that have a mature macrogamete within (Fig. 16.10, no. 14), and fertilization occurs. The regulatory mechanisms that control whether a merozoite will transform into a macro- or microgamont, the ability of microgametes to distinguish and select cells with developed macrogametes, and the actual fertilization process, which happens very quickly, are all areas that warrant further study.

UNSPORULATED OOCYST. As development continues, two types of wall-forming bodies develop within the cytoplasm of the macrogamont (Scholtyseck 1973). After fertilization, a delicate fertilization membrane is formed, and the wall-forming bodies migrate toward and then fuse with the surface membranes of the zygote (Kheysin 1967). Finally, a resistant oocyst wall composed of two to four layers is formed (Speer et al. 1979;

Duszynski et al. 1981), endogenous development is completed, and it is time for the oocyst to leave the host (Fig. 16.10, no. 15). In most *Eimeria* and *Isospora* spp., the oocysts are discharged from their host in an undeveloped (unsporulated) state (Fig. 16.10, no. 16). The time period between when the host first ingested a sporulated oocyst and when the first unsporulated oocysts leave the host in its feces is called the prepatent period. The length of time that oocysts are passed in the host's feces is termed the patent period. These time intervals vary greatly between coccidian species and are dependent, in part, on parasite genome, the size of the inoculating dose, the number of endogenous stages, depth within the tissues where gamogony and fertilization was initiated, concurrent infections with other parasites, host age, the immune and nutritional status of the host, and to some degree, biotic and abiotic environmental factors.

SPORULATION. Once outside the host, oxygen, temperature, moisture, and lack of direct exposure to ultraviolet (UV) radiation are key elements in the survival of the oocyst and its ability to sporulate (Fig. 16.10, nos. 16-19). The cellular material within the oocyst (zygote, 2N) is called the sporoplasm. It generally is agreed that the first nuclear division that occurs in the sporoplasm is meiotic (Fig. 16.10, no. 17) (Canning and Anwar 1968; Canning and Morgan 1975; Wang 1982) and that subsequent divisions leading to sporocyst and sporozoite formation are mitotic. As soon as the meiotic division is completed, a second (mitotic) division follows quickly to form four nuclei, at which time four protrusions often appear on the surface of the zygote. These protrusions transform into pyramid-shaped structures (Fig. 16.10, no. 18) that eventually become rounded to form smaller cyst structures, the sporocysts. A single mitotic division of the nucleus later occurs within each sporocyst, after which the cytoplasm divides into two sporozoites (Fig. 16.10, no. 19). The process described is for *Eimeria* spp.; *Cyclospora* spp. have two sporocysts with two sporozoites each, and *Isospora* spp. have two sporocysts, each with four sporozoites, and both undergo a process similar in principle. The sporozoites within the sporulated oocyst are the actual infective units, and most sporulated oocysts are resistant to environmental extremes and are immediately infective to the next hosts that chance to ingest them.

Finally, within the last two decades, we have learned that there may be another mode of transmission for members of these monoxenous genera. At least a few species of *Isospora* have been shown to use paratenic (transport) hosts (Frenkel and Dubey 1972; Dubey and Fayer 1976; Matsui 1991), and extraintestinal tissue stages have been shown experimentally to be able to transfer/transmit a successful infection in some mammalian *Eimeria* species (Mayberry et al. 1989; Mottalei et al. 1992). Sporozoites excyst from oocysts ingested by these paratenic hosts, infect cells in various places within the body, and become dormant. If the infected host is eaten by the appropriate predator, these dormant sporozoites become active, infect enterocytes of the predator, and initiate a typical coccidian life cycle.

Epizootiology. *Eimeria* and *Isospora* spp. are ubiquitous, found in all orders of mammals that have been sampled for them. Unfortunately, many parasite surveys of mammals have concentrated only on helminth and/or arthropod companions and largely have ignored the coccidia and other protista. Nonetheless, there are about 869 *Eimeria* spp. and about 132 *Isospora* spp. described from all mammals to date (Table 16.11). This must be only a fraction of the number of species that occur in mammals and clearly points to the urgent need for more work in this area, especially given the alarming rate of habitat destruction and species extinctions.

For the purpose of this chapter, we divide the class Mammalia into five groups: humans, domesticated mammals [e.g., cattle, camels, sheep, goats, horses, pigs, dogs, cats, lab animals (mice, guinea pigs, rats), lagomorphs (rabbits), mink, etc.], game mammals (e.g., deer, antelope, moose, elk, bighorn sheep), zoo mammals (mostly exotics), and wild mammals (all others); obviously, there is overlap among the latter four groups. Most of our knowledge about life cycles, pathology and clinical disease, physiology, biochemistry, cell culture, immunology, and drug therapy comes from work on the *Isospora* and *Eimeria* spp. that infect humans and domesticated mammals (e.g., Long 1982; Lindsay and Todd 1993), but these are not the purview of this series. Information about the other three groups (game mammals, other wild mammals, and zoo mammals) is germane to our discussion, and each is addressed briefly below.

Game mammals. Most game mammals are in two orders, Artiodactyla and Lagomorpha, and species in each group have both economic (food, clothing) and recreational (hunting) value. Unfortunately, with the exception of deer (Cervidae, 25 *Eimeria* spp.) and the chamois (*Rupicapra*, 6 *Eimeria* spp.), only the coccidia of domestic Artiodactyla (Table 16.11) have been studied extensively (Levine and Ivens 1986). The literature on game hosts consists almost entirely of surveys (e.g., Beaudoin et al. 1970; Penzhorn et al. 1994; Gōmez-Bautista et al. 1996), descriptions of new species (e.g., Inoue and Inura 1991; Hussein and Mohammed 1992; Wilber et al. 1996) or redescriptions of named species (e.g., Todd et al. 1967), and experimental infections, usually in young animals given artificially massive doses of sporulated oocysts (15–100 x 10^3) (Abbas and Post 1980; Conlogue and Foreyt 1984; Lindsay and Blagburn 1985). Only rarely is any pathology (usually mild to severe diarrhea) reported under natural conditions (McCully et al. 1970). However, we often keep herding species in semicaptive conditions (preserves, ranches); such conditions of limited habitat and crowding may lead to occasional case reports about outbreaks of coccidiosis (Hussein and Mohammed 1992), although sometimes they do not (Penzhorn et al. 1994).

There are 13 genera of lagomorphs, and 65 *Eimeria* and two *Isospora* spp. have been named from 10 of them (Table 16.11). This host-parasite association is unique in many ways. Surveys have shown that all species are infected with coccidia when examined; the prevalence of infection has been reported from as low as 4% (Soveri and Valtonen 1983) to as high as 100% (Duszynski and Marquardt 1969), and infected animals usually are infected with from two to nine species. A number of species, *Eimeria intestinalis, E. piriformis, E. coecicola* (intestinal forms), *E. stiedai* (liver, bile duct), and a few others, are known to be highly pathogenic (Kheysin 1947, 1948; Pellérdy and Dürr 1970; Coudert et al. 1993), but these are found primarily in the Old World rabbit (*Oryctolagus cuniculus*). The 3 lagomorph genera from which 70% of their coccidia species are described are *Lepus, Oryctolagus,* and *Sylvilagus* (Levine and Ivens 1972, D.W. Duszynski, unpublished data). Although numerous surveys for coccidia and helminth parasites have been done on species in these genera, Andrews and Davidson (1980) noted a lack of salient coccidiosis lesions in conjunction with an absence of any cases of clinical coccidiosis in numerous surveys of wild rabbits. This suggested to them "that the pathogenicity of coccidian parasites in wild cottontails has been overestimated." Although some of the *Eimeria* that infect these genera have been shown by cross-infection experiments to be species specific (e.g., *E. sculpta:* see Carvalho 1943) other species (e.g., *E. neoleporis:* see Carvalho 1942, 1944; *E. stiedai:* Jankiewicz 1941) can be transmitted between genera. Other interesting work has been done with rabbit coccidia that has biological implications beyond the individual organisms used. Licois et al. (1990) were able to develop a precocious line of *E. intestinalis* by selection for early developmental oocysts after six consecutive passages in rabbits (*Oryctolagus*); more recently, Pakandl et al. (1996), developed a precocious strain of *E. media.* Such studies may lead to the development of immunity via attenuated pathogenicity in highly pathogenic strains (see Jeffers 1975; McDonald et al. 1986). Aly (1993) was able to infect dexamethaxone-treated mice with *E. stiedai* and achieve a patent infection in 20 of 25 mice; the prepatent period was 30–35 days, and patency lasted at least until 60 days postinfection. Perhaps host transfer occurs more often than we know under natural conditions where many random cross-transmission events must occur daily among syntopic hosts, especially those that have similar nutritional requirements and can provide coccidia with intestinal milieus similar to one another. Finally, molecular tools have begun to be used for diagnosis of coccidia species in veterinary parasitology (for review see Comes et al. 1996). Among the first to demonstrate this use with mammalian coccidia were Cere et al. (1995) who studied inter- and intraspecific variation of *Eimeria* spp. in rabbits using random amplified polymorphic DNA (RAPD) assays. Although profiles differed signifi-

cantly among nine eimerian species, species-specific fingerprints were obtained that might prove useful in species diagnosis.

Other wild mammals. The major orders (numbers of species) of other wild mammals include rodents (Rodentia, 2015 spp.), bats (Chiroptera, 925 spp.), moles and shrews (Insectivora, 428 spp.), marsupials (orders Dasyuromorphia, Didelphiomorphia, Diprodontia, Microbiotheria, Notoryctemorphia, Paucituberculata, Peramelemorphia, 272 spp.), carnivores (Carnivora, 271 spp.), and primates (Primates, 233 spp.) (Table 16.11). The final order we will mention (Cetacea, 78 spp.) includes the world's largest and most endangered species.

When most people think about wild mammals, they generally do not think about rodents, which comprise the most specious order of mammals. Yet we know more about the coccidia of rodents than we do about those of any other mammalian order (Table 16.11). Levine and Ivens (1965) published the first comprehensive review on the coccidian parasites from rodents, a treatise they later revised and updated (1990). Their first review (1965) included 204 *Eimeria* and 10 *Isospora* spp., and their second (1990) listed 374 *Eimeria* and 39 *Isospora* spp., an increase of 199 described (named) species (93%) in 25 years (note their addendum). Even with this "plethora" of species, there remains an enormous void in our knowledge. To wit: (a) an additional 32 *Eimeria* and *Isospora* spp. are listed in Levine and Ivens (1990) without complete names because information is insufficient to justify species names; (b) < 15% of all 2015 rodent species (Wilson and Reeder 1993) have been examined for coccidia, and it is most likely that those named coccidia do not include all the coccidia species to be found in each host species; (c) most of the descriptions of sporulated oocysts are far from complete; (d) the complete life cycles of < 10 named species are known, and even the general location of endogenous development in the host is known for < 20% of the named species; (e) information about the molecular genetics (*e.g.,* gene sequences) is virtually nonexistent. Clearly, this is an area that deserves enormous research effort in the future.

Bats are the second most diverse order of mammals with > 900 species (Table 16.11). Surprisingly, however, there are only 30 valid *Eimeria* spp. described from bats worldwide (Duszynski 1997; Scott and Duszynski 1997; D.W. Duszynski, unpublished data) in comparison to > 400 eimerians described from rodents [Levine and Ivens (1990) listed 372]. Ubelaker et al. (1977) suggested that this low diversity of *Eimeria* in bats is due primarily to a lack of searching for them when bats are surveyed for parasites. However, examination of additional bats for coccidia by several authors since 1977 suggests that their overall prevalence is generally lower in bats than in rodents. Marinkelle (1968) found only 2 of 400 bats (< 1%) infected, and Scott and Duszynski (1997) found 28 of 548 (5%) infected with *Eimeria* spp. However, Yang-Xian and Fu-Qiang

(1983) reported 105 of 151 (70%) infected, so the prevalence of coccidia in bat species also can be quite variable. The factors that contribute to the prevalence of coccidia in vertebrates include, but are not limited to, host specificity, acquired immunity, and several abiotic factors (Marquardt et al. 1960; Todd and Hammond 1968a,b; Wilber et al. 1994a,b). Although no one has demonstrated it empirically, the abiotic factors most likely to contribute to the infection of bats by coccidia are the stability of the roost microclimate (e.g., relative humidity, temperature) and roosting behavior by bats (i.e., colonial vs. solitary). For example, bats that prefer crowded roosts with stable microclimates (e.g., maternity colonies in attics, caves) may be more likely to ingest sporulated oocysts than bats that prefer to roost alone where microclimates may be highly variable (e.g., trees, leaf litter). Compact roost types (attics, crevices) may bring bats into contact with feces more often than large, open roosts (caves). Also, increased grooming (maternity colonies) may contribute to a greater chance of bats ingesting infective oocysts (Scott and Duszynski 1997). No *Isospora* spp. have been found in bats, and all infected bats found to date have been infected only with a single species; no multiple species infections have been recorded. Finally, Gruber et al. (1996) recently examined 14 bats belonging to six different insectivorous species, and 4 bats, each a different species (*Pipistrellus pipistrellus, Myotis mystacinus, M. nattereeri,* and *Nyctalus noctula*), had renal coccidiosis with cystic tubular dilatation. Previously, Kusewitt et al. (1977) reported *Klossiella* sp. in the kidneys of two *Myotis sodalis.* However, the asexual and sexual developmental stages shown in the tubular epithelium and lumina and a "suggested unsporulated oocyst" demonstrated in a collecting duct were typical of *Eimeria* or *Isospora* infections (Eimeriidae), which look quite different than those of *Klossiella* (Klossiellidae). But since no sporulated oocysts were available for study, the genus of this coccidian organism is unknown. Most of those who have studied bats for coccidia have looked for oocysts only in bat feces. The possibility exists that many more coccidian species may have been found if the kidneys and urine also had been examined.

The insectivores have been described as a zoological catchall into which a number of ancient and seemingly distantly related taxa have been placed. Some insectivores are considered to be pests (e.g., moles on golf courses), while others (e.g., shrews) are important in human agriculture in the control of insect, slug and snail pests. Only about 8.6% (37/428) of insectivore species have been examined for coccidia, but these have produced a wealth of named species including about 48 *Eimeria,* 22 *Isospora,* and 5 *Cyclospora* spp. (Table 16.11); this is a significant increase in the number of species (24, 10, and 2, respectively) since Levine and Ivens (1979) last reviewed the coccidia of insectivores. The vast majority of these species are known only from the description of sporulated oocysts that have been studied in fecal samples from their hosts

(e.g., Duszynski 1989; Duszynski and Upton 2000). A few of the endogenous stages of *Cyclospora caryolytica, C. talpae,* and *Eimeria goussevi* (Pellérdy and Tanyi 1968; Entzeroth and Scholtyseck 1984) from the European mole (*Talpa europaea*) and of *E. darjeelingensis, E. murinus,* and *E. suncus* (Ahluwalia et al. 1979; Sinha and Sinha 1980; Bandyopadhyay and Dasgupta 1985) from the house shrew (*Suncus murinus*) have been documented. To our knowledge, however, there are no complete life cycles known. This is certainly an area ripe for future study, especially given the interesting observation of Cable and Conway (1953) discussing endogenous stages of a coccidian parasite in the mammary tissues of a shrew.

The marsupials now occupy seven orders in the newest systematic treatise on mammals (Wilson and Reeder 1993), but only two orders have coccidia described from them. By far, the great majority of species live in Australia; most are herbivores, but a few are predators. To date, 56 *Eimeria* and only 2 *Isospora* spp. have been recorded from sporulated oocysts (Table 16.11). Of these, details of gamogony have been recorded for 4 *Eimeria* spp., only a few merogonous stages have been seen, and no complete life cycles are known. Beveridge (1993) reported that coccidiosis was a major disease of large kangaroos, but that continuous, simultaneous infection with several species of *Eimeria* make it impossible to determine which of the species present is the major pathogen. The eastern gray kangaroo (*Macropus giganteus*) seems to be particularly susceptible to developing pathology, and *E. wilcanniensis* (syn. *E. kogoni*) is thought to be the major pathogen. Barker et al. (1979) documented obvious intestinal tissue pathology due to *Eimeria arundeli* in wombats (*Vombatus ursinus*), and Beveridge (1993) mentioned that coccidia present in the echidna (*Tachyglossus aculetaus*) appear to cause a mild enteritis. However, coccidia found in many Australian marsupials (e.g., platypus, *Ornithorhynchus anainus*) either cause no obvious pathology or have not been formally described, or both (Beveridge 1993). For example, Beveridge (1993) reported that an undescribed *Eimeria* sp. was totally nonpathogenic in the bush-tailed opossum (*Trichosurus vulpecula*).

Levine and Ivens (1981) reviewed the coccidia [including *Besnoitia, Frenkelia, Sarcocystis,* and *Toxoplasma* (Sarcocystidae), which we do not cover] of carnivores and listed 78 named species of *Eimeria* (39) and *Isospora* (39) in 46 host species in 26 genera (7 families); these names included at least one *nomen nudum* and many species of questionable validity [e.g., 5 *Eimeria* spp. from *Felis* and 3 from *Leo* may be pseudoparasites; also see Arther and Post (1977), for pseudoparasites in *Canis*]. Wilson and Reeder (1993) lump the former mammalian order Pinnipedia (seals, sea cows) within the Carnivora (canids, felids, bears, raccoons, mustelids, etc.). Even 15 years after Levine and Ivens (1981), only 20% (55/271) of the carnivore species have been examined for coccidia, and about 107 species have been named (many of dubious distinction), divided evenly between *Eimeria* and *Isospora* spp. (Table 16.11). The coccidia of domesticated *Canis* and *Felis* spp. were reviewed recently (Lindsay and Todd 1993; Lindsay et al. 1997a), and because of their importance to humans as companion animals it is their coccidia about which we have the most knowledge concerning life cycles, immunity, cross-transmission, and similar matters. Despite a few erroneous reports to the contrary, neither dogs nor cats (Lindsay and Todd 1993; Lindsay et al. 1997a) serve as hosts for *Eimeria* spp.; as far as is known, only *Isospora* spp. parasitize these hosts. In addition, both genera develop solid immunity following primary infection, and cross-infection work, to date, suggests that cats and dogs do not share their *Isospora* spp. Within the Canidae, however, cross-transmission can bridge generic boundaries; Bledsoe (1976), for example, demonstrated that *Isospora vulpina* from the silver fox (*Vulpes vulpes*) could be transmitted to beagle dogs (*Canis familiaris*). Within other Carnivora families and/or genera, only oocyst descriptions are known for the majority of reported species (many of these are questionable), with two exceptions. Within the Mustelidae, enteric (Blankenship-Paris et al. 1993), respiratory and urinary (Jolley et al. 1994), and biliary (Williams 1996) coccidiosis have been documented histologically in ferrets (*Mustela* spp.); and in the Phocidae, endogenous development of *Eimeria phocae* was reported in both asymptomatic and clinically ill harbor seals (*Phoca vitulina*) (McClelland 1993).

The most accepted taxonomic scheme divides the primates into two suborders, Prosimii (the lower primates) and the Anthropoidea (higher primates) (Nowak 1991); there are 7 *Eimeria* (natural) and 1 *Isospora* (experimental) spp. described from the former and 7 *Isospora* and 1 *Cyclospora* spp. from the latter (Duszynski et al. 1999). Lindsay and Todd (1993) and Lindsay et al. (1997a) recently reviewed the *Isospora* spp. from the higher primates. Only four valid species are known from wild, higher primates (excluding humans which have *Isospora belli* and two questionable species, *I. chilensis* and *I. natalensis*): *I. arctopitheci*, *I. callimico*, *I. endocallimici*, and *I. saimirae*; the latter three species are known only from the structure of their sporulated oocysts. Hsu and Melby (1974) described *I. callimico* from the feces of captive Goeldi's marmoset (*Callimico goeldi*) at a primate facility in Baltimore, Maryland. At almost the same time, *Isospora endocallimici* was described from five captive *C. goeldii* at the Tulane University Delta Regional Primate Research Center, Covington, Louisiana (Duszynski and File 1974). Two of these animals were born at the Center, the other three were born in the wild and imported from Peru. All animals were passing oocysts when examined, so it was not possible to state in which one(s) the infection originated. *Isospora saimirae* was described from the feces of a squirrel monkey, *Saimiri sciureus*, from Tocantins Island, Pará State, Brazil (Lainson and Shaw 1989). Ironically, the type locality now lies beneath the Tucu-

rui Reservoir, a man-made lake built shortly after 1989. There are other isosporan species that have been named based on the structure of sporulated oocysts found in the feces of higher primates (e.g., *Isospora cebi*, *Isospora paponis*), but careful analysis (see Lindsay et al. 1997a) suggests these are likely oocysts of *Sarcocystis* spp. Finally, *I. arctopitheci* was described by Rodhain (1933) from a captive marmoset (*Callithrix penicillata*) that had died in France. He saw no connection between the presence of the parasite and death of the marmoset. *Isospora arctopitheci* is the most studied of the higher primate species. It has a broad host range, having been transmitted to members of six genera of New World primates, four families of carnivores and one marsupial species (according to Hendricks 1977). Its life cycle was described by Olcott et al. (1982) and is unusual in that asexual reproduction takes place by a process called endodyogeny rather than by merogony. In heavy experimental infections (1–2 x 10^5 oocysts), 4 of 13 experimental titi marmosets (*Saguinus geoffroyi*) died 3 to 5 days after inoculation (Olcott et al. 1982). In all other reports of *Isospora* spp. from higher primates, infections do not show clinical symptoms under normal circumstances.

Finally, it is of interest that there are 7 *Eimeria* spp. described from lower primates, but only 1 *Isospora* sp. (experimentally). In general, our knowledge of primate coccidia is poor: *Eimeria*, *Isospora*, and *Cyclospora* spp. have been reported from 7 of 13 (54%) of the families (listed in Wilson and Reeder 1993), but only from 14 (23%) of the 60 genera and 18 (8%) of the 233 species (see Duszynski et al. 1999).

There are no coccidia described from cetaceans (whales); however, this is not because no one has looked. Dailey and Vogelbein (1991) published a parasite survey on 176 whales, including 35 sei whales (*Balaenoptera borealis* Lesson, 1828), 106 minke whales (*B. acutorostrata* Lacépede, 1804) and 35 sperm whales (*Physeter catodon* L., 1758). We examined the feces of these and about a dozen other cetaceans (D.W. Duszynski, unpublished), but were unable to find any structures resembling coccidian oocysts. Recently, Kuttin and Kaller (1996) described a species they named *Cystoisospora delphini* as the cause of enteritis in a captive bottle-nosed dolphin (*Tursiops truncatus*) at the Laboratory for Marine Mammals Research, Tel-Aviv University, Israel. They placed the oocysts of the organism they saw in the genus *Cystoisospora* because they believed that the dolphin, which had been in captivity 5 years, acquired the infection from (frozen, whole) fish it had been fed, but they did not present evidence of parasitic cysts in the presumed intermediate hosts. We believe that *Cystoisospora* is best considered a junior synonym of *Isospora*.

Zoo mammals. There is an increased interest in the diseases of zoo/captive animals worldwide (Fowler 1978, 1986, 1996a,b; Modl et al. 1995; Artois et al. 1996; Cubas 1996; Porter 1996; Schultz et al. 1996; Williams and Thorne 1996). Most mammals in zoos are

TABLE 16.11—The number of mammalian orders and species (Wilson and Reeder, 1993) showing the approximate number of host species that have coccidia described from them and the approximate numbers of *Eimeria, Isospora,* and *Cyclospora* spp. described from each order.

Order (Common Names)	No. of spp.	No. Host spp. with Coccidia	No. of spp. *Eimeria*	No. of spp. *Isospora*	No. of spp. *Cyclospora*
Artiodactyla (pigs, deer, sheep)	220	54	170	7	0
Carnivora (cats, dogs, seals)	271	55	56	51	0
Cetacea (whales, dolphins)	78	0	0	0	0
Chiroptera (bats)	925	26	30	0	0
Dasyuromorphia (Tasmanian devil)	63	0	0	0	0
Dermoptera (flying lemurs)	2	0	0	0	0
Didelphimorpha (American opossums)	63	6	6	2	0
Diprodontia (koala, kangaroos)	117	35	50	0	0
Hyracoidea (hyraxes)	6	0	0	0	0
Insectivora (shrews, moles)	428	37	48	22	5
Lagamorpha (rabbits, hares)	80	20	65	2	0
Macroscelidae (elephant shrews)	15	0	0	0	0
Microbiotheria (Monito del Monte)	1	0	0	0	0
Monotremata (spiny anteaters)	3	2	1	0	0
Notoryctemorphia (marsupial moles)	2	0	0	0	0
Paucituberculata (shrew opossums)	5	0	0	0	0
Peramelemorphia (bandicoots)	21	0	0	0	0
Perissodactyla (horses, zebras)	18	5	3	0	0
Pholidota (scaly anteaters)	7	1	1	0	0
Primates (monkeys, humans)	233	18	7	8	1
Proboscidea (elephants)	2	0	0	0	0
Rodentia (mice, rats, squirrels)	2015	280	415	40	1
Scadentia (tree shrews)	19	4	4	0	0
Sirenia (manatees, dugongs)	5	3	3	0	0
Tubulidentata (aardvarks)	1	0	0	0	0
Xenarthra (armadillos)	29	10	10	0	0
26	4629	556	869	132	7

large, exotic wild mammals. They present unique problems to zoo managers, veterinarians, and biologists alike for many reasons: (a) it is impossible to reproduce the abiotic environmental conditions of their native habitat (e.g., photoperiod, temperature and humidity extremes, space requirements); (b) it is impossible to duplicate the biotic conditions or interactions of their natural environment (e.g., seasonal dietary needs, coevolved invertebrates and vertebrates); (c) the presence of nonnative cohorts of other captive animals, crowding, and proximity of large numbers of people are "unnatural" and likely produce various levels of stress; (d) stress likely predisposes zoo mammals to parasitic diseases, especially those, like coccidia, with direct life cycles that do not require specialized intermediate hosts; and (e) captive/zoo animals have the potential to act as vectors of zoonoses. In addition, the concentration of like or nearly like mammals into small areas and the ability of parasites with direct life cycles to greatly increase the number of transmission propagules via asexual reproduction, combined with the above factors, create conditions ideal for serious disease consequences due to parasites in zoo mammals and/or their keepers. Such disease manifestations may occur often, but they are seldom reported (e.g., Schillhorn van Veen 1986) or, if reported, often are not attributed to coccidian parasites. Sometimes, new species of coccidia are described from zoo mammals (e.g. Rastegaãeff 1930; Yakimoff and Matschoulsky 1940; Agrawal et al. 1981; Flach et al. 1991), but these reports must be interpreted with caution, given the conditions unique to zoos (above).

PREVALENCE IN WILD MAMMALS. Using the clear definitions given by Margolis et al. (1982), the prevalence (number hosts infected/number individuals examined) of coccidial infection in a given population of wild mammals may vary from 0% (e.g., bats) to 100% (e.g., cottontail rabbits), whereas the incidence (number new cases of infection/number uninfected individuals in the population) of infection usually is impossible to determine in feral mammal populations. Likewise, terms like intensity, density, abundance, and infrapopulation that are applicable to helminth infections have no meaning in coccidial infections. Even when one samples a large, representative number of individuals in a natural population, the prevalence determined is only a guess of the real prevalence of that coccidian species in the population. The reason(s) have to do with the transient nature of the coccidian infection. Suppose you sample an animal and no oocysts are found in its feces; that animal is considered negative for coccidia. However, it may be infected with one or more coccidia that are only in an asexual reproductive phase (merogony), not yet making oocysts or, because gamogony, fertilization, and oocyst discharge are relatively rapid events in most cycles, the last oocysts in the cycle may have been in the animal's fecal discharge just prior to its collection. Also, the first and last days of patency may have so few oocysts in the feces that they can be missed in routine fecal examinations, especially if the oocysts are small (< 10 μm). Other biotic (size of the infecting dose; age, nutritional, and immune status of the host; location where the feces are deposited) and abiotic (season, temperature, moisture, altitude, direct UV radiation, longitude) factors all influence the real incidence of coccidial parasites in a host population. Sometimes, less obvious environmental factors such as radon-rich soils may have a significant effect on both the prevalence and the survival of a coccidian parasite in its natural host population (Wilber et al. 1994b). Finally, repeated removal of host animals from a site will cause immigration rates high enough to mask or alter previous patterns of prevalence (Wilber and Patrick 1997). Thus, determining the true prevalence of coccidial infection in populations of wild mammals is tricky and inaccurate, at best.

SURVIVAL OF OOCYSTS. This is an area that deserves future, critical study, because most of what we know has been observed in the laboratory working with four species of chicken and two species of rabbit coccidia. Although we know that temperature, moisture and direct exposure to UV radiation (sunlight) all have an influence on the ability of oocysts to sporulate once discharged from the host to the external environment, the importance of these, and perhaps other, factors (e.g., mechanical vectors) and their interactions have not been precisely determined. In general, oocysts sporulate more slowly at lower temperatures and faster at higher temperatures (Becker and Crouch 1931; Edgar 1954). If maintained in an aqueous medium at < 10° C or > 50° C, oocysts will degenerate and die (Becker and Crouch 1931). Between these extremes, the percent of oocysts that will sporulate in a field-collected sample depends on the species, the time between collection and getting the sample to the laboratory, the temperature at which the sample was kept during that time (D.W. Duszynski, unpublished), the medium in which the fecal sample was stored (Duszynski and Wilber 1997), the rate of putrification of the sample, the amount of molecular oxygen available to the stored oocysts (Duszynski and Conder 1977), and possibly other factors such as the proximity of other, sporulating oocysts (Duszynski and Conder 1977). Once a field-collected fecal sample is in the laboratory and maintained under optimal conditions (Duszynski and Wilber 1997), sporulation of most mammalian coccidia occurs best between 20°C–23° C. Exceptions include some tropical species such as *Cyclospora cayetanensis,* which sporulates best at 37° C. Once sporulated, the oocysts of some mammalian species can remain viable and infective in 2% $K_2Cr_2O_7$ 4–5 years (D.W. Duszynski, personal observation). When oocysts are exposed to the natural conditions of their external environment, they remain viable and infective from as little as 49 days up to 86 weeks, dependent upon the species and the interplay of sunlight, shade, and vegetation (Warner 1933; Farr and Wehr 1949; Koutz 1950; Dorney 1962; Wilber et al. 1994a).

The role that naturally occurring soil organisms (e.g., mites, insects, earthworms) may play as mechanical vectors is virtually unknown. Recently, however, Goodwin and Waltman (1996) demonstrated that darkling beetles (*Alphitobius diaperinus*) collected directly from chicken broiler house soils could transmit viable coccidial infections to 6 of 7 SPF (specific pathogen free) chicks inoculated with homogenates from 75 beetles. Another area in desperate need of further study is the mechanisms coccidian species use to overwinter in hibernating mammals (Anderson 1971) and the importance of those mechanisms to the maintenance of coccidian populations in such hosts.

HOST SPECIFICITY. Host specificity is defined (Roberts and Janovy 1996) as the "degree to which a parasite is able to mature in more than one host species." Strict specificity means that one coccidian species will only infect one host species. In reality, this condition rarely, if ever, exists in nature because it would not be to the advantage of the parasite to so limit its reproductive opportunities, and most coccidia probably are infective to different species, at least within the same host genus. Complicating the issue, the degree of specificity seems to vary from host group to host group. For example, *Eimeria* from goats cannot be transmitted to sheep and vice versa (Lindsay and Todd 1993), but the *Eimeria* from cattle (*Bos*) often are found to infect American bison (*Bison*) (Ryff and Bergstrom 1975; Penzhorn et al. 1994), and *Eimeria* that infect certain rodents (Sciuridae) seem to easily cross host generic boundaries (Todd and Hammond 1968a,b; Wilber et al. 1998). Some coccidia even have been reported to cross familial lines, but this is rare. De Vos (1970) demonstrated that *E. chinchillae,* originally isolated from the chinchilla, could be experimentally transmitted to seven genera of wild rodents (two families), and Hendricks (1977) said that *Isospora arctopitheci,* a parasite of New World primates, could infect six genera of primates (two families), four genera of carnivores (four families) and one genus of marsupial. We also know that *E. separata* from rats will infect certain genetic strains of mice (Mayberry and Marquardt 1973; Mayberry et al. 1982) and that genetically altered (Rose and Millard 1985) or immunosuppressed mammals (Todd et al. 1971; Todd and Lepp 1972; Nowell and Higgs 1989; Aly 1993) are susceptible to infection with *Eimeria* spp. to which they otherwise might be naturally resistant. Thus, numerous biotic interactions between host and parasite must contribute, in concert, to the host specificity (or lack thereof) in the coccidia, especially the genetic constitution of both participants.

Clinical Signs. Most mammals pass oocysts in their feces, sometimes in large numbers under natural conditions, with no apparent ill effects. Mention of obvious signs of illness due to coccidiosis in wild mammals is rare in the literature (e.g., Tanabe 1938; Beveridge 1993). Almost all the information known about the disease state, coccidiosis, comes either from experimental work with domestic or laboratory mammals or from wild, zoo, or domestic stocks where overcrowding, stress, and easy fecal-oral contamination are factors. Both experimentally driven coccidiosis and that resulting from overcrowded conditions result in hosts becoming exposed to massive numbers of sporulated oocysts, which they are unlikely to acquire under natural conditions, but which can graphically demonstrate the clinical symptoms associated with heavy coccidial infections: fever, diarrhea (sometimes with blood), weight loss, abdominal tenderness and cramping, nervous distress, dehydration, anorexia, emaciation, and weakness. Symptoms occur because coccidia first change the integrity of the host enterocyte in which they live and reproduce asexually (Sheppard 1974), thus interfering with digestion and absorption (Stein and Marquardt 1973; Duszynski et al. 1982). In modest to heavy infections they can change the architecture of

the intestinal villi themselves and/or the length of the crypts (Fernando and McCraw 1973; Duszynski et al. 1978a); they later destroy the host's intestinal cells, sometimes whole sections of epithelial lining, making the host more susceptible to bacterial invasion (Li et al. 1996) and allowing increased flow of tissue fluid and blood into the intestinal lumen (Bailey 1994).

Pathology and Pathogenesis. Factors that affect the pathogenesis of coccidial infections in wild mammals include at least the following: the number, strain, age (=viability), and species of sporulated oocysts ingested; the age, sex, strain/breed of host; the site of development within the host; the nutritional and immune status of the host; occupation by other parasites and microbes that may compete for space or other host resources with the endogenous stages of the parasite; the behavior and feeding habits of the host; and the coevolutionary process of host and parasites that unite all of these factors and their interactions. Many of these factors have been discussed elsewhere (Fernando 1982; Duszynski 1986; Lindsay and Todd 1993; Li et al. 1996).

The endogenous development of mammalian coccidia usually takes place within specific sites and cells of the gastrointestinal tract of their host. Since merogony is multiplicative, the number of viable oocysts ingested and the location of meronts within the gut are important early determinants of pathology in naive or susceptible hosts. Although most coccidia develop in villus enterocytes, some can develop in crypt enterocytes or cells within the lamina propria (e.g., *E. bovis* in cattle); it is these species that can cause the most damage to the intestinal mucosa. Development in villus enterocytes may result in villus atrophy (Fernando 1982) or elongation (Duszynski et al. 1978a), often accompanied by changes in crypt depth and abnormal epithelial differentiation such as hyperplasia. Such response is common to a wide variety of unrelated intestinal pathogens, leading to the suggestion that altered morphology is an inherent, nonspecific response of the mucosa to damaging agents (Sprinz 1962; Fernando 1982).

As noted, pathology due to coccidia in wild mammals usually is documented in captive wild animals or domesticated (formerly wild) mammals, but seldom in wild mammals under natural circumstances. A few selected examples can serve to illustrate pathogenesis during coccidial infection. In Australia, Barker et al. (1979) documented intestinal pathology when they examined histological sections of small intestine from three wombats (*Vombatus ursinus*) infected with *E. arundeli.* Some of the hosts were wild, some captive; unfortunately, the animal from which the pathology was described was not noted. They found villi over extensive areas of the lower small intestine to be hypertrophied, projecting above uninfected mucosa. The lamina propria also was distended, and many mononuclear inflammatory cells were dispersed among the gametocytes. Although the changes in gross appearance and histological changes associated with gamogony were striking, "none of the animals had diarrhea or other signs of gastrointestinal disease. The intestinal epithelium was intact and inflammatory infiltrates were moderate and chronic, indicating little pathogenicity in animals examined." However, *E. arundeli* is able to cause disease in captive wombats. Hum et al. (1991) documented disease in two captive juveniles (*V. ursinus*) infected with the parasite. One animal had diarrhea and the second had soft feces, lost weight, and later died. Postmortem tissue sections showed massive gametocytes in hypertrophic cells of the lamina propria, distended villi, and grossly visible, thickened regions of the mucosa over extensive areas of the small intestine. The authors concluded, "heavy infections may be pathogenic under some circumstances." In several species of the larger kangaroos in Australia, coccidiosis frequently takes a peracute form in which the animal is found dead after few premonitory signs. At necropsy, severe hemorrhagic enteritis is found, with blood throughout the small intestine, but contents of the large intestine seem unusually normal (Beveridge 1993).

Not all coccidia are limited to cells of the gastrointestinal tract. The ubiquitous *Eimeria stiedai,* for example, undergoes its endogenous development in epithelial cells of the bile duct and in parenchymal cells of the liver of rabbits. Light infections tend to be unapparent, but heavy infections can result in serious morbidity and mortality, especially in younger animals. Similarly, endogenous stages of *Cyclospora talpae* occur in the liver of the European mole, *Talpa europaea* (Pellérdy and Tanyi 1968). Dubey (1986) found meronts, gamonts, and oocysts in the villous epithelium and submucosal glands of the gall bladder of a commercial dairy goat in Montana that was infected by an unidentified *Eimeria* sp. The infection was localized and did not extend into the liver, no stages were seen in sections of intestine, and no oocysts were found in the feces. Other mammalian coccidia also are known to develop outside the gut, including a coccidium affecting the placenta of the hippopotamus (McCully et al. 1967; Kuttin et al. 1982); a species found in the epididymus of elk (Hrudka et al. 1983); *E. neitzi,* which causes uterine coccidiosis in the impala (McCully et al. 1970); *E. genitalia,* reported by Arcay (1994) to have developmental stages in the epididymis, seminal vesicles, vagina, uterus, and oviducts of hamsters (*Cricetus cricetus*); meronts of *E. riedmuelleri* reported in the bile ducts of chamois (*Rupicapra rupicapra*) by Desser (1978) and later confirmed by Brunnett et al. (1992); and a goat reported by Mahmoud et al. (1994) that died of liver failure attributed to lesions due to coccidiosis. Meronts, gamonts, and oocysts were seen in bile duct epithelium. Granulomas in the liver were composed of oocysts and macrophages encapsulated in a fibrous capsule. Hepatic lymph nodes had oocysts and macrophages diffusely scattered in them. Oocysts of *Eimeria caprina* and *E. alijevi* were identified in the bile, but only oocysts of *E. christenseni* were seen in the feces. In Australian marsupials, hepatic coccidiosis occurs in the Tammar wallaby (*M. eugenii*), and in the western gray kangaroo (*M. fuliginosus*), large meronts associated with focal hemorrhage were found in the pyloric antrum (Beveridge 1993). This opens a related issue that may be pertinent to the discussion on pathogenesis. Unlike the gut, which is a highly plastic, adaptable organ (Dowling and Riecken 1974), other tissues and cells may be more susceptible to pathogenesis by coccidia developing in them.

Diagnosis. In most instances when the host is not to be killed, the diagnosis of a coccidial infection in a wild mammal depends upon demonstration of oocysts in the feces. Initial handling of the sample in the field is critical so that oocysts, if present, can be brought back to the laboratory and allowed to sporulate under favorable conditions (see Duszynski and Wilber 1997). It is necessary for the oocysts to sporulate completely before a specific identification can be made. Once this has been accomplished, sporulated oocysts must be separated from the fecal debris and studied in detail. There are many ways to do this, and there is a rich and lengthy literature, comparing various concentration techniques (sedimentation, flotation) in a variety of fluids, on how to best isolate oocysts from feces (Faust et al. 1939; Farr and Luttermoser 1941; Gill 1954; Ryley et al. 1976; Greve 1989; Moitineo and Ferreira 1992; Arjomandzadeh and Dalimi 1994); methods for cleaning, purifying, and concentrating oocysts (Sharma et al. 1963; Wagenbach et al. 1966; Vetterling 1969; Smith and Ruff 1975; Dulski and Turner 1988); suggestions on how best to count oocysts (Long and Rowell 1958; Dorney 1964); and even methods for staining oocysts (Crouch and Becker 1931; Berland and Højgaard 1981; Markus and Bush 1987; Ashraf and Nepote 1990). Recently, Price (1994) compiled a comprehensive manual of techniques that can be used to isolate the transmission stages, including coccidian oocysts, of intestinal parasites from host fecal material.

In our experience, especially when processing small amounts of feces from large numbers of mammals, sporulated oocysts can be conveniently and efficiently separated from potassium dichromate (2% w/v $K_2Cr_2O_7$ in water) solution by suspending a 1–3-ml aliquot in a modified Sheather's sugar solution (500 g sucrose, 350 ml tap water, 5 ml phenol) and centrifuging 5 minutes at 1500 rpm (= 225 g) (see Duszynski and Wilber 1997, for details).

Recently, modern molecular tools [e.g., polymerase chain reaction (PCR), random amplified polymorphic DNA (RAPD)] that are used to study phylogenetic relationships among the coccidia (e.g., Relman et al. 1996; Barta et al. 1997; Pieniazek and Herwaldt 1997) have been employed to detect and identify coccidia, which are important in veterinary and human parasitology (Comes et al. 1996; Yoder et al. 1996). The nested PCR assay, for example, is reported to be able to detect as few as 10–50 oocysts of *Cyclospora cayetanensis* in human stools (Yoder et al. 1996).

The endogenous (asexual and/or sexual) stages in a coccidian life cycle often can be visualized in cells from an intestinal biopsy that has been properly fixed, embedded, sectioned, stained, and mounted on microscope slides. However, there are inherent dangers in the interpretation of such material. First, the endogenous stages of the vast majority of mammalian coccidia (98%) are unknown and thus cannot be directly linked to most species' oocysts; second, stages of merogony found in enterocytes are not necessarily the progenitors of the oocysts seen in the feces—they may represent the stages of another coccidium that has not yet reached gamont formation and oocyst production; and third, we now know that certain endogenous stages of a growing number of coccidian species may not be completely confined to the gastrointestinal tract. For example, Lotze et al. (1964) infected both sheep and goats with sporulated oocysts of *Eimeria arloingi, E. faurei,* and *E. ninaekohlyakimovi* of sheep origin; 13–18 days postinfection they found schizonts (= meronts), presumably of coccidial origin, in the enlarged mesenteric lymph nodes of both sheep and goats. This raises the question whether or not coccidial stages commonly occur in areas of the host's body besides the "regular" sites of their development in gut epithelium (also see Mottalei et al. 1992). Such stages have been well documented for the isosporan spp. of dogs and cats (see review, Lindsay et al. 1997a), for *Isospora belli* in humans (Lindsay et al. 1997b), and for at least one rodent *Eimeria* (Mayberry et al. 1989). In an intriguing note that has never been substantiated or followed up, Cable and Conway (1953) reported gametocytes of a coccidium in the mammary glands of a shrew (*Sorex paulustris*). The confirmed existence of this variety of tissue stages raises additional questions concerning the biology of the coccidia. Are such stages capable of producing, or responsible for, relapse when the host becomes stressed or immunosuppressed? Can the coccidia also be transmitted vertically? These are very fertile areas for future studies on mammalian coccidia.

Immunity. Infection of wild mammals by species of coccidia generally will result in a protective immune response that is specific to that coccidian species. Thus, if a host is infected for the first time with coccidia A, the parasite should go through normal endogenous development in the epithelium of the host, and oocysts will be discharged in the feces. The number of oocysts discharged and the length of time they are shed (the patent period) are dependent upon the number of sporulated oocysts in the initial infective dose, among other things. Later, if the same host becomes exposed again to A and also to coccidia B, there will be some protective immunity against A, but not against B. This protective response can be judged by the reduction or absence of oocyst production for species A and a general lack of clinical signs after challenge. Since wild mammals are probably exposed to thousands of oocysts of many different coccidian species on a daily

basis, the immunity that develops as a result of such regular exposure probably is the most important factor in keeping animals in their natural environment free of disease. The literature on immunity to coccidia in general, and on immunity in mammals specifically, is voluminous, with most of the work done either with the bovine coccidium, *E. bovis,* or with several rodent coccidia that can be manipulated easily in the laboratory in either rats (*E. nieschulzi*) or mice (*E. falciformis, E. ferrisi, E. papillata*).

Both the sporozoites that excyst from an oocyst/ sporocyst propagule to infect endothelial cells and the merozoites that develop intracellularly via multiple fission and then infect yet other endothelial cells are antigenic and stimulate the host's immune response; in fact, sporozoites and merozoites from the same parasite species seem to share many antigens (for review, see Lindsay and Todd 1993). Both arms of the immune system, humoral (serum antibodies) and cellular immunity, are manifested in the host's response to these foreign invaders (Rose 1974; Rose 1984, 1987; Rose et al. 1984; J.B. Rose et al. 1988; Lindsay and Todd 1993).

Although most coccidial infections induce a strong humoral response, circulating serum antibodies are thought to play only a minor role in impacting coccidial infections. However, locally produced antibodies (IgA-containing cells in the villi under the epithelium and IgM-containing cells deeper in the lamina propria) may present a more meaningful response to the parasite, although the exact mechanism of this effect is not understood. During infections in mice with *E. falciformis,* the locally produced IgA was found to be reactive with other stages in the life cycle (e.g., sporocysts, oocysts), but was parasite-specific in that antibodies failed to cross-react with stages of a second species, *E. ferrisi* (Douglas and Speer 1985). This, despite the fact that Lindsay et al. (1991), Tilahun and Stockdale (1982) Hughes et al. (1989), and others have shown there are surface antigens that are common among some mammalian eimerias.

The evidence is strong that immunity following infection with coccidia (at least *Eimeria* spp.) is cell-mediated (Rose and Hesketh 1979; Rose et al. 1979, 1985; Stockdale et al. 1985); this evidence comes primarily from studies with immune-deficient animals, such as nude (athymic) mice, and with T- and B-cell depleted animals (Lindsay and Todd 1993). Athymic animals have more severe primary infections than wild type animals and have little or no resistance to challenge infections. In mice, immunity can be adoptively transferred using either splenic or, more optimally, mesenteric lymphocytes (M.E. Rose et al. 1988a,b). In addition, depletion of CD4+ cells following administration of anti-Thy-1.2 antibodies abrogates the protective immunity to challenge *E. falciformis* infections (see M.E. Rose et al. 1988b; Stiff and Vasilakos 1990). These results imply that immunity to coccidiosis, at least in rodents, is mediated through CD4+ cells.

Depletion of CD8+ cells in mice infected with *E. vermiformis* had no effect on oocyst production during primary infections, and there was only a slight increase in oocyst production during secondary infections. However, identical experiments in mice during *E. pragensis* infections resulted in a slight decrease in oocyst production during the primary infection and significant increases in oocyst production during the secondary infection (Rose et al. 1992). Although the exact mechanism by which this phenomenon occurs is unknown, Lillehoj and Trout (1994) suggested that CD8+ cell depletion may increase the severity of challenge infections by eliminating cytotoxic cells that would normally target the infected cells and limit parasite replication.

Neutralization of endogenous IFN-γ (interferon-gamma) by treating mice with anti-IFN-γ has been shown to have a variety of effects that depend, in part, on the species of coccidium studied. Following administration of anti-IFN-γ, enhanced oocyst output was observed during primary *E. vermiformis* infections, whereas no difference was noted during *E. pragensis* infections (M.E. Rose et al. 1989, 1991). Whichever coccidium was studied, however, anti-IFN-γ treatment was not found to prevent development of resistance to challenge, nor did it affect previously established immunity. These data imply that even though IFN-γ may sometimes modulate the intensity of primary infections, other types of immune mechanisms that may affect the intensity of a coccidial infection appear unaffected.

In nature, parasites tend to be overdispersed; that is, a few individuals in a host population bear a majority of the parasites (Roberts and Janovy 1996). Thus, coccidia in wild mammals often are found infecting hosts that also are infected with other parasites; the question arises whether there will be interactions, mediated by the immune response, among the several parasite species. Intrageneric interactions between two eimerias have been documented only once (Duszynski 1972), but intergeneric interactions have been demonstrated between coccidia and nematodes. Duszynski et al. (1978b) were the first to demonstrate that *Eimeria nieschulzi* could suppress the rejection of *Trichinella spiralis* in immunized rats that were concurrently infected. Suppression of the immune response to *Nippostrongylus brasiliensis,* another nematode, also has been demonstrated during concurrent infections with *E. nieschulzi* (Bristol et al. 1983, 1989) and with *E. separata* (Mayberry et al. 1985). Castro and Duszynski (1984) showed that *E. nieschulzi* has the ability to reduce the systemic inflammatory response by interfering with some phase of directed leukocyte migration. Conversely, Stewart et al. (1980) reported that rats inoculated with *T. spiralis* during primary infections with *E. nieschulzi* expelled these nematodes more rapidly than in comparable control animals. Thus, the ability to modulate a host's immune and/or inflammatory response may be a generalized phenomenon, at least in rodents infected concurrently with nematodes and *Eimeria* spp. This is an area of experimental parasitology that deserves attention.

Prevention and Control. A discussion on the prevention and/or control of access to sporulated oocysts does not seem applicable to wild mammals in their natural habitats, under most circumstances. However, over coevolutionary time, hosts may have evolved behavioral adaptations within their specific microenvironments that help them prevent or control contact with infective oocysts. To our knowledge, there is only one reference to lend credibility to this notion. Doran (1953), in a detailed and intriguing survey in California, livetrapped, over 3 years, 611 kangaroo rats (*Dipodomys* spp.) representing 6 species and 11 subspecies: *D. agilis agilis* (12 rats); *D. deserti deserti* (10); *D. heermanni morroensis* (19); *D. h. swarthi* (10); *D. h. tularensis* (15); *D. merriami merriami* (197); *D. nitratoides brevinasus* (21); *D. panamintinus caudatus* (20); *D. p. leucogenys* (33); *D. p. mohavensis* (251); and *D. p. panamintinus* (23). Only 22/251 (9%) *D. p. mohavensis* were found to be infected, all with a single species, *Eimeria mohavensis.* However, when 150–270 sporulated oocysts of *E. mohavensis* were administered to between 9 and 42 uninfected rats of each of the 11 subspecies under laboratory conditions, all 11 subspecies became infected. In addition, interestingly, the 20 *D. m. merriami* that were cross-infected produced almost twice as many oocysts during patency as did the 42 *D. p. mohavensis* when inoculated with equivalent numbers of oocysts. In other words, in this very large survey, only 1 of 11 subspecies was infected naturally with *E. mohavensis,* but all 11 subspecies were susceptible under laboratory conditions, and 1 subspecies, never found to be infected naturally (0/197 *D. m. merriami*), was more susceptible to the parasite than its presumed normal host. Is it possible that the other 10 subspecies have evolved a behavioral mechanism to avoid contact with sporulated oocysts in their natural environment and thus prevent/control infection? This is another area that deserves further study.

Treatment. Most or all of the drugs marketed for use against coccidia infections in mammals were first used to treat avian coccidiosis (McDougald 1982). Anticoccidials function by biochemically altering an important chemical pathway in the metabolism of the parasite without affecting a similar chemical pathway in the host to the same degree. The drugs most often used to treat coccidiosis in mammals (domestic, zoo, and captive animals) include the ionophores (interfere with membrane function by altering ionic gradients) such as monensin, lasalocid, and salinomycin; the sulfonamides (interfere with folic acid synthesis) such as trimethoprim; amprolium (thiamine-antagonist that interferes with cofactor synthesis); clopidol (a pyridone compound that interferes with energy metabolism in sporozoites or merozoites); robenidine [a bis-(benzylidineamino) guanidine that interferes with energy metabolism by inhibiting oxidative phosphorylation in the mitochondria (Wong et al. 1972)]; and decoquinate (blocks mitochondrial electron transport) (McDougald 1982; Gutteridge 1993). Drug resistance to anticoccidials is a major problem in controlling potential disease-producing species (e.g., *E. arlongi, E. bovis, E. stiedai*). Since drug resistant forms sometimes can be selected out in the absence of the drug to which they are resistant, diet-formulating companies often rotate the coccidiostats they incorporate into their diets to minimize this problem (Gutteridge 1993). Providing medicated feed or water is the most reliable means of control when mammals are contained in some way, but seems impractical for most wild mammals.

Public Health Concerns. Unlike *Cryptosporidium,* which can be a serious zoonosis (see below), there is no evidence that *Eimeria* or *Isospora* spp. of wild mammal origin can infect humans; not even *I. arctopitheci,* which seems to have the broadest host range for any known species in these three genera (Hendricks 1977). However, since 1985 there has been a growing literature on "cyanobacterium-like bodies" (CLBs) identified worldwide in the feces of immunocompetent and immunocompromised humans with diarrhea. In 1993, these CLBs were finally identified as coccidian oocysts in the genus *Cyclospora* (Ortega et al. 1993). Recently, Smith et al. (1996) found *Cyclospora* oocysts in the feces of all 37 baboons (*Papio*) and in 1 of 15 chimpanzees (*Pan*) in Gombe National Park, Tanzania. They stated that Dr. R.W. Ashford, Liverpool School of Tropical Medicine, confirmed that the oocysts they found "were identical to those described previously in human beings" as *C. cayetanensis.* If true, this suggests that in East Africa, higher primates may be an animal reservoir for human infection. However, the opposite also may be true since Smith et al. (1996) said that previous studies in Gombe suggested that the number of parasite species isolated from baboons and chimps in the park was greatest in those groups that had the most frequent human contact.

Domestic Animal Health Concerns. The importance of mammalian wildlife in their natural habitat has only recently begun to be appreciated. However, as human population continues to increase and agricultural development accelerates, attempting to keep pace, the potential for domestic animals to become infected by coccidian parasites maintained in wild reservoir hosts always remains a possibility (Roth 1972). For example, elk, deer, or bison can serve as reservoirs of coccidia or other parasites (helminths, mites, ticks, fleas, lice) for domestic livestock (Worley et al. 1969; Penzhorn et al. 1994); wild canids and felids can serve as reservoirs for domestic dog and cat parasites (Davidson et al. 1992a,b), including *Isospora* spp.; opossums may serve as hosts for parasites and diseases known to occur in ruminants in specialized, confined environments such as Kangaroo Island near Adelaide, South Australia (O'Callaghan and Moore 1986); and cottontail (*Sylvilagus* spp.) and jack (*Lepus* spp.) rabbits can serve as reservoirs for domesticated rabbit (*Oryctolagus* sp.) coccidia.

Management Implications. All natural populations of wild mammals surveyed for coccidia are found to be infected with at least one, but usually several, species unique to that host group, but the vast majority are not pathogenic under such conditions. The application of management practices to prevent outbreaks of coccidiosis in wild mammals should be focused on zoo and/or captive mammal situations. New animals should be quarantined several weeks before being introduced into a closed, captive environment with conspecifics or congenerics, and their feces should be monitored for the presence of (generally unsporulated) oocysts on a daily basis or at least several times each week. They should not be placed with other captive hosts until oocysts are no longer found in their feces. Oocysts also can be transferred to, and introduced into, captive mammal populations mechanically by flying vertebrates or invertebrates. Mammals in such situations should never be kept under crowded conditions to avoid potential outbreaks of disease.

FAMILY CRYPTOSPORIDIIDAE

Life History. Currently, seven named *Cryptosporidium* spp. are recognized as valid, four of which occur in mammals (Fayer et al. 1997) (Table 16.12). However, additional isolates are certain to be assigned names in the future, including at least two from mammals. *Cryptosporidium parvum* (Tyzzer 1912) primarily targets the ileum of humans and neonate animals and is responsible for > 99% all reported cases of diarrheal illness due to cryptosporidiosis in mammals. At least 79 mammalian species were reported recently as suitable hosts for the parasite (O'Donoghue 1995), and this list grows monthly.

More is known about the development and life cycle (Fig. 16.11) of *C. parvum* than about any other member of the genus. Infection begins with ingestion of the environmentally resistant oocysts, which are small, measure 5.2 x 4.6 μm (4.8–5.6 x 4.2–4.8 μm), and have a shape index of 1.2 (1.0–1.3) (Tilley et al. 1991). Each oocyst contains four sporozoites, which exit from a suture located along one side of the oocyst. The preferred site of infection is the ileum, although other sites also can be colonized. Sporozoites penetrate individual epithelial cells and become enclosed by a thin layer of host cell cytoplasm and membranes. A desmosome-like attachment organelle and accessory foldings of the parasite membranes develop at the interface between the parasite proper and the host cell cytoplasm (Fig. 16.11). This attachment organelle is sometimes referred to as the "feeder organelle." Merogony occurs, resulting in the formation of eight merozoites within the meront. These meronts are termed Type I meronts, and they rupture open to release free merozoites. These merozoites penetrate new cells and undergo another merogony. Type I merozoites are thought to be capable of recycling indefinitely; thus, the potential exists for new Type I meronts to arise continuously.

TABLE 16.12—Known species of *Cryptosporidium* (and synonyms) from mammals[a]

Valid Named and Unnamed Species [Synonyms]	Principal Hosts	Site of Infection	Select Key References
felis sensu lato Iseki, 1979	*Felis catus* (domestic cat)	Small intestine	Asahi et al. 1991, Iseki 1979
muris Tyzzer, 1907	*Mus musculus* (house mouse)	Stomach	Iseki 1986
	Rattus spp. (old world rats)		Iseki et al. 1989; Moriya 1989; Rhee et al. 1991b; Tyzzer 1907, 1910
parvum Tyzzer, 1912	> 90 known mammalian spp.	Small intestine	Current and Reese 1986, Fayer et al. 1997, Tyzzer 1912
[*agni* Barker & Carbonnel, 1974] [*bovis* Barker & Carbonnel, 1974] [*cuniculus* Inman & Takeuchi, 1979] [*enteritides* Qadripur & Klose, 1985] [*enteritidis* Müller, 1986] [*garnhami* Bird, 1981] [*rhesi* Levine, 1980] [*vobis* Iseki, 1979 *lapsus*]			
sp. of Upton and Current, 1985 [*muris* of Upton & Current, 1985]	*Bos taurus* (cattle)	Abomasum	Anderson 1987, 1988, 1990, 1991a; Esteban and Anderson 1995
wrairi Vetterling, Jervis, Merrill & Sprinz, 1971	*Cavia porcellus* (guinea pig)	Small intestine	Angus et al. 1985; Chrisp et al. 1990, 1992; Tilley et al. 1991; Vetterling et al. 1971a,b

[a]*C.* sp Bearup, 1954 from *Canis familiaris* (a dingo), *C.* sp. Dubey and Pande, 1963 from *Felis chaus* (jungle cat), and *C. vulpis* Wetzel, 1938 from *Vulpes vulpes* (fox) are misidentifications of *Sarcocystis* spp.; *C. curyi* Oggassawara, Benassi, Larsson and Hagiwara, 1986 from *Felis catis* (cat) is most likely a misidentification of nematode eggs.

Some Type I merozoites are triggered into forming a second type of meront, the Type II meront, which contains only four merozoites. Once liberated, the Type II merozoites appear to form the sexual stages. Some Type II merozoites enter cells, enlarge into the macrogametocyte, and then form macrogametes. Others enter cells to become the microgametocyte that undergoes multiple fission to form 16 nonflagellated microgametes. Microgametes rupture from the microgametocyte and penetrate macrogametes, forming a zygote. Sporogony occurs, resulting in the production of four sporozoites; thus, sporulated oocysts are passed in the feces into the environment.

About 20% of the oocysts produced in the gut fail to form an oocyst wall, and only a series of membranes surround the developing sporozoites. These "oocysts," devoid of a true wall, are sometimes termed "thin-walled oocysts." It is believed that the sporozoites produced from these thin-walled oocysts can excyst while still within the gut and infect new cells. Thus, *C. parvum* appears to have two autoinfective cycles: (1) continuous recycling of Type I merozoites and (2) sporozoites rupturing from thin-walled oocysts.

Development of *C. parvum* occurs more rapidly than many textbooks imply, and each generation can develop and mature in as little as 14–16 hours. Due to the rapidity of the life cycle and to the autoinfective cycles, huge numbers of organisms can colonize the intestinal tract in several days. The ileum soon becomes crowded, and secondary sites, such as the duodenum and large intestine, are often infected. In immunosup-

pressed individuals, parasites sometimes can be found in the stomach, biliary and pancreatic ducts, and respiratory tract. The prepatent period of *C. parvum* is generally 4 days, and patency generally lasts 7–10 days in immunocompetent hosts, but may become prolonged in immunosuppressed animals.

A morphologically similar species, *C. wrairi* Vetterling, Jervis, Merrill, and Sprinz 1971 *sensu lato,* also infects the small intestine, but has a high degree of specificity for the guinea pig, *Cavia porcellus.* Oocysts of this species are virtually identical to those of *C. parvum,* and measure 5.4 x 4.6 μm (4.8–5.6 x 4.0–5.0 μm) with a shape index of 1.2 (1.0–1.3) (Tilley et al. 1991). Although the parasite readily infects guinea pigs, it is weakly transmissible to ruminants and suckling mice (Angus et al. 1985; Tilley et al. 1991; Chrisp et al. 1992, 1995); it never has been reported from natural populations of guinea pigs in the wild, however. The life cycle was studied in detail by Vetterling et al. (1971a,b), and it appears nearly identical to that of *C. parvum.*

A third intestinal species, *C. felis* (Iseki 1979) *sensu lato,* also infects the small intestine and has oocysts similar in size to, and perhaps slightly smaller than, *C. parvum.* Iseki (1979) studied the life cycle in detail and reported oocysts to measure about 5 x 4.5 μm. Asahi et al. (1991) reported oocysts as 4.5 μm in diameter and Arai et al. (1990) as 4.7 x 4.3 μm. The life cycle appears virtually identical to that of *C. parvum* (Iseki 1979). Both Iseki (1979) and Asahi et al. (1991) were successful in transmitting feline-derived oocysts back

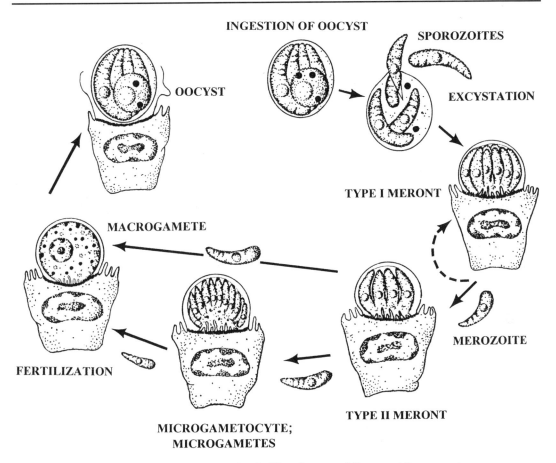

FIG. 16.11—Line drawing showing the life-cycle stages of *Cryptosporidium parvum.*

to cats, but failed to infect other animals including adult, suckling, or immunosuppressed mice, rats, guinea pigs, or dogs. These data suggest that this parasite may be specific only for felids and, if so, probably deserves true specific status. Prepatency appears to be 5–6 days, and some cats develop chronic infections and shed oocysts over long periods (Iseki 1979; Asahi et al. 1991). Mtambo et al. (1996) stated that they were able to infect two lambs, but not suckling mice, with oocysts derived from cats, but control lambs were lacking in the study. The wide range in prepatency in the two lambs (3 and 10 days) is unusual, and infections may simply have been spurious.

Cryptosporidium muris (Tyzzer 1907), the type species, develops in the gastric glands of Old World mice and rats (Tyzzer 1907, 1910; Iseki 1986; Moriya 1989; Aydin 1991; Rhee et al. 1991a,b; Chalmers et al. 1994; özkul and Aydin 1994). It also has been reported from *Phodopus roborovskii,* the desert hamster (Pavlásek and Lávika 1995). Oocysts are infective for both juvenile and adult animals and are larger than *C. parvum, C. wrairi,* or *C. felis,* measuring 8.4 x 6.3 μm

(7.5–9.8 x 5.5–7.0 μm) with a shape index of about 1.3 (Iseki 1986). Although it is likely that more than one type of asexual stage occurs, Tyzzer (1907, 1910) only reported a single autoinfective merogonous generation from the gastric mucosa, and no one yet has reported additional types. Both juvenile and adult rodents can be infected, and prepatency approaches 6 days (Rhee et al. 1991b). Peak oocyst production occurs between 15 and 31 days, with patency exceeding 2 months (Rhee et al. 1995). Experimental transmission studies have shown that some animals in addition to rodents also can become infected; these include dogs, guinea pigs, rabbits, and especially cats (Iseki et al. 1989; Aydin 1991). *Cryptosporidium* spp. from camels and rock hyrax also may represent *C. muris* as they both are similar in size to the type species and are transmissible to rodents (Anderson 1991b; Fayer et al. 1991; Esteban and Anderson 1995).

A large, abomasal form commonly found in juvenile and adult cattle and water buffalo sometimes is called *C. muris* or *C. muris*–like (Upton and Current 1985; Anderson 1987, 1988, 1990, 1991a; Esteban and

Anderson 1995; Nagy 1995; Pavlásek 1995; Araújo et al. 1996; Bukhari and Smith 1996). However, oocysts are slightly smaller and less elongate than *C. muris* and measure 7.4 x 5.6 μm (6.6–7.9 x 5.3–6.5 μm), with a shape index of 1.3 (1.1–1.5) (Upton and Current 1985). Experimental transmission studies in cattle result only in a limited number of successful infections (Anderson 1988). Pavlásek (1994) suggested that the parasite may be transmissible to mice, but other investigators have not been able to reproduce these data (Esteban and Anderson 1995). One study suggested that horses also may pass this parasite (da Silva et al. 1996). The life cycle of this parasite is unknown.

Epizootiology. *Cryptosporidium parvum* has been reported to occur worldwide on all continents except Antarctica. Fayer et al. (1997) list 95 countries where human cryptosporidiosis has been reported to be common in both humans and domestic animals, especially ruminants. Little epizootiology data are available for the parasite in wildlife, and most information is confined to sporadic case reports or outbreaks in captive herds, but evidence suggests that the organism is widespread throughout wildlife populations.

Epidemiologic studies suggest that major outbreaks of cryptosporidiosis occur during increased rainfall and/or high humidity (D'Antonio et al. 1985; Mathan et al. 1985; Shahid et al. 1985, 1987; Mata 1986; Cruickshank et al. 1988; Brown et al. 1989; Hayes et al. 1989; Pal et al. 1989; Steele et al. 1989; Mølbak et al. 1990, 1993; Skeels et al. 1990; Mangini et al. 1992; Leland et al. 1993; MacKenzie et al. 1994; Gennari-Cardoso et al. 1996). This often correlates with birthing of animals in the spring, although differences in local climate and rainfall, or point source contamination, can affect results. Dagan et al. (1991) noted *Cryptosporidium* to be more prevalent during the hot and dry season in southern Israel, but Clavel et al. (1996) found no seasonal variation. Generally, however, numbers of viable oocysts in wildlife populations in the Western Hemisphere should be highest in the spring because of the increased numbers of neonates and increased rainfall.

Spontaneous or experimental infections can result in diarrhea in neonate and immunosuppressed primates. Known hosts include baboon (Miller et al. 1990), *Cercopithecus* spp. (Gomez et al. 1992), lemur (Gomez et al. 1992), marmosets (Kalishman et al. 1996), *Macaca* spp. (Kovatch and White 1972; Cockrell et al. 1974; Wilson et al. 1984; Russell et al. 1987; Miller et al. 1990), mangabey (Gomez et al. 1992), orangutan (Wang and Liew 1990), patas monkeys (Gomez et al. 1992), spider monkeys (Gomez et al. 1992), squirrel monkeys (Bryant et al. 1983), and tamarins (Heuschele et al. 1986). Cryptosporidiosis has not been reported in immunocompetent, adult primates, nor have infections from wild populations been reported.

Cervids appear to be highly susceptible to *C. parvum,* and significant morbidity and mortality can occur. Infections have been reported in axis (*Axis axis*), Barasingha (*Cervus duvauceli*), Eld's deer (*Cervus*

eldi*), fallow deer (*Dama dama*), mule deer (*Odocoileus hermionus*), red deer (*Cervus elephus*), roe (*Capreolus capreolus*), sika (*Cervus nippon*), and white-tailed deer (*Odocoileus virginianus*). Most reports of severe diarrhea involve neonates and domestically reared or captive animals (Tzipori et al. 1981a; Angus et al. 1982; Korsholm and Henriksen 1984; Mason 1985; Orr et al. 1985; van Winkle 1985; Heuschele et al. 1986; Angus 1988, 1989; Blewett 1989; Simpson 1992; Fayer et al. 1996a). One study reported a captive white-tailed doe and her fawn passed oocysts, but neither had clinical illness (Fayer et al. 1996a).

In addition to deer, numerous other wild, captive artiodactyls, predominately neonates, have been reported to harbor *C. parvum.* Most reports involve incidental findings, and hosts include addax (*Addax nasomaculatus*), antelope (*Connochaetes taurinus, Hippotragus niger, Kobus ellipsiprymmus*), Barbary sheep (*Ammotragus lervia*), blackbuck (*Antilope cervicapra*), eland (*Taurotragus oryx*), gazelle (*Gazella dama, G. dorcas, G. leptoceros, G. subgutterosa, G. thomsoni*), giraffe (*Giraffa camelopardalis*), impala (*Aepyceros melampus*), llama (*Llama glama*), mouflon (*Ovis orientalis*), nilgai (*Boselaphus tragocamelus*), oryx (*Oryx gazella*), springbok (*Antidorcas marsupialis*), Turkomen markhor (*Capra falconeri*), and buffalo (*Bubalus bubalis, Syncerus caffer*) (Canestri-Trotti and Quesada 1983; Ducatelle et al. 1983; Fenwick 1983; Canestri-Trotti et al. 1984; van Winkle 1985; Heuschele et al. 1986; Crawshaw and Mehren 1987; Iskander et al. 1987; Canestri-Trotti 1989; Hovda et al. 1990; Rodriguez-Diego et al. 1991; Dubey et al. 1992; Gomez et al. 1996). Significant morbidity and some mortality in water buffalo calves have been reported. In Italy, 7% of 229 neonates with diarrhea passed oocysts (Canestri-Trotti and Quesada 1983), and 20%–21% of the neonates in Cuba and Egypt were reported to be infected (Iskander et al. 1987; Rodriguez-Diego et al. 1991).

Equids and other Perissodactyla, including the rhinoceros, also acquire *C. parvum.* Again, diarrheal illness generally is associated only with neonates or immunodeficient animals (Snyder et al. 1978; Tzipori and Campbell 1981; Gibson et al. 1983; Soule et al. 1983; Canestri-Trotti and Visconti 1985; Gajadhar et al. 1985; Lengronne et al. 1985; Carneiro et al. 1987; Chermette et al. 1987, 1989; DiPietro et al. 1988; Fernández et al. 1988; Coleman et al. 1989; Poonacha and Tuttle 1989; Mair et al. 1990; Wang and Liew 1990; Bjorneby et al. 1991b; Eydal 1994; Xiao and Herd 1994a,b; Gomez et al. 1996; Netherwood et al. 1996; da Silva et al. 1996). The parasite was first reported in equids by Snyder et al. (1978), who noted five of six immunodeficient Arabian foals that died of adenoviral infection also harbored *C. parvum.* However, a high percentage of immunocompetent foals also acquire the parasite. Infection rates vary from 2%–60% (Xiao and Herd 1994a,b), and foals seem to be most susceptible between 5 and 20 weeks of age (Xiao and Herd 1994b). Although most studies suggest the prevalence of infection in older horses is low (Coleman et al. 1989; Xiao and Herd 1994a,b), adult animals can pass oocysts, and a study in France suggested that mares may serve as a source of infection for foals (Chermette et al. 1989). A similar study in North America came to the opposite conclusion (Xiao and Herd 1994b).

Incidental findings of *C. parvum* in other wild, captive, or zoo mammals include reports documenting the parasite in ferrets (Rehg et al. 1988; Gómez-Villamandos et al. 1995); grey fox (Davidson et al. 1992a,b), insectivores (Sinski 1993; Sinski et al. 1993), leopard (Wang and Liew 1990), Malayan bear (Wang and Liew 1990), marsupials (Barker et al. 1978; O'Donoghue 1995; Fayer et al. 1997), monotremes (O'Donoghue 1995), rabbits (Ryan et al. 1986), raccoon (Carlson and Neilsen 1982; Snyder 1988; Martin and Zeidner 1992), and various rodents (Elton et al. 1931; Sundberg et al. 1982; Davis and Jenkins 1986; Yamini and Raju 1986; Isaac-Renton et al. 1987; Yamaura et al. 1990; Pavlásek and Kozakiewicz 1991; Elangbam et al. 1993; Sinski 1993; Sinski et al. 1993; Laakkonen et al. 1994; O'Donoghue 1995; Pavlásek and Lávicka 1995). Nearly all data on *Cryptosporidium* spp. in wild populations is confined to rodent studies. Oocysts were found in 1 of 131 (0.8%) *Microtus agrestis* and 1 of 41 (2%) *Cleithrionomys glareolus* in Finland (Laakkonen et al. 1994). Chalmers et al. (1994) found 19 of 58 (33%) wild mice trapped near Moreton Morrell, United Kingdom, to be passing oocysts, and Elangbam et al. (1993) found developmental stages in the intestinal tract of 1 of 9 (11%) *Sigmodon hispidus* from Pryor, Oklahoma. In Poland, in the district of Mazury Lake, 55 of 275 (20%) *C. glareolus,* 6 of 39 (15%) *Apodemus flavicoliis,* and 5 of 16 (31%) *Sorex araneus* were positive (Sinski et al. 1993). Of 115 *Mus musculus* live-trapped near a calving site in Auburn, Alabama, and placed in captivity 2–3 weeks, 35 (30%) were passing oocysts (Klesius et al. 1986).

Although the majority of reports of *Cryptosporidium* spp. in wildlife appear to be due to *C. parvum,* some information is available about other *Cryptosporidium* spp. Of the two named intestinal species, *C. felis* and *C. wrairi,* only the former is known to occur in natural populations, with the latter reported only from laboratory-reared guinea pigs. Iseki (1979) found 5 of 13 (38%) cats infected in Osaka. Five of 608 (4%) felids were passing oocysts in Tokyo (Arai et al. 1990), and 35 of 871 (4%) cats were shedding oocysts in Austria (Supperer and Hinaidy 1986). In Glasgow, 19 of 235 (8%) and 7 of 57 (12%) cats were found to be passing oocysts (Mtambo et al. 1991; Nash et al. 1993). Because oocysts of *C. parvum* and *C. felis* are indistinguishable and because both have been shown to infect cats, some of the prevalence data actually may represent infections with *C. parvum.*

Several studies suggest that the *Cryptosporidium* sp. from the abomasum of juvenile and adult cattle is widespread. Bukhari and Smith (1996) found 23% of 109 dairy cattle in Scotland to be infected. In the Czech Republic, 4 of 96 (4%) cows were passing oocysts

(Pavlásek 1994), and 1.4% of 95,874 randomly collected bovine fecal samples from 12 states in the United States were infected (Anderson 1991a). Overall, samples collected from dairy herds were found to have twice the prevalence of feedlot samples (Anderson 1991a). A total of 4.5% of 887 Holstein-Friesian breed heifers entering the Czech Republic from France and 7.9% of those imported from Germany were passing oocysts (Pavlásek 1995). Although this coccidium may be specific for bovids, Pospischil et al. (1987) reported that captive Mountain gazelles (*Gazella cuvieri*) from the Munich Zoo were infected by an abomasal *Cryptosporidium* sp. similar in size to that reported in cattle.

Cryptosporidium muris has not been reported from natural populations of rodents in the Western Hemisphere, but it is known to occur naturally in Europe and Asia. This includes 3 of 64 (5%) *Rattus* spp. in Osaka (Iseki 1979) and 15 of 58 (26%) mice on a farm in Moreton Morrell, United Kingdom (Chalmers et al. 1994). A *C. muris*–like organism was reported from a Bactrian camel (*Camelus bactrianus*) from the National Zoological Park in Virginia (Anderson 1991b; Fayer et al. 1991). Experimental transmission studies demonstrated that mice, but not calves, could acquire the infection, suggesting that the parasite may truly be *C. muris.* Similar-sized oocysts passed by a rock hyrax at the National Zoological Park also were infective for mice (Esteban and Anderson 1995), and da Silva et al. (1996) reported what may be this parasite from equids in Brazil.

Clinical Signs. Significant illness due to *C. parvum* rarely has been reported from wild-caught animals, but it is common once the animals become captive, when crowding and additional stress become factors. Acute cryptosporidiosis manifests itself in moderate to severe diarrhea, weight loss, abdominal cramping, lethargy, inappetence, and occasionally fever. Severe dehydration may occur, occasionally resulting in electrolyte imbalance and death. In bovids, the disease is typically characterized by high morbidity, but low mortality, and cases involving significant mortality generally involve a second pathogen such as rotavirus or ETEC-K99+ (Fayer et al. 1985; 1997). Cases involving high mortality in the absence of secondary pathogens usually can be traced to an immunodeficient host population or to misdiagnoses (Heine et al. 1984b; Fayer et al. 1997). However, other animals may be more susceptible to the parasite, and significant mortality may occur, especially if additional stress on the animals is incurred.

Immunocompetent animals reported to have significant illness include chinchilla (Yamini and Raju 1986), fawns (Tzipori et al. 1981a; Korsholm and Henriksen 1984; Orr et al. 1985; Heuschele et al. 1986), foals (Gajadhar et al. 1985; DiPetro et al. 1988; Fernández et al. 1988; Coleman et al. 1989; Browning et al. 1991; Xiao and Herd 1994a,b; Netherwood et al. 1996), hamsters (Davis and Jenkins 1986; Orr 1988), primates (Kovatch and White 1972; Cockrell et al. 1974; Wilson et al. 1984; Russell et al. 1987; Miller et al. 1990), water buffalo (Canestri-Trotti and Quesada 1983; Iskander et al. 1987), and other ruminants (Fenwick 1983; Heuschele et al. 1986; Hovda et al. 1990).

Infections with *C. wrairi* in guinea pigs may range from subclinical to acute, similar to that reported for *C. parvum* in other animals. Clinical signs include diarrhea, dehydration, and weight loss (Angus et al. 1985; Gibson and Wagner 1986). Morbidity and mortality associated with cryptosporidiosis in guinea pig colonies of various suppliers was reported to range from 0%–50% (Gibson and Wagner 1986).

Since both *C. parvum* and *C. felis* are capable of infecting neonate and immunosuppressed cats, and because multiple types of immunosuppressive viruses exist in felids, reports of diarrheal illness due to cryptosporidiosis in cats must be viewed cautiously. It is known, however, that juvenile and adult cats are highly susceptible to *C. felis*. Infections in adult animals generally are chronic and subclinical, even when large numbers of oocysts are shed in the feces (Arai et al. 1990; Asahi et al. 1991).

In mammals, infections with the large species of *Cryptosporidium* infecting the gastric mucosa often are chronic and subclinical. Neither Iseki (1986) or Iseki et al. (1989) noted clinical signs in animals infected with *C. muris*, and Anderson (1987, 1988) reported cattle infected with the abomasal *Cryptosporidium* sp. also were subclinical. However, some animals infected with the latter species had depressed weight gain (Anderson 1987; Esteban and Anderson 1995). One study suggested that dairy cows shedding oocysts may produce less milk than uninfected cohorts, although these differences were not found to be statistically significant (Esteban and Anderson 1995).

Pathology and Pathogenesis. The primary site of infection by *C. parvum* is the distal region of the small intestine, although the cecum, colon, and duodenum also support development. Sometimes parasites can be found in the pancreatic and biliary ducts, as well as the urogenital and respiratory tracts (Sanford and Josephson 1982; Heine et al. 1984a; Pavlásek 1984; Pavlásek and Nikitin 1987; Kaup et al. 1994; Mascaró et al. 1994). However, only in rare instances are these latter sites colonized to any degree in immunocompetent animals. Infections have been associated with villus atrophy and villus fusion, infiltration of the lamina propria by inflammatory cells, and sloughing and degeneration of individual enterocytes (Panciera et al. 1971; Pearson and Logan 1978; Howerth 1981; Tzipori et al. 1981b,c; Angus et al. 1982; Sanford and Josephson 1982; Heine et al. 1984b; Vítovec and Koudela 1988, 1992). Metaplasia of the surface epithelium to cuboidal or low columnar cells has been observed (Howerth 1981; Heine et al. 1984b), and crypts may become dilated and fill with necrotic debris (Powell et al. 1976; Sanford and Josephson 1982). These changes result in reduced absorption of vitamins and sugars (Argenzio et al. 1990; Holland et al. 1992; Nappert et al. 1993; Clark

and Sears 1996), and it is likely that enterocyte damage results in impaired glucose-stimulated Na+ and H$_2$O absorption (Clark and Sears 1996). Since disaccharidase activity is thought to decrease due to the loss of mature enterocytes, it has been postulated that the undegraded sugars also may allow for bacterial overgrowth and a change in osmotic pressure due to the formation of volatile free fatty acids (Holland et al. 1989). Alternatively, the accumulation of nonabsorbed nutrients may lead to a hypertonic condition that also contributes to diarrhea (Holland et al. 1989). Argenzio et al. (1993) suggested that at least some of the diarrhea in piglets experimentally infected with *C. parvum* can be attributed to local prostanoid production. Although the presence of an enterotoxin has been postulated (Garza et al. 1986; Guarino et al. 1994), no definitive evidence exists to conclusively demonstrate that the parasite produces an enterotoxin.

Experimental infections of immunocompetent cats with *C. felis* results in a notable lack of gross pathology and histopathology associated with the digestive tract (Iseki 1979; Asahi et al. 1991). However, infections of guinea pigs with *C. wrairi* induce a pathology similar to that of *C. parvum,* and results range from subclinical to fatal. Angus et al. (1985) noted that infections occur throughout the small intestine and cecum, but are heaviest in the ileum where severe villus stunting and fusion occur. The lamina propria becomes infiltrated with macrophages and eosinophils, and the mucosa becomes covered by a thick, flat layer of cuboidal cells. Similar results have been reported by other researchers (Jervis et al. 1966; Kunstý and Naumann 1981; Gibson and Wagner 1986; Chrisp et al. 1990). Gibson and Wagner (1986) described such macroscopic findings as emaciation, intestinal hyperemia, and serosal edema of the cecal wall.

Although *Cryptosporidium* spp. developing in the stomach generally produce few clinical signs, infections are persistent, and pathology has been observed. Abomasal cryptosporidiosis in cattle results in an abomasum that is enlarged and thickened by ~10%, an increase in the depth of the gastric glands and widening of the gland lumen, and dilation and atropy of some glandular cells (Anderson 1987, 1988). Plasma pepsinogen concentrations also have been reported to be above normal (Anderson 1988). Pathological findings associated with *C. muris* in rodents include enlargement of the lumens of the gastric glands, flattening and atrophy of epithelial cells, and reduction in the number of microvilli (Aydin 1991; Yoshikawa and Iseki 1992; Özkul and Aydin 1994).

Diagnosis. Early diagnostic procedures for *Cryptosporidium* spp. often involved histological processing of biopsy materials, but identification of oocysts passed in the feces is now the primary method of diagnosis. These assays fall under three general categories: microscopic, which includes flotations, smears, stains, and immunofluorescent antibody (IFA) probes; enzyme immunoassays (EIA), usually based on binding of an antibody to the outer oocyst wall followed by colorimetric detection; and molecular, which include polymerase chain reaction (PCR) and derivitives.

Proper collection and storage of feces is critical for any diagnostic method involving antibodies. Many fixatives and storage solutions change outer-wall antigenicity and must be avoided. Aqueous solutions of potassium dichromate and sodium acetate are known to affect binding of some antibodies (Nichols et al. 1991; Upton 1997), and sedimentation techniques using diethyl ether or chloroform should be strictly avoided whenever IFA or EIA are used. Most commercially available antibody-based tests are designed for parasites that have been either frozen or preserved in 10% formalin.

Chermette and Boufassa-Ouzrout (1988) list 18 published staining techniques for oocysts of *Cryptosporidium* in fecal smears. Arrowood (1997) lists 28 different microscopic techniques, which predominately consist of staining and indirect or direct IFA assays. The techniques that have gained the most popularity for field use are modifications of the original acid-fast technques, which stain the contents of oocysts with a compromised outer wall bright red, often against a bluish-green background. These techniques are relatively quick and inexpensive and allow for differentiation of *Cryptosporidium* oocysts from yeast spores (Henriksen and Pohlenz 1981; Garcia et al. 1983; Ma and Soave 1983; Bronsdon 1984; Casemore et al. 1984; Pohjola et al. 1985; Ma 1986; Chermette and Boufassa-Ouzrout 1988; Ridley and Olsen 1991; Entrala et al. 1995; Arrowood 1997). Numerous other conventional and fluorescent staining methods exist, however, and include acridine orange, aniline-carbol-methyl violet and tartrazine, auramine O, auramine-rhodamine, auramine-carbol-fuchsin, 4',6-diamidino-2-phenylindole (DAPI), Giemsa, hemacolor, mepacrine, modified Kohn's, modified Koster, negative staining, safranine-methylene blue, propridium iodide, and others (Heine 1982; Current 1983; Payne et al. 1983; Baxby et al. 1984; Kageruka et al. 1984; Ma et al. 1984; Pohjola 1984; Casemore et al. 1985; Milácek and Vítovec 1985; Kawamoto et al. 1987; Asahi et al. 1988; Chermette and Boufassa-Ouzrout 1988; Arrowood and Sterling 1989; Chichino et al. 1991; Cozon et al. 1992; Ungureanu and Dontu 1992; Grimason et al. 1994; Kang and Mathan 1996). In these techniques, differentiation of species is accomplished based on knowing which *Cryptosporidium* sp. occurs in which host species and on the relative oocyst sizes (see above).

Immunofluorescent antibody (IFA) assays require the use of a primary monoclonal or polyclonal antibody directed against one or more epitopes on the outer oocyst wall, followed by some form of fluorescent detection. Although a number of variables, including aging of oocysts, storage and fixation media, and cross-reacting epitopes from contaminants can compound the assays, the IFA assay tends to be more specific and sensitive than staining fecal smears (Casemore et al. 1985; Sterling and Arrowood 1986; Stibbs and Ongerth 1986;

Garcia et al. 1987, 1992; McLauchlin et al. 1987; Stetzenbach et al. 1988; Arrowood and Sterling 1989; J.B. Rose et al. 1989; Rusnak et al. 1989; Tsaihong and Ma 1990; MacPherson and McQueen 1993; Tee et al. 1993; Grigoriew et al. 1994; Rodríguez-Hernandez et al. 1994; Kehl et al. 1995; LeChevallier et al. 1995; Rodgers et al. 1995; Zimmerman and Needham 1995). Although most diagnostic tests have been developed specifically to detect *C. parvum*, several companies market tests that identify oocysts of multiple *Cryptosporidium* spp. (Garcia et al. 1987; Arrowood and Sterling 1989; J.B. Rose et al. 1989; Vesey et al. 1994; Graczyk et al. 1996a). None of the IFA assays are known to be entirely species specific.

A variety of commericaly available EIAs are available for detection of *C. parvum* in feces. These have been shown repeatedly to be superior to acid-fast staining, but generally cannot be performed using routine laboratory reagents. Arrowood (1997) provides a summary of the sensitivity and specificities of five commercially available test kits that have been studied in peer reviewed journals. Several others have been examined since his chapter was written. Sensitivities range from 66% to 100% and specificities from 93% to 100% (Siddons et al. 1992; Newman et al. 1993; Rosenblatt and Sloan 1993; Aarnaes et al. 1994; Dagan et al. 1995; Kehl et al. 1995; McCluskey et al. 1995; Parisi and Tierno 1995; Zimmerman and Needham 1995; Graczyk et al. 1996a; Garcia and Shimizu 1997). Graczyk et al. (1996a) examined multiple *Cryptosporidium* spp. collected from mammals, birds, and reptiles and concluded that the EIA was less specific and less sensitive for non–*C. parvum* isolates than direct and indirect IFA-based tests. Again, none of these tests are species specific.

The techniques that are now gaining in popularity for typing *Cryptosporidium* spp. are molecular-based assays. PCR-based assays have the potential not only to detect the presence of single oocysts in samples, but also to determine the exact species of *Cryptosporidium* in question. DNA probes specific for *C. parvum* and several other *Cryptosporidium* spp. have been developed in many laboratories and include assays using both specific and random primers (Laxer et al. 1991, 1992; Johnson et al. 1993, 1995; Webster et al. 1993, 1996; Awad-El-Kariem et al. 1994; Filkorn et al. 1994; Morgan et al. 1995, 1996; Wagner-Wiening and Kimmig 1995; Balatbat et al. 1996; Laberge et al. 1996a; Leng et al. 1996; Mayer and Palmer 1996; Stinear et al. 1996; Gobet et al. 1997; Rochelle et al. 1997a,b). The main disadvantage of PCR-based diagnostic tests is that a certain degree of expertise as well as expensive reagents and equipment are currently required. In the near future, however, it appears that some versions will allow for rapid, colorimetric diagnosis of *Cryptosporidium* infections without the need for elaborate equipment or expertise.

Immunity. *Cryptosporidium parvum* appears to make little effort to evade the immune system of the host.

Many of the surface proteins, glycoproteins, and phospholipids are strongly immunogenic, and many surface molecules on both sporozoites and merozoites are antigenically cross-reactive. The success of the parasite appears to be in its ability to develop rapidly and flood the environment with oocysts. If this parasite were not efficiently eliminated from the body in a reasonable amount of time, it would soon kill many animals through dehydration and electrolyte imbalance, rapidly eliminating host species from the environment. Indeed, the severe effects of the parasite on immunosuppressed animals and humans clearly demonstrate the need for an effective immune response.

Cryptosporidiosis is primarily a disease of neonates. Although some adults become infected and shed low numbers of oocysts intermittently for long periods of time, clinical signs are generally absent except for unusual strains. Only in humans do adults commonly become acutely infected and have clinical disease, and this makes immunological studies difficult because of the lack of immunocompetent animal models. The mechanism by which age affects parasite development in the intestine is not yet known. However, this age-related susceptibility has been clearly documented (Mead et al. 1991; Novak and Sterling 1991; Harp et al. 1992; Kuhls et al. 1992; Harp and Sacco 1996; Upton and Gillock 1996), and Harp et al. (1992) suggested that this effect is mediated, in part, by the type of intestinal microflora. Upton and Gillock (1996) reported that developmentally expressed antigens may be the reason why neonates are more susceptible to infections than most adult animals.

Although infections with *C. parvum* generate an active humoral immune response, it is unclear whether these antibodies play a significant role in reducing the parasite burden. Antibody responses to both the 15–20 kDa antigen and 25–30 kDa antigen appear to be good indicators of infection (Mead et al. 1988; Hill et al. 1990; Répérant et al. 1992, 1994; Arnault et al. 1994; El-Shewy et al. 1994a,b; Moss et al. 1994; Ortega-Mora et al. 1994; Lorenzo et al. 1995; Tilley and Upton 1997), and both serum and mucosal antibodies generally are elevated at the time diarrhea and oocyst production wane (Tzipori and Campbell 1981; Lazo et al. 1986; Ungar and Nash 1986; Casemore 1987; Williams 1987; Mead et al. 1988; Hill et al. 1990; Whitmire and Harp 1991; Mosier et al. 1992; Peeters et al. 1992; Ortega-Mora et al. 1993). A number of studies also have shown that infected animals or individuals given antibodies orally often have lowered levels of infections, indicating a significant effect of antibody on parasite levels (Tzipori et al. 1986, 1987; Lopez et al. 1988; Arrowood et al. 1989; Fayer et al. 1989a,b, 1990; Bjorneby et al. 1990, 1991a; Nord et al. 1990; Ungar et al. 1990a; Cama and Sterling 1991; Perryman and Bjorneby 1991; Plettenberg et al. 1993; Watzl et al. 1993; Heaton 1994; Naciri et al. 1994; Riggs et al. 1994; Kuhls et al. 1995; Greenberg and Cello 1996). Nevertheless, there is no apparent correlation between exact serum or fecal antibody titers and elimination of

the parasite, and numerous examples of individuals or animals with high anticryptosporidial antibody titers and persistent infections can be found (Ungar et al. 1986; Kassa et al. 1991; Kapel et al. 1993; Cozon et al. 1994; Benhamou et al. 1995; Favennec et al. 1995).

A variety of studies have demonstrated clearly the importance of CD4 cells, IFN-γ, IL-5, and IL-12 in the immune response (Ungar et al. 1990b, 1991; Gardner et al. 1991; McDonald et al. 1992, 1994; Chen et al. 1993a,b; Aguirre et al. 1994; Perryman et al. 1994; Gomez-Morales et al. 1995, 1996; Tilley et al. 1995; Huang et al. 1996; Urban et al. 1996; Riggs 1997; Wyatt et al. 1997). Studies involving major histocompatibility deficient class I (MHC class I) or class II (MHC class II) rodents have shown CD4 lymphocytes, but not CD8 lymphocytes, are required to prevent persistent infections (Aguirre et al. 1994). Alpha/beta-T-cells appear more important than γ/δ-T-cells in controlling the level of infection. Both neonate and adult αβ-T-cell–deficient mice develop persistent infections, whereas only γ/δ-T-cell–deficient neonates, not adults, develop slightly higher levels of infections over controls (Waters and Harp 1996). In immune calves, challenge infections result in a T-lymphocyte response favoring αβ-T-cells over γδ-T-cells (Abrahamsen et al. 1997).

Depletion of IFN-γ reduces prepatency, enhances oocyst output, and prolongs oocyst shedding in experimentally infected mice (Ungar et al. 1991; McDonald et al. 1992; Chen et al. 1993b; Kuhls et al. 1994; McDonald and Bancroft 1994; Tzipori et al. 1995; Urban et al. 1996). Depletion of IL-5, but apparently not IL-2 or IL-4, also significantly increases the level of infection (Ungar et al. 1991; Enriquez and Sterling 1993). Studies on activated intestinal T lymphocytes in calves have shown tumor necrosis factor alpha (TNF-α) to be elevated (Wyatt et al. 1997), but depletion of TNF-α in severe combined immunodeficiency disease (SCID) mice does not appear to increase susceptibility to infection (Chen et al. 1993a; McDonald et al. 1994).

Prevention and Control. Because all infections with *Cryptosporidium* spp. are initiated through ingestion of environmentally resistant oocysts, control of this stage is the single most important factor limiting the spread of cryptosporidiosis. As host density nearly always determines whether coccidial infections become epizootic, it is important to keep captive herd sizes sparse. The numbers and intensity of neonate calves infected with *C. parvum* have been shown to be proportional to herd size (Garber et al. 1994), and it is likely that a similar situation will be shown for other animals. Infected animals will contaminate the environment with oocysts; thus, animals producing detectable levels of oocysts should be isolated from uninfected cohorts to prevent spread of the disease. However, recent studies suggest many adult animals may periodically shed low numbers of oocysts into the environment, thus serving as reservoirs of the parasite (Villacorta et al. 1991;

Lorenzo-Lorenzo et al. 1993a; Xiao et al. 1993; Scott et al. 1995; Quílez et al. 1996; Tacal et al. 1987).

Animal husbandry, disinfection regimes, and hygiene are important factors that limit the spread of *Cryptosporidium*. In addition, animal handlers should be considered an important source of infection as they pass oocysts from enclosure to enclosure. Oocysts and feces containing oocysts will adhere to any surface, including skin, clothing, shoes, water bottles, feed, bedding, and tools. It is possible that insects, birds, or other animals that freely move between enclosures also carry infective oocysts mechanically. Wallace (1971, 1972) showed that both flies and cockroaches are capable of disseminating oocysts of *Toxoplasma gondii* in the environment, and both arthropods have been implicated in dissemination of *C. parvum* (Zerpa and Huicho 1994). Oocysts of *C. parvum* passing through the intestine of experimentally inoculated waterfowl remain viable and infective for laboratory rodents, even when feces are collected 6–7 days postinfection (Graczyk et al. 1996b, 1997). No reasonable technique will eliminate 100% of the viable oocysts or keep all animals from becoming infected. For instance, oocysts were still passed in the feces several days after calves were removed in plastic bags at birth to new stalls (Heine et al. 1984b). Cryptosporidiosis, however, can become a manageable disease.

Fayer et al. (1997) lists 26 commercially available disinfectants, employed by various investigators, that had little or no effect on parasite infectivity, even when *C. parvum* oocysts were exposed at intervals ranging from 30 minutes to 24 hours. At least some oocysts remain infective even after exposure to 15,000 mW/sec ultraviolet light for 2, but not 2.5, hours (Lorenzo-Lorenzo et al. 1993b); -15° C for 24 hours, but not 1 week (Fayer 1994); -20° C for 8, but not 24, hours (Fayer 1994); and +59.7° C for 5 minutes, but not +60° C for 6 minutes (Fayer and Nerad 1996). Typically, 100% of the encysted parasites are killed only when extreme and unpractical measures are employed. These include exposure to 1 J/cm² pulsed light (Dunn et al. 1995), 100% bromomethane gas for 24 hours (Fayer et al. 1996b), 28,000 mg/l chlorine for 24 hours (Smith et al. 1990), 10% formol saline for 18 hours (Campbell et al. 1982), 5% ammonia for 18 hours (Campbell et al. 1982), and 100% ethylene dioxide gas for 24 hours (Fayer et al. 1996b). Lengthy exposures to gaseous or aqueous solutions of ammonia, hydrogen peroxide, high concentrations of chlorine and related compounds, and short-term exposure to ozone significantly reduce numbers of viable *C. parvum* oocysts, but only rarely result in 100% efficacy (Fayer 1995; Fayer et al. 1997; Rose et al. 1997).

Perhaps the most effective and economic method to reduce the numbers of oocysts in the environment is desiccation. Using dye exclusion to measure viability, Robertson et al. (1992) found viability of a population of air-dried *C. parvum* oocysts to be reduced by 97% after 2 hours and 100% after 4 hours. Feces containing *C. parvum* oocysts that were air dried for 1 day were

found to be noninfectious for suckling mice in another study (Anderson 1986). These data imply that application of aqueous disinfectant solutions, which keep feces moist, may result in prolonging parasite survival in feces rather than reducing parasite numbers.

Treatment. Dozens of compounds have undergone various in vivo evaluations for efficacy against *C. parvum* infections, and testing has included both rodent and, occasionally, ruminant animal models. Virtually all of the traditional anticoccidials and other antimicrobials consistently fail to eliminate infections entirely at nontoxic levels, although some reduce parasite numbers significantly. Blagburn and Soave (1997) provide an extensive list of in vivo drug trials against this parasite, and results suggest the most effective compounds to be ionophores (alborixin, halofuginone, lasalocid, and maduramicin), the aminoglycoside paromomycin, the nucleoside analog arprinocid, the macrolide azithromycin, the steroid dehydroepiandrosterone, the sulfonamide sulfadimethoxine, and the immune modulator diethyldithiocarbamate. In ruminants, paromomycin and the ionophores have received the greatest attention. In one experiment, calves fed 25–100 mg/kg body weight paromomycin in their milk twice daily for 11 consecutive days prior to oral inoculation had significantly fewer parasites in the feces and less diarrhea than unmedicated controls (Fayer and Ellis 1993). Mancassola et al. (1995) used paromomycin prophylactically in kid goats at 100 mg/kg body weight daily to delay and dramatically lower oocyst shedding in experimentally infected animals. In calves, Naciri et al. (1993) found halofuginone at concentrations of 60 and 120 μg/kg body weight daily delayed oocyst shedding and reduce signs of clinical disease in a dose-dependent manner. Halofuginone at 500 μg/kg body weight daily also was shown to reduce and delay oocyst shedding in experimentally infected lambs (Naciri and Yvoré 1989).

Because treatment regimes for *C. parvum* largely are ineffective, current therapy for severe cryptosporidiosis involves oral or parenteral rehydration using fluids and electrolytes. Although most reports involve humans or calves, Hovda et al. (1990) described success using parenteral therapy to reverse weight loss, electrolyte imbalance, and cachexia associated with prolonged diarrhea in a llama severely infected with *C. parvum.*

Public Health Concerns. Because so many mammalian species can be infected with *C. parvum,* a large potential zoonotic reservoir exists. Numerous studies have demonstrated or correlated transmission of the parasite from animals to humans, especially to children. These cases generally involve direct exposure to infected animals or their feces or exposure to contaminated raw milk, food, or water (Babb et al. 1982; Blagburn and Current 1983; Rahman et al. 1984; Casemore et al. 1986; Pohjola et al. 1986; Ribeiro and Palmer 1986; Biggs et al. 1987; Shahid et al. 1987; Hamoudi et al. 1988; Levine et al. 1988; Casemore 1989, 1990;

Palmer and Biffin 1990; Shield et al. 1990; Miron et al. 1991; Nouri and Karami 1991; Nouri and Toroghi 1991; Lengerich et al. 1993; Smith 1993; Millard et al. 1994; Nimri and Batchoun 1994; Sanchez-Mejorada and Ponce-de-Leon 1994; Dawson et al. 1995; Laberge et al. 1996b). One study suggested a case of airborne transmission (Højlyng et al. 1987).

Although wildlife may, at first, appear to be obvious sources of oocysts in surface waters, it is difficult to determine the degree to which wild animals actually contribute to overall numbers of infections. Ruminants, especially cattle, sometimes are implicated when high parasite numbers are detected (Ongerth and Stibbs 1987, 1989; J.B. Rose et al. 1988; Hansen and Ongreth 1991; Ong et al. 1996), but most studies fail to pinpoint the source of contamination. Ong et al. (1996) were able to correlate higher numbers of oocysts downstream from a cattle range with calving activity. Because cervids (above), beaver (Isaac-Renton et al. 1987), and rodents (above) are known to harbor the parasite and frequently are associated with watersheds, it is likely that at least some oocysts originate from these hosts in North America.

Domestic Animal Health Concerns. The role by which wildlife contribute to infections in domestic animals has not been elucidated. Occasional introduction of the parasite into domestic animal populations from wildlife such as deer, medium-sized mammals, or rodents probably occurs regularly. However, since the majority of information on prevalence of *C. parvum* worldwide demonstrates a high prevalence in cattle and other ruminants, it is likely that domestic animals themselves are responsible for most cases of domestic animal cryptosporidiosis.

Management Implications. Natural infections in wildlife with the various species of *Cryptosporidium,* especially *C. parvum,* will continue to occur despite the best of management practices. In some instances, severely infected animals probably can be removed from wild populations to reduce numbers of oocysts in a local area. This may be especially important in the spring when birthing occurs, although it is impractical under most conditions. However, as stated above, recent evidence has suggested that high numbers of adult animals continue to shed low numbers of oocysts into the environment, thus serving as reservoirs for neonates.

ACKNOWLEDGEMENTS. This work was supported by NSF grant DEB-95216876. We are grateful to Ms. L.A. Hertel and Dr. T.L. Vance for the line drawings.

LITERATURE CITED

Aarnaes, S.L., J. Blanding, S. Speier, D. Forthal, L.M. De La Masa, and E.M. Peterson. 1994. Comparison of the ProSpecT and Color Vue enzyme-linked immunoassays for the detection of *Cryptosporidium* in stool specimens. *Diagnostic Microbiology and Infectious Diseases* 19:221–225.

Abbas, B., and G. Post. 1980. Experimental coccidiosis in mule deer fawns. *Journal of Wildlife Diseases* 16:565–570.

Abrahamsen, M.S., C.A. Lancto, B. Walcheck, W. Layton, and M.A. Jutila. 1997. Localization of α/β and γ/δ-T lymphocytes in *Cryptosporidium parvum*–infected tissues in naive and immune calves. *Infection and Immunity* 65:2428–2433.

Agrawal, R.D., S.S. Ahluwalia, B.B. Bhatia, and P.P.S. Chauhan. 1981. Note on mammalian coccidia at Lucknow Zoo. *Indian Journal of Animal Science* 51:125–128.

Aguirre, S.A., P.H. Mason, and L.E. Perryman. 1994. Suscepibility of major histocompatibility complex (MHC) class I- and MHC class II-deficient mice to *Cryptosporidium parvum* infection. *Infection and Immunity* 62:697–699.

Ahluwalia, S.S., R.V. Singh, G.S. Arora, A.K. Mandal, and N.C. Sarkar. 1979. *Eimeria suncus* sp. nov. (Sporozoa: Eimeriidae) from the common house shrew, *Suncus murinus* Linnaeus. *Acta Protozoologica* 18:451–451.

Aly, M.M. 1993. Development of *Eimeria stiedae* in a nonspecific host. *Journal of the Egyptian Society of Parasitology* 23:95–99.

Anderson, B.C. 1986. Effect of drying on infectivity of cryptosporidia-laden calf feces for 3- to 7-day-old mice. *American Journal of Veterinary Research* 47:2272–2273.

———. 1987. Abomasal cryptosporidiosis in cattle. *Veterinary Pathology* 24:235–238.

———. 1988. Gastric cryptosporidiosis of feeder cattle, beef cows, and dairy cows. *Bovine Practitioner* 23:99–101.

———. 1990. A preliminary report on prevalence of *Cryptosporidium muris* oocysts in dairy cattle. *California Veterinarian* 44:11–12.

———. 1991a. Prevalence of *Cryptosporidium muris*–like oocysts among cattle populations of the United States: Preliminary report. *Journal of Protozoology* 38:14s–15s.

———. 1991b. Experimental infection in mice of *Cryptosporidium muris* isolated from a camel. *Journal of Protozoology* 38:16s–17s.

Anderson, L.C. 1971. Experimental coccidian infections in captive hibernating and non-hibernating Uinta ground squirrels, *Spermophilus armatus*. Ph.D. Dissertation, Utah State University, Logan, Utah, 147 pp.

Andrews, C.L., and W.R. Davidson. 1980. Endoparasites of selected populations of cottontail rabbits (*Sylvilagus floridanus*) in the southeastern United States. *Journal of Wildlife Diseases* 16:395–401.

Angus, K.W. 1988. Cryptosporidiosis in red deer. *Publication of the Veterinary Deer Society* 3:3–10.

———. 1989. Mammalian cryptosporidiosis: A veterinary perspective. In *Cryptosporidiosis,* Proceedings of the 1st International Workshop. Ed. K.W. Angus and D.A. Blewett. Edinburgh: Moredun Research Institute, pp. 43–53.

Angus, K.W., G. Hutchison, H.M.C. Munro. 1985. Infectivity of a strain of *Cryptosporidium* found in the guinea-pig (*Cavia porcellus*) for guinea-pigs, mice and lambs. *Journal of Comparative Pathology* 95:151–165.

Angus, K.W., S. Tzipori, and E.W. Gray. 1982. Intestinal lesions in specific-pathogen-free lambs associated with a *Cryptosporidium* from calves with diarrhea. *Veterinary Pathology* 19:67–78.

Arai, H., Y. Fukuda, T. Hara, Y. Funakoshi, S. Kaneko, T. Yoshiday, H. Asahi, M. Kumada, K. Kato, and T. Koyama. 1990. Prevalence of *Cryptosporidium* infection among domestic cats in the Tokyo metropolitan district, Japan. *Japanese Journal of Medical Science and Biology* 43:7–14.

Araújo, F.A.P., M.G.S. Paiva, R.L. Antunes, E.L. Chaplin, and N.R.S. da Silva. 1996. Occurrence of *Cryptosporidium parvum* and *Cryptosporidium muris* in buffalos (*Bubalus bubalis*) at Amapá state, Brazil. *Arquivos Faculdade de Veterinaria UFRGS Porto Alegro* 24:85–90.

Arcay, L. 1994. Genital coccidiosis in the golden hamster (*Cricetus cricetus*) produced for *Eimeria genitali* sp. nova. *Revista de la Facultad de Ciencias Veterinarias,* pp. 111–134.

Argenzio, R.A., J.A. Liacos, M.L. Levy, D.J. Meuten, J.G. Lecce, and D.W. Powell. 1990. Villous atropy, crypt hyperplasia, cellular infiltration, and impaired glucose-Na absorption in enteric cryptosporidiosis of pigs. *Gastroenterology* 98:1129–1140.

Argenzio, R.A., J. Lecce, and D.W. Powell. 1993. Prostanoids inhibit intestinal NaCl absorption in experimental porcine cryptosporidiosis. *Gastroenterology* 104:440–447.

Arjomandzadeh, K., and A. Dalimi. 1994. Comparison of 12 techniques for detection of *Cryptosporidium* oocysts. *Archives Institut RAZI* 44/45:31–38.

Arnault, I., J.M. Répérant, and M. Naciri. 1994. Humoral antibody response and oocyst shedding after experimental infection of histocompatible newborn and weaned piglets with *Cryptosporidium parvum. Veterinary Research* 25:371–383.

Arrowood, M.J. 1997. Diagnosis. In Cryptosporidium *and* Cryptosporidiosis. Ed. R. Fayer. Boca Raton, FL: CRC Press, pp. 43–64.

Arrowood, M.J., and C.R. Sterling. 1989. Comparison of conventional staining methods and monoclonal antibody-based methods for *Cryptosporidium* oocyst detection. *Journal of Clinical Microbiology* 27:1490–1495.

Arrowood, M.J., J.R. Mead, J.L. Mahrt, and C.R. Sterling. 1989. Effects of immune colostrum and orally administered antisporozoite monoclonal antibodies on the outcome of *Cryptosporidium parvum* infections in neonatal mice. *Infection and Immunity* 57:2283–2288.

Arther, R.G., and G. Post. 1977. Coccidia of coyotes in Eastern Colorado. *Journal of Wildlife Diseases* 13:97–100.

Artois, M., F. Claro, M. Rémond, and J. Blancou. 1996. Pathologie infectieuse des Canidés et Félidés des parcs zoologiques. *Revue Scientifique et Technique-Office International des épizooties* 15:15–140.

Asahi, H., T. Koyama, H. Arai, Y. Funikoshi, H. Yamaura, R. Shirasaka, and K. Okutomi. 1991. Biological nature of *Cryptosporidium* sp. isolated from a cat. *Parasitology Research* 77:237–240.

Asahi, H., M. Kumada, K. Kato, and T. Koyana. 1988. A simple staining method for cryptosporidian oocysts and sporozoites. *Japanese Journal of Medical Science and Biology* 41:117–121.

Ashraf, M., and K.H. Nepote. 1990. A new coccidial staining technique. *Small Ruminant Research* 3:187–190.

Awad-el-Kariem, F.M., D.C. Warhurst, and V. McDonald. 1994. Detection and species identification of *Cryptosporidium* oocysts using a system based on PCR and endonuclease restriction. *Parasitology* 109:19–22.

Aydin, Y. 1991. Experimental cryptosporidiosis in laboratory animals: Pathological findings and cross-transmission studies. *Ankara üniversitesi Veteriner Fakültesi Dergisi* 38:465–482.

Babb, R.R., J.T. Differding, and M.L. Trollope. 1982. Cryptosporididia enteritis in a healthy professional athelete. *American Journal of Gastroenterology* 77:833–834.

Bailey, K. 1994. Coccidiosis in farmed ruminants. *Surveillance* 21:27–28.

Balatbat, A.B., G.W. Jordan, Y.J. Tang, and J. Silva. 1996. Detection of *Cryptosporidium parvum* DNA in human feces by nested PCR. *Journal of Clinical Microbiology* 34:1769–1772.

Bandoni, S.M., and D.W. Duszynski. 1988. A plea for improved presentation of type material for coccidia. *The Journal of Parasitology* 74:519–523.

Bandyopadhyay, S., and B. Dasgupta. 1985. A new coccidium, *Eimeria murinusi* n. sp., from a grey musk shrew, *Suncus murinus murinus* (Linnaeus), in west Bengal, India. *Indian Journal of Parasitology* 9:101–103.

Barker, I.K., I. Beveridge, A.J. Bradley, and A.K. Lee. 1978. Observations on spontaneous stress-related mortality among males of the dasyurid marsupial *Antechinus stuartii* Macleay. *Australian Journal of Zoology* 26:435–447.

Barker, I.K., B.L. Munday, and P.J.A. Presidente. 1979. Coccidia of wombats: Correction of host-parasite relationships. *Eimeria wombati* (Gilruth and Bull 1912) comb. nov. and *Eimeria ursini* Supperer, 1957 from the hairy-nosed wombat and *Eimeria arundeli* sp. n. from the common wombat. *The Journal of Parasitology* 65:451–456.

Barta, J.R., D.S. Martin, P.A. Liberator, M. Dashkevicz, J.W. Anderson, S.D. Feighner, A. Elbrecht, A. Perkins-Barrow, M.C. Jenkins, H.H. Danforth, M.D. Ruff, and H. Profous-Juchelka. 1997. Phylogenetic relationships among eight *Eimeria* species infecting domestic fowl inferred using complete small subunit ribosomal DNA sequences. *Journal of Parasitology* 83:262–271.

Baxby, C., B. Getty, N. Blundell, and S. Ratcliff. 1984. Recognition of whole *Cryptosporidium* oocysts in feces by negative staining and electron microscopy. *Journal of Clinical Microbiology* 19:566–567.

Beaudoin, R.L., W.M. Samuel, and P.A. Strome. 1970. A comparative study of the parasites in two populations of white-tailed deer. *Journal of Wildlife Diseases* 6:56–63.

Becker, E.R., and H.B. Crouch. 1931. Some effects of temperature upon development of the oocysts of coccidia. *Proceedings of the Society for Experimental Biology and Medicine* 18:529–530.

Benhamou, Y., N. Kapel, C. Hoabng, H. Matta, D. Meillet, D. Magne, M. Raphael, M. Gentilini, P. Opolon, and J.-G. Gobert. 1995. Inefficacy of intestinal secretory immune response to *Cryptosporidium* in acquired immunodeficiency syndrome. *Gastroenterology* 108:627–635.

Berland, B., and D.P. Højgaard. 1981. IKI-solution used for flotation of coccidia (*Eimeria* sp.) and precipitation of oil from fish liver. *The Journal of Parasitology* 67:598–599.

Beveridge, I. 1993. Marsupial parasitic diseases. In *Zoo and wild animal medicine,* vol. 3. Ed. M.E. Fowler. Philadelphia, PA: W.B. Saunders Company, pp. 288–293.

Biggs, B.-A., R. Megna, S. Wickremesinghe, and B. Dwyer. 1987. Human infection with *Cryptosporidium* spp.: Results of a 24-month survey. *Medical Journal of Australia* 147:175–177.

Bjorneby, J.M., M.W. Riggs, and L.E. Perryman. 1990. *Cryptosporidium parvum* merozoites share neutralization-sensitive epitopes with sporozoites. *Immunology* 145:298–304.

Bjorneby, J.M., B.D. Hunsaker, M.W. Riggs, and L.E. Perryman. 1991a. Monoclonal antibody immunotherapy in nude mice persistently infected with *Cryptosporidium parvum. Infection and Immunity* 59:1172–1176.

Bjorneby, J.M., D.R. Leach, and L.E. Perryman. 1991b. Persistent cryptosporidiosis in horses with severe combined immunodeficiency. *Infection and Immunity* 59:3823–3826.

Blagburn, B.L., and W.L. Current. 1983. Accidental infection of a researcher with human *Cryptosporidium. Journal of Infectious Diseases* 148:772–773.

Blagburn, B.L., and R. Soave. 1997. Prophylaxis and chemotherapy: Human and animal. In Cryptosporidium and Cryptosporidiosis. Ed. R. Fayer. Boca Raton, FL: CRC Press, pp. 111–128.

Blankenship-Paris, T.L., J. Chang, and C.R. Bagnell. 1993. Enteric coccidiosis in a ferret. *Laboratory Animal Science* 43:361–363.

Bledsoe, B. 1976. *Isospora vulpina* Nieschulz and Bos 1933: Description and transmission from the fox (*Vulpes vulpes*) to the dog. *Journal of Protozoology* 23:365–367.

Blewett, D.A. 1989. Quantitative techniques in *Cryptosporidium* research. In *Cryptosporidiosis*, Proceedings of the 1st International Workshop. Ed. K.W. Angus and D.A. Blewett. Edinburgh: Moredun Research Institute, pp. 85–95.

Box, E.D., A.A. Marchiondo, D.W. Duszynski, and C.P. Davis. 1980. Ultrastructure of sarcocystis sporocysts from passerine birds and opossums: Comments on classification of the genus *Isospora*. *The Journal of Parasitology* 66:68–74.

Bristol, J.R., A.J. Piñon, and L.F. Mayberry. 1983. Interspecific interactions between *Nippostrongylus brasiliensis* and *Eimeria nieschulzi* in the rat. *The Journal of Parasitology* 69:372–374.

Bristol, J.R., S.J. Upton, L.F. Mayberry, and E.D. Rael. 1989. Suppression of phytohemagglutinin induced splenocyte proliferation during concurrent infection with *Eimeria nieschulzi* and *Nippostrongylus brasiliensis*. *Experientia* 45:762–763.

Bronsdon, M.A. 1984. Rapid dimethyl sulfoxide-modified acid-fast stain of *Cryptosporidium* oocysts in stool specimens. *Journal of Clinical Microbiology* 19:952–953.

Brooks, D.R. 1993. Extending the symbiotype concept to host voucher specimens. *The Journal of Parasitology* 79:631–633.

Brooks, D.R., and D.A. McLennan. 1993. Parascript: Parasites and the language of evolution. Washington, DC: Smithsonian Institution University Press, 429 pp.

Brown, E.A.E., D.P. Casemore, A. Gerkin, and I.F. Greatorex. 1989. Cryptosporidiosis in Great Yarmouth-the investigation of an outbreak. *Public Health* 103:3–9.

Browning, G.F., R.M. Chalmers, D.R. Snodgrass, R.M. Batt, C.A. Hart, S.E. Ormarod, T.J. Leadon, S.J. Stoneham, and P.D. Rossdale. 1991. The prevalence of enteric pathogens in diarrhoeic thoroughbred foals in Britan and Ireland. *Equine Veterinary Journal* 23:405–409.

Brunnett, S.R., S.B. Cintino, A.J. Herron, and N.H. Altman. 1992. Hepatic coccidiosis in chamois (*Rupicapra rupicapra*). *Journal of Zoo and Wildlife Medicine* 23:276–280.

Bryant, J.L., H.F. Sills, and C.C. Middleton. 1983. Cryptosporidia in squirrel monkeys (*Saimiri sciureus*). *Laboratory Animal Science* 33:482.

Bukhari, Z., and H.V. Smith. 1996. Detection of *Cryptosporidium muris* oocysts in the faeces of adult dairy cattle in Scotland. *Veterinary Record* 138:207–208.

Cable, R.M. and C.H. Conway. 1953. Coccidiosis of mammary tissue in the water shrew *Sorex palustris navigator*. *The Journal of Parasitology* 39(Supplement): 30.

Cama, V.A., and C.R. Sterling. 1991. Hyperimmune hens as a novel source of anti-*Cryptosporidium* antibodies suitable for passive immune transfer. *Journal of Protozoology* 38:42s–43s.

Campbell, I., S. Tzipori, G. Hutchison, and K.W. Angus. 1982. Effect of disinfectants on survival of *Cryptosporidium* oocysts. *Veterinary Record* 111:414–415.

Canestri-Trotti, G. 1989. Studies on *Cryptosporidium* sp. In *Cryptosporidiosis*, Proceedings of the 1st International Workshop. Ed. K.W. Angus, and D.A. Blewett. Edinburgh: Moredun Research Institute, p. 118.

Canestri-Trotti, G., and A. Quesada. 1983. Primo reporto di *Cryptosporidium* sp. in bufali italiani (*Bubalus bubalis*). *Atti della Societa Italiana delle Scienze Veterinarie* 37:737–740.

Canestri-Trotti, G., and S. Visconti. 1985. Inagine parassitologica su protozoi intestinali in quini del'escerito italiano. *Atti della Societa Italiana delle Scienze Veterinarie* 39: 758–761.

Canestri-Trotti, G., A. Quesada, and S. Visconti. 1984. Ricerche sulla fauna protozoaria intestinale del bufalo (*Bubalus bubalis*). *Atti della Societa Italiana di Buitaria* 16:433–450.

Canning, E.U., and M. Anwar. 1968. Studies on meiotic division in coccidial and malarial parasites. *Journal of Protozoology* 15:290–298.

Canning, E.U., and K. Morgan. 1975. DNA synthesis, reduction and elimination during life cycles of the Eimeriine coccidian, *Eimeria tenella* and the Haemogregarine, *Hepatozoon domerguei*. *Experimental Parasitology* 38:217–227.

Carlson, B.L., and S.W. Nielson. 1982. Cryptosporidiosis in a raccoon. *Journal of the American Veterinary Medical Association* 181:1405–1406.

Carneiro, C.S., C. Tarnau, and R. Chermette. 1987. Essais de transmission experimentale de cryptosporidies d'origine equine aux souriceaux et aus poussins. *Revista Ecuatoriana de higiene y Medicina Tropical* 37:37–46.

Carvalho, J. 1942. *Eimerian neoleporis* n. sp., occurring naturally in the cottontail and transmissible to the tame rabbit. *Iowa State College Journal of Science* 16:409–410.

———. 1943. The coccidia of wild rabbits of Iowa. I. Taxonomy and host-specificity. *Iowa State College Journal of Science* 18:103–134.

———. 1944. The coccidia of wild rabbits of Iowa. II. Experimental studies with *E. neoleporis* Carvalho, 1942. *Iowa State College Journal of Science* 18:177–189.

Casemore, D.P. 1987. The antibody response to *Cryptosporidium:* Development of a seological test and its use in a study of immunologiclly normal persons. *Journal of Infection* 14:125–134.

———. 1989. Sheep as a source of human cryptosporidiosis. *Journal of Infection* 19:101–104.

———. 1990. Foodborne protozoal infection. *Lancet* 336:1427–1432.

Casemore, D.P., M. Armstrong, and B. Jackson. 1984. Screening for *Cryptosporidium* in stools. *Lancet* 311:734–735.

Casemore, D.P., M. Armstrong, and R.L. Sands. 1985. Laboratory diagnosis of *Cryptosporidium*. *Journal of Clinical Pathology* 38:1337–1341.

Casemore, D.P., E.G. Jessop, D. Douce, and F.B. Jackson. 1986. *Cryptosporidium* plus *Campylobacter:* An outbreak in a semi-rural population. *Journal of Hygiene (Cambridge)* 96:95–105.

Castro, G.A., and D.W. Duszynski. 1984. Local and systemic effects on inflammation during *Eimeria nieschulzi* infection. *Journal of Protozoology* 31:283–287.

Cere, N., D. Licois, and J.F. Humbert. 1995. Study of the inter- and intraspecific variation of *Eimeria* spp. from the rabbit using random amplified polymorphic DNA. *Parasitology Research* 81:324–328.

Chalmers, R.M., A.P. Sturdee, D.P. Casemore, A. Curry, A. Miller, N.D. Parker, and T.M. Richmond. 1994. *Cryptosporidium muris* in wild house mice (*Mus musculus*): First report in the UK. *European Journal of Protistology* 30:151–155.

Chen, W., J.A. Harp, and A.G. Harmsen. 1993a. Requirements for CD4+ cells and gamma interferon in resolution of established *Cryptosporidium parvum* infection in mice. *Infection and Immunity* 61:3928–3932.

Chen, W., J.A. Harp, A.G. Harmsen, and E.A. Havell. 1993b. Gamma interferon functions in resistance to *Cryptosporidium parvum* infection in severe combined immunodeficient mice. *Infection and Immunity* 61:3548–3551.

Chermette, R., and S. Boufassa-Ouzrout 1988. *Cryptosporidiosis: A cosmopolitan disease in animals and in man,* 2nd ed. Paris: Office International des Epizooties, 122 pp.

Chermette, R., S. Boufassa, C. Squle, C. Tarnau, O. Courder, and D. Lengronne. 1987. La cryptosporidiose équine: Une parasitose méconnue. *Bulletin du Cereopa* 13:81–94.

Chermette, R., C. Tarnau, S. Boufassa-Ouzrout, and O. Couder. 1989. Survey on equine cryptosporidiosis in Normandy. In *Coccidia and intestinal coccidomorphs.* Proceedings of the 5th International Coccidiosis Conference, Tours, France. Ed. P. Yvore. Versailles, France: Les Colloques de Institut National de la Recherche Agronomique No. 49, pp. 493–498.

Chichino, G., A. Bruno, C. Cevini, C. Atzori, S. Gatti, and M. Scaglia. 1991. New rapid staining methods for *Cryptosporidium* oocysts in stools. *Journal of Protozoology* 38:212s–214s.

Chobotar, B., and E. Scholtyseck. 1982. Ultrastructure. In *The biology of the coccidia.* Ed. P.L. Long. Baltimore, MD: University Park Press, pp. 101–165.

Chrisp, C.E., W.C. Reid, H.G. Rush, M.A. Suckow, A. Bush, and M.J. Thomann. 1990. Cryptosporidiosis in guinea pigs: An animal model. *Infection and Immunity* 58:674–679.

Chrisp, C.E., M.A. Suckow, R. Fayer, M.J. Arrowood, M.C. Healey, and C.R. Sterling. 1992. Comparison of the host ranges and antigenicity of *Cryptosporidium parvum* and *Cryptosporidium wrairi* from guinea pigs. *Journal of Protozoology* 39:406–409.

Chrisp, C.E., P. Mason, and L.E. Perryman. 1995. Comparison of *Cryptosporidium parvum* and *Cryptosporidium wrairi* by reactivity with monoclonal antibodies and ability to infect severe combined immunodeficient mice. *Infection and Immunity* 63:360–362.

Christie, E., P.W. Pappas, and J.P. Dubey. 1978. Ultrastructure of excystment of *Toxoplasma gondii* oocysts. *Journal of Protozoology* 25:438–443.

Clark, D.P., and C.L. Sears. 1996. The pathogenesis of cryptosporidiosis. *Parasitology Today* 12:221–225.

Clavel, A., J.L. Olivares, J. Fleta, J. Castillo, M. Varea, F.J. Ramos, A.C. Arnal, and J. Quílez. 1996. Seasonality of cryptosporidiosis in children. *European Journal of Clinical Microbiology and Infectious Diseases* 15:77–80.

Cockrell, B.Y., M.G. Valior, and F.M. Garner. 1974. Cryptosporidiosis in the intestines of Rhesus monkeys (*Macaca mulatta*). *Laboratory Animal Science* 24:881–887.

Coleman, S.U., T.R. Klei, D.D. French, M.R. Chapman, and R.E. Corstvet. 1989. Prevalence of *Cryptosporidium* spp. in equids in Louisiana. *American Journal of Veterinary Research* 50:575–577.

Comes, A.M., J.F. Humbert, J. Cabaret, and L. Élard. 1996. Using molecular tools for diagnosis in veterinary parasitology. *Veterinary Research* 27:333–342.

Conlogue, G.C., and W.J. Foreyt. 1984. Experimental infections of *Eimeria mccordocki* (Protozoa, Eimeriidae) in white-tailed deer. *Journal of Wildlife Diseases* 20:31–33.

Coudert, P., D. Licois, F. Provôt, and F. Drouet-Viard. 1993. *Eimeria* sp. from the rabbit (*Oryctolagus cuniculus*): Pathogenicity and immunogenicity of *Eimeria intestinalis. Parasitology Research* 79:186–190.

Cozon, G., D. Cannella, F. Biron, M.-A. Piens, M. Jeanne, and J.-P. Revillard. 1992. *Cryptosporidium parvum* sporo-

zoite staining by propidium iodide. *International Journal for Parasitology* 22:385–389.

Cozon, G., F. Biron, M. Jeannin, D. Cannella, and J.P. Revillard. 1994. Secretory IgA antibodies to *Cryptosporidium parvum* in AIDS patients with chronic cryptosporidiosis. *Journal of Infectious Diseases* 169:696–699.

Crawshaw, G.J., and K.G. Mehren. 1987. Cryptosporidiosis in zoo and wild animals. In *Erkrankungen der Zootiere.* Verhandlungsbericht des 29. Internationalen Symposiums über die Erkrankungen der Zootiere, 20–24 May 1987 in Cardiff. Ed. R. Ippen, H. D. Schröder. Berlin: Akademie-Verlag, pp. 353–362.

Crouch, H.B., and E.R. Becker. 1931. A method of staining the oocysts of coccidia. *Science* 73:212–213.

Cruickshank, R., L. Ashdown, and J. Croese. 1988. Human cryptosporidiosis in North Queensland. *Australian New Zealand Journal of Medicine* 18:582–586.

Cubas, Z.S. 1996. Special challenges of maintaining wild animals in captivity in South America. *Revue Scientifique et Technique-Office International des épizooties* 15:267–287.

Current, W.L. 1983. Human cryptosporidiosis. *New England Journal of Medicine* 309:1326–1327.

Current, W.L., and N.C. Reese. 1986. A comparison of endogenous development of three isolates of *Cryptosporidium* in suckling mice. *Journal of Protozoology* 33:98–108.

Dagan, R., Y. Bar-David, I. Kassis, B. Sarov, D. Greenberg, Y. Afflalo, M. Katz, C.Z. Margolis, and J. El-On. 1991. *Cryptosporidium* in Bedouin and Jewish infants and children in southern Israel. *Israel Journal of Medical Sciences* 27:380–385.

Dagan, R., D. Fraser, J. El-On, I. Kassis, R. Deckelbaum, and S. Turner. 1995. Evaluation of an enzyme immunoassay for the detection of *Cryptosporidium* spp. in stool specimens from infants and young children in field studies. *American Journal of Tropical Medicine and Hygiene* 52:134–138.

Dailey, M.D., and W.K. Vogelbein. 1991. Parasite fauna of three species of Antarctic whales with reference to their use as potential stock indicators. *Fishery Bulletin of the United States* 89:355–265.

D'Antonio, R.G., R.E. Winn, J.P. Taylor, T.L. Gustafson, W.L. Current, M.M. Rhodes, G.W. Gary, and R.A. Zajac. 1985. A waterborne outbreak of cryptosporidiosis in normal hosts. *Annals of Internal Medicine* 103:886–888.

Davidson, W.R., M.J. Appel, G.L. Doster, O.E. Baker, and J.F. Brown. 1992a. Diseases and parasites of red foxes, gray foxes, and coyotes from commercial sources selling to fox-chasing enclosures. *Journal of Wildlife Diseases* 28:581–589.

Davidson, W.R., V.F. Nettles, L.E. Hayes, E.W. Howerth, and C.E. Couvillion. 1992b. Diseases diagnosed in gray foxes (*Urocyon cinereoargenteus*) from the southeastern United States. *Journal of Wildlife Diseases* 28:28–33.

Davis, A.J., and S.J. Jenkins. 1986. Cryptosporidiosis and proliferative ileitis in a hamster. *Veterinary Pathology* 23:632–633.

Dawson, A., R. Griffin, A. Fleetwood, and N.J. Barrett. 1995. Farm visits and zoonoses. *Public Health Laboratory Service, Communicable Disease Report (Rev.)* 5:R81.

Desser, S.S. 1978. Extraintestinal development of eimeriid coccidia in pigs and chamois. *Journal of Parasitology* 64:933–935.

De Vos, A.J. 1970. Studies on the host range of *Eimeria chinchillae* (De Vos and Van der Westhuizen 1968). *Ondersteeport Journal of Veterinary Research* 37:29–36.

DiPietro, J.A., C.E. Kirkpatrick, T.V. Baszler, K.S. Todd, and S.M. Austin. 1988. *Cryptosporidium* spp. infection of pony foals (abstract 212). Proceedings of the 69th annual meeting of the Conference of Research Workers in Animal Diseases, Chicago, November 14–15, 1988, p. 38.

Dobell, C. 1932. The discovery of the coccidia. *Parasitology* 14:342–348.

Doran, D.G. 1953. Coccidiosis in the kangaroo rats of California. *University of California Publications in Zoology* 59:31–60.

Doran, D.J. 1982. Behavior of coccidia in vitro. In *The biology of the coccidia.* Ed. P.L. Long. Baltimore, MD: University Park Press, pp. 229–285.

Dorney, R.S. 1962. Coccidiosis in Wisconsin cottontail rabbits in winter. *The Journal of Parasitology* 48:276–279.

———. 1964. Evaluation of a microquantitative method for counting coccidial oocysts. *The Journal of Parasitology* 50:518–522.

Douglas, T.G., and C.A. Speer. 1985. Effects of intestinal contents from normal and immunized mice on sporozoites of *Eimeria falciformis. Journal of Protozoology* 32:156–163.

Dowling, R.H., and E.O. Riecken (eds.). 1974. *Intestinal adaptation.* Proceedings of an international conference on the anatomy, physiology and biochemistry of intestinal adaptation. Stuttgart, Germany: F.K. Schattauer Verlag, 271 pp.

Dubey, J.P. 1986. Coccidiosis in the gallbladder of a goat. *Proceedings of the Helminthological Society of Washington* 53:277–281.

Dubey, J.P., and R. Fayer. 1976. Development of *Isospora bigemina* in dogs and other mammals. *Parasitology* 73:371–380.

Dubey, J.P., R. Fayer, and J.R. Rao. 1992. Cryptosporidial oocysts in feces of water buffalo and Zebu calves in India. *Journal of Veterinary Parasitology* 6:55–56.

Ducatelle, R., D. Maenhout, G. Charlier, C. Miry, W. Coussement, and J. Horrens. 1983. Cryptosporidiosis in goats and mouflon sheep. *Vlaams Diergeneeskundig Tijdschrift* 52:7–17.

Dulski, P., and M. Turner. 1988. The purification of sporocysts and sporozoites for *Eimeria tenella* oocysts using Percoll density gradients. *Avian Diseases* 32:235–239.

Dunn, J., T. Ott, and W. Clark. 1995. Pulsed light treatment of food and packaging. *Food Technology* 49:95–98.

Duszynski, D.W. 1971. Increase in size of *Eimeria separata* oocysts during patency. *The Journal of Parasitology* 57:948–952.

———. 1972. Host and parasite interactions during single and concurrent infections with *Eimeria nieschulzi* and *E. separata* in the rat. *Journal of Protozoology* 19:82–88.

———. 1986. Host specificity in the coccidia of small mammals: Fact or fiction? In *Advances in protozoological research.* Ed. M. Bereczky. *Symposia Biologica Hungarica,* vol. 33. Budapest: Akademiai Kiado, pp. 325–337.

———. 1989. Coccidian parasites (Apicomplexa: Eimeriidae) from insectivores. VIII. Four new species from the star-nosed mole, *Condylura cristata. The Journal of Parasitology* 75:514–518.

———. 1997. Coccidia from bats (Chiroptera) of the World: A new *Eimeria* species in *Pipistrellus javanicus* from Japan. *The Journal of Parasitology* 83:280–282.

Duszynski, D.W., and G.A. Conder. 1977. External factors and self-regulating mechanisms which may influence the sporulation of oocysts of the rat coccidium, *Eimeria nieschulzi. International Journal of Parasitology* 7:83–88.

Duszynski, D.W., and S.K. File. 1974. Structure of the oocyst and excystation of sporozoites of *Isospora endocallimici* n. sp. from the marmoset *Callimico goeldii. Transactions of the American Microscopical Society* 93:403–408.

Duszynski, D.W., and S.L. Gardner. 1991. Fixing coccidian oocysts in not an adequate solution to the problem of pre-

serving protozoan type material. *The Journal of Parasitology* 77:52–57.

Duszynski, D.W., and W.C. Marquardt. 1969. *Eimeria* (Protozoa: Eimeriidae) of the cottontail rabbit *Sylvilagus audubonii* in northeastern Colorado, with descriptions of three new species. *Journal of Protozoology* 16:128–137.

Duszynski, D.W., and C.A. Speer. 1976. Excystation of *Isospora arctopitheci* Rodhain, 1933 with notes on a similar process in *Isospora bigemina* (Stiles, 1891) Lühe, 1906. *Zeitschrift für Parasitenkunde* 48:191–197.

Duszynski, D.W., and S.J. Upton. 2000. Coccidia (Apicomplexa: Eimeriidae) of the mammalian order Insectivora. Special Publications of the Museum of Southwestern Biology, No. 4. Albuquerque: University of New Mexico Printing Services, pp. 1–67.

Duszynski, D.W. and P.G. Wilber. 1997. A guideline for the preparation of species descriptions in the Eimeriidae. *The Journal of Parasitology* 83:333–336.

Duszynski, D.W., M.J. Altenbach, A.A. Marchiondo, and C.A. Speer. 1977. *Eimeria crotalviridis* sp. n. from prairie rattlesnakes, *Crotalus viridis viridis* in New Mexico with data on excystation of sporozoites and ultrastructure of the oocyst wall. *Journal of Protozoology* 24:359–361.

Duszynski, D.W., S.A. Roy, and G.A. Castro. 1978a. Intestinal dissaccharidase and peroxidase deficiencies during *Eimeria nieschulzi* infections in rats. *Journal of Protozoology* 25:226–231.

Duszynski, D.W., D. Russell, S.A. Roy, and G.A. Castro. 1978b. Suppressed rejection of *Trichinella spiralis* in immunized rats concurrently infected with *Eimeria nieschulzi. The Journal of Parasitology* 64:83–88.

Duszynski, D.W., C.A. Speer, B. Chobotar, and A.A. Marchiondo. 1981. Fine structure of the oocyst wall and excystation of *Eimeria procyonis* from the American raccoon (*Procyon lotor*). *Zeitschrift für Parasitenkunde* 65:131–136.

Duszynski, D.W., K. Ramaswamy, and G.A. Castro. 1982. Intestinal absorption of b-methyl-D-glucoside in rats infected with *Eimeria nieschulzi. The Journal of Parasitology* 68:727–729.

Duszynski, D.W., W.D. Wilson, S.J. Upton, and N.D. Levine. 1999. Coccidia (Apicomplexa: Eimeriidae) in the Primates and the Scandentia. *International Journal of Primatology* 20:761–797.

Edgar, S.A. 1954. Effect of temperature on the sporulation of oocysts of the protozoan, *Eimeria tenella. Transactions of the American Microscopical Society* 73:237–242.

Elangbam, C.S., C.W. Qualls, S.A. Ewing, and R.L. Lochmiller. 1993. Cryptosporidiosis in a cotton rat (*Sigmodon hispidus*). *Journal of Wildlife Diseases* 29:161–164.

El-Shewy, K., P.C. Kibsey, and W.M. Wenman. 1994a. Development of an enzyme-linked immunosorbent assay and counterimmunoelectrophoresis for the detection of *Cryptosporidium parvum* copro-antigens. *Serodianosis and Immunotherapy of Infectious Diseases* 6:82–86.

El-Shewy, K., R.T. Kilani, M.M. Hegazi, L.M. Makhlouf, and W.M. Wenman. 1994b. Identification of low-molecular-mass coproantigens of *Cryptosporidium parvum. Journal of Infectious Diseases* 169:460–463.

Elton, C., E.B. Ford, and J.R. Baker. 1931. The health and parasites of a wild mouse population. *Proceedings of the Zoological Society of London* 1931:657–721.

Enriquez, F.J., and C.R. Sterling. 1993. Role of CD4+ TH1- and TH2-cell-secreted cytokines in cryptosporidiosis. *Folia Parasitologica* 40:307–311.

Entrala, E., M. Rueda-Rubio, D. Janssen, and C. Mascaró. 1995. Influence of hydrogen peroxide on acid-fast staining of *Cryptosporidium parvum* oocysts. *International Journal for Parasitology* 25:1473–1477.

Entzeroth, R., and E. Scholtyseck. 1984. Ultrastructural study of intestinal coccidia of the European mole (*Talpa europaea*). *Zentrablatt für Bakteriologie und Hygiene A* 256:280–285.

Ernst, J.V., and B. Chobotar. 1978. The endogenous stages of *Eimeria utahensis* (Protozoa: Eimeriidae) in the kangaroo rat, *Dipodomys ordii. The Journal of Parasitology* 64:27–34.

Esteban, E., and B.C. Anderson. 1995. *Cryptosporidium muris:* Prevalence, persistency, and detrimental effect on milk production in a drylot dairy. *Journal of Dairy Science* 78:1068–1072.

Eydal, M. 1994. Parasites of horses in Iceland. *Livestock Production Science* 40:85.

Farr, M.M., and G.W. Luttermoser. 1941. Comparative efficiency of zinc sulfate and sugar solutions for the simultaneous flotation of coccidial oöcysts and helminth eggs. *The Journal of Parasitology* 27:417–424.

Farr, M.M., and E.E. Wehr. 1949. Survival of *Eimeria acervulina, E. tenella,* and *E. maxima* oocysts on soil under various field conditions. *Annals of the New York Academy of Sciences* 52:468–472.

Faust, E.C., W. Sawitz, J. Tobie, V. Odom, C. Perks, and D.R. Lincicome. 1939. Comparative efficiency of various technics for the diagnosis of protozoa and helminths in feces. *The Journal of Parasitology* 25:241–262.

Favennec, L., E. Comby, J.J. Ballet, and P. Brasseur. 1995. Serum IgA antibody response to *Cryptosporidium parvum* is mainly represented by IgA1. *Journal of Infectious Diseases* 171:256.

Fayer, R. 1994. Effect of high temperature on infectivity of *Cryptosporidium parvum* oocysts in water. *Applied and Environmental Microbiology* 60:2732–2735.

———. 1995. Effect of sodium hypochlorite exposure on infectivity of *Cryptosporidium parvum* oocysts for neonatal BALB/c mice. *Applied and Environmental Microbiology* 61:844–846.

Fayer, R., and W. Ellis. 1993. Paromomycin is effective as prophylaxis for cryptosporidiosis in dairy calves. *The Journal of Parasitology* 79:771–774.

Fayer, R., and T. Nerad. 1996. Effects of low temperatures on viability of *Cryptosporidium parvum* oocysts. *Applied and Environmental Microbiology* 62:1431–1433.

Fayer, R., J.V. Ernst, R.G. Miller, and R.G. Leek. 1985. Factors contributing to clinical illness in calves experimentally infected with a bovine isolate of *Cryptosporidium. Proceedings of the Helminthological Society of Washington* 52:64–70.

Fayer, R., C. Andrews, B.L.P. Ungar, and B.L. Blagburn. 1989a. Efficacy of hyperimmune bovine colostrum for prohylaxis of cryptosporidiosis in neonatal calves. *The Journal of Parasitology* 75:393–397.

Fayer, R., L.E. Perryman, and M.W. Riggs. 1989b. Hyperimmune bovine colostrum neutralizes *Cryptosporidium* sporozoites and protects mice against oocyst challenge. *The Journal of Parasitology* 75:151–153.

Fayer, R., A. Guidry, and B.L. Blagburn. 1990. Immunotherapeutic efficacy of bovine colostral immunoglobulins from a hyperimmunized cow against cryptosporidiosis in neonatal mice. *Infection and Immunity* 58:2962–2965.

Fayer, R., L. Phillips, B.C. Anderson, and M. Bush. 1991. Chronic cryptosporidiosis in a bactrian camel (*Camelus bactrianus*). *Journal of Zoo and Wildlife Medicine* 22:228–232.

Fayer, R., J.R. Fischer, C.T. Sewell, D.M. Kavanaugh, and D.A. Osborn. 1996a. Spontaneous cryptosporidiosis in captive white-tailed deer (*Odocoileus virginianus*). *Journal of Wildlife Diseases* 32:619–622.

Fayer, R., T.K. Graczyk, M.R. Cranfield, and J.M. Trout. 1996b. Gaseous disinfection of *Cryptosporidium parvum*

oocysts. Applied and Environmental Microbiology 62:3908–3909.

Fayer, R., C.A. Speer, and J.P. Dubey. 1997. The general biology of *Cryptosporidium.* In Cryptosporidium *and Cryptosporidiosis.* Ed. R. Fayer. Boca Raton, FL: CRC Press, pp. 1–41.

Fenwick, B.W. 1983. Cryptosporidiosis in a neonatal gazella. *Journal of the American Veterinary Medical Association* 183:1331–1332.

Fernández, A., S.C. Gómez-Villamandos, L. Carrasco, A. Perea, M. Quezada, and M.A. Gómez. 1988. Brote diarréico en potros asociado a cryptosporidios. *Medicina Veterinaria* 5:311–313.

Fernando, M.A. 1982. Pathology and pathogenicity. In *The biology of the coccidia.* Ed. P.L. Long. Baltimore: University Park Press, pp. 287–327.

Fernando, M.A., and B.M. McCraw. 1973. Mucosal morphology and cellular renewal in the intestine of chickens following a single infection of *Eimeria acervulina. The Journal of Parasitology* 59:493–501.

Filkorn, R., A. Wiedenmann, and K. Botzenhart. 1994. Selective detection of viable *Cryptosporidium* oocysts by PCR. *Zentrablatt für Hygiene und Umweltmedizin* 195:489–494.

Flach, E.J., D.A. Blewett, and K.W. Angus. 1991. Coccidial infections of captive red lechwe (*Kobus leche leche*) at Edinburgh Zoo, with a note on concurrent *Trichuris* sp. infections. *Journal of Zoo and Wildlife Medicine* 22:446–452.

Fowler, M.E. 1978. *Zoo and wild animal medicine.* Vol. *Zoo animals—Diseases.* Philadelphia, PA: W.B. Saunders Company.

———. 1986. *Zoo and wild animal medicine.* Vol. 2. *Wildlife diseases.* Philadelphia, PA: W.B. Saunders Company.

———. 1996a. An overview of wildlife husbandry and diseases in captivity. *Review Scientifique et Technique-Office International des épizooties* 15:15–42.

———. 1996b. Husbandry and diseases of camelids. *Review Scientifique et Technique-Office International des épizooties* 15:155–169.

Frenkel, J.K., and J.P. Dubey. 1972. Rodents as vector hosts for feline coccidia, *Isospora felis* and *I. rivolta. Journal of Infectious Diseases* 125:69–72.

Frey, J.K., T.L. Yates, D.W. Duszynski, W.L. Gannon, and S.L. Gardner. 1992. Designation and curatorial management of type host specimens (symbiotypes) for new parasite species. *The Journal of Parasitology* 78:930–932.

Frizzell, D.L. 1933. Terminology of types. *The American Midland Naturalist* 14:637–668.

Gajadhar, A.A., J.P. Caron, and J.R. Allen. 1985. Cryptosporidiosis in two foals. *Canadian Journal of Veterinary Research* 26:132–134.

Garber, L.P., M.D. Salman, H.S. Hurd, T. Keele, and J.L. Schlater. 1994. Potential risk factors for *Cryptosporidium* infection in dairy calves. *Journal of the American Veterinary Medical Association* 205:86–91.

Garcia, L.S., and R.Y. Shimizu. 1997. Evaluation of nine immunoassay kits (enzyme immunoassay and direct fluorescence) for detection of *Giardia lamblia* and *Cryptosporidium parvum* in human fecal sepcimens. *Journal of Clinical Microbiology* 35:1526–1529.

Garcia, L.S., D.A. Bruckner, T.C. Brewer, and R.Y. Shimizu. 1983. Tehniques for the recovery and identification of *Cryptosporidium* oocysts from stool specimens. *Journal of Clinical Microbiology* 18:185–190.

Garcia, L.S., T.C. Brewer, and D.A. Bruckner. 1987. Fluorescence detection of *Cryptosporidium* oocysts in human fecal specimens by using monoclonal antibodies. *Journal of Clinical Microbiology* 25:119–121.

Garcia, L.S., A.C. Shum, and D.A. Bruckner. 1992. Evaluation of a new monoclonal antibody combination reagent for direct immunofluorescence detection of *Giardia* cysts and *Cryptosporidium* oocysts in human fecal specimens. *Journal of Clinical Microbiology* 30:3255–3257.

Gardner, S.L., and D.W. Duszynski. 1990. Polymorphism of eimerian oocysts can be a problem in naturally infected hosts: An example from subterranean rodents in Bolivia. *The Journal of Parasitology* 76:805–811.

Gardner, A.L., J.K. Roche, C.S. Weikel, and R.L. Guerrant. 1991. Intestinal cryptosporidiosis: Pathophysiologic alterations and specific cellular and humoral immune responses in RNU/+ and RNU/RNU (athymic) rats. *American Journal of Tropical Medicine and Hygiene* 44:49–62.

Garza, D.H., R.N. Fedorak, and R. Soave. 1986. Enterotoxin-like activity in cultured cryptosporidia: Role of diarrhea. *Gastroenterology* 90:1424.

Gennari-Cardoso, M.L., J.M. Costa-Cruz, E. de Castro, L.M.F.S. Lima, and D.V. Prudente. 1996. *Cryptosporidium* sp. in children suffering from acute diarrhea at Uberlândia City, state of Minas Gerais, Brazil. *Memorias do Instituto Oswaldo Cruz* 91:551–554.

Gibson, J.A., M.W.M. Hill, M.J. Huber. 1983. Cryptosporidiosis in Arabian foals with severe combined immunodeficiency. *Australian Veterinary Journal* 60:378–379.

Gibson, S.V., and J.E. Wagner. 1986. Cryptosporidiosis in guinea pigs: A retrospective survey. *Journal of the American Veterinary Medical Association* 189:1033–1034.

Gill, B.S. 1954. Comparative floating efficiency of copper nitrate, common salt and zinc sulphate solutions as levitating media in a modified Lane's (1923–24) D.C.F. technique for poultry coccidia. *Indian Journal of Veterinary Science and Animal Host* 24:249–257.

Gobet, P., J.C. Buisson, O. Vagner, M. Naciri, M. Grappin, S. Comparot, G. Garly, D. Aubert, I. Varga, P. Camerlynck, and A. Bonnin. 1997. Detection of *Cryptosporidium parvum* DNA in formed human feces by a sensitiv PCR-based assay including uracil-N-glycosylase inactivation. *Journal of Clinical Microbiology* 35:254–256.

Gomez, M.S., M. Gracenea, P. Gosalbez, C. Feliu, C. Enseñat, and R. Hidalgo. 1992. Detection of oocysts of *Cryptosporidium* in several species of monkeys and one prosimian species at the Barcelona Zoo. *Parasitology Research* 78:619–620.

Gomez, M.S., T. Vila, C. Feliu, I. Montoliu, M. Gracenea, and J. Fernández. 1996. A survey for *Cryptosporidium* spp. in mammals at the Barcelona Zoo. *International Journal for Parasitology* 26:1331–1333.

Gómez-Bautista, M., M. Luzón-Peña, J. Santiago-Moreno, A.G. de Buines, and A. Meana. 1996. Coccidial infection in mouflon, *Ovis musimon*, in central Spain. *Journal of Wildlife Diseases* 32:125–129.

Gomez-Morales, M.A., C.M. Ausiella, F. Urbani, and E. Pozio. 1995. Crude extract and recombinant protein of *Cryptosporidium parvum* oocysts induce proliferation of human peripheral blood mononuclear cells in vitro. *Journal of Infectious Diseases* 172:211–216.

Gomez-Morales, M.A., C.M. Ausiella, A. Guarino, F. Urbani, M.I. Spagnulolo, C. Pignata, and E. Pozio. 1996. Severe, protracted intestinal cryptosporidiosis associated with interferon g deficiency: Pediatric case report. *Clinical Infectious Diseases* 22:848–850.

Gómez-Villamandos, J.C., L. Carrasco, E. Mozos, and J. Hervás. 1995. Fatal cryptosporidiosis in ferrets (*Mustela putorius furo*): A morphopathologic study. *Journal of Zoo and Wildlife Medicine* 26:539–544.

Goodwin, M.A., and W.D. Waltman. 1996. Transmission of *Eimeria,* viruses, and bacteria to chicks: Darkling beetles (*Alphitobius diaperinus*) as vectors of pathogens. *Journal of Applied Poultry Research* 5:51–55.

Graczyk, T.K., M.R. Cranfield, and F. Fayer. 1996a. Evaluation of commercial enzyme immunoassay (EIA) and immunofluorescent antibody (IFA) test kits for detection of *Cryptosporidium* oocysts of species other than *Cryptosporidium parvum*. *American Journal of Tropical Medicine and Hygiene* 54:274–279.

Graczyk, T.K., M.R. Cranfield, R. Fayer, and M.S. Anderson. 1996b. Viability and infectivity of *Cryptosporidium parvum* oocysts are retained upon intestinal passage through a refractory avian host. *Applied and Experimental Microbiology* 62:3234–3237.

Graczyk, T.K., M.R. Cranfield, R. Fayer, J. Trout, and H.J. Goodale. 1997. Infectivity of *Cryptosporidium parvum* oocysts is retained upon intestinal passage through a migratory water-fowl species (Canada goose, *Branta canadensis*). *Tropical Medicine and International Health* 2:341–347.

Greenberg, P.D., and J.P. Cello. 1996. Treatment of severe diarrhea caused by *Cryptosporidium parvum* with oral bovine immunoglobulin concentrate in patients with AIDS. *Journal of Acquired Immune Deficiency Syndromes and Human Retrovirology* 13:348–354.

Greve, J.H. 1989. Comparison of sugar and sodium nitrate flotation methods for detection of parasites in dog feces. *Iowa State University Veterinarian* 51:76.

Grigoriew, G.A., S. Walmsley, L. Law, S.L. Chee, J. Yang, J. Keystone, and M. Krajden. 1994. Evaluation of the Merifluor immunofluoresent assay for the detection of *Cryptosporidium* and *Giardia* in sodium acetate formalin-fixed stools. *Diagnostic Microbiology and Infectious Diseases* 19:89–91.

Grimason, A.M., H.V. Smith, J.F.W. Parker, Z. Bukhari, A.T. Campbell, and L.J. Robertson. 1994. Application of DAPI and immunofluorescence for enhanced identification of *Cryptosporidium* spp. oocysts in water samples. *Water Research* 28:733–736.

Gruber, A.D., C.A. Schulze, M. Brügmann, and J. Pohlenz. 1996. Renal coccidiosis with cystic tubular dilatation in four bats. *Veterinary Pathology* 33: 442–225.

Guarino, A., R.B. Canani, E. Pozio, L. Terracciano, F. Albano, and M. Mazzeo. 1994. Enterotoxic effect of stool supernatant of *Cryptosporidium*-infected calves on human jejunum. *Gastroenterology* 106:28–34.

Gutteridge, W.E. 1993. Chemotherapy (Chapter 9). In *Modern parasitology*. Ed. F. E. G. Cox. Oxford, UK: Blackwell Scientific Publications, pp. 219–242.

Hammond, D.M., F.L. Anderson, and M.L. Miner. 1963. The occurrence of a second asexual generation in the life cycle of *Eimeria bovis*. *The Journal of Parasitology* 32:428–434.

Hamoudi, A.C., S.J. Qualman, M.J. Marcon, M. Hribar, H.J. McClung, R.D. Murray, and H.J. Cannon. 1988. Do regional variations in prevalence of cryptosporidiosis occur? The central Ohio experience. *American Journal of Public Health* 78:273–275.

Hansen, J.S., and J.E. Ongerth. 1991. Effects of time and watershed characteristics on the concentration of *Cryptosporidium* oocysts in river water. *Applied and Environmental Microbiology* 57:2790–2795.

Harp, J.A., and R.E. Sacco. 1996. Development of cellular immune functions in neonatal to weanling mice: Relationship to *Cryptosporidium parvum* infection. *The Journal of Parasitology* 82:245–249.

Harp, J.A., W. Chen, and A.G. Harmsen. 1992. Resistance of severe combined immunodeficient mice to infection with *Cryptosporidium parvum*: The importance of intestinal microflora. *Infection and Immunity* 60:3509–3512.

Hayes, E.B., T.D. Matte, T.R. O'Brien, T.W. McKinley, G.S. Logsdon, J.B. Rose, B.L.P. Ungar, D.M. Word, P.F. Pinsky, M.L. Cummings, M.A. Wilson, E.G. Long, E.S.

Hurwitz, and D.D. Juranek. 1989. Large community outbreak of cryptosporidiosis due to contamination of a filtered public water supply. *New England Journal of Medicine* 320:1372–1376.

Heaton, P. 1994. Bovine colostrum immunoglobulin concentrate for cryptosporidiosis in AIDS. *Archives of Diseases in Childhood* 70:356–357.

Heine, J. 1982. An easy technique for the demonstration of cryptosporidia in faeces. *Zentralblatt für Veterinarmedizin Reiche B* 29:324–327.

Heine, J., H.W. Moon, D.B. Woodmansee, and J.F.L. Pohlenz. 1984a. Experimental tracheal and conjunctival infections with *Cryptosporidium* sp. in pigs. *Veterinary Parasitology* 17:17–25.

Heine, J., J.F.I. Pohlenz, H.W. Moon, and G.N. Woode. 1984b. Enteric lesions and diarrhea in gnotobiotic calves monoinfected with *Cryptosporidium* species. *Journal of Infectious Diseases* 150:768–775.

Hendricks, L.D. 1977. Host range characteristics of the primate coccidian *Isospora arctopitheci* Rodhain, 1933 (Protozoa: Eimeriidae). *The Journal of Parasitology* 63:32–35.

Henriksen, S.A., and J.F.L. Pohlenz. 1981. Staining of cryptosporidia by a modified Ziehl-Neelsen technique. *Acta Veterinaria Scandinavica* 22:594–596.

Heuschele, W.P., J. Oosterhuis, D. Janssen, P.T. Robinson, P.K. Ensley, E. Meier, T. Olson, M.P. Anderson, and K. Benirschke. 1986. Cryptosporidial infections in captive wild animals. *Journal of Wildlife Diseases* 22:493–496.

Hill, B.D., D.A. Blewett, A.M. Dawson, and S. Wright. 1990. Analysis of the kinetics, isotype and specificity of serum and coproantibody in lambs infected with *Cryptosporidium parvum. Research in Veterinary Science* 48:76–81.

Højlyng, N., W. Holten-Anderson, and S. Jepsen. 1987. Cryptosporidiosis: A case of airborne transmission. *Lancet* 325:271–272.

Holland, R.E., T.H. Herdt, and K.R. Refsal. 1989. Pulmonary excretion of H$_2$ in calves with *Cryptosporidium*-induced malabsorption. *Digestive Diseases and Sciences* 34:1399–1404.

Holland, R.E., S.M. Boyle, T.H. Herdt, S.D. Grimes, and R.D. Walker. 1992. Malabsorption of vitamin A in preruminating calves infected with *Cryptosporidium parvum. American Journal of Veterinary Research* 53:1947–1952.

Hovda, L.R., S.M. McGuirk, and D.P. Lunn. 1990. Total parenteral nutrition in a neonatal llama. *Journal of the American Veterinary Medical Association* 196:319–322.

Howerth, E.W. 1981. Bovine cryptosporidiosis. *Journal of the South African Veterinary Association* 52:251–253.

Hrudka, F., R.J. Cawthorn, and J.C. Haigh. 1993. The occurrence of coccidia (Eimeriidae) in epdiidymal semen of a wapiti (*Cervus canadensis nelsoni*). *Canadian Journal of Zoology* 61:1693–1699.

Hsu, C., and E.C. Melby. 1974. *Isospora callimico* n. sp., (Coccidia: Eimeriidae) from Goeldi's marmoset (*Callimico goeldii*). *Laboratory Animal Science* 24:476–477.

Huang, D.S., M.C. Lopez, J.Y. Wang, F. Martinez, and R.R. Watson. 1996. Alterations of the mucosal immune system due to *Cryptosporidium parvum* infection innormal mice. *Cellular Immunology* 173:176–182.

Hughes, H.P.A., W.M. Whitmire, and C.A. Speer. 1989. Immunity patterns during acute infection by *Eimeria bovis. The Journal of Parasitology* 75:86–91.

Hum, S., N.J. Barton, D. Obendorf, and I.K. Barker. 1991. Coccidiosis in common wombats (*Vombatus ursinus*). *Journal of Wildlife Diseases* 27:697–700.

Hussein, H.S., and O.B. Mohammed. 1992. *Eimeria rheemi* sp. n. (Apicomplexa: Eimeriidae) from the Arabian sand gazelle, *Gazella subgutturosa marica* (Artiodactyla:

Bovidae) in Saudi Arabia. *Journal of the Helminthological Society of Washington* 59:190–194.

Isaac-Renton, J.L., M.M. Moricz, and E.M. Proctor. 1987. A *Giardia* survey of fur-bearing water mammals in British Columbia, Canada. *Journal of Environmental Health* 50:80–83.

Iseki, M. 1979. *Cryptosporidium felis* sp. n. (Protozoa, Eimeriorina) from the domestic cat. *Japanese Journal of Parasitology* 28:285–307.

———. 1986. Two species of *Cryptosporidium* naturally infecting house rats, *Rattus norvegicus. Japanese Journal of Parasitology* 35:521–526.

Iseki, M., T. Maekawa, K. Moriya, S. Uni, and S. Takada. 1989. Infectivity of *Cryptosporidium muris* (strain RN 66) in various laboratory animals. *Parasitology Research* 75:218–222.

Iskander, A.R., A. Tawfeek, and A.F. Farid. 1987. Cryptosporidial infection among buffalo calves in Egypt. *Indian Journal of Animal Sciences* 57:1057–1059.

Jankiewicz, H.A. 1941. Transmission of the liver coccidium, *Eimeria stiedae* from the domestic to the cottontail rabbit. *The Journal of Parasitology* 27(Supplement): 28.

Jeffers, T.K. 1975. Attenuation of *Eimeria tenella* through selection for precociousness. *The Journal of Parasitology* 61:1083–1090.

Jervis, H.R., T.G. Merrill, and H. Sprinz. 1966. Coccidiosis in the guinea pig small intestine due to *Cryptosporidium. Journal of Veterinary Research* 27:408–414.

Johnson, D.W., N.J. Pieniazek, and J.B. Rose. 1993. DNA probe hybridization and PCR detection of *Cryptosporidium* compared to immunofluoresence assay. *Water Science Technology* 27:77–84.

Johnson, D.W., N.J. Pieniazek, D.W. Griffin, L. Misener, and J.B. Rose. 1995. Development of a PCR protocol for sensitive detection of *Cryptosporidium* oocysts in water samples. *Applied and Environmental Microbiology* 61:3849–3855.

Jolley, W.R., N. Kingston, E.S. Williams, and C. Lynn. 1994. Coccidia, *Giardia* sp., and a physalopteran nematode parasite from black-footed ferrets (*Mustela nigripes*) in Wyoming. *Journal of the Helminthological Society of Washington* 61:89–94.

Joyner, L.P. 1982. Host and site specificity. In *The biology of the coccidia*. Ed. P.L. Long. Baltimore, MD: University Park Press, pp. 35–62.

———. 1985. The development of knowledge on the speciation of coccidia. In *Research in avian coccidiosis*. Proceedings of the Georgia Coccidiosis Conference. Ed. L.R. McDougald, L.P. Joyner, and P.L. Long. Athens, GA: University of Georgia, pp. 1–12.

Kageruka, P., J.R.A. Brandt, H. Taelman, and C. Jonas. 1984. Modified koster staining method for the diagnosis of cryptosporidiosis. *Annales de la Société Belge de Médécine Tropicale* 64:171–175.

Kalishman, J., J. Paul-Murphy, J. Scheffler, and J.A. Thomson. 1996. Survey of *Cryptosporidium* and *Giardia* spp. in a captive population of common marmosets. *Laboratory Animal Science* 46:116–119.

Kang, G., and M.M. Mathan. 1996. A comparison of five staining methods for detection of *Cryptosporidium* oocysts in faecal specimens from the field. *Indian Journal of Medical Research* 103:264–266.

Kapel, N., D. Meillet, M. Buraud, L. Favennec, D. Magne, and J.G. Gobert. 1993. Determination of anti-*Cryptosporidium* coproantibodies by time-resolved immunofluorometric assay. *Transactions of the Royal Society of Tropical Medicine and Hygiene* 87:330–332.

Kassa, M., E. Comby, D. LEmeteil, P. Brasseur, and J.-J. Ballet. 1991. Characterization of anti-*Cryptosporidium* IgA antibodies in sera from immunocompetent individuals and HIV-infected patients. *Journal of Protozoology* 38:179s–180s.

Kaup, F.J., E.M. Kuhn, B. Makoschey, and G. Hunsmann. 1994. Cryptosporidiosis of liver and pancreas in rhesus monkeys with experimental SIV infection. *Journal of Medical Primatology* 23:304–308.

Kawamoto, F., S. Mizuno, H. Fujioka, N. Kumada, E. Sugiyama, T. Takuchi, S. Kobayashi, M. Iseki, M. Yamada, Y. Matsumoto, T. Tegoshi, and Y. Yoshida. 1987. Simple and rapid staining for detection of *Entamoeba* cysts and other protozoans with fluorochromes. *Japanese Journal of Medical Science and Biology* 40:35–46.

Kehl, K.S.C., H. Cicirello, and P.L. Havens. 1995. Comparison of four different methods for detection of *Cryptosporidium* species. *Journal of Clinical Microbiology* 33:416–418.

Kheysin, Y.M. 1947. New species of rabbit intestinal coccidium *Eimeria coecicola* [In Russian]. *Doklady Akademii Nauk SSSR* 55:181–183.

———. 1948. Development of two intestinal coccidia of the rabbit—*Eimeria piriformis* Kotlán and Popech and *Eimeria intestinalis* nom nov. [In Russian]. *Uchenye Zapiski Karelo-Finskogo Gosudarstvennogo Universiteta Biologicheskie Nauki* 3:179–187.

———. 1967. Life cycles of coccidia of domestic animals [translated from Russian]. Ed. K.S. Todd, Jr. Baltimore, MD: University Park Press, 264 pp.

Klesius, P.H., T.B. Haynes, and L.K. Malo. 1986. Infectivity of *Cryptosporidium* sp. isolated form wild mice for calves and mice. *Journal of the American Veterinary Medical Association* 189:192–193.

Korsholm, H., and S.A. Henriksen. 1984. Infection with *Cryptosporidium* in roe deer (*Capreolus capreolus* L.). A preliminary report. *Nordisk Veterinaermedicin* 36:266.

Koutz, F.R. 1950. The survival of oocysts of avian coccidia in the soil. *The Speculum* 3:1–5.

Kovatch, R.M., and J.D. White. 1972. Cryptosporidiosis in two juvenile Rhesus monkeys. *Veterinary Pathology* 9:426–440.

Kuhls, T.L., D.A. Mosier, V.L. Abrams, D.L. Crawford, and R.A. Greenfield. 1994. Inability of interferon-gamma and aminoguanidine to alter *Cryptosporidium parvum* infection in mice with severe combined immunodeficiency. *The Journal of Parasitology* 80:480–485.

Kuhls, T.L., R.A. Greenfield, D.A. Mosier, D.L. Crawford, and W.A. Joyce. 1992. Cryptosporidiosis in adult and neonatal mice with severe combined immunodeficiency. *Journal of Comparative Pathology* 106:399–410.

Kuhls, T.L., S.L. Orlicek, D.A. Mosier, D.L. Crawford, V.L. Abrams, and R.A. Greenfield. 1995. Enteral human serum immunoglobulin treatment of cryptosporidiosis in mice with severe combined immunodeficiency. *Infection and Immunity* 63:3582–3586.

Kunstýř, I., and S. Naumann. 1981. Coccidiosis in guinea pigs; with emphasis on diagnosis. *Zeitschriff für Vesuchstierkunde* 23:255–257.

Kusewitt, D.F., J.E. Wagner, and P.D. Harris. 1977. *Klossiella* sp. in the kidneys of two bats (*Myotis sodalis*). *Veterinary Parasitology* 3:365–369.

Kuttin, E.S., and A. Kaller. 1996. *Cystoisospora delphini* n. sp. causing enteritis in a bottlenosed dolphin (*Tursiops truncatus*). *Aquatic Mammals* 22:57–60.

Kuttin, E.S., G. Loupal, H. Köhlor, and R. Supperer. 1982. über eine Plazentarkokzidiose bei einem Flubpferd (*Hippopotamus amphibius*). *Zentralblatt für Veterinari Medicine B* 29:153–159.

Laakkonen, J., T. Soveri, and H. Henttonen. 1994. Prevalence of *Cryptosporidium* sp. in peak density *Microtus agrestis*, *Microtus oeconomus* and *Clethrionomys glareolus* populations. *Journal of Wildlife Diseases* 30:110–111.

Laberge, I., A. Ibrahin, J.R. Barta, and M.W. Griffiths. 1996a. Detection of *Cryptosporidium parvum* in raw milk by PCR and oligonucleotide probe hybridization. *Applied and Environmental Microbiology* 62:3259–3264.

Laberge, I., M.W. Griffiths, and M.W. Griffiths. 1996b. Prevalence, detection and control of *Cryptosporidium parvum* in food. *International Journal of Food Microbiology* 31:1–16.

Lainson, R., and J.J. Shaw. 1989. Two new species of *Eimeria* and three new species of *Isospora* (Apicomplexa: Eimeriidae) from Brazilian mammals and birds. *Bulletin du Museum (National) d'Histoire Naturelle, Paris* 11:349–365.

Laxer, M.A., B.K. Timblin, and R.J. Patel. 1991. DNA sequences for the specific detection of *Cryptosporidium parvum* by the polymerase chain reaction. *American Journal of Tropical Medicine and Hygiene* 45:688–694.

Laxer, M.A., M.E. D'Nicuola, and R.J. Patel. 1992. Detection of *Cryptosporidium parvum* DNA in fixed, paraffin-embedded tissue by the polymerase chain reaction. *American Journal of Tropical Medicine and Hygiene* 47:450–455.

Lazo, A., O.O. Barriga, D.R. Redman, and S. Bech-Nielsen. 1986. Identification by transfer blot of antigens reactive in the enzyme-linked immunosorbent assay (ELISA) in immunized and a calf infected with *Cryptosporidium* sp. *Veterinary Parasitology* 21:151–163.

LeChevallier, M.W., W.D. Norton, J.E. Siegel, and M. Abbaszadegan. 1995. Evaluation of the immunofluorescence procedure for detection of *Giardia* cysts and *Cryptosporidium* oocysts in water. *Applied and Environmental Microbiology* 61:690–697.

Leland, D., J. McAnulty, W. Keene, and G. Stevens. 1993. A cryptosporidiosis outbreak in a filtered-water supply. *Journal of the American Water Works Association* 85:34–42.

Leng, X., D. Mosier, and R.D. Oberst. 1996. Simplified method for recovery and PCR detection of *Cryptosporidium* DNA from bovine feces. *Applied and Environmental Microbiology* 62:643–647.

Lengerich, E.J., D.G. Addiss, J.J. Marx, B.L.P. Ungar, and D.D. Juranek. 1993. Increased exposure to cryptosporidia among dairy farmers in Wisconsin. *Journal of Infectious Diseases* 167:1252–1255.

Lengronne, D., G. Regnier, P. Veau, R. Chermette, S. Boufassa, and C. Soule. 1985. Cryptosporidiose chez les poulains diarrhoiques. *Le Point Vétérinaire* 17:528–529.

Levine, J.F., M.G. Levy, R.L. Walker, S. Crittenden. 1988. Cryptosporidiosis in veterinary students. *Journal of the American Veterinary Medical Association* 193:1413–1414.

Levine, N.D. 1962. Protozoology today. *Journal of Protozoology* 9:1–6.

———. 1973a. Historical aspects of research on coccidiosis. In *Proceedings of the symposium on coccidia and related organisms*. Guelph, Ontario: University of Guelph, pp. 1–10.

———. 1973b. Introduction, history, and taxonomy. In *The coccidia*. Eimeria, Isospora, Toxoplasma, *and related genera*. Ed. D.M. Hammond and P.L. Long. Baltimore, MD: University Park Press, pp. 1–22.

Levine, N.D., and V. Ivens. 1965. *The coccidian parasites (Protozoa, Sporozoa) of rodents*. Illinois Biological Monograph No. 33. Urbana: University of Illinois Press, 365 pp.

———. 1972. Coccidia of the Leporidae. *Journal of Protozoology* 19:572–581.

———. 1979. The coccidia (Protozoa, Apicomplexa) of insectivores. *Revista Iberica de Parasitologia* 39:261–297.

———. 1981. *The coccidian parasites (Protozoa, Apicomplexa) of carnivores*. Illinois Biological Monograph No. 51. Urbana: University of Illinois Press, 205 pp.

————. 1986. *The coccidian parasites (Protozoa, Apicomplexa) of Artiodactyla.* Illinois Biological Monograph No. 55. Urbana: University of Illinois Press, 265 pp.

————. 1990. *The coccidian parasites of rodents.* Boca Raton, FL: CRC Press, 228 pp.

Li, Xiantang, J. Pang, and J.G. Fox. 1996. Coinfection with intracellular *Desulfovibrio* species and coccidia in ferrets with proliferative bowel disease. *Laboratory Animal Science* 46:569–571.

Licois, D., P. Coudert, M. Boivin, F. Drouet-Viard, and F. Provôt. 1990. Selection and characterization of a precocious line of *Eimeria intestinalis,* an intestinal rabbit coccidium. *Parasitology Research* 76:192–198.

Lillehoj, H.S., and J.M. Trout. 1994. CD8+ T cell-coccidia interactions. *Parasitology Today* 10:10–14.

Lindsay, D.S., and B.L. Blagburn. 1985. Experimental coccidiosis (*Isospora suis*) in a litter of feral piglets. *Journal of Wildlife Diseases* 21:309–310.

Lindsay, D.S., and K.S. Todd, Jr. 1993. Coccidia of mammals. In *Parasitic protozoa,* vol. 4. New York: Academic Press, Inc., pp. 89–131.

Lindsay, D.S., J.P. Dubey, and R. Fayer. 1991. Demonstration that monoclonal antibodies generated against *Eimeria bovis* sporozoites recognize common antigens on meronts and sexual stages of *E. bovis* and other eimeria (sic) species. *American Journal of Veterinary Research* 51:239–242.

Lindsay, D.S., J.P. Dubey, and B.L. Blagburn. 1997a. Biology of *Isospora* spp. from humans, nonhuman primates and domestic animals. *Clinical Microbiology Reviews* 10:19–34.

Lindsay, D.S., J.P. Dubey, M.A. Toivio-Kinnucan, J.F. Michiels, and B.L. Blagburn. 1997b. Examination of extraintestinal tissue cysts of *Isospora belli. Journal of Parasitology* 83:620–625.

Lom, J., and J.R. Arthur. 1989. A guideline for the preparation of species descriptions in Myxosporea. *Journal of Fish Diseases* 12:151–156.

Long, P.L. (ed.). 1982. *The biology of the coccidia.* Baltimore, MD: University Park Press, 502 pp.

Long, P.L., and L.P. Joyner (eds.). 1996. Profiles of coccidiologists, 2nd ed. London, UK: Academic Services, St. George's Hospital Medical School, pp. 1–2.

Long, P.L., and J.G. Rowell. 1958. Counting oocysts of chicken coccidia. *Laboratory Practice* 7:515–534.

Lopez, J.W., S.D. Allen, J. Mitchell, and M. Quinn. 1988. Rotavirus and *Cryptosporidium* shedding in dairy calf feces and its relationship to colostrum immune transfer. *Journal of Dairy Science* 71:1288–1294.

Lorenzo, M.J., B. Ben, F. Mendez, I. Villacorta, and M.E. Ares-Mazás. 1995. *Cryptosporidium parvum* oocyst antigens recognized by sera from infected asymptomatic adult cattle. *Veterinary Parasitology* 60:17–25.

Lorenzo-Lorenzo, M.J., M.E. Ares-Mazás, and I. Villa Corta Martínez de Maturana. 1993a. Detection of oocysts and IgG antibodies to *Cryptosporidium parvum* in asymptomatic adult cattle. *Veterinary Parasitology* 47:9–15.

Lorenzo-Lorenzo, M.J., M.E. Ares-Mazás, I. Villa Corta, and D. Duran-Oreiro. 1993b. Effect of ultraviolet disinfection of drinking water on the viability of *Cryptosporidium parvum* oocysts. *The Journal of Parasitology* 79:67–70.

Lotze, J.C., W.T. Shalkop, R.G. Leek, and R. Behin. 1964. Coccidial schizonts in mesenteric lymph nodes of sheep and goats. *Journal of Parasitology* 50:205–208.

Ma, P. 1986. *Cryptosporidium*-biology and diagnosis. *Advances in Experimental Biology and Medicine* 202:135–152.

Ma, P., and R. Soave. 1983. Three-step stool examination for cryptosporidiosis in ten homosexual men with protracted watery diarrhea. *Journal of Infectious Diseases* 147:824–828.

Ma, P., T.G. Villanueva, D. Kaufman, and J.F. Gillooley. 1984. Respiratory cryptosporidiosis in the acquired immune deficiency syndrome. Use of modified cold Kinyoun and hemacolor stains for rapid diagnosis. *Journal of the American Medical Association* 252:1298–1301.

MacKenzie, W.R., N.J. Hoxie, M.E. Proctor, M.S. Gradus, K.A. Blair, D.E. Peterson, J.J. Kazmierczak, D.G. Addiss, K.R. Fox, J.B. Rose, and J.P. Davis. 1994. A massive outbreak in Milwaukee of *Cryptosporidium* infection transmitted through the public water supply. *New England Journal of Medicine* 331:161–167.

MacPherson, D.W., and R. McQueen. 1993. Cryptosporidiosis: Multiattribute evaluation of six diagnostic methods. *Journal of Clinical Microbiology* 31:198–202.

Mahmoud, O.M., E.M. Haroun, and A. Sulman. 1994. Hepato-biliary coccidiosis in a dairy goat. *Veterinary Parasitology* 53:15–21.

Mair, T.S., F.G.R. Taylor, D.A. Harbour, and G.R. Pearson. 1990. Concurrent *Cryptosporidium* and coronavirus infections in an Arabian foal with combined immunodeficiency syndrome. *Veterinary Record* 126:127–130.

Mancassola, R., J.-M. Répérant, M. Naciri, and C. Chartier. 1995. Chemoprophylaxis of *Cryptosporidium parvum* infection with paromomycin in kids and immunological study. *Antimicrobial Agents and Chemotherapy* 39:75–78.

Mangini, A.C.S., R.M.D.S. Dias, S.J.F.E. Grisi, A.M.U. Escobar, D.M.A.G.V. Torres, I.P.R. Zuba, C.M.S. Quadros, and P.P. Chieffi. 1992. Parasitismo por *Cryptosporidium* sp. Em crianças com diarréia aguda. *Revista de Instituto Medicine Tropicale São Paulo* 34:341–345.

Margolis, L., G.W. Esch, J.C. Holmes, A.M. Juris, and G.A. Schad. 1982. The use of ecological terms in parasitology (Report of an *ad hoc* committee of the American Society of Parasitologists). *The Journal of Parasitology* 68:131–133.

Marinkelle, C.J. 1968. *Eimeria eumops* n. sp. from a Colombian bat *Eumops trumbulli. Journal of Protozoology* 15:57–58.

Martin, H.D., and N.S. Zeidner. 1992. Concomitant cryptosporidia, coronavirus, and parvovirus in a raccoon (*Procyon lotor*). *Journal of Wildlife Diseases* 28:113–115.

Markus, M.B., and J.B. Bush. 1987. Staining of coccidial oocysts. *The Veterinary Record* 118:329.

Marquardt, W.C. 1966. The living, endogenous stages of the rat coccidium, *Eimeria nieschulzi. Journal of Protozoology* 13:509–514.

Marquardt, W.C., C.M. Senger, and L. Seghetti. 1960. The effect of physical and chemical agents on the oocyst of *Eimeria zurnii* (Protozoa, Coccidia). *Journal of Protozoology* 7:186–189.

Mascaró, C., T. Arnedo, and J. Rosales. 1994. Respiratory cryptosporidiosis in a bovine. *The Journal of Parasitology* 80:334–336.

Mason, P.C. 1985. Cryptosporidia and other protozoa in deer. *New Zealand Veterinary Association, Deer Branch Course* 2:52–59.

Mata, L. 1986. *Cryptosporidium* and other protozoa in diarrheal disease in less developed countries. *Pediatric Infectious Disease* 5:s117–s130.

Mathan, M.M., S. Venkatesan, R. George, and M. Mathew. 1985. *Cryptosporidium* and diarrhoea in southern Indian children. *Lancet* 318:1172–1175.

Matsui, T. 1991. The tissue stages of *Isospora heydorni* in guinea pig as an intermediate host. *Japanese Journal of Parasitology* 40:581–586.

Mayberry, L.F., and W.C. Marquardt. 1973. Transmission of *Eimeria separata* from the normal host, *Rattus,* to the mouse, *Mus musculus. The Journal of Parasitology* 59:198–199.

Mayberry, L.F., W.C. Marquardt, D.J. Nash, and B. Plan. 1982. Genetic dependent transmission of *Eimeria separata* from *Rattus* to three strains of *Mus musculus,* an abnormal host. *The Journal of Parasitology* 68:1124–1126.

Mayberry, L.F., J.R. Bristol, and V.M. Villalobos. 1985. Intergeneric interactions between *Eimeria separata* (Apicomplexa) and *Nippostrongylus brasiliensis* (Nematoda) in the rat. *Experientia* 41:689–690.

Mayberry, L.F., O. Gaytán, and J.R. Bristol. 1989. Transfer of *Eimeria nieschulzi* using extraintestinal tissue. *The Journal of Parasitology* 75:470–472.

Mayer, C.L., and C.J. Palmer. 1996. Evaluation of PCR, nested PCR, and fluorescent antibodies for detection of *Giardia* and *Cryptosporidium* species in wastewater. *Applied and Environmental Microbiology* 62:2081–2085.

Mayr, E., E.G. Linsley, and R.L. Usinger. 1953. *Methods and principles of systematic zoology.* New York: McGraw-Hill Book Company, Inc.

McClelland, G. 1993. *Eimeria phocae* (Apicomplexa: Eimeriidae) in harbour seals *Phoca vitulina* from Sable Island, Canada. *Diseases of Aquatic Organisms* 17:1–8.

McCully, R.M., J.W. van Niekerk, and S.P. Kruger. 1967. Observations on the pathology of bilharziasis and other parasitic infestations of *Hippopotamus amphibus* Linnaeus, 1758, from the Kruger National Park. *Onderstepoort Journal of Veterinary Research* 34:563–618.

McCully, R.M., P.A. Basson, V. DeVos, and A.J. DeVos. 1970. Uterine coccidiosis of the impala caused by *Eimeria neitzi* spec. nov. *Onderstepoort Journal of Veterinary Research* 37:45–58.

McCluskey, B.J., E.C. Greiner, and G.A. Donovan. 1995. Patterns of *Cryptosporidium* oocyst shedding in calves and a comparison of two diagnostic methods. *Veterinary Parasitology* 60:185–190.

McDonald, V., and G.J. Bancroft. 1994. Mechanisms of innate and acquired resistence to *Cryptosporidium parvum* infection in SCID mice. *Parasite Immunology* 16:315–320.

McDonald, V., M.W. Shirley, and M.A. Bellatti. 1986. *Eimeria maxima:* Characteristics of attenuated lines obtained by selection for precocious development in the chicken. *Experimental Parasitology* 61:192–200.

McDonald, V., R. Deer, S. Uni, M. Iseki, and G.J. Bancroft. 1992. Immune responses to *Cryptosporidium muris* and *Cryptosporidium parvum* in adult immunocompetent or immunocompromised (Nude and SCID) mice. *Infection and Immunity* 60:3325–3331.

McDonald, V., H.A. Robinson, J.P. Kelly, and G.J. Bancroft. 1994. *Cryptosporidium muris* in adult mice: Adoptive transfer of immunity and protective roles of CD4 vs. CD8 cells. *Infection and Immunity* 62:2289–2294.

McDougald, L.R. 1982. Chemotherapy of coccidiosis. In *The biology of the coccidia.* Ed. P.L. Long. Baltimore, MD: University Park Press, pp. 373–427.

McLauchlin, J., D.P. Casemore, T.G. Harrison, P.J. Geron, D. Samuel, and A.G. Taylor. 1987. Identification of *Cryptosporidium* oocysts by monoclonal antibody. *Lancet* 323:51.

Mead, J.R., M.J. Arrowood, and C.R. Sterling. 1988. Antigens of *Cryptosporidium* sporozoites recognized by immune sera of infected animals and humans. *The Journal of Parasitology* 74:135–143.

Mead, J.R., M.J. Arrowood, R.W. Sidwell, and M.C. Healey. 1991. Chronic *Cryptosporidium parvum* infection in congenitally immunodeficient SCAID and nude mice. *Journal of Infectious Diseases* 163:1297–1304.

Milácek, P., and Vítovec, J. 1985. Differential staining of cryptosporidia by aniline-carbol-methyl violet and tartrazine in smears and faeces and scrapings of intestinal mucosa. *Folia Parasitologica* 32:50.

Millard, P.S., K.F. Gensheimer, D.G. Addiss, D.M. Sosin, G.A. Beckett, A. Houck-Jankoski, and A. Hudson. 1994. An outbreak of cryptosporidiosis from fresh-pressed apple cider. *Journal of the American Medical Association* 272:1592–1596.

Miller, R.A., M.A. Bronsdon, L. Kuller, and W.R. Morton. 1990. Clinical and parasitologic aspects of cryptosporidiosis in nonhuman primates. *Laboratory Animal Science* 40:42–46.

Miron, D., J. Kenes, and R. Dagan. 1991. Calves as a source of an outbreak of cryptosporidiosis among young children in an agricultural closed community. *Pediatric Infectious Disease Journal* 10:438–441.

Modl, G.S., B.N. Prasad, A.K. Sinha, and B.K. Sinha. 1995. Parasitic infections in herbivorous zoo animals. *Indian Journal of Veterinary Research* 4:45–50.

Moitineo, M. de L.R., and C.S. Ferreira. 1992. Sedimentation in parasitological coproscopy. *Revista do Instituto Medicina tropicos Sáo Paulo* 34:255–258.

Mølbak, K., N. Højlyng, L. Ingholt, A.P.J. da Silva, S. Jepsen, and P. Aaby. 1990. An epidemic outbreak of cryptosporidiosis: a prospective community study from Guinea Bissau. *Pediatric Infectious Disease Journal* 9:566–570.

Mølbak, K., N. Højlyng, A. Gottschau, J.C.C. Sá, L. Ingholt, A.P.J. da Silva, and P. Aaby. 1993. Cryptosporidiosis in infancy and childhood mortality in Guinea Bissau, West Africa. *British Medical Journal* 307:417–420.

Morgan, U.M., C.C. Constantine, P. O'Donoghue, B.P. Meloni, P.A. O'Brien, and R.C.A. Thompson. 1995. Molecular characterization of *Cryptosporidium* isolates from humans and other animals using random amplified polymorphic DNA analysis. *American Journal of Tropical Medicine and Hygiene* 52:559–564.

Morgan, U.M., P.A. O'Brien, and R.C.A. Thompson. 1996. The development of diagnostic PCR primers for *Cryptosporidium* using RAPD-PCR. *Molecular and Biochemical Parasitology* 77:103–108.

Moriya, K. 1989. Ultrastructural observations on oocysts, sporozoites and oocyst residuum of *Cryptosporidium muris* (strain RN 66). *Journal of the Osaka City Medical Center* 38:177–201.

Mosier, D.A., T.L. Kuhls, K.R. Simons, and R.D. Oberst. 1992. Bovine humoral immune response to *Cryptosporidium parvum. Journal of Clinical Microbiology* 30:3277–3279.

Moss, D.M., S.N. Bennett, M.J. Arrowood, M.R. Hurd, P.J. Lammie, S.P. Wahlquist, and D.G. Addiss. 1994. Kinetic and isotypic analysis of specific immunoglobulins from crew members with cryptosporidiosis on a U.S. Coast Guard cutter. *Journal of Eukaryotic Microbiology* 41:52s–55s.

Mottalei, F., L.F. Mayberry, and J.R. Bristol. 1992. Localization of extraintestinal *Eimeria nieschulzi* (Apicomplexa: Eimeriidae) stages in the rat utilizing an indirect immunofluorescence technique. *Transactions of the American Microscopical Society* 111:61–64.

Mtambo, M.M., A.S. Nash, D.A. Blewett, H.V. Smith, and S. Wright. 1991. *Cryptosporidium* infection in cats: Prevalence of infection in domestic and feral cats in the Glasgow area. *Veterinary Record* 129:502–504.

Mtambo, M.M., S.E. Wright, A.S. Nash, and D.A. Blewett. 1996. Infectivity of *Cryptosporidium* species isolated from a domestic cat (*Felis domestica*) in lambs and mice. *Research in Veterinary Science* 60:61–63.

Naciri, M., and P. Yvoré. 1989. Efficacite due lactate d'halofuginone dans le traitement de la cryptosporidiose chez l'agneau. *Recueil de Médecine Vétérinaire* 165:823–826.

Naciri, M., R. Mancassola, P. Yvoré, and J.E. Peeters. 1993. The effect of halofuginone lactate on experimental *Cryp-*

tosporidium parvum infections in calves. *Veterinary Parasitology* 45:199–207.

Naciri, M., R. Mancassola, J.M. Répérant, O. Canivez, B. Quinque, and P. Yvoré. 1994. Treatment of experimental ovine cryptosporidiosis with ovine or bovine hyperimmune colostrum. *Veterinary Parasitology* 53:173–190.

Nagy, B. 1995. Epidemiologic data on *Cryptosporidium parvum* infection of mammalian domestic animals in Hungary. *Magyar Állatorvosok Lapja* 50:139–144.

Nappert, G., D. Hamilton, L. Petrie, and J.M. Naylor. 1993. Determination of lactose and xylose malabsorption in preruminant calves. *Canadian Journal of Veterinary Research* 57:152–158.

Nash, A.S., M.M.A. Mtambo, and H.A. Gibbs. 1993. *Cryptosporidium* infection in farm cats in the Glasgow area. *Veterinary Record* 133:576–577.

Netherwood, T., J.L.N. Wood, H.G.G. Townsend, J.A. Mumford, and N. Chanter. 1996. Foal diarrhea between 1991 and 1994 in the United Kingdom associated with *Clostridium perfringens,* rotavirus, *Strongyloides westeri* and *Cryptosporidium* spp. *Epidemiology and Infection* 117:375–383.

Newman, R.D., K.L. Jaeger, T. Wuhib, A.A.M. Lima, R.L. Guerrant, and C.L. Sears. 1993. Evaluation of an antigen capture enzyme-linked immunosorbent assay for detection of *Cryptosporidium* oocysts. *Journal of Clinical Microbiology* 31:2080–2084.

Nichols, G.L., J. McLauchlin, and D. Samuel. 1991. A technique for typing *Cryptosporidium* isolates. *Journal of Protozoology* 38:237s–240s.

Nimri, L.F., and R. Batchoun. 1994. Prevalence of *Cryptosporidium* species in elementary school children. *Journal of Clinical Microbiology* 32:1040–1042.

Nord, J., P. Ma, D. Dijohn, S. Tzipori, and C.O. Tacket. 1990. Treatment with bovine hyperimmune colostrum of cryptosporidial diarrhea in AIDS patients. *AIDS* 4:581–584.

Nouri, M., and M. Karami. 1991. Asymptomatic cryptosporidiosis in nomadic shepherds and their sheep. *Journal of Infection* 23:331–333.

Nouri, M., and R. Toroghi. 1991. Asymptomatic cryptosporidiosis in cattle and humans in Iran. *Veterinary Record* 128:358–359.

Novak, S.M., and C.R. Sterling. 1991. Susceptibility dynamics in neonatal BALB/c mice infected with *Cryptosporidium parvum. Journal of Protozoology* 38:102s–104s.

Nowak, R.M. 1991. Walker's Mammals of the World, 5th ed., vol. 1. Baltimore, MD: Johns Hopkins University Press, pp. 400–514.

Nowell, F., and S. Higgs. 1989. *Eimeria* species infecting wood mice (genus *Apodemus*) and the transfer of two species to *Mus musculus. Parasitology* 98:329–336.

O'Callaghan, M.G., and E. Moore. 1986. Parasites and serological survey of the common bushtail possum (*Trichosurus vulpecula*) from Kangaroo Island, South Australia. *Journal of Wildlife Diseases* 22:589–591.

O'Donoghue, P.J. 1995. *Cryptosporidium* and cryptosporidiosis in man and animals. *International Journal for Parasitology* 25:139–195.

Olcott, A.T., C.A. Speer, and L.D. Hendricks. 1982. Endogenous development of *Isospora arctopitheci* Rodhain, 1933 in the marmoset *Saguinus geoffroyi. Proceedings of the Helminthological Society of Washington* 49:118–126.

Ong, C., W. Moorehead, A. Ross, and J. Isaac-Renton. 1996. Studies on *Giardia* spp. and *Cryptosporidium* spp. in two adjacent watersheds. *Applied and Environmental Microbiology* 62:2798–2805.

Ongerth, J.E., and H.H. Stibbs. 1987. Identification of *Cryptosporidium* oocysts in river water. *Applied and Environmental Microbiology* 53:672–676.

———. 1989. Prevalence of *Cryptosporidium* infection in dairy calves in western Washington. *American Journal of Veterinary Research* 50:1069–1070.

Orr, J.P. 1988. *Cryptosporidium* infection associated with proliferative enteritis (wet tail) in Syrian hamsters. *Canadian Veterinary Journal* 29:843–844.

Orr, M.B., C.G. MacKintosh, and J.M. Suttie. 1985. Cryptosporidiosis in deer calves. *New Zealand Veterinary Journal* 33:151–152.

Ortega, Y.R., C.R. Sterling, R.H. Gilman, V.A. Cama, and F. Díaz. 1993. *Cyclospora* species—A new protozoan pathogen of humans. *New England Journal of Medicine* 328:1308–1312.

Ortega-Mora, J.M., J.M. Troncoso, F.A. Rojo-Vázquez, and M. Gómez-Bautista. 1993. Serum antibody response in lambs naturally and experimentally infected with *Cryptosporidium parvum. Veterinary Parasitology* 50:45–54.

———. 1994. Identification of *Cryptosporidium parvum* oocyst/sporozoite antigens recognized by infected and hyperimmune lambs. *Veterinary Parasitology* 53:159–166.

Özkul, I.A., and Y. Aydin. 1994. Natural *Cryptosporidium muris* infection of the stomach in laboratory mice. *Veterinary Parasitology* 55:129–132.

Pakandl, M., K. Gaca, D. Licois, and P. Coudert. 1996. *Eimeria media* Kessel, 1929: Comparative study of endogenous development between precocious and parental strains. *Veterinary Research* 27:465–472.

Pal, S., S.K. Bhattacharya, P. Das, P. Chaudhuri, P. Dutta, S.P. De, D. Sen, M.R. Saha, G.B. Nair, and S.C. Pal. 1989. Occurrence and significance of *Cryptosporidium* infection in Calcutta. *Transactions of the Royal Society for Tropical Medicine and Hygiene* 83:520–521.

Palmer, S.R., and A.H. Biffon. 1990. Cryptosporidiosis in England and Wales: prevalence and clinical and epidemiological features. *British Medical Journal* 300: 774–777.

Panciera, R.J., R.W. Thomassen, and F.M. Garner. 1971. Cryptosporidial infection in a calf. *Veterinary Pathology* 8:479–484.

Parisi, M.T., and P. M. Tierno. 1995. Evaluation of new rapid commercial enzyme immunoassay for detection of *Cryptosporidium* oocysts in untreated stool specimens. *Journal of Clinical Microbiology* 33:1963–1965.

Parker, B.B., and D.W. Duszynski. 1986. Coccidiosis of sandhill cranes (*Grus canadensis*) wintering in New Mexico. *Journal of Wildlife Diseases* 22:25–35.

Pavlásek, I. 1984. First record of developmental stages of *Cryptosporidium* sp. in various organs of experimentally infected mice and spontaneously infected calves. *Folia Parasitologica* 31:191–192.

———. The first cases of spontaneous infection of cattle by *Cryptosporidiummuris* Tyzzer (1907), 1910 in the Czech Republic. *Veterinarni Medicina-Czech* 39:279–286.

———. 1995. Findings of cryptosporidia and of other endoparasites in heifers imported into the Czech Republic. *Veterinarni Medicina-Czech* 40:333–336.

Pavlásek, I., and B. Kozakiewicz. 1991. Coypus (*Myocastor coypus*) as a new host of *Cryptosporidium parvum* (Apicomplexa: Cryptosporidiidae). *Folia Parasitologica* 38:90.

Pavlásek, I., and M. Lavička. 1995. The first findings of natural *Cryptosporidium* infection of stomach in desert hamsters (*Phodopus roborovskii* Satunin, 1903). *Veterinarni Medicina-Czech* 40:261–263.

Pavlásek, I., and V.F. Nikitin. 1987. Finding of coccidia of the genus *Cryptosporidium* in the organs of calf excretory system. *Folia Parasitologica* 34:197–198.

Payne, P., L.A. Lancaster, M. Heinzman, and J.A. McCutchan. 1983. Identification of *Cryptosporidium* in patients with the acquired immunodeficiency syndrome. *New England Journal of Medicine* 309:613–614.

Pearson, G.R., and E.F. Logan. 1978. Demonstration of cryptosporidia in the small intestine of a calf by light, transmission electron and scanning electron microscopy. *Veterinary Record* 103:212–213.

Peeters, J.E., I. Villacorta, E. Vanopdenbosch, D. Vandergheynst, M. Naciri, E. Ares-Mazás, and P. Yvoré. 1992. *Cryptosporidium parvum* in calves: kinetics and immunoblot analysis of specific serum and local antibody responses (immunoglobulin A [IgA], IgG, and IgM) after natural and experimental infections. *Infection and Immunity* 60:2309–2316.

Pellérdy, L.P., and U. Dürr. 1970. Orale und parenterale übertragungsversuche von Kokidien auf nicht specifische Wirte. *Acta Veterinaria Academiae Scientarum Hungaricae* 19:253–268.

Pellérdy, L.P., and J. Tanyi. 1968. *Cyclospora talpae* sp. n. (Protozoa: Sporozoa) from the liver of *Talpa europaea*. *Folia Parasitologica (Praha)* 15:275–277.

Penzhorn, B.L., S.E. Knapp, and C.A. Speer. 1994. Enteric coccidia in free-ranging American bison (*Bison bison*) in Montana. *Journal of Wildlife Diseases* 30:267–269.

Perryman, L.E., and J.M. Bjorneby. 1991. Immunotherapy of cryptosporidiosis in immunodeficient animal models. *Journal of Protozoology* 38:98s–100s.

Perryman, L.E., P.H. Mason, and C.E. Chrisp. 1994. Effect of spleen cell populations on resolution of *Cryptosporidium parvum* infection in SCID mice. *Infection and Immunity* 62:1474–1477.

Pieniazek, N.J., and B.L. Herwaldt. 1997. Reevaluating the molecular taxonomy: Is human-associated *Cyclospora* a mammalian *Eimeria* species? *Emerging Infectious Diseases* 3:381–383.

Plettenberg, A., A. Stoehr, H.-J. Stellbrink, H. Albrecht, and W. Meigal. 1993. A preparation from bovine colostrum in the treatment of HIV-positive patients with chronic diarrhea. *Clinical Investigation* 71:42–45.

Pohjola, S. 1984. Negative staining method with nigrosin for the detection of cryptosporidial oocysts: a comparative study. *Research in Veterinary Science* 36:217–219.

Pohjola, S., L. Jokippi, and A.M.M. Jokippi. 1985. Demethylsulphoxide-Ziehl-Neelsen staining technique for detection of cryptosporidial oocysts. *Veterinary Record* 116:442–443.

Pohjola, S., A.M.M. Jokippi, and L. Jokipii. 1986. Sporadic cryptosporidiosis in a rural population is asymptomatic and associated with contact to cattle. *Acta Veterinaria Scandinavica* 27:1–12.

Poonacha, K.B., and P.A. Tuttle. 1989. Intestinal cryptosporidiosis in two Thoroughbred foals. *Equine Practice* 11:6–8.

Porter, S.L. 1996. Dealing with infections and parasitic diseases in safari parks, roadside menageries, exotic animal auctions and rehabilitation centres. *Revue Sccientifique et Technique-Office International des épizooties* 15:227–236.

Pospischil, A., M.T. Stiglmair-Herb, G. von Hegel, and H. Wiesner. 1987. Abomasal cryptosporidiosis in mountain gazelles. *Veterinary Record* 121:379–380.

Powell, H.S., M.A. Hoscher, J.E. Heath, and F.F. Beasley. 1976. Bovine cryptosporidiosis. *Veterinary Medicine/Small Animal Clinician* 71:205–207.

Price, D.L. 1994. *Diagnosis of intestinal parasites*. Boca Raton, FL: CRC Press, 263 pp.

Price, P. 1980. *The evolutionary biology of parasites*. Princeton, NJ: Princeton University Press, 237 pp.

Quílez, J., C. Sánchez-Acedo, E. del Cacho, A. Clavel, and A.C. Causapé. 1996. Prevalence of *Cryptosporidium* and *Giardia* infections in cattle in Aragón (northern Spain). *Veterinary Parasitology* 66:139–146.

Rahman, A.S.M.H., S.C. Sanyal, K.A. Al-Mahmud, A. Sobhan, K.S. Hossain, and B.C. Anderson. 1984. Cryptosporidiosis in calves and their handlers in Bangladesh. *Lancet* 313:221.

Rastegaïeff, E.F. 1930. Zur Frage über Coccidien wilder Tiere. *Archive für Protistenkunde* 71:377–404.

Rehg, J.E., F. Gigliotti, and D.C. Stokes. 1988. Cryptosporidiosis in ferrets. *Laboratory Animal Science* 38:155–158.

Relman, D.A., T.M. Schmidt, A. Gajadhar, M. Sogin, J. Cross, K. Yoder, O. Sethabutr, and P. Echeverria. 1996. Molecular phylogenetic analysis of *Cyclospora*, the human intestinal pathogen, suggests that it is closely related to *Eimeria* spp. *The Journal of Infectious Diseases* 173:440–445.

Répérant, J.-M., M. Naciri, T. Chardes, and D.T. Bout. 1992. Immunological characterization of a 17-kDa antigen from *Cryptosporidium parvum* recognized early by mucosal IgA antibodies. *FEMS Microbiology Letters* 99:7–14.

Répérant, J.-M., M. Naciri, S. Iochmann, M. Tilley, and D.T. Bout. 1994. Major antigens of *Cryptosporidium parvum* recognized by serum antibodies from different infected animal species and man. *Veterinary Parasitology* 55:1–13.

Rhee, J.K., Y.S. Seu, and B.K. Park. 1991a. Isolation and identification of *Cryptosporidium* from various animals in Korea. I. Prevalence of *Cryptosporidium* in various animals. *Korean Journal of Parasitology* 29:139–148.

———. 1991b. Isolation and identification of *Cryptosporidium* from various animals in Korea. II. Identification of *Cryptosporidium muris* from mice. *Korean Journal of Parasitology* 29:149–159.

Rhee, J.K., S.Y. Yook, and B.K. Park. 1995. Oocyst production and immunogenicity of *Cryptosporidium muris* (strain MCR) in mice. *Korean Journal of Parasitology* 33:377–383.

Ribeiro, C.D., and S.R. Palmer. 1986. Family outbreak of cryptosporidiosis. *British Medical Journal* 292:377.

Ride, W.D.L., C.W. Sabrosky, G. Bernardi, and R.V. Melville (eds.). 1985. *International code of zoological nomenclature*, 3rd ed. Huddersfield, England: H. Charlesworth and Co. Ltd. Huddersfield, England, 338 pp.

Ridley, R.K., and R.M. Olsen. 1991. Rapid diagnosis of bovine cryptosporidiosis with a modified commercial acid-fast staining procedure. *Journal of Veterinary Diagnostic Investigation* 3:182–183.

Riggs, M.W. 1997. Immunology: Host response and development of passive immunotherapy and vaccines. In *Cryptosporidium and Cryptosporidiosis*. Ed. R. Fayer. Boca Raton, FL: CRC Press, pp. 129–162.

Riggs, M.W., V.A. Cama, H.L. Leary, and C.R. Sterling. 1994. Bovine antibody against *Cryptosporidium parvum* elicits a circumsporozoite precipitate-like reation and has immunotherapeutic effect against persistent cryptosporidiosis in SCID mice. *Infection and Immunity* 62:1927–1939.

Roberts, L.S., and J. Janovy, Jr. 1996. Foundations of parasitology, 5th ed. Dubuque, IA: William C. Brown Publishers, 659 pp.

Robertson, L.J., A.T. Campbell, and H.V. Smith. 1992. Survival of *Cryptosporidium parvum* oocysts under various environmental pressures. *Applied and Environmental Microbiology* 58:3494–3500.

Rocehlle, P., R. de Leon, M.H. Stewart, and R.L. Wolfe. 1997a. Comparison of primers and optimization of PCR conditions for detection of *Cryptosporidium parvum* and *Giardia lamblia* in water. *Applied and Environmental Microbiology* 63:106–114.

Rochelle, P., D.M. Ferguson, T.J. Handojo, R. de Leon, M.H. Stewart, and R.L. Wolfe. 1997b. An assay combining cell culture with reverse transcriptase PCR to detect and determine the infectivity of waterborne *Cryptosporidium parvum. Applied and Environmental Microbiology* 63:2029–2037.

Rodgers, M.R., D.J. Flanigan, and W. Jakubowski. 1995. Identification of algae which interfere with the detection of *Giardia* cysts and *Cryptosporidium* oocysts and a method for alleviating this interference. *Applied and Environmental Microbiology* 61:3759–3763.

Rodhain, J. 1933. Sur une coccidie de l'intestin de l'ouistiti, *Hepale jaechus penicillatus* (Goeffroy). *Comptes Rendus Société Biologie (Paris)* 114:1357–1358.

Rodriguez-Diego, J., J.R. Abreu, E. Perez, E. Rogue, and O. Cartas. 1991. Presenciade *Cryptosporidium* sp. en bufalos (*Bubalus bubalis*) en Cuba. *Revista deSalud Animal* 13:78–80.

Rodríguez-Hernandez, J., A. Canut-Blasco, M. Ledesma-Garcia, and A.M. Martin-Sánchez. 1994. *Cryptosporidium* oocysts in water for human consumption. *Comparison of staining methods. European Journal of Epidemiology* 10:215–218.

Rose, J.B., H. Darbin, and C.P. Gerba. 1988. Correlations of the protozoa, *Cryptosporidium* and *Giardia,* with water quality variables in a watershed. *Water Science Technology* 20:271–276.

Rose, J.B., L.K. Landeen, K.R. Riley, and C.P. Gerba. 1989. Evaluation of immunofluoresence techniques for detection of *Cryptosporidium* oocysts and Giardia cysts from environmental samples. *Applied and Environmental Microbiology* 55:3189–3196.

Rose, J.B., J.T. Lisle, and M. LeChevallier. 1997. Waterborne cryptosporidiosis: Incidence, outbreaks and treatment strategies. In Cryptosporidium *and cryptosporidiosis.* Ed. R. Fayer. Boca Raton, FL: CRC Press, pp. 93–110.

Rose, M.E. 1974. Immune responses to the *Eimeria:* Recent observations. In *Proceedings of the symposium on coccidia and related organisms.* Guelph, Ontario: University of Guelph, pp. 92–118.

———. 1984. Cell-mediated immunity in coccidiosis. In *Cell-mediated immunity.* Ed. P.J. Quinn. Luxembourg: Commission of the European Communities, pp. 288–297.

———. 1987. Immunity to *Eimeria* infections. *Veterinary Immunology and Immunopathology* 17:333–343.

Rose, M.E., and P. Hesketh. 1979. Immunity to coccidiosis: T-lymphocyte- or B-lymphocyte-deficient animals. *Infection and Immunity* 26:630–637.

Rose, M.E., and B.J. Millard, Jr. 1985. Host specificity in eimerian coccidia: Development of *Eimeria vermiformis* of the mouse, *Mus musculus,* in *Rattus norvegicus. Parasitology* 90:557–563.

Rose, M.E., B.M. Ogilvie, P. Hesketh, and M.F. Festing. 1979. Failure of nude (athymic) rats to become resistant to reinfection with the intestinal coccidian parasite *Eimeria nieschulzi* or the nematode *Nippostrongylus brasiliensis. Parasite Immunology* 1:125–132.

Rose, M.E., J.V. Peppard, and S.M. Hobbs. 1984. Coccidiosis: Characterization of antibody responses to infection with *Eimeria nieschulzi. Parasite Immunology* 6:1–12.

Rose, M.E., D. Wakelin, and P. Hesketh. 1985. Susceptibility to coccidiosis: Contrasting course of primary infections with *Eimeria vermiformis* in BALB/c and C57/BL/6 mice is based on immune response. *Parasite Immunology* 7:557–566.

Rose, M.E., H.S. Joysey, P. Hesketh, R.K. Grencis, and D.W. Wakelin. 1988a. Mediation of immunity to *Eimeria vermiformis* in mice by L3T4+ T cells. *Infection and Immunity* 56:1760–1765.

Rose, M.E., D. Wakelin, H.S. Joysey, and P. Hesketh. 1988b. Immunity to coccidiosis: Adoptive transfer in NIH mice challenged with *Eimeria vermiformis. Parasite Immunology* 10:59–69.

Rose, M.E., D. Wakelin, and P. Hesketh. 1989. Gamma interferon controls *Eimeria vermiformis* primary infection in BALB/c mice. *Infection and Immunity* 57:1599–1603.

Rose, M.E., D. Wakelin, and P. Hesketh. 1991. Interferon-gamma-mediated effects upon immunity to coccidial infections in the mouse. *Parasite Immunology* 13:63–74.

Rose, M.E., P. Hesketh, and D. Wakelin. 1992. Immune control of murine coccidiosis: CD4+ and CD8+ lymphocytes contribute differently in resistance to primary and secondary infections. *Parasitology* 105:349–354.

Rosenblatt, J.E., and L.M. Sloan. 1993. Evaluation of an enzyme-linked immunosorbent assay for detection of *Cryptosporidium* spp. in stool specimens. *Journal of Clinical Microbiology* 31:1468-1471.

Roth, H.H. 1972. Needs, priorities and development of wildlife disease research in relation to agricultural development in Africa. *Journal of Wildlife Diseases* 8:369–374.

Roudabush, R.L. 1937. The endogenous phases of the life cycle of *Eimeria nieschulzi, Eimeria separata,* and *Eimeria miyairii* coccidian parasites of the rat. *Iowa State College Journal of Science* 11:135–163.

Rusnak, J., T.L. Hadfield, M.M. Rhodes, and J.K. Gaines. 1989. Detection of *Cryptosporidium* oocysts in human fecal specimens by an indirect immunofluoresence assay with monoclonal antibodies. *Journal of Clinical Microbiology* 27:1135–1136.

Russell, R.G., S.L. Rosenkranz, L.A. Lee, H. Howard, R.F. DiGiacomo, M.A. Bronsdon, G.A. Blakely, C-C. Tsai, and W.R. Morton. 1987. Epidemiology and etiology of diarrhea in colony-born *Macaca nemestrina. Laboratory Animal Science* 37:309–316.

Ryan, M.J., J.P. Sundberg, R.J. Sauerschell, and K.S Todd, Jr. 1986. *Cryptosporidium* in a wild cottontail rabbit (*Sylvilagus floridanus*). *Journal of Wildlife Diseases* 22:267.

Ryff, K.L., and R.C. Bergstrom. 1975. Bovine coccidia in American bison. *Journal of Wildlife Diseases* 11:412–414.

Ryley, J.F., R. Meade, J. Hazelhurst, and T.E. Robinson. 1976. Methods in coccidiosis research: separation of oocysts from faeces. *Parasitology* 73:311–326.

Sam-Yellowe, T.Y. 1996. Rhoptry organelles of the Apicomplexa: Their role in host cell invasion and intracellular survival. *Parasitology Today* 12:308–315.

Sanchez-Mejorada, G., and A. Ponce-de-Leon. 1994. Clinical patterns of diarrhea in AIDS: Etiology and prognosis. *Revista de Investigacion Clinica* 46:187–196.

Sanford, S.A., and G.K.A. Josephson. 1982. Bovine cryptosporidiosis: Clinical and pathological findings in forty-two scouring neonatal calves. *Canadian Veterinary Journal* 23:343–347.

Schillhorn van Veen, T.W., A.L. Trapp, D. Daunt, and N.A. Richter. 1986. Coccidiosis in a kudu antelope. *Journal of the American Veterinary Medical Association* 189:1178–1179.

Scholtyseck, E. 1973. Ultrastructure. In *The coccidia,* Eimeria, Isospora, Toxoplasma, *and related genera.* Ed. D.M. Hammond and P.L. Long. Baltimore, MD: University Park Press, pp. 81–144.

Schultz, D.J., I.J. Hough, and W. Boardman. 1996. Special challenges of maintaining wild animals in captivity in Australia and New Zealand: Prevention of infections and parasitic diseases. *Revue Scientifique et Technique-Office International des épizootie* 15:289–308.

Scott, C.A., H.V. Smith, M.M.A. Mtambo, and H.A. Gibbs. 1995. An epidemiological study of *Cryptosporidium parvum* in two herds of adult beef cattle. *Veterinary Parasitology* 57:277–288.

Scott, D.T., and D.W. Duszynski. 1997. *Eimeria* from bats of the World: Two new species from *Myotis* spp. (Chiroptera: Vespertilionidae). *The Journal of Parasitology* 83:495–501.

Shahid, N.S., A.S.M.H. Rahman, B.C. Anderson, L.J. Mata, and S.C. Sanyal. 1985. Cryptosporidiosis in Bangladesh. *British Medical Journal* 290:114–115.

Shahid, N.S., A.S.M.H. Rahman, and S.C. Sanyal. 1987. *Cryptosporidium* as a pathogen for diarrhoea in Bangladesh. *Tropical and Geographical Medicine* 39:265–270.

Sharma, N.N., W.M. Reid, and J.W. Foster. 1963. A cleaning method for coccidial oocysts using density-gradient sedimentation. *Journal of Parasitology* 49:159–160.

Sheather, A.L. 1923. The detection of intestinal protozoa and mange parasites by a flotation technique. *Journal of Comparative Pathology* 36:266–275.

Sheppard, A.M. 1974. Ultrastructural pathology of coccidial infection. *The Journal of Parasitology* 60:369–371.

Shield, J., J.H. Baumer, J.A. Dawson, and P.J. Wilkinson. 1990. Cryptosporidiosis—an educational experience. *Journal of Infection* 21:297–301.

Siddons, C.A., P.A. Chapman, and B.A. Rush. 1992. Evaluation of an enzyme immunoassay kit for detecting *Cryptosporidium* in faeces and environmental samples. *Journal of Clinical Pathology* 45:479–482.

da Silva, N.R.S., G.L. Braccini, E.L. Chaplin, and F.A.P. Araújo. 1996. *Cryptosporidium muris* in equine. Pôrto Alegre Area, RS, Brazil. *Arquivos Faculdade de Veterinaria UFRGS, Pôrto Alegre* 24:81–84.

Simpson, V.R. 1992. Cryptosporidiosis in newborn red deer (*Cervus elaphus*). *Veterinary Record* 130:116–118.

Sinha, C.K. and S. Sinha. 1980. *Eimeria darjeelingensis* sp. n. from a house-shrew, *Suncus murinus soccatus* (Hodgson*). Acta Protozoologica* 19:293–296.

Sinski, E. 1993. Cryptosporidiosis in Poland: Clinical, epidemiologic and parasitologic aspects. *Folia Parasitologica* 40:297–300.

Sinski, E., E. Hlebowicz, and M. Bednarska. 1993. Occurrence of *Cryptosporidium parvum* infection in wild small mammals in district of Mazury Lake (Poland). *Acta Parasitologica Polonica* 38:59–61.

Skeels, M.R., R. Sokolow, C.V. Hubbard, J.K. Andrus, and J. Baisch. 1990. *Cryptosporidium* infection in Oregon public health clinic patients 1985–88: The value of statewide laboratory surveillance. *American Journal of Public Health* 80:305–308.

Smith, J.L. 1993. *Cryptosporidium* and *Giardia* as agents of foodborne disease. *Journal of Food Protection* 56:451–461.

Smith, H.V., A.L. Smith, R.W.A. Girdwood, and E.G. Carrington. 1990. The effect of free chlorine on the viability of *Cryptosporidium* oocysts isolated from human feces. In Cryptosporidium *in water supplies*. Ed. J. Badenoch. London, UK: Her Majesty's Stationary Office, pp. 185–204.

Smith, H.V., C.A. Paton, R.W.A. Girdwood, and M.M.A. Mtambo. 1996. *Cyclospora* in non-human primates in Gombe, Tanzania. *Veterinary Record* 33:528.

Smith, R.R., and M.D. Ruff. 1975. A rapid technique for the cleaning and concentration of *Eimeria* oocysts. *Poultry Science* 54:2081–2086.

Snyder, D.E. 1988. Indirect immunofluorescent detection of oocysts of *Cryptosporidium parvum* in the feces of naturally infected raccoons (*Procyon lotor*). *The Journal of Parasitology* 74:1050–1052.

Snyder, S.P., J.J. England, and A.E. McChesney. 1978. Cryptosporidiosis in immunodeficient Arabian foals. *Veterinary Pathology* 15:12–17.

Soule, C., E. Plateau, C. Perret, R. Chermette, and M.M. Feton. 1983. Observation de cryptosporidies chez le poulain. Note preliminaire. *Recueil de Medecine Veterinaire de l'Ecole d'Alfort* 159:719–720.

Soveri, T., and M. Valtonen. 1983. Endoparasites of hares (*Lepus timidus* L. and *L. europaeus* Pallas) in Finland. *Journal of Wildlife Diseases* 19:337–341.

Speer, C.A., and D.W. Duszynski. 1975. Fine structure of the oocyst walls of *Isospora serini* and *Isospora canaria* and excystation of *Isospora serini* from the canary, *Serinus canarius* L. *Journal of Protozoology* 22:476–481.

Speer, C.A., D.M. Hammond, J.L. Mahrt, and W.L. Roberts. 1973. Structure of the oocyst and sporocyst walls and excystation of sporozoites of *Isospora canis. The Journal of Parasitology* 59:35–40.

Speer, C.A., A.A. Marchiondo, and D.W. Duszynski. 1976. Ultrastructure of the sporocyst wall during excystation of *Isospora endocallimici. The Journal of Parasitology* 62:984–987.

Speer, C.A., A.A. Marhiondo, B. Mueller, and D.W. Duszynski. 1979. Scanning and transmission electron microscopy of the oocyst wall of *Isospora lacazei. Zeitschrift für Parasitenkunde* 59:219–225.

Sprinz, H. 1962. Morphological response of intestinal mucosa to enteric bacteria and its implication for sprue and Asiatic cholera. *Federation Proceedings* 21:57–64.

Steele, A.D., E. Gove, and P.J. Meewes. 1989. Cryptosporidiosis in white patients in South Africa. *Journal of Infection* 19:281–285.

Stein, A.S., and W.C. Marquardt. 1973. *Eimeria nieschulzi:* Glucose absorption in infected rats. *Experimental Parasitology* 34:262–267.

Sterling, C.R., and M.J. Arrowood. 1986. Detection of *Cryptosporidium* sp. infections using a direct immunofluorescent assay. *Pediatric Infectious Disease* 5:s139–s142.

Stetzenbach, L.D., M.J. Arrowood, M.M. Marshall, and C.R. Sterling. 1988. Monoclonal antibody based immunofluorescent assay for *Giardia* and *Cryptosporidium* detection in water samples. *Water Science Technology* 20:193–198.

Stewart, G.L., J.J. Reddington, and A.M. Hamilton. 1980. *Eimeria nieschulzi* and *Trichinella spiralis:* Analysis of concurrent infection in the rat. *Experimental Parasitology* 50:115–122.

Stibbs, H.H., and J.E. Ongerth. 1986. Immunofluoresence detection of *Cryptosporidium* oocysts in fecal smears. *Journal of Clinical Microbiology* 24:517–521.

Stiff, M.I., and J.P. Vasilakos. 1990. Effect of in vivo T-cell depletion on the effector T-cell function of immunity to *Eimeria falciformis. Infection and Immunity* 58:1496–1499.

Stinear, T., A. Matusan, K. Hines, and M. Sandery. 1996. Detection of a single viable *Cryptosporidium parvum* oocyst in environmental water concentrates by reverse transcription-PCR. 1996. *Applied and Environmental Microbiology* 62:3385–3390.

Stockdale, P.H.G., M.J. Stockdale, M.D. Rickard, and G.F. Mitchell. 1985. Mouse strain variation and effects of oocyst dose in infection of mice with *Eimeria falciformis*, a coccidian parasite of the large intestine. *International Journal of Parasitology* 15:447–452.

Sundberg, J.P., D. Hill, and M.J. Ryan. 1982. Cryptosporidiosis in a gray squirrel. *Journal of the American Veterinary Medical Association* 181:1420–1422.

Supperer, R., and H.K. Hinaidy. 1986. On the parasitic infections of dogs and cats in Austria. *Deutsche Tierärztliche Wochenschrift* 93:383–386.

Tacal, J.V., M. Sobieh, and A. El-Ahraf. 1987. *Cryptosporidium* in market pigs in southern California, USA. *Veterinary Record* 120:615–617.

Tanabe, M. 1938. On three species of coccidia of the mole, *Mogera wogura coreana* Thomas, with special reference to the life history of *Cyclospora caryolitica. Keijo Journal of Medicine* 9:21–52.

Tee, G.H., A.H. Moody, A.H. Cooke, and P.L. Chiodini. 1993. Comparison of technqiues for detecting antigens of *Giardia lamblia* and *Cryptosporidium parvum* in faeces. *Journal of Clinical Pathology* 46:555–558.

Tilahun, G., and P.H.G. Stockdale. 1982. Sensitivity and specificity of the indirect fluorescent antibody test in the study of four murine coccidia. *Journal of Protozoology* 29:124–132.

Tilley, M., and S.J. Upton. 1997. Biochemistry of *Cryptosporidium*. In Cryptosporidium *and cryptosporidiosis*. Ed. R. Fayer. Boca Raton, FL: CRC Press, pp. 163–180.

Tilley, M., S.J. Upton, and C.E. Chrisp. 1991. A comparative study on the biology of *Cryptosporidium* sp. from guinea pigs and *Cryptosporidium parvum* (Apicomplexa). *Canadian Journal of Microbiology* 37:949–952.

Tilley, M., V. McDonald, and G.J. Bancroft. 1995. Resolution of cryptosporidial infection in mice correlates with parasite-specific lymphocyte proliferation associates with both T_h1 and T_h2 cytokine secretion. *Parasite Immunology* 17:459–464.

Todd, K.S., Jr., and D.M. Hammond. 1968a. Life cycle and host specificity of *Eimeria callospermophili* Henry, 1932 from the Uinta ground squirrel *Spermophilus armatus*. *Journal of Protozoology* 15:1–8.

———. 1968b. Life cycle and host specificity of *Eimeria larimerensis* Vetterling, 1964, from the Uinta ground squirrel *Spermophilus armatus*. *Journal of Protozoology* 15:268–275.

Todd, K.S., Jr., and D.L. Lepp. 1972. Completion of the life cycle of *Eimeria vermiformis* Ernst, Chobotar, and Hammond, 1971 from the mouse *Mus musculus*, in dexamethasone-treated rats, *Rattus norvegicus*. *The Journal of Parasitology* 58:400–401.

Todd, K.S., Jr., D.M. Hammond, and B.W. O'Gara. 1967. Redescription and incidence of *Eimeria antelocaprae* Huizinga, 1942 in the pronghorn antelope, *Antilocapra americana* (Ord, 1815). *Journal of Wildlife Diseases* 3:71–73.

Todd, K.S., Jr., D.L. Lepp, and C.V. Trayser. 1971. Development of the asexual cycle of *Eimeria vermiformis* Ernst, Chobotar, and Hammond, 1971, from the mouse, *Mus musculus*, in dexamethasone-treated rats, *Rattus norvegicus*. *The Journal of Parasitology* 57:1137–1138.

Tsaihong, J.C., and P. Ma. 1990. Comparison of an indirect flourescent antibody test and stool examination for the diagnosis of cryptosporidiosis. *European Journal of Microbiology and Infectious Diseases* 9:770–774.

Tyzzer, E.E. 1907. A sporozoan found in the peptic glands of the common mouse. *Proceedings of the Society for Experimental Biology and Medicine* 5:12–13.

———. 1910. An extracellular coccidium, *Cryptosporidium muris* (gen. et sp. nov.), of the gastric glands of the common mouse. *Journal of Medical Research* 23:487–509.

———. 1912. *Cryptosporidium parvum* (sp. nov.), a coccidium found in the small intestine of the common mouse. *Archiv für Protistenkunde* 26:394–418.

Tzipori, S., and I. Campbell. 1981. Prevalence of *Cryptosporidium* antibodies in 10 animals species. *Journal of Clinical Microbiology* 14:455–456.

Tzipori, S., K.W. Angus, I. Campbell, and D. Sherwood. 1981a. Diarrhea in young red deer associates with infection with *Cryptosporidium*. *Journal of Infectious Diseases* 144:170–175.

Tzipori, S., K.W. Angus, E.W. Gray, I. Campbell, and F. Allan. 1981b. Diarrhea in lambs experimentally infected with *Cryptosporidium* isolated from calves. *American Journal of Veterinary Research* 42:1400–1404.

Tzipori, S., E. McCartney, G.H.K. Lawson, A.C. Rowland, and I. Campbell. 1981c. Experimental infection of piglets with *Cryptosporidium*. *Research in Veterinary Science* 31:358–368.

Tzipori, S., D. Roberton, and C. Chapman. 1986. Remission of diarrhoea due to cryptosporidiosis in an immunodeficient child treated with hyperimmune bovine colostrum. *British Medical Journal* 293:1276–1277.

Tzipori, S., D. Roberton, D.A. Cooper, and L. White. 1987. Chronic cryptosporidial diarrhoea and hyperimmune cow colostrum. *Lancet* 325:344–345.

Tzipori, S., W. Rand, and C. Theodos. 1995. Evaluation of two-phase SCID mouse model preconditioned with anti-interfereon-g monoclonal antibody for drug testing against *Cryptosporidium parvum*. *Journal of Infectious Diseases* 172:1160–1164.

Ubelaker, J.E., R.D. Specian, and D.W. Duszynski. 1977. Endoparasites. In *Biology of bats of the New World family Phyllostomatidae*, part 2. Ed. R.J. Baker, J.K. Jones, and D.C. Carter. Lubbock, TX: Special Publications, The Museum, Texas Tech University Press, pp. 7–56.

Ungar, B.L.P., and T. E. Nash. 1986. Quantification of specific antibody response to *Cryptosporidium* antigens by laser densitometry. *Infection and Immunity* 53:124–128.

Ungar, B.L.P., R. Soave, R. Fayer, and T.E. Nash. 1986. Enzyme immunoassay detection of immunoglobulin M and G antibodies to *Cryptosporidium* in immunocompetent and immunocompromised persons. *Journal of Infectious Diseases* 153:570–578.

Ungar, B.L.P., D.J. Ward, R. Fayer, and C.A. Quinn. 1990a. Cessation of *Cryptosporidium*-associated diarrea in an acquired immunodeficiency syndrome patientafter treatment with hyperimmune bovine colostrum. *Gastroenterology* 98:486–489.

Ungar, B.L.P., J.A. Burris, C.A. Quinn, and F.D. Finkelman. 1990b. New mouse models for chronic *Cryptosporidium* infection in immunodeficient hosts. *Infection and Immunity* 58:961–969.

Ungar, B.L.P., T.-C. Kao, J.A. Burris, and F.D. Finkelman. 1991. *Cryptosporidium* infection in an adult mouse model. Independent roles for IFN-γ and CD4+ lymphocytes in protective immunity. *Journal of Immunology* 147:1014–1022.

Ungureanu, E.M., and G. Dontu. 1992. A new staining technique for the identification of *Cryptosporidium* oocysts in faecal smears. *Transactions of the Royal Society for Tropical Medicine and Hygiene* 86:638.

Upton, S.J. 1997. In vitro cultivation. In Cryptosporidium *and cryptosporidiosis*. Ed. R. Fayer. Boca Raton, FL: CRC Press, pp. 181–207.

Upton, S.J., and W.L. Current. 1985. The species of *Cryptosporidium* (Apicomplexa: Cryptosporidiidae) infecting mammals. *The Journal of Parasitology* 71:625–629.

Upton, S.J., and H.H. Gillock. 1996. Infection dynamics of *Cryptosporidium parvum* in ICR outbred suckling mice. *Folia Parasitologica* 43:101–106.

Urban, J.F., R. Fayer, S–J. Chen, W.C. Gause, M.K. Gately, and F.D. Finkelman. 1996. IL-12 protects immunocompetent and immunodeficient neonatal mice against infection with *Cryptosporidium parvum*. *Journal of Immunology* 156:263–268.

Van Winkle, T.J. 1985. Cryptosporidiosis in young artiodactyls. *Journal of the Veterinary Medicine Association* 187:1170–1172.

Vesey, G., P. Hutton, A. Champion, N. Ashbolt, K.L. Williams, A. Warton, and D. Veal. 1994. Application of flow cytometric methods for the routine detection of *Cryptosporidum* and *Giardia* in water. *Cytometry* 16:1–6.

Vetterling, J.M. 1969. Continuous-flow differential density flotation of coccidial oocysts and a comparison with other methods. *The Journal of Parasitology* 55:412–417.

Vetterling, J.M., H.R. Jervis, T.G. Merrill, and J. Sprinz. 1971a. *Cryptosporidium wrairi* sp. n. from the guinea pig *Cavia porcellus*, with an emendation of genus. *Journal of Protozoology* 18:243–247.

Vetterling, J.M., A. Takeuchi, and P.A. Madden. 1971b. Ultrastructure of *Cryptosporidium wrairi* from the guinea pig. *Journal of Protozoology* 18:248–260.

Villacorta, I., E. Ares-Mazás, and M.J. Lorenzo. 1991. *Cryptosporidium parvum* in cattle, sheep and pigs in Galicia (N.W. Spain). *Veterinary Parasitology* 38:249–252.

Vítovec, J., and B. Koudela. 1988. Location and pathogenicity of *Cryptosporidium parvum* in experimentally infected mice. *Zeitschrift für Veterinarmedizin Reihe B* 35:515–524.

———. 1992. Pathogenesis of intestinal cryptosporidiosis in conventional and gnotobiotic piglets. *Veterinary Parasitology* 43:25–36.

Wagenbach, G.E., J.R. Challey, and W.C. Burns. 1966. A method for purifying coccidian oocysts employing Clorox and sulfuric acid-dichromate solution. *The Journal of Parasitology* 52:1222.

Wagner-Wiening, C., and P. Kimmig. 1995. Detection of viable *Cryptosporidium parvum* oocysts by PCR. *Applied and Environmental Microbiology* 61:4514–4516.

Wallace, G.D. 1971. Experimental transmission of *Toxoplasma gondii* by filth-flies. *American Journal of Tropical Medicine and Hygiene* 20:411–413.

———. 1972. Experimental transmission of *Toxoplasma gondii* by cockroaches. *Journal of Infectious Diseases* 126:545–547.

Wang, C.C. 1982. Biochemistry and physiology of coccidia. In *The biology of the coccidia.* Ed. P.L. Long. Baltimore, MD: University Park Press, pp. 167–228.

Wang, J.S., and C.T. Liew. 1990. Prevalence of *Cryptosporidium* spp. in birds in Taiwan. *Taiwan Journal of Veterinary Medicine and Animal Husbandry* 56:45–57.

Warner, D.E. 1933. Survival of coccidia of the chicken in soil and on the surface of eggs. *Poultry Science* 12:343–348.

Wash, C.D., D.W. Duszynski, and T.L. Yates. 1985. Eimerians from different karyotypes of the Japanese wood mouse (*Apodemus* spp.), with descriptions of two new species and a redescription of *Eimeria montgomeryae* Lewis and Ball, 1983. *The Journal of Parasitology* 71:808–814.

Waters, W.R., and J.A. Harp. 1996. *Cryptosporidium parvum* infection in T-cell receptor (TCR)-a and TCR-d deficient mice. *Infection and Immunity* 64:1854–1857.

Watzl, B., D.S. Huang, J. Alak, H. Darban, E.M. Jenkins, and R.R. Watson. 1993. Enhancement of resistance to *Cryptosporidium parvum* by pooled bovine colostrum during murine retroviral infection. *American Journal of Tropical Medicine and Hygiene* 48:519–523.

Webster, K.A., J.D.E. Pow, M. Giles, J. Catchpole, and M.J. Woodward. 1993. Detection of *Cryptosporidium parvum* using a specific polymerase chain reaction. *Veterinary Parasitology* 50:35–44.

Webster, K.A., H.V. Smith, M. Giles, L. Dawson, and L.J. Robertson. 1996. Detection of *Cryptosporidium parvum* oocysts in faeces: Comparison of conventional coproscopical methods and the polymerase chain reaction. *Veterinary Parasitology* 61:5–13.

Wenyon, C.M. 1926. Protozoology. London: Bailliere, Tyndall and Cox, pp. 803–869.

Whitmire, W.M., and J.A. Harp. 1991. Characterization of bovine cellular and serum antibody responses during infection by *Cryptosporidium parvum*. *Infection and Immunity* 59:990–995.

Wilber, P.G., and M.J. Patrick. 1997. Mark-recapture vs. simulated removal trapping for assessing temporal patterns in ecological communities: An example using coccidian parasites of two species of rodents. *American Midland Naturalist* 137:112–123.

Wilber, P.G., B. Hanelt, B. VanHorne, and D.W. Duszynski. 1994a. Two new species and temporal changes in the prevalence of eimerians in a free-living population of Townsend's ground squirrels (*Spermophilus townsendii*) in Idaho. *The Journal of Parasitology* 80:251–259.

Wilber, P.G., K. McBee, D.J. Hafner, and D.W. Duszynski. 1994b. A new coccidian (Apicomplexa: Eimeriidae) in the northern pocket gopher (*Thomomys talpoides*) and a comparison of oocyst survival in hosts from radon-rich

and radon-poor soils. *Journal of Wildlife Diseases* 30:359–364.

Wilber, P.G., E.C. Hellgren, and T.M. Gabor. 1996. Coccidia of the collared peccary (*Tayassu tajacu*) in southern Texas with descriptions of three new species of *Eimeria* (Apicomplexa: Eimeriidae). *The Journal of Parasitology* 82:624–629.

Wilber, P.G., D.W. Duszynski, S.J. Upton, R.S. Seville, and J.O. Corliss. 1998. A revision of the taxonomy and nomenclature of the *Eimeria* spp. (Apicomplexa: Eimeriidae) from rodents in the tribe Marmotini (Sciuridae). *Systematic Parasitology* 39:113–135.

Williams, B.H. 1996. Biliary coccidiosis in a ferret (*Mustela putorius furo*). *Veterinary Pathology* 33:437–439.

Williams, E.S., and E.T. Thorne. 1996. Infectious and parasitic diseases of captive carnivores, with special emphasis on the black-footed ferret (*Mustela nigripes*). *Revue Scientifique et Technique-Office International des épizooties* 15:91–114.

Williams, R.O. 1987. Measurement of class specific antibody against *Cryptosporidium* in serum and faeces from experimentally infected calves. *Research in Veterinary Science* 43:264–265.

Wilson, D.E., and D.M. Reeder (eds.). 1993. *Mammal species of the world,* 2nd ed. Washington, DC: Smithsonian Institution Press, 1207 pp.

Wilson, D.W., P.A. Day, and M.E.G. Brummer. 1984. Diarrhea associated with *Cryptosporidium* sp. in juvenile macaques. *Veterinary Pathology* 21:447–450.

Wong, D.T., J.S. Horng, and J.R. Wilkinson. 1972. Robenzidine, an inhibitor of oxidative phosphorylation. *Biochemical and Biophysical Research Communications* 46:621–627.

Worley, D.E., R.E. Barrett, P.J.A. Presidente, and R.H. Jacobson. 1969. The Rocky Mountain elk as a reservoir host for parasites of domestic animals in western Montana. *Bulletin of the Wildlife Disease Association* 5:348–350.

Wyatt, C.R., E.J. Brackett, L.E. Perryman, A.C. Rise-Ficht, W.C. Brown, and K.I. O'Rourke. 1997. Activation of intestinal intraepithelial T lymphocytes in calves infected with *Cryptospordium parvum*. *Infection and Immunity* 65:185–190.

Xiao, L., and R.P. Herd. 1994a. Review of equine *Cryptosporidium* infection. *Equine Veterinary Journal* 26:9–13.

———. 1994b. Epidemiology of equine *Cryptosporidium* and *Giardia* infections. *Equine Veterinary Journal* 26:14–17.

Xiao, L., R.P. Herd, and D.M. Rings. 1993. Diagnosis of *Cryptosporidium* on a sheep farm with neonatal diarrhea by immuno fluorescence assays. *Veterinary Parasitology* 47:17–23.

Yakimoff, W.L., and S.N. Matschoulsky. 1940. Coccidia of animals from the Tashkente Zoological Gardens [in Russian]. *Parasitologicheski sbornik Zoologicheskogo instituta Akademii Nauk SSSR* 8:236–248.

Yamaura, H., R. Shirasaka, H. Asahi, T. Koyama, M. Motoki, and H. Ito. 1990. Prevalence of *Cryptosporidium* infection among house rats, *Rattus rattus* and *R. norvegicus,* in Tokyo, Japan and experimental cryptosporidiosis in roof rats. *Japanese Journal of Parasitology* 39:439–444.

Yamini, B., and N.R. Raju. 1986. Gasroenteritis associated with a *Cryptosporidium* sp. in a chinchilla. *Journal of the Veterinary Medical Association* 189:1158–1159.

Yang-Xian, Z., and C. Fu-Qiang. 1983. A new species of the genus *Eimeria* (Sporozoa: Eimeriidae) from *Myotis ricketti* Thomas. *Acta Zootaxonomica Sinica* 8:1–3.

Yoder, K.E., O. Sethabutr, and D.A. Relman. 1996. PCR-based detection of the intestinal pathogen *Cyclospora*. In *PCR protocols for emerging infectious diseases.* Ed. D.H. Persing. Washington, DC: ASM Press, pp. 169–175.

Yoshikawa, H., and M. Iseki. 1992. Freeze-fracture study of the site of attachement of *Cryptosporidium muris* in gastric glands. *Journal of Protozoology* 39:539–544.

Zerpa, R., and L. Huicho. 1994. Childhood diarrhea associated with identification of *Cryptosporidium* sp. in the cocroach *Periplaneta americana. Pediatric Infectious Diseases* 13:546–548.

Zimmerman, S.K., and C.A. Needham. 1995. Comparison of concentional stool concentration and preserved-smear methods with Merifluor *Cryptosporidium/Giardia* direct immunofluorescence assay and ProSpecT *Giardia* EZ microplate assay for detection of *Giardia lamblia. Journal of Clinical Microbiology* 33:1942–1943.

17

TISSUE-INHABITING PROTOZOANS

OPPORTUNISTIC AMOEBAE

DAVID T. JOHN

ETIOLOGIC AGENT(S). Under most conditions, free-living amoebae of the genera *Naegleria, Balamuthia,* and *Acanthamoeba* live as phagotrophs in ponds, rivers, and lakes, feeding mainly on bacteria. However, under specific conditions they are able to cause disease and even death in numerous animals, including humans. Infections with *Naegleria fowleri* can result in primary amoebic meningoencephalitis (PAM), a rapidly fatal infection involving the central nervous system . Human infections are usually associated with swimming in freshwater. Infections with *Balamuthia* and *Acanthamoeba* may result, respectively, in granulomatous amoebic encephalitis (GAE), a chronic central nervous system infection, or *Acanthamoeba* keratitis, an ocular infection. The reader is referred to reviews by John (1993) and Martinez (1985) for information on infections by pathogenic free-living amoebae in humans.

EPIZOOTIOLOGY. Amoebae of the genera *Naegleria, Acanthamoeba,* and *Balamuthia* have a worldwide distribution in soil and freshwater, while *Acanthamoeba* has been recorded from both freshwater and marine environments. The life cycle includes a motile feeding trophozoite or amoeba stage, a resting cyst stage, and in *Naegleria,* an intermittent flagellate stage. The invasive stage of *Naegleria* is the trophozoite (amoeba) stage, with infection occurring by intranasal instillation of amoebae, often associated with freshwater. The amoebae invade the nasal mucosa, cribriform plate, and olfactory bulbs of the brain. Only the trophozoite form has been recovered from tissues or cerebrospinal fluid in *Naegleria* infections. *Acanthamoeba* infections involve the central nervous system, eye, and other organs. Invasion of the central nervous system appears to be via the circulation, with the initial focus of amoebic infection occurring elsewhere in the body. Ocular infections are by direct invasion of the cornea through trauma or contamination. Unlike *Naegleria* infections, both cysts and trophozoites (amoebae) can occur in tissues in *Acanthamoeba* infections. *Balamuthia* causes a chronic central nervous system infection similar to that produced by *Acanthamoeba.*

These organisms have been reported from many mammals (Table 17.1). Although not a human pathogen, *Hartmannella* is listed in the table since the initial citations probably resulted from a confusion with *Acanthamoeba.* Although there are few reports of naturally occurring infections in wild or domestic animals by pathogenic free-living amoebae, it appears that *Acanthamoeba* may be more likely to produce disease in animals than *Naegleria.* Although *Naegleria* organisms are rarely recovered from mammalian tissues other than humans, they have been recovered from the gills and intestinal contents of fish and from the feces of snakes. The only report of *N. fowleri* infecting a nonhuman animal under natural conditions is that of a South American tapir (*Tapirus terrestris*) in an Arizona zoo (Lozano-Alarcon et al. 1997)

Naturally occurring cases of acanthamoebiasis have been reported in domestic canines, especially greyhounds, with respiratory distress and neurologic signs being common (Pearce et al. 1985).

Fatal experimentally induced infections in mice have been achieved with *Naegleria, Acanthamoeba,* and *Balamuthia* organisms. The clinical course of infection appears to be related to both the route of administration and the dosage. Experimental infections in guinea pigs, sheep, rabbits, and monkeys have been reported for *Naegleria,* and experimental *Acanthamoeba* infections in monkeys have also been documented. Ocular *Acanthamoeba* infections have been experimentally induced in rabbits.

Studies designed to determine wild species susceptibility to *N. fowleri* indicate that of seven species evaluated, only rodents are susceptible to intranasal inoculations (John and Hoppe 1990). Susceptible species include the gray squirrel, cotton rat, muskrat, and house mouse. Mammals not susceptible to similar inoculations are opossum, raccoon, and cottontail rabbit. Recent cases of fatal meningoencephalitis caused by free-living amoebae other than *Naegleria* and *Acanthamoeba* have been described. The amoeba, *Balamuthia mandrillaris,* which belongs to the family Leptomyxidae, has been implicated in fatal cases in humans, a baboon, a gorilla, and a sheep (Visvesvara et al. 1993). Additionally, the free-living amoeba

TABLE 17.1—Naturally occurring pathogenic free-living amoeba infections in wild and domestic mammals

Mammalian Host	Location	Amoeba	Geographic Location
Beaver	Kidney, liver, muscle	*Hartmannella*	Switzerland
Rabbit	Liver	*Acanthamoeba*	Czechoslovakia
Water buffalo	Lung	*Acanthamoeba*	India
Cattle	Lung	*Hartmannella*	Azores
	Prepuce	*Acanthamoeba*	Czechoslovakia
	Vagina	*Acanthamoeba*	Czechoslovakia
Baboon	Brain	*Balamuthia*	USA
Gorilla	Brain	*Balamuthia*	USA
Colobus monkey	Brain, mammary gland, lung, kidney	*Balamuthia*	USA
Gibbon	Brain, spinal cord	*Balamuthia*	USA
Domestic dogs	Brain, lungs, kidney, heart, liver	*Acanthamoeba*	USA
	Pancreas	*Acanthamoeba*	Vietnam
	Lungs	*Hartmannella*	Czechoslovakia
Domestic sheep	Brain	*Balamuthia*	USA
Tapir	Brain, lungs	*Naegleria fowleri*	USA

Vahlkampfia has been suggested as a cause of animal and human disease. An animal reservoir or carrier state involving wild species and potentially pathogenic free-living amoebae is not presently known.

PATHOLOGY AND PATHOGENESIS. Primary amoebic meningoencephalitis is routinely associated with aquatic exposure. The disease is rapidly fatal, usually resulting in death within 72 hours of the onset of symptoms. Although well documented in humans and experimentally infected mice, the naturally occurring disease in other mammals is unknown. The known cycle involves invasion by amoebae of the nasal mucosa and cribiform plate with subsequent infection of the olfactory bulbs of the brain. Amoebae first invade the olfactory bulbs and eventually spread posteriorly. Inflammation and extensive tissue destruction in brain tissue follow infection. In humans, symptoms include headache, anorexia, nausea, vomiting, fever, and neck stiffness.

Granulomatous amoebic encephalitis can be subacute or chronic and is characterized by focal granulomatous lesions of the brain. Infections probably occur through the lower respiratory tract or through cutaneous lesions. Invasion of the central nervous system is thought to be by spread from primary foci, probably via the bloodstream. Headache, seizures, neck stiffness, and an altered mental state are the prominent human symptoms. Human cases are primarily in debilitated or immunosuppressed individuals.

Pathologic findings in primary amoebic meningoencephalitis (PAM) include edema and swelling of the cerebral hemispheres. The meninges are hyperemic, with a slight purulent exudate. Hemorrhage, necrosis, and purulent exudate are common in the olfactory bulbs. Amoebae can be found microscopically in the subarachnoid and perivascular spaces. By comparison, GAE is

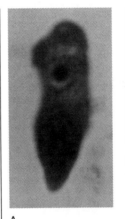 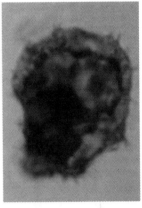

A   B

FIG. 17.1—(**A**) *Naegleria* trophozoite with a blunt pseudopodium (hematoxylin stain); (**B**) *Acanthamoeba* trophozoite with a broad pseudopodium having tiny acanthopodia (Greek a*canth* = spine or thorn), tapering spike-like projections. (Hematoxylin stain)

characterized as a focal granulomatous encephalitis. Central nervous system lesions are characterized by necrosis with hemorrhagic foci and localized leptomeningitis. The leptomeninges contain purulent exudate. The cerebral hemispheres show edema and hemorrhagic necrosis. The olfactory bulbs are not involved.

DIAGNOSIS. Diagnosis of PAM is by microscopic detection of living or stained amoebae in cerebrospinal fluid or by culture (Fig. 17.1). Granulomatous amoebic encephalitis is diagnosed by microscopic detection of trophozoites in cerebrospinal fluid or by detection of trophozoites or cysts in brain tissue. *Acanthoamoeba is more difficult to culture from infected animals than is*

Naegleria. Corneal infections can be diagnosed by microscopic detection of amoebae from corneal scrapings or by histologic examination of corneal tissue.

TREATMENT. There is no satisfactory treatment for PAM or GAE. All known survivors of PAM have received amphotericin B therapy. Corneal infections can be treated with topical propamidine, topical miconazole, and neosporin, with epithelial debridement and systemic ketoconazole.

PUBLIC HEALTH CONCERNS. Infections are known to result from environmental exposure, and animal-to-animal transmission is unknown. Although presently poorly understood, the role of naturally infected wild mammals in the maintenance and transmission of pathogenic free-living amoebae to domestic animals or humans is also unknown. Similarly, the rate of infection and the potential impact of disease on individuals or populations of susceptible wild animals are not known. The fact that numerous wild and domestic mammals are susceptible to infection with several species of pathogenic free-living amoebae does warrant evaluation for amoebic infections, especially in fatalities with unknown central nervous system symptomology.

LITERATURE CITED

John, D.T. and K.L. Hoppe. 1990. Susceptibility of wild mammals to infections with *Naegleria fowleri. The Journal of Parasitology* 76:865–868.
———. 1993. Opportunistically pathogenic free-living amoebae. In *Parasitic protozoa,* vol 3. Ed. J.P. Krier and J.R. Baker. New York: Academic Press, pp. 143–246.
Lozano-Alarcon, F., G.A. Bradley, B.S. Houser, and G.S. Visvesvara. 1997. Primary amebic meningoencephalitis due to *Naegleria fowleri* in a South American tapir. *Veterinary Pathology* 34:239–243.
Martinez, A.J. 1985. Free-living amoebas: Natural history, prevention, diagnosis, pathology, and treatment of disease. Boca Raton FL: CRC Press, 156 pp.
Pearce, J.R., H.S. Powell, F.W. Chandler, and G.S. Visvesvara. 1985. Amebic meningoencephalitis caused by *Acanthamoeba castellani* in a dog. *Journal of the American Medical Association* 187:951–952.
Visvesvara, G.S., F.L. Schuster, A.J. Martinez. 1993. *Balamuthia mandrillaris* NG, N. Sp., agent of amebic meningoencephalitis in humans and other animals. *Journal of Eukaryotic Microbiology* 40:504–514.

HEPATOZOON SPP. AND HEPATOZOONOSIS

THOMAS M. CRAIG

INTRODUCTION

Members of the genus *Hepatozoon* are apicomplexan parasites that infect all classes of terrestrial vertebrates, which by definition—see Life History section, below—are intermediate hosts, while using a variety of arthropods as definitive hosts. Transmission to the vertebrate host occurs by the ingestion of infected arthropods or by predation of other infected vertebrates. Smith (1996) reviewed the biology of *Hepatozoon* spp. that occur in amphibians, reptiles, and various arthropods, and Vincent-Johnson et al.(1997a) reviewed the disease in dogs. However, the disease manifestations of *Hepatozoon* species that infect other mammals have not been reviewed recently and will be the focus of this discussion.

The taxonomic designation of the various species within this genus has historically been based on the morphology of the gamonts and the systematic relationship of the host(s) in which they are observed (Wenyon 1910; Krampitz 1982). Recently, a new species, *Hepatozoon americanum,* was described from domestic dogs using clinical signs, organ predilection, serologic reaction, and histopathologic changes as the defining features (Vincent-Johnson et al. 1997b). Identification of species in this genus will be difficult until a criterion based on genetic composition is accepted.

ETIOLOGIC AGENTS. *Hepatozoon* spp. apicomplexan parasites belong to the suborder Adeleina, family Haemogregarinidae (Smith 1996). Schizogony occurs in various tissues of the intermediate (vertebrate) host, and gamonts are found in blood cells. Oocysts, which contain numerous sporocysts and sporozoites, are found in the hemocoel of the invertebrate (definitive) host.

LIFE HISTORY. In the life cycle of *Hepatozoon* spp. parasites, the isogamonts, found within leukocytes of the vertebrate host, are ingested by arthropods during blood-feeding activities. In the arthropod, isogametes enter the hemocoel, and oocyst formation occurs. There is no apparent mechanism for the resulting sporozoites to enter the salivary glands of the arthropod, so transmission requires the ingestion of the arthropod containing the sporulated oocyst.

In the mammalian host, schizogony occurs in various tissues, ultimately giving rise to gamonts or cysts. A tissue stage (cyst) may represent a stage of the life cycle which can be transmitted by predation (Desser 1990). A large cystic form has been described from naturally infected dogs (Craig et al. 1984); this form may constitute a mechanism for evading the host immune response so that gamonts will be available for seasonal arthropod activity (Murata et al. 1993a) or for vertical transmission among vertebrate hosts (Murata et al. 1993b).

EPIZOOTIOLOGY. *Hepatozoon* spp. infections have been reported from a wide range of terrestrial vertebrates, with reptiles being the most commonly infected. Among susceptible mammalian hosts, infec-

TABLE 17.2—*Hepatozoon* **spp. reported from carnivores**

Scientific Name	Common Name	Reference
Canidae		
Canis familiaris	Domestic dog	Bentley 1905, Christophers 1906, Vincent-Johnson et al. 1997b
Canis adustus	Jackal	Nuttal 1910
Canis latrans	Coyote	Davis et al. 1978
Canis aureus	Jackal	Patton, 1910
Canis mesomelas	Jackal	Basson et al. 1971
Cerdocyon thous	Crab-eating fox	Alencar et al. 1997
Vulpes vulpes	Red fox	Maede et al. 1982, Conceicao-Silva et al. 1988
Felidae		
Acinonyx jubatus	Cheetah	Keep 1970
Felis catus	Domestic cat	Klopfer et al. 1973
Felis pardalis	Ocelot	Mercer et al. 1988
Lynx rufis	Bobcat	Lane and Kocan 1983
Panthera leo	Lion	Brocklesby and Vidler 1963
Panthera pardus	Leopard	Brocklesby and Vidler 1963
Hyaenidae		
Crocuta crocuta	Spotted hyena	Krampitz et al. 1968
Mustelidae		
Martes foiva	Stone marten	Geisel et al. 1979
Martes martes	Pine marten	Geisel et al. 1979
Martes melampus	Japanese marten	Yanai et al. 1995
Mustela erminea	Weasel	Geisel et al. 1979
Mustela eversmanni	Siberian polecat	Novilla et al. 1980
Mustela vison	Mink	Presidente and Karstad 1975
Procyonidae		
Procyon cancrivorus	Crab-eating raccoon	Schneider 1968
Procyon lotor	Raccoon	Richards 1961
Viverridae		
Genetta felina	Genet	
Paradoxurus hermaphroditus	Palm civit	Laird 1959

TABLE 17.3—*Hepatozoon* **spp. reported from ungulates**

Scientific Name	Common Name	Reference
Redunca arundinum	Reed buck	McCully et al. 1975
Giraffa camelopordalis	Giraffe	McCully et al. 1975
Aepyceros melampus	Impala	Basson et al. 1971
Tragelaphus angasi	Nyala	McCully et al. 1975
Tragelaphus scriptus	Bush buck	McCully et al. 1975
Odocoileus virginianus	White-tailed deer	Clark et al. 1973

tions have been reported from carnivores, ungulates, rodents, lagomorphs (Tables 17.2–17.4), marsupials, and insectivores. The importance, if any, of predator-prey relationships in transmission of this parasite among mammals is presently poorly understood. Should this method of transmission prove to be a common occurrence, our present understanding of the epizootiology of this parasite would be significantly altered.

A wide variety of arthropods, especially ticks and mites, have been implicated in the transmission of *Hepatozoon* spp. to mammalian hosts. Again, the range of suitable hosts is unknown since only a few of the possible candidate arthropods have been evaluated.

Turner (1986) found that *H. erhardovae* in wild-caught bank voles (*Clethrionomys glareolus*) in the United Kingdom varied with the season of the year and the age of the host. Young animals developed parasitemias early in life, with a high prevalence of infection occurring in summer and autumn while no transmission occurred during the winter. In experimental exposures, where infected fleas were fed to captive 4-month-old voles, 2–6 infected fleas were sufficient to cause death that was characterized by an exudative pneumonia (Krampitz and Haberkorn 1988). These findings indicate that the level of exposure in young voles may be a determining factor in the production of a disease state.

CLINICAL SIGNS AND PATHOLOGY. The clinical signs associated with *Hepatozoon* spp. infection vary from being inapparent to those of lethargy, anemia, anorexia, and occasionally death. Miller (1908), studying *H. perniciosum* in white rats, reported that individuals with high parasitemias became anemic, anorexic, and depressed, and developed a leukocytosis of more than 100,000 cells/μl[3]; half died. Schizogony was only observed in the lungs. Hemorrhages on the surface of the lungs and splenomegaly were common. Only young rats had signs of disease in the presence of large numbers of vectors.

TABLE 17.4—*Hepatozoon* spp. reported from rodents and lagomorphs

Hepatozoon spp.	Scientific Name, Host	Reference
H. balfouri	Jaculus jaculus	Wenyon 1926
H. citellicolum	Spermophilus beechege	Wellman and Wherry 1910
H. criceti	Cricetus frumentarius	Wenyon 1926
H. cuniculi	Oryctolagus cuniculus	Wenyon 1926
H. erhardovae	Clethrionomys glareolus	Krampitz 1981
H. leporis	Lepus nigricollis	Wenyon 1926
H. funambuli	Funambulus pennanti	Wenyon 1926
H. peromysci	Peromyscus spp.	Levine 1982
H. kramptizi	Microtus oeconomus	Ohbayashi 1971
H. microti	Allactaga spp.	Wenyon 1926
	Microtus agrestis	Smith 1996
H. muris	Rattus spp.	Wenyon 1926
H. musculi	Mus musculus	Porter 1908
H. gerbilli	Meriones erythrourus	Christophers 1905
	Rhombomys opimus	Smith 1996
	Tatera indicus	Smith 1996
H. dolichomorphon	Idiurus macrotis	Killick-Kendrick 1984
H. normani	Idiurus macrotis	Killick-Kendrick 1984
H. leptosoma	Peromyscys maniculatus	Wood 1962
H. gaetulum	Atlantoxerus getulus	Clark 1958
H. griseisciuri	Sciurus carolinensis	Clark 1958
H. sciuri	Sciurus spp.	Coles 1914
H. sylvatici	Apodemus	Wenyon 1926
	Clethrionomys glareolus	Smith 1996
H. mereschkowskii	Spermophilus spp.	Smith 1996

In the various *Hepatozoon* species that infect rodents, schizogony occurs in a variety of organs, with the associated clinical signs being reflective of the organ(s) affected. For example, schizogony occurs in the bone marrow of *Mus musculus* with *H. musculi* (Porter 1908); in the lungs of *Sciurus carolinensis* and *C. glareolus* infected with *H. griseisciuri* and *H. erhardovae*, respectively (Davidson and Calpin 1976; Krampitz and Haberkorn 1988); and in the liver of *Rattus rattus* and *Jaculus* spp. infected with *H. perniciosum* and *H. balfouri*, respectively (Miller 1908; Hoogstraal 1961).

In *Hepatozoon* infections in raccoons, an intense granulomatous response has been reported associated with merozoites released from schizonts within myofibers, although a similar response was not associated with immature schizonts (Clark et al. 1973). When raccoons were concomitantly infected with canine distemper virus, focal myocardial necrosis was seen at the site of the former schizont. In infections in coyotes, inflammatory cells were seen in the myocardium, but it was not certain that this response was solely due to the *Hepatozoon* sp. infection (Davis et al. 1978) (Fig. 17.2).

Hepatozoon spp. schizonts, thought to be *H. canis*, were reported in the cardiac muscle of a leopard (Keymer 1971), lion (Brocklesby 1971; Dubey and Bwangamoi 1994), cheetah, and spotted hyena (Keep 1970) without an apparent host response. However, schizonts in the skeletal muscles of jackals, *Canis mesomelas*, were associated with severe focal myositis (McCully et al. 1975). Alencar et al. (1997) reported an anemia, neutrophilia (19,000/µl³) accompanied by diarrhea, and anorexia in a crab-eating fox, *Cerdocyon*

thous, that was presented after being struck by an automobile. Circulating gamonts, described as *H. canis*, were also detected. On postmortem examination there was hepatic degeneration and hyperplasia of splenic white pulp. It could not be determined if the changes observed in the fox were due to the *Hepatozoon* sp. infection alone or a combined effect of the infection and trauma.

Schizonts and nodules consisting of phagocytic cells and gamonts have been reported from the cardiac muscle of various mustelids (Presidente and Karstad 1975; Giesel et al. 1979; Yanai et al. 1995). Grossly visible lesions measuring 50 to 400 µm in diameter have also been reported from the cardiac muscle of naturally infected Japanese martins (Yanai et al. 1995). Nodules that consisted of neutrophils and macrophages containing merozoites appeared to be a host response to ruptured schizonts. Focal microgranulomas resembled those seen in naturally infected domestic dogs in North America (Craig et al. 1984; Vincent-Johnson et al. 1997b) and in naturally infected raccoons (Richards 1961; Clark et al. 1973). Mortalities have been reported in naturally infected 17–20-day-old Siberian polecat kits. Postmortem evaluation revealed extensive lesions in the liver, skin, cardiac, and skeletal muscles. The kits were concurrently infected with *Encephalitozoon cuniculi*. It was hypothesized that the kits were infected congenitally and that the concurrent infection was a factor in the resulting death (Novilla et al. 1980).

Mild focal hepatitis and lymphadenitis has been described in impala (*Aepycaros melampus*) infected with *Hepatozoon*-like organisms in South Africa (Basson et al. 1967). Parasites thought to be a single merozoite schizont were seen in the livers of 7% of the

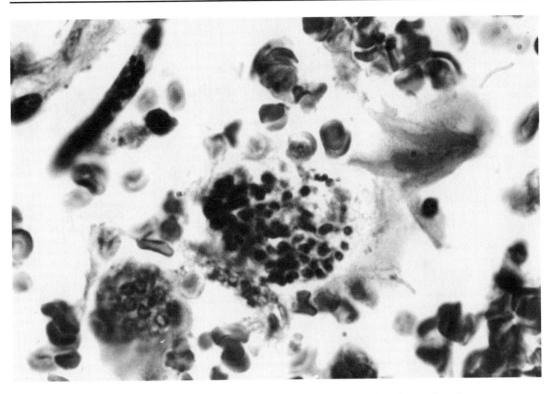

FIG. 17.2—*Hepatozoon* sp. schizont in the cardiac muscle of a coyote *Canis latrans,* from Texas.

impala examined. The lesions were similar to those observed in dogs naturally infected with *H. canis* in North America.

Hepatozoon-like gamonts were seen in hepatic mononuclear cells associated with a notable granulomatous infiltration in young Nabezuru cranes (*Grus monacha*) (Shimizu et al. 1987). Organisms were observed free in the plasma, in circulatory monocytes, and in focal areas of the spleen. Numerous schizonts were found in the liver of one juvenile bird, and a few were seen in older birds. Shimizu et al. (1987) were uncertain if the schizonts were those of *Hepatozoon* sp. or another apicomplexan parasite.

These reports seem to indicate that *Hepatozoon* spp. can be virulent agents, but concomitant infection or other factors may be necessary for clinical disease to occur.

IMMUNITY. The observation that disease associated with *Hepatozoon* spp. infections occurs most commonly in younger animals indicates either that vertical transmission is associated with increased virulence or that disease is more likely to occur in a naive host, and older animals become resistant to superinfection while remaining chronic carriers (Krampitz 1981). In areas where *H. canis* is endemic, infections can be detected

in animals of all ages, although the number of dogs with a circulating parasitemia far exceeds the number of animals with notable clinical signs of infection (Ezeokoli et al. 1983). Additionally, serologic studies have shown that, although one-third of dogs tested had detectable antibody activity to *H. canis*, only 1% were parasitemic (Baneth et al. 1996). It does not appear that antibody activity is of any protective value against infection in dogs, and this assumption probably applies for other species as well.

DIAGNOSIS. Infection with *Hepatozoon* is most commonly diagnosed either by microscopic identification of gamonts in Giemsa-stained preparations of whole blood (Fig. 17.3) or by microscopic detection of schizonts in histologic preparations of various tissues. Specific antibody activity has been demonstrated with *H. canis* in dogs.

CONTROL AND TREATMENT. A number of authors have described the clinical use of various compounds in the treatment of *H. canis* in naturally occurring infections in domestic dogs (Vincent-Johnson et al. 1997a). The consensus seems to be that there is no single therapy that universally works or even that, in

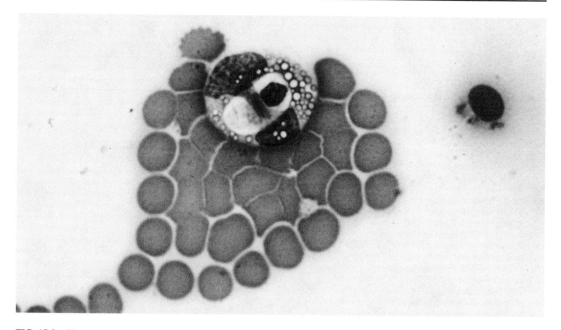

FIG. 17.3—*Hepatozoon* sp. gamont in a leukocyte of an ocelot *Felis pardalis,* from Texas. The host was a wild caught animal with no observed clinical signs of disease.

most cases, there is a need for treatment. The variability in the virulence of the organism in different geographic areas and among infected individuals makes evaluation of treatment difficult if not impossible. The only controlled trials evaluating the efficiency of chemotherapy were those of Krampitz and Haberkorn (1988), who demonstrated that toltrazuril would control the clinical signs of disease in voles, but therapy did not eliminate the infection.

PUBLIC HEALTH CONCERNS. Except for a single report of a human case of hepatozoonosis in an individual with malaria-like signs in the Philippines (Carlos et al. 1971), there is no evidence that *Hepatozoon* spp. infect human beings.

DOMESTIC ANIMAL HEALTH CONCERNS AND MANAGEMENT IMPLICATIONS. Although hepatozoonosis is primarily a disease of domestic canids, it is realistic to believe that wildlife reservoirs may be involved in the numerous cases reported from throughout the world (Mercer et al. 1988; McCully et al. 1975). The disease in dogs is represented by two distinct geographic syndromes which are outlined by Vincent-Johnson et al. (1997a,b). Because accurate identification of the various species of *Hepatozoon* is difficult and the host range of most species is poorly understood, control, at present, may be impossible. Adding to the problem is an incomplete understanding

of the role of vector ingestion as compared to "cyst" ingestion in the overall epidemiology of the disease in both domestic and wild animals. Based on the understanding that disease due to *Hepatozoon* spp. is apparently unusual whereas infection may be common in many wild animal populations, it appears that this parasite is one that will attract considerably more attention in future years from both the veterinary and wildlife communities.

LITERATURE CITED

Alencar N.X., A.A. Kohayagawa, and V.A. Santaren. 1997. *Hepatozoon canis* infection in a crab-eating fox (*Cerdocydon thous*) from Brazil. *Veterinary Parasitology* 70:279–282.

Baneth, G., V. Shkap, B.Z. Presemtey, and E. Pipano. 1996. *Hepatozoon canis:* The prevalence of antibodies and gametocytes in dogs in Israel. *Veterinary Research Communications* 20:41–46.

Basson, P.A., R.M. McCully, R.D. Bigalke, and J.W. Van Niekerk. 1967. Observations on a *Hepatozoon*-like parasite in the impala. *Journal of the South African Veterinary Medical Association* 38:12–16.

Basson, P.A., R.M. McCully, S.P Kruger, J.W. Van Niekerk, E. Young, V. Devos, M.E. Keep, and H. Ebedes. 1971. Disease and conditions of game in southern Africa. *Recent miscellaneous findings. Veterinary Medical Review* 2/3:313–340.

Bentley, C.A. 1905. Preliminary note upon a *Leukocytoon* of the dog. *British Medical Journal* 1:988.

Brocklesby, D.W. 1971. Illustrations of a *Hepatozoon* species in the heart of a lion. *Journal Zoological Society of London* 164:525–528.

Brocklesby, D.W., and B.O. Vidler. 1963. Some new host records for *Hepatozoon* species in Kenya. *The Veterinary Record* 75:1265.

Carlos, E.T., F.B. Cruz, and C.C. Cabiles. 1971. *Hepatozoon* sp. in the WBC of a human patient. *University of the Philippines Veterinarian* 15:5–7.

Christophers, S.R. 1905. *Haemogregarina gerbilli. Scientific Memoirs by Officers of the Medical and Sanitary Departments of the Government of India* 18:1–15.

———. 1906. *Leukocytozoon canis. Scientific Memoirs by Officers of the Medical and Sanitary Departments of the Government of India* 26:1–18.

Clark, G.M. 1958. *Hepatozoon griseisciuri* n. sp. in a new species of *Hepatozoon* from the grey squirrel (*Sciurus carolinensis* Gnelin, 1788), with studies on the life cycle. *The Journal of Parasitology* 44:52–63.

Clark, K.A., R.M. Robinson, L.L. Weishuhn, T.J. Galvin, and K. Horvath. 1973. *Hepatozoon procyonis* infections in Texas. *Journal of Wildlife Diseases* 9:182.

Coles, A.C. 1914. Blood parasites found in mammals, birds and fishes in England. *Parasitology* 7:17–61.

Conceicao-Silva, F.M., P. Abranches, M.C.D. Silv-Pereira, and J.G. Janz. 1988. Hepatozoonisis in foxes from Portugal. *Journal of Wildlife Diseases* 24:344–347.

Craig, T.M., L.P. Jones, and R. M. Nordgren. 1984. Diagnosis of *Hepatozoon canis* by muscle biopsy. *Journal of the American Animal Hospital Association* 20:301–303.

Davidson, W.R., and J.P. Calpin. 1976. *Hepatozoon griseisciuri* infection in gray squirrels of the southeastern United States. *Journal of Wildlife Diseases* 12:72–76.

Davis, D.S., R.M. Robinson, and T.M. Craig. 1978. Naturally occurring hepatozoonosis in a coyote. *Journal of Wildlife Diseases* 14:44–246.

Desser, S. S. 1990. Tissue "cysts" of *Hepatozoon griseisciuri* in the grey squirrel, *Sciurus carolinesis:* The significance of these cysts in species of *Hepatozoon. The Journal of Parasitology* 76:257–259.

Dubey, J.P., and O. Bwangamoi. 1994. *Microbesnoitia leoni* Bwangamoi, 1989, from the African lion (*Panthera leo*) redetermined as a junior synonym of *Hepatozoon canis* (James, 1905) Wenyon, 1926. *The Journal of Parasitology* 80:333–334.

Ezeokoli, C.D., B. Ogunkoya, R. Abullahi, L.B. Tekdek, A. Sannusi, and A.A. Ilemobade. 1983. Clinical and epidemiological studies on canine hepatozoonosis in Zaria, Nigeria. *Journal of Small Animal Practice* 24:455–460.

Geisel O. Von, H. E. Krampitz, and A. Pospischil. 1979. Zur Pathomorphologie eina *Hepatozoon* infektion bei Musteliden. *Berlin Münchener Tierärztlichen Wochenschrift* 92:421–425.

Hoogstraal, H. 1961. The life cycle and incidence of *Hepatozoon balfouri* (Laveran, 1905) in Egyptian Jerboas (*Jaculus* spp.) and mites (*Haemolaelaps aegyptius* Keegan, 1956). *The Journal of Protozoology* 8:231–248.

Keep, M.E. 1970. Hepatozoonosis in some wild animals in Zululand. *Lammergeyer* 12:70–71.

Keymer, I.F. 1971. Blood protozoa of wild carnivores in central Africa. *Journal Zoological Society of London* 164:513–524.

Killick-Kendrick, R. 1984. Parasitic protozoa of the blood of rodents. VI. Two new hemogregarines of the pigmy flying squirrel *Idiurus macrotis* (Rodentia: Theridomyomorpha: Anomaluridae) in West Africa. *The Journal of Protozoology* 3:532–535.

Klopfer, U., T.A. Nobel, and F. Neumann. 1973. *Hepatozoon*-like parasite (schizonts) in the myocardium of the domestic cat. *Veterinary Pathology* 10:185–190.

Krampitz, H.E. 1981. Development of *Hepatozoon erherdovae*. Krampitz, 1964 (Protozoa: Haemogregarinidae) in experimental mammalian and arthropod hosts. II. Sexual development in fleas and sporozoite indices in xen-

odiagnosis. *Transactions of the Royal Society of Tropical Medicine and Hygiene* 75:155–157.

———. 1982. Long term experimental research of *Hepatozoon* species in rodents: Taxonomic and phyletic considerations. 5th International Congress for Parasitology Toronto, August.

Krampitz, H.E., and A. Haberkorn. 1988. Experimental treatment of *Hepatozoon* infections with the anticoccidial agent Toltrazuril. *Journal of Veterinary Medicine* B35:131–137.

Krampitz, H.E., R. Sachs, G.B. Schaller, and R. Schindler. 1968. Sur verbreitung von Parcesiten der guttug *Hepatozoon* Miller, 1908 (Protozoa, Adeleidae) in Ostrafrikanischen wildsaugetieren. *Zeitschreift für Parasitenkunde* 31:203–210.

Laird, M. 1959. Malayan protozoa 2. *Hepatozoon* Miller (Sporozoa: Coccidia), with and unusual host record for *H. canis* (James). *The Journal of Protozoology* 6:316–319.

Lane, J.R., and A.A. Kocan. 1983. *Hepatozoon* sp. infection in bobcats. *Journal American Veterinary Medical Association* 183:1323–1324.

Levine, N.D. 1982. Some corrections in haemogregarines (Apicomplexa: Protozoa) Nomenclature. *The Journal of Protozoology* 29:601–603.

Maede, Y., T. Ohsugi, and N. Ohotaoshi. 1982. *Hepatozoon* infection in a wild fox (*Vulpes vulpes schrencki* Kishida) in Japan. *Japanese Journal of Veterinary Science* 44:137–142.

McCully, R.M., P.A. Basson, R.D. Bigalke, V. De Vos, and E. Young. 1975. Observations on naturally acquired hepatozoonosis of wild carnivores and dogs in the Republic of South Africa. *Onderstepoort Journal of Veterinary Research* 42:117–134.

Mercer, S.H., L.P. Jones, J.H. Rappole, D. Twedt, L.L. Laack, and T.M. Craig. 1988. *Hepatozoon* sp. in wild carnivores in Texas. *Journal of Wildlife Diseases* 24:574–576.

Miller, W.W. 1908. *Hepatozoon perniciosum* (N.G., N. Sp.)— A Haemogregarine pathogenic for white rats; with a description of the sexual cycle in the intermediate host, a mite (*Lelaps echidninus* Berlese). Public Health and Marine Hospital Service of United States, Bulletin 46.

Murata, T., K. Shimoda, M. Inoue, K. Shiramizu, M. Kanoe, Y. Taura, and S. Nakama. 1993a. Seasonal periodical appearance of *Hepatozoon canis* gamont in the peripheral blood. *Journal of Veterinary Medical Science* 55:877–879.

Murata, T., M. Inoue, S. Tateyama, Y. Taura, and S. Nakama. 1993b. Vertical transmission *of Hepatozoon canis* in dogs. *Journal of Veterinary Medical Science* 55:867–868.

Novilla, M.A., J.W. Carpenter, and R.P. Kwapein. 1980. Dual infection of Siberian polecats with *Encephalitozoon cuniculi* and *Hepatozoon mustelis* n. sp. In *Symposium on the comparative pathology of zoo animals.* National Zoological Park, Smithsonian Institution, 1978. Ed. R. J. Montali. Washington, DC: Smithsonian Institution Press, pp. 353–363.

Nuttal, G.H.F. 1910. On haematozoa occurring in wild animals in Africa. *Parasitology* 3:108–116.

Ohbayashi, M. 1971. *Hepatozoon* sp. in Northern voles. *Microtus oeconomus,* on St. Lawrence Island, Alaska. *Journal of Wildlife Diseases* 7:49–51.

Patton, W.S. 1910. Preliminary report on a new piroplasm (*Piroplasma gibsoni* sp. Nov.) in the blood of the hounds of the Modrashunt and subsequently discovered in the blood of the jackal (*Canis aureus*). *Bulletin of the Society of Pathology Exotic* 3:274–281.

Porter, A. 1908. *Leucocytozoon musculi* sp. n., a parasitic protozoon from the blood of white mice. *Proceedings of the Zoological Society of London* 3:703–716.

Presidente, P.J.A., and L.H. Karstad. 1975. *Hepatozoon* sp. infection in mink from southwestern Ontario. *Journal of Wildlife Diseases* 11:479–481.

Richards, C.S. 1961. *Hepatozoon procyonis,* n. sp., from the raccoon. *The Journal of Protozoology* 8:360–362.

Schneider, C.R. 1968. *Hepatozoon procyonis* Richards, 1961 in a Panamanian raccoon, *Procyon cancrivorus panamensis* (Goldman). *Review Biological Tropical* 15:123–135.

Shimizu, T., N. Yasuda, I. Kono, and T. Koyama. 1987. Fatal infection of *Hepatozoon*-like organisms in the young captive cranes (*Grus monacha*). *Memories of the Faculty of Agriculture Kagoshima University* 23:99–107.

Smith, T.G. 1996. The genus *Hepatozoon* (Apicomplexa: Adeleina). *The Journal of Parasitology* 82:565–585.

Turner, C.M.R. 1986. Seasonal and age distributions of *Babenia, Hepatozoon, Trypanosoma,* and *Grahamella* species in *Clethrionomys glareolus* and *Apodenus sylvaticus* populations. *Parasitology* 93:279–289.

Vincent-Johnson, N., D.K. Macintire, and G. Baneth. 1997a. Canine hepatozoonosis: Pathophysiology, diagnosis, and treatment. *Compendium of Continuing Education* 19:51–65.

Vincent-Johnson, N., D.K. Macintire, and G. Baneth. 1997b. A new *Hepatozoon* species from dogs: Description of the causative agent of canine hepatozoonosis in North America. *The Journal of Parasitology* 83:1165–1172.

Wellman, C., and W.B. Wherry. 1910. Some new internal parasites of the California ground squirrel (*Otspermophilus beecheyi*). *Parasitology* 3:417–422.

Wenyon, C.M. 1910. Some remarks on the genus *Leucocytozoon. Parasitology* 3:63–72.

Wenyon, C.M. 1926. *Protozoology: A manual for medical men, veterinarians, and zoologists.* London: Bailliere, Tindall, and Cassel Ltd., 1563 pp.

Wood, S.F. 1962. Blood parasites of mammals of the Californian Sierra Nevada Foothills, with special reference to *Trypanosoma cruzi* and *Hepatozoon leptosoma* sp. n. *Bulletin of the Southern California Academy of Science* 61:161–176.

Yanai, T., A. Tomita, T. Masegi, K. Ishikawa, T. Iwasake, K. Yamazoe, and K. Ueda. 1995. Histopathologic features of naturally occurring hepatozoonosis in wild martins (*Martes melampus*) in Japan. *Journal of Wildlife Diseases* 31:233–237.

BESNOITIA SPP. AND BESNOITIOSIS

**FREDERICK A. LEIGHTON
AND ALVIN A. GAJADHAR**

INTRODUCTION. Species of the Genus *Besnoitia* are parasitic protozoa belonging to the group of cyst-forming coccidia. A two-host life cycle that is typical of other members of this group is known to occur in some species of *Besnoitia*. The principle distinguishing morphological characteristic of the genus is the large zoite-filled cyst that occurs in the connective tissues of the intermediate (herbivore) hosts. Disease caused by *Besnoitia* spp. (besnoitiosis) has been recognized only in intermediate hosts. Little is known about the life cycle, taxonomy, epidemiology, or ecology of most of the species of *Besnoitia,* nor is their relationship to the health or effect on the population dynamics of their hosts understood. Prevalence of infection is high in some host populations, and clinical disease does occur. Cross-infections among wild and domestic animals occur in some species, and besnoitiosis in cattle is of considerable economic importance in some parts of the world. Concern about possible infection of wild populations transmitted by infected animals of the same or of different species translocated to new geographic areas has resulted in controversial management decisions that have, variously, restricted agricultural pursuits or placed wild populations at risk.

In this chapter, general information that is broadly applicable to all species of *Besnoitia* will be presented, followed by brief accounts of each currently recognized species.

ETIOLOGIC AGENT. *Besnoitia* belong to the Family Sarcocystidae, Phylum Apicomplexa. Synonyms from earlier classifications include *Gastrocystis, Globidium, Fibrocystis, Isospora,* and *Sarcocystis.* Seven species of *Besnoitia* have been named, and there are additional reported occurrences in which the species have not been named (Table 17.5). The primary basis for the classification of species of *Besnoitia* is the species of naturally infected intermediate host(s); therefore, this taxonomy should be considered provisional, pending more rigorous assessment. Molecular approaches to classification have not yet been applied to this genus. The sporulated oocysts of *Besnoitia* spp., when recognized, have been small (> 20 mm) and contained two sporocysts, each with four sporozoites. Thus, oocysts of *Besnoitia* spp. cannot reliably be distinguished from oocysts of other coccidia such as *Toxoplasma gondii, Hammondia* spp., and *Isospora* spp., which are similar in size and have the same sporocyst-sporozoite configuration. Two characteristic features of *Besnoitia* in the intermediate host that distinguish it from other cyst-forming coccidia are that a primary cyst wall is absent and that the cyst is within a greatly enlarged host cell with multiple nuclei.

The genus and type species was named by Henry (1913), apparently in recognition of the first description of infection with a species of this genus by Besnoit and Robin (1912), who recognized a *Sarcocystis*-like protozoan cyst in muscle-free connective tissue of the skin of a cow from the south of France. Pronunciation of the names of the genus and the disease is problematic in English. French colleagues indicate that the "s" in Dr. Besnoit's name was pronounced, not silent. The suggested pronunciation is "bez-nwáh-tee-ya" and "bez-nwáh-tee-óh-sis".

SPECIES OF *BESNOITIA*. Despite the large number of species of wild and domestic animals infected with *Besnoitia* throughout the world, very little is known about the number of species of *Besnoitia* that exist or of the relationships among them. Based on specificity to intermediate hosts and, in some cases, on cross-transmission studies, seven species were named as of

TABLE 17.5—Natural hosts and geographic distribution of *Besnoitia*

Species of *Besnoitia*	Host Species	Location	References
B. bennetti	Zebra	Africa	Bigalke and Prozesky 1994
	Burro	United States	Terrel and Stookey 1973
		Unstated	Gorlin et al. 1959
	Horse	Sudan	Bennett 1939
		South Africa	Pols 1960, Van Heerden et al. 1993
		France	Gorlin et al. 1959
B. besnoiti	Impala	South Africa	McCully et al. 1966
	Kudu	South Africa	McCully et al. 1966
	Wildebeest	South Africa	McCully et al. 1966
	Cattle	Africa	Bigalke and Prozesky 1994
		Europe	Besnoit and Robin 1912, Bigalke and Prozesky 1994, Uvaliev et al. 1979
		Israel	Neuman and Nobel 1960
		Kazakhstan	Vsevolodov 1961, Peteshev et al. 1974
		Korea	Lee et al. 1979
		Venezuela	Bigalke and Prozesky 1994
B. caprae	Wild goat	Iran	Cheema and Toofanian 1979
	Goat	Kenya	Heydorn et al. 1984, Bwangamoi et al. 1989, Njenga et al. 1993
B. darlingi	Opossum	Panama	Darling 1910, Schneider 1967a
		United States	Smith and Frenkel 1977, 1984, Jack et al. 1989
B. jellisoni	Opossum	United States	Stabler and Welch 1961
	Peromyscus	United States	Frenkel 1953
	Dipodomys	United States	Ernst et al. 1968
	Rodents	South America	Jellison et al. 1960
B. tarandi	Caribou	North America	Hadwen 1922, Choquette et al. 1967, Wobeser 1976, Lewis 1989
	Reindeer	North America	Lewis 1989, Glover et al. 1990
		Europe	Rehbinder et al. 1981, Nikolaevskii 1961
		Asia	Nikolaevskii 1961
	Mule deer	Canada	Glover et al. 1990
	Muskox	Canada	Fig. 17.9, this chapter, data of A. Gunn and F.A. Leighton
B. wallacei	Cat	Australia	Mason 1980
		Hawaii	Wallace and Frenkel 1975
		Japan	Ito et al. 1978
		Kenya	Ng'ang'a et al. 1994
Besnoitia spp. Mammalian Hosts	Various	Kazakhstan	Peteshev and Polomoshnov 1976
	Rabbit	Kenya	Mbuthia et al. 1993
	Lion	Kenya	Bwangamoi et al. 1990
	Blue duiker	USA	Foley et al. 1990
	Chamois	Switzerland	Burgisser 1975
	Warthog	South Africa	Keep and Basson 1973
	Buffalo	India	Kharole et al. 1989
	Camel	India	Kharole et al. 1984
	Sheep	India	Kharole et al. 1979
Non-Mammalian Hosts	Flamingo	Africa	Karstad et al. 1981
	Chicken	India	Kharole et al. 1979
	Knot	United States	Simpson et al. 1977
	Sparrow	Kazakhstan	Peteshev and Polomoshnov 1976
	Snake	Africa	Matuschka and Häfner 1984
	Lizard	Madeira	Frank and Frenkel 1981

1997: *B. bennetti*, *B. besnoiti*, *B. caprae*, *B. darlingi*, *B. jellisoni*, *B. tarandi*, and *B. wallacei*. This classification should be regarded as provisional until better data are available upon which to base taxonomy of the genus.

Besnoitia bennetti. Bennett (1939) described besnoitiosis in horses in the Sudan, and now all occur-rences of *Besnoitia* infection in equids are attributed to *B. bennetti*, simply on the basis of the intermediate host. As such, *B. bennetti* has been seen in horses, don-keys, and zebra in Africa, Asia, Europe, and North America (Table 17.5). The first record of besnoitiosis in an equid was of a horse in France described by Henry and Masson in 1922 (Pols 1960). The life cycle of *B. bennetti* is not known; infections have been recognized only in intermediate hosts. Infections have ranged from inapparent, recognized only fortuitously, to severe, with generalized clinical manifestations in the skin. Van Heerden et al. (1993) compared the ultrastructure of bradyzoites from a horse with that described for *B. besnoiti* and for *B. jellisoni,* and concluded that the structural differences justified classification of *B. bennetti* as a separate species.

Besnoitia besnoiti. This is the most studied species of *Besnoitia,* and most of what is known about the genus was learned from studies of this species (reviewed by Bigalke and Prozesky 1994). The ungulate intermediate hosts include domestic cattle and free-ranging blue wildebeest (*Connochaetes taurinus*), impala (*Aepyceros melampus*), and kudu (*Tragelaphus strepsiceros*) (McCully et al. 1966; Bigalke et al. 1967; Table 17.5). The strains of *B. besnoiti* in wild ungulates appear to be different from those in domestic cattle in that they have been of low pathogenicity when tested in cattle, and cysts form predominantly in the connective tissues of the cardiovascular system rather than in the skin (Le Blancq et al. 1986; Bigalke and Prozesky 1994). Thus, wild ungulates are not considered important reservoirs of infection for domestic cattle. Clinical disease has not been reported in wild ungulates. There is some evidence that cats may be a definitive, carnivore host for *B. besnoiti* (Peteshev et al. 1974; Diesing et al. 1988), but infection also can be transmitted among intermediate hosts by biting arthropods (Bigalke 1968). Experimental infections (cysts) have been produced in rabbits (*Oryctolagus cuniculus*) and rats (*Rattus norvegicus*).

Besnoitia caprae. Wild goats (*Capra aegagrus*) and domestic goats (*C. hircus*) are the only known intermediate hosts for this species; no definitive host has been recognized. Besnoitiosis in goats was first reported in Kenya (Bwangamoi 1967) and then in Iran (Cheema and Toofanian 1978). Information on *B. caprae* in wild animals is limited to a description of the disease in two wild goats (Cheema and Toofanian 1978). There were severe skin lesions and vascular obstruction of arteries and veins in the testis and epididymis, accompanied by testicular atrophy and, probably, sterility. Experimental and epidemiological data indicate that *B. caprae* is distinct from *B. besnoiti* (Bwangamoi et al. 1989; Njenga et al. 1993; Ng'ang'a and Kasigazi 1994; Njenga et al. 1995).

Besnoitia darlingi. Cysts in the tissue of an opossum (*Didelphis marsupialis*) in Panama were described by S.T. Darling in 1910, and subsequently, were found in central American lizards (*Basiliscus, Ameiva*) and opossums (Schneider 1967a,b; Smith and Frenkel 1977). The domestic cat was shown to be a definitive host for *B. darlingi* by Smith and Frenkel (1977, 1984). Laboratory mice also can serve as intermediate hosts. Opossums could be infected with oocysts from cats and by feeding tissue that contains cysts. Thus, transmis-

sion among intermediate hosts by predation or cannibalism is possible. The importance of this parasite to the health of wild animals has not been evaluated.

Besnoitia jellisoni. Tissue cysts attributed to this species have been found in deer mice (*Peromyscus maniculatus*) and kangaroo rats (*Dipodomys* spp.). Cysts found in opossums also were attributed to this species; it is not clear whether two species (*B. darlingi and B. jellisoni*) or only one occurs in opossums. *Besnoitia jellisoni* caused severe natural disease in kangaroo rats captured in the wild (Chobotar et al. 1970). Vast numbers of cysts were found in the skin and in internal organs. The species also produces severe disease in laboratory mice (Kaggwa et al. 1979; Tadros and Laarman 1982). Experimental infections also have been produced in rabbits, rats, and hamsters (*Mesocricetus auratus*). Transmission among rodent intermediate hosts by cannibalism has been reported (Frenkel 1953, 1965; Jellison et al. 1956). No definitive host is known.

Besnoitia tarandi. Tissue cysts are commonly found in reindeer and caribou (Hadwen 1922; Choquette et al. 1967; Wobeser 1976; Rehbinder et al. 1981; Lewis 1989). Cysts also occur commonly in the skin of musk-ox (*Ovibos moschatus*) in the western Canadian Arctic (Fig. 17.9; A. Gunn, F.A. Leighton, and A.A. Gajadhar, unpublished) and are assumed to be the same species as occurs in sympatric caribou. Disease, manifest as skin lesions and blood vessel occlusion, occurs occasionally in these species. Mule deer at two zoos in western Canada developed severe besnoitiosis that was attributed to transmission by biting insects from nearby groups of infected caribou and reindeer. No definitive host has been identified for *B. tarandi* (Glover et al. 1990, Ayroud et al. 1995).

Besnoitia wallacei. This species was discovered fortuitously as oocysts in the feces of domestic cats in Hawaii during a survey for *Toxoplasma* (Wallace and Frenkel 1975) and was named by Frenkel in 1977. Three rodent species, the Polynesian rat (*Rattus exulans*), laboratory rats, and mice (*R. norvegicus* and *Mus musculus*) were infected with sporulated oocysts, and cats were infected with tissue cysts from these species. *Rattus exulans* developed tissue cysts when cyst material from an infected individual was injected into a naive individual. Such intermediate host–to–intermediate host infection did not occur with the other two rodent species; only oocysts were infective for them. *Besnoitia wallacei* also has been reported from domestic cats in Africa, Japan, and Australia (Table 17.5.). Little is known about the occurrence or dynamics of this species in wild animal populations.

Other Species of Besnoitia. It is likely that other species of *Besnoitia* exist. Table 17.5 lists references to occurrences of infections with *Besnoitia* that were not assigned to any of the species listed above. Even designation of *B. besnoiti* in African wild ungulates is uncertain, because clear differences in pathogenicity and tissue predilection have been documented between the form in wild ungulates and the form in cattle.

LIFE HISTORY. After nearly a century of study and speculation, the life history of *Besnoitia* spp. in wild animals remains largely unknown. A carnivore-herbivore, two-host life cycle and developmental stages typical of the family Sarcocystidae have been demonstrated for *B. darlingi* and *B. wallacei,* one unnamed species, and possibly also for *B. besnoiti* (Peteshev et al. 1974; Smith and Frenkel 1977, 1984; Wallace and Frenkel 1975; Frenkel 1977; Matuschka and Häfner 1984; Diesing et al. 1988). Intermediate hosts ingest sporulated oocysts that release sporozoites in the alimentary tract. These penetrate host cells and undergo generations of asexual reproduction, known as merogony. The first generation of merozoites develops in endothelial cells of blood vessels. Subsequent generations of merogony occur in various organs and tissues, particularly in fibroblasts; the number of asexual generations is believed to be fixed for each species. The final generation of merogony yields very large (up to 1 mm) intracellular cysts (also called pseudocysts) without subdivisions that contain numerous small bradyzoites. When cyst-containing tissues are eaten by a definitive carnivore host, the bradyzoites are released, invade endothelial cells or enterocytes, and undergo merogony, presumably a single generation. The resulting merozoites enter intestinal epithelial cells and differentiate into male or female gamonts. Female gamonts are fertilized in situ by male gametocytes released from male gamonts and develop into oocysts. The infected intestinal cells rupture, and the oocysts are excreted with feces. Sporulation of oocysts occurs in the external environment, and the sporulated oocysts are infective for intermediate hosts.

The period from ingestion of sporulated oocysts to the occurrence of infective cysts in the intermediate host cells is 1–3 weeks, depending on the species of *Besnoitia.* The time between ingestion of cysts by the definitive host and shedding of oocysts in the feces (the "prepatent" period) ranges from 4 days to 4 weeks. Oocysts from a single experimental infection have been shed up to 21 days. Freshly passed oocysts require a week or more in a sufficiently warm and moist environment to sporulate and become infective for intermediate hosts.

Only two genera of definitive (carnivore) host have been recognized for any species of *Besnoitia.* The cat (*Felis catus*) is known to be the definitive host for *B. darlingi* and *B. wallacei.* There is evidence both for and against cats (*F. catus, F. lybica*) as definitive hosts for *B. besnoiti* (Peteshev et al. 1974; Diesing et al. 1988), perhaps indicating that this taxon, as currently defined, actually consists of more than one species. Snakes of the genus *Bitis* are the definitive host for an unnamed African species of *Besnoitia* (Matuschka and Häfner

1984). For the other species of *Besnoitia,* no definitive host has been identified, despite considerable effort to infect a wide range of potential carnivores (Uvaliev et al. 1979; Diesing et al. 1988; Glover et al. 1990; N'gang'a and Kasigazi 1994).

EPIZOOTIOLOGY. The population dynamics of *Besnoitia* that have an obligate two-host life cycle are influenced by the population dynamics of both host species and by environmental conditions. However, some species may be able to exist at high prevalence in populations of intermediate hosts through direct transmission among intermediate hosts, independent of definitive hosts. Transmission among intermediate hosts by arthropods, particularly biting flies acting as mechanical vectors, has been demonstrated for *B. besnoiti* (Cuillé et al. 1936; Bigalke 1960, 1967; Pols 1960) and suspected for *B. tarandi* (Glover et al. 1990). For *B. besnoiti,* cysts in the intermediate host remain viable up to 9 years (Bigalke 1967), thus representing a constant source of bradyzoites for mechanical transmission by biting arthropods. In both *B. besnoiti* in cattle and *B. tarandi* in reindeer, caribou (*Rangifer tarandus*), and mule deer, (*Odocoileus hemionus*), high densities of cysts have been found in the dermis and subcutis of the skin of the lower limbs and face and in the nasal cavity, possible predilection sites for potential arthropod vectors (Bigalke and Prozesky 1994, Wobeser 1976; Glover et al. 1990; Ayroud et al. 1995). *Besnoitia jellisoni* is transmissible among rodent intermediate hosts through scavenging or cannibalism (Frenkel 1953; Jellison et al. 1956).

CLINICAL SIGNS. Infection and disease in wild animals have been recognized only in intermediate (herbivore) hosts and never in definitive (carnivore) hosts. Clinical disease is well described for *B. besnoiti* in cattle and *B. bennetti* in horses (Bigalke and Prozesky 1994) and for *B. caprae* in domestic goats (Bwangamoi et al. 1989). Clinical signs in wild animal species, when described, have been similar. Most infections are entirely inapparent and are not associated with any form of clinical disease. In cattle, two phases of clinical disease are recognized: (1) acute febrile disease associated with merogony in endothelial cells and (2) chronic disease associated with the presence of large intracellular cysts in connective tissues. Acute disease has not been described in wild animals. In cattle, it consists of sudden onset of fever (40°C–41° C) 4 days after experimental infection with sporulated oocysts or 13 days after experimental infection with biting flies (Bigalke and Prozesky 1994). Affected animals stop eating and avoid bright light. Within a few days, subcutaneous swelling due to accumulation of fluid (edema) develops in localized areas or over the entire body. This edema can range from inapparent to severe and generalized. Fever subsides after a week or so, and edema generally disappears within 3 weeks.

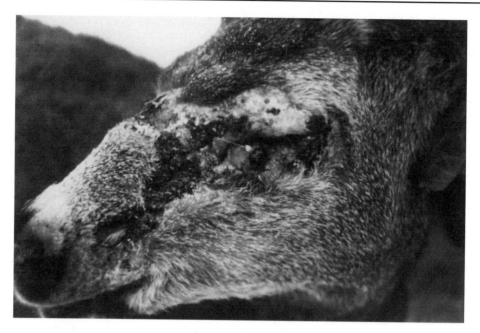

FIG. 17.4—Captive mule deer with severe besnoitiosis. The skin of the face is thickened and inflamed, with loss of hair and superficial crusts of exudate. (Courtesy of Dr. Gordon Glover, Winnipeg, Manitoba.)

Occasionally, acute disease is fatal; more often, it is not evident at all.

Chronic disease results from the development of cysts in tissue. Cysts in high density can increase the thickness and decrease the pliability of the skin. Cracks and fissures in the skin are a frequent consequence, and these then become secondarily infected with bacteria. The result is an area of thickened skin with hair loss and varying amounts of inflammatory exudate and hemorrhage on the surface. Lesions of this kind are most common over joints, but often also occur on the face and elsewhere on the body (Figs. 17.4 and 17.5). Thickening of the mucosa of the nasal cavity can obstruct breathing. Tissue cysts sometimes can be seen in the scleral conjunctiva of the eyes as glistening pale spheres 0.5–1 mm in diameter. Their appearance is quite characteristic, particularly when the cysts are present in large numbers (Choquette et al. 1967; Chobotar et al. 1970; Wobeser 1976; Cheema and Toofanian 1979; Rehbinder et al. 1981; Glover et al. 1990; Ayroud et al. 1995); however, small nodules of lymphoid tissue can look similar.

Male sterility is an outcome of besnoitiosis regularly reported in cattle. It is due to a combination of reduced blood supply from cysts obstructing the lumens of arteries and inflammation of the testicles. Lesions compatible with this clinical outcome have been seen in wild goats (*Capra aegagrus*) (Cheema and Toofanian 1979) and captive mule deer (Diagnostic records, Western College of Veterinary Medicine, Saskatoon). Thus, it is possible that male sterility is a common outcome of severe chronic besnoitiosis.

PATHOLOGY. Acute disease in cattle is associated with redness of the skin and edema and, histologically, with endothelial cells distended with small organisms. Acute disease has not been recognized in wild animals. In animals suffering chronic clinical disease, the skin lesions, described above as clinical signs of besnoitiosis, are the gross lesions of importance (Figs. 17.4 and 17.5). In these, and also in infected but clinically normal animals, the tiny 0.5–1.0-mm cysts often can be seen in a variety of locations. At necropsy, they are most evident in subcutaneous tissue, on the periosteum (Fig. 17.6), and on the connective tissue fascia of muscle. In cattle, reindeer, caribou, and muskox, they are particularly numerous in tissues of the distal limbs. The cysts are very firm in texture; when a heavily infected lower limb bone is skinned and palpated, a finely rough texture is readily apparent, which Hadwen (1922) likened to a surface sprinkled with ground maize (corn meal). Cysts often develop on or in blood vessel walls and thus can be seen in linear chains along vessel tracts in the subcutaneous tissue (Fig. 17.6). Wild African ungulates infected with *B. besnoiti* are reported to have cysts in the connective tissue of the cardiovascular system more than at other sites (Bigalke et al. 1967). Histologically, cysts can be found in connective tissues anywhere in the body. Locations include the bone, where the cysts form small pits in the bone surface and also develop entirely within bone, and the walls of blood vessels, where cysts in the intima can protrude into the lumen and reduce blood flow through the vessel (Fig 17.7). Cysts can also develop in the connective

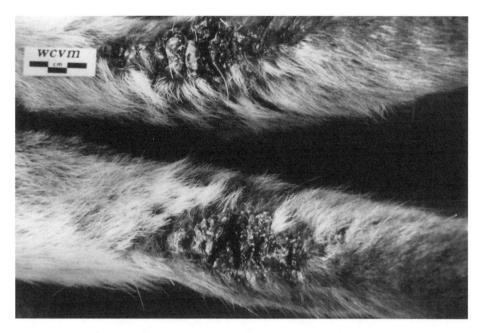

FIG. 17.5—Flexure surfaces of tarsal (hock) joints of a barren-ground caribou from the central Canadian Arctic with locally severe besnoitiosis. The skin is thickened, inflamed, and has multiple, deep, fissure-like lacerations through which abundant exudate has reached the surface to form a superficial crust. (Courtesy of Dr. Gary Wobeser, Saskatoon, Saskatchewan.)

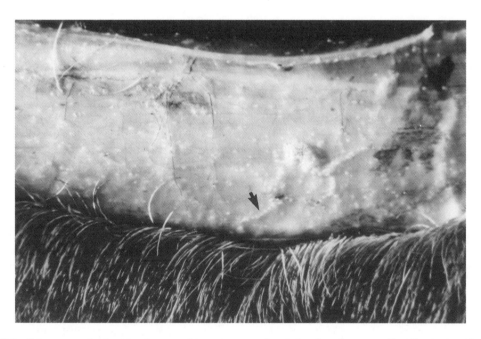

FIG. 17.6—Subcutaneous fascia and periosteum of the metacarpus of a reindeer from the western Canadian Arctic with subclinical infection with *B. tarandi*. Numerous bead-like spherical cysts, singly and in small chains along blood vessels (arrow), are visible in the connective tissue. (Courtesy of Dr. Ron Lewis, Abbotsford, British Columbia.)

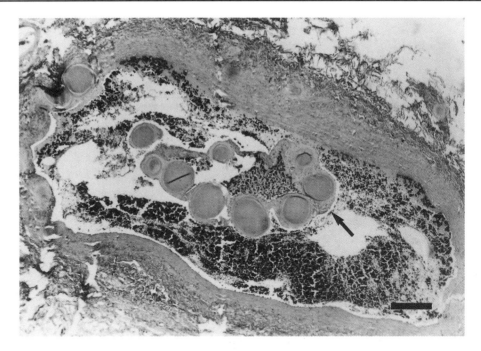

FIG. 17.7—Histological section of an artery from a mule deer. Large round cysts of *Besnoitia* (arrow) are in the arterial wall and in a polyp-like mass that partially occludes the lumen. (Stained with hematoxylin and eosin.) (Bar = 300 μm)

tissue stroma of any organ or tissue and thus can be found within muscle, testicle, spleen, kidney, etc. They are not present in the parenchymal cells of these tissues, however, but rather in the supporting connective tissue. Most cysts provoke no inflammatory reaction in the host, but some are surrounded by a granulomatous inflammatory reaction consisting of multinucleated giant cells, macrophages, and lymphocytes. Such reactions often appear associated with cysts that are damaged and degenerating. When the skin is heavily infected, the dermis is greatly thickened by the presence of numerous cysts (Figs. 17.5 and 17.8), and there may be considerable acute and chronic inflammation associated with breaks in the epidermis and consequent bacterial infection.

The morphology of the zoite-filled cyst in the intermediate host and its location exclusively in connective tissue is unique and is the principle criterion used to identify the genus. Each cyst consists of a very thick extracellular capsule of hyaline material that surrounds a large parasitized cell (Fig.17.9). The cell has multiple nuclei that are pressed flat against the peripheral cell membrane. A huge mass of very small zoites that are tightly packed together in a large parasitophorus vacuole occupies most of the cell volume. Electron microscopic observations indicate that the capsule consists of collagen and amorphous matrix material, and the zoites are contained within a membrane-bound parasitophorous vacuole that is not subdivided (Fig. 17.10). The host cell cytoplasm forms a thin layer between the

capsule and the mass of parasites (Glover et al. 1990; Ayroud et al. 1995).

DIAGNOSIS. Diagnosis usually is based on finding cysts of typical morphology in infected tissues viewed histologically. For this, a section of skin fixed in formalin is required. Cysts can be recognized grossly with some confidence by those who regularly examine infected animals (Lewis 1989). Such cysts can be minced in buffered physiological saline solution and the fluid examined for the presence of zoites. It is possible to diagnose infection in live animals by identifying the cysts on the scleral conjunctiva. However, the sensitivity of this diagnostic approach to identifying infected animals is very low; many, perhaps most, infected animals will have no scleral cysts. The sensitivity of histological detection of cysts also is of unknown but, probably, quite low sensitivity. For most species of *Besnoitia,* there is no sensitive and specific method available to identify live animals that are infected. Immunological tests (ELISA and immunofluorescence) of low sensitivity have been developed for *B. besnoiti* in cattle (Janitschke et al. 1984). Recent advances in molecular biology offer new opportunities to develop sensitive and specific diagnostic tests. However, mild infections may continue to elude detection, particularly in individual live animals; the cysts within host cells may provoke no detectable immune response that would permit serological detection, and their usual

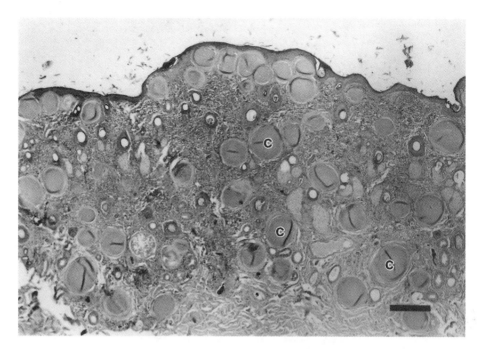

FIG. 17.8—Histological section of skin from a mule deer heavily infected with *Besnoitia*. Numerous cysts (**c**) are present in the dermis and subcutaneous connective tissue. There is moderate inflammation. Fold lines across cysts are artifacts of processing. (Stained with hematoxylin and eosin.) (Bar = 300 μm)

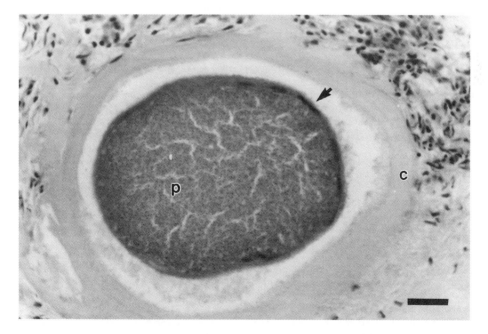

FIG. 17.9—Histological section of a single cyst of *Besnoitia* in the skin of a muskox from the central Canadian Arctic. There is a thick capsule (**c**) surrounding a large host cell with multiple, peripheral nuclei (arrow) and a large parasitophorous vacuole (**p**) filled with bradyzoites. The space between the cell and the capsule is an artifact of fixation and processing. (Stained with hematoxylin and eosin.) (Bar = 30 μm)

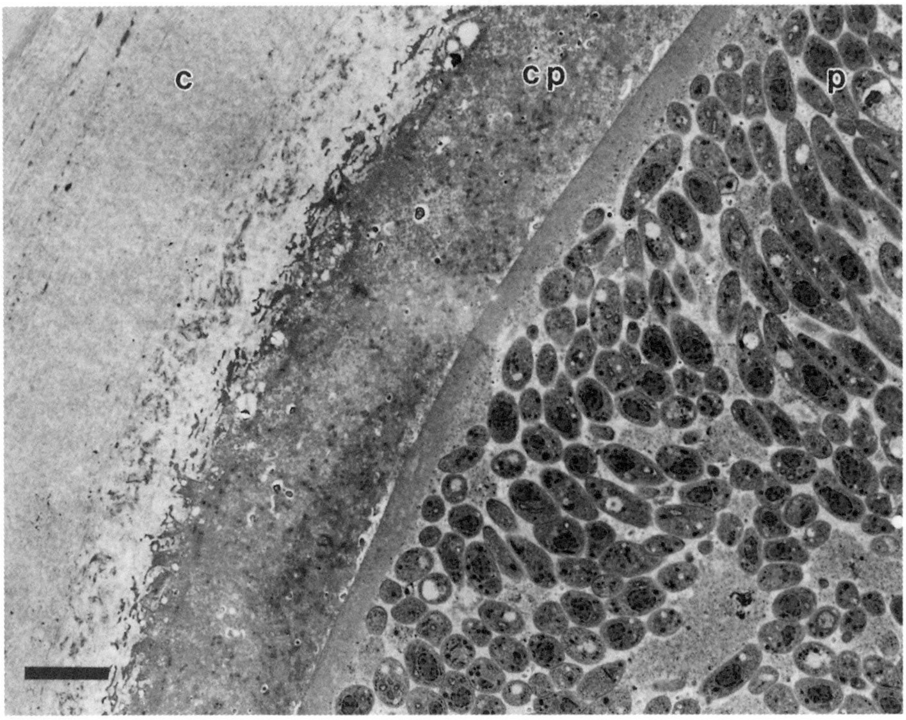

FIG. 17.10—Electron micrograph of a section of a cyst of *B. tarandi* in the skin of a reindeer: extracellular capsule (**c**), cytoplasm of host cell (**cp**), parasitophorus vacuole (**p**) containing many bradyzoites. (Bar = 5 μm) (Courtesy of Dr. Mejid Ayroud, Airdrie, Alberta.)

wide but sparse distribution throughout the body may defy detection methods that require inclusion of at least one organism in a tissue sample.

Skin lesions that resemble those caused by *Besnoitia* can be caused by other agents, particularly the bacterium *Dermatophilus congolense,* mange mites, and "dermatophyte" fungi ("ringworm").

IMMUNITY AND CONTROL. Almost nothing is known about the immunological response of the intermediate host to *Besnoitia.* A live vaccine has been developed for cattle and is reported to reduce the occurrence or severity of clinical disease, but not to prevent infection (Bigalke and Prozesky 1994). No effective pharmaceutical treatment for besnoitiosis has been reported. Successful establishment of a disease-free herd of captive reindeer from an infected herd, by exclusion of biting flies for a period of reproduction and removal of offspring to a separate facility, has been reported (Glover et al. 1990). Control of the disease in wild populations has not been contemplated.

PUBLIC HEALTH CONCERNS. There is no evidence that any species of *Besnoitia* infects humans.

MANAGEMENT IMPLICATIONS. Besnoitiosis has been a management issue in western Canada because of the desire of agriculturists to translocate reindeer from the Arctic to southern agricultural zones for commercial production. Arctic reindeer and caribou have a high prevalence of infection with *B. tarandi.* The management issue has been the disease risk such translocation might pose for wild populations of mule deer and other native cervids. Severe besnoitiosis in mule deer has occurred in two zoos in western Canada, each occurrence associated with the presence nearby of infected reindeer or caribou (Glover et al. 1990; Diagnostic Laboratory of the Western College of Veterinary Medicine, Saskatoon, unpublished reports). No data exist upon which to base an accurate assessment of this risk. Three Canadian provinces have responded differently to this issue. British Columbia undertook preliminary studies of the prevalence of *Besnoitia* in woodland caribou, moose (*Alces alces*), and mule deer in areas where these species are broadly sympatric in the province and permitted limited importation of Arctic reindeer on the basis of these findings (Lewis 1989). Alberta and Saskatchewan initially barred all importation, but subsequently have permitted importation of calves derived from the limited importation into British Columbia. It is not known whether or not these calves are infected. In South Africa, there appear to be two distinct strains of *B. besnoiti,* one in cattle and one in wild ungulates. The wild ungulate strain is of low pathogenicity to cattle (Bigalke and Prozesky 1994).

LITERATURE CITED

Ayroud, M., F.A. Leighton, and S.V. Tessaro. 1995. The morphology and pathology of *Besnoitia* sp. in reindeer (*Rangifer tarandus tarandus*). *Journal of Wildlife Disease* 31:319-326.

Bennett, S. 1939. Besnoitiosis in the Sudan. Annual Report of the Sudan Veterinary Service, p. 37.

Besnoit, C., and V. Robin. 1912. Sarcosporidiose cutanée chez une vache. *Revue Vétérinaire* 37:649-663.

Bigalke, R.D. 1960. Preliminary observations on the mechanical transmission of cyst organisms of *Besnoitia besnoiti* (Marotel, 1912) from a chronically infected bull to rabbits by *Glossina brevipalpis* Newstead. 1910. *Journal South African Veterinary Medicine Association* 31:37-44.

Bigalke, R.D. 1967. The artificial transmission of *Besnoitia besnoiti* (Marotel, 1912) from chronically infected to susceptible cattle and rabbits. *Onderstepoort Journal of Veterinary Research* 34:303-316.

———. 1968. New concepts on the epidemiological features of besnoitiosis as determined by laboratory and field investigations. *Onderstepoort Journal of Veterinary Research* 35:3-138.

Bigalke, R.D. and L. Prozesky. 1994. Besnoitiosis. In *Infectious diesease of livestock with special reference to South Africa,* vol 1., ch. 18. Ed. J.A.W. Coetzer, G.R. Thomson and R.C. Tustin. Cape Town: Oxford University Press, pp. 245-252.

Bigalke, R.D., J.W. Van Niekerk, P.A. Basson, and R.M. McCully. 1967. Studies on the relationship between *Besnoitia* of blue wildebeest and impala, and *Besnoitia besnoiti* of cattle. *Onderstepoort Journal of Veterinary Research* 34:7-28.

Burgisser, H. 1975. Compte-rendu sur les maladies des animaux sauvages (1973-1974). *Schweizer Archiv für Tierheilkunde* 117:397-400.

Bwangamoi, O. 1967. A preliminary report on the finding of *Besnoitia besnoitii* in goat skins affected with dimple in Kenya. *Bulletin of Epizootic Diseases of Africa* 15:263.

Bwangamoi, O., A.B. Carles and J.G. Wnadera. 1989. An epidemic of besnoitiosis in goats in Kenya. *Veterinary Record* 125:461.

Bwangamoi, O., D. Rottcher and C. Wekesa. 1990. Rabies, microbesnoitiosis and sarcocystosis in lion. *Veterinary Record* 127:411.

Cheema, A.H. and F. Toofanian. 1979. Besnoitiosis in wild and domestic goats in Iran. *Cornell Veterinarian* 69:159-168.

Chobotar, B., L.C. Anderson, J.V. Ernst, and D.M. Hammond. 1970. Pathogenicity of *Besnoitia jellisoni* in naturally infected kangaroo rats (*Didodomys ordii*) in northwestern Utah. *The Journal of Parasitology* 56:192-193.

Choquette, L.P.E., E. Broughton, F.L. Miller, H.C. Gibbs and J.G. Cousineau. 1967. Besnoitiosis in barren-ground caribou in northern Canada. *Canadian Veterinary Journal* 8:282-287.

Cuillé, J., P. Chelle, and F. Berlureau. 1936. Transmission expérimentale de la maladie dénommée "sarcosporidiose cutanée" du boeuf (Besnoit et Robin) et déterminée par *Globidium besnoiti. Bulletin Academy Medicine* 115:161-163.

Darling, S.T. 1910. Sarcosporidiosis in the opossum and its experimental production in the guinea pig by the intra-muscular injection of sporozoites [in French]. *Bulletin de la Société de Pathologie Exotique* 3:513-518.

Diesing, L., A.O. Heydorn, F.R. Matuschka, C. Bauer, E. Pipano, D.T. De Waal, and F.T. Potgieter. 1988. *Besnoitia besnoiti:* Studies on the definitive host and experimental infections in cattle. *Parasitology Research* 75:114-117.

Ernst, J.V., B. Chobotar, E.C. Oaks, and D.M. Hammond. 1968. *Besnoita jellisoni* (Sporozoa: Toxoplasmea) in rodents from Utah and California. *The Journal of Parasitology* 54:545-549.

Foley, G.L., W.I. Anderson and H. Steinberg. 1990. Besnoitiosis of the reproductive tract of a blue duiker (*Cephalophus monticola*). *Veterinary Pathology* 36:157-163.

Frank, W., and J.K. Frenkel. 1981. *Besnoitia* in a Palearctic lizard (*Lacerta dugesii*) from Madeira. *Parasitology Research* 64:203-206.

Frenkel, J.K. 1953. Infections with organisms resembling *Toxoplasma,* together with the description of a new organism: *Besnoitia jellisoni. Atti del VI Congress of International Microbiology* 5:426-434

———. 1965. The development of the cyst of *Besnoitia jellisoni:* Usefulness of this infection as a biological model. *Progress of Protozoology; Excerpta Medica Foundation International Congress Series* 91:122-124.

———. 1977. *Besnoitia wallacei* of cats and rodents: With a reclassification of other cyst-forming isosporoid coccidia. *The Journal of Parasitology* 63:611-628.

Glover, G.J., M. Swendrowski and R.J. Cawthorn. 1990. An epizootic of besnoitiosis in captive caribou (*Rangifer tarandus caribou*), reindeer (*Rangifer tarandus tarandus*) and mule deer (*Odocoileus hemionus hemionus*). *Journal of Wildlife Diseases* 26:186-195.

Gorlin, R.J., C.N. Barron, A.P. Chandhry and J.J. Clark. 1959. The oral and pharyngeal pathology of domestic animals: A study of 487 cases. *American Journal of Veterinary Research* 20:1032-1061.

Hadwen, S. 1922. Cyst-forming protozoa in reindeer and caribou, and a sarcosporidian parasite of the seal (*Phoca ricardi*). *Journal of the American Veterinary Medical Association* 61:374-382.

Henry, A. 1913. Analyse d'un travail de Besnoit et Robin, 1912. *Recueil de Médecine Vétérinaire* 90:327-328.

Heydorn, A.O., J. Sénaud, and H. Mehlhorn. 1984. *Besnoitia* sp. from goats in Kenya. *Parasitology Research* 70:709-713.

Ito, S., K. Tsunoda and K. Shimura. 1978. Life cycle of the large type of *Isospora bigemina* of the cat. *National Institute of Animal Health Quarterly* 18:69-82.

Jack, S.W., W.G. Van Alstine, and J. Swackhammer. 1989. Besnoitiasis in Indiana opossums. *Journal of Veterinary Diagnostic Investigation* 1:189-191.

Janitschke, K., A.J. De Vos and R.D. Bigalke. 1984. Serodiagnosis of bovine besnoitiosis by ELISA and immunofluorescense tests. *Onderstepoort Journal of Veterinary Research* 51:239-243.

Jellison, W.L., W.J. Fullerton, and H. Parker. 1956. Transmission of the protozoan *Besnoitia jellisoni* by ingestion. *Annuals of New York Academy of Science* 64:271.

Jellison, W.L., L. Glesne, and R.S. Peterson. 1960. *Emmonsia,* a fungus, and *Besnoitia,* a protozoan, reported from South America. *Boletin Chileno de Parasitologia* 15:46-47.

Kaggwa, E., G. Weiland, and M. Rommel. 1979. *Besnoitia besnoiti* and *Besnoitia jellisoni:* A comparison of indirect flourescent antibody test (IFAT) and the enzyme-linked immunosorbent assay (ELISA) in diagnosis of *Besnoitia* infections in rabbits and mice. *Bulletin Animal Health and Production in Africa* 27:127-137.

Karstad, L., L. Sileo, and W.J. Hartley. 1981. A *Besnoitia*-like parasite associated with arteritis in flamingos. In *Wildlife* diseases of the pacific basin and other countries. Ed. M.E. Fowler. Proceedings 4th International Conference Wildlife Disease Association, Sydney, Australia, pp. 98-101.

Keep, M.E., and P.A. Basson. 1973. Besnoitiosis in a warthog (*Phacochoerus aethiopicus* Curvier 1922). *Journal of the South African Veterinary Association* 44:237.

Kharole, M.U., D.S. Kalra, and B.M. Dutta. 1979. A note on Besnoitiosis in animals and chicken. *Indian Veterinary Journal* 56:969-971

Kharole, M.U., S.K. Gupta, and J. Singh. 1984. Note on besnoitiosis in a camel. *Indian Journal of Animal Science* 51:802-804.

Le Blancq, S.M., S.S. Desser, and V. Shwap. 1986. *Besnoitia* strain differentiation using Isoenzyme electrophoresis. *The Journal of Parasitology* 72:475-476.

Lee, H.S., H.B. Lee, and M.H. Moon. 1979. Studies on control and therapeutics of *Besnoitia besnoiti* (Marotel, 1912) infection in Korean native cattle. *Suwon, Korean Society of Animal Sciences* 21:281-288.

Lewis, R.J. 1989. Cross-Canada disease report: *Besnoitia* infection in woodland caribou. *Canadian Veterinary Journal* 30:436.

Mason, R.W. 1980. The discovery of *Besnoitia wallacei* in Australia and the identification of a free-living intermediate host. *Parasitology Research* 61:173-178.

Matuschka, F.R., and U. Häfner. 1984. Cyclic transmission of an African *Besnoitia* species by snakes of the genus *Bitis* to several rodents. *Parasitology Research* 70:471-476.

Mbuthia, P.G., P.K. Gathumbi, and O. Bwangamoi. 1993. Natural *besnoitiosis* in a rabbit. *Veterinary Parasitology* 45:191-198.

McCully, R.M., P.A. Basson, J.W. Van Niekerk and R.D. Bigalke. 1966. Observations of *besnoitia* cysts in the cardiovascular system of some wild antelopes and domestic cattle. *Onderstepoort Journal of veterinary Research* 33:245-276.

Neuman, M., and T.A. Nobel. 1960. Globidiosis of cattle and sheep in Israel. *Refuah Veterinarith* 17:101-103.

N'gang'a, C.J., and S. Kasigazi. 1994. Caprine besnoitiosis: Studies on the experimental intermediate hosts and the role of the domestic cat in transmission. *Veterinary Parasitology* 52:207-210.

N'gang'a, C., P.W. Kanyari and W.K. Munyua. 1994. Isolation of *Besnoitia wallacei* in Kenya. *Veterinary Parasitology* 52:203-206.

Nikolaevskii, L.D. 1961. Diseases of reindeer [In Russian]. In *Reindeer husbandry*. Ed. P.S. Zhignnov. Moscow, USSR. [Washington, DC: Israel Program for Scientific Translations, pp. 266-268.]

Njenga, J. M., O. Bwangamoi, E. R. Mutiga, E. K. Kangethe, and G. M. Mugera. 1993. Preliminary findings from an experimental study of caprine besnoitiosis in Kenya. *Veterinary Research Communications* 17:203-208.

Njenga, J.M., O. Bwangamoi, and E.K. Kangethe. 1995. Comparative ultrastructural studies on *Besnoitia besnoiti* and *Besnoitia caprae*. *Veterinary Research Communications* 19:295-308.

Peteshev, V.M., I.G. Galuzo, and A.P. Polomoshnov. 1974. Cats—Definitive host of *Besnoitia (Besnoitia besnoiti)*[In Russian]. *Isvestiya Akademii Nauka Kazakhskoi SSR. Seria Biologicheskiya* 1:33-38.

Peteshev, V.M., and A.P. Polomoshnov. 1976. Role of small animals in the circulation of *Besnoitia* in nature [In Russian]. In *Prirodnoochagovye antropozoonozy*, National Conference on Diseases of Man and Animals, 18-21 May, Omsk, pp. 222-223.

Pols, J.W. 1960. Studies on bovine besnoitiosis with special reference to the aetiology. *Onderstepoort Journal of Veterinary Research* 28:265-356.

Rehbinder, C., M. Elvander, and M. Nordkvist. 1981. Cutaneous Besnoitiosis in a Swedish reindeer (*Rangifer tarandus* t.). *Nordisk Veterinaer Medicin* 33:270-272.

Schneider, C.R. 1967a. *Besnoitia darlingi* (Brumpt, 1913) in Panama. *Journal of Protozoology* 14:78-82.

Schneider, C. R. 1967b. The distribution of lizard besnoitiosis in Panama, and its transfer to mice. *Journal of Protozoology* 14:674-678.

Simpson, C.F., J.C. Woodard and D.J. Forrester. 1977. An epizootic among knots (*Calidris canutus*) in Florida. II. Ultrastructure and the causative agent, a besnoitia-like organism. *Veterinary Pathology* 14:351-360.

Smith, D.D., and J.K. Frenkel. 1977. *Besnoitia darlingi* (Protozoa: Toxoplasmatinae): Cyclic transmission by cats. *The Journal Parasitology* 63:1066-1071.

———. 1984. *Besnoitia darlingi* (Apicomplexa, Sarcocystidae, Toxoplasmatinae): Transmission between opossums and cats. *Journal of Protozoology* 31:584-587.

Stabler, R.M., and K. Welch. 1961. *Besnoitia* from an opossum. *The Journal of Parasitology* 47:576.

Tadros, W., and J.J. Laarman. 1982. Current concepts on the biology, evolution and taxonomy of tissue cyst-forming Eimeriid coccidia. *Advances in Parasitology* 20:293-468.

Terrell T.G., and J.L. Stookey. 1973. *Besnoitia bennetti* in two Mexican burros. *Veterinary Pathology* 10:177-184.

Uvaliev I.U., Y.U.A. Popov, and T.T. Susleimenov. 1979. Experimental infection of kittens with *Besnoitia*. *Protozoological Abstract* 7:2450.

Van Heerden, J., H.J. Els, E.J. Raubenheimer, and J.H. Williams. 1993. *Besnoitiosis* in a horse. *Journal of the South African Veterinary Association* 64:92-95.

Vsevolodov, B.P. 1961. On besnoitiosis of cattle in Kazakhstan. Natural foci of diseases and problems in parasitology. *Academy of Sciences of Kazakh SSR* 3:196-206.

Wallace, G.D. and J.K. Frenkel. 1975. *Besnoita* sp. (Protozoa, Sporozoa, Toxoplasmatidae): Recognition of cyclic transmission by cats. *Science* 188:369-371.

Wobeser, G. 1976. Besnoitiosis in a woodland caribou. *Journal of Wildlife Diseases* 12:566-571.

TOXOPLASMOSIS AND RELATED INFECTIONS

JITENDER P. DUBEY AND KLAUS ODENING

Discussed in this chapter are *Toxoplasma, Neospora, Sarcocystis,* and *Frenkelia,* which are classified as coccidia.

INTRODUCTION AND TAXONOMY. The four genera of parasites discussed in this chapter, are classified as coccidia. They belong to phylum Apicomplexa, Levine 1970; class Sporozoasida, Leuckart 1879; subclass Coccidiasina, Leuckart 1879; order Eimeriorina, Leger 1911. Opinions differ regarding further classification of these coccidia into families and subfamilies; here they are classified in the families Sarcocystidae or Toxoplasmatidae.

The four genera are closely related. Infections by the protozoan parasites *Toxoplasma* and *Sarcocystis* are widespread in both domestic and wild animals. Therefore most of the chapter will be devoted to the biology of these parasites. The genus *Neospora* is so closely

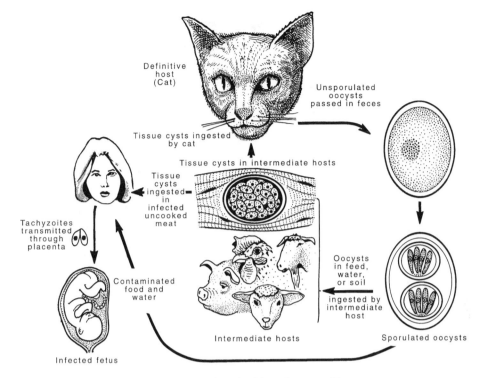

FIG. 17.11—Life cycle of *Toxoplasma gondii.*

related to *Toxoplasma* that they were considered the same parasites until 1988. It will be mentioned briefly. The genus *Frenkelia* is discussed here briefly because structurally it is very similar to *Sarcocystis.*

TOXOPLASMA GONDII AND TOXOPLASMOSIS

Etiologic Agent. *Toxoplasma gondii* (Nicolle and Manceaux 1908) Nicolle and Manceaux, 1909, is a coccidian with felids as definitive hosts and with an unusually wide range of intermediate hosts. Infection by this parasite is prevalent in many warm-blooded animals including humans. The name *Toxoplasma* (*toxon* = arc, *plasma* = form) is derived from the crescent shape of the tachyzoite stage. *Toxoplasma gondii* was first discovered by Nicolle and Manceaux in 1908 in a rodent, *Ctenodactylus gundi.*

Structure and Life Cycle. There are three infectious stages of *T. gondii* (Fig. 17.11): the tachyzoites (in groups or clones), the bradyzoites (in tissue cysts), and the sporozoites (in oocysts). Tachyzoite (in Greek *tachos* = speed) is the stage that rapidly multiplies inside the body. Tachyzoites and endodyozoites are the same. The tachyzoite is often crescent-shaped and is approximately 2 x 6 μm (Fig. 17.12). Its anterior end is

pointed, and its posterior end is round. Ultrastructurally, it has a pellicle (outer covering), polar ring, conoid, rhoptries, micronemes, mitochondria, subpellicular microtubules, endoplasmic reticulum, Golgi apparatus, ribosomes, rough surface endoplasmic reticulum, micropore, apicoplast, and a well-defined nucleus. The nucleus is usually situated toward the posterior end or in the central area of the cell. Twenty-two subpellicular microtubules originate from the anterior end and run longitudinally almost the entire length of the cell. Terminating within the anterior end (conoid) are eight to ten club-shaped organelles called rhoptries (Fig. 17.13). The rhoptries are glandlike structures, often labyrinthine.

The tachyzoite enters the host cell by active penetration of the host cell membrane. After entering the host cell the tachyzoite becomes ovoid in shape and becomes surrounded by a parasitophorous vacuole (PV). It has been suggested that the PV is derived from both the parasite and the host. Numerous intravacuolar tubules connect the parasitophorous vacuolar membrane (Fig. 17.13).

The tachyzoite multiplies asexually within the host cell by repeated endodyogeny. Endodyogeny is a specialized form of reproduction in which two progeny form within the parent parasite, consuming it. In endodyogeny, anterior membranes of the progeny cells

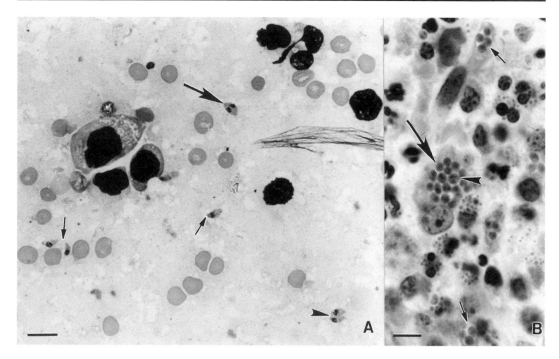

FIG. 17.12—Tachyzoites of *T. gondii*. (Bar = 10 μm) (**A**) Individual (small arrows), binucleate (large arrow), and divided (arrowhead) tachyzoites. Impression smear of lung. Compare size with red blood cells and leukocytes. (Giemsa stain.) (**B**) Tachyzoites in a group (large arrow) and in pairs (small arrows) in section of a mesenteric lymph node. Note organisms are located in parasitophorous vacuoles and some are dividing (arrowhead). (Hematoxylin and eosin stain.)

appear as dome-shaped structures anteriorly. The parasite nucleus becomes horseshoe-shaped, and portions of the nucleus move into the dome-shaped anterior ends of the developing progeny. The progeny continue to grow until they reach the surface of the parent. The inner membrane of the parent disappears, and its outer membrane joins the inner membrane of the progeny cells. Tachyzoites continue to divide by endodyogeny until the host cell is filled with parasites. Organisms of a group rarely divide simultaneously, so the progeny are usually arranged at random. On occasion, rosettes may be formed by synchronous division of the progeny cells. Tachyzoites in sections are often oval, and 2–3 μm in diameter (Fig. 17.12B).

Tissue cysts grow and remain intracellular (Fig. 17.14) as the bradyzoites (in Greek *bradys* = slow) divide by endodyogeny. Tissue cysts vary in size (Fig. 17.14). Young tissue cysts may be as small as 5 μm and contain only two bradyzoites, while older ones may contain hundreds of organisms. Tissue cysts in the brain are often spheroidal and rarely reach a diameter of 60 μm, whereas intramuscular cysts are elongated and may be 100 μm long in formalin-fixed histologic sections. Although tissue cysts may develop in visceral organs, including lungs, liver, and kidneys, they are more prevalent in the neural and muscular tissues, including the brain, eye, and all types of muscles.

Intact tissue cysts probably do not cause any harm and may persist for the life of the host. The tissue cyst wall is elastic, thin (< 0.5 μm), and argyrophilic and encloses hundreds of crescent-shaped slender bradyzoites. The bradyzoites are ~7 x 1.5 μm.

Bradyzoites differ structurally only slightly from tachyzoites. They have a nucleus situated toward the posterior end, whereas the nucleus in tachyzoites is more centrally located. The contents of rhoptries in bradyzoites are electron dense (Fig. 17.15). They contain several glycogen granules which stain red with periodic acid–Schiff (PAS) reagent; such material is either small or absent in tachyzoites. Bradyzoites are more slender than are tachyzoites. Bradyzoites are less susceptible to destruction by proteolytic enzymes than are tachyzoites (Jacobs et al. 1960a).

Cats shed oocysts after ingesting any of the three infectious stages of *T. gondii* (i.e., tachyzoites, bradyzoites, and sporozoites) (Dubey and Frenkel 1976). Prepatent periods (time to the shedding of oocysts after initial infection) and frequency of oocyst shedding vary according to the stage of *T. gondii* ingested. Prepatent periods are 3–10 days after ingesting tissue cysts, 18 days or more after ingesting oocysts, and 13 days or more after ingesting tachyzoites. Less than 50% of cats shed oocysts after ingesting tachyzoites or oocysts, whereas nearly all cats shed oocysts after ingesting tissue cysts.

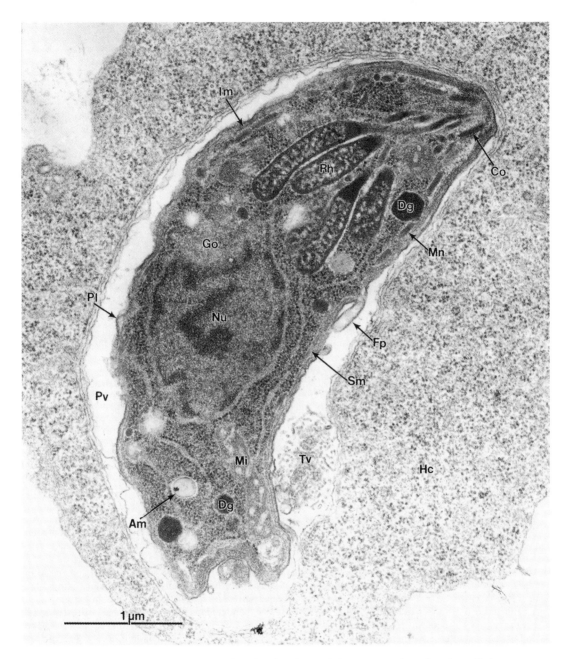

FIG. 17.13—Transmission electron micrograph of a tachyzoite of *T. gondii* in a mouse peritoneal exudate cell; **Am,** amylopectin granule; **Co,** conoid; **Dg,** electron-dense granule; **Fp,** finger-like projection of tachyzoite plasmalemma; **Go,** Golgi complex; **Hc,** host cell cytoplasm; **Im,** inner membrane complex; **Mi,** mitochondrion; **Mn,** microneme; **Nu,** nucleus; **Pl,** plasmalemma; **Pv,** parasitophorous vacuole; **Rh,** rhoptry; **Sm,** subpellicular microtubule; **Tv,** tubulovesicular membranes. (Bar = 1 μm) (Courtesy of Dr. C.A. Speer, Montana State University, Bozeman, Montana).

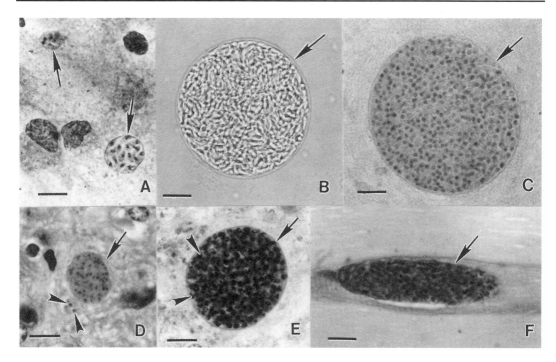

FIG. 17.14—Tissue cysts of *T. gondii.* (Bar = 10 μm) (**A**) Two tissue cysts (arrows). Note thin cyst wall enclosing brady-zoites. Impression smear of mouse brain. (Silver impregnation and Giemsa stain.) (**B**) A tissue cyst freed from mouse brain by homogenization in saline. Note thin cyst wall (arrow) enclosing many bradyzoites. (Unstained.) (**C**) A large tissue cyst in section of rat brain 14 months post-infection. Note thin cyst wall (arrow). (Hematoxylin and eosin stain.) (**D**) A small tissue cyst (arrow) with intact cyst wall (arrow) and four bradyzoites (arrowheads) with terminal nuclei adjacent to it. Section of mouse brain 8 months postinfection. (Hematoxylin and eosin stain.) (**E**) A tissue cyst in section of mouse brain. Note PAS-negative cyst wall (arrow) enclosing many PAS-positive bradyzoites (arrowheads). The bradyzoites stain bright red with PAS, but they appear black in this photograph. (Periodic acid Schiff hematoxylin.) (**F**) An elongated tissue cyst (arrow) in section of skeletal muscle of a mouse. (Periodic acid Schiff hematoxylin.)

After the ingestion of tissue cysts by cats, the cyst wall is dissolved by proteolytic enzymes in the stomach and small intestine. The released bradyzoites penetrate the epithelial cells of the small intestine and initiate asexual development of numerous generations of *T. gondii* (Dubey and Frenkel 1972). Five morphologically distinct types (schizonts) of *T. gondii* develop in intestinal epithelial cells before gametogony (Figs. 17.15–17.17) begins. These stages are designated types A to E instead of generations because there are several generations within each *T. gondii* type.

Merozoites (Fig. 17.16) released from meronts (probably types D and E) initiate gamete formation. Gamonts occur throughout the small intestine but most commonly in the ileum, 3–15 days after infection. The female gamont is subspherical and contains a single centrally located nucleus and several PAS-positive granules.

Mature male gamonts are ovoid to ellipsoidal in shape. When microgametogenesis takes place, the nucleus of the male gamont divides to produce 10 to 21 nuclei (Dubey and Frenkel 1972). The nuclei move toward the periphery of the parasite, entering protuber-ances formed in the pellicle of the mother parasite. One or two residual bodies are left in the microgamont after division into microgametes. Each microgamete is a biflagellate organism (Fig. 17.16B). The microgametes swim to and penetrate a mature macrogamete. After penetration, oocyst wall formation begins around the fertilized gamete.

Unsporulated oocysts are subspherical to spherical and are 10 x 12 μm in diameter (Fig. 17.16C). The oocyst wall contains two colorless layers. The sporont almost fills the oocyst, and sporulation occurs outside the cat within 1–5 days depending upon aeration and temperature.

Sporulated oocysts are subspherical to ellipsoidal and are 11 x 13 μm in diameter (Fig. 17.16D). Each sporulated oocyst contains two ellipsoidal sporocysts without a Stieda body. Sporocysts measure 6 x 8 μm; each contains four sporozoites (Fig. 17.11). The sporozoites are 2 x 6–8 μm in size with a subterminal to central nucleus and a few PAS-positive granules in the cytoplasm.

As the enteroepithelial cycle progresses, bradyzoites penetrate the lamina propria of the feline intestine and

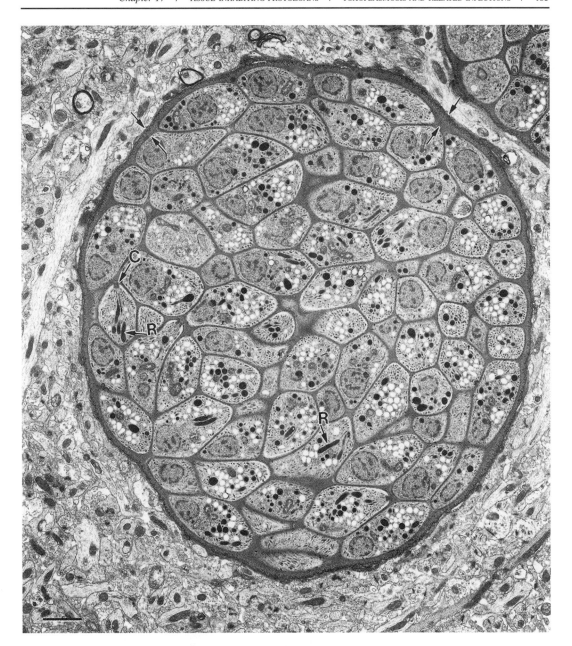

FIG. 17.15—Transmission electron micrograph of a tissue cyst in brain of a mouse 6 months postinfection. Note thin cyst wall (opposing arrows); numerous bradyzoites, each with a conoid (**C**); and electron-dense rhoptries (**R**). (Bar = 3.0 μm)

multiply as tachyzoites. Within a few hours after infection of cats, *T. gondii* may disseminate to extraintestinal tissues. *Toxoplasma gondii* persists in intestinal and extraintestinal tissues of cats at least several months, if not for the life of the cat.

Host-Parasite Relationships. *Toxoplasma gondii* usually parasitizes the host (both definitive and inter-mediate) without producing clinical signs. Only rarely does it cause severe clinical manifestations. The majority of natural infections are probably acquired by ingestion of tissue cysts in infected meat or oocysts in food or water contaminated with cat feces. The bradyzoites from the tissue cysts or sporozoites from the oocyst penetrate the intestinal epithelial cells and multiply in the intestine as tachyzoites within 24 hours of

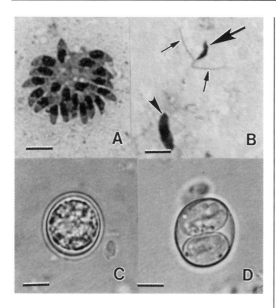

FIG. 17.16—Enteroepithelial stages of *T. gondii* in smears. (Bar = 5 μm) (**A**) A type D schizont from intestinal epithelium of a cat. (Giemsa stain.) (**B**) A microgamete (large arrow) with 2 flagella (small arrows), and a merozoite (arrowhead). Impression smear of cat intestine. (Giemsa stain.) (**C**) Unsporulated oocyst in cat feces. (Unstained.) (**D**) Sporulated oocyst from cat feces. (Unstained.)

infection. *Toxoplasma gondii* may spread first to mesenteric lymph nodes and then to distant organs by invasion of lymphatics and blood. An infected host may die because of necrosis of intestine and mesenteric lymph

nodes (Figs. 17.12, 17.17) before other organs are severely damaged. Focal areas of necrosis may develop in many organs. The clinical picture is determined by the extent of injury to organs, especially vital organs such as the eye, heart, and adrenals. Necrosis is caused by the intracellular growth of tachyzoites (Fig. 17.18). *Toxoplasma gondii* does not produce a toxin.

In those hosts with disease the host may die due to acute toxoplasmosis but much more often recovers with the acquisition of immunity. Inflammation usually follows the initial necrosis. By about the third week after infection, *T. gondii* tachyzoites begin to disappear from visceral tissues and may localize as tissue cysts in neural and muscular tissues. Tachyzoites may persist longer in the spinal cord and brain because immunity is less effective in neural organs than in visceral tissues (Fig. 17.18). How *T. gondii* is destroyed in immune cells is not completely known. All extracellular forms of the parasite are directly affected by antibody, but intracellular forms are not. It is believed that cellular factors including lymphocytes and lymphokines are more important than humoral ones in mediation of effective immunity against *T. gondii*.

Immunity does not eradicate infection. Tissue cysts persist several years after acute infection. The fate of tissue cysts is not fully known. It has been proposed that tissue cysts may at times rupture during the life of the host. The released bradyzoites may be destroyed by the host's immune responses. The reaction may cause local necrosis accompanied by inflammation. Hypersensitivity plays a major role in such reactions. However, after such events, inflammation usually subsides with no local renewed multiplication of *T. gondii* in the tissue, but occasionally there may be formation of new tissue cysts.

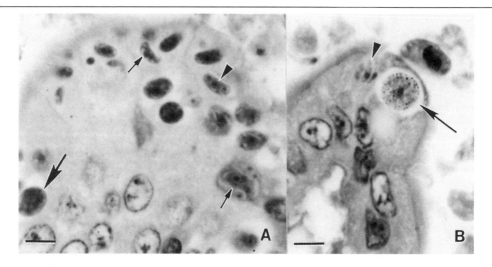

FIG. 17.17—Enteroepithelial stages of *T. gondii* in small intestine of a naturally infected Pallas cat. (Hematoxylin and eosin stain.) (Bar = 10 μm) (**A**) Numerous parasites at the tip of the villous. Note two immature female gamonts (small arrows), a three-nucleated schizont (arrowhead), and probably a microgamont (large arrow). (**B**) An oocyst (large arrow) and merozoites (arrowhead) at the tip of the villus.

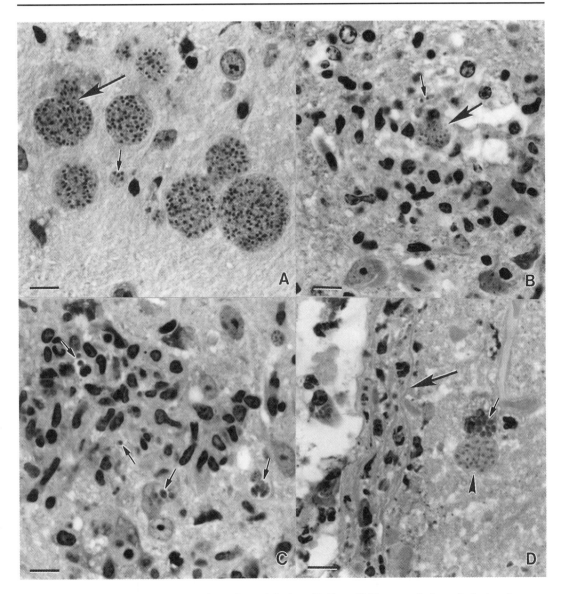

FIG. 17.18—Severe encephalitis in a mouse 8 months postinfection with *T. gondii*. The mouse had neurologic signs for several weeks. (Hemotoxylin and eosin stain.) (Bar = 10 μm) (**A**) A cluster of tissue cysts of varying sizes. Note a small cyst (small arrow) with four bradyzoites, each with a terminal nucleus. Also note a tissue cyst with bradyzoites adjacent to it (large arrow). (**B**) A glial nodule around a degenerating tissue cyst (large arrow). Note two bradyzoites (small arrow), each with a terminal nucleus near the degenerating tissue cyst. (**C**) Glial nodule with tachyzoites (arrows). (**D**) Necrosis of a meningeal blood vessel (large arrow), a tissue cyst (arrowhead), and a group of tachyzoites (small arrow) in the necrotic tissue.

In immunosuppressed patients, such as those given large doses of immunosuppressive agents in preparation for organ transplants and those with acquired immunodeficiency syndrome (AIDS), rupture of a tissue cyst may result in transformation of bradyzoites into tachyzoites and then renewed multiplication. The immunosuppressed host may die from toxoplasmosis unless treated. It is not known how corticosteroids cause relapse, but it is unlikely that they directly cause rupture of the tissue cysts.

Pathogenicity of *T. gondii* is determined by the pathogenicity of the strain and the susceptibility of the host species. *Toxoplasma gondii* strains may vary in their pathogenicity in a given host. Certain species are genetically resistant to clinical toxoplasmosis. For example, adult rats do not become ill, while the young rats can die because of toxoplasmosis. Mice of any age are susceptible to clinical *T. gondii* infection. Adult dogs, like adult rats, are resistant, whereas puppies are fully susceptible. Cattle and horses are among the hosts more resistant to *T. gondii,* whereas certain marsupials and New World monkeys are the most susceptible to *T. gondii* infection (Dubey and Beattie 1988).

Various factors vaguely classified as stress may affect *T. gondii* infection in a host. More severe infections are found in pregnant or lactating mice than in nonlactating mice. Concomitant infection may make the host more susceptible or resistant to *T. gondii* infection. Clinical toxoplasmosis in dogs and other canids is often associated with canine distemper virus infection.

Public Health Concerns. *Toxoplasma gondii* infection is widespread among humans, and its prevalence varies widely from place to place (Dubey and Beattie 1988). In the United States and the United Kingdom it is estimated that about 9%–40% of people are infected, whereas in Central and South America and continental Europe estimates of infection range from 50% to 80%. Most infections in humans are asymptomatic, but at times the parasite can produce devastating disease. Infection may be congenitally or postnatally acquired. Congenital infection occurs only when a woman becomes infected during pregnancy, and severity of disease may depend upon the stage of pregnancy when infection occurs. While the mother rarely has symptoms of infection, she does have a temporary parasitemia. Focal lesions develop in the placenta, and the fetus may become infected. At first there is generalized infection in the fetus. Later, infection is cleared from visceral tissues and may localize in the central nervous system. A wide spectrum of clinical disease occurs in congenitally infected children. Mild disease may consist of slightly diminished vision, whereas severely diseased children may have the full tetrad of signs: retinochoroiditis, hydrocephalus, convulsions, and intracerebral calcification.

By far the most common sequel of congenital toxoplasmosis is ocular disease. Except for occasional involvement of an entire eye, in virtually all cases the disease is confined to the posterior chamber. *Toxoplasma gondii* proliferates in the retina, and this leads to inflammation in the choroid. Therefore, the disease is correctly designated as retinochoroiditis. Although severe infections may be detected at birth, milder infections may not flare up until adulthood. The socioeconomic impact of toxoplasmosis on human suffering and the cost of care of sick children, especially those with mental retardation and blindness, are enormous (Roberts et al. 1994). The testing of all pregnant women for *T. gondii* infection is compulsory in France. The cost benefits of such mass screening are being debated in many countries.

Postnatally acquired infection may be localized or generalized. Oocyst-transmitted infections may be more severe than tissue cyst–induced infections. Lymphadenitis is the most frequently observed clinical form of toxoplasmosis in man. Lymphadenopathy may be associated with fever, malaise, and fatigue; muscle pains and sore throat; and headaches. Although the condition may be benign, its diagnosis is vital in pregnant women because of the risk to the fetus.

Encephalitis is the most important manifestation of toxoplasmosis in immunosuppressed patients, although any organ may be involved. In the brain, the predominant lesion is necrosis, especially of the thalamus. Clinically, patients may have headache, disorientation, drowsiness, hemiparesis, reflex changes, and convulsions, and many may become comatose. Encephalitis is now recognized with great frequency in patients treated with immunosuppressive agents. Toxoplasmosis ranks high in the list of diseases that lead to death of patients with AIDS.

Domestic Animal Health Concerns. *Toxoplasma gondii* is capable of causing severe disease in animals other than humans. Among livestock, the greatest losses occur in sheep and goats. *Toxoplasma gondii* causes early embryonic death and resorption, fetal death and mummification, abortion, stillbirth, and neonatal death. Disease is more severe in goats than in sheep (Dubey and Beattie 1988). Outbreaks of toxoplasmosis in pigs have been reported from several countries, especially Japan. Mortality in young pigs is more common than mortality in adult pigs. Pneumonia, myocarditis, encephalitis, and placental necrosis have been reported. Cattle and horses are more resistant to clinical toxoplasmosis than any other species of livestock. Cats, like nonfeline hosts, also suffer from clinical toxoplasmosis. Affected cats may appear depressed and anorexic and die suddenly with no obvious clinical signs. Pneumonia is the most important clinical manifestation of feline toxoplasmosis. Other common clinical manifestations are hepatitis, pancreatic necrosis, myositis, myocarditis, and encephalitis.

Toxoplasmosis in Wild Animals. Clinical and subclinical toxoplasmosis have been reported in many host species. Only a few examples are given in this chapter. Reports earlier than 1988 were reviewed by Dubey and Beattie (1988) and Siim et al. (1963).

SUBCLINICAL INFECTIONS IN WILD GAME. Wild game can be a source of infection in humans, cats, and other carnivores. Serologic data (Table 17.6) show that a significant population of feral pigs, bears, and cervids are exposed to *T. gondii*. Viable *T. gondii* was demonstrated in edible tissues of red deer in New Zealand (Collins 1981) and roe deer in Germany (Entzeroth et al. 1981). In the United States, *T. gondii* was isolated from pronghorn, moose, and mule deer (Dubey 1981, 1982c) white-tailed deer (Lindsay et al. 1991), and black bears (Dubey et al. 1994, 1995a). Wapiti, pronghorn, bison, red deer, mule deer, and reindeer were also susceptible to *T. gondii* oral infection with oocysts. Thus, the potential for human infections after eating undercooked wild game appears to be high. Indeed,

TABLE 17.6—Serologic prevalence of *T. gondii* in wild game in the United States

Species	Locality	No. of Animals Examined	% Positive	Serologic Test and Titer	Reference
Black bears	Alaska	40	15	LAT (1:64)	Chomel et al. 1995
(*Ursus americanus*)	Pennsylvania	665	80	MAT (1:25)	Briscoe et al. 1993
	Pennsylvania	28	79	MAT (1:25)	Dubey et al. 1995a
	North Carolina	143	84	MAT (1:25)	Nutter et al. 1998
Grissly bears	Alaska	480	18	LAT (1:64)	Chomel et al. 1995
(*Ursus arctos*)	Alaska	892	25	MAT (1:25)	Zarnke et al. 1997
White-tailed deer	Kansas	106	44	MAT (1:25)	Brillhart et al. 1994
(*Odocoileus virginianus*)	Minnesota	1367	30	MAT (1:25)	Vanek et al., 1996
	Pennsylvania	593	60	MAT (1:25)	Humphreys et al. 1995
	Alabama	16	44	MAT (1:25)	Lindsay et al. 1991
Feral Pigs (*Sus scofa*)	Georgia	170	18.2	MAT (1:25)	Dubey et al. 1997
	California	135	13	IHAT (1:64)	Clark et al. 1983
	North and South Carolina	257	34.2	MAT (1:32)	Diderrich et al. 1996
	Florida	457	2.6	IHAT (1:64)	Burridge et al. 1979
Moose (*Alces alces*)	Nova Scotia, Canada	125	15	IHAT (1:64)	Siepierski et al. 1990
	Alaska	110	23	IHA (1:64)	Kocan et al. 1986
Bison (*Bison bison*)	Montana	93	2	MAT (1:128)	Dubey (1985)

Jordan et al. (1975) reported both *T. gondii* and *Trichinella spiralis* infections in a patient who had eaten wild bear meat, and Sacks et al. (1983) reported acute toxoplasmosis in three deer hunters in the United States, probably acquired by ingesting undercooked venison. Unpublished reports from Australia have linked toxoplasmosis in humans to eating uncooked kangaroo meat. Recently, Choi et al. (1997) reported an outbreak of toxoplasmosis in humans in Korea acquired by eating meat from a feral pig. Edelhofer et al. (1996) found indirect hemagglutination test (IHAT) antibodies in 19% of 264 wild pigs from Austria, and Dubey et al. (1997) found similar prevalence (18% of 170) in feral pigs from the United States.

FURBEARING CARNIVORES. Serologic surveys indicate that *T. gondii* infections are common in carnivores (Table 17.7). Fatal toxoplasmosis was diagnosed in animals submitted for necropsy, often for rabies examination. Most animals had concurrent distemper virus infection, which is immunosuppressive (Helmboldt and Jungherr 1955). Clinical toxoplasmosis has been reported in chinchillas from the United States (Keagy 1949; Gorham and Farrell 1955), mink from Denmark (Momberg-Jørgensen 1956) and Canada (Pridham and Belcher 1958; Pridham 1961), ferrets (*Mustela putorius furo*) from New Zealand (Thornton and Cook 1986; Thornton 1990), red fox (*Vulpes vulpes*) from Denmark (Møller 1952) and the United States (Dubey et al. 1990a; Dubey and Lin 1994), raccoons (*Procyon lotor*) from the United States (Møller and Nielsen 1964; Dubey et al. 1992d), a skunk from the United States (Diters and Nielsen 1978), and raccoon-dogs from Japan (Hirato 1939).

Clinical toxoplasmosis was diagnosed in a 6-day-old polar bear (*Thalarctos maritimus*) in Hungary (Kiss and Graf 1989). Lesions were seen in the liver, skeletal muscles, heart, retina, and brain. Pinhead-sized, grey-white foci were seen in the parenchyma of liver, pancreas, and thymus. The hepatitis was characterized by necrosis associated with protozoal tachyzoites. Organisms were also seen in the heart and skeletal muscles in association with lesions. Tissue cysts were seen in the retina and brain. Kiupel et al. (1987) reported toxoplasmosis in 9 living bears (*Ursus arctos*) from Germany; 2 of 20 other bears that died had acute primary toxoplasmosis. Necrotizing pancreatitis associated with *T. gondii* was a constant finding. In some bears only tissue cysts were seen in the brain. However, in the light of the discovery of fatal sarcocystosis in black bears and polar bears in the United States (Zeman et al. 1993; Garner et al. 1997), the diagnosis is not definitive.

Furbearing animals can often harbor live *T. gondii* without clinical signs as evidenced by serologic prevalence (Table 17.7) and by isolation of *T. gondii* from apparently normal animals (Watson and Beverley 1962; Walton and Walls 1964; Bigalke et al. 1966; Dubey et al. 1993; Smith and Frenkel 1995). Therefore, care should be taken while pelting to avoid infection with *T. gondii* because of the presence of viable organisms in subclinically infected animals (Dubey 1982d, 1983e; Dietz et al. 1993).

TOXOPLASMOSIS IN WILD FELIDS. Serologic surveys indicate widespread infection in feral cats in North America (Table 17.8) and probably other countries (Pizzi et al. 1978). Clinical toxoplasmosis rarely has

TABLE 17.7—Serologic prevalence of *T. gondii* antibodies in wild carnivorous animals

Species	Test (titer)	No. Examined	% Positive	Reference	Country
Mink (*Mustela vison*)	LAT 1:64	195	3	Henriksen et al. 1994	Denmark
	DT (?)	161	24.8	Starzyk et al. 1973	Czechoslovakia
	DT 1:16	24	54.2	Smith and Frenkel 1995	USA
	DT 1:8	29	66	Watson and Beverley 1962	England
Raccoon (*Procyon lotor*)	MAT 1:25	427	50.3	Dubey et al. 1992d	USA
	MAT 1:25	379	48.5	Mitchell et al. 1999	USA
	DT 1:16	77	23.4	Jacobs et al. 1962	USA
	MAT 1:25	20	70	Brillhart et al. 1994	USA
	MAT 1:25	188	67.0	Dubey et al. 1995b	USA
	DT 1:4	67	33	Walton and Walls 1964	USA
	DT 1.8	52	13	Smith and Frenkel 1995	USA
Coyote (*Canis latrans*)	DT 1:8	13	62	Smith and Frenkel 1995	USA
	DT 1:8	87	26	Marchiondo et al. 1976	USA
	MAT 1:25	52	62	Lindsay et al. 1996	USA
	MAT 1:25	222	59	Dubey et al. 1999b	USA
Fox, red (*Vulpes vulpes*)	DT 1:8	10	90	Smith and Frenkel 1995	USA
	MAT 1:25	283	85.9	Dubey et al. 1999b	USA
Fox, gray (*Urocyon cinereoargenteus*)	DT 1:8	4	25	Smith and Frenkel 1995	USA
	MAT 1:25	97	75.3	Dubey et al. 1999b	USA
Skunk (*Mephitis mephitis*)	DT 1:8	4	50	Smith and Frenkel 1995	USA
Opposum (*Didelphis marsupialis*)	DT 1:8	38	13	Smith and Frenkel 1995	USA

TABLE 17.8—Serologic prevalence of *T. gondii* in large feral cats in Canada and the United States

Species	No. Examined	Test	Titer	% Positive	Locality	Reference
Bob cat (*Lynx rufus*)	2	DT	1:8	50	Kansas	Smith and Frenkel 1995
	12	IHAT	1:64	72	California	Riemann et al. 1975
	15	DT	1:4	73	Georgia	Walton and Walls 1964
	86	IHAT	1:64	69	California	Franti et al. 1975
	27	DT	1:8	44	New Mexico	Marchiondo et al. 1976
	150	IHAT	1:16	18	West Virginia and Georgia	Oertley and Walls 1980
	3	IHAT	1:64	66	Florida	Burridge et al. 1979
Cougar (*Felis concolar*)	36	LAT	1:64	58	California	Paul-Murphy et al. 1994
	5	IHAT	1:64	100	British Columbia	Stephen et al. 1996
	12	MAT	1:25	92	British Columbia	Aramini et al. 1998
Panther (*Felis concolor coryi*)	56	KELA	1:48	9	Florida	Roelke et al. 1993

been diagnosed in wild felids, mostly from animals in zoos. These reports include two 4–6-month-old lions (*Panthera leo*) in captivity at the Jos Zoological Gardens, Nigeria (Ocholi et al. 1989); a 6-year-old captive pallas cat (*Felis manul*) from Milwaukee County Zoo, Milwaukee, Wisconsin (Dubey et al. 1988b); a colony of pallas cats in a California zoo (Riemann et al. 1974); a 6-month-old bobcat from Georgia (Smith et al. 1995); a 1-week-old bobcat from Montana (Dubey et al. 1987); a 9-month-old cheetah from South Africa (Van Rensburg and Silkstone 1984); and a cheetah from a Texas zoo (Cannon 1974). The bobcat from Montana was probably congenitally infected. The pallas cat from Wisconsin probably became infected by eating tissue cysts because enteroepithelial stages (Fig. 17.17A) were found in sections of small intestine. A typical finding in the pallas cat was severe *T. gondii*–associated enteritis.

Oocysts of *T. gondii* were reported from feces of naturally infected iriomote cats (*Prionailurus iriomoten-*

sis) (Akuzawa et al. 1987), jaguar (*Panthera onca*), ocelots (*Felis pardalis*), (Patton et al. 1986), cheetah (*Acinonyx jubatus*), bobcats (*Lynx rufus*) (Marchiondo et al. 1976), and Canadian lynx (*L. canadensis*) (Aramini et al. 1998). An outbreak of acute toxoplasmosis in humans was attributed to contamination of a water reservoir by oocysts shed by feral cats (Bell et al. 1995; Bowie et al. 1997).

TOXOPLASMOSIS IN MARINE MAMMALS. Migaki et al. (1977) reported toxoplasmosis in the heart and stomach of a sea lion (*Zalophus californianus*) housed in a fresh water tank, and Ratcliffe and Worth (1951) found toxoplasmosis in 1 of 43 sea lions that died in the Philadelphia Zoo. Holshuh et al. (1985) found *T. gondii* in a northern fur seal (*Callorhinus ursinus*) that died of encephalitis.

Recently toxoplasmosis has been diagnosed in Atlantic bottlenose dolphins (*Tursiops truncatu*s) from Canada (Cruickshank et al. 1990) and the United States

(Inskeep et al. 1990), two dolphins (*Stenella coeruleoalba*) from Spain (Domingo et al. 1992), and a spinner dolphin (*Stenella longirostris*) from the United States (Migaki et al. 1990).

TOXOPLASMOSIS IN WILD CERVIDS. Fatal toxoplasmosis was reported in Saiga antelope (*Saiga tatarica*) by Bulmer (1971) and Ippen et al. (1981). Burgisser (1960) reported fatal toxoplasmosis in two unnamed deer. Although fatal toxoplasmosis has not been reported in the pronghorn (*Antilocapra americana*), the pronghorn is highly susceptible to infection (Dubey et al. 1982). Generalized visceral toxoplasmosis was reported in naturally infected antelopes (Ippen et al. 1981) as well as in experimentally infected pronghorns (Dubey et al. 1982) and reindeer (Oksanen et al. 1996).

TOXOPLASMOSIS IN OTHER UNGULATES. Clinical toxoplasmosis has been reported from ungulates and nondomestic ruminants: a 1-year-old gazelle (*Gazella leptoceros*), two gerenuk (*Litocranius walleri*), and one dama gazelle (*Gazalle dama*) from White Oak Plantation, Florida (Stover et al. 1990). Junge et al. (1992) diagnosed fatal disseminated toxoplasmosis in a Cuvier's gazelle (*Gazella cuvieri*) from a zoo in St. Louis, Missouri. Results of histopathologic examination suggested that the animal had recently acquired toxoplasmosis. Stiglmair-Herb (1987) reported toxoplasmosis in four gazelles that died in Germany.

TOXOPLASMOSIS IN SMALL MAMMALS. Asymptomatic *T. gondii* infections are widely prevalent in many small mammals including rats (Dubey 1983g; Dubey and Beattie 1988; Dubey and Frenkel 1998), various species of mice (Dubey and Beattie 1988; Brillhart et al. 1994; Smith and Frenkel 1995; Dubey et al. 1995b), and rabbits (Cox et al. 1981; Dubey and Beattie 1988), but clinical toxoplasmosis is relatively rare. We are not aware of any reports of clinical toxoplasmosis in naturally infected rats and mice. Epizootics of toxoplasmosis have been reported from rabbits and hares, mainly from Scandinavia (Christiansen and Siim 1951; Møller 1958; Andersson and Andersson 1963; Siim et al. 1963; Gustafsson et al. 1988), and there are occasional reports from other countries (Shimizu 1958; Harcourt 1967; Nobel et al. 1969; Dubey et al. 1992a; Leland et al. 1992). Gustafsson and Uggla (1994) did not find antibodies to *T. gondii* in 176 brown hares (*Lepus europaeus*) from Sweden, suggesting that this animal is highly susceptible to *T. gondii* and that perhaps the disease is fatal in most of them.

Other reports of fatal toxoplasmosis include neurologic disease in a porcupine (*Erethizon dorsatum*) (Medway et al. 1989), tree hyrax (*Dendrohyrax robustus*) (Olubayo and Karstad 1981), chinchillas (Keagy 1949; Ratcliffe and Worth 1951), guinea pigs (Markham 1937; Rodaniche and Pinzon 1949; Green and Morgan 1991), squirrels (Soave and Lennette 1959; Van Pelt and Dieterich 1972; Roher et al. 1981), and a penguin from New Zealand (Mason et al. 1991).

TOXOPLASMOSIS IN MONKEYS. New World monkeys are highly susceptible to clinical toxoplasmosis, whereas Old World monkeys are resistant. Reports up to 1987 were summarized by Dubey and Beattie (1988) and are not repeated here. Recent reports of acute toxoplasmosis in New World monkeys are those of Dietz et al. (1997) from Denmark and Cunningham et al. (1992) from England.

TOXOPLASMOSIS IN MARSUPIALS. Toxoplasmosis is a serious disease of Australasian marsupials, and there are numerous reports of deaths in zoos (see Table 17.9). Even animals in the wild can die of toxoplasmosis (Attwood et al. 1975; Obendorf and Munday 1983, 1990). Animals can die suddenly, without clinical signs, or have neurological signs, loss of vision, diarrhea, and respiratory distress. Virtually any organ of the body can be affected. Clinical signs and necropsy findings in a variety of marsupials can be found in the report of Canfield et al. (1990). In addition to reports summarized in Table 17.9, Hartley (1993) found *T. gondii* encephalitis in an unknown number of brush-tail possum in eastern Australia. *Toxoplasma gondii* has been isolated from tissues of a number of Australian marsupials, including bandicoots (*Thylacis obestus*) (Cook and Pope 1959; Pope et al. 1957a,b). Gibb et al. (1966) found *T. gondii* infection in 32 apparently normal quokkas (*Setonix brachurus*) on Rottnest Island. Attwood et al. (1975) found *T. gondii* infection in 122 of 240 (51%) dasyurids from Australia. Most of these animals were not ill at the time of examination; 4 had lesions in the eyes, and 14 had difficulty in walking. In general, kangaroos are able to survive with toxoplasmosis, whereas wallabies often die because of toxoplasmosis. Recently Bourne (1997) found that a population of Bennett's wallabies in a zoological park in England had high antibody titers to *T. gondii* without obvious illness.

Antibodies to *T. gondii* were found in certain species of wallabies. Attwood et al. (1975) found dye test antibodies (1:4 to 1:4096) in 13 of 15 dasyurids (*Dasyuroides byrnei* and *Dasycercus cristicauda*). High levels of *T. gondii* antibodies were found in adult black-faced kangaroos in a zoo (Dubey et al. 1988c), indicating that not all exposed wallabies die of toxoplasmosis. The type of serologic test used and the dilution of the serum tested are important. Jakob-Hoff and Dunsmore (1983) found antibodies in 2 of 25 tammar wallabies but not in any of 26 black-flanked rock wallabies or 3 bandicoots using the indirect hemagglutination test (IHAT). Because the IHAT is insensitive for the diagnosis of toxoplasmosis in animals in general, it is not known if these differences in seroprevalence of *T. gondii* in various species of kangaroos were real.

Little is known of the specificity and sensitivity of different serologic tests for the detection of antibodies to *T. gondii* in kangaroos. Johnson et al. (1988) evaluated ELISA in naturally infected animals. They isolated *T. gondii* from brains of 4 of 17 Tasmanian pademelons and 6 of 17 Bennett's wallabies, and they

TABLE 17.9—Summary of reports of clinical toxoplasmosis in Australasian marsupials

Country/Location	No. and Type of Marsupials	Main Findings	Reference
Australia			
Taronga Zoo, Sydney, and Zoo Pathology Registry	43 Macropods, 2 wombats, 2 koalas, 6 possums, 15 dasyurids, 2 numbats, 8 bandicoots, 1 bilby	Clinical signs, lesions, immunohistochemistry (IHC)	Canfield et al. 1990
Melbourne area	122 Dasyurids (several genera) (17 clinical signs)	Histologic, serologic, bioassay	Attwood and Wooley 1970; Attwood et al. 1975
Queensland	1 Yellow-footed rock wallaby (*Petrogale xanthopus*)	Histology	Phillips 1986
Sydney	2 Koalas (*Phascolarctos cinereus*)	Histologic, IHC	Hartley et al. 1990
Victoria	1 Wombatt (*Vombattus ursinus*)	Histology, serology	Skerratt et al. 1997
Victoria	1 Bandicoot (*Perameles gunnii*)	Histology	Lenghaus et al. 1990
Tasmania	2 Tasmanian pademelons (*Thylogale billardierii*)	Clinical signs in wild animals, histology	Obendorf and Munday 1983
Tasmania	3 Eastern barred bandicoots (*Perameles gunnii*)	Clinical signs, histology	Obendorf and Munday 1990
	8 Eastern barred bandicoots (*Perameles gunnii*)	Clinical signs, histology, serology	Obendorf et al. 1996 Johnson et al. 1989
	4 Tasmanian pademelons (*Thylogale billardierii*)	Clinical signs, histology, serology	
Austria	1 Macropod *(Macropus rufogriseus)*	Histologic	Grünberg 1959
Germany			
(Berlin-Friedrichsfelde Zoo) Berlin Zoo	4 Bennett's wallaby (*Macropus rufogriseus*)	Clinical signs, lesions, histology	Hilgenfeld 1965
	1 Bennett's wallaby (*Macroopus rufogriseus*)	Histology	Schmidt 1975
	15 Red kangaroos (*Macroopus rufus*)	Histology, isolation	Schröder and Ippen 1976
	3 Bennett's wallabies (*Macroopus rufogrieseus*)	Histology, isolation	
	2 Tammar wallabies (*Macropus eugenii*)		Kronberger and Schüppel 1976
	3 Kangaroos	Histology	
Dresden Zoo	Tammar wallabies (*Macropus eugenii*) also called Derby Kangaroos	Histology	Schneider et al. 1976
Thüringer Zoo Park, Erfurt	5 Bennett's wallabies (*Macropus rufogrieseus*)	Histology	Altmann and Schüppel 1988
Hungary (Budapest Zoo)	3 Derby kangaroos or Tammar wallabies (*Thylogale eugenii* or *Macropus eugenii*)	Clinical signs, histologic, epidemiologic	Dobos-Kovács et al. 1974a,b
Italy	3 Bennett's wallabies (*Macropus rufogriseus*)	Clinical signs, lesions, bioassay, serology	Mandelli et al. 1966
USA			
California Zoo	4 Wallaroos (*Macropus robustus*)	Histologic, serologic	Boorman et al. 1977
Chicago, Illinois Brookfield Zoo	1 infant black-faced kangaroo (*macropus fuliginosus melanops*)	Clinical signs, serology, histology	Dubey et al. 1988c
Tennessee Knoxville Zoo	5 long-nosed rat kangaroos (*Potorous tridactylus*), 3 Tammar wallabies (*Wallabia eugenii* or *Macropus eugenii*), 3 grey kangaroos (*Macropus giganteus*), 2 red kangaroos (*Macropus rufus*)	Clinical signs, lesions, chemotherapy	Patton et al. 1986, Jensen et al. 1985
Missouri (Exotic farm)	7 Bennett's wallabies (*Macropus rufogriseus*)	Clinical signs, histology, IHC, treatment	Miller et al. 1992
San Francisco Zoo	1 Koala (*Phascolarctos cinereus*)	Disseminated infection, histology, IHC	Dubey et al. 1991b
	1 Parma wallaby (*Macropus parma*)	Histologic lesions	Wilhelmsen and Montali 1980
	1 swamp wallaby (*Protemnodon bicolor* or *Wallabia bicolor*)	Histology	Thompson and Reed 1957
United Kingdom			
Zoological Garden, London, and Whipsnade Wild Animal Park	3 Mitchell's wombat or common wombat (*Phascolom mitchelli* or *Vambatus ursinus*)	Histologic	Hamerton 1932, 1933, 1934; Coutelen 1932
Whipsnade Wild Animal Park,	3 Bennett's wallabies (*Macropus rufugriseus*)	Ocular	Ashton 1979
Bedfordshire, England	21 Bennett's wallabies (*Macropus rufogriseus*)	Clinical signs, lesions IHC, histology, cytology	Bourne 1997

used sera from *T. gondii*–infected animals to standard-ize their ELISA. They found antibodies in 5 of 151 *Macropus rufogriseus* and 15 of 85 *Thylogale bil-lardierii*. They further evaluated the direct agglutina-tion test (DAT) in experimentally infected animals (Johnson et al. 1989).

Although the modified direct agglutination test (MAT) is a sensitive and specific test, it only measures IgG antibodies. Therefore, MAT may be falsely nega-tive during acute toxoplasmosis because the 2M mer-captoethanol used in the test destroys both specific and nonspecific IgM. Therefore, a direct agglutination test (DAT) without mercaptoethanol has been used by some researchers to measure IgM-associated serologic response. In experimentally infected eastern grey kan-garoo (*Macropus giganteus*) (Johnson et al. 1989) and tammar wallaby (*Macropus eugenii*) (Lynch et al. 1993), antibodies (presumably specific IgM) to *T. gondii* were detected 7 to 10 days after infection in the DAT but not in the MAT. Thus, some macropods may die of acute toxoplasmosis without detectable IgG anti-bodies (Obendorf et al. 1996). Skerratt et al. (1997) diagnosed acute toxoplasmosis in a wombat without MAT antibodies in serum; the diagnosis was confirmed histologically.

Obendorf et al. (1996) compared survival and trapa-bility in 150 *T. gondii* seropositive and seronegative eastern barred bandicoots (*Perameles gunnii*) trapped at two sites in Tasmania. Sera were screened both by DAT and MAT in 1:64 serum dilution. Antibodies to *T. gondii* were not detected by DAT and MAT in sera from 133 (89%) bandicoots and 68% of seronegative animals that were retrapped. Seven (4.6%) animals were classified as suspicious because they were posi-tive by DAT but not by MAT, and none of these animals were retrapped. Ten (6.7%) animals were positive by both DAT and MAT. Five of these were not retrapped, but the other 5 bandicoots had antibodies on two bleed-ings 3 months apart. One bandicoot with a DAT and a MAT titer of 1:256 died in a trap and had histologically proven *T. gondii* infection in the brain, heart, lung, and skeletal muscles. One seropositive bandicoot devel-oped neurologic signs but was not available for necropsy. The authors concluded that most *T. gondii* infected bandicoots die in nature, but occasionally they remain asymptomatic. They also found that some bandicoots with low or moderate titers (not specified) in DAT but negative by MAT became seronegative by DAT on subsequent samplings. Thus, DAT can give false positive results.

Little is known of treatment and prophylaxis. Treat-ment with standard antitoxoplasmic therapy (sulfadi-azine and pyrimethamine) had some success in treating clinical toxoplasmosis in a zoo (Jensen et al. 1985). However, there has not been any controlled study of treatment in marsupials. Treatment with atovaquine was recently reported to have saved wallabies from imminent death and to have restored health, including recovery from blindness (Crutchley et al. 1997).

Vaccination with a live, modified, nonpersistent strain of *T. gondii* (e.g., S-48 strain used for vaccine in sheep) was lethal in tammar wallabies (Lynch et al. 1993). Some success was achieved in vaccination with the related coccidian *Hammondia hammondi* (Redda-cliff et al., 1993a,b). However, it is unlikely that there will be enough commercial interest in this vaccine. Therefore, the only rational approach is to prevent con-tamination of food and water *with T. gondii* oocysts.

Diagnosis. Diagnosis is made by biologic, serologic, or histologic methods or by some combination of them. Clinical signs of toxoplasmosis are nonspecific and cannot be depended upon for a definite diagnosis because toxoplasmosis mimics several other infectious diseases.

The isolation of *T. gondii* from patients by inocula-tion of laboratory animals and tissue cultures is a defin-itive way of diagnosis. Secretions, excretions, body flu-ids, and tissues taken by biopsy antemortem or tissues with macroscopic lesions taken postmortem are all pos-sible specimens from which to attempt isolation of *T. gondii*.

Mice are highly susceptible to *T. gondii* infection, and *T. gondii* grows virtually in all cell lines (Fig. 17.18A,B). Finding *T. gondii* antibody can aid diagnosis. There are numerous serologic procedures used to detect humoral antibodies (Dubey and Beattie 1988); these include the Sabin-Feldman dye test (DT), the indirect hemagglutination test (IHAT), the indirect fluorescent antibody test (IFAT), the modified direct agglutination test (MAT), the latex agglutination test (LAT), the enzyme-linked immunoabsorbent assay (ELISA), and the immunoabsorbent agglutination assay test (IAAT). Of these, IFAT, IAAT, and ELISA have been modified to detect IgM antibodies. The IgM anti-bodies appear sooner than the IgG antibodies, but IgM antibodies also disappear faster than IgG antibodies.

One positive serum sample only establishes that the host has been infected at some time in the past. It is best to collect two samples on the same individual. A 16-fold higher antibody titer in a serum taken 2–4 weeks after the first serum was collected indicates an acutely acquired infection. A high antibody titer some-times persists for months, and a rise may not be associ-ated with clinical signs.

Diagnosis can be made by finding *T. gondii* in host tissue removed by biopsy or at necropsy. A rapid diag-nosis may be made by making impression smears of lesions on glass slides. After drying 10–30 minutes, the smears are fixed in methyl alcohol and stained with Giemsa. Well-preserved *T. gondii* are crescent-shaped and stain well with any of the Romanowsky stains (Fig. 17.19C). However, degenerating organisms, which are commonly found in lesions, usually appear oval, and their cytoplasm stains poorly as compared to their nuclei. Diagnosis should not be made unless organisms with typical structure are located because degenerating host cells may resemble degenerating *T.*

gondii. In sections, the tachyzoites usually do not stain differently from host cells. Electron microscopy can aid diagnosis. *Toxoplasma gondii* tachyzoites are always located in vacuoles and have a few (usually four) rhoptries, often with honeycomb structure (Fig. 17.13). Tissue cysts are without septa and have a thin cyst wall butted against the host cell plasmalemma (Fig. 17.13). Occasionally, tissue cysts might be found in areas with lesions. Tissue cysts are usually spherical and have silver positive walls, and the bradyzoites are strongly PAS positive (Fig. 17.14). The immunohistochemical staining of parasites with *T. gondii* antiserum can aid in diagnosis (Fig. 17.19C).

Treatment. Sulfadiazine and pyrimethamine (Daraprim) are two drugs widely used for therapy of toxoplasmosis. These two drugs act synergistically by blocking the metabolic pathway involving aminobenzoic acid and the folic-folinic acid cycle, respectively. These drugs are usually well tolerated, but sometimes thrombocytopenia or leukopenia may develop. These effects can be overcome by administering folinic acid and yeast without interfering with treatment because the vertebrate host can utilize presynthesized folinic acid while *T. gondii* cannot. While these drugs have a beneficial action when given in the acute stage of the disease process when there is active multiplication of the parasite, they will not usually eradicate infection and are not effective in the chronic phase.

Because pyrimethamine is toxic, some clinicians use a combination of trimethoprim and sulfamethoxazole as possible alternatives to pyrimethamine and sulfadiazine.

Epidemiology. The relative frequency of acquisition of postnatal toxoplasmosis due to eating raw meat and that due to ingestion of food contaminated by oocysts from cat feces is not known and is difficult to investigate. *Toxoplasma gondii* infection is common in many animals used for food. Sheep, pigs, and rabbits are commonly infected throughout the world. Infection in cattle is less prevalent than in sheep or pigs (Jacobs et al. 1960b; Dubey and Beattie 1988; Dubey et al. 1992b). Infection is common in rabbits throughout the world (Dubey 1982c, 1983f; Reed and Turk 1985; Williamson et al. 1980). *Toxoplasma gondii* tissue cysts survive years in live food animals (Dubey 1988; Dubey and Beattie 1988). As stated earlier, humans can acquire infection by eating raw or undercooked meat.

Oocysts are shed by cats, not only by the domestic cat but also by other cats like ocelots, jaguars, marguays, jaguarundi, bobcats, and Bengal tigers and by iriomote and Pallas cats. Oocyst formation, however, is greatest in the domestic cat. Widespread natural infection is possible since a cat may excrete millions of oocysts after ingesting one infected mouse. Oocysts are resistant to most ordinary environmental conditions and can survive months or years in moist conditions.

Invertebrates like flies, cockroaches, dung beetles, and earthworms can mechanically spread oocysts.

Only a few cats may be involved in the spread of *T. gondii* at any given time: as few as 1% of the domestic cat population may be shedding oocysts at any given time.

Prevention and Control. To prevent infection of human beings by *T. gondii,* hands should be washed thoroughly with soap and water after handling meat. All cutting boards, sink tops, knives, and other materials coming in contact with uncooked meat should be washed with soap and water. This is effective because the stages of *T. gondii* in meat are killed by soap and water. Meat of any animal should be cooked to 67° C before consumption, and tasting meat while cooking or seasoning homemade sausages should be avoided. Pregnant women, especially, should avoid contact with cats, soil, raw meat, and aborted animals. Pet cats should be fed only dry, canned, or cooked food. The cat litter box should be emptied daily, preferably not by a pregnant woman. Gloves should be worn while gardening. Vegetables should be washed thoroughly before eating because they may have been contaminated with cat feces. Expectant mothers should be aware of the dangers of toxoplasmosis.

Cats should never be fed uncooked meat, viscera, or bones, and efforts should be made to keep cats indoors to prevent hunting. Because cats cannot utilize plant sources of vitamin A, some owners feed raw liver to improve their cat's coat. This practice should be discontinued because (1) *T. gondii* tissue cysts frequently are found in the liver of food animals, and (2) cat foods contain most essential nutrients cats need. Trash cans also should be covered to prevent scavenging. Although freezing can kill most *T. gondii* tissue cysts, it cannot be relied on to kill them all.

Cats should be neutered to control the feline population on farms. Dead animals should be removed promptly to prevent cannibalism by animals and scavenging by cats.

To prevent infection of zoo animals with *T. gondii,* cats, including all wild Felidae, should be housed in a building separate from other animals, particularly marsupials and New World monkeys. Cats as a rule should not be fed uncooked meat. However, if a choice has to be made, frozen meat is less likely to contain live *T. gondii* than fresh meat, and beef is less likely to contain *T. gondii* than is horse meat, pork, or mutton. Dissemination of *T. gondii* oocysts in zoos should be prevented because of potential exposure of children. Brooms, shovels, and other equipment used to clean cat cages and cat enclosures should be autoclaved or heated to 67° C at least 10 minutes at regular intervals. Animal caretakers should wear masks and protective clothing while cleaning cages. Feline feces should be removed daily to prevent sporulation of oocysts.

At present there is no vaccine to control toxoplasmosis in humans, cats, or wild animals.

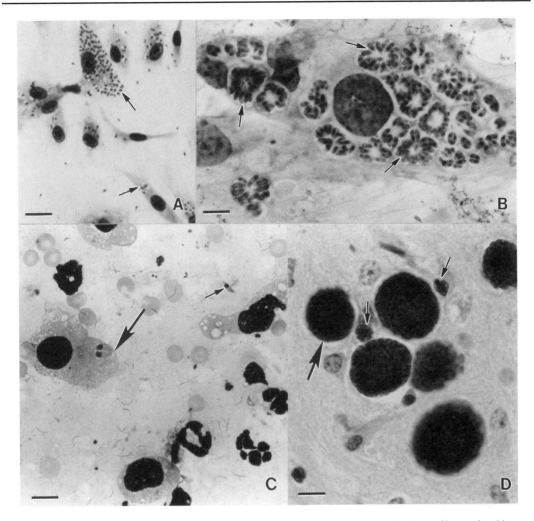

FIG. 17.19—*Toxoplasma gondii* stages in in vitro and in vivo preparations. (**A**) Tachyzoites in culture of human foreskin fibroblasts cells. Smear. (Giemsa stain.) (Bar = 25 μm) (**B**) Rosettes of tachyzoites in human foreskin fibroblasts. Smear. (Immunohistochemical stain with anti-tachyzoite specific antibody.) (Bar = 10 μm) (**C**) Tachyzoites in a cytospin smear of pleural fluid from a cat with pneumonia. Compare the size of tachyzoites (arrow) with host cells. (Giemsa stain.) (Bar = 10 μm) (**D**) Tachyzoites (small arrows) and tissue cysts (large arrow) in section of mouse brain. (Immunohistochemical stain with *T. gondii*-specific antibody.) (Bar = 10 μm)

NEOSPORA CANINUM AND NEOSPOROSIS. *Neospora caninum* is a recently recognized organism, structurally and biologically similar to *T. gondii* (Dubey 1999; Dubey et al. 1988a, 1999a,b; Dubey and Lindsay 1996). Until 1988, it was misdiagnosed as *T. gondii*. Its life cycle was unknown until recently. In 1998 dogs were found to be the defintive hosts *N. caninum*. *Neospora caninum* oocysts are structurally identical with *T. gondii* (McAllister et al. 1998). Congenital transmission is the only recognized route of infection in nature. It can cause neurologic and other signs in cattle, sheep, goats, horses, and dogs, and experimentally

the parasite has a wide host range (Dubey and Lindsay 1996).

There are two reports of clinical neosporosis in wild deer. *Neospora caninum* were found in sections of lung, liver, and kidneys in a 2-month-old female black-tailed deer (*Odocoileus hemionus columbianus*) found dead in California (Woods et al. 1994). Tachyzoites were most numerous in lung tissue and were associated with interstitial pneumonia. The nephritis was characterized by interstitial inflammation and tubular necrosis, and tachyzoites were seen in tubular epithelium and tubular lumina. In the liver,

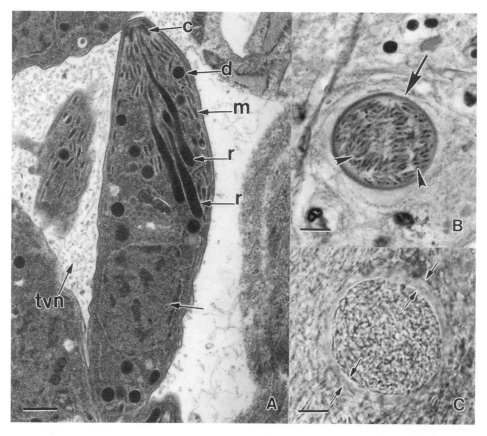

FIG. 17.20—Stages of *Neospora caninum*. (**A**) Transmission electron micrograph of a tachyzoite in cell culture. Note a conoid (**c**), electron-dense rhoptries (**r**), dense granules (**d**), nucleus (**n**), and tubulovesicular network (**tvn**) in the parasitophorous vacuole. (Photo courtesy of Dr. D.S. Lindsay, Virginia Polytech, Blacksburg, Virginia) (Bar = 0.4 μm). (**B**) A tissue cyst in section of spinal cord of a naturally infected calf. Note cyst wall (arrow) thicker than the bradyzoites (arrowheads). (Hematoxylin and eosin stain.) (Bar = 10 μm) (**C**) A tissue in squash preparation of brain of an experimentally infected mouse. Note thick cyst wall (opposing arrows). (Unstained.) (Bar = 10 μm)

tachyzoites were within hepatocytes and Kupffer cells and in sinusoids.

The second report is from France in a full-term stillborn deer (*Cervus eldi siamensis*) from the Paris Zoo (Dubey et al. 1996a). *Neospora caninum* tissue cysts were found associated with nonsuppurative encephalitis. Neosporosis was thought to be the main disease affecting the decline of this endangered species in the zoo. Recently, antibodies to *N. caninum* were found in 40.5% of 400 white-tailed deer from Illinois (Dubey et al. 1999a).

Neospora caninum tachyzoites are structurally identical to *T. gondii* under the light microscope. Ultrastructurally, the rhoptries in *N. caninum* are more numerous and are electron dense (Fig. 17.20), whereas those of *T. gondii* are honeycombed. Tissue cysts of *N. caninum* have thicker walls than those of *T. gondii* (Fig. 17.20). Immunohistochemical tests and serologic tests can distinguish between *N. caninum* and *T. gondii* (Dubey and Lindsay 1996).

SARCOCYSTIS AND SARCOCYSTOSIS

Etiologic Agent. *Sarcocystis* Lankester, 1882 was first reported by Miescher (1843), who described "milky white threads" in the skeletal muscle of a house mouse *M. musculus* (Dubey 1991, 1993) (Fig. 17.21), in Switzerland.

Sarcocysts (in Greek *Sarkos* = flesh, *kystis* = bladder) are the terminal asexual stage and are found encysted, primarily in striated muscles of mammals, birds, marsupials, and poikilothermic animals. These animals are the intermediate hosts. The numbers and distribution of sarcocysts in the body vary greatly from host to host. In addition to their presence in skeletal muscle, sarcocysts occur in the central nervous system, and in Purkinje fibers of the heart, and in muscle bundles.

Sarcocysts vary in size and shape, depending on the species of the parasite. Some always remain microscopic (Fig. 17.22), whereas others become macro-

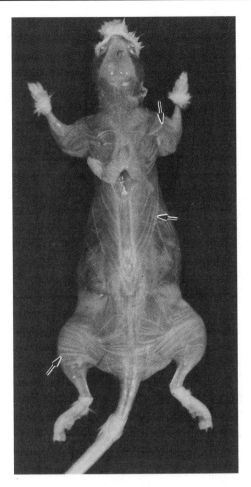

FIG. 17.21—Carcass of a mouse infected with *Sarcocystis muris*. Note macroscopic (arrows) thread-like sarcocysts. Sarcocysts may occupy as much as 25% of the muscle mass yet the mouse may show no obvious clinical signs.

scopic. Microscopic sarcocysts vary from very long and narrow to short and wide. Macroscopic sarcocysts appear filamentous, like rice grains, or globular.

Sarcocystis has an obligatory prey-predator, two-host, life cycle (Fig. 17.23). Asexual stages develop only in the intermediate host, which in nature is often a prey animal. Sexual stages develop only in the definitive host, which is carnivorous. There are different intermediate and definitive hosts for each species of *Sarcocystis*. For example, there are three named species of *Sarcocystis* in cattle: *S. cruzi, S. hirsuta,* and *S. hominis*. The definitive host for these species are Canidae, Felidae, and primates, respectively. In the following description of the life cycle and structure of *Sarcocystis, S. cruzi* will serve as the example.

Dogs, coyotes, and foxes and possibly wolves, jackals, and raccoons are the definitive hosts, whereas bison (*Bison bison*) and cattle (*Bos taurus*) are the

intermediate hosts for *S. cruzi*. The definitive host becomes infected by ingesting muscular or neural tissue containing mature sarcocysts. Bradyzoites liberated from the sarcocyst by digestion in the stomach and intestine penetrate the mucosa of the small intestine and transform into male (micro) and female (macro) gamonts. Within 6 hours after ingestion of infected tissue, gamonts are found within a parasitophorous vacuole (PV) in goblet cells near the tips of villi. Macrogamonts are ovoid to round, are 10 to 20 μm in diameter, and contain a single nucleus. Microgamonts are ovoid to elongated and contain one to several nuclei. The microgamont nucleus divides into several nuclei (usually up to 15), and as the microgamont matures the nuclei move toward the periphery of the gamont. In *S. cruzi,* mature microgamonts which are about 7 x 5 μm, contain 3 to 11 slender gametes. The microgametes, which are about 4 x 0.5 μm in size, consist of a compact nucleus and two flagella. Microgametes liberated from the microgamont actively move to the periphery of the macrogamont. After fertilization, a wall develops around the zygote, and the oocyst is formed. The entire process of gametogony and fertilization can be completed within 24 hours, and gamonts and oocysts may be found at the same time. The location of gametogony and the type of cell parasitized varies with species of *Sarcocystis* and the stage of gametogenesis.

Sarcocystis oocysts sporulate in the lamina propria. The inner mass of the oocyst (sporont) divides into two sporocysts. Four sporozoites are formed in each sporocyst. Because sporulation is asynchronous, unsporulated and sporulated oocysts are found simultaneously (Fig. 17.24). Sporulated oocysts are generally colorless and thin-walled (< 1 μm) and contain two elongate sporocysts. Each sporocyst contains four elongated sporozoites and a granular sporocyst residuum, which may be compact or dispersed. There is no Stieda body. Each sporozoite has a central to terminal nucleus, several cytoplasmic granules, and a crystalloid body, but there is no refractile body.

The oocyst wall is thin and often ruptures. Free sporocysts, released into the intestinal lumen, are passed in the feces. Occasionally unsporulated and partially sporulated oocysts are shed in the feces. The prepatent and patent periods vary, but for most *Sarcocystis* species oocysts are first shed in feces between 7 and 14 days after sarcocyst ingestion.

The intermediate host becomes infected by ingesting sporocysts in food or water. Sporozoites excyst from sporocysts in the small intestine. The fate of the sporozoite from the time of ingestion of the sporocyst until initial development in the mesenteric lymph node arteries is not known. First-generation merogony begins in endothelial cells as early as 7 days postinoculation and may be completed as early as 15 days postinoculation. Second-generation meronts have been seen in endothelium from 19 to 46 days postinoculation, predominantly in capillaries but also in small arteries, virtually throughout the body.

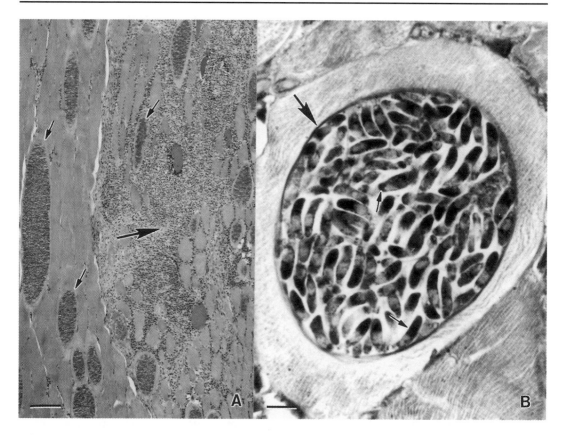

FIG. 17.22—*Sarcocystis muris* in sections of muscles of a mouse. (**A**) An area of granulomatous myositis (large arrow) around sarcocysts and several intact sarcocysts (small arrows). (Hematoxylin and eosin stain.) (Bar = 100 μm) (**B**) A sarcocyst in a myocyte. Note thin cyst wall (arrow) and numerous banana-shaped bradyzoites (small arrows). (Giemsa stain.) (Bar = 10 μm)

The meronts divide by endopolygeny. The nucleus becomes lobulated and divides into several nuclei (up to 37). Merozoites form at the periphery. The shape and size of schizonts (meronts) vary considerably (Fig. 17.25). Meronts in skeletal muscle are longer than those in other tissues. Both first and second generation meronts are located within the host cytoplasm and are not surrounded by a PV. *Sarcocystis* sp. merozoites have the same organelles as *T. gondii* tachyzoites, except that there are no rhoptries (Fig. 17.26).

Merozoites are found in peripheral blood 24 to 46 days postinoculation, coincident with the maturation of second generation meronts. Merozoites in blood are extracellular or located within unidentified mononuclear cells. Intracellular merozoites contain one or two nuclei, and some divide into two, apparently by endodyogeny.

The number of generations of merogony and the type of host cell in which merogony may occur vary with each species of *Sarcocystis,* but trends are apparent. For example, all species of *Sarcocystis* of large domestic animals (sheep, goats, cattle, pigs, horses) form first and second generation meronts in vascular endothelium, whereas only a single precystic generation of merogony has been found in *Sarcocystis* species of small mammals (mice, deer mice) and this is generally in hepatocytes.

Merozoites liberated from the terminal generation of merogony initiate sarcocyst formation. The intracellular merozoite surrounded by a PV becomes round to ovoid, forming a metrocyte that undergoes repeated divisions. Eventually the sarcocyst is filled with bradyzoites, which are the infective stage for the predator. Sarcocysts generally become infectious at about 75 days postinoculation, but in this there is considerable variation among species of *Sarcocystis.* Immature sarcocysts containing only metrocytes, and meronts are not infectious for the definitive host. There is no lactogenous transmission.

Sarcocysts are always located within a PV in the host cell cytoplasm. More than one sarcocyst may be found in one host cell. The sarcocyst consists of a cyst wall that surrounds the parasitic metrocyte or zoite stages. The structure and thickness of the cyst wall differs among species of *Sarcocystis* and within each species as the sarcocyst matures. A connective tissue wall (sec-

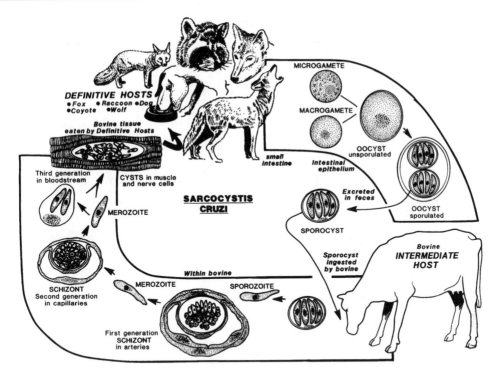

FIG. 17.23—Life cycle of *Sarcocystis cruzi.*

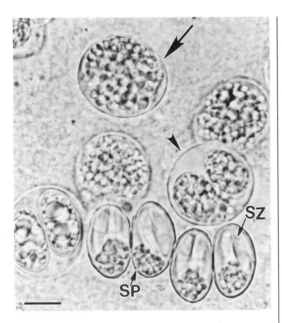

FIG. 17.24—Sporogony of *S. cruzi* in the intestine of a coyote. Note an unsporulated oocyst (large arrow), an oocyst with two sporocysts (arrowhead), and two sporulated oocysts containing mature sporocysts (**sp**) and sporozoites (**sz**). (Unstained) (Bar = 10 μm)

ondary sarcocyst wall) surrounds the *S. gigantea, S. moulei, S. hardangeri,* and *S. rangiferi* sarcocysts. Histologically, the sarcocyst wall may be smooth, striated, or hirsute or may possess complex branched protrusions (Fig. 17.27). Internally, groups of zoites are divided among compartments by septa that originate from the sarcocyst wall. Septa are present in all but a few species of *Sarcocystis.* The structure of the parasites within the sarcocysts changes with the maturation of the sarcocyst. Immature sarcocysts contain metrocytes (mother cells). Each metrocyte produces two progeny metrocytes by endodyogeny. After what appear to be several such generations, some of the metrocytes, through the process of endodyogeny, produce banana-shaped zoites called bradyzoites (also called cystozoites). The bradyzoites contain prominent amylopectin granules that stain bright red when treated with the PAS reagents. Even mature sarcocysts may contain some peripherally arranged metrocytes (Fig. 17.27).

Sarcocystis species have the organelles that are characteristic of the phylum Apicomplexa such as apical rings (also called conoidal or preconoidal rings), polar rings, conoid pellicle, subpellicular microtubules, micropores, and micronemes. The ultrastructure of the mature sarcocyst wall is of taxonomic value. The structure of the sarcocyst wall may vary with stage of development. Sarcocyst development begins when a merozoite enters a muscle or nerve cell. The merozoite

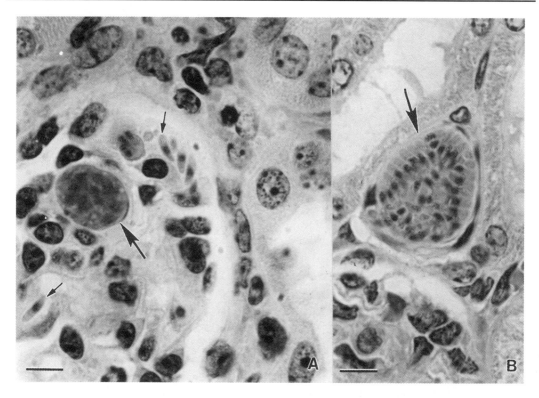

FIG. 17.25—Second generation schizonts of *S. cruzi* in sections of an experimentally infected calf. (Hematoxylin and eosin stain.) (Bar = 10 μm) **(A)** Glomerulus with an immature multinucleated schizont (large arrow), and free merozoites (small arrows). **(B)** A schizont in a capillary endothelium in between renal tubules.

resides in a PV and is surrounded by a parasitophorous vacuolar membrane (PVM) which appears to develop into a primary sarcocyst wall. The primary sarcosyst wall consists of a PVM plus an underlying electron-dense layer. A granular layer is immediately beneath the primary sarcocyst wall. Septa which arise from the granular layer traverse the sarcocyst, separating it into compartments which contain bradyzoites and metrocytes. Dubey et al. (1989b) categorized sarcocyst walls into 24 types to aid species determination (Fig. 17.28).

Species of *Sarcocystis* are generally more specific for their intermediate hosts than for their definitive hosts (Dubey et al. 1989b). For example, for *S. cruzi* ox and bison are the only intermediate hosts, whereas dog, wolf, coyote, raccoon, jackal, and foxes can act as definitive hosts. Coyotes and foxes also serve as efficient definitive hosts for other dog-transmitted species such as *S. tenella* and *S. capracanis*. However, none of the species infective for dogs are infective for cats and vice versa.

Pathogenesis and Clinical Signs. Only some species of *Sarcocystis* are pathogenic for the intermediate hosts (Dubey et al. 1989b). Generally, species transmitted by canids are more pathogenic than those transmitted by felids. For example, of the three species in cattle, *S. cruzi* is the most pathogenic, whereas *S. hirsuta* and *S. hominis* are only mildly pathogenic.

Depending on the number of sporocysts ingested, animals may develop mild to severe anorexia, diarrhea, weight loss, weakness, muscle twitching, or prostration. Larger doses may sometimes cause death. Pregnant animals may undergo a premature parturition or abortion or produce a stillborn fetus. Some or all of those clinical signs may last for from a few days to several weeks. Clinical laboratory findings indicate that anemia, tissue damage, and clotting dysfunctions occur in infected animals.

The most striking gross lesion seen in acutely ill animals is hemorrhage. Hemorrhage may be generalized and often not associated with inflammation. Necrosis may be found in many organs, especially in skeletal muscles, heart, and kidneys, probably associated with vasculitis. The overall predominant lesions in sarcocystosis are inflammatory rather than degenerative.

Degenerating sarcocysts may be surrounded by mononuclear cells, neutrophils, eosinophils, giant cells, or a combination of these cells (Fig. 17.22). In livestock of most species, the cellular response is mainly mononuclear. A presumptive diagnosis of acute

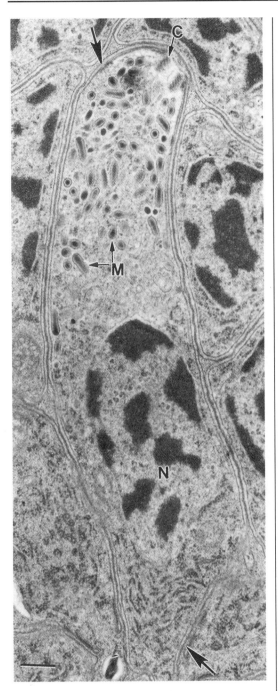

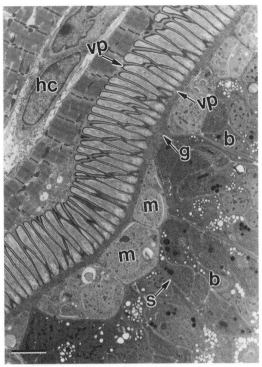

FIG. 17.27—Transmission electron micrograph of *S. hominis* showing a sarcocyst in a myocyte. Note the thick sarcocyst wall consisting of villar protrusions (**vp**) and the ground substance (**g**) projecting into the matrix as septa (**s**), few metrocytes (**m**), and several bradyzoites (**b**). Note that the villar protrusions are butted against the host cell (**hc**). (Bar = 2.9 μm)

FIG. 17.26—Transmission electron micrograph of a merozoite (arrows) from a second generation schizont of *S. cruzi* in glomerular capillary of a calf. Note an anteriorly located conoid (**C**), and micronemes (**M**) anterior to the nucleus (**N**). Note absence of rhoptries. (Bar = 0.7 μm) (Courtesy of Dr. C.A. Speer, Montana State University, Bozeman, Montana.)

sarcocystosis can be made if there is anemia, anorexia, fever, excessive salivation, abortion, and loss of body hair.

Sarcocystis generally does not cause illness in definitive hosts. Dogs, cats, coyotes, foxes, and raccoons fed tissues infected with numerous species of *Sarcocystis* shed sporocysts but were otherwise normal. However, human volunteers who ingested beef and pork infected with *S. hominis* or *S. suihominis,* respectively, developed symptoms including vomition, diarrhea, and respiratory distress. These symptoms were more pronounced in volunteers who ate infected pork than in those who ate infected beef.

Sarcocystosis in Wild Mammals. Tables 17.10–17.20 show the hosts and the geographical occurrence of *Sarcocystis* species in different groups of mammalian hosts. For each species one or a few essential references are indicated, thus providing the most factual information. Where known, the diagnostically important transmission electron micrograph (TEM) types of the sarcocyst wall are added, following the classification by Dubey et al. (1989b). Some species

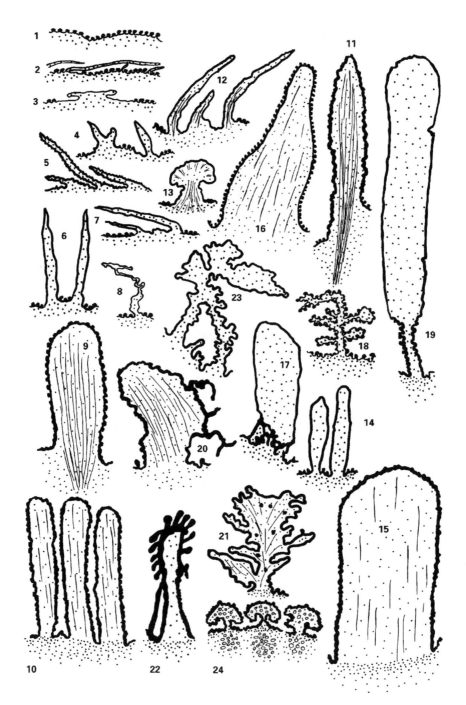

FIG. 17.28—Line drawings of the 37 transmission electron micrograph types of the cyst wall of corresponding reference species of *Sarcocystis*. **Type 1** is the basic type in which the cyst wall is devoid of any villar protrusions; its surface is provided with regularly arranged small invaginations and can be undulated (*S. muris*). In **types 2-37**, the cyst wall is folded resulting in specific villar protrusions projecting into the remnant of the host cell, as follows: **type 2** (*S. wapiti*) thread-like with a smooth surface, parallel to the cyst wall surface and invisible by light microscopy; **type 3** (*S. ferovis*) flattened and mushroom-like with a dsmooth surface; **type 4** (*S. sigmodontis*) irregularly to club-shaped and loosely arranged; **type 5** (*S. sulawesiensis*) hair-like with small invaginations on the surface; **type 6** (*S. capreolicanis*) and **type 7** (*S. arieticanis*) hair-like and labile with smooth surface; **type 8** (*S. grueneri*) like type 2 but with distal ends branched; **type 9** (*S. campestris*) widely spaced and tongue-like with small invaginations on the surface and microtubules in the core, reaching into the ground substance of the cyst wall; **type 10** (*S. odoi*) tightly packed and finger-like with microtubules in the core and small invaginations on the surface; **type 11** (*S. fayeri*) cone- or club-shaped with small invaginations on the surface and microtubules in the interior, penetrating the ground substance as a tightly packed bundle up to the bradyzoites; **type 12** (*S. sybillensis*) tightly packed and hair-like with a smooth surface and microtubules in the proximal third; **type 13** (*S. mucosa*) widely spaced and mushroom-like with microtubules in the proximal half which reach into the ground substance; **type 14** (*S. tenella*) palisade-like and

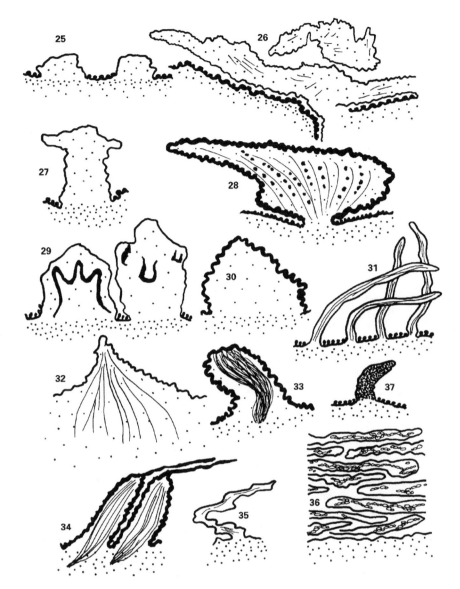

cylindrical with smooth surface; **type 15** (*S. rangiferi*) palisade-like and tombstone-shaped with microtubules in the core and small invaginations on the surface; **type 16** (*S. youngi*) palisade-like and pyramidal with microtubules in the interior and small invaginations on the surface; **type 17** (*S. odocoileocanis*) palisade-like and rectangular to tombstone-like with a smooth surface; **type 18** (*S. zamani*) irregularly branched, T-shaped to cauliflower-like, with small invaginations on the surface; **type 19** (*S. singaporensis*) club-shaped with a cylindrical stalk and a long sausage-shaped distal segment; **type 20** (*S. medusiformis*) irregularly rectangular with microtubules in the interior and snakelike projections; **type 21** (*S. gigantea*) cauliflower-like with microtubules and large osmophilic granules in the core; **type 22** (*S. villivillosi*) cocklebur-like with radiating projections; **type 23** (*S. rileyi*) consisting of an anastomosing, cauliflower-like structure; **type 24** (*S. cornagliai*) club-shaped with small invaginations on the surface, two longitudinal grooves, and a bundle of microtubules reaching into the ground substance, being mushroom-like in the cross section; **type 25** (*S. gracilis*) widely spaced and irregularly dome-shaped with a smooth surface; **type 26** (*S. hardangeri*) flattened and very irregularly linguiform with small invaginations on the surface and microtubules in the interior; **type 27** (*S. capricornis*) palisade-like and thickly T-shaped with a smooth surface; **type 28** (*S. hirsuta*) palisade-like and rhombic with microtubules and large osmiophilic granules in the interior and an undulated surface, arising with a stalklet from the cyst wall; **type 29** (*S. danzani*) tightly arranged and tooth-like with a smooth surface and cord-like condensations in the interior; **type 30** (*S. dubeyella*) irregularly semicircular or rectangular with indented margins; **type 31** (*S. suihominis*) labile, thickly hair-like with microtubules in the core and a smooth surface; **type 32** (*S. ippeni*) thorn-like with microtubules or filaments radiating into the ground substance; **type 33** (*S. hippopotami*) thumb-like with a compact central bundle of microtubules in the core and with small invaginations on the surface; **type 34** (*S. giraffae*) finger-like with microtubules penetrating the ground substance, small invaginations on the surface, and a hair-like projection at the tip; **type 35** (*S. klaseriensis*) kinked finger-like with scattered microtubules or filaments in the interior; **type 36** (*S. camelopardalis*) parallel to the cyst wall surface and strap-like with chain-like osmophilic structures in the interior; **type 37** (*S. dugesii*) spine-like with irregularly indented margins and condensed matrix.

could not be attributed to these types. We give new numbers 25–37 to these additional types.

Some marsupials, primates, and carnivores can act both as intermediate (Tables 17.18–17.20) and definitive hosts, but usually not for the same species of *Sarcocystis*. The life cycles of *Sarcocystis* species that form sarcocysts in carnivorous animals are not known. In certain carnivores muscular sarcocysts are quite common. For example, *S. felis* was found in 11 of 14 Florida panthers (*Felis concolor coryi*), 30 of 60 Florida bobcats (*Felis rufus floridanus*), and 4 of 6 bobcats from Arkansas.

Besides the species listed in Tables 17.10–17.20, all with mammals as intermediate hosts, there are five cases in which birds act as intermediate and mammals as definitive hosts. The sarcocysts (TEM type 9 or 10) (Orazalinova et al. 1986) of *Sarcocystis alectorivulpes* (Pak et al. 1989b), with slim fusiform cystozoites, occur in the skeletal musculature of 18.8% of the chukar partridge (*Alectoris chukar*) (Galliformes) in Kazakhstan. The red fox and the corsac (*Alopex corsac*) (Canidae) serve as definitive hosts. *Sarcocystis falcatula*, with fat macrocysts (TEM type 11) (Dubey et al. 1989b), uses birds of the orders Passeriformes, Cuculiformes, Columbiformes, and Psittaciformes as intermediate hosts in the Americas. The opossum (*Didelphis virginiana*) is the definitive host. The grossly visible sarcocysts (TEM type 23) of *S. rileyi* occur in anseriform birds in North America. The striped skunk *Mephitis mephitis* (Mustelidae) acts as definitive host (see Dubey et al. 1989b). *Sarcocystis wenzeli* from domestic fowl in Europe uses dog and cat as definitive hosts; *S. peckai* from *Phasianus colchicus* only the dog (Odening 1997).

Little is known of the life cycle, pathogenicity, and clinical significance of sarcocystosis in wild mammals. More is known of *S. hemionilatrantis* of mule deer where canids (coyotes, dogs) are the definitive hosts. *Sarcosystis hemionilatrantis* is pathogenic for mule deer under experimental conditions. Mule deer fed 50,000 or more sporocysts became ill and some died, depending on the dose (Koller et al. 1977). Histopathologic data on naturally infected mule deer suggest that *S. hemionilatrantis* affects growth of fawns and predisposes them to predation (Dubey and Kistner 1985).

Diagnosis. *Sarcocystis* antibodies have been detected by IHAT, ELISA, dot-ELISA, and IFAT. At present these tests are not standardized. Because antigen is obtained from sarcocysts in muscles of experimentally infected animals and consists of a lysate of the bradyzoites, variations in preparative methods yield antigens varying greatly from one batch to another. Although antigen obtained from in vitro cultured merozoites may be more suitable for serologic diagnosis of acute sarcocystosis than antigen from bradyzoites, merozoite antigen has not been utilized for diagnostic purposes. Recent studies on the proteins, antigens, and nucleic acids of *Sarcocystis* are likely to improve the serological diagnosis of sarcocystosis in future.

Finding of vascular meronts in biopsy specimens of muscles and lymph nodes or in tissues obtained postmortem may aid diagnosis. However, meronts are often too few to be found in histologic sections. Meronts may disappear by the time clinical disease is obvious. Immunohistochemical staining with anti-*S. neurona* serum can aid diagnosis. Finding large numbers of immature or mature sarcocysts all at the same stage of development suggests a diagnosis of sarcocystosis.

For diagnosis of sarcocystosis based on examination of histologic sections, *Sarcocystis* must be differentiated from *T. gondii* and other closely related coccidians. *Sarcocystis* meronts develop in the endothelium of blood vessels. The immature meronts are basophilic structures with or without differentiated nuclei. *Sarcocystis* schizonts occur within the host cell cytoplasm without a parasitophorous vacuole (PV), whereas all stages of *T. gondii* are separated from the host cell cytoplasm by a PV and can develop in virtually any cell in the body. Electron microscopy is needed to determine these characteristics. In the intermediate host, *T. gondii* divides into two, whereas *Sarcocystis* meronts (schizonts) divide into more than four, merozoites by endopolygeny.

Epizootiology. *Sarcocystis* infection is common in many species of animals worldwide. Virtually 100% of adult cattle in the United States are infected with this parasite. A variety of conditions exist that permit such an unusually high prevalence. A host, for example, may harbor any of several species of *Sarcocystis*. Sheep may become infected with as many as six species, and cattle may have as many as three species. In addition, many definitive hosts are involved in transmission. For example, cattle sarcocystosis is transmitted by Felidae, Canidae, and primates. Wild carnivores such as coyotes spread the parasite over long distances during their forays for food. *Sarcocystis* oocysts and sporocysts develop in the lamina propria and are discharged over a period of many months.

Sporocysts or oocysts remain viable many months in the environment. They may be further spread or protected by invertebrate transport hosts. Large numbers of sporocysts may be shed. There is little or no immunity to reshedding of sporocysts. Therefore, each meal of infected meat can initiate a new round of production of sporocysts. Oocysts or sporocysts are resistant to freezing and, thus, can overwinter on the pasture. Apparently, sporocysts can be killed by drying and by a 10-minute exposure at 56° C. However, they are resistant to disinfectants. Unlike any other species of coccidia, *Sarcocystis* is passed in feces in the infective form and is not dependent on weather conditions for maturation and infectivity.

Control. There is no vaccine to protect livestock against clinical sarcocystosis. Shedding of *Sarcocystis* in feces of definitive hosts is the key factor in the spread of *Sarcocystis* infection. Therefore, to interrupt this cycle, carnivores should be excluded from animal

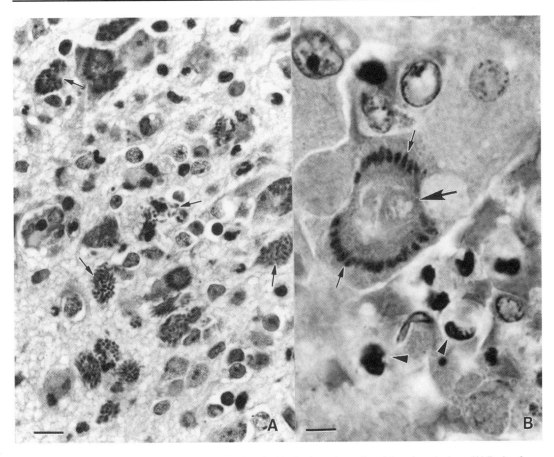

FIG. 17.29—Stages of *Sarcocystis neurona*–like organisms in histologic sections of a mink and a polar bear. (**A**) Brain of a mink from Oregon. Note numerous schizonts (arrows) in neurons. (Hematoxylin and eosin stain.) (Bar = 10 μm) (**B**) Liver of a polar bear. Note a nearly mature schizont (arrow) with merozoites (arrows) radiating from a faint residual body. Few hepatocytes are degenerating (arrowheads). (Hematoxylin and eosin stain.) (Bar = 5 μm)

houses and from feed, water, and bedding for livestock. Uncooked meat or offal should never be fed to carnivores. As freezing can drastically reduce or eliminate infectious sarcocysts in meat, meat should be frozen if not cooked. Exposure to heat at 55° C for 20 minutes kills sarcocysts and sporocysts, so only limited cooking or heating is required to kill sporocysts. Dead livestock should be buried or incinerated. Dead animals should never be left in the field for vultures and carnivores to eat.

Sarcocystosis-like Acute Fatal Disease in Wild Mammals. In 1990 a *Sarcocystis neurona*-like organism was recognized to cause a neurologic disease in a raccoon in the United States (Dubey et al. 1990b). Since then, a similar disease has been reported from mink, skunk, Pacific harbor seals and southern sea otters (Table 17.21). Another unidentified *Sarcocystis*-like infection causes hepatitis in bears, sea lions, and chinchillas (Table 17.21). Only a schizont stage has been recognized (Fig. 17.29).

Life cycles of these organisms are not known. In all three infected raccoons (Dubey et al. 1990b; Stoffregen and Dubey 1991; Thulin et al. 1992) there was a concomitant distemper virus infection, and the monkey was infected with an immunodepressive virus (Klumpp et al. 1994). The organism and the lesions in raccoons most closely resembled that of *S. neurona* infection of horses (Dubey et al. 1991a) with equine protozoal myeloencephalitis (EPM). The etiologic organism of EPM (*S. neurona*) can be grown in cell culture, and a serologic test is available for antemortem diagnosis of EPM. The opossum is the definitive host (Fenger et al. 1997); intermediate hosts and sarcocysts are unknown (Dubey and Lindsay 1998; Dubey et al. 1998). The horse appears to be a dead-end aberrant intermediate host; sarcocysts are not found in the horse. The opossum is the definitive host for at least three species of *Sarcocystis: S. falcatula, S. neurona,* and *S. speeri* (Dubey and Lindsay 1999).

TABLE 17.10—Cervids as intermediate and canids as definitive hosts of *Sarcocystis* spp

Intermediate Host	Definitive Host	*Sarcocystis* spp. (TEM type)	Distribution
Alces alces	*Canis latrans,* dog	*alceslatrans*[1,2,3] (2/8)	North America, Europe
Cervus elaphus + probably other cervids	Dog	*cervicanis*[4] (2/8)	Europe
Cervus elaphus, Rangifer tarandus + probably other cervids	*Alopex lagopus:* blue fox; dog, *Nyctereutes procyonoides, Vulpes vulpes:* silver fox	*grueneri*[4,5] (2/8)	Eurasia
Cervus elaphus	*Canis latrans,* dog	*wapiti*[2] (2/8)	North America
Capreolus capreolus + probably other cervids	Dog, *Vulpes vulpes*	*capreolicanis*[6,11] (6/7)	Europe
Rangifer tarandus	*?Alopex lagopus, Vulpes vulpes*	*rangi*[2,5](6/7)	Europe
Cervus elaphus	Dog	*sybillensis*[2,7,12] (12)	North America
Capreolus capreolus, C. pygargus	Dog, *Vulpes vulpes*	*gracilis*[6] (25)	Eurasia
Rangifer tarandus	*Alopex lagopus:* blue fox; *Nyctereutes procyonoides* + probably dog, *Vulpes vulpes:* silver fox	*tarandivulpes*[2,5] (17 or 25)	Europe
Odocoileus hemionus	*Canis latrans,* dog	*hemionilatrantis*[2,8] (17)	North America
Odocoileus virginianus + probably *Cervus nippon*	*Canis latrans, C. lupus:* dog/wolf; *Vulpes vulpes, Urocyon cinereoargenteus*	*odocoileocanis*[2,9] (17)	North America
Capreolus capreolus, Cervus elaphus, C. nippon, Dama dama	Dog, *Nyctereutes procyonoides*	cf. *hofmanni*[4,6,10,11] (10/15/16)	Eurasia

[1]Dubey 1980a,b; [2]Dubey et al. 1989b; [3]Sedlaczek and Zipper 1986; [4]Wesemeier and Sedlaczek 1995a, b; [5]Gjerde 1986; [6]Sedlaczek and Wesemeier 1995; [7]Dubey et al. 1983a; [8]Dubey and Speer 1985, 1986; [9]Atkinson et al. 1993; [10]Saito et al. 1995; [11]Odening et al. 1999; [12]Foreyt et al. 1995.

TABLE 17.11—Cervids as intermediate hosts of *Sarcocystis* spp., definitive hosts uncertain or unknown

Intermediate Host	Definitive Host	*Sarcocystis* spp. (TEM type)	Distribution
Rangifer tarandus	Unknown	*tarandi*[1,2](10)	Europe
Odocoileus hemionus	Unknown	*hemioni*[2,3](10)	North America
Odocoileus virginianus	Probably Felidae: cat	*odoi*[2] (10)	North America
Odocoileus hemionus	Unknown	*youngi*[2,3](16)	North America
Rangifer tarandus	Unknown	*rangiferi*[1,2](15)	Europe
Dama dama	Unknown	*jorrini*[4] (15)	Europe
Rangifer tarandus; probably *Alces alces*	Unknown	*hardangeri*[1,2]; probably = sp. type B[5] (26)	Europe + probably North America
Odocoileus hemionus	Unknown	*americana*[2]	North America
Odocoileus virginianus	Unknown	sp.[6] (15)	North America
Cervus unicolor	Unknown	sp.[7]	India
Pudu pudu	Unknown	sp.[8]	South America

[1] Gjerde 1986; [2]Dubey et al. 1989b; [3]Dubey and Speer 1985; [4]Hernández-Rodríguez 1992; [5]Colwell and Mahrt 1981; [6]Dubey and Lozier 1983; [7]Gangadharan et al. 1992;, [8]Rioseco et al. 1976.

***FRENKELIA* AND FRENKELIAOSIS.** Structurally and biologically this genus is related to *Sarcocystis. Frenkelia* species form thin-walled cysts in the brains of small mammals (field voles, meadow mice, chinchillas, muskrats, bank voles). There are two species, *F. microti* and *F. glareoli. Frenkelia microti* tissue cysts are up to 1 mm in diameter, lobulated, and thin walled (Figs. 17.30, 17.31), and they occur in the brains of field voles (*Microtus agrestis*), meadow mice (*M. modestus*), muskrats (*Ondatra zibethicus*), and numerous other rodents and small mammals (Rommel and Krampitz 1975; Krampitz and Rommel 1977; Dubey 1977; Dubey et al. 1989b). *Frenkelia glareoli* cysts are spherical and occur in the brain of bank voles (*Clethrionomys glareolus*). Tissue cysts of *Frenkelia* can be seen through the skull. Ultrastructurally, the tissue cyst contains three types of cells, metrocytes at the periphery, intermediary cells, and endodyocytes (bradyzoites) in the center (Fig. 17.31). The metrocytes and bradyzoites structurally resemble those of *Sarcocystis.*

The buzzard (*Buteo buteo*) is the definitive host for *F. glareoli* and *F. microti.* The red-tailed hawk (*Buteo jamaicensis*) is the definitive host for *F. microti* in the United States (Upton and McKown 1992; Lindsay et al. 1992b). Gametogony and sporogony occur in the lamina propria of the small intestine of the buzzard after the ingestion of cysts from the brain of mice.

The intermediate host becomes infected by ingesting sporocysts. Meronts occur in the liver of mice as early

TABLE 17.12—Caprinae as intermediate hosts of *Sarcocystis* spp.

Intermediate Host	Definitive Host	*Sarcocystis* spp. (TEM type)	Distribution
Ovis canadensis	Canidae: *Canis latrans*	*ferovis*[1,2](3)	North America
Ovis ammon/aries (wild and domestic)	Canidae: dog	*arieticanis*[2,3](6/7)	Worldwide
Capra hircus; wild and feral goats probable	Canidae: dog	*hircicanis*[2] (6/7)	Worldwide
Capra hircus; wild and feral goats probable	Canidae: *Alopex corsac, Canis latrans, C. lupus:* dog/wolf; *Cerdocyon thous, Vulpes vulpes*	*capracanis*[2] (14)	Worldwide
Ovis ammon/aries (wild and domestic)	Canidae: *Canis latrans,* dog, ?dingo, *Vulpes vulpes*	*tenella*[2,3](14)	Worldwide
Ovis ammon/aries	Canidae: dog	*micros*[4,5](27)	China
Capricornis crispus	Unknown	*capricornis*[5] (27)	East Asia
Ovis ammon/aries; wild bovids probable	Felidae: cat	*medusiformis*[2] (20)	Australia/ New Zealand/ ?Europe
Ovis ammon/aries; wild sheep probable	Felidae: cat	*gigantea*[2] (21)	Worldwide
Capra hircus; wild and feral goats probable	Felidae: cat	*moulei*[2,6](21)	Europe, North Africa, West Asia
Rupicapra rupicapra	Unknown	*cornagliai*[7] (24)	Europe
Oreamnos americanus	Unknown	sp.[8] (24)	North America
Capra sibirica	Unknown	*orientalis*[5]	Central Siberia
Ovis ammon/aries, wild sheep probable	Canidae: dog	*mihoensis*[9] (24)	Japan

[1]Dubey 1983b; [2]Dubey et al. 1989b; [3]Odening et al. 1995a; [4]Wang et al. 1988; [5]Odening et al. 1996a; [6]Ghaffar et al. 1989; [7]Odening et al. 1996b; [8]Foreyt 1989; [9]Saito et al. 1997.

TABLE 17.13—Bovinae as intermediate hosts of *Sarcocystis* spp.

Intermediate Host	Definitive Host	*Sarcocystis* spp. (TEM type)	Distribution
Bos frontalis, B. javanicus, B. taurus, Bison bison, B. bonasus, Bubalus bubalis	Canidae: *Canis latrans, C. lupus:* dog/wolf; *Vulpes vulpes, Nyctereutes procyonoides.* Probably Procyonidae: *Procyon lotor*	*cruzi*[1,2,3,4](6/7)	Worldwide
Bos grunniens	Canidae: dog	*poephagicanis*[2] (6/7)	China
Bos frontalis, B. javanicus, B. taurus, Bison bison, B. bonasus, Bubalus bubalis; ?Taurotragus oryx	Primates: man. Experimentally *Chimpansee troglodytes, Macaca mulatta, Papio cynocephalus*	*hominis*[2,3,5,6](10)	World-wide
Bubalus bubalis,?Syncerus caffer	Felidae: cat	*fusiformis*[2,6](21)	Asia, Brazil, Southeast Europe, Africa
Bos frontalis, B. javanicus, B. taurus, Bison bison, B. bonasus	Felidae: *Felis catus* (wild and domestic)	*hirsuta*[2,3,5](28)	World-wide
Bos grunniens	Unknown	*poephagi*[2] (28)	China
Bubalus bubalis	Canidae: dog	*levinei*[8] (7)	Asia, Brazil
Bubalus bubalis	Felidae: cat	*buffalonis*[7] (28)	SE Asia
Bubalus bubalis	Unknown	*Dubeyi* (9)	

[1]Dubey 1980a,b, 1982a,b; [2]Dubey et al. 1989b; [3]Odening et al. 1995c, 1999; [4]Xiao et al. 1993; [5]Dubey et al. 1989a; [6]Dubey et al. 1989c; Quandt et al. 1997; [7] Huong et al. 1997a; [8] Huong et al. 1997b; Huong and Uggla 1999.

TABLE 17.14—Antelopes and giraffe as intermediate hosts of *Sarcocystis* spp.

Intermediate Host	Definitive Host	*Sarcocystis* spp. (TEM type)	Distribution
Procapra gutturosa	Unknown	*danzani*[1] (29)	Mongolia
Antidorcas marsupialis, Gazella granti	Unknown	*woodhousei*[2] (29)	Africa
Gazella rufifrons, probably *G. granti, G. thomsoni, Antidorcas marsupialis*	Unknown	*gazellae*[2] (4, or 14)	Africa
Antidorcas marsupialis	Unknown	sp.[6]	Africa
Procapra gutturosa	Unknown	*mongolica*[1] (1)	Mongolia
Antilocapra americana	Unknown	sp.[3]	North America
Alcelaphus buselaphus cokii	Unknown	*bubalis*[2]	Africa
Kobus ellipsiprymnus defassa; probably *K. e. ellipsiprymnus, K. kob, K. vardonii*	Unknown	*nelsoni*[2]	Africa
Saiga tatarica	Unknown	*saiga*[4]	Kazakhstan
Giraffa camelopardalis	Unknown	*giraffae*[5] (34)	Africa
Giraffa camelopardalis	Unknown	*klaseriensis*[5] (35)	Africa
Giraffa camelopardalis	Unknown	*camelopardalis*[5] (36)	Africa
Aepyceros melampus	Unknown	*melampi*[6](6/7)	Africa
Tragelaphus strepsiceros	Unknown	*hominis*[6] (10/15/16)	Africa

[1]Odening et al. 1996c; [2]Mandour and Keymer 1970; [3]Dubey 1980a; [4]Pak et al. 1991; [5]Bengis et al. 1998; [6]Odening et al. 1998b.

TABLE 17.15—Equids, suids, hippopotamids, and camelids as intermediate hosts of *Sarcocystis* spp.

Intermediate Host	Definitive Host	*Sarcocystis* spp. (TEM type)	Distribution
Equidae			
Equus caballus (wild, feral, and domestic), *E. asinus somalicus, E. burchellii antiquorum, E. kiang holdereri;* ass	Canidae: dog	*bertrami*[1,2](11)	Worldwide
ass, *Equus b. burchellii, E. burchellii chapmani, E. onager kulan, E. zebra hartmannae,* horse	Canidae: dog	*fayeri*[1,2](11)	Worldwide
Suidae			
Sus scrofa (wild, feral, and domestic)	Canidae: *Canis aureus, C. lupus:* dog/wolf; *Vulpes vulpes, Nyctereutes procyonoides.* Probably Procyonidae: *Procyon lotor*	*miescheriana*[1,4] (10)	Worldwide
Pig	Felidae: cat	*porcifelis*[1]	Russia
Sus scrofa (wild, feral, and domestic)	Primates: man. Experimentally *Chimpansee troglodytes, Macaca fascicularis, M. mulatta*	*suihominis*[1,4](31)	Worldwide
Phacochoerus aethiopicus	Unknown	*dubeyella*[5] (30)	Africa
Phacochoerus aethiopicus	Unknown	*phacochoeri*[5] (29)	Africa
Hippopotamidae			
Hippopotamus amphibius	Unknown	*hippopotami*[6] (33)	Africa
Hippopotamus amphibius	Unknown	*africana*[6] (30)	Africa
Camelidae			
Lama glama (alpaca, guanaco, and llama)	Canidae: dog	*aucheniae*[1,3] (21; syns. *tilopodi, guanicoe-canis*)	South America
Lama glama (llama)	Unknown	sp.[1]	South America
Camelus bactrianus, C. dromedarius	Canidae: dog	*cameli*[1] (9)	Africa, Asia
Camelus dromedarius	Unknown	*ippeni*[7] (32)	Africa

[1]Dubey et al. 1989b; [2]Odening et al. 1995b; [3]Gorman et al. 1984; [4]Tadros and Laarman 1982; [5]Stolte et al. 1998; [6]Odening et al. 1997; [7]Odening 1997.

TABLE 17.16—Rodents: Caviidae, Cricetidae, and Cricetidae + Muridae as intermediate hosts of *Sarcocystis* spp.

Intermediate Host	Definitive Host	*Sarcocystis* spp. (TEM type)	Distribution
Caviidae			
Cavia porcellus	Unknown	*caviae* [2, 3]	South America
Cricetidae			
Gerbillus gerbillus, G. perpallidus, Meriones shawi isis, Psammomys obesus, Pachyuromys duprasi natronensis	Serpentes: *Echis coloratus*	*gerbilliechis*[1] (1)	Egypt
Microtus arvalis	Accipitriformes: *Falco tinnunculus*	*cernae*[4] (1)	Europe
Microtus ochrogaster, M. pennsylvanicus, probably *M. longicaudus*	Serpentes: *Agkistrodon c. contortix*	*montanaensis*[3, 5, 6](1)	North America
Neotoma micropus	Felidae: cat	*neotomafelis*[7] (1)	Mexico
Dicrostonyx richardsoni	Strigiformes: *Nyctea scandiaca*	*rauschorum*[3, 8](1)	North America
Rhombomys opimus	Canidae: *Vulpes vulpes*	*rhombomys*[9] (1)	Kazakhstan
Rhombomys opimus	Unknown	*fedoseenkoi*[17] (9)	Kazakhstan
Sigmodon hispidus	Unknown	*sigmodontis*[3, 10] (4)	North America
Clethrionomys glareolus, Microtus arvalis, M. guentheri, M. oeconomus	Serpentes: *Elaphe longissima;* experimentally *E. dione, E. guttata, E. obsoleta, E. quatuorlineata, E. scalaris*	*clethrionomyelaphis*[3] (9)	Europe, Middle East, possibly also North America
Microtus pennsylvanicus, M. longicaudus	Unknown	*microti*[3, 6](9)	North America
Microtus agrestis, M. arvalis	Mustelidae: *Mustela erminea, M. nivalis, Putorius putorius:* ferret and polecat	*putorii*[4] (9, or 10)	Europe
Oryzomys capito	Unknown	*azevedoi*[2, 3]	South America
Clethrionomys rufocanus bedfordiae	Unknown	*clethrionomysi*[11]	Japan
Oryzomys capito	Unknown	*oryzomyos*[2, 3]	South America
Peromyscus maniculatus	Unknown	*peromysci*[3, 12]	North America
Peromyscus maniculatus	Serpentes: *Pituophis melanoleucus*	*roudabushi*[3, 12] (syn. *idahoensis*[13])	North America
Peromyscus maniculatus	Strigiformes: *Aegolius acadicus*	*espinosai*[7] (1)	North America
Cricetidae + Muridae			
Cricetidae: *Gerbillus perpallidus, Meriones unguiculatus, Mesocricetus auratus, Phodopus sungorus* Muridae: *Mus musculus, Praomys natalensis*	Serpentes: *Bitis arietans, B. caudalis, B. gabonica, B. nasicornis*	*dirumpens*[14] (1)	Africa
Cricetidae: *Gerbillus perpallidus, Mesocricetus auratus, Meriones unguiculatus, Phodopus sungorus* Muridae: *Mastomys natalensis, Mus musculus*	Serpentes: *Bitis arietans, B. nasicornis;* experimentally *B. caudalis, B. gabonica*	*hoarensis*[15] (18, or 1)	Africa
Cricetidae: *Clethrionomys glareolus* Muridae: *Mus musculus, Rattus norvegicus*	Felidae: cat	*rodentifelis*[16] (probably 1)	East Europe

[1]Jäkel 1995; [2]Levine 1988; [3]Dubey et al. 1989b; [4]Tadros and Laarman 1982; [5]Lindsay et al. 1992a; [6]Dubey 1983c; [7]Galavíz-Silva et al. 1991; [8]Friesen et al. 1989; [9]Institute of Zoology, Kazakh Academy of Science 1984; [10]Dubey and Sheffield 1988; [11]Inoue et al. 1990; [12]Dubey 1983d; [13]Daszak and Cunningham 1995; [14]Häfner and Matuschka 1984; [15]Matuschka et al. 1987; [16]Grikienienée et al. 1993; [17]Odening 1997.

TABLE 17.17—Rodents: Echimyidae, Muridae, Sciuridae, and Erethizontidae as intermediate hosts of *Sarcocystis* spp.

Intermediate Host	Definitive Host	*Sarcocystis* spp. (TEM type)	Distribution
Echimyidae			
Proechimys guyannensis	Unknown	*proechimyos*[1, 2]	South America
Muridae			
Mus musculus	Serpentes: *Crotalus s. scutulatus*	*crotali*[2] (1)	North America
Rattus norvegicus, R. rattus	Felidae: cat	*cymruensis*[1, 2](1)	World-wide
Mus musculus	Felidae: cat; Mustelidae: *Putorius putorius:* ferret	*muris*[1, 2](1)	World-wide
Mus musculus	Strigiformes: *Strix aluco*	*scotti*[3] (1)	Europe
Apodemus sylvaticus, Mus musculus. Perhaps *Lepus europaeus* (Leporidae), *Meles meles, Mustela nivalis* (Mustelidae), and *Procyon lotor* (Procyonidae)	Strigiformes: *Strix aluco*	*sebeki*[3, 4](1)	Europe
Mus musculus	Strigiformes: *Asio otus, Tyto alba, T. novaehollandiae*	*dispersa*[3] (18, or 1)	Europe, ? Australia
Mus musculus	Serpentes: *Vipera palaestinae* + 5 species from Israel	*muriviperae*[2] (18)	Middle East
Bandicota indica, Rattus annandalei, R. rattus diardii, R. exulans, R. norvegicus, R. rattus	Serpentes: *Python reticulatus*	*zamani*[1, 2](18)	Asia
Mastacomys fuscus, Pseudomys higginsi, Rattus fuscipes, R. lutreolus, R. norvegicus, R. rattus	Serpentes: *Notechis ater*	*murinotechis*[1, 2] (4)	Australia
Bunomys chrysocomus, B. fratrorum, Paruromys dominator	Unknown	*sulawesiensis*[1, 2] (5)	Indonesia
Bandicota indica, B. savilei, Bunomys chrysocomus, B. fratrorum, Maxomys bartelsii, M. musschenbroekii, Paruromys dominator, Rattus argentiventer, R. colletti, R. exulans, R. fuscipes, R. jalorensis, R. losea, R. norvegicus, R. rattus, R. rattus diardii, R. tiomanicus, R. villosissimus, R. xanthurus	Serpentes: *Aspidites melanocephalus, Python reticulatus, P. sebae, P. timorens*	*singaporensis*[1, 2] (19)	Asia
Bandicota bengalensis, B. indica, B. svilei, Rattus argentiventer, R. colletti, R. exulans, R. losea, R. norvegicus, R. rattus, R. tiomanicus, R. villosissimus	Serpentes: *Aspidites melanocephalus, Python reticulatus, P. timorensis, P. zebae*	*villivillosi*[1, 2] (22)	Asia
Sciuridae			
Marmota baibacina, M. bobac, M. caudata	Canidae: *Canis lupus:* dog/wolf; *Vulpes vulpes*	*baibacinacanis*[1, 2, 5]	Kazakhstan
Citellus richardsoni	Unknown	*bozemanensis*[2, 6](1)	North America
Citellus richardsoni	Mustelidae: *Taxidea taxus*	*campestris*[2, 6](9)	North America
Citellus fulvus	Acciptriformes: *Buteo buteo*	*citellibuteonis*[8] (1)	Kazakhstan
Citellus fulvus	Canidae: *Alopex corsac, Vulpes vulpes;* Mustelidae: *Mustela eversmanni*	*citellivulpes*[2, 5](9)	Kazakhstan
Citellus undulatus	Canidae: *Alopex corsac, Vulpes vulpes;* Mustelidae: *Mustela eversmanni*	*undulati*[5]	Kazakhstan
Tamias striatus, Tamiasciurus	Unknown *hudsonicus*	sp.[7] (1)	North America
Erethizontidae			
Erethizon dorsatum	Unknown	*sehi*[9]	North America

[1]Levine 1988; [2]Dubey et al. 1989b; [3]Tadros and Laarman 1982; [4]Odening et al. 1994a, 1996d, Odening 1997, Stolte et al. 1996; [5]Institute of Zoology, Kazakh Academy of Science 1984; [6]Dubey 1983a; [7]Entzeroth et al. 1983a, b; [8]Pak et al. 1989a; [9]Dubey et al. 1992c.

TABLE 17.18—Marsupials, Edentata, and insectivores as intermediate hosts of *Sarcocystis* spp.

Intermediate Host	Definitive Host	*Sarcocystis* spp. (TEM type)	Distribution
Marsupialia			
Didelphis marsupialis	Unknown	*didelphidis*[1, 2]	South America
Didelphis marsupialis; perhaps *D. virginiana, Metachirops opossum*	Unknown	*garnhami*[1, 2, 3] (presumably 9)	America
Marmosa murina	Unknown	*marmosae*[1, 2]	South America
Macropus rufogriseus, Petrogale assimilis, P. penicillata	Unknown	*mucosa*[2] (13; syn. *macropodis*)	Australia
Edentata			
Dasypodidae: *Dasypus novemcinctus*	Unknown	*dasypi*[1, 2, 4] (between 9 and 11)	America
Dasypodidae: *Dasypus novemcinctus*	Unknown	*diminuta*[1, 2, 4] (between 9 and 11)	America
Myrmecophagidae: *Tamandua tetradactyla*	Unknown	tamanduae[1, 2]	South America
Insectivora			
Erinaceidae: *Echinosorex gymnurus*	Unknown	*booliati*[1, 2](1)	Asia

[1]Levine 1988; [2]Dubey et al. 1989b; [3]Scholtyseck et al. 1982; [4]Lindsay et al. 1996.

TABLE 17.19—Lagomorphs and primates as intermediate hosts of *Sarcocystis* spp.

Intermediate Host	Definitive Host	*Sarcocystis* spp. (TEM type)	Distribution
Lagomorpha (Leporidae)			
Oryctolagus cuniculus; probably *Lepus europaeus*	Felidae: cat	*cuniculorum*[1] (9; syn. *cuniculi*)	Europe, Australia, New Zealand
Ochotona sp.	Unknown	*ochotonae*[2] (1)	China
Ochotona daurica, O. alpina	Unknown	*dogeli*[3, 4]	Siberia Kazakhstan
Ochotona alpina	Unknown	*galuzoi*[4]	Kazakhstan
Sylvilagus floridanus, S. nuttalli, S. palustris	Felidae: cat. Procyonidae: *Procyon lotor*	*leporum*[1, 5, 6](10)	North America
Primates			
Cercopithecus mitis, Erythrocebus patas, Macaca mulatta; probably *Cercocebus atys, Macaca radiata, and Miopithecus talapoin*	Unknown	*kortei*[3, 5]	Asia, Africa
Macaca mulatta; probably *M. fascicularis, Cercocebus atys, Papio papio, P. cynocephalus,* man	Unknown	*nesbitti*[3, 5, 7, 8] (probably 1)	Asia,
Africa			
Oedipomidas oedipus	Unknown	sp.[8] (1)	South America
Cercopithecus pygerythrus	Unknown	*markusi*[9] (9)	Africa

[1]Odening et al. 1994c, 1996d; [2]Odening et al. 1998a; [3] Levine 1988; [4]Institute of Zoology, Kazakh Academy of Science 1984; [5]Dubey et al. 1989b; [6]Elwasila et al. 1984; [7]Wong and Pathmanathan 1994; [8]Mehlhorn et al. 1977; [9]Odening 1997.

as 7 days after sporocyst ingestion. Meronts contain 20 to 30 merozoites. Tissue cysts are formed in the brain, beginning 18 days after infection. They are 326 μm in diameter 120 days after infection.

Frenkelia microti and *F. glareoli* are only mildly pathogenic for their intermediate hosts. Although *Frenkelia* cysts may occupy as much as 3.6% of the brain, clinical signs, except diuresis, are rarely observed. Experimentally infected voles (*M. agrestis*) only developed mild disease.

ACKNOWLEDGEMENTS. The authors are grateful to Dr. Debra Bourne, Royal Veterinary College, London, for her help with data on toxoplasmosis in wallabies in Table 17.9.

TABLE 17.20—Carnivores and whales as intermediate hosts of *Sarcocystis* spp.

Intermediate Host	Definitive Host	*Sarcocystis* spp. (TEM type)	Distribution
Fissipedia			
Felidae: *Acinonyx jubatus,* cat, *Felis concolor, F. rufus, Panthera leo.* Probably Canidae: dog	Unknown	*felis*[1,2,3,4,5] (4)	North America, Africa
Procyonidae: *Procyon lotor*	Unknown	*kirkpatricki*[6,7] (between 9 and 11)	North America
Mustelidae: *Meles meles;* probably *Procyon lotor* (Procyonidae)	Unknown	*hofmanni*[8] (10/15/16)	Europe
Mustelidae: *Meles meles*	Unknown	*melis*[8] (?1)	Europe
Mustelidae: *Lutra lutra*	Unknown	sp. [15] (1)	Norway, Sweden
Mustelidae: *Mephitis mephitis*	Canidae: dog	*erdmanae*[8]	North America
Canidae: *Alopex corsac*	Canidae: *Alopex corsac*	*corsaci*[1,9]	Kazakhstan
Canidae: *Canis mesomelas*	Unknown	sp. 1 (10), sp. 2 (3?)[10]	Africa
Pinnipedia			
Otariidae: *Zalophus californianus*	Unknown	*hueti*[1,11,14]	East Pacific
Phocidae: *Hydrurga leptonyx*	Unknown	*hydrurgae*[11,12,13] (1)	Antarctic
Phocidae: *Phoca richardi*	Unknown	*richardii*[1,11,13]	Bering Sea
Cetacea			
Balaenopteridae: *Balaenoptera borealis*	Unknown	*balaenopteralis*[1,13] (1)	Pacific
Delphinidae: *Lagenorhynchus acutus*	Unknown	sp.[14] (1)	St. Lawrence estuary
Monodontidae: *Delphinapterus leucas*	Unknown	sp.[14] (1)	St. Lawrence estuary
Physeteridae: *Physeter catadon*	Unknown	sp.[13,14] (1)	Near Australia

[1]Dubey et al. 1989b; [2]Dubey et al. 1992e; [3]Greiner et al. 1989; [4]Anderson et al. 1992; [5]Dubey and Bwangamoi 1994; [6]Snyder et al. 1990; [7]Kirkpatrick et al. 1987; [8]Odening et al. 1994a,b; Odening 1997; [9]Institute of Zoology, Kazakh Academy of Science 1984; [10]Wesemeier et al. 1995; [11]Odening 1983; [12]Odening and Zipper 1986; [13]Odening 1986; [14]De Guise et al. 1993; [15]Wahlström et al. 1999.

TABLE 17.21—Summary of reports of fatal acute sarcocystosis in wild mammals in the United States

Animal Species	Locality	Reference	Main Findings	No. of Animals
Raccoon (*Procyon lotor*)	New York	Stoffregen and Dubey 1991	Weak, seizures, *S. neurona*-like meronts in brain	1
	Illinois	Thulin et al. 1992	Ataxia	1
	Ohio	Dubey et al. 1990b, 1991b	Ataxia	1
Monkey (*Macaca mulata*)	Atlanta	Klumpp et al. 1994	Neurologic	1
Pacific harbor seals (*Phoca vitalina richardsi*)	California	Lapointe et al. 1998	Encephalitis	7
Southern sea otters	Alaska	Rosonke et al. 1999	Encephalitis	
Mink (*Mustela vison*)	Oregon	Dubey and Hedstrom 1993	Ataxia	2
Skunk (*Mephitis mephitis*)	Massachusetts	Dubey et al. 1996b	Paralysis	1
Black bear (*Ursus americanus*)	South Dakota	Zeman et al. 1993	Hepatitis	1
Polar bears (*Ursus maritimus*)	Alaska	Garner et al. 1997	Hepatitis, acute disease	2
Chinchilla	Georgia	Rakich et al. 1992	Sudden death, hepatitis	1
Sea lion (*Zalophus californianus*)	Florida	Mense et al. 1992	Hepatitis	1

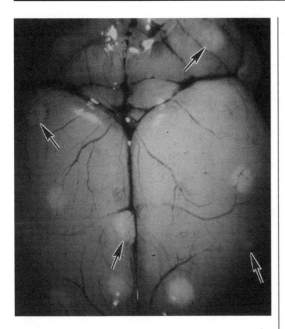

FIG. 17.30—Macroscopic *Frenkelia microti* cysts (arrows) in the brain of a vole (*Microtus agrestis*). [Courtesy of M. Rommel].

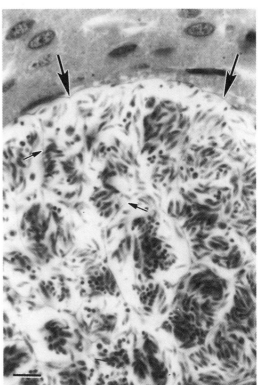

FIG. 17.31—*Frenkelia microti* cysts (arrows) in the brain of *Microtus modestus.* (**A**) Numerous lobulated cysts. 32X. (**B**) Higher magnification to show smooth, thin cyst wall (arrows). (Hemotoxylin and eosin stain.) (Bar = 10 μm)

LITERATURE CITED

Akuzawa, M., M. Mochizuki, and N. Yasuda. 1987. Hematological and parasitological study of the iriomote cat (*Prionailurus iriomotensis*). *Canadian Journal of Zoology* 65:946–949.

Altmann, D., and K. F. Schüppel. 1988. Ein Beitrag zur Therapie und Pathologie der Toxoplasmose bei Bennettkänguruhs. Verhandlungsbericht des 30. Internationalen Symposiums über die Erkrankungen der Zoo und Wildtiere vom 11 Mai bis 15 Mai 1988 in Sofia, Bulgaria, pp. 407–411.

Anderson, A. J., E.C. Greiner, C.T. Atkinson, and M.E. Roelke. 1992. Sarcocysts in the Florida bobcat (*Felis rufus floridanus*). *Journal of Wildlife Diseases* 28:116–120.

Andersson, P., and A. S. Garry-Andersson. 1963. Eläinten toksoplasmoosista suomessa. *Finsk Veterinartidskrift.* 69:59–166.

Aramini, J.J., C. Stephen, and J.P. Dubey. 1998. *Toxoplasma gondii* in Vancouver Island cougars (*Felis concolor vancoverensis*): Serology and oocyst shedding. *The Journal of Parasitology* 84:438–440.

Ashton, N. 1979. Ocular toxoplasmosis in wallabies (*Macropus rufogriseus*). *American Journal of Ophthalmology* 88:322–332.

Atkinson, C.T., S.D. Wright, S.R. Telford Jr., G.S. McLaughlin, D.J. Forrester, M.E. Roelke, and J.W. McCown. 1993. Morphology, prevalence, and distribution of *Sarcocystis* spp. in white-tailed deer (*Odocoileus virginianus*) from Florida. *Journal of Wildlife Diseases* 29:3–84.

Attwood, H.D., and P.A. Woolley. 1970. Toxoplasmosis in dasyurid marsupials. *Pathology* 2:77–78.

Attwood, H.D., P.A. Woolley, and M.D. Rickard. 1975. Toxoplasmosis in dasyurid marsupials. *Journal of Wildlife Diseases* 11:543–551.

Bell, A., J. Isaac-Renton, A. King, L. Martinez, D. Roscoe, D. Werker, S. Eng, T. Johnstone, R. Stanwick, W.R. Bowie, S. Marion, C. Stephen, A. Burnett, J. Cadham, F. Jagdis, P. MacLeod, K. Barnard, J. Millar, S. Peck, and J. Hull. 1995. Outbreak of toxoplasmosis associated with municipal drinking water—British Columbia. *Canada Communicable Disease Report* 21–18:161–163.

Bengis, R.G., K. Odening, M. Stolte, S. Quandt, and I. Bockhardt. 1998. Three new *Sarcocystis* species, *Sarcocystis giraffae, S. klaseriensis,* and *S. camelopardalis* (Protozoa: Sarcocystidae) from the giraffe in South Africa. *The Journal of Parasitology* 84: 562–565

Bigalke, R.D., R.C. Tustin, J.L. Du Pleissis, P.A. Basson, and R.M. McCully. 1966. The isolation of *Toxoplasma gondii* from ferrets in South Africa. *Journal South Africa Veterinary Medical Association* 37:243–247.

Boorman, G.A., G.V. Kollias, and R.F. Taylor. 1977. An outbreak of toxoplasmosis in wallaroos (*Macropus robustus*) in a California zoo. *Journal of Wildlife Diseases* 13:64–68.

Bourne, D.C. 1997. Disease and mortality in Bennett's wallabies (*Macropus rufogriseus rufogriseus*) at Whipsnade Wild Animal Park, with special reference to toxoplasmosis. PhD. Thesis. University of London, London, 280 pp.

Bowie, W.R., A.S. King, D.H. Werker, J.L. Isaac-Renton, A. Bell, S.B. Eng, S.A. Marion. 1997. Outbreak of toxoplasmosis associated with municipal drinking water. *Lancet* 350:173–177.

Brillhart, D.B., L.B. Fox, J.P. Dubey, and S.J. Upton. 1994. Seroprevalence of *Toxoplasma gondii* in wild mammals in Kansas. *Journal of the Helminthological Society of Washington* 61:117–121.

Briscoe, N., J.G. Humphreys, and J.P. Dubey. 1993. Prevalence of *Toxoplasma gondii* infections in Pennsylvania black bears, *Ursus americanus. Journal of Wildlife Diseases* 29:599–601.

Bulmer, W.S. 1971. Toxoplasmosis in captive Saiga antelope. *Journal of Wildlife Diseases* 7:310–316.

Burgisser, H. 1960. Toxoplasmose chez le chevreuil. *Pathologia et Microbiologia* 23:415–417.

Burridge, M.J., W.J. Bigler, D.J. Forrester, and J.M. Hennemann. 1979. Serologic survey for *Toxoplasma gondii* in wild animals in Florida. *Journal of the American Veterinary Medical Association* 175:964–967.

Canfield, P.J., W.J. Hartley, and J.P. Dubey. 1990. Lesions of toxoplasmosis in Australian marsupials. *Journal of Comparative Pathology* 103:159–167.

Cannon, J. 1974. Case report: Toxoplasmosis in cheetahs. *American Association of Zoo Veterinarians, Annual Proceedings* 225:225–227.

Choi, W.-Y., H.W. Nam, N.H. Kwak, W. Huh, Y.R. Kim, M.W. Kang, S.Y. Cho, and J.P. Dubey. 1997. Foodborne outbreaks of human toxoplasmosis. *Journal of Infectious Diseases* 175:1280–1282.

Chomel, B.B., R.L. Zarnke, R.W. Kasten, P.H. Kass, and E. Mendes. 1995. Serologic survey of *Toxoplasma gondii* in grizzly bears (*Ursus arctos*) and black bears (*Ursus americanus*), from Alaska, 1988 to 1991. *Journal of Wildlife Diseases* 31:472–479.

Christiansen, M., and J.C. Siim. 1951. Toxoplasmosis in hares in Denmark. Serological identity of human and hare strains of *Toxoplasma. Lancet* 1: 1201–1203.

Clark, R.K., D.A. Jessup, D.W. Hird, R. Ruppanner, and M.E. Meyer. 1983. Serologic survey of California wild hogs for antibodies against selected zoonotic disease angents. *Journal of the American Veterinary Medical Association* 183:1248–1251.

Collins, G.H. 1981. Studies in *Sarcocystis* species. VII. *Sarcocystis* and *Toxoplasma* in red deer (*Cervus elaphus*). *New Zealand Veterinary Journal* 29:126–127.

Colwell, D.D., and J.L. Mahrt. 1981. Ultrastructure of the cyst wall and merozoites of *Sarcocystis* from moose (*Alces alces*) in Alberta, Canada. *Zeitschrift für Parasitenkunde* 65:317–329.

Cook, I., and J.H. Pope. 1959. *Toxoplasma* in Queensland. III. A preliminary survey of animal hosts. *Australian Journal of Experimental Biology* 37:253–262.

Coutelen, F. 1932. Existence d'une encéphalite toxoplasmique spontanée chez les wombats. Un toxoplasme nouveau, *Toxoplasma wenyoni* n. sp. parasite de *Phascolomys mitchelli* (Australie). *Comptes Rendus des Séances de la Societé de Biologie* 110:1245–1247.

Cox, J.C., J.W. Edmonds, and R.C. Shepherd. 1981. Toxoplasmosis and the wild rabbit *Oryctolagus cuniculus* in Victoria, Australia, with suggested mechanisms for dissemination of oocysts. *Journal of Hygiene, Cambridge* 87:331–337.

Cruickshank, J.J., D.M. Haines, N.C. Palmer, and D.J. Staubin. 1990. Cysts of a *Toxoplasma*-like organims in an Atlantic Bottlenose-Dolphin. *Canadian Veterinary Journal* 31:213–215.

Crutchley, C.A., J.P. Dubey, and D.S. Adams. 1997. Recovery from blindness caused by toxoplasmosis in Bennett's Wallabies (*Macropus rufogriseus*). Proceedings of the 42nd Annual Meeting of the American Association of Veterinary Parasitologist, Reno, Nevada, July 19–22, 1997, p. 42.

Cunningham, A.A., D. Buxton, and K.M. Thomson. 1992. An epidemic of toxoplasmosis in a captive colony of squirrel-monkeys (*Saimiri sciureus*). *Journal of Comparative Pathology* 107:207–219.

Daszak, P., and A. Cunningham. 1995. A report of intestinal sarcocystosis in the bullsnake (*Pituophis melanoleucos sayi*) and a re-evaluation of *Sarcocystis* sp. from snakes of the genus *Pituophis. Journal of Wildlife Diseases* 31:400–403.

De Guise, S., A. Lagacé, C. Girard, and P. Béland. 1993. Intramuscular *Sarcocystis* in two beluga whales and an Atlantic white-sided dolphin from the St. Lawrence estuary, Quebec, Canada. *Journal of Veterinary Diagnostic Investigation* 5:296–300.

Diderrich, V., J.C. New, G.P. Noblet, and S. Patton. 1996. Serologic survey of *Toxoplasma gondii* antibodies in free-ranging wild hogs (*Sus scrofa*) from the Great Smoky Mountains National Park and from sites in South Carolina. *Journal of Eukaryotic Microbiology* 43:122S.

Dietz, H.H., P. Henriksen, M. Lebech, and S.A. Henriksen. 1993. Experimental infection with *Toxoplasma gondii* in farmed mink (*Mustela visons*). *Veterinary Parasitology* 47:1–7.

Dietz, H.H., P. Henriksen, V. Bille-Hansen, and S.A. Henriksen. 1997. Toxoplasmosis in a colony of New World monkeys. *Veterinary Parasitology* 68:299–304.

Diters, R.W., and S.W. Nielsen. 1978. Toxoplasmosis, distemper, and herpesvirus infection in a skunk (*Mephitis mephitis*). *Journal of Wildlife Diseases* 14:132–136.

Dobos-Kovács, M., J. Meszaros, L. Pellerdy, and A. Balsai. 1974a. Studies on the source of *Toxoplasma* infection in captive kangaroos. *Acta Veterinaria Academiae Scientiarum Hungaricae* 24:293–301.

———. 1974b. Toxoplasmose bei Känguruhs (*Thylogale eugenii*) verursacht durch *Toxoplasma*-Oozysten enthaltendes Futter. *Parasitologia Hungarica* 7:85–90.

Domingo, M., J. Visa, M. Pumarola, A.J. Marco, L. Ferrer, R. Rabanal, and S. Kennedy. 1992. Pathologic and immunocytochemical studies of morbillivirus infection in striped dolphins (*Stenella coeruleoalba*). *Veterinary Pathology* 29:1–10.

Dubey, J.P. 1977. *Toxoplasma, Hammondia, Besnoitia, Sarcocystis,* and other tissue cyst-forming coccidia of man and animals. In *Parasitic protozoa,* vol. 3. Ed. J.P. Kreier. New York: Academic Press, pp. 101–237.

———. 1980a. *Sarcocystis* species in moose (*Alces alces*), bison (*Bison bison*), and pronghorn (*Antilocapra americana*) in Montana. *American Journal of Veterinary Research* 41:2063–2065.

———. 1980b. Coyote as a final host for *Sarcocystis* species of goats, sheep, cattle, elk, bison, and moose in Montana. *American Journal of Veterinary Research* 41:1227–1229.

———. 1981. Isolation of encysted *Toxoplasma gondii* from musculature of moose and pronghorn in Montana. *American Journal of Veterinary Research* 42:126–127.

———. 1982a. Development of ox-coyote cycle of *Sarcocystis cruzi. Journal of Protozoology* 29:591–601.

———. 1982b. Sarcocystosis in neonatal bison fed *Sarcocystis cruzi* sporocysts derived from cattle. *Journal of the American Veterinary Medical Association* 181:1272–1274.

———. 1982c. Isolation of encysted *Toxoplasma gondii* from muscles of mule deer in Montana. *Journal of the American Veterinary Medical Association* 181:1535.

———. 1982d. Induced *Toxoplasma gondii, Toxocara canis,* and *Isospora canis* infection in coyotes. *Journal of the American Veterinary Medical Association* 181:1268–1269.

———. 1983a. *Sarcocystis bozemanensis* sp. nov. (Protozoa: Sarcocystidae) and *S. campestris* from the Richardson's ground squirrel (*Spermophilus richardsonii*) in Montana, USA. *Canadian Journal of Zoology* 61:942–946.

———. 1983b. *Sarcocystis ferovis* sp. n. from the bighorn sheep (*Ovis canadensis*) and coyote (*Canis latrans*). *Pro-

ceedings of the Helminthological Society of Washington 50:153–158.

———. 1983c. *Sarcocystis montanaensis* and *S. microti* sp. n. from the meadow vole (*Microtus pennsylvanicus*). *Proceedings of the Helminthological Society of Washington* 50:318–324.

———. 1983d. *Sarcocystis peromysci* n. sp. and *S. idahoensis* in deer mouse (*Peromyscus maniculatus*) in Montana. *Canadian Journal of Zoology* 61:1180–1182.

———. 1983e. Experimental infections of *Sarcocystis cruzi, Sarcocystis tenella, Sarcocystis capracanis* and *Toxoplasma gondii* in red foxes (*Vulpes vulpes*). *Journal of Wildlife Diseases* 19:200–203.

———. 1983f. Experimental infection of a bison with *Toxoplasma gondii* oocysts. *Journal of Wildlife Diseases* 19:148–149.

———. 1983g. *Toxoplasma gondii* infection in rodents and insectivores from Montana. *Journal of Wildlife Diseases* 19:149–150.

———. 1985. Serologic prevalence of toxoplasmosis in cattle, sheep, goats, pigs, bison, and elk in Montana. *Journal of the American Veterinary Medical Association* 186:969–970.

———. 1988. Long-term persistence of *Toxoplasma gondii* in tissues of pigs inoculated with *T. gondii* oocysts and effect of freezing on viability of tissue cysts in pork. *American Journal of Veterinary Research* 49:910–913.

———. 1991. Sarcocystosis of the skeletal and cardiac muscle, mouse. In *Cardiovascular and musculoskeletal systems*. Ed. T.C. Jones, U. Mohr, and R.D. Hunt. New York: Springer-Verlag, pp. 165–169.

———. 1993. *Toxoplasma, Neospora, Sarcocystis,* and other tissue cyst-forming coccidia of humans and animals. In *Parasitic protozoa*, vol. 6. Ed. J.P. Kreier. New York: Academic Press, pp. 1–158.

———. 1999. Recent advances in *Neospora* and neosporosis. *Veterinary Parasitology* 85:349–367.

Dubey, J.P., and C.P. Beattie. 1988. *Toxoplasmosis of animals and man.* Boca Raton, FL: CRC Press, 220 pp.

Dubey, J.P., and O. Bwangamoi. 1994. *Sarcocystis felis* (Protozoa: Sarcocystidae) from the African lion (*Panthera leo*). *Journal of the Helminthological Society of Washington* 61:113–114.

Dubey, J.P., and J.K. Frenkel. 1972. Cyst-induced toxoplasmosis in cats. *Journal of Protozoology* 19:155–177.

———. 1976. Feline toxoplasmosis from acutely infected mice and the development of *Toxoplasma* cysts. *Journal of Protozoology* 23:537–546.

———. 1998. Toxoplasmosis of rats: A review, with considerations of their value as an animal model and their possible role in epidemiology. *Veterinary Parasitology* 77:1–32.

Dubey, J.P., and D. Hedstrom. 1993. Meningoencephalitis in mink associated with a *Sarcocystis neurona*–like organism. *Journal of Veterinary Diagnostic Investigation* 5:467–471.

Dubey, J.P., and T.P. Kistner. 1985. Epizootiology of *Sarcocystis* infections in mule deer fawns in Oregon. *Journal of the American Veterinary Medical Association* 187:1181–1186.

Dubey, J.P., and T.L. Lin. 1994. Acute toxoplasmosis in a gray fox (*Urocyon cinereoargenteus*). *Veterinary Parasitology* 51:321–325.

Dubey, J.P., and D.S. Lindsay. 1996. A review of *Neospora caninum* and neosporosis. *Veterinary Parasitology* 67:1–58.

———. 1998. Isolation in immunodeficient mice of *Sarcocystis neurona* from opossum (*Didelphis virginiana*) faeces, and its differentiation from *Sarcocystis falcatula*. *International Journal for Parasitology* 29:1823–1828

———. 1999. *Sarcocystis speeri,* n. sp. (Protozoa: Sarcocystidae) from the opossum (*Didelphis virginiana*). *The Journal of Parasitology* 85:903–909.

Dubey, J.P., and S.M. Lozier. 1983. *Sarcocystis* infection in the white-tailed deer (*Odocoileus virginianus*) in Montana: Intensity and description of *Sarcocystis odoi* n. sp. American *Journal of Veterinary Research* 44:1738–1743.

Dubey, J.P., and H.G. Sheffield. 1988. *Sarcocystis sigmodontis* n. sp. from the cotton rat (*Sigmodon hispidus*). *The Journal of Parasitology* 74:889–891.

Dubey, J.P., and C.A. Speer. 1985. Prevalence and ultrastructure of three types of *Sarcocystis* in mule deer, *Odocoileus hemionus* (Rafinesque), in Montana. *Journal of Wildlife Diseases* 21:219–228.

———. 1986. *Sarcocystis* infections in mule deer (*Odocoileus hemionus*) in Montana and the description of three new species. *American Journal of Veterinary Research* 47:1052–1055.

Dubey, J.P., E.T. Thorne, and E.S. Williams. 1982. Induced toxoplasmosis in pronghorns and mule deer. *Journal of the American Veterinary Medical Association* 181:1263–1267.

Dubey, J.P., W.R. Jolley, and E.T. Thorne. 1983a. *Sarcocystis sybillensis* sp. nov. from the North American elk (*Cervus elaphus*). *Canadian Journal of Zoology* 61:737–742.

Dubey, J.P., T.P. Kistner, and G. Callis. 1983b. Development of *Sarcocystis* in mule deer transmitted through dogs and coyotes. *Canadian Journal of Zoology* 61:2904–2912.

Dubey, J.P., W.J. Quinn, and D. Weinandy. 1987. Fatal neonatal toxoplasmosis in a bobcat (*Lynx rufus*). *Journal of Wildlife Diseases* 23:324–327.

Dubey, J.P., J.L. Carpenter, C.A. Speer, M.J. Topper, and A. Uggla. 1988a. Newly recognized fatal protozoan disease of dogs. *Journal of the American Veterinary Medical Association* 192:1269–1285.

Dubey, J.P., A.P. Gendron-Fitzpatrick, A.L. Lenhard, and D. Bowman. 1988b. Fatal toxoplasmosis and enteroepithelial stages of *Toxoplasma gondii* in a Pallas cat (*Felis manul*). *Journal of Protozoology* 35:528–530.

Dubey, J.P., J. Ott-Joslin, R.W. Torgerson, M.J. Topper, and J.P. Sundberg. 1988c. Toxoplasmosis in black-faced kangaroos (*Macropus fuliginosus melanops*). *Veterinary Parasitology* 30:97–105.

Dubey, J.P., C.A. Speer, and W.A.G. Charleston. 1989a. Ultrastructural differentiation between sarcocysts of *Sarcocystis hirsuta* and *Sarcocystis hominis*. *Veterinary Parasitology* 34:153–157.

Dubey, J.P., C.A. Speer, and R. Fayer. 1989b. Sarcocystosis of animals and man. Boca Raton, FL: CRC Press, 215 pp.

Dubey, J.P., C.A. Speer, and H.L. Shaw. 1989c. Ultrastructure of sarcocysts from water buffalo in India. *Veterinary Parasitology* 34:149–152.

Dubey, J.P., A.N. Hamir, and C.E. Rupprecht. 1990a. Acute disseminated toxoplasmosis in a red fox (*Vulpes vulpes*). *Journal of Wildlife Diseases* 26:286–290.

Dubey, J.P., A.N. Hamir, C.A. Hanlon, M.J. Topper, and C.E. Rupprecht. 1990b. Fatal necrotizing encephalitis in a raccoon associated with a *Sarcocystis*-like protozoon. *Journal of Veterinary Diagnostic Investigation* 2:345–347.

Dubey, J.P., G.W. Davis, C.A. Speer, D.D. Bowman, D.E. de Lahunta, M.J. Granstrom, M.J. Topper, A.N. Hamir, J.F. Cummings, and M.M. Suter. 1991a. *Sarcocystis neurona* n. sp. (Protozoa: Apicomplexa), the etiological agent of equine protozoal myeloencephalitis. *The Journal of Parasitology* 77:212–218.

Dubey, J.P., D. Hedstrom, C.R. Machado, and K.G. Osborn. 1991b. Disseminated toxoplasmosis in a captive koala (*Phascolarctos cinereus*). *Journal of Zoo and Wildlife Medicine* 22:348–350.

Dubey, J.P., C.A. Brown, J.L. Carpenter, and J.J. Moore. 1992a. Fatal toxoplasmosis in domestic rabbits in the USA. *Veterinary Parasitology* 44:305–309.

Dubey, J.P., H.R. Gamble, A. Rodrigues, and P. Thulliez. 1992b. Prevalence of antibodies to *Toxoplasma gondii* and *Trichinella spiralis* in 509 pigs from 31 farms in Oahu, Hawaii. *Veterinary Parasitology* 43:57–63.

Dubey, J.P., A.N. Hamir, C. Brown, and C.E. Rupprecht. 1992c. *Sarcocystis sehi* sp. n. (Protozoa: Sarcocystidae) from the porcupine (*Erethizon dorsatum*). *Journal of the Helminthological Society of Washington* 59:127–129.

Dubey, J.P., A.N. Hamir, C.A. Hanlon, and C.E. Rupprecht. 1992d. Prevalence of *Toxoplasma gondii* infection in raccoons. *Journal of the American Veterinary Medical Association* 200:534–536.

Dubey, J.P., A.N. Hamir, C.E. Kirkpatrick, K.S. Todd, and C.E. Rupprecht. 1992e. *Sarcocystis felis* sp. n. (Protozoa: Sarcocystidae) from the bobcat (*Felis rufus*). *Journal of the Helminthological Society of Washington* 59:227–229.

Dubey, J.P., A.N. Hamir, S.K. Shen, P. Thulliez, and C.E. Rupprecht. 1993. Experimental *Toxoplasma gondii* infection in raccoons (*Procyon lotor*). *The Journal of Parasitology* 79:548–552.

Dubey, J.P., N. Briscoe, R. Gamble, D. Zarlenga, J.G. Humphreys, and P. Thulliez. 1994. Characterization of *Toxoplasma* and *Trichinella* isolates from muscles of black bears in Pennsylvania. *American Journal of Veterinary Research* 55:815–819.

Dubey, J.P., J.G. Humphreys, and P. Thulliez. 1995a. Prevalence of viable *Toxoplasma gondii* tissue cysts and antibodies to *T. gondii* by various serologic tests in black bears (*Ursus americanus*) from Pennsylvania. *The Journal of Parasitology* 81:109–112.

Dubey, J.P., R.M. Weigel, A.M. Siegel, P. Thulliez, U.D. Kitron, M.A. Mitchell, A. Mannelli, N.E. Mateus-Pinilla, S.K. Shen, O. C.H. Kwok, and K.S. Todd. 1995b. Sources and reservoirs of *Toxoplasma gondii* infection on 47 swine farms in Illinois. *The Journal of Parasitology* 81:723–729.

Dubey, J.P., J. Rigoulet, P. Lagourette, C. George, L. Longeart, and J.L. LeNet. 1996a. Fatal transplacental neosporosis in a deer (*Cervus eldi siamensis*). *The Journal of Parasitology* 82:338–339.

Dubey, J.P., C. A. Speer, M. Niezgoda, and C. E. Rupprecht. 1996b. A *Sarcocystis neurona*–like organism associated with encephalitis in a striped skunk (*Mephitis mephitis*). *The Journal of Parasitology* 82:172–174.

Dubey, J.P., E.A. Rollor, K. Smith, O.C.H. Kwok, and P. Thulliez. 1997. Low seroprevalence of *Toxoplasma gondii* in feral pigs from a remote island lacking cats. *The Journal of Parasitology* 83:839–841.

Dubey, J.P., E.A. Rollor, and D.S. Lindsay. 1998. Isolation of a third species of *Sarcocystis* in immunodeficient mice fed feces from opossums (*Didelphis virginiana*) and its differentiation from *Sarcocystis falcatula* and *Sarcocystis neurona*. *The Journal of Parasitology* 84:1158–1164.

Dubey, J.P., K. Hollis, S. Romand, P. Thulliez, O.C.H. Kwok, L. Hungerford, C. Anchor, and D. Etter. 1999a. High prevalence of antibodies to *Neospora caninum* in white-tailed deer (*Odocoileus virginianus*). *International Journal of Parasitology* 29:1709–1711.

Dubey, J.P., S.T. Storandt, O.C.H. Kwok, P. Thulliez, and K.R. Kazacos. 1999b. *Toxoplasma gondii* antibodies in naturally exposed wild coyotes, red foxes and gray foxes, and serologic diagnosis of toxoplasmosis in red foxes fed *T. gondii* oocysts and tissue cysts. *The Journal of Parasitology* 85:240–243.

Edelhofer, R., H. Prosl, and E. Kutzer. 1996. Zur Trichinellose und Toxoplasmose der Wildschweine in Ostösterreich. *Wiener Tierärztliche Monatsschrift* 83:225–229.

Elwasila, M., R. Entzeroth, B. Chobotar, and E. Scholtyseck. 1984. Comparison of the structure of *Sarcocystis cuniculi* of the European rabbit (*Oryctolagus cuniculus*) and *Sar-*
cocystis leporum of the cottontail rabbit (*Sylvilagus floridanus*) by light and electron microscopy. *Acta Veterinaria Hungarica* 32:71–78.

Emerson, H. R., and W. T. Wright. 1970. Correction. *Journal of Wildlife Disease* 6:519.

Entzeroth, R., E. Scholtyseck, and B. Chobotar. 1983a. Ultrastructure of *Sarcocystis* sp. from the eastern chipmunk (*Tamias striatus*). *Zeitschrift für Parasitenkunde* 69:823–826.

Entzeroth, R., B. Chobotar, and E. Scholtyseck. 1983b. Ultrastructure of a *Sarcocystis* species from the red squirrel (*Tamiasciurus hudsonicus*) in Michigan. *Protistologica* 19:91–94.

Entzeroth, R., G. Piekarski, and E. Scholtyseck. 1981. Fine structural study of a *Toxoplasma* strain from the Roe deer. *Zeitschrift für Parasitenkunde* 66:109–112.

Fenger, C.K., D.E. Granstrom, A.A. Gajadhar, N.M. Williams, S.A. McCrillis, S. Stamper, J.L. Langemeier, and J.P. Dubey. 1997. Experimental induction of equine protozoal myeloencephalitis in horses using *Sarcocystis* sp. sporocysts from the opossum (*Didelphis virginiana*). *Veterinary Parasitology* 68:199–213.

Foreyt, W.J. 1989. *Sarcocystis* sp. in mountain goats (*Oreamnos americanus*) in Washington: Prevalence and search for the definitive host. *Journal of Wildlife Diseases* 25:619–622.

Foreyt, W.J., T.J. Baldwin, and J.E. Lagerquist. 1995. Experimental infections of *Sarcocystis* spp. in Rocky Mountain elk (*Cervus elaphus*) calves. *Journal of Wildlife Diseases* 31:462–466.

Franti, C.E., G.E. Connolly, H.P. Riemann, D.E. Behymer, R. Ruppanner, C.M. Willadsen, and W. Longhurst. 1975. A survey for *Toxoplasma gondii* antibodies in deer and other wildlife on a sheep range. *Journal of the American Veterinary Medical Association* 167:565–568.

Friesen, D.L., R.J. Cawthorn, C.A. Speer, and R.J. Brooks. 1989. Ultrastructural development of the sarcocyst of *Sarcocystis rauschorum* (Apicomplexa: Sarcocystidae) in the varying lemming *Dicrostonyx richardsoni*. *The Journal of Parasitology* 75:422–427.

Galavíz-Silva, L., R. Mercado-Hernández, E. Ramírez-Bon, J.M. Arredondo-Cantú, and D. Lazcano-Villarreal. 1991. *Sarcocystis neotomafelis* sp. n. (Protozoa; Apicomplexa) from the woodrat *Neotoma micropus* in Mexico. *Revista Latinoamericana de Microbiologia* 33:313–322.

Galuszka, J. 1963. Toksoplazmoza ptaków. *Medycyna Weterynaryjna* 19:151–152.

Gangadharan, B., K.V. Valsala, M.G. Nair, and A. Rajan. 1992. Sarcocystosis in a sambar deer (*Cervus unicolor*). *Indian Journal of Animal Sciences* 62:127–128.

Garner, M.M., B.C. Barr, A.E. Packham, A.E. Marsh, K.A. Burek-Huntington, R.K. Wilson, and J.P. Dubey. 1997. Fatal hepatic sarcocystosis in two polar bears (*Ursus maritimus*). *The Journal of Parasitology* 83:523–526.

Ghaffar, F.A., A.O. Heydorn, and H. Mehlhorn. 1989. The fine structure of cysts of *Sarcocystis* moulei from goats. *Parasitology Research* 75:416–418.

Gibb, D.G.A., B.A. Kakulas, D.H. Perret, and D.J. Jenkyn. 1966. Toxoplasmosis in the Rottnest Quokka (*Setonix brachyurus*). *Australian Journal of Experimental Biology and Medical Science* 44:665–672.

Gjerde, B. 1986. Scanning electron microscopy of the sarcocysts of six species of *Sarcocystis* from reindeer (*Rangifer tarandus tarandus*). *Acta Pathologica, Microbiologica et Immunologica Scandinavica, Sect. B* 94:309–317.

Gorham, J.R., and K. Farrell. 1955. Diseases and parasites of Chinchillas. *Proceedings of the American Veterinary Medical Association,* 92nd Annual Meeting, Minneapolis, MN, August 15–18, pp. 228–234.

Gorman, T.R., H.A. Alcaino, H. Munoz, and C. Cunazza. 1984. *Sarcocystis* sp. in guanaco (*Lama guanicoe*) and effect of temperature on its viability. *Veterinary Parasitology* 15:95–101.

Green, L.E., and K.L. Morgan. 1991. *Toxoplasma* abortion in a guinea pig. *Veterinary Record* 129:266–267.

Greiner, E.C., M.E. Roelke, C.T. Atkinson, J.P. Dubey, and S.D. Wright. 1989. *Sarcocystis* sp. in muscles of free-ranging Florida panthers and cougars (*Felis concolor*). *Journal of Wildlife Diseases* 25:623–628.

Grikieniené, J., T. Arnastauskiené, and L. Kutkiené. 1993. On some disregarded ways of sarcosporidians' circulation and remarks about systematics of the genus *Sarcocystis* Lankester, 1882 with the description of the new species from rodents [in Russian]. *Ekologija (Vilnius)* 1:16–22.

Grünberg, W. 1959. Toxoplasmose beim Bennett-Känguruh (*Makropus bennetti* Gould) und einem Klippschilefer (*Hyrax syriacus* Schreb). *Wiener Tierärztliche Monatsschrift* 46:586–593.

Gustafsson, K., and A. Uggla. 1994. Serologic survey for *Toxoplasma gondii* infection in the brown hare (*Lepus europaeus* P.) in Sweden. *Journal of Wildlife Diseases* 30:201–204.

Gustafsson, K., and A. Uggla, T. Svensson, and L. Sjöland. 1988. Detection of *Toxoplasma gondii* in liver tissue sections from brown hares (*Lepus europaeus* P.) and mountain hares (*Lepus timidus* L) using the peroxidase antiperoxidase technique as a complement to conventional histopathology. *Journal of Veterinary Medicine B* 35:402–407.

Häfner, U., and F.R. Matuschka. 1984. Life cycle studies on *Sarcocystis dirumpens* sp. n. with regard to host specificity. *Zeitschrift für Parasitenkunde* 70:715–720.

Hamerton, A.E. 1932. Report on the deaths occurring in the Society's Gardens during the year 1931. *Proceedings of the Zoological Society of London,* pp. 613–638.

———. 1933. Report on deaths occurring in the Society's Gardens during the year 1932. *Proceedings of the Zoological Society of London,* pp. 451–482.

———. 1934. *Toxoplasma wenyoni* in the brain of a Mitchell's wombat (*Phasocolom mitchell*). *Transactions of the Royal Society of Tropical Medicine* 28:2.

Harcourt, R.A. 1967. Toxoplasmosis in rabbits. *Veterinary Record* 81:191–192.

Hartley, W.J. 1993. Central nervous system disorders in the brush-tail possum in Eastern Australia. *New Zealand Veterinary Journal* 41:44–45.

Hartley, W.J., J.P. Dubey, and D.S. Spielman. 1990. Fatal toxoplasmosis in Koalas (*Phascolarctos cinereus*). *The Journal of Parasitology* 76:271–272.

Helmboldt, C.F., and E.L. Jungherr. 1955. Distemper complex in wild carnivores simulating rabies. *American Journal of Veterinary Research* 16:463–469.

Henriksen, P., H.H. Dietz, A. Uttenthal, and M. Hansen. 1994. Seroprevalence of *Toxoplasma gondii* in Danish farmed mink (*Mustela vison* S.). *Veterinary Parasitology* 53:1–5.

Hernández-Rodríguez, S., I. Acosta, and I. Navarrete. 1992. *Sarcocystis jorrini* sp. nov. from the fallow deer *Cervus dama*. *Parasitology Research* 78:557–562.

Hilgenfeld, M. 1965. Toxoplasmose bei Zootieren. *Zoologische Garten (Berlin)* 30:262–270.

Hirato, K. 1939. Notes on two cases of *Toxoplasma* observed among raccoon-dogs in the vicinity of Sapporo. *Japanese Journal of Veterinary Science* 1:544–552.

Holshuh, H.J., A.E. Sherrod, C.R. Taylor, B.F. Andrews, and E.B. Howard. 1985. Toxoplasmosis in a feral northern fur seal (tech. note). *Journal of the American Veterinary Medical Association* 187:1229–1230.

Humphreys, J.G., R.L. Stewart, and J.P. Dubey. 1995. Prevalence of *Toxoplasma gondii* antibodies in sera of hunter-killed white-tailed deer in Pennsylvania. *American Journal of Veterinary Research* 56:172–173.

Huong, L.T.T., and A. Uggla. 1999. *Sarcocystis dubeyi* n. sp. (Protozoa: Sarcocystidae) in the water buffalo (*Bubalis bubalis*). *The Journal of Parasitology* 85:102–104

Huong, L.T.T., J.P. Dubey, T. Nikkilä, and A. Uggla. 1997a. *Sarcocystis buffalonis* n. sp. (Protozoa: Sarcocystidae) from the water buffalo (*Bubalus bubalis*) in Vietnam. *The Journal of Parasitology* 83:471–474.

Huong, L.T.T., J.P. Dubey, and A. Uggla. 1997b. Redescription of *Sarcocystis levinei* Dissanaike and Kan, 1978 (Protozoa: Sarcocystidae) of the water buffalo (*Bubalus bubalis*). *The Journal of Parasitology* 83:1148–1152.

Inoue, I., M. Yamada, Y. Yoshimi, Y. Imai, I. Utsugi, R. Suzuki, S. Nogami, E. Fujita, K.-I. Takahashi, K. Tsuchiya, K. Miyamoto, and K. Takagi. 1990. Prevalence of *Sarcocystis* (Protozoa, Apicomplexa) in voles in Japan. *Japanese Journal of Parasitology* 39:415–417.

Inskeep, W., II, C.H. Gardiner, R.K. Harris, J.P. Dubey, and R.T. Goldston. 1990. Toxoplasmosis in Atlantic bottle-nosed dolphins (*Tursiops truncatus*). *Journal of Wildlife Diseases* 26:377–382.

Institute of Zoology, Kazakh Academy of Sciences (ed.). 1984.*Sarcosporidians of animals in Kazakhstan* [in Russian]. Alma-Ata: Nauka, 258 pp.

Ippen, R., J. Jíra, and K. Blazek. 1981. Toxoplasmose als Todesursache bei Saiga-Antilopen (*Saiga tatarica*). Verhandlungsbericht des 23. Internationaler Symposiums über die Erkrankungen der Zootiere vom 24 Juni bis 28 Juni 1987 in Halle, Germany, pp. 185–191.

Jacobs, L., J.S. Remington, and M.L. Melton. 1960a. The Resistance of the encysted form of *Toxoplasma gondii*. *The Journal of Parasitology* 4:11–21.

Jacobs, L., J.S. Remington, and M.L. Melton. 1960b. A survey of meat samples from swine, cattle, and sheep for the presence of encysted *Toxoplamsa*. *Journal of Parasitology* 46:23–28.

Jacobs, L., A.M. Stanley, and C.M. Herman. 1962. Prevalence of *Toxoplasma* antibodies in rabbits, squirrels, and raccoons collected in and near the Patuxent wildlife research center. *The Journal of Parasitology* 48:550

Jäkel, T. 1995. Cyclic transmission of *Sarcocystis gerbilliechis* n. sp. by the Arabian saw-scaled viper, *Echis coloratus*, to rodents of the subfamily Gerbillinae. *The Journal of Parasitology* 81:626–631.

Jakob-Hoff, R.M., and J.D. Dunsmore. 1983. Epidemiological aspects of toxoplasmosis in southern Western Australia. *Australian Veterinary Journal* 60:217–218.

Jensen, J.M., S. Patton, B.G. Wright, and D.G. Loeffler. 1985. Toxoplasmosis in marsupials in a zoological collection. *Journal of Zoo Animal Medicine* 16:129–131.

Johnson, A.M., H. Roberts, and B.L. Munday. 1988. Prevalence of *Toxoplasma gondii* antibody in wild macropods. *Australian Veterinary Journal* 65:199–201.

Johnson, A.M., H. Roberts, P. Statham, and B.L. Munday. 1989. Serodiagnosis of acute toxoplasmosis in macropods. *Veterinary Parasitology* 34:25–33.

Jordan, G.W., J. Theis, C.M. Fuller, and P.D. Hoeprich. 1975. Bear meat trichinosis with a concomitant serologic response to *Toxoplasma gondii*. *American Journal of Medical Sciences* 269:251–257.

Junge, R.E., J.R. Fischer, and J.P. Dubey. 1992. Fatal disseminated toxoplasmosis in a captive Cuvier's gazelle (*Gazella cuvieri*). *Journal of Zoo and Wildlife Medicine* 23:342–345.

Keagy, H.F. 1949. *Toxoplasma* in the chinchilla. *Journal of the American Veterinary Medical Association* 114:15.

Kirkpatrick, C.E., A.N. Hamir, J.P. Dubey, and C.E. Rupprecht. 1987. *Sarcocystis* in muscles of raccoons (*Procyon lotor* L.). *Journal of Protozoology* 34:445–447.

Kiss, G., and Z. Graf. 1989. Perinatale Toxoplasmose bei einem Eisbären (*Thalarctos maritimus*). Internationalen Symposium über die Ekrankungen der Zoo- und Wildtiere, 24 Mai bis 28 Mai 1989 in Dortmund, Germany, pp. 433–435.

Kiupel, H., D. Ritscher, and G. Fricke. 1987. Toxoplasmose bei jungen Kodiakbären (*Ursus arctos middendorffi*). Verhandlungsbericht des 29. Internationalen Symposiums über die Erkrankungen der Zootiere vom 20 Mai bis 24 Mai 1987 in Cardiff, UK, pp. 335–340.

Klumpp, S.A., D.C. Anderson, H.M. McClure, and J.P. Dubey. 1994. Encephalomyelitis due to a *Sarcocystis neurona*-like protozoan in a rhesus monkey (*Macaca mulatta*) infected with simian immunodeficiency virus. *American Journal of Tropical Medicine and Hygiene* 51:332–338.

Kocan, A.A., S.J. Barron, J.C. Fox, and A.W. Franzmann. 1986. Antibodies to *Toxoplasma gondii* in moose (*Alces alces L.*) from Alaska. *Journal of Wildlife Diseases* 22:432.

Koller, L.D., T.P. Kistner, and G.G. Hudkins. 1977. Histopathologic study of experimental *Sarcocystis hemionilatrantis* infection in fawns. *American Journal of Veterinary Research* 38:1205–1209.

Krampitz, H.E., and M. Rommel. 1977. Experimentelle Untersuchungen über das Wirtsspektrum der Frenklien der Erdmaus. *Berliner und Münchener Tierärztliche Wochenschrift* 90:17–19.

Kronberger, H., and K.F. Schüppel. 1976. Todesursachen von Känguruhs—Durchsicht der Sekionsprotokolle von 1853 bis 1975. Verhandlungsbericht des 18 Internationalen Symposiums über die Erkrankungen der Zootiere vom 16 Juni bis 20 Juni 1976 in Innsbruck, Austria, pp. 27–30.

Lapointe, J.-M., P.J. Duigman, A.E. Marsh, F.M. Gulland, B.C. Barr, D.K. Naydan, D.P. King, C.A. Farman, K.A. Burek Huntington, and L.J. Lowenstine. 1998. Meningoencephalitis due to a *Sarcocystis neurona*-like protozoan in pacific harbor seals (*Phoca vitulina richardsi*). *Journal of Parasitology* 84:1184–1189

Leland, M.M., G.B. Hubbard, and J.P. Dubey. 1992. Clinical toxoplasmosis in domestic rabbits. *Laboratory Animal Science* 42:318–319.

Lenghaus, C., D.L. Obendorf, and F.H. Wright. 1990. Veterinary aspects of *Perameles gunnii* biology with special reference to species conservation. In *Management and conservation of small populations* Ed. T.W. Clark and J.H. Seebeck. Chicago: Chicago Zoological Society, pp. 89–108.

Levine, N.D. 1988. *The protozoan phylum Apicomplexa*, vols. 1 and 2. Boca Raton, FL: CRC Press, Inc.

Lindsay, D.S., B.L. Blagburn, J.P. Dubey, and W.H. Mason. 1991. Prevalence and isolation of *Toxoplasma gondii* from white-tailed deer in Alabama. *The Journal of Parasitology* 77:62–64.

Lindsay, D.S., S.J. Upton, B.L. Blagburn, M. Toivio-Kinnucan, J.P. Dubey, C.T. McAllister, and S.E. Trauth. 1992a. Demonstration that *Sarcocystis montanaensis* has a speckled kingsnake-prairie vole life cycle. *Journal of the Helminthological Society of Washington* 59:9–15.

Lindsay, D.S., S.J. Upton, M. Toivio-Kinnucan, R.D. McKown, and B.L. Blagburn. 1992b. Ultrastructure of *Frenkelia microti* in praire voles inoculated with sporocysts from red-tailed hawks. *Journal of the Helminthological Society of Washington* 59:170–176.

Lindsay, D.S., R. McKown, S.J. Upton, C.T. McAllister, M. Toivio-Kinnucan, J.K. Veatch, and B.L. Blackburn. 1996. Prevalence and identity of *Sarcocystis* infections in armadillos (*Dasypus novemcinctus*). *The Journal of Parasitology* 82:518–520.

Lynch, M. J., D. L. Obendorf, P. Statham, and G. L. Reddacliff. 1993. An evaluation of a live *Toxoplasma gondii* vaccine in tammar wallabies (*Macropus eugenii*) (technical note). Australian Veterinary Journal 70:352–353.

Mandelli, G., A. Cerioli, E.E.A. Hahn, and F. Strozzi. 1966. Osservazioni anatomo-istologiche e parassitologiche su di un episodio di toxoplasmosi nel canguro di Bennett (*Macropis Bennetti* Gould). *Bollettino del Istituto Sieroterapico Milanese* 45:177–192.

Mandour, A.M., and I.F. Keymer. 1970. *Sarcocystis* infection in African antelopes. *Annals of Tropical Medicine and Parasitology* 64:513–523.

Marchiondo, A.A., D.W. Duszynski, and G.O. Maupin. 1976. Prevalence of antibodies to *Toxoplasma gondii* in wild and domestic animals of New Mexico, Arizona and Colorado. *Journal of Wildlife Diseases* 12:226–232.

Markham, F.S. 1937. Spontaneous *Toxoplasma* encephalitis in the guinea pig. *American Journal of Hygiene* 26:193–196.

McAllister, M.M., J.P. Dubey, D.S. Lindsay, W.R. Jolley, R.A. Wills, and A.M. McGuire. 1998. Dogs are definitive hosts of *Neospora caninum*. *International Journal for Parasitology* 28:1473–1478.

Mason, R.W., W.J. Hartley, and J.P. Dubey. 1991. Lethal toxoplasmosis in a little penguin (*Eudyptula minor*) from Tasmania. *The Journal of Parasitology* 77:328.

Matuschka, F.R., H. Mehlhorn, and Z. Abd-Al-Aal. 1987. Replacement of *Besnoitia* Matuschka and Häfner 1984 [sic] by *Sarcocystis hoarensis*. *Parasitology Research* 74:94–96.

Medway, W., D.L. Skand, and C.F. Sarver. 1989. Neurologic signs in American porcupines (*Erethizon dorsatum*) infected with *Baylisascaris* and *Toxoplasma*. *Journal of Zoo and Wildlife Medicine* 20:207–211.

Mehlhorn, H., A.O. Heydorn, and K. Janitschke. 1977. Light and electron microscopical study on sarcocysts from muscles of the rhesus monkey (*Macaca mulatta*), baboon (*Papio cynocephalus*) and tamarin [*Saguinus* (= *Oedipomidas*) *oedipus*]. *Zeitschrift für Parasitenkunde* 51:165–178.

Mense, M.G., J.P. Dubey, and B.L. Homer. 1992. Acute hepatic necrosis associated with a *sarcocystis*-like protozoa in a sea lion (*Zalophus californianus*). *Journal of Veterinary Diagnostic Investigation* 4:486–490.

Miescher, F. 1843. Uber eigenthumliche Schläuche in den Muskeln einer Hausmaus. *Bericht über die Verbandlungen der Naturforschenden Gesellschaft* in Basel. Vol. 5, pp. 198–202. Illustration in *Zeitschrift für wissenschaftliche Zoologie* 5: plate X, 1854.

Migaki, G., J.F. Allen, and H.W. Casey. 1977. Toxoplasmosis in a California sea lion (*Zalophus californianus*). *American Journal of Veterinary Research* 38:135–136.

Migaki, G., T.R. Sawa, and J.P. Dubey. 1990. Fatal disseminated toxoplasmosis in a spinner dolphin (*Stenella longirostris*). *Veterinary Pathology* 27:463–464.

Miller, M.A., K. Ehlers, J.P. Dubey, and K. van Steenbergh. 1992. Outbreak of toxoplasmosis in wallabies on an exotic animal farm. *Journal of Veterinary Diagnostic Investigation* 4:480–483.

Mitchell, M.A., L.L. Hungerford, C.M. Nixon, T.L. Esker, J.B. Sullivan, R. Koerkenmeier, and J.P. Dubey. 1999. Serologic survey for *Leptospira spp.*, canine distemper virus, pseudorabies virus, and *Toxoplasma gondii* in raccoons from west–central Illinois. *Journal of Wildlife Diseases*, 35:347–355.

Møller, T. 1952. Toxoplasmosis *Vulpis vulpis*. *Acta Pathologica Microbiologica Scandinavica Supplement* 93:308–320.

———. 1958. *Toxoplamosis cuniculi*. Verificering af diagnosen, patologisk-anatomiske og serologiske undersogelser. *Nordisk Veterinärmedicin* 10:1–56.

Møller, T., and S.W. Nielsen. 1964. Toxoplasmosis in distemper-susceptible carnivora. *Pathologia Veterinaria* 1:189–203.

Momberg-Jørgensen, H.C. 1956. Toxoplasmose i forbindelse med hvalpesyge hos minken. *Nordisk Veterinärmedicin* 8:239–242.

Nobel, T.A., U. Klopfer, and F. Neuman. 1969. Toxoplasmosis in wild animals in Israel. *Journal of Comparative Pathology* 79:127–129.

Nutter, F.B., J.F. Levine, M.K. Stoskopf, H.R. Gamble, and J.P. Dubey. 1998. Seroprevalence of *Toxoplasma gondii* and *Trichinella spiralis* in North Carolina black bears (*Ursus americanus*). *The Journal of Parasitology* 84:1048–1050.

Obendorf, D.L., and B.L. Munday. 1983. Toxoplasmosis in wild Tasmanian wallabies. *Australian Veterinary Journal* 60:62.

———. 1990. Toxoplasmosis in wild eastern barred bandicoots, *Perameles gunnii*. In *Bandicoots and bilbies; Australian mammal society symposium*. Ed. J.H. Seebeck, P.R. Brown, R.L. Wallis, and C.M. Kemper. Sydney, Australia: Surrey Beatty and Sons, pp. 193–197.

Obendorf, D.L., P. Statham, and M. Driessen. 1996. Detection of agglutinating antibodies to *Toxoplasma gondii* in sera from free-ranging eastern barred bandicoots (*Perameles gunnii*). *Journal of Wildlife Diseases* 32:623–626.

Ocholi, R.A., J.O. Kalejaiye, and P.A. Okewole. 1989. Acute disseminated toxoplasmosis in two captive lions (*Panthera leo*) in Nigeria. *Veterinary Record* 124:515–516.

Odening, K. 1983. Sarkozysten in einer antarktischen Robbe. *Angewandte Parasitologie* 24:197–200.

———. 1986. Tissue cyst-forming Coccidia in Antarctic vertebrates. In *Advances in Protozoological Research/Symposia Biologica Hungaricae (Budapest)* 33:351–355.

———. 1997. Die *Sarcocystis*-Infektion: Wechselbeziehungen zwischen freilebenden Wildtieren, Haustieren und Zootieren, Der Zoologische Garten N.F. 67:317–340.

Odening, K., and J. Zipper. 1986. Zur Ultrastruktur von *Sarcocystis hydrurgae* n. sp. (Apicomplexa: Sporozoea) aus *Hydrurga leptonyx* (Carnivora: Phocidae). *Archiv für Protistenkunde* 131:27–32.

Odening, K., M. Stolte, G. Walter, and I. Bockhardt. 1994a. The European badger (Carnivora: Mustelidae) as intermediate host of further three *Sarcocystis* species (Sporozoa). *Parasite (Paris)* 1:23–30.

Odening, K., M. Stolte, G. Walter, I. Bockhardt, and W. Jakob. 1994b. Sarcocysts (*Sarcocystis* sp.: Sporozoa) in the European badger *Meles meles*. *Parasitology* 108:421–424.

Odening, K., H.H. Wesemeier, M. Pinkowski, G. Walter, and I. Bockhardt. 1994c. European hare and European rabbit (Lagomorpha) as intermediate hosts of Sarcocystis species (Sporozoa) in central Europe. *Acta Protozoologica* 33:177–189.

Odening, K., M. Stolte, G. Walter, and I. Bockhardt. 1995a. Cyst wall ultrastructure of two *Sarcocystis* species from European mouflon (*Ovis ammon musimon*) in Germany compared with domestic sheep. *Journal of Wildlife Diseases* 31:550–554.

Odening, K., H.H. Wesemeier, G. Walter, and I. Bockhardt. 1995b. Ultrastructure of sarcocysts from equids. *Acta Parasitologica* 40:12–20.

———. 1995c. On the morphological diagnostics and host specificity of the *Sarcocystis* species of some domesticated and wild Bovini (cattle, banteng and bison). *Applied Parasitology* 36:161–178.

Odening, K., M. Stolte, and I. Bockhardt. 1996a. Sarcocysts in exotic Caprinae (Bovidae) from zoological gardens. *Acta Parasitologica* 41:67–75.

———. 1996b. On the diagnostics of *Sarcocystis* in chamois (*Rupicapra rupicapra*). *Applied Parasitology* 37:153–160.

Odening, K., M. Stolte, E. Lux, and I. Bockhardt. 1996c. The Mongolian gazelle (*Procapra gutturosa,* Bovidae) as an intermediate host of three *Sarcocystis* species in Mongolia. *Applied Parasitology* 37:54–65.

Odening, K., H.H. Wesemeier, and I. Bockhardt. 1996d. On the sarcocysts of two further *Sarcocystis* species being new for the European hare. *Acta Protozoologica* 35:69–72.

Odening, K., S. Quandt, R.G. Bengis, M. Stolte, and I. Bockhardt. 1997. *Sarcocystis hippopotami* sp. n. and *S. africana* sp. n. (Protozoa: Sarcocystidae) from the hippopotamus in South Africa. *Acta Parasitologica* 42:187–191.

Odening, K., A. Aue, A. Ochs, and M. Stolte. 1998a. *Emmonsia crescens* (Ascomycotina) und *Sarcocystis ochotonae* n. sp. bei Pfeifhasen (*Ochotona*) aus China im Zoologischen Garten Berlin. *Der Zoologische Garten* N.F. 68:80–94.

Odening, K., M. Rudolph, S. Quandt, R.G. Bengis, I. Bockhardt, D. Viertel. 1998b. *Sarcocystis* spp. in antelopes from southern Africa. *Acta Protozoologica* 37:149–158.

Odening, K., A. Aue, and A. Ochs. 1999. Einheimische *Sarcocystis*-Arten (Sporozoa) in exotischen Zoosäugetieren (Gayal, Cerviden, Cameliden, Ozelot). *Der Zoologische Garten* N.F. 69:109–125.

Oertley, K.D., and K.W. Walls. 1980. Prevalence of antibodies to *Toxoplasma gondii* among bobcats of West Virginia and Georgia. *Journal of the American Veterinary Medical Association* 177:852–853.

Oksanen, A., K. Gustafsson, A. Lundén, J.P. Dubey, P. Thulliez, and A. Uggla. 1996. Experimental *Toxoplasma gondii* infection leading to fatal enteritis in reindeer (*Rangifer tarandus*). *The Journal of Parasitology* 82:843–845.

Olubayo, R.O., and L.H. Karstad. 1981. Fatal toxoplasmosis in a tree hyrax (*Dendrohyrax arboreus*). *Bulletin of Animal Health and Production in Africa* 29:263–264.

Orazalinova, V.A., V.M. Fedoseenko, and O.N. Sklyarova. 1986. The ultrastructure of the cyst of *Sarcocystis* sp. from *Alectoris chukar* [in Russian]. *Izvestiya Akademii Nauk Kazakhskoi SSR, Seriya Biologicheskaya* 6:43–48.

Pak, S.M., L.S. Pak, and O.N. Sklyarova. 1989a. *Sarcocystis citellibuteonis* n. sp. of Sarcosporidia from the large-toothed suslik *Citellus fulvus* [in Russian]. *Izvestiya Akademii Nauk Kazakhskoi SSR, Seriya Biologicheskaya* (3):30–33.

Pak, S.M., O.N. Sklyarova, and L.S. Pak. 1989b. *Sarcocystis alectorivulpes* and *Sarcocystis alectoributeonis*—New sarcosporidian species of *Alectoris chugar* [in Russian]. *Izvestiya Akademii Nauk Kazakhskoi SSR, Seriya Biologicheskaya* 6:25–30.

Pak, S.M., O.N. Sklyarova, and N.D. Dymkova. 1991. Sarcocysts (Sporozoa, Apicomplexa) of some species of wild mammals (in Russian). *Izvestiya Akademii Nauk Kazakhskoi SSR, Seriya Biologicheskaya* 5:35–40.

Patton, S., S.L. Johnson, D.G. Loeffler, B.G. Wright, and J.M. Jensen. 1986. Epizootic of toxoplasmosis in kangaroos, wallabies, and potaroos: Possible transmission via domestic cats. *Journal of the American Veterinary Medical Association* 189:1166–1169.

Paul-Murphy, J., T. Work, D. Hunter, E. McFie, and D. Fjelline. 1994. Serologic survey and serum biochemical reference ranges of the free-ranging mountain lion (*Felis concolor*) in California. *Journal of Wildlife Diseases* 30:205–215.

Phillips, P. 1986. Toxoplasmosis in yellow footed rock wallabies, *Veterinary Pathology Report, Australian Registry Veterinary Pathology* 11:211–216.

Pizzi, H.L., C.M. Rico, and O.A.M. Pessat. 1978. Hallazgo del circlo ontogenico selvatic o del *Toxoplasma gondii* en felidos salvajes (*Oncifelis geofroyi, Felis colocolo y Felis eira*) de la Provincia de Cordoba. *Revista Militar de Veterinaria* 25:293–300.

Pope, J.H., E.H. Derrick, and I. Cook. 1957a. *Toxoplasma* in Queensland. I. Observations on a strain of *Toxoplasma gondii* isolated from a bandicoot, *Thylacis obesulus. Australian Journal of Experimental Biology* 35:467–480.

Pope, J.H., V.A. Bicks, and I. Cook. 1957b. *Toxoplasma* in Queensland. II. Natural infections in bandicoots and rats. *Australian Journal of Experimental Biology* 35:481–490.

Pridham, T.J. 1961. An outbreak of toxoplasmosis in ranch mink. *Canadian Journal of Public Health* 52:389–393.

Pridham, T.J., T.J., and J. Belcher. 1958. Toxoplasmosis in mink. *Canadian Journal of Comparative Medicine* 22:99–106.

Quandt, S., R.G. Bengis, M. Stolte, K. Odening, and I. Bockhardt. 1997. *Sarcocystis* infection of the African buffalo (*Syncerus caffer*) in the Kruger National Park, South Africa. *Acta Parasitologica* 42:68–73.

Rakich, P.M., J.P. Dubey, and J.K. Contarino. 1992. Acute Hepatic sarcocystosis in a chinchilla. *Journal of Veterinary Diagnostic Investigation* 4:484–486.

Ratcliffe, H.L., and C.B. Worth. 1951. Toxoplasmosis of captive wild birds and mammals. *American Journal of Pathology* 27:655–667.

Reddacliff, G.L., W.J. Hartley, J.P. Dubey, and D.W. Cooper. 1993a. Pathology of experimentally-induced, acute toxoplasmosis in macropods. *Australian Veterinary Journal* 70:4–6.

Reddacliff, G.L., S.J. Parker, J.P. Dubey, P.J. Nicholls, A.M. Johnson, and D.W. Cooper. 1993b. An attempt to prevent acute toxoplasmosis in macropods by vaccination with *Hammondia hammondi. Australian Veterinary Journal* 70:33–35.

Reed, W.M., and J.J. Turek. 1985. Concurrent distemper and disseminated toxoplasmosis in a red fox. *Journal of the American Veterinary Medical Association* 187:1264–1265.

Riemann, H.P., M.E. Fowler, T. Schulz, J.A. Lock, J. Thilsted, L.T. Pulley, R.V. Henrickson, A.M. Henness, C.E. Franti, and D.E. Behymer. 1974. Toxoplasmosis in pallas cats. *Journal of Wildlife Diseases* 10:471–477.

Riemann, H.P., M.E. Meyer, J.H. Theis, G. Kelso, and D.E. Behymer. 1975. Toxoplasmosis in an infant fed unpasteurized goat milk. *Pediatrics* 87:573–576.

Rioseco, H.B., V. Cubillos, G. González, Q., and L.C. Díaz. 1976. Sarcosporidiosis en pudues (*Pudu pudu,* Molina, 1782). *Archivos de Medicina Veterinaria (Valdivia)* 8:122–123.

Roberts, R., K.D. Murrell, and S. Marks. 1994. Economic losses caused by foodborne parasitic diseases. *Parasitology Today* 10:419–423.

Rodaniche, E. de, and T. de Pinzon. 1949. Spontaneous toxoplasmosis in the guinea-pig in Panama. *The Journal of Parasitology* 35:152–154.

Roelke, M.E., D.J. Forrester, E.R. Jacobson, G.V. Kollias, F.W. Scott, M.C. Barr, J.F. Evermann, and E.C. Pirtle. 1993. Seroprevalence of infectious-disease agents in free-ranging Florida panthers (*Felis concolor coryi*). *Journal of Wildlife Diseases* 29(1):36–49.

Roher, D.P., M.J. Ryan, S.W. Neilsen, and D.E. Roscoe. 1981. Acute fatal toxoplasmosis in squirrels. *Journal of the American Veterinary Medical Association* 179:1099–1101.

Rommel, M., and H.E. Krampitz. 1975. Beiträge zum Lebeszyklus der *Frenkelien.* I. Die Identität von *Isospora buteonis* aus dem Mäusebussard mit einer Frenkelienart (*F. clethrionomyobuteonis* sp. n.) aus der Rötelmaus. *Berliner und Münchener Tierärztliche Wochenschrift* 88:338–340.

Rosonke, B.J., S.R. Brown, S.J. Tornquist, S.P. Snyder, M.M. Garner, and L.L. Blythe. 1999. Enchephalomyelitis associated with a *Sarcocystis neurona*–like organism in a sea otter. *Journal of the American Veterinary Medical Association* 215:1849–1842.

Sacks, J.J., D.G. Delgado, H.O. Lobel, and R.L. Parker. 1983. Toxoplasmosis infection associated with eating undercooked venison. *American Journal of Epidemiology* 118:832–838.

Saito, M., T. Itagaki, Y. Shibata, and H. Itagaki. 1995. Morphology and experimental definitive hosts of *Sarcocystis* sp. from sika deer, *Cervus nippon centralis,* in Japan. *Japanese Journal of Parasitology* 44:218–221.

Saito, M., Y. Shibata, M. Kubo, and H. Itagaki. 1997. *Sarcocystis mihoensis* n. sp. from sheep in Japan. *Journal of Veterinary Medical Science* 59:103–106.

Schmidt, V. 1975. Todesursachen bei Känguruhs. Verhandlungsbericht des XVII. Internationalen Symposiums über die Erkrankungen der Zootiere vom 4 Juni bis 8 Juni 1975 in Tunis, Tunisia, pp. 321–325.

Schneider, H.E., G. Berger, F. Dathe, and W. Gensch. 1976. Erkrankungen australischer Tiere im Zoologischen Garten Dresden. Verhandlungsbericht des XVIII. Internationalen Symposiums über die Erkrankungen der Zootiere vom 16 Juni bis 20 Juni 1976 in Innsbruck, Austria, pp. 5–12.

Scholtyseck, E., R. Entzeroth, and B. Chobotar. 1982. Light and electron microscopy of *Sarcoccystis* sp. in the skeletal muscle of an opossum (*Didelphis virginiana*). *Protistologica* 18:527–532.

Schröder, H.D., and R. Ippen. 1976. Beitrag zu den Erkrankungen der Känguruhs. Erkrankungen der Zootiere. Verhandlungsbericht des XVIII. Internationalen Symposiums über die Erkrankungen der Zootiere vom 16 Juni bis 20 Juni 1976 in Innsbruck, Austria, pp. 21–26.

Sedlaczek, J., and H.-H. Wesemeier. 1995. On the diagnostics and nomenclature of *Sarcocystis* species (Sporozoa) in roe deer (*Capreolus capreolus*). *Applied Parasitology* 36:73–82.

Sedlaczek, J., and J. Zipper. 1986. *Sarcocystis alceslatrans* (Apicomplexa) bei einem palärktischen Elch (Ruminantia). *Angewandte Parasitologie* 27:137–144.

Shimizu, K. 1958. Studies on toxoplasmosis. I. An outbreak of toxoplasmosis among hares (*Lepus timidus ainu*) in Sapporo. *Japanese Journal of Veterinary Research* 6:157–166.

Siepierski, S.J., C.E. Tanner, and J.A. Embil. 1990. Prevalence of antibody to *Toxoplasma gondii* in the moose (*Alces alces americana* Clinton) of Nova Scotia, Canada. *The Journal of Parasitology* 76:136–138.

Siim, J.C., U. Biering-Sorensen, and T. Moller. 1963. Toxoplasmosis in domestic animals. *Advances in Veterinary Science* 8:335–429.

Skerratt, L.F., J. Phelan, R. McFarlane, and R. Speare. 1997. Serodiagnosis of toxoplasmosis in a common wombat. *Journal of Wildlife Diseases* 33:346–351.

Smith, D.D., and J.K. Frenkel. 1995. Prevalence of antibodies to *Toxoplasma gondii* in wild mammals of Missouri and east central Kansas: Biologic and ecologic considerations of transmission. *Journal of Wildlife Diseases* 31:15–21.

Smith, K.E., J.R. Fischer, and J.P. Dubey. 1995. Toxoplasmosis in a bobcat (*Felis rufus*). *Journal of Wildlife Diseases* 31:555–557.

Snyder, D.E., G.C. Sanderson, M. Toivio-Kinnucan, and B.L. Blagburn. 1990. *Sarcocystis kirkpatricki* n. sp. (Apicomplexa: Sarcocystidae) in muscles of raccoons (*Procyon lotor*) from Illinois. *The Journal of Parasitology* 76:495–500.

Soave, O.A., and E.H. Lennette. 1959. Naturally acquired toxoplasmosis in the gray squirrel, *Sciurus griseus,* and its bearing on the laboratory diagnosis of rabies. *Journal of Laboratory and Clinical Medicine* 53:163–166.

Starzyk, J., B. Pawlik, and Z. Pawlik. 1973. Studies on the frequency of occurrence of *Toxoplasma gondii* in fur-bearing animals. *Acta Biologica Cracoviensia, Series Zoologia* 16:229–233.

Stephen, C., D. Haines, T. Bollinger, K. Atkinson, and H. Schwantie. 1996. Serological evidence of *Toxoplasma* infection in cougars on Vancouver Island, British Columbia. *Canadian Veterinary Journal* 37:241.

Stiglmair-Herb, M.T. 1987. Microparasitosis (toxoplasmosis) in moutain gazelles (*Gazella g. curvieri*). *Berliner und Münchener Tierärztliche Wochenschrift* 100:273–277.

Stoffregen, D.A., and J.P. Dubey. 1991. A *Sarcocystis* sp.–like protozoan and concurrent canine distemper virus infection associated with encephalitis in a raccoon (*Procyon lotor*). *Journal of Wildlife Diseases* 27:688–692.

Stolte, M., K. Odening, G. Walter, and I. Bockhardt. 1996. The raccoon as intermediate host of three *Sarcocystis* species in Europe. *Journal of the Helminthological Society of Washington* 63:145–149.

Stolte, M., K. Odening, S. Quandt, R.G. Bengis, and I. Bockhardt. 1998. *Sarcocystis dubeyella* n. sp. and *Sarcocystis phacochoeri* n. sp. (Protozoa: Sarcocystidae) from the warthog (*Phacochoerus aethiopicus*) in South Africa. *Journal of Eukaryotic Microbiology* 45:101–104.

Stover, J., E.R. Jacobson, J. Lukas, M.R. Lappin, and C.D. Buergelt. 1990. *Toxoplasma gondii* in a collection of nondomestic ruminants. *Journal of Zoo and Wildlife Medicine* 21:295–301.

Tadros, W., and J.J. Laarman. 1982. Current concepts on the biology, evolution and taxonomy of tissue cyst-forming eimeriid Coccidia. *Advances in Parasitology* 20:293–468.

Thompson, S.W., and T.H. Reed. 1957. Toxoplasmosis in a swamp wallaby. *Journal of the American Veterinary Medical Association* 131:545–549.

Thornton, R.N. 1990. Toxoplasmosis in ferrets. *New Zealand Veterinary Journal* 38:123.

Thornton, R.W., and T.G. Cook. 1986. A congenital *Toxoplasma*-like disease in ferrets (*Mustela putorius furo*). *New Zealand Veterinary Journal* 34:31–33.

Thulin, J.D., D.E. Granstrom, H.B.Gelberg, D.G. Morton, R.A. French, and R.C. Giles. 1992. Concurrent protozoal encephalitis and canine distemper virus infection in a raccoon (*Procyon lotor*). *Veterinary Record* 130:162–164.

Upton, S.J., and R.D. McKown. 1992. The red-tailed hawk, *Buteo jamaicensis,* a native definitive host of *Frenkelia microti* (apicomplexa) in North America. *Journal of Wildlife Diseases* 28:85–90.

Vanek, J.A., J.P. Dubey, P. Thulliez, M.R. Riggs, and B.E. Stromberg. 1996. Prevalence of *Toxoplasma gondii* antibodies in hunter-killed white-tailed deer (*Odocoileus virginianus*) in four regions of Minnesota. *The Journal of Parasitology* 82:41–44.

van Pelt, R.W., and R.A. Dieterich. 1972. Toxoplasmosis in thirteen-lined ground squirrels. *Journal of the American Veterinary Medical Association* 161:643–647.

van Rensburg, I.B.J., and M.A. Silkstone. 1984. Concomitant feline infectious peritonitis and toxoplasmosis in a cheetah (*Acinonyx jubatus*). *Journal of the South African Veterinary Association* 55:205–207.

Wahlström, K., T. Nikkilä, and A. Uggla. 1999. *Sarcocystis* species in skeletal muscle of otter (*Lutra lutra*). *Parasitology* 118:59–62

Walton, B.C., and K.W. Walls. 1964. Prevalence of toxoplasmosis in wild animals from Fort Stewart, Georgia, as indicated by serological tests and mouse inoculation. *American Journal of Tropical Medicine and Hygiene* 13:530–533.

Wang, G.L., T. Wei, X.Y. Wang, W.Y. Li, P.C. Zhang, M.X. Dong, and H. Xiao. 1988. The morphology and life cycle of *Sarcocystis micros* n. sp. (in Chinese). *Chinese Journal of Veterinary Science and Technology* 6:9–11.

Watson, W.A., and J.K.A. Beverley. 1962. Toxoplasmosis in mink. *Veterinary Record* 74:1027.

Wesemeier, H.H., and J. Sedlaczek. 1995a. One known *Sarcocystis* species and two found for the first time in red deer and wapiti (*Cervus elaphus*) in Europe. *Applied Parasitology* 36:245–251.

———. 1995b. One known *Sarcocystis* species and one found for the first time in fallow deer (*Dama dama*). *Applied Parasitology* 36:299–302.

Wesemeier, H.H., K. Odening, G. Walter, and I. Bockhardt. 1995. The black-backed jackal (Carnivora: Canidae) in Namibia as intermediate host of two *Sarcocystis* species (Protozoa: Sarcocystidae). *Parasite (Paris)* 2:391–394.

Wilhelmsen, C.L., and R.J. Montali. 1980. Toxoplasmosis in a parma wallaby. *Annual Proceedings of the American Association of Zoo Veterinarians,* pp. 141–143.

Williamson, J.M., H. Williams, and G.A. Sharman. 1980. Toxoplasmosis in farmed red deer (*Cervus elaphus*) in Scotland. *Research in Veterinary Science* 29:36–40.

Wong, K.T., and R. Pathmanathan. 1994. Ultrastructure of the human skeletal muscle sarcocyst. *The Journal of Parasitology* 80:327–330.

Woods, L.W., M.L. Anderson, P.K. Swift, and K.W. Sverlow. 1994. Systemic neosporosis in a California black-tailed deer (*Odocoileus hemionus columbianus*). *Journal of Veterinary Diagnostic Investigation* 6:508–510.

Xiao, B.N., D.I. Zeng, C.G. Zhang, M. Wang, Y. Li, and Z.F. Gong. 1993. Development of *Sarcocystis cruzi* in buffalo (*Bubalus bubalis*) and cattle (*Bos taurus*). *Acta Veterinaria et Zootechnica Sinica* 24:185–192.

Zarnke, R.L., J.P. Dubey, O.C.H. Kwok, and J.M. Ver Hoef. 1997. Serologic survey for *Toxoplasma gondii* in grizzly bears from Alaska. *Journal of Wildlife Diseases* 33:267–270.

Zeman, D.H., J.P. Dubey, and D. Robison. 1993. Fatal hepatic sarcocystosis in an American black bear. *Journal of Veterinary Diagnostic Investigation* 5:480–483.

18

BLOOD-INHABITING PROTOZOANS

BLOOD-INHABITING PROTOZOAN PARASITES

A. ALAN KOCAN

***PLASMODIUM* SPP. (MALARIA).** The most significant of the blood-inhabiting haemosporidian parasites of mammals and birds are those of the genus *Plasmodium*. Although the disease they cause, malaria, is unquestionably one of the most important parasitic diseases of human beings, infection and disease in free-ranging mammals is poorly understood. This, in spite of the fact that *Plasmodium* spp. infections in laboratory rodents have been one of the most intensely studied group of protozoan parasites. In fact, information on naturally occurring disease and the impact of infections on wild rodent populations is virtually unknown. Similarly, information on malaria infections of nonhuman primates is primarily laboratory derived and unrelated to any presently known significance in free-ranging populations. This is most interesting when one considers that human forms of malaria are generally thought to have arisen from simian ancestors. For a more extensive review of human, rodent, and nonhuman primate infections see Cox (1993), Collins and Aikawa (1993), and Lopez-Antunano and Schmunis (1993).

TRYPANOSOMA SPP. AND *LEISHMANIA* SPP.

The flagellated protozoan parasites (hemoflagellates) that inhabit the blood and/or tissues of their hosts are of considerable medical and veterinary medical importance. North American species of the genera *Trypanosoma* and *Leishmania* will be covered here.

Trypanosomiasis is a disease resulting from infection with one of many kinetoplastid flagellated protozoan organisms that have a geographic range covering most of the tropical and subtropical regions of the world. Most infections are benign, although some, especially those that involve human beings and domestic animals, often result in severe pathogenic disease.

Species within the genus *Trypanosoma* are divided into those that develop in the midgut or hindgut of their insect vectors (Stercoraria) and those that develop in the midgut and mouth parts or the mouth parts alone of their insect vectors (Salivaria). With the exception of *T. cruzi*, all pathogenic species of trypanosomes belong to

TABLE 18.1—Epidemiological grouping of trypanosomal diseases of man and domestic animals

Disease	Grouping	Species
Nagana	Salivaria	*T. vivax, T. congolense* *T. brucei brucei* *T. simiae*
Sleeping sickness	Salivaria	*T. brucei gambiense* *T. brucei rhodesiense*
Surra	Salivaria	*T. evansi,* *T. equinum*
Dourine	Salivaria	*T. equiperdum*
Chagas' disease	Stercoraria	*T. cruzi*

the Salivaria group (metacyclic forms are in the insect saliva; inoculative transmission). Epidemiological grouping of pathogenic trypanosomes into trypanosomal diseases is often used to simplify the understanding of the pathogenic trypanosomes (Table 18.1). For example, Chagas' disease of human beings and other mammals in South and Central America is caused by *T. cruzi* and is transmitted by ruduvid bugs. Sleeping sickness is the *Glossina*-transmitted disease of Africa; surra is the infection in domestic animals in South and Central America, North Africa, and Asia; and dourine is the sexually transmitted disease of horses. Most if not all of these diseases involve infections in wild animals.

Trypanosomal infections of man, domestic animals, and wild animals are both a common and an important problem throughout much of tropical Africa. Even today, an estimated 10,000 new cases of human African trypanosomiasis occur annually. Additionally, animal trypanosomiasis, both in and outside sub-Saharan Africa, is responsible for an annual loss of millions of dollars in livestock production and costs related to treatment, prevention programs, and vector control efforts. The fact that wildlife can and often do serve as reservoir hosts for many of the trypanosomes has further complicated control efforts. Beyond a doubt, trypanosomiasis is the most important disease of livestock on the African continent (Logan-Henfrey et al. 1992). The volumes of literature related to the diseases caused by these organisms in human beings, domestic animals, and African wildlife and the limited scope of this chapter makes it impossible to adequately cover this subject here. The reader is referred to the many references available on these important areas (Ashcroft 1959; Baker 1968; Hoare 1967; Beck 1976; Mulla and Rickman 1988; Gardiner and Mahmoud 1992; Seed and Hall 1992; Logan-Henfrey et al. 1992; Bowman 1995; Hide et al. 1997).

Even today, classification (Wells and Lumsden 1968) within the family Trypanosomatidae remains controversial. A history of classification based on definitive hosts has resulted in numerous subgenera and subspecies designations. Modern techniques such as isoenzyme analysis have helped clarify some of the problems, but considerable confusion still exists.

Trypanosomes of North American Mammals

ETIOLOGIC AGENTS. *Trypanosoma theileri* occurs in the blood of bovids and appears to be worldwide in occurrence. Various tabanid flies including several species of *Tabanus* and *Haematopota* are known vectors for this organism. Infection is generally by contamination of mucus membranes by hindgut-developing metacyclic trypomastigotes, although intrauterine infections are also reported. Infections are routinely nonpathogenic, although abortions and even deaths have been noted in stressed animals. A similar species, *T. cervi*, is known from several cervids in North America including white-tailed deer (*Odocoileus virginianus*), mule deer (*Odocoileus hemionus*), elk (*Cervus canadensis*), moose (*Alces alces*), and reindeer (*Rangifer tarandus*) (Kingston and Morton 1973; Kingston et al. 1975, 1981, 1982, 1985; Kingston and Crum 1977; Matthews et al. 1977; Kingston 1981). Additional *Trypanosoma* sp. have been recovered from black-tailed deer (*Odocoileus hemionus columbianus*) (Morton and Kingston 1976), pronghorn antelope (*Antilocapra americana*) and bison (*Bison bison*) (Kingston et al. 1981, 1986), and woodland caribou (*Rangifer tarandus caribou*) (Lefebvre et al. 1997). These organisms appear to be nonpathogenic under normal conditions. Infection levels with these species are generally low and are seldom detected by microscopic examination of stained blood films (Dusanic 1991; Lefebvre et al. 1997). *Trypanosoma melophagium* of sheep, *T. lewisi* of rats, and *T. musculi* of mice are also nonpathogenic species infecting their respective hosts throughout the world (D'Alesandro and Behr 1991).

Trypanosoma rangeli is a parasite of man, domestic and wild animals, and triatomine insects in the New World. It is typically harmless to its mammalian host but often damaging to its vector. The distribution of *T. rangeli* overlaps with that of *T. cruzi*. Since both *T. cruzi* and *T. rangeli* use the same vector(s) and parasitize the same hosts, differentiation is an important problem. D'Alessandro-Bacigalupo and Saravia (1992) review this subject.

Because of their morphological similarity to *T. cruzi*, trypanosomal parasites of bats, especially those of the subgenus *Schizotrypanum* have been studied extensively. Although isolates from bats have been used as models for *T. cruzi* studies, the inability of these organisms to infect common laboratory animals restrict their use. Most studies on bat trypanosomes in the New World have been hampered by the costs of field studies and difficulties related to the identification of parasitic organisms, vectors, and the hosts that they infect. At present, it does not appear that trypanosomal infections in bats play any role in host population dynamics, and there is no evidence of pathogenicity for any species infecting bats. Molyneux (1991) provides a more complete review of this area.

Trypanosoma (Schizotrypanum) cruzi (**American Human Trypanosomiasis, Chagas' Disease**). *Trypanosoma cruzi* occurs throughout southern the United States, Central America, and South America from Argentina north. It has been reported in > 100 species of mammals, including man. Although humans are considered the most significant host, many species of domestic and wild mammals are important reservoir hosts for this infection.

LIFE HISTORY. The trypomastigote form, which is common in the peripheral blood during early stages of infection, does not multiply. Instead, this form enters cells within the reticuloentherlial system, heart muscle, and occasionally striated muscle and turn into the amastigote form. It multiplies by binary fission. Variations exist in different strains related to both morphologic stages present and virulence of infection. In most cases, amastigotes transform into additional trypomastigotes and reenter the circulating blood.

The vector becomes infected by ingesting trypomastigotes, which transform into epimastigotes in the gut of the vector. Multiplication is by binary fission. Epimastigotes transform into trypomastigotes in the hindgut of the vector prior to being passed in the feces.

EPIZOOTIOLOGY. Transmission of *T. cruzi* is influenced by a number of factors, including the presence of vector(s), reservoir animals, the parasite, and a susceptible host species. Vector behavior also influences transmission, with some species preferring human habitation and others being more sylvatic. In the United States the two principal vectors (*Triatoma protracta* and *T. sanguisuga*) tend not to infest human dwellings and have behavioral traits involving both feeding and defecation that result in a low prevalence. Prevalence in wild animals in the United States is highest in raccoons (16%), opossums (38%), and armadillos. Infections in wild animal hosts are reported from most southern states including Florida, Georgia, Alabama, Louisiana, Texas, Oklahoma, New Mexico, Arizona, and southern California. Although appearing to be quite prevalent, little information exists on the role of this parasite in mortality of wild species or the role that it might play in population regulation.

PATHOLOGY AND PATHOGENESIS. Once introduced, trypomastigotes enter the blood and soon thereafter enter host cells. There they multiply and are transported within macrophages throughout the body. A parasitemia develops in a few days and peaks at 2–3 weeks after the initial exposure. Acute disease is noted in 2–5 weeks. In acute cases, lesions are generally confined to the right side of the heart. Subepicardial hemorrhages and white myocardial spots are generally associated with the coronary groove. Hepatic, splenic, and renal congestion with pulmonary edema are often present but are secondary to cardiac failure. Cardiomyopathy may occur due to toxic parasite products. Mechanical damage to myofibrils due to the presence of the parasite is often associated with acute cases. Disease in naturally infected wildlife reservoirs is poorly understood, and little information is available. Infection in domestic dogs usually occurs in young animals and is characterized by acute myocarditis with sudden collapse and death. Dogs that do not die suddenly often develop secondary problems related to right-heart failure. Anorexia, diarrhea, and neuralgic signs are also reported.

THERAPY. Only an experimental drug (Nifurtimox) (Bayer 2502, Bayer AG, Leverkusen-Bayerwerk, West Germany) is available for treatment of human cases. Availability is through the Centers for Disease Control.

DIAGNOSIS. Serologic testing is available using indirect fluorescent antibody (IFA), compliment fixation, and direct hemagglutination tests. Although used routinely in the United States, these tests show considerable cross-reactivity with other similar species as well as with most *Leishmania* organisms. Direct isolation of trypomastigotes or amastigotes can be accomplished with inoculation of blood agar slants overlaid with liver or veal infusion tryptose. Vero cell monolayer inoculation is also effective, as is direct inoculation of young laboratory mice. Detection of trypomastigotes (Fig. 18.1) by microscopic examination of stained blood films is generally only practical during the early acute phase of infection. Giemsa-stained samples of lymph node aspirates or impression smears are often useful when parasitemias are low.

PUBLIC HEALTH CONCERNS. The presence of this disease in domestic canines and wildlife species is of considerable public health concern. Although the number of naturally acquired human cases in the United States is low, the risk of human exposure from handling or treating infected domestic or wildlife hosts poses a considerable human health threat.

***Leishmania* spp. (Leishmaniasis).** Members of this genus are primarily parasites of mammals in both the Old and New Worlds. Natural infections are reported in humans, dogs, and several species of rodents. Historically, classification has been based on clinical symptoms and pathogenesis of the disease as well as geographic distribution of the parasite. Although modern laboratory techniques have shown that the relationships may be more complex than originally thought, most authors still use an Old World and New World classification. For a review on *Leishmania* taxonomy, see Williams and Coelho (1978).

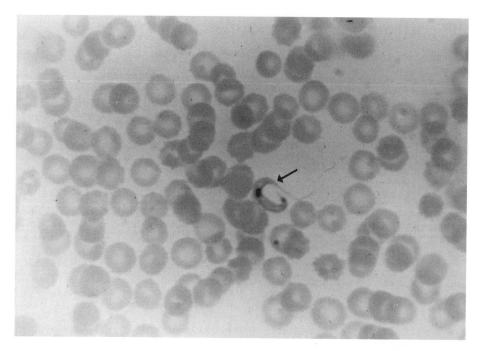

FIG. 18.1—Trypomastigote of *Trypanosoma cruzi* (arrow) in stained erythrocyte preparation. Note curved shape, long free flagellum, and darkly stained central nucleus and kinetoplast. (200X magnification)

In the New World, humans and canines are the primary hosts. *Leishmania donovani* complex parasites are considered the primary viscerotropic subspecies in the Americas, although cutaneous lesions in both humans and canines also occur. Endemic regions include South and Central America and isolated areas in Mexico. Isolated foci have also been reported in Texas, Oklahoma, and Ohio. Although of considerable significance in human medicine and perhaps of increasing concern to veterinary medicine, few if any reports implicate wild animal reservoirs in North America, and little information exists on the impact of infection by parasites of this genus on wild animal populations.

PUBLIC HEALTH CONCERNS. Leishmaniasis, especially the visceral form, is an important health problem in humans. In endemic areas, exposure to infected vectors (sand flies) poses a health threat. In these regions, dogs are presumably the most significant reservoir, although dog-to-dog transmission appears to be more common than dog-to-human transmission. Even in areas without vectors, infected domestic dogs may pose a risk of accidental human exposure. In the United States, wild species do not, at present, appear to be involved in the transmission of leishmaniasis to either domestic animal or human hosts. However, this situation may be different in other parts of the world (Mancianti et al. 1994)

Persons handling biological material in endemic areas or dealing with animals with compatible clinical signs should consider the seriousness and potential for accidental exposure.

LITERATURE CITED

Ashcroft, M.T. 1959. The importance of African wild animals as reservoirs of trypanosomes. *East African Medical Journal* 36:289–297.
Baker, J.R. 1968. Trypanosomes of wild mammals in the neighborhood of the Serengeti National Park. In *Diseases of free-living animals.* Ed. A. McDiarmid. London: Academic Press, pp. 147–158.
Beck, J.W., and J.E. Davies. 1976. *Medical parasitology,* 2nd ed. St. Louis: C.V. Mosby Co.
Bowman, D.D. 1995. *Parasitology for veterinarians,* 6th ed. Philadelphia, PA: W.B. Saunders Co.
Collins, W.E., and M. Aikawa. 1993. Plasmodia of nonhuman primates. In *Parasitic protozoa,* vol. 5. Ed. J.P. Kreier. New York: Academic Press, pp. 105–132.
Cox, F.E.G. 1993. Plasmodia of rodents. In *Parasitic protozoa,* vol. 5. Ed. J.P. Kreier. New York: Academic Press, pp. 49–102.
D'Alesandro, P.A., and M.A. Behr. 1991. *Trypanosoma lewisi* and its relatives. In *Parasitic protozoa,* vol. 1. Ed. J.P. Kreier and J.R Baker. New York: Academic Press, pp. 225–263.
D'Alessandro-Bacigalupo, A. and N.G. Saravia. 1992. *Trypanosoma rangeli.* In *Parasitic protozoa,* vol. 2. Ed. J.P. Kreier and J.R. Baker. New York: Academic Press, pp. 1–54.
Dusanic, D.G. 1991. *Trypanosoma (Schizotrypanum) cruzi.* In *Parasitic protozoa,* vol. 1. Ed. J.P. Kreier and J.R. Baker. New York: Academic Press, pp. 137–194.
Gardiner, P.R., and M.M. Mahmoud. 1992. Salvarian trypanosomes causing disease in livestock outside sub-Saharan Africa. In *Parasitic protozoa,* vol. 2. Ed. J.P.

Kreier and J.R. Baker. New York: Academic Press, pp. 277–314.
Hide, G., J.C. Mottram, G.H. Coombs, and P.H. Holmes (eds.). 1997. Trypanosomiasis and leishmaniasis: Biology and control. Wallingford, UK: CAB International, 266 pp.
Hoare, C.A. 1967. Evolutionary trends in mammalian trypanosomes. *Advances in Parasitology* 5:47–91.
Kingston, N. 1981. Protozoan parasites. In *Diseases and parasites of white-tailed deer.* Ed. W.R. Davidson, F.A. Hayes, V.F. Nettles, and F.E. Kellogg. Miscellaneous Publication No. 7. Tallahassee, FL: Tall Timbers Research Station, pp. 193–236.
Kingston, N., and J. Crum. 1977. *Trypanosoma cervi* Kingston and Morton, 1975 in white-tailed deer, *Odocoileus virginianus,* in the southeastern United States. *Proceedings of the Helminthological Society of Washington* 44:179–184.
Kingston, N., and J.K. Morton. 1973. Trypanosomes from elk (*Cervus canadensis*) in Wyoming. *The Journal of Parasitology* 59:1132–1133.
Kingston, N., J. K. Morton, and M. Matthews. 1975. Trypansomes from mule deer, *Odocoileus hemionus,* in Wyoming. *Journal of Wildlife Diseases* 11:519–521.
Kingston, N., E.T. Thorne, G.H. Tyomas, L. McHolland, and M.S. Trueblood. 1981. Further studies on trypanosomes in game animals in Wyoming II. *Journal of Wildlife Diseases* 17:539–564.
Kingston, N., J.K. Morton, and R. Dieterich. 1982. *Trypanosoma cervi* from Alaskan reindeer, *Rangifer tarandus. The Journal of Protozoology* 29:588–591.
Kingston, N., A. Franzmann, and L. Maki. 1985. Redescription of *Trypanosoma cervi* (Protozoa) in moose (*Alces alces),* from Alaska and Wyoming. *Proceedings of the Helminthological Society of Washington* 52:54–59.
Kingston, N., G. Thomas, L. McHolland, E.S. Williams, M.S. Trueblood, and L. Maki. 1986. Experimental transmission of *Trypanosoma theileri* to bison. *Proceedings of the Helminthological Society of Washington* 53:198–203.
Lefebvre, M.F., S.S. Semalulu, A.E. Oatway, and J.W. Nolan. 1997. Trypanosomiasis in woodland caribou of northern Alberta. *Journal of Wildlife Diseases* 33:271–277.
Logan-Henfrey, L.L., P.R. Gardiner, and M.M. Mahmoud. 1992. Animal trypanosomiasis in sub-Sahara Africa. In *Parasitic protozoa,* vol. 2. Ed. J.P. Kreier and J.R. Baker. New York: Academic Press, pp. 157–276.
Lopez-Antunano, F.J., and G.A. Schmunis. 1993. Plasmodia of humans. In *Parasitic protozoa,* vol. 5. Ed. J.P. Kreier. New York: Academic Press, pp. 135–266.
Mancianti, F., W. Mignone, and F. Galastri. 1994. Serologic survey for leishmaniasis in free-ranging red foxes (*Vulpes vulpes*) in Italy. *Journal of Wildlife Diseases* 30:454–456.
Matthews, M.J., N. Kingston, and J.K. Morton. 1977. *Trypanosoma cervi,* Kingston and Morton, 1975 from mule deer, *Odocoileus hemionus,* in Wyoming. *Journal of Wildlife Diseases* 13:33–39.
Molyneux, D.H. 1991. Trypanosomes of bats. In *Parasitic protozoa,* vol. 1. Ed. J.P. Krier and J.R. Baker. New York: Academic Press, pp. 195–223.
Morton, J.K., and N. Kingston. 1976. Further studies on trypanosomes in game animals in Wyoming. *Journal of Wildlife Diseases* 12:233–236.
Mulla, A.F., and L.R. Rickman. 1988. How do African game animals control trypanosome infections? *Parasitology Today* 4:352–354.
Seed, J.R., and J.E. Hall. 1992. Trypanosomes causing disease in man in Africa. In *Parasitic protozoa,* vol. 2. Ed. J.P. Kreier and J.R. Baker. New York: Academic Press, pp. 85–155.

Wells, E.A.,, and W.H. Lumsden. 1968. Trypanosome infections of wild mammals in relation to trypanosome diseases of man and his domestic animals. In *Diseases in free-living wild animals*. Ed. A. McDiarmid. Symposium of the Zoological Society of London (24). London: Academic Press, pp. 135–145.

Williams, P., and M. Coelho. 1978. Taxonomy and transmission of Leishmania. *Advances in Parasitology* 16:1–42.

PIROPLASMS (*THEILERIA* SPP., *CYTAUXZOON* SPP., AND *BABESIA* SPP.)

A. ALAN KOCAN AND KENNETH A. WALDRUP

***THEILERIA* SPP. (THEILERIOSIS) AND *CYTAUXZOON* SPP. (CYTAUXZOONOSIS).** Members of the genera *Theileria* and *Cytauxzoon* are tick-transmitted protozoan parasites that affect a variety of wild and domestic mammals. They are distinguished from members of the closely related genus *Babesia* by several important developmental characters: Asexual multiplication (schizogony) occurs in both erythrocytes and other cells, while no extraerythrocytic development is known for members of the genus *Babesia*. Also, only transstadial transmission (across stages of the tick vector life cycle) is known for members of *Theileria* and *Cytauxzoon*, while transovarial transmission occurs in the genus *Babesia*. Although numerous species of *Theileria* and *Cytauxzoon* occur in a variety of mammals throughout the world, only *Theileria cervi* and *Cytauxzoon felis* are known from wild mammals in North America.

Etiologic Agents. *Theileria* and *Cytauxzoon* belong to the phylum Apicomplexa, class Aconoidasida, order Piroplasmorida, family Theileridae. However, taxonomy for this group is not uniformly agreed upon. Levine (1971) proposed a classification of piroplasms in which *Cytauxzoon* was placed in synonymy with *Theileria*. This was based on the determination that the site where schizogony occurs was either unknown or was in cells other than erythrocytes. Barnett (1977) retained the genus *Cytauxzoon* in his classification scheme primarily because (1) schizogony did occur in different cells and (2) *Cytauxzoon* schizonts were multiple in aggregations within the host cell, while those in *Theileria* were single or in small aggregations within lymphocytes. Other findings that strengthen the case for the separation of these two genera include the fact that although naphthoquinones have been shown to have both in vitro and in vivo activity against members of the genus *Theileria*, treatment with two different naphthoquinones had little effect on *C. felis* in experimentally infected cats (Motzel and Wagner 1990). Additionally, members of *Theileria* are unique in that the exoerythrocytic schizont stage that infects lymphoid cells induces the host cell to transform to a lymphoblast, thus promoting continuous proliferation.

Life History. *Theileria* and *Cytauxzoon* infections are initiated when an infected tick introduces sporozoites into a susceptible host at the time of feeding (usually 3–5 days after attachment). Light and electron microscopic observations of infected endothelial macrophages and/or lymphocytes indicate a similarity in developmental sequence in the vertebrate host for these two genera. During merogony, the parasite first appears as a multinucleated syncytium in which nuclear proliferation is evident. As the syncytium develops, it begins to branch with interconnected processes of parasite cytoplasm. Merozoite formation occurs as a rapid sequential fission along the margins of the multinucleated sporont in the cytoplasm of the host cell (Schein et al. 1978; Simpson et al. 1985; Kocan et al. 1992). Merozoites enter erythrocytes 8–14 days after the initial infection. The intraerythrocytic piroplasms are described as pleomorphic, being round, oval, bipolar, and rod-shaped. Maltese crosses and paired forms are also common. Electron micrographic observations indicate that the process of intraerythrocytic multiplication is similar to that by which merozoites are formed and that intraerythrocytic schizogony is a general feature of these infections (Conrad et al. 1985). Sporogony in the tick vector has also been observed to be similar for several species of *Theileria* and *Cytauxzoon* (Fawcett et al. 1985; Hazen-Karr et al. 1987; Kocan et al. 1988).

Epizootiology: Distribution and Host Range. In domesticated animals, bovine theileriosis occurs on all continents and is caused by at least six species. Numerous reports and reviews are available on bovine theileriosis, and the reader is referred to these for specifics related to bovine theileriosis (Groutenhuis and Young 1981; Mehlhorn and Schein 1984; Conrad and Waldrup 1993; Mehlhorn et al. 1994).

Many species of *Theileria* and *Cytauxzoon* have been reported from wild mammals (Conrad and Waldrup 1993). Of the numerous species (or subspecies) of *Theileria* that affect bovines throughout the world, the African cape buffalo (*Syncerus caffer*) appears to be the original host for *T. parva*, *T. mutans*, and *T. velifera*, and the eland antelope (*Taurotragus oryx*) appears to be the host for *T. (Cytauxzoon) taurotragus*. The Asian water buffalo is considered to be the original host for *T. annulata* and *T. orientalis*. In North America only *T. cervi*, *T. annulata*, and *C. felis* have been reported (Table 18.2).

Theileria parva infections occur as several clinically distinct biological types. The original parasite of Cape buffalo, *T. parva lawrenci*, the causative agent of "corridor disease" of cattle, is typified by having few lymphocyte schizonts and few intraerythrocytic piroplasms. By comparison, *T. parva parva*, the causative agent of East Coast fever, has large numbers of lymphocyte-infected schizonts and intraerythrocytic piroplasms in acute cases. Infections with the so-called Zimbabwean malignant theileriosis (*T. parva bovis*) result in parasite numbers intermediate between the two.

TABLE 18.2—*Theileria* and *Cytauxzoon* parasites of wild mammals from North America

Parasite Species	Mammalian Host
Theileria cervi	White-tailed deer (*Odocoileus virginianus*)
	Mule deer (*O. hemionus*)
	Sika deer (*Cervus nippon*)[a]
	Fallow deer (*Dama dama*)[a]
	Axis deer (*Axis axis*)[a]
	Wapiti (*Cervus elaphus*)
Theileria annulata	American bison (*Bison bison*)
Cytauxzoon felis	Bobcat (*Lynx rufus*)
	Florida panther (*Felis concolor coryi*)
	Texas cougar (*Felis concolor stanleyana*)

[a]Denotes nonindigenous (introduced) hosts.

Theileria parva is found from the southern Sudan to South Africa and from the Indian Ocean west to Zaire. Its distribution is probably related to the distribution of its primary vector *Rhipicephalus appendiculatus* and related species such as *R. zambeziensis*. *Theileria p. parva* has been eradicated from most of southern Africa, but *T. p. lawrenci* persists in wild Cape buffalo. Strains of *T. p. bovis* occur in Zimbabwe and as far north as Rwanda. *Theileria annulata* is found in North Africa from Morocco to Egypt to the Sudan, in southern Europe, in Asia, the Near East and Middle East, the Indian peninsula, and western China. *Theileria orientalis* (*T. sergenti*) occurs in Asia, Iran, India, Myalaysia, Vietnam, Indonesia, Korea, Japan, and eastern Australia and New Zealand, and there are other reports from northern Africa, Latin America, and the United States. *Theileria mutans* is limited to sub-Saharan Africa, islands near Africa, Guadeloupe, and the Caribbean area, with a single report from the United States (Splitter 1950). *Theileria* (*Cytauxzoon*) *taurotragi* is known to exist as far north as Kenya and as far south as South Africa. It is probably distributed anywhere its natural host, the eland antelope, and its vectors, *R. appendiculatus* and *R. pulchellus,* coexist. Areas are recognized, however, where the parasite exists independently of the eland host, but in association with its tick vector(s). *Theileria velifera* has a distribution similar to that of *T. mutans*.

Theileria cervi is the only species confirmed in wildlife in North America and has been reported from white-tailed deer, *Odocoileus virginianus,* and perhaps mule deer (*Odocoileus hemionus*), sika deer (*Cervus nippon*), fallow deer (*Dama dama*), and wapiti (*Cervus elaphus*) (Davidson et al. 1985; Waldrup et al. 1989b). It was first recognized in 1961 and reported from a splenectomized white-tailed deer that was a part of an anaplasmosis research project (Krier et al. 1962). The parasite was initially called *T. mutans* but was later renamed *T. cervi* to correspond with an earlier report of a *Theileria* organism in fallow deer from Portugal (Bettencourt et al. 1907). However, experimental trials using a confirmed infective North American stabilate

of *T. cervi* sporozoites were unsuccessful in infecting captive fallow deer in the United States, indicating some variability in the ability of this species to infect different deer (Kocan et al. 1987). *Theileria cervi* occurs in white-tailed deer in the southern and southeastern United States (Fig. 18.2) and parallels the distribution of its only known vector, the lone star tick, *Amblyomma americanum* (Krier et al. 1962; Kuttler et al. 1967; Robinson et al. 1968; Emerson 1969; Hair and Bowman 1986; Laird et al. 1988).

Neitz and Thomas (1948) first reported the genus *Cytauxzoon* from a gray duiker (*Sylvicaprae grimmia*) in South Africa. Numerous additional reports of cytauxzoonosis in other African ungulates have since occurred. The first report of a *Cytauxzoon*-like parasite in felids outside of Africa occurred in 1976 and described two fatal cases in domestic cats in Missouri (Wagner 1976). Numerous reports have since occurred that indicate infections in domestic and wild felids including possible cases in captive cheetahs and wild and semicaptive cougars (Zinkl et al. 1981; Butt et al. 1991; Rostein et al. 1999). In North America, the distribution of *C. felis* appears to correspond to that of its only known tick vector, *Dermacentor variabilis* (Blouin et al. 1984) (Fig. 18.3).

Clinical Signs. Clinical signs associated with the African species of *Theileria* vary according to the species involved. In *T. p. parva* infections in domestic bovines, the acute disease is characterized by large numbers of schizont-infected lymphocytes that cause a generalized leukosis-like disease with dissemination of infected lymphocytes leading to a generalized hyperplasia of lymph nodes and lymphoid tissue. Severe leukopenia is common in late stages of infection with severe immunosuppression. Most cattle with *T. p. lawrenci* die, even when numbers of schizonts or piroplasms are few. Infections with *T. mutans* and *T. orientalis* are characterized by a high rate of multiplication of intraerythrocytic piroplasms resulting in an anemia and icterus. Hemoglobinuria is not a common sign.

Fatalities in European cattle infected with *T. p. parva* often reach 90%, while those associated with *T. annulata* infections have been reported to be as high as 70% in European dairy herds. African zebu cattle born and maintained in endemic areas where calfhood infection is common appear to be resistant to disease. *Theileria orientalis* is generally nonpathogenic, but strain variations are known. *Theileria mutans* and *T. taurotragi* are similarly nonpathogenic in areas with endemic stability.

The incubation period varies depending on the species involved. It usually is 10–15 days. Fever is associated with the schizonic phase in both *T. parva* and *T. annulata* infections, often lasting until death. Regional lymph nodes, often associated with tick attachment sites, become enlarged, leading to a generalized swelling of all superficial lymph glands. In *T. parva* and *T. annulata,* symptoms of acute septicemia develop, with labored breathing occurring during the

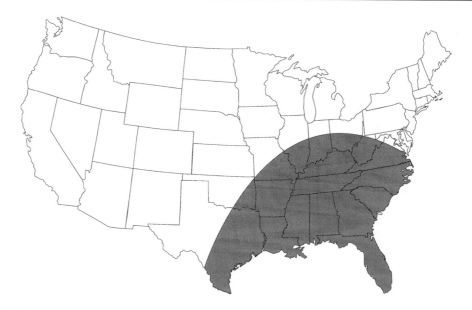

FIG. 18.2—Approximate reported distribution of *Theileria cervi* in white-tailed deer from North America.

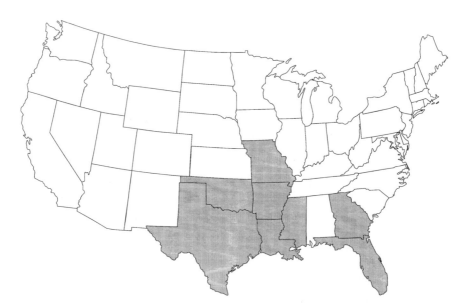

FIG. 18.3—Distribution of *Cytauxzoon felis* by state in North America, based on reported cases in domestic felines.

terminal phase. Death is due to asphyxia following edema of the lungs. In *T. mutans* and *T. orientalis* infections, febrile periods are short, followed by anemia and icterus. Cerebral forms with central nervous system signs are known for *T. parva, T. annulata,* and *T. (C.) taurotragi.*

Clinical signs of *T. cervi* in naturally infected white-tailed deer are rare, and only mild to nonapparent ane-

mia has been reported. Prepatent periods of 14–21 days are reported for infections initiated by experimental tick feeding. Robinson et al. (1967) showed that infections with *T. cervi* could cause death or disease in immunosuppressed or malnourished deer. Barker et al. (1973) indicated that little change was evident in experimentally infected fawns unless the deer was concurrently infested with large numbers of ticks. When noted, clinical signs include fever, anemia, pale membranes, emaciation, weakness, and general debilitation.

Clinical signs of infection with *C. felis* include pallor and icterus, although the stage of the disease will determine the presenting signs. Initially, anemia and depression are observed, followed by high fever, dehydration, pallor and icterus, splenomegaly, and hepatomegaly. After the fever peaks, the body temperature usually falls to subnormal. The prepatent period is between 14 and 20 days. Hematologic manifestations include a regenerative anemia with a mild increase in metarubricytes. Splenic, mesenteric, and renal veins are distended from parasite development. The spleen is also enlarged and dark in color, while the lungs contain petechial hemorrhages. The pericardial sac is distended and gelatinous and contains icteric fluid accompanied by petechial and ecchymotic hemorrhaging of the epicardium (Whiteman et al. 1977; Glenn and Stair 1984). Similar lesions, although milder in nature, have been observed in experimentally infected bobcats (Glenn et al. 1982, 1983; Kocan et al. 1985).

Pathogenesis and Pathology. Gross lesions related to *T. parva* and *T. annulata* infections include hyperplasia of lymphoid tissue, edema of the lungs, and foci of infected lymphoid tissue in the renal cortex and in cellular walls around ulcers in the abomasal mucosa. Lesions in fatal cases of *T. mutans* and *T. orientalis* are usually associated with anemia and icterus.

Pathogenesis of *C. felis* is not well understood, although erythrocyte hemolysis and circulatory failure are likely. Obstruction of venous blood flow by infected and distended macrophages appears to be responsible for circulatory impairment. Microscopic lesions include numerous large, parasitized, mononuclear phagocytes filled with schizonts within the lumen of veins and venous channels of the lungs, liver, lymph nodes, and spleen (Fig. 18.4A). Ultrastructural changes associated with merogony have been previously described (Simpson et al. 1985; Kocan and Kocan 1991; Kocan et al. 1992).

Diagnosis. Theilerial infections, suspected on clinical grounds, must be confirmed by microscopic demonstration of piroplasms in Giemsa-stained blood (Fig. 18.4B) or schizonts in smears of lymph node biopsy material. Presence of *C. felis* can also be confirmed by demonstration of piroplasms in stained blood films (Fig. 18.4C) and by microscopic detection of infected mononuclear phagocytes containing schizonts from blood films and impression smears (Fig. 18.4D) or histologic preparations (Fig. 18.4A). Natural existing infection with *C. felis* in the bobcat is usually < 2%, while death in domestic cats frequently occurs without piroplasm parasitemias being detectable. A piroplasm carrier state exists in *C. felis*–infected bobcats, although schizogonous tissue stages cannot be detected beyond 30 days postexposure (Blouin et al. 1987). Serologic comparison of *C. felis* and various other

African piroplasms indicated little or no direct relationship (Uilenberg et al. 1987).

Only intraerythrocytic piroplasms are known in *T. cervi* infections, and as such, diagnosis must be based on their recognition. Again, parasitemia is usually < 1% in adult deer but is frequently greater in fawns.

Indirect fluorescent antibody tests (IFAT) are used as a serologic test to identify infected animals and may have some value in differentiating between piroplasms of different genera (Waldrup et al. 1989a). Recently, gene sequence comparisons have proven to be useful in detecting piroplasm infections in wild cervids (Chae et al. 1999).

Immunity. Immunity to *Theileria* and *Cytauxzoon* appears to be dependent on the animal having experienced the exoerythrocytic phase of parasite development. In natural infections, recovery, resulting in premunity, appears to be protective, although variations exist among geographic and antigenic isolates. Piroplasm infections alone do not appear to afford protection to challenge in the absence of a previously occurring exoerythrocytic infection. Willadsen and Jongejan (1999) review immune mechanisms to ticks and tick-borne diseases.

Control and Treatment. Treatment of domestic bovines with theilerial infections has been accomplished with parvoquone (Burroughs Wellcome, 20 mg/kg IM), buparvoquone (Butales, Pittman-Moore, 2.5 mg/kg IM), and oxytetracycline (Pfizer, Terramycin LA, 20 mg/kg IM) (Mutugi et al. 1988a,b). It is conceivable that these products would be effective in free-ranging species.

Control of bovine theileriosis and other tick-borne diseases in endemic areas of the world has historically been dependent on arachnicidal treatment of the mammalian host in an attempt to prevent infection. In addition to being costly and labor intensive, this approach has been shown to be effective only if administered adequately and used continuously. New efforts at immunization against bovine *Theileria* infections using an infection and treatment method with sporozoite stabilates and treatment with oxytetracyclines or parvaquone are promising (Mutugi et al. 1988a,b). Use of varying concentrations of *T. p. parva* and *T. p. lawrenci* stabilates, particularly low concentration dosages, has been successful in producing subclinical theileriosis that was controlled by the use of both long- and short-acting formulations of oxytetracyclines. Immunized cattle were immune to homologous and heterologous challenges, often resulting in a persisting carrier state. However, the widespread application of these procedures will require that the economics, efficacy, and safety of the products make them feasible for general use. Additionally, a better understanding of both the role of parasite endemic stability and the importance of host breed resistance will help to provide a more integrated approach to widespread control efforts (Young et al. 1986). At present, the best approach appears to

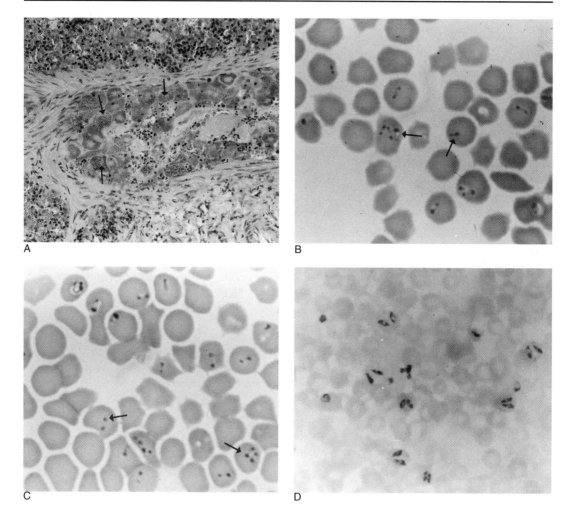

FIG. 18.4—Piroplasms of mammals from North America. (**A**) Pulmonary vessels of a *Cytauxzoon felis* infected domestic cat containing large schizont-laden macrophages associated with the intimal lining of the vessel (arrows). (Hematoxylin and eosin stain) (200X) (**B**) The piroplasms (arrows) of *Theileria cervi* in erythrocytes of white-tailed deer appear as ring, comma, and dumbbell forms. (200X) (**C**) The piroplasms of *C. felis* in feline erythrocytes appear as ring, rod, or maltese cross forms. (200X magnification) (**D**) *Cytauxzoon felis* schizont in circulating macrophage. (200X magnification)

include intermittent acaricide treatment based on minimizing specific tick damage, immunization that either preserves or reestablishes enzootic stability, and use or improvement on the use of animals with natural host resistance to both tick infestations and susceptibility to disease. Important in this approach will be the continued development of immunization methods against tick infestations. Presently, antigens from saliva and midgut fractions of select ticks are used to immunize mammalian hosts against infestations. Other approaches using boluses that release compounds in order to give long-term control against tick attachment also show promise. This type of control appears best suited to situations where 100% control of tick infestation is not sought and/or where tick control is used in conjunction with or separately from control of tick-borne disease control.

The use or application of these procedures in free-ranging species has not been evaluated and may not be feasible. Buparvaquone treatment of captive white-tailed deer infected with *T. cervi* was effective in reducing circulating piroplasm numbers but only for a short period (Mitema et al. 1991). Likewise, treatment of experimentally infected domestic cats exposed to *C. felis* stabilates was not successful in preventing or eliminating the parasite or disease (Motzel et al. 1990).

Public Health Concerns. There are no known species of either *Theileria* or *Cytauxzoon* that infect humans. Of interest, however, are recent findings that several species of small *Babesia* including *B. microti, B. equi, B. gibsoni,* and a newly identified piroplasm infectious for humans in Washington state (*Babesia* sp.-WA1) may be phylogenetically related to *Theileria* (Thomford et al. 1994; Persing and Conrad 1995). Clearly, further studies related to the zoonotic potential of many of the known and yet-to-be-described piroplasms of domestic and wild animals is warranted.

Domestic Animal Health Concerns. Since *Theileria* parasites are known from numerous species of mammals from throughout the world, the importation of infected carrier animals or the introduction of exotic species of ticks should always be a concern. Although infections in wild artiodactyls are usually nonclinical, the potential for both mechanical and biological transmission to other captive or domestic species should not be overlooked. Wild species that harbor *Theileria* can serve as a source of infection for domestic bovines. Eland, for example, are a natural host for *T. (C.) taurotragi,* which is capable of infecting cattle and splenectomized goats and sheep. The African Cape buffalo can harbor nonclinical infections of *T. p. lawrenci,* which is highly pathogenic for domestic cattle. Additionally, it is more difficult to immunize domestic cattle against buffalo-derived *T. parva* than against the organism derived from cattle. Cape buffalo can also carry *T. mutans,* which is more pathogenic to cattle than the cattle-derived strain of this organism. In general, the potential for carrying a wide variety of antigenically and geographically derived parasites makes wild hosts a far more important reservoir for this organism than are domestic animals.

Infections with *Cytauxzoon* or *Cytauxzoon*-like organisms in wild antelope are more likely to result in clinically ill animals or fatalities than do infections with *Theileria* sp. parasites. Reports of fatal infections in eland, gray duiker, greater kudu, sable, roan, and tsessebe antelope have been documented. In many instances, stress, including capture and captivity or nutritional deficiencies, may increase the likelihood of clinical disease resulting from these infections.

In North America, clinical disease in white-tailed deer due to infections with *T. cervi* is rare and probably occurs only under conditions of stress, immunosuppression, or concurrent conditions. *Cytauxzoon felis* infections in free-ranging bobcats appear to be nonclinical under natural conditions, although fatalities in animals with concurrent infections and in animals under captive conditions are not uncommon. By comparison, *C. felis* in domestic cats is generally fatal.

Management Implications. Control of *Theileria* and *Cytauxzoon* in wild animals is probably best accomplished by tick control. Therapeutic treatment of free-ranging animals is not yet feasible, and in general, little or no information is available on the efficacy of known therapeutic agents effective against these organisms in wild species. Although tick control methods aimed at wild species that inhabit large areas may

not be either feasible or effective, other measures that would minimize tick populations might be advisable. Certainly, preventing the introduction of nonindigenous species of ticks to new areas is always advisable. Arachnicidal treatments including dips, sprays, and quarantine are advisable for all animals of exotic origin and in cases where animals are being relocated or transplanted from different geographic regions. Perhaps equally important is the management of wild and captive species in such a manner as to minimize potentially immunosuppressive factors such as excess population numbers, stress, and poor nutrition. The role of endemic stability resulting from early and frequent exposure to parasites of these genera may be of more significance than presently recognized. It is known that the introduction of new species of parasites into a herd or situation where the endemic population has not been previously exposed can and often does result in severe clinical infections. This is compounded by the fact that many animals carry low-level piroplasm parasitemias and that new or previously unrecognized tick-borne parasites are being described with an alarming frequency. Compounding the problem is the fact that the potential host range of many species of parasites varies more than was previously thought and that the exact host range for other species has not yet been determined.

BABESIA SPP. (BABESIOSIS)

Etiologic Agents. Members of the genus *Babesia* that infect mammals are obligate intraerythrocytic, pyriform-shaped, protozoan parasites. Individual organisms may be pyriform, round, or elongate in shape. Individual species are grouped into "small *Babesia*" with pyriform bodies measuring 1.0 to 2.5 µm in size or "large *Babesia*" that are greater than 2.5 µm long. *Babesia* spp. are transmitted by numerous species of ixodid ticks, with sexual reproduction of the parasite occurring in the gut and hemolymph of the specific tick vector.

Life History. Within infected red blood cells of the mammalian host, the *Babesia* piroplasm stage divides asexually by binary fission to form two or four individuals. The parasitized cell eventually ruptures, liberating the newly formed merozoites, which penetrate new red blood cells. There are two types of development in the tick vector: transovarial and transstadial. Although the next sequence of development is not completely understood, it appears that when the appropriate tick ingests the parasitized blood cells, the sexual stage of the life cycle is initiated in the tick gut, followed by schizogony. In transovarial transmission, the resultant stages migrate to the tissues of the tick, especially the ovary, where further multiplication occurs. Once within the tick ovary, the parasite invades the tick egg(s) in order to multiply in the tissue of newly formed larvae. When a newly hatched larva first feeds, the parasite moves to and enters the salivary acini and multiplies further, with the eventual production of infective sporozoites. These sporozoites are inoculated into a new host at the time of feeding, whereupon they enter red blood cells directly. In transstadial transmission, development of sporozoites in tick salivary glands occurs in the next stage of the tick life cycle, once again following the initiation of feeding activity. For a review of the development of this parasite, see Ristic and Lewis (1977), Purnell (1981), Mehlhorn and Schein (1984), Telford et al. (1993), and Kakoma and Mehlhorn (1994).

Epizootiology

BABESIA BOVIS IN NORTH AMERICAN UNGULATES. *Babesia bovis* is one of the "small *Babesia*" and is the species that is most often associated with clinical disease in domestic cattle in southern Europe, Africa, Asia, and the Middle East. The hemolytic disease caused by this piroplasm in bovine hosts is called "cattle fever".

The ixodid tick vector is the tropical cattle tick, *Boophilus microplus*. It is a one-host tick which preferentially feeds on domestic cattle but has also been found on white-tailed deer (Park et al. 1966). The piroplasm survives transstadial and transovarial development in the tick. Infection in cattle may develop into a "cerebral" form characterized by sequestration of infected erythrocytes in cerebral capillaries (Potgieter and Els 1979).

The susceptibility of white-tailed deer to infection with *B. bovis* is not completely understood. Clark (1918) reported that white-tailed deer in Panama were infected with a piroplasm that caused sequestration of infected erythrocytes and was transmissible to domestic cattle. Unfortunately, since *B. bovis* had not yet been separately characterized, this piroplasm was reported as *Babesia bigemina*, another piroplasm of cattle that does not demonstrate this sequestration. It appears, however, that these deer in Panama, identified as *Odocoileus chiriquensis*, were infected with a *Babesia* organism that was transmissible to cattle, and these deer could have been reservoirs of that organism (Clark and Zetek 1925). Subsequent experiments in the United States have not shown the same relationship with white-tailed deer (*O. v. texanus*) from Texas. Experimental exposures by both tick feeding and inoculation of *B. bovis*–infected blood did not produce disease in white-tailed deer nor was subsequent blood transfer from deer to cattle successful in transmitting the infection (Kuttler et al. 1972). *Babesia bovis* can be cultured in vitro in white-tailed deer erythrocytes (Holman et al. 1993), but only with bovine serum in the culture media. It therefore seems unlikely that white-tailed deer are reservoirs of *B. bovis* infections in the United States. While white-tailed deer in Texas may not be susceptible to *B. bovis*, they can be maintenance hosts for the tropical fever tick, *B. microplus* (Park et al. 1966).

Reviews dealing with host susceptibility to *B. bovis* have maintained that red deer (*Cervus elaphus*) are hosts of *B. bovis*, based on an original report of bovine hemoglobinuria in Rumania caused by *Hematococcus bovis*. Starcovici (1893) subsequently renamed the parasite *Babesia bovis*. Kuttler (1988) has indicated that the described parasite may not have been the parasite that is now known as *B. bovis* since *Boophilus* spp. tick vectors are not present in Rumania. Based on these observations, it is not likely that red deer are a host for *B. bovis* and that the organism was probably *Babesia divergens*, which closely resembles *Babesia capreoli*, known to routinely infect European deer.

BABESIA BIGEMINA IN NORTH AMERICAN UNGULATES. *Babesia bigemina* is a "large" *Babesia* commonly associated with infections in domestic cattle. The ixodid tick vector is the one-host tick *Boophilus annulatus*. In addition to cattle, this tick has been shown to readily infest white-tailed deer (Cooksey et al. 1989), nilgai (*Boselaphus tragocamelus*) (Gray and Schubert 1979, Davey 1993), and wapiti (George 1996).

Repeated attempts to infect white-tailed deer with *B. bigemina* by both tick feeding and blood inoculation have proven unsuccessful (Kuttler et al. 1972). Experimental inoculations of *B. bigemina* into American plains bison (*Bison b. bison*) have demonstrated that these animals are susceptible to a severe parasitic, hemolytic anemia (Zaugg and Kuttler 1987).

BABESIA ODOCOILEI IN NORTH AMERICAN DEER. The original description of a *Babesia* species from a deer in North America was from New Mexico (Spindler et al. 1958). Since that initial description, there have been no further records of babesial infections from deer in that area. *Babesia odocoilei* was later described from white-tailed deer in Texas (Emerson and Wright 1968) and has since been isolated from deer in Virginia, Oklahoma, and perhaps other southern states (Perry et al. 1985; Waldrup et al. 1989a) (Fig. 18.5). Successful transmission of this piroplasm to susceptible white-tailed deer was accomplished with *Ixodes scapularis* but not with *Boophilus annulatus* (Waldrup et al. 1990). Transstadial transmission occurs in the tick host, but apparently transovarial transmission does not. Attempts to transmit this organism to domestic cattle, sheep, and goats by blood transfer have also been unsuccessful (Emerson and Wright 1968).

In endemic areas, the prevalence of infection in deer > 1 year of age is usually > 50% and may approach 100%. Seroconversion of white-tailed deer in eastern Texas occurs in late autumn, which coincides with the activity of *I. scapularis* adults (Waldrup et al. 1992). Experimental inoculation of *B. odocoilei* into immunocompetent deer rarely produces clinical signs or mortality. However, the infection in immunocompromised (by splenectomy or corticosteriod treatment) deer is quite virulent, with mortality approaching 90%. Mortality is due to a severe hemolytic anemia with observed parasitemia approaching 50%.

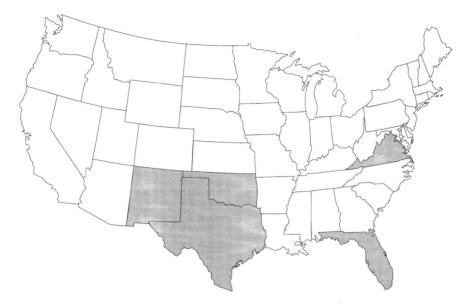

FIG. 18.5—Reported distribution of *Babesia odocoilei* by state in white-tailed deer from North America.

In natural infections with *B. odocoilei,* the parasitemia in circulating erythrocytes is low, often < 0.01%. In addition, the detection of *B. odocoilei* in Giemsa-stained blood smears is often complicated by the presence of concurrent infections with *T. cervi* piroplasms. Prevalence of the infection is best established using a serologic test such as the indirect fluorescent antibody test (IFAT) or by in vitro erythrocyte cultivation (Waldrup et al. 1989a; Holman et al. 1988).

At the ultrastructural level, *B. odocoilei* shares characteristics with *B. capreoli,* found in European deer, and *B. divergens,* a *Babesia* parasite of cattle of Europe and Asia (Droleskey et al. 1993). The cell membrane of *B. odocoilei* has a close association with the deer erythrocyte membrane, a characteristic that also occurs with *B. capreoli* and *B. divergens,* but not with *B. bigemina* or *B. bovis.* Serologic cross-reactivity has also been noted among *B. odocoilei, B.capreoli,* and *B. divergens,* but not with *B. bigemina* or *B. bovis* (Goff et al. 1993).

Caribou (*Rangifer tarandus caribou*) in North America have been diagnosed with severe hemolytic anemia associated with babesial infection (Holman et al. 1994a; Petrini et al., 1995) in captive herds in Minnesota and Oklahoma. The etiologic agents of these infections have not been completely characterized, but they appear to share significant characteristics with *B. odocoilei* (Goff et al. 1993, Holman et al. 1994a*).*

BABESIA IN WILD SHEEP AND DEER IN THE WESTERN UNITED STATES. A *Babesia* organism was first isolated from desert bighorn sheep (*Ovis canadensis nelsoni*) in 1993 (Goff et al. 1993). The isolation was made from blood collected from nonclinical free-

ranging sheep and inoculated into a captive bighorn sheep. The erythrocyte parasitemia reached 12% in this animal, although clinical signs of anemia were minimal. Blood from this sheep was further inoculated into both a spleen-intact and a splenectomized white-tailed deer. Microscopic evaluation detected parasitized erythrocytes after 5 days postinoculation in both deer. The spleen-intact deer showed no clinical signs and remained a carrier for at least 87 days. The splenectomized deer developed a more severe anemia (hematocrit as low as 15%) but showed signs of recovery (increase in hematocrit and reticulocytes) after 12 days postinoculation. On day 21 postinoculation, the splenectomized deer died of cerebral babesiosis. A second splenectomized white-tailed deer was inoculated from the original spleen-intact recipient and died of cerebral babesiosis on day 22 postinoculation. A second spleen-intact deer was inoculated and became infected with no clinical signs to day 25 postinoculation. The animal was euthanized on day 25 postinoculation, and no cerebral sequestration of infected erythrocytes was noted.

Additional isolations of *Babesia* organisms have been made from mule deer and black-tailed deer (*O. h. columbianus*) in California and elk (*Cervus elaphus nelsoni*) in Texas (Holman et al. 1994b). Additionally, a high prevalence of seroreactivity in free-ranging mule deer and bighorn sheep has been reported in California (Kjemtrup et al. 1995). It is possible that these *Babesia* species from sheep and deer in the western United States are strains of the same organism. This is especially true since asymptomatic infections with *B. capreoli* are known from domestic sheep in Europe (Purnell et al. 1981). Further characterization, including vector identification, will be necessary to clarify this situation.

BABESIA IN WILD CARNIVORES. *Babesia canis* has been described from experimentally infected coyotes (*Canis latrans*) (Ewing et al. 1964; Roher et al. 1985). To date, isolations of *Babesia* have not been reported from free-ranging coyotes, although seroreactivity in coyotes to *B. gibsoni* antigen has been documented in California (Conrad et al. 1991; Yamane et al. 1994).

BABESIA LOTORI IN RACCOONS (*PROCYONIS LOTOR*). *Babesia lotori* is a small intraerythrocytic piroplasm which has been found in raccoons in Connecticut (Anderson et al. 1981), Maryland (Frerichs and Holbrook 1970), Florida (Telford and Forrester 1991), Tennessee, Virginia, West Virginia, Georgia, Texas (Schaffer et al. 1978), and California (Woods 1952). Many researchers believe that the distribution of this parasite may be more widespread than these reports indicate. Some early reports incorrectly describe the parasite in raccoons as *B. procyonis,* but these two species should be considered synonymous (Anderson et al. 1981). Experimental studies have indicated that infections can be established in hamsters via inoculation of infected whole blood.

The tick vector for this species is unknown, but studies in Florida have shown a seasonal variation, with the greatest prevalence occurring between September and December (Telford and Forrester 1991). Naturally occurring cases are generally nonclinical, with parasitemias of < 1%.

BABESIA MEMPHITIS IN THE STRIPED SKUNK (*MEPHITIS MEPHITIS*). *B. memphitis* is a large intraerythrocytic parasite that is typically seen as a double pyriform. Natural infections have been reported from striped skunks in Maryland (Frerichs and Holbrook 1970). Infections appear to be subclinical in naturally infected hosts, and cross-species transmission trials have not been successful.

BABESIA IN RODENTS. In the United States several rodents appear to be susceptible to infection with *B. microti,* with the white-footed mouse, *Peromyscus leucopus,* being the most frequently infected. Various aspects of the host-parasite-vector relationship have been identified in enzootic areas of Massachusetts; the most significant is the association between rodent babesial infections and large deer populations (Spielman et al. 1981). Infections with *B. microti* have not been shown to have any known effect on rodent health or population dynamics in enzootic areas.

Clinical Signs and Pathology. Infection by *Babesia* piroplasms in the erythrocytes of mammalian hosts causes changes to the erythrocyte membrane that can result in changes in membrane fragility (Droleskey at al. 1993). The primary clinical sign of disease is a hemolytic anemia, with severe anemia often being the

only apparent clinical sign (Holman et al. 1988; Gray et al. 1991). In some species, hemoglobinemia, hemoglobinuria, and fever accompany the rapid red blood cell destruction. Necropsy findings generally show a carcass that is pale and jaundiced with subepicardial and subendocardial hemorrhages. In some hosts, infection with some species of *Babesia* may result in neurological signs due to a cerebral form of the disease. The cerebral form of *Babesia* infection in mammalian hosts is caused by sequestration of infected erythrocytes in the cerebral capillaries (Potgieter and Els 1979, Goff et al. 1993). This sequestration blocks the capillaries and creates an anoxic condition in the cerebrum, resulting in neurological signs such as ataxia. In infections with less pathogenic species of *Babesia* or in hosts that are resistant, infections may be subclinical and characterized by fever, anorexia, and slight jaundice (Gray et al. 1991, Goff et al. 1993). Babesiosis is often less of a clinical disease problem in free-ranging animals than in domestic animals, even though prevalence may be high in some free-ranging populations (Waldrup et al. 1989a).

Diagnosis. Clinical signs and history of tick exposure are often sufficient for a tentative diagnosis of babesiosis. However, a definitive diagnosis is based on microscopic visualization of piroplasms in Giemsa-stained whole blood (Fig. 18.6). Care must be exercised, however, since in many species of *Babesia,* piroplasms are difficult to find once the acute phase of the infection has passed.

Immunity. In general, infections with most species of *Babesia* result in an inverse age resistance, with young animals being more resistant to disease than older animals. It is thought that most young animals in endemic areas acquire immunity passively from the colostrum of the dam. The resultant exposure and infection is usually mild with transient clinical signs. In most cases, the infections that are acquired by young animals that are passively immunized in enzootic areas are sufficient to stimulate active immunity. This immunity may or may not be dependent on a persisting carrier state and/or continuous exposure. Often, enzootic stability that is dependent on a high rate of infection and large numbers of infected ticks is important in maintaining a high level of immunity in susceptible herds.

Control and Treatment. Historically, immunity to *Babesia* infections has been through exposure of the host to live agents. More recently, attenuated agents and nonliving agents have proven useful in stimulating and perhaps maintaining the host's immune status. This area has been thoroughly reviewed as it relates to bovine infections (Kakoma and Mehlhorn 1994). Likewise, chemotherapy and chemoprophylaxis have been used to reduce the severity the clinical signs and minimize the parasitemia, although the treatment of severely infected white-tailed deer with Imidicarb was unsuccessful (K.A. Waldrup and P.A. Conrad, unpub-

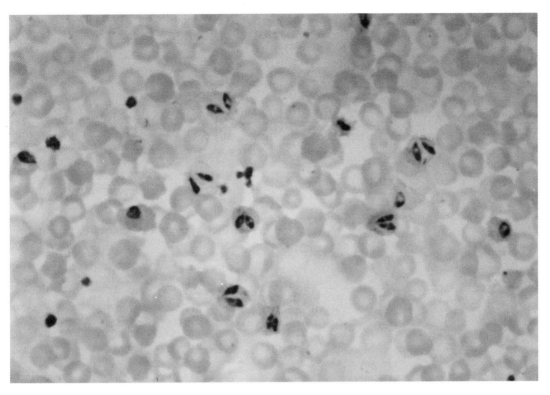

FIG. 18.6—*Babesia bigemina* piroplasms in erythrocytes of a domestic bovine. (200X magnification)

lished). The specific drugs used often depend on the species of *Babesia* involved and on the availability of the compounds in the individual countries. Although many compounds, especially Imidicarb (2.8 mg/kg SQ), have been evaluated as means of chemoprophylaxis, complete elimination of the infection may not be possible. An integrated approach involving tick control combined with chemoprophylaxis and chemotherapy offer the best long-term control. A similar effort in free-ranging animals appears to have been poorly evaluated and many not be practical (see Kakoma and Mehlhorn 1994).

Public Health Concerns. Until recently, only two babesial organisms have been associated with infections in humans. *Babesia microti,* a parasite of rodents, has been responsible for human cases in the northeastern and upper-Midwestern states. In most cases, nonspecific "malaria"-like symptoms are associated with infection, although a few fatalities and severe clinical cases are reported. *Peromyscus leucopus* is the normal host for *B. microti,* and the vector is *Ixodes scapularis.* Human cases in Europe are attributed to infection with the bovine parasite *B. divergens* that appears to run a more severe clinical course, especially in splenectomized hosts. More recently, a genetically and antigenically distinct *Babesia* organism was reported from

humans in Washington state. This organism is closely related to the canine parasite *B. gibsoni* and also appears closely related to members of the genus *Theileria* (Persing and Conrad 1995; Persing et al. 1995).

Domestic Animal Health Concerns. In the United States, *Babesia* spp. of wild ungulates do not appear to be capable of infecting domestic animals, although the reverse is apparently not true. The role of *Babesia* species that infect domestic canids is less clear, especially in light of the recent identification of naturally occurring *B. gibsoni* infections is the Pacific Northwest (Yamann et al., 1994), North Carolina (Birkenheuer et al. 1999), and Oklahoma (A.A. Kocan, unpublished).

Management Implications. It is important to minimize exposure of susceptible animals to infections with *Babesia* spp. parasites. Host specificity and naturally occurring infections should be considered when potentially infected domestic animals and wild species are placed in contact. Just as important are tick vectors that can inadvertently be introduced into new areas and nonindigenous ticks that can accompany animal introductions. Because our present understanding of vector competence and host susceptibility to babesial infections is inadequate, care should be taken to reduce the spread of these infections and their tick vectors.

LITERATURE CITED

Anderson, J.F., L. Magnarelli, and A. Sulzer. 1981. Raccoon babesiosis in Connecticut, USA: *Babesia lotori* sp. N. *The Journal of Parasitology* 67:417-425.

Barker, R.W., A.L. Hoch, R.G Buckner, and J.A. Hair. 1973. Hematological changes in white-tailed deer fawns, *Odocoileus virginianus,* infested with *Theileria* infected lone star ticks. *The Journal of Parasitology* 59:1091-1098.

Barnett, S.F. 1977. *Theileria.* In *Parasitic protozoa,* vol. 4. Ed. J.P. Krier. New York: Academic Press, pp. 77-113.

Bettencourt, A., C. Franca, and J. Borges. 1907. Un cas de piroplasmose bacilliforme chez le daim. *Arquivas do Instituto Bacteriologico Camara Pestana* 1:341-349.

Birkenheuer, A.J., M. Levy, K. Savary, R. Gager, and E. Breitschwerdt. 1999. *Babesia gibsoni* infections in dogs from North Carolina. *Journal of the American Animal Hospital Association* 35:125-128.

Blouin, E.F., A.A. Kocan, K.M. Kocan, and J.A. Hair. 1984. Transmission of *Cytauxzoon felis* Kier, 1979 from bobcats, *Felis rufus* (Schreber) to domestic cats by *Dermacentor variabilis* (Say). *Journal of Wildlife Diseases* 20:241-242.

———. 1987. Evidence of a limited schizogenous cycle for *Cytauxzoon felis* in bobcats following exposure to infected ticks. *Journal of Wildlife Diseases* 23: 409-501.

Butt, M.T., D. Bowman, M.C. Barr, and M.E. Roelke. 1991. Latrogenic transmission of *Cytauxzoon felis* from a Florida panther (*Felix concolor coryi*) to a domestic cat. *Journal of Wildlife Diseases* 27:342-347.

Chae, J., S. Waghela, T. Craig, A. Kocan, G. Wagner, and P. Holman. 1999. Two *Theileria cervi* SSU RRNA gene sequence types found in isolates from white-tailed deer and elk in North America. *Journal of wildlife Diseases* 35:458-465.

Clark, H.C. 1918. Piroplasmosis of cattle in Panama. *Journal of Infectious Diseases* 22:159-168.

Clark, H.C., and J. Zetek. 1925. Tick biting experiments in bovine and cervine piroplasms. *American Journal of Tropical Medicine* 5:17-26.

Conrad, P.A., and K.A. Waldrup. 1993. Babesiosis and theileriosis in free-ranging and captive artiodactylids. In *Zoo and wild animal medicine.* Vol. 3, *Current therapy.* Ed. M.E. Fowler. Philadelphia, PA: W.B. Saunders Co., pp. 506-511.

Conrad, P.A., B. G. Kelly, and C. G. D. Brown. 1985. Intraerythrocytic schizogony of *Theileria annulata. Parasitology* 91:67-82.

Conrad, P.A., J. Thomford, I. Yamane, J. Whiting, L. Bosma, T. Uno, H.J. Holshuh, and S. Shelly. 1991. Hemolytic anemia caused by *Babesia gibsoni* infection in dogs. *Journal of the American Veterinary Medical Association* 199:601-605.

Cooksey, L.M., R. Davey, E. Ahrens, and J. George 1989. Suitability of white-tailed deer as hosts for cattle fever ticks (Acari: Ixodidae). *Journal of Medical Entomology* 26:155-158.

Davey, R.B. 1993. Stagewise mortality, ovipositional biology, and egg viability of *Boophilus annulatus* (Acari: Ixodidae) on *Boselaphus tragocamelus* (Artiodactyla: Bovidae). *Journal of Medical Entomology* 30:997-1002.

Davidson, W.R., J.M. Crum, J.L. Blue, D.W. Sharp, and J.H. Phillips. 1985. Parasites, diseases and health status of sympatric populations of fallow deer and white-tailed deer in Kentucky. *Journal of Wildlife Diseases* 21:153-159.

Droleskey, R.E., P.J. Holman, K.W. Waldrup, D.E. Corrier, and G.G. Wagner. 1993. Ultrastructural characteristics of *Babesia odocoilei* in vitro. *The Journal of Parasitology* 79:424-434.

Emerson, H.R. 1969. A comparison of parasitic infections of white-tailed deer (*Odocoileus virginianus*) from central and east Texas. *Bulletin of the Wildlife Disease Association* 5:137-139.

Emerson, H.R., and W.T. Wright. 1968. Isolation of a *Babesia* in white-tailed deer. *Bulletin of the Wildlife Disease Association* 4:142–143.

Ewing, S.A., R. Buckner, and B. Stringer. 1964. The coyote, a potential host for *Babesia canis* and *Ehrlichia* sp. *The Journal of Parasitology* 50:704.

Fawcett, D.W., A.S. Young, and B.L. Leitch. 1985. Sporogony in *Theileria* (Apicomplexa: Piroplasmida). A comparative ultrastructural study. *Journal of Submicroscopic Cytology* 17:299-314.

Frerichs, W.M. and A. Holbrook. 1970. *Babesia* sp. and *Haemobartonella* sp. in wild mammals trapped at the Agricultural Research Center, Beltsville, Maryland. *The Journal of Parasitology* 56:130.

George, J.E. 1996. The campaign to keep *Boophilus* ticks out of the United States: Technical problems and solutions. *Proceedings of the United States Animal Health Association* 100:196-206.

Glenn, B.L., and E.L. Stair. 1984. Cytauxzoonosis in domestic cats: Report of two cases in Oklahoma with a review and discussion of the disease. *Journal of the American Veterinary Medical Association* 184:822-825.

Glenn, B.L., R.E. Rolley, and A.A. Kocan. 1982. *Cytauxzoon*-like piroplasms observed in erythrocytes of wild-tapped bobcats (*Lynx rufus rufus*) in Oklahoma. *Journal of the American Veterinary Medical Association* 181:1251-1253.

Glenn, B.L., A.A. Kocan, and E.F. Blouin. 1983. Cytauxzoonosis in bobcats. *Journal of the American Veterinary Medical Association* 183:1155-1158.

Goff, W., D. Jessup, K. Waldrup, J. Gorham, and G. Wagner. 1993. The isolation and partial characterization of a *Babesia* spp. from desert bighorn sheep (*Ovis canadensis nelsoni*). *Journal of Eukaryotic Microbiology* 40:237-243.

Gray, J.H., and G.O. Schubert. 1979. Report of the Committee on parasitic diseases and parasiticides tick eradication program. *Proceedings of the United States Animal Health Association* 83:347-349.

Gray, J.S., T.M. Muphy, K.A. Waldrup, G.G. Wagner, D.A. Blewett, and R. Harrington. 1991. Comparative studies of *Babesia* spp. from white-tailed and sika deer. *Journal of Wildlife Diseases* 27(1):86–91.

Grootenhuis, J.G., and A.S. Young. 1981. The involvement of wildlife in *Theileria* infections of domestic animals in East Africa. In *Advances in the control of theileriosis.* Ed. A.D. Irvin, M.P. Cunningham, and A.S. Young. Boston: Martinus Nijhoff, pp. 71-73.

Hair, J.A., and J.L. Bowman. 1986. Behavioral ecology of *Amblyomma americanum* (L). In *Morphology. physiology, and behavioral biology of ticks.* Ed. J. Sauer and J. Hair. New York: Ellis Horwood Limited, pp. 406-420.

Hazen-Karr, C.G., A.A. Kocan, K.M. Kocan, and J.A. Hair. 1987. The ultrastructure of sporogony in *Theileria cervi* (Bettencourt et al., 1907) in salivary glands of female *Amblyomma americanum* (L.) ticks. *The Journal of Parasitology* 73:1182-1188.

Holman, P.J., K. Waldrup, and G. Wagner. 1988. In vitro cultivation of a *Babesia* isolate from a white-tailed deer (*Odocoileus virginianus*). *The Journal of Parasitology* 74:111-115.

Holman, P.J., K.A. Waldrup, E. Droleskey, D.E. Corrier, and G.G. Wagner. 1993. In vitro growth of *Babesia bovis* in white-tailed deer (*Odocoileus virginianus*) erythrocytes. *The Journal of Parasitology* 79:233-237.

Holman, P.J., K. Petrini, J. Rhyan, and G. Wagner. 1994a. In vitro isolation and cultivation of a *Babesia* sp. from an

American woodland caribou (*Rangifer tarandus caribou*). *Journal of Wildlife Diseases* 30:195-200.

Holman, P.J., T. Craig, D. Crider, K. Petrini, J. Rhyan, and G. Wagner. 1994b. Culture, isolation and partial characterization of a B*abesia* sp. from a North American elk (*Cervus elaphus*). *Journal of Wildlife Diseases* 30:460-465.

Kakoma, I., and H. Mehlhorn. 1994. Babesia in domestic animals. In *Parasitic protozoa*, vol. 7. Ed. J.P. Krier. New York: Academic Press, pp. 147-216.

Kjemtrup, A.M., J.W. Thomford, I.A. Gardner, P.A. Conrad, D.A. Jessup, and W.M. Boyce. 1995. Seroprevalence of two *Babesia* spp. isolated in selected bighorn sheep (*Ovis canadensis*) and mule deer (*Odocoileus hemionus*) populations in California. *Journal of Wildlife Diseases* 31:467-471.

Kocan, A.A., and K.M. Kocan. 1991. Tick-transmitted diseases of wildlife in North America. *Bulletin of the Society of Vector Ecology* 16:94-108.

Kocan, A.A., E.F. Blouin, and B.L. Glenn. 1985. Hematologic and serum chemical values for free-ranging bobcats *Felis rufus* (Schreber), with reference to animals with natural infections of *Cytauxzoon felis* Kier, 1979. *Journal of Wildlife Diseases* 21:190-192.

Kocan, A.A., S. W. Mukolwe, and S. J. Laird. 1987. The inability to infect fallow deer (*Cervis dama*) with *Theileria cervi*. Journal of Wildlife Diseases 23: 674-676.

Kocan, A.A., K. M. Kocan, C. Hazen-Karr, and J. A. Hair. 1988. Electron microscopic observations of *Theileria cervi* in salivary glands of male *Amblyomma americanum*. Proceedings of the Helminthological Society of Washington 55: 55-57.

Kocan, A.A., K.M. Kocan, E.F. Blouin, and S.W. Mukolwe. 1992. A redescription of schizogony of *Cytauxzoon felis* in the domestic cat. *Annals New York Academy of Sciences* 653:161-167.

Krier, J.P., M. Ristic, and A.M. Watrach. 1962. *Theileria* sp. in a deer in the United States. *American Journal of Veterinary Research* 23:657-662.

Kuttler, K. 1988. World wide impact of babesiosis. *In Babesiosis of domestic animals and man*. Ed. M. Ristic. Boca Raton, FL: CRC Press, pp. 1-22.

Kuttler, K., R.M. Robinson, and R.R. Bell. 1967. Tick transmission of theileriosis in white-tailed deer. *Bulletin of the Wildlife Disease Association* 3:182-183.

Kuttler, K., O.H. Graham, S.R. Johnson, and J.L. Trevino. 1972. Unsuccessful attempts to establish cattle *Babesia* infections in white-tailed deer. *Journal of Wildlife Diseases* 8:63-66.

Laird, J.S., A.A. Kocan, K.M. Kocan, S.M Presley, and J.A. Hair. 1988. Susceptibility of *Amblyomma americanum* to natural and experimental infections with *Theileria cervi*. *Journal of Wildlife Diseases* 24:679-683.

Levine, N.D. 1971. Taxonomy of the piroplasms. *Transactions of the American Microscopic Society* 90:2-33.

Mehlhorn, H. and E. Schein. 1984. The piroplasms: Life cycle and sexual stages. *Advances in Parasitology* 23:37-102.

Mehlhorn, H., E. Schein, and J.S. Ahmed. 1994. *Theileria*. In *Parasitic protozoa*, vol. 7. Ed. J.P. Kreier. New York: Academic Press, pp. 217-304.

Mitema, E.S., A.A. Kocan, S.W. Mukolwe, S. Sangiah, and D. Sherban. 1991. Activity of buparvaquone against *Theileria cervi* in white-tailed deer. *Veterinary Parasitology* 38:49-53.

Motzel, S. and J.E. Wagner. 1990. Treatment of experimentally induced cytauxzoonosis in cats with parvaquone and buparvaquone. *Veterinary Parasitology* 35:131-138.

Mutugi, J.J., A.S. Young, A.C. Maritim, S.G. Ndungu, D.A. Stagg, J.G. Grootenhuis, and B.L. Leitch. 1988a. Immunization of cattle against theileriosis using varying

dosages of *Theileria parva lawrencei* and *T. Parva parva* sporozoites and oxytetracycline treatments. *International Journal of Parasitology* 18(4): 453-461.

Mutugi, J.J., A.S. Young, A.C. Maritim, A. Linyoni, S.K. Mbogo, and B.L. Leitch. 1988b. Immunization of cattle using varying infective dosages of *Theileria parva lawrencei* sporozoites derived from an African buffalo (*Syncerus caffer*) and treatment with buparvaquone. *Parasitology* 96:391-402.

Neitz, W.O., and A.D. Thomas. 1948. *Cytauxzoon sylvicaprae* gen. nov., spec. nov., a piroplasm responsible for the hitherto undescribed disease of the duiker (*Sylvicaprae grimmia*). *Onderstepoort Journal of Veterinary Science and Animal Industry* 23:63-76.

Park, R.L., O. Skov, G.A. Seaman, and R.M. Bondl. 1966. Deer and cattle fever ticks. *The Journal of Wildlife Management* 30:202-203.

Perry, B.D., D.K. Nickols, and E.S. Cullom. 1985. *Babesia odocoilei* Emerson and Wright, 1970, in white-tailed deer, *Odocoileus virginianus*, in Virginia. *Journal of Wildlife Diseases* 21:149-152.

Persing, D.A., and P.C. Conrad. 1995. Babesiosis: New insight from phylogenetic analysis. *Infectious Agents and Disease* 4:182-195.

Persing, D.A., B. Herwaldt, C. Glaser, R. Lane, J. Thomford, D. Mathiesen, P. Krause, D. Phillip, and P. Conrad. 1995. Infection with a *Babesia*–like organism in Northern California. *The New England Journal of Medicine* 332:298-303.

Petrini, K.R., P.J. Holman, J.C. Rhyan, S.J. Jenkins, and G.G. Wagner. 1995. Fatal babesiosis in an American woodland caribou (*Rangifer tarandus caribou*). *Journal of Zoo and Wildlife Medicine* 26(2): 298–305.

Potgieter, F.T., and H.J. Els. 1974. An electron microscopic study of intra-erythrocytic stage of *Babesia bovis* in the brain capillaries of infected splenectomized calves. *Onderstepoort Journal of Veterinary Research* 46:41-49.

Purnell, R.E. 1981. Babesiosis in various hosts. In *Babesiosis*. Ed. M. Ristic and J.P. Krier. New York: Academic Press, pp. 25-63.

Purnell, R.E., D. Lewis, M. R. Holman, and E. R. Young. 1981. Investigations on a *Babesia* isolated from Scottish sheep. *Parasitology* 83:347-356.

Ristic, M., and G.E. Lewis. 1977. *Babesia* in man and wild and laboratory-adapted mammals. In *Parasitic protozoa*, vol. 4. Ed. J.P. Krier. New York: Academic Press, pp. 53-76.

Robinson, R.M., K.L. Kuttler, J.W. Thomas, and R.G. Marburger. 1967. Theileriosis in Texas white-tailed deer. *The Journal of Wildlife Management* 31:455-549.

Robinson, R.M., K.L. Kuttler, H.R. Emerson, L.P. Jones, and R.G. Marburger. 1968. Blood parasites in Texas deer. *Transactions 33rd North American Wildlife Natural Resource Conference* 33:359-364.

Roher, D.P., J.F. Anderson, and S.W. Nielson. 1985. Experimental babesiosis in coyotes and coydogs. *American Journal of Veterinary Research* 46:256-262.

Rostein, D.S., S. Taylor, J. Harvey, and J. Bean. 1999. Hematologic effects of cytauxzoonosis in Florida panthers and Texas cougars in Florida. *Journal of Wildlife Diseases* 35:613-617.

Schaffer, G.D., W. Hanson, W. Davidson, and V. Nettles. 1978. Haematotropic parasites of translocated raccoons in the southeast. *Journal of the American Veterinary Medical Association* 173:1148-1151.

Schein, E., H. Mehlhorn, and M. Warnecke. 1978. Electron microscopic studies of the schizogony of four *Theileria* species of cattle (*T. parva, T. lawrenci, T. annulata*, and *T. mutans*). *Parasitologica* 14:337-348.

Simpson, C.F., J.W. Harvey, M.J. Lawman, J. Murray, A.A. Kocan, and J.C. Carlisle. 1985. Ultrastructure of schizonts in the liver of cats with experimentally induced cytauxzoonosis. *American Journal of Veterinary Research* 46:384-390.

Spielman, A., P. Etkind, J. Piesman, T. Ruebush, D. Jaranek, and M. Jacobs. 1981. Reservoir hosts of human babesiosis on Nantucket Island. *American Journal of Tropical Medicine and Hygiene* 30:560-565.

Spindler, L.A., R.W. Allen, L.S. Diamond, and J.C. Lotz. 1958. *Babesia* in white-tailed deer. *Journal of Protozoology* 5:8.

Splitter, E.J. 1950. *Theileria mutans* associated with bovine anaplasmosis in the United States. *Journal of the American Medical Association* 117:134-135.

Starcovici, C. 1893. Bemerkungen uber den durch Babes entdeckten Blutparasiten und die durch denselben hervoügebrachten Krankheiten, die seuchenhafte Hämoglobinurie des Rinds (Babes), des Texasfieber (Th. Smith), und der Carceag der Schafe (Babes). *Zentralblatt für Bakteriologie, Parasitenkunde, Infektionskrankheiten und Hygiene, Abteilung I: Medizinisch-Hygienische Bakteriologie, Virusforschung und Parasitologie, Originale* 14:1-8.

Telford, S., and D.J. Forrester. 1991. Haemoparasites of raccoons (*Procyon lotor*) in Florida. *Journal of Wildlife Diseases* 27:486-490.

Telford, S., A. Gorenflot, P. Brasseur, and A. Spielman. 1993. Babesial infections in humans and wildlife. In *Parasitic protozoa*, vol. 5. New York: Academic Press, pp. 1-27.

Thomford, J.W., P. A. Conrad, S. R. Thelford, D. Mathiesen, B. H. Bowman, A. Spielman, M. L. Eberhard, B. L. Herwaldt, R. E. Quick, and D. H. Persing. 1994. Cultivation and phylogenetic characterization of a newly recognized human pathogenic protozoan. *Journal of Infectious Diseases* 169:1050-1056.

Uilenberg, G., F.F. Franssen, and N.M. Perie. 1987. Relationships between *Cytauxzoon felis* and African piroplasms. *Veterinary Parasitology* 26:21-28.

Wagner, J.E. 1976. A fatal cytauxzoonosis-like disease in domestic cats. *Journal of the American Veterinary Medical Association* 168:585-588.

Waldrup, K., A.E. Collisson, S.E. Bentsen, C.K. Winkler, and G.G. Wagner. 1989a. Prevalence of erythrocytic protozoa and serologic reactivity to selected pathogens in deer in Texas. *Preventative Veterinary Medicine* 7:49-58.

Waldrup, K., A.A. Kocan, T. Quereshi, D.S. Davis, D. Baggett, and G.G. Wagner. 1989b. Serologic prevalence and isolation of *Babesia odocoilei* among white-tailed deer (*Odocoileus virginianus*) in Texas and Oklahoma. *Journal of Wildlife Diseases* 25:194-201.

Waldrup, K., A.A. Kocan, R.W. Barker, and G.G. Wagner. 1990. Transmission of *Babesia odocoilei* in white-tailed deer (*Odocoileus virginianus*) by *Ixodes scapularis* (Acari: Ixodidae). *Journal of Wildlife Diseases* 26:390-391.

Waldrup, K.A., J. Moritz, D. Baggett, S. Magyar, and G.G. Wagner. 1992. Monthly incidence of *Theileria cervi* and seroconversion to *Babesia odocoilei* in white-tailed deer(*Odocoileus virginianus*) in Texas. *Journal of Wildlife Diseases* 28(3): 457–459.

Whiteman, S.R., A.B. Kier, and J.E. Wagner. 1977. Clinical features of feline cytauxzoonosis, a newly described blood parasitic disease. *Feline Practice* 7:23-26.

Willadsen, P., and F. Jongejan. 1999. Immunology of the tick-host interaction and the control of ticks and tick-borne diseases. *Parasitology Today* 15:258-262.

Woods, S.F. 1952. Mammal blood parasite records from the southwestern United States and Mexico. *The Journal of Parasitology* 38:85-86.

Yamane, I., I. Gardner, C. Ryan, M. Levy, J. Urrico, and P.A. Conrad. 1994. Serosurvey of *Babesia canis, Babesia gibsoni,* and *Ehrlichia canis* in pound dogs in California, USA. *Preventative Veterinary Medicine* 18:293-304.

Young, A.S., B.L. Leitch, R.M. Newson, and M.P. Cunningham. 1986. Maintenance of *Theileria parva parva* infection in an endemic area of Kenya. *Parasitology* 93:9-16.

Zaugg, J.L., and K. Kuttler. 1987. Experimental infections of *Babesia bigemina* in American bison. *Journal of Wildlife Diseases* 23:99-102.

Zinkl J.G., S.W. McDonald, A.B. Keir, and S.S. Cippa. 1981. *Cytauxzoon*–like organisms in erythrocytes of two cheetahs. *Journal of the American Veterinary Medical Association* 179:1261-1262.

CONTRIBUTORS

Sandra A. Allan, M.Sc., Ph.D.
Department of Pathobiology
College of Veterinary Medicine
University of Florida
Gainesville, FL

Roy C. Anderson M.A., Ph.D.
Department of Zoology
University of Guelph
Guelph, Ontario, Canada

Lora G. Rickard, M.S., D.V.M.
College of Veterinary Medicine
Mississippi State University
Mississippi State, MS

Set Bornstein, D.V.M., Ph.D.
Department of Parasitology
National Veterinary Institute
Uppsala, Sweden

Andre G. Buret, M.Sc., Ph.D.
Department of Biological Sciences
University of Calgary
Calgary, Alberta, Canada

Douglas D. Colwell, M.Sc., Ph.D.
Agriculture and Agri-Food Canada
Lethbridge Research Centre
Lethbridge, Alberta, Canada

Thomas M. Craig, D.V.M., Ph.D.
Department of Veterinary Pathobiology
College of Veterinary Medicine
Texas A&M University
College Station, TX

Terry A. Dick, M.Sc., Ph.D.
Department of Zoology
University of Manitoba
Winnipeg, Manitoba, Canada

Jitender P. Dubey, M.V.Sc., Ph.D.
Parasite Biology and Epidemiology Laboratory
Livestock and Poultry Sciences Institute
Agricultural Research Service
U.S. Department of Agriculture
Beltsville, MD

Lance A. Durden, Ph.D.
Institute of Arthropodology and Parasitology
Georgia Southern University
Statesboro, GA

Donald W. Duszynski, M.S., Ph.D.
Department of Biology
The University of New Mexico
Albuquerque, NM

Alvin A. Gajadhar, M.Sc., Ph.D.
Centre for Animal Parasitology
Canadian Food Inspection Agency
Saskatoon, Saskatchewan, Canada

Eric C. Hoberg, M.S., Ph.D.
Biosystematics and National Parasite Collection Unit
Agricultural Research Service
U.S. Department of Agriculture
Beltsville, MD

David T. John, M.S.P.H., Ph.D.
Department of Biochemistry and Microbiology
College of Osteopathic Medicine
Oklahoma State University
Tulsa, OK

Arlene Jones, Ph.D.
Department of Zoology
The Natural History Museum
London, United Kingdom

Kevin R. Kazacos, Ph.D.
Department of Veterinary Pathology
School of Veterinary Medicine
Purdue University
West Lafayette, IN

537

A. Alan Kocan, M.S.P.H., Ph.D.
Department of Veterinary Pathobiology
College of Veterinary Medicine
Oklahoma State University
Stillwater, OK

Murray W. Lankester, M.Sc., Ph.D.
Department of Biology
Lakehead University
Thunder Bay, Ontario, Canada

Frederick. A. Leighton, D.V.M., Ph.D.
Canadian Cooperative Wildlife Health Centre
Department of Veterinary Pathology
Western College of Veterinary Medicine
University of Saskatchewan
Saskatoon, Saskatchewan, Canada

Lena N. Measures, M.Sc., Ph.D.
Maurice Lamontagne Institute
Fisheries and Oceans
Mont-Joli, Quebec, Canada

Torsten Mörner, D.V.M., Ph.D
Department of Wildlife
National Veterinary Institute
Uppsala, Sweden

Klaus Odening, Ph.D.
Institute for Zoo Biology and Wildlife
Berlin, Germany

Merle E. Olson, M.Sc., D.V.M.
Department of Microbiology and Infectious Diseases
University of Calgary
Calgary, Alberta, Canada

Edoardo Pozio, Ph.D.
Laboratory of Parasitology
Instituto Superiore di Sanito
Rome, Italy

Margo J. Pybus, M.Sc., Ph.D.
Alberta Natural Resource Services
Department of Environment
Edmonton, Alberta, Canada

William M. Samuel, M.Sc., Ph.D.
Department of Biological Sciences
University of Alberta
Edmonton, Alberta, Canada

Grant R. Singleton, Ph.D.
CSIRO Wildlife and Ecology
Canberra, Australia

David M. Spratt, Ph.D.
CSIRO Wildlife and Ecology
Canberra, Australia

Steve J. Upton, M.S., Ph.D.
Division of Biology
Kansas State University
Manhattan, KS

Kenneth A. Waldrup, D.V.M., Ph.D.
Texas Animal Health Commission
Cleburne, TX

INDEX

Aardvarks
  coccidia and, 427
  sucking lice and, 7
Aardwolfs, *Sarcoptes scabiei*
  (mange) and, 110
Abrocomaphthirus, 7
Abrocomophaga, 10
Acanthamoeba
  diagnosis/treatment, 461–462
  epizootiology, 460–461
  pathology/pathogenesis, 461
  public health concerns, 462
Acanthamoebiasis. *See*
  Acanthamoeba
Acarina. *See* Hard ticks; Soft ticks
Addax, *Cryptosporidium parvum*
  and, 436
Aedes
  abserratus, 19
  aegypi, 19
  albopictus, 19–20
  atlanticus, 20
  canadensis, 20
  canator, 19
  communis, 20
  dorsalis, 19
  hendersoni, 19
  hexodontus, 19–20
  impiger, 19
  infirmatus, 20
  melanimon, 20
  nigripes, 19
  provocans, 20
  sollicitans, 19–20
  stimulans, 19–20
  stricticus, 20
  taeniorhynchus, 20
  triseriatus, 19–20
  trivittatus, 19–21
  vexans, 19–21
  vigilax, 20
African buffalo
  liver flukes (*Fasciola gigantica*)
    and, 137
  Taenia acinonyxi and, 151
  Taenia crocutae and, 153
  Theileria spp. and, 524
African swine fever, 74–75
African wild cats, *Echinococcus*
  granulosus and, 176–177
Alectorobius. See Ornithodoros
Allergic reactions
  to biting midges, 22
  lice and, 9

Alouattamyia baeri, 48, 51, 53, 66–67
Alpacas, *Sarcoptes scabiei* (mange)
  and, 111
Amblycera
  Boopiidae, 10
  Gyropidae, 10
  Trimenoponidae, 10
Amblyomma
  americanum, 83–88
  cajennense, 83–88
  dissimile, 83
  imitator, 83–88
  inornatum, 83–88
  maculatum, 83–88
  rotundatum, 83
  tuberculatum, 83–88
Amebiasis. *See* Protozoans (enteric
  parasites)
American Human Trypanosomiasis,
  521–522
American liver flukes. *See* Liver
  flukes (*Fascioloides magna*)
Amoebic diseases, 460–462
Anaphylaxis, 29
Anaplasma, 29
Anaplasmosis, 79, 90–91, 93
Ancistroplax, 7
Ancylostomatoidea. *See* Strongylate
  nematodes
Anopheles
  punctipennis, 20–21
  quadrimaculatus, 19–21
Anophelinae. *See* Mosquitos
Anoplura. *See* Sucking lice
Antarctophthirus, 7
  trichechi, 8
Anteaters, coccidia and, 427
Antelope
  biting midges as vectors of
    bluetongue virus (BT), 23
  epizootic hemorrhagic disease
    (EHD), 23
  Camelostrongylus mentulatus and,
    214
  Cryptosporidium parvum and, 436
  Cytauxzoon spp. and, 529
  hard ticks and, 85, 91
  muscoid flies and, 33
  nose/pharyngeal bots (Oestrinae)
    and, 59
  Parelaphostrongylosis tenuis and,
    245
  Sarcoptes scabiei (mange) and,
    110

Setaria labiatopalillosa and, 21
strongylate nematodes and,
  196–197
sucking lice and, 9
Taenia acinonyxi and, 151
Taenia crocutae and, 153
Taenia hyaenae and, 155–157
Taenia olnojinei and, 162
Theileria spp. and, 524
Toxoplasma gondii and, 489
Trypanosoma spp. and, 521
Anthelmintic therapy in free-ranging
  ruminants, 208
Anthericidae, *Suragina,* 27
Anthrax
  muscoid flies as vectors for,
    33–34
  tabanids and snipe flies as vectors
    for, 28–29
Antricola coprophilus, 73–74
Aotiella, 10
Apteragia
  odocoilei, 211
  pursglovei, 211
  quadrispiculata, 213
Argas
  miniatus, 72
  persicus, 72
  polonicus, 75
  radiata, 72
  sanchezi, 72
  vespertilionis, 72, 74–75
Armadillos
  coccidia and, 427
  hard ticks and, 85
  Trichinella spiralis and, 390
Artiodactyls, 6–7
Ascarids (Ascaridoidea). *See*
  Baylisascaris
Ascaris
  filicollis, 215
  renales, 357
  renalis, 357
  visceralis, 357
Ashworhius sidemi, 207
Ass, *Sarcoptes scabiei* (mange) and,
  111. *See also* Donkeys
Ataxia, 252
Atopophthirus, 9
Atylotus, 27
Axis deer
  lice and, 9
  Theileria spp. and, 523–529